KLINE & HUDSON'S

NERVE INJURIES

OPERATIVE RESULTS FOR MAJOR NERVE INJURIES, ENTRAPMENTS, AND TUMORS

Commissioning Editor: **Susan Pioli**
Development Editor: **Alexandra Mortimer**
Project Manager: **Bryan Potter**
Design Manager: **Charles Gray**
Illustration Manager: **Merlyn Harvey**
Illustrator: **Tecmedi, Chartwell**
Marketing Manager(s) (UK/USA): **Clara Toombs/Catalina Nolte**

KLINE & HUDSON'S

NERVE INJURIES

OPERATIVE RESULTS FOR MAJOR NERVE INJURIES, ENTRAPMENTS, AND TUMORS

SECOND EDITION

Daniel H. Kim MD
Professor
Spinal Neurosurgery and Reconstructive
Peripheral Nerve Surgery
Baylor College of Medicine
Houston, TX

Rajiv Midha MD, MSc, FRCS(C)
Professor and Chief
Division of Neurosurgery, Department of Clinical Neurosciences
University of Calgary
Calgary, AB

Judith A. Murovic MD
Instructor, Neurosurgery
Department of Neurosurgery
Stanford University Medical Center
Stanford, CA

Robert J. Spinner MD
Professor of Neurologic Surgery, Orthopedics and Anatomy
Mayo Clinic
Rochester, MN

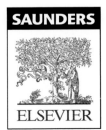

SAUNDERS

ELSEVIER

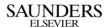

SAUNDERS
ELSEVIER

An imprint of Elsevier Inc

© 1995 W.B. Saunders Company
© 2008, Elsevier Inc. All rights reserved.

First published 1995
First edition 1995
Second edition 2008

EAD: 978-0-7216-9537-2

British Library Cataloguing in Publication Data
A catalogue record for this book is available from the British Library

Library of Congress Cataloging in Publication Data
A catalog record for this book is available from the Library of Congress

Notice
Medical knowledge is constantly changing. Standard safety precautions must be followed, but as new research and clinical experience broaden our knowledge, changes in treatment and drug therapy may become necessary or appropriate. Readers are advised to check the most current product information provided by the manufacturer of each drug to be administered to verify the recommended dose, the method and duration of administration, and contraindications. It is the responsibility of the practitioner, relying on experience and knowledge of the patient, to determine dosages and the best treatment for each individual patient. Neither the Publisher nor the authors assume any liability for any injury and/or damage to persons or property arising from this publication.

The Publisher

ELSEVIER your source for books, journals and multimedia in the health sciences
www.elsevierhealth.com

Working together to grow libraries in developing countries

www.elsevier.com | www.bookaid.org | www.sabre.org

ELSEVIER   BOOK AID International   Sabre Foundation

Printed in China

Last digit is the print number: 9 8 7 6 5 4 3 2 1

The publisher's policy is to use **paper manufactured from sustainable forests**

Contents

Foreword to the First Edition

Although peripheral nerve surgery has been done since the 19th century, significant progress was not demonstrated until the use of the operating microscope in the mid-1960s, accompanied by appropriate suture materials and instruments. A second major advance has been the utilization of electrophysiologic testing for the evaluation of peripheral nerve injury and repair.

The senior author of this text has been in the vanguard of these technical advances as well as of many other aspects of patient care. I have enjoyed a professional relationship with David G Kline since we met at the Walter Reed Army Medical Center more than 30 years ago. During that two year period, he published eight research papers and participated in routine patient care activities. Subsequently, David Kline developed productive research facilities and a neurosurgical postgraduate education program at the Louisiana State University in New Orleans. He has achieved worldwide recognition for his research in peripheral nerve injuries, neurophysiology of nerve regeneration and nerve tumors. In these efforts, he has published more than 165 medical articles and has served on the editorial boards of 11 medical journals. David Kline is Professor of Neurosurgery and Head of the Department of Neurosurgery at the Louisiana State University. His many administrative activities in education have included appointments as Chairman of the American Board of Neurologic Surgeons and as President of the Sunderland Society for International Peripheral Nerve Study.

Alan R Hudson completed his neurosurgical postgraduate training program at the University of Toronto in Ontario, where he is Professor of Neurosurgery and was Chairman of the Division of Neurosurgery. His research activities have produced more than 120 medical articles. During his tenure at the University of Toronto, he has received international recognition for his professional and research activities, including the presidency of the Canadian Neurosurgical Society. Professor Hudson has held the McCutcheon Chair as Surgeon in Chief of the Toronto Hospital from 1989 to 1991; in 1991 he was made President and Chief Executive Officer of that hospital, Canada's largest for acute care.

In 1970, Alan Hudson established a peripheral nerve research laboratory and received a Clinical Traineeship Award from the Royal College of Surgeons. He chose to spend the Award with David Kline in New Orleans. From that experience grew a very productive relationship for ongoing research, and these two physicians have collaborated on more than 30 published medical articles. This text is the result of their agreed upon approach to major problems and brings together two experts with international reputations in the field of peripheral nerve surgery.

This book discusses in detail the varied etiologic mechanisms, the appropriate clinical and laboratory evaluation, and the operative techniques, including intraoperative electrophysiologic studies and their potential complications, that are involved in the treatment of major peripheral nerve injuries, entrapments, and the tumors of both the upper and lower extremities.

The text of this book is unique in that it presents not only a comprehensive review but also attempts to portray in some detail results of treatment. It has been written by only two authors, in contrast to the usual text by multiple authors. The result is a presentation of personal experiences with proven approaches to very complex problems. Further, the statistical conclusions are based on a single database from the Louisiana State University Medical Center, which documents actual experience in a single practice location.

This book will be of great assistance to all medical personnel who have taken up the challenge of managing major problems of the peripheral nervous system.

GEORGE E OMER, JR, MD, MS, FACS
Professor and Chairman Emeritus
Department of Orthopaedics and Rehabilitation
The University of New Mexico

Preface to the First Edition

When we began work on this book more than nine years ago, there were already several excellent texts available on nerve injuries and entrapments. In the interim, several more books have been published. We set to work on a relatively comprehensive manuscript because we wished to present results from a large personal series of major injuries and other nerve lesions. We believe that outcome analysis will be demanded by society in general and by third-party payers in particular in the last decade of the twentieth century or in the early years of the twenty-first century. Analysis of such results was thought to be necessary to provide future directions for patient care and for research and development concerning nerve lesions. A comprehensive and yet readable analysis of results in this field appeared to be indicated and had not been done since publication of the VA Monograph, *Peripheral Nerve Injury*, in 1957. Although correcting loss caused by nerve injury is very demanding, analysis of outcomes in a usable fashion proved to be even more difficult.

The series of cases presented here come primarily from one institution (Louisiana State University Medical Center and related hospitals such as Charity, Ochsner, and University), but we have tried to reflect upon and extrapolate from the data. We have similar philosophies concerning clinical investigation, timing for operations, and techniques used. The information presented represents our joint and current recommendations for care of these difficult lesions.

We are presenting these data in the hope that they will be improved upon in future years. We expect that others who follow us will contribute in a fashion that will lead to better results than ours. Rather than editing a multi-authored book, we have tried to consolidate the personal experiences of two clinicians who have been involved in the surgery of nerve injuries and repairs for the last thirty years, including major nerve injuries, entrapments, and tumors. Not included in this text are injuries to the cranial nerves. The only exception is the eleventh cranial or accessory nerve, because this is an important part of shoulder and upper limb function. Several excellent texts already exist on the facial nerve and some of the other cranial nerves less frequently involved in injury.

We both feel strongly that workers in this field need to have a thorough background in the gross anatomy and microanatomy of the limbs; therefore each chapter has this background as a core. We also believe that there is a great need for clinicians to have good grasp of the basic physiologic principles involved in both the intact and injured or regenerating nerve. There are advantages as well as drawbacks to the various electrophysiologic tests used to help guide the care of a patient with a peripheral nerve problem, and these are commented upon throughout the text. Neither of us are electromyographers but we have tried to weight such information and to provide some detail especially about intraoperative electrical studies. There is also great value to laboratory research, but this is primarily a clinical book, so only selected basic scientific findings related to nerve repair are presented.

The outline for each chapter in this book, even those on individual nerves, is not the same. We tried to mold each section along selected and important areas to be addressed for each nerve or region of anatomy. The book is not intended to provide answers for the many variations in anatomy and function of each nerve and the many things that can occur connected with it but rather to emphasize major injury, an area with which we do have experience. Our efforts for this text have focused on providing detail about major nerve injury management and especially about degree of recovery. The tables presenting the data analyzed and their outcomes in terms of results are central to the book and require close and repetitive study. In this regard, an initial survey of the chapters on mechanisms of injury, clinical evaluation, and grading of loss and subsequent recovery is very important, especially if the tables are to be used to apply the lessons gained from these outcomes to future problems.

Preface to the Second Edition

When asked to do a Second Edition of this back 4 or 5 years ago both of us were reluctant, because the First Edition had required almost a decade of work. This is because the principal basis for the book is to provide outcomes of nerve injuries, entrapments, and tumors and collecting new data and updating the various chapters with this in mind would be very time consuming. In the meantime however, two fortuitous events came about: Dr. Daniel Kim and his colleagues at that time from Stanford began to travel to New Orleans and to systematically "mine" the LSUHSC office files for pertinent data for a series of papers published mainly in *Neurosurgery* and the *Journal of Neurosurgery*. These efforts then provided much of the updated data needed for a Second Edition. In addition, we decided to ask a small group of younger workers in the field of peripheral nerve surgery to either rewrite or re-edit many of the chapters. Since all concerned are busy people, this has been a slow process but it is now complete. Thus, we are indebted to not only to Daniel Kim but also his former colleague from Stanford Judith Murovic and their many colleagues there and now here in New Orleans but also Raj Midha of Calgary, Canada; and Robert Spinner from Rochester, Minnesota for their contributions. Ron Tasker of Toronto has also provided his unique perspective on Pain of Neuropathic Origin and for this we are thankful. Various residents and fellows helped with some chapters particularly Chris Winfrey with Anesthetic and Positional Palsies; Rashid Janjua with Thoracic Outlet Syndrome; and Shaun O'Leary with Plexus Birth Palsies. New chapters were added on Iatrogenic Nerve Injuries and Anesthetic and Positional Palsies while the chapter on Reconstructive Procedures underwent substantial revision as did those on Birth Palsies and Thoracic Outlet Syndromes. New sections under lower extremity lesions include those on the ilioinguinal and iliohypogastric nerves and the genitofemoral nerve while the suprascapular nerve and its lesions has been split away from the chapters on plexus lesions and is now a "stand alone" chapter. Modern surgical practice is more and more evidence-based, and more and more oriented to quality and safety of patient care. This book is offered alongside the contributions of other authors around the world, as a contribution to these fundamental principles of modern surgery.

Hurricane Katrina of course complicated and slowed the process down, but our editors, Susan Pioli and Rebecca Gaertner, and their assistants at Elsevier have been extremely patient as well as helpful in this process and for that we are especially grateful. The hard work of Tim Kimber, Alex Mortimer, Bryan Potter and others at Elsevier made much of this Second Edition possible.

D.G.K
A.R.H

List of Contributors

Alan R. Hudson OC, MB, ChB, FRCS (Ed), FRCSC, FCSSA (Hon)
Professor Emeritus
University of Toronto
Toronto, ON

Daniel H. Kim MD
Professor
Spinal Neurosurgery and Reconstructive Peripheral Nerve Surgery
Baylor College of Medicine
Houston, TX

David G. Kline AB, MD
Boyd Professor
Neurosurgery Department
Louisiana State University School of Medicine in New Orleans
New Orleans, LA

Rajiv Midha MD, MSc, FRCS(C)
Professor and Chief
Division of Neurosurgery, Department of Clinical Neurosciences
University of Calgary
Calgary, AB

Judith A. Murovic MD
Instructor, Neurosurgery
Department of Neurosurgery
Stanford University Medical Center
Stanford, CA

Robert J. Spinner MD
Professor of Neurologic Surgery, Orthopedics and Anatomy
Mayo Clinic
Rochester, MN

Ron R. Tasker MD, MA, FRCS(C)
Professor Emeritus
Division of Neurosurgery
Toronto Western Hospital
Toronto, ON

Acknowledgments

A large debt is owed to Judith Hickey, RN who has faithfully and thoroughly collected records and made arrangements for patients to be seen and operated upon for many years and our LSUHSC of Neurosurgery Administrator, Latricia Jackson who has recently moved to another department post-Katrina. Willie Coleman our Laboratory technician passed away shortly after Hurricane Katrina and we miss him. The work for this edition could not have been completed without the constant diligence of Dr. Kline's secretary, Vanissia Prout. Dr. Leo Happel our neurophysiologist has also provided advice and sometimes directions for the operative recordings used in many of the patients reported upon. Especial thanks are also due our medical artist for the First Edition, Eugene New and to Barbara Seide for some drawings used in the Second Edition.

Of course, especial thanks to our patients and their referring physicians our residents and fellows and other faculty, especially Austin Sumner, and of course our own families without whom this Second Edition would not be possible.

David G. Kline, M.D.

Alan R. Hudson, M.D.

DEDICATION TO SYDNEY SUNDERLAND

Dedication
SIR SYDNEY SUNDERLAND
December 31, 1910 – August 27, 1993

Sir Sydney Sunderland was born in 1910 in Brisbane, Australia, an received his MB, DSc, MD and LLD (Honorary) degrees from the University of Melbourne, where he began his career as a Lecturer in Anatomy and Neurology in 1937. He was influenced greatly by work with Frederick Wood Jones, Professor of Anatomy; with Dr. Leonard Cox, who established a neurologic clinic in Australia; and subsequently with Hugh Cairns, a neurosurgeon in Oxford, England. Sydney Sunderland was appointed to the Chair of Anatomy when he was only 27 years of age. He became Professor of Anatomy and then of Experimental Neurology at the same institution, publishing a remarkably large volume of original experimental work concerning the anatomy and regeneration of the peripheral nervous system. He was a Visiting Specialist in Peripheral Nerve Injuries at the 115th Australasian Hospital Unit from 1941 to 1945, working with Mr. Hugh Trumble, a neurosurgeon. He served as Dean of the University of Melbourne from 1953 to 1971, worked as a member and eventually Chairman of the Royal Australasian College of Surgeons Certification Committee between 1945 and 1969, and served on many governmental and academic councils in Australia and New Zealand. In addition to being knighted by the Queen of England in 1971, Sir Sydney worked as a Demonstrator in Anatomy at Oxford, as a Visiting Professor in Anatomy at Johns Hopkins, and as a Fogarty Scholar at the National Institutes of Health in Washington DC, gave a number of honorary lectures, and had an international peripheral nerve society named after him. His professional life's work was with peripheral nerve, and this was highlighted by publication of a reference text of encyclopedic proportions, *Nerves and Nerve Injuries*, in 1968. He extensively revised, updated, and republished this large reference work in 1978.

In 1991, Sir Sydney published a book entitled *Nerve Injuries and their Repair: A Critical Appraisal.* This work is based on his lifetime study of nerves and reflects on selected and, at times, controversial topics concerning nerve injury and repair. He is best known for his work with fascicular anatomy and the changing topography of these intraneural structures. He also made singular contributions to our understanding of oculomotor function and its involvement by uncal herniation and of the mechanisms involved in nerve root or spinal nerve stretch and avulsion. He was married for 53 years to Nina Gwendoline, or "Lady Gwen." This wonderful woman was educated as a lawyer and yet helped Sir Sydney type and edit his many manuscripts. They had one son, who has served as Deputy Medical Director at the Alfred Hospital in Melbourne, the same hospital at which his father had his medical roots. Sir Sydney died in Melbourne on August 27, 1993, at the age of 82, having had a very full life.

1

Selected basic considerations

David G. Kline

SUMMARY

The purpose of this chapter is to present selected and hopefully practical basic considerations concerning the anatomy, physiology and molecular biology of intact and injured nerve. Peripheral nerves provide the final motor pathway for impulses to the trunk and extremities as well as that for the sympathetic fibers. Axons also provide the afferent pathways for position sense, pressure, touch, temperature perception, and pain. These axons are extensions of the central nervous system (CNS) and have an active axoplasmic flow.

The majority of nerve volume is, however, composed of connective tissue (Fig. 1-1), and not axons and their covering with myelin. These connective tissue layers, including the endoneurium, perineurium, interfascicular epineurium, and epineurium, and their attendant fibroblasts, respond to serious injury with a proliferative and disorganized pattern. Thus, despite a rich and forgiving blood supply and a substantial neuronal ability to reform axons, serious injury to nerve results in poor spontaneous recovery.

A firm understanding of both the Wallerian process of degeneration and the human nerves' ability to recover from a given injury, as well as some method to graduate damage are, therefore, extremely important. Appreciation of some of the recent information developed concerning neuronal response to injury, neurotropism, and axonal metabolism is necessary, but not without a firm understanding of the more basic elements of a nerve's response to serious injury.

SELECTED BASIC CONSIDERATIONS

The successful peripheral nerve surgeon requires a wide portfolio of skills. These include knowledge of peripheral nerve anatomy and physiology, manual dexterity, clinical acumen, and many others. An essential skill is a comprehension of basic pathological, biochemical, and microscopic knowledge of peripheral nerve in health and disease, as this underlies much of the decision-making required both in the clinic and the operating room.

It is not our intent to review the large literature available in this area, but rather to present the more important basic information needed by the clinician caring for patients with nerve lesions. In many cases, many other publications provide more basic detail.

CONNECTIVE TISSUE LAYERS

The major tissue component of peripheral nerve is connective tissue.[120,130] This provides the skeleton or framework for the conductive elements, the axons, and their Schwann cells. The connective tissue layers help to protect as well as to provide nutrition for their enclosed nerve fibers (axons and their attendant Schwann cells). Estimates as to the amount of connective tissue in nerve vary, but its volume is greater than that for axons and their coverings.[58,135] The comparative areas occupied by fascicles versus epineurium and interfascicular epineurium vary from nerve to nerve as well as at given levels or cross-sectional areas in the same nerve (Fig. 1-2).[128] For example, close to 85% of the cross-sectional area of the sciatic nerve at the level of the hip is connective tissue.

The outer covering of nerve is provided by epineurium which is connective tissue containing both collagen and elastic fibers. The epineurium is a loose collection of areolar connective tissue with longitudinally oriented collagen fibrils.[90] The connective tissue tends to be increased where nerve crosses joints. The epineurial vessels are abundant, longitudinal, and tend to be arterioles and venules.[1] The microvessels between these arterioles and venules have relatively fenestrated endothelial cells which are leakier than the endoneurial ones which have tight junctions.[79] The epineurial vessels communicate with the endoneurial ones via oblique vessels in the perineurium. This layer serves to invest the fascicles and also provides a slight undulation to nerve. This undulation provides some longitudinal mobility, relative fixation being provided by neural branches entering musculature and the subcutaneous spaces.[130] Some investigators feel that there is a mesoneurium external to the epineurium.[69,131] In health, this connective tissue layer is filmy and transparent and helps to tether or secure nerve to adjacent structures such as tendons, vessels, muscles, and fascial planes.

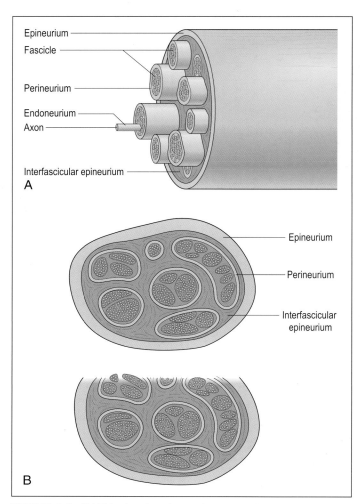

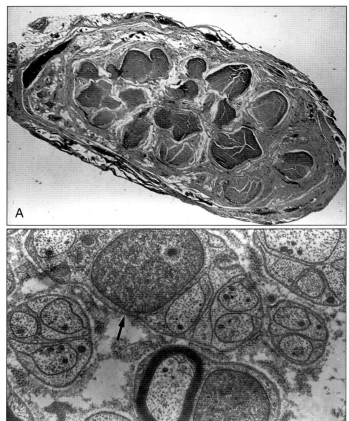

FIGURE 1-1 **(A)** This drawing shows the connective tissue layers of nerve. The epineurium is more compact than the interfascicular epineurium but not as compact as the more tightly woven three layers of the perineurium. Endoneurium surrounds each myelinated fiber and groups of unmyelinated or poorly myelinated fibers. **(B)** This drawing of a cross-section of nerve shows the disposition of the connective tissue layers from another perspective *(top)* and with a portion of epineurium and perineurium resected with resultant changes in fascicular structure *(bottom)*.

FIGURE 1-2 **(A)** Cross-section of a large nerve to show its fascicular disposition. This is a healthy primate nerve, and yet one can see the extensive connective tissue components at an epineurial and interfascicular level. Masson stain ×12. **(B)** Electron micrograph of normal nerve showing a myelinated nerve fiber with attendant Schwann cell *(lower arrow)* and surrounding endoneurium at the lower right. In the upper portion of the picture is a group of unmyelinated fibers and a Schwann cell *(upper arrow)* surrounded by an endoneurial envelope. A similar grouping of three small fibers is seen to the left.

Epineurial connective tissue is continuous with that between and surrounding the fascicles, which is termed the interfascicular epineurium. The latter is not as compact as the epineurium itself, and its volume varies from nerve to nerve and level to level in the same nerve. Vessels communicating between the epineurial and endoneurial levels travel in this compartment.

FASCICLES

Fascicles vary in number as well as size, depending on a given nerve as well as the level of the nerve examined. Each fascicle is encircled by perineurium which consists of oblique, circular, and longitudinal collagen fibrils dispersed amongst perineurial cells.[100] The latter have some morphological features in common with Schwann cells, including the presence of a basement lamella.[77,135] The polygonal cells of the perineurium have a laminated structure.[100] The outer lamellae have a high density of endocytotic vesicles which may play

a role in transport of some molecules such as glucose.[45] The inner lamellae have tight junctions between contiguous cells which may block the intercellular transport of macromolecules. The perineurium is an important site for a blood–nerve barrier since the perineurial cells have tight junctions.[82,99] Interruption of the perineurium can affect the function of the axons which it encloses (Fig. 1-3).[119,120,123] Thus, injury to the perineurium alone, such as resection of a portion of it, has an adverse effect on nerve function.[67] Such damage can be prolonged because the perineurium does not reconstitute itself well.[12,134] The conductive properties of axons will be dampened (Fig. 1-4), and, in some cases, the fibers will undergo partial demyelination as well as loss of axonal diameter.[61,67] The perineurium is the major source of tensile strength for nerve and also seems to constrain pressure within the fascicle since a sizable opening in the perineurium will cause some herniation of fascicular structure.[63]

Perineurium is traversed by vessels which carry a perineurial sleeve of connective tissue with them to mingle somewhat with the endoneurium.[77] The perineurial sleeves have close approximation to vessel walls. This anatomic feature may provide a potential

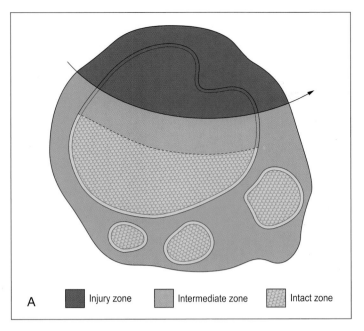

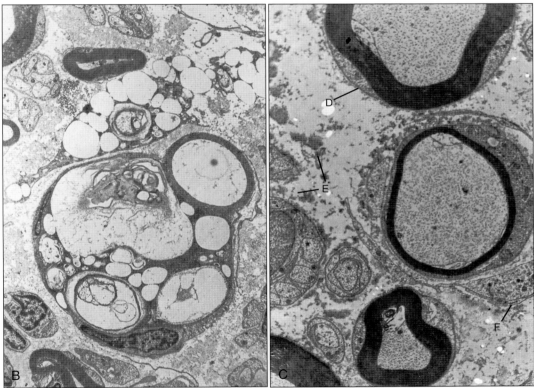

FIGURE 1-3 **(A)** The effect on a nerve of a partial injury in which the perineurium has been interrupted. Initial physical injury in this case leads to an area of complete axonal destruction and subsequent scar formation. **(B)** In the intermediate zone, some axons undergo degeneration amid ones that are maintained. **(C)** In other areas of the intermediate zone, axons may lose caliber and have decreased myelination. D, basement lamella; E, collagen fibers; F, endoneurial fibroblast.

vascular communication between the connective tissues of the epineurium and those of the endoneurium.[80] Endoneurium as well as the basal lamina encircles each myelinated axon and groups of unmyelinated or poorly myelinated axons. Endoneurium is a matrix of small-diameter collagen fibrils which are predominantly longitudinally oriented. Microvessels with tight junctions are found at this level, and the endothelium of these capillaries probably serves as another blood–nerve barrier along with the endoneurial tissue itself (Fig. 1-5).[90,130] These endoneurial microvessels are morphologically similar to the capillaries and their related astrocytic connections seen in the central nervous system (CNS). Changes in the permeability of these vessels frequently occur, even after relatively mild

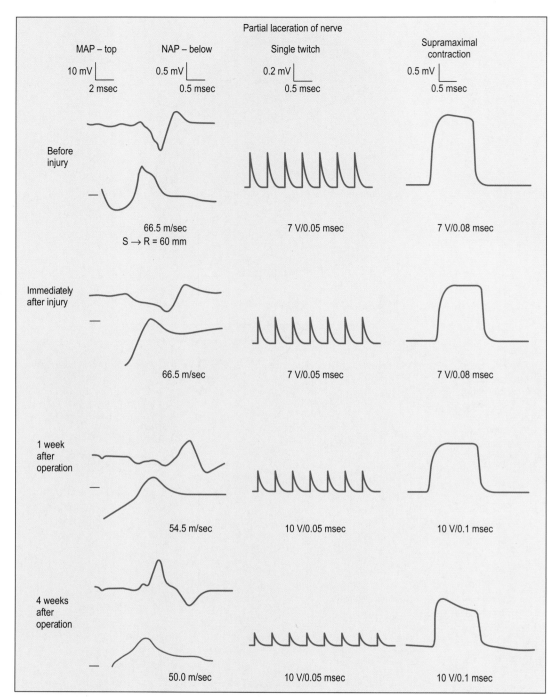

FIGURE 1-4   Progression of a partial nerve injury is documented by electrophysiologic studies. Baseline nerve action potential (NAP) and evoked muscle action potential (MAP), single twitch, and supramaximal contraction traces are at the top followed by traces made immediately after injury and recordings made at 1 and 4 weeks postoperatively. Settings for recordings were kept constant, but the amplitudes of the supramaximal single-twitch contraction as well as the tetanic contraction decreased with time. (From Kline D: Primate laboratory models for peripheral nerve repair. In: Omer G and Spinner M, Eds. Management of Peripheral Nerve Injuries, Philadelphia, WB Saunders, 1980.)

nerve trauma.[111] Endoneurial fibroblasts occasionally can be seen in the connective tissues between the nerve fibers of normal nerve.

Endoneurium is the final protective investiture of the axon and protects it when the nerve is mildly elongated or stretched.[76,131] Endoneurium also provides a constraint for the intracellular pressure provided by the axon and its myelin sheath much as the perineurium does for the intrafascicular contents.

NERVE FIBERS AND SCHWANN CELLS

The neural structure is comprised of axons and their accompanying Schwann cells. In a healthy nerve, these nerve fibers reside within the fascicular structure. Axons and their Schwann cells are surrounded not only by ground substance but by collagen fibrils which have some degree of condensation immediately superficial to the

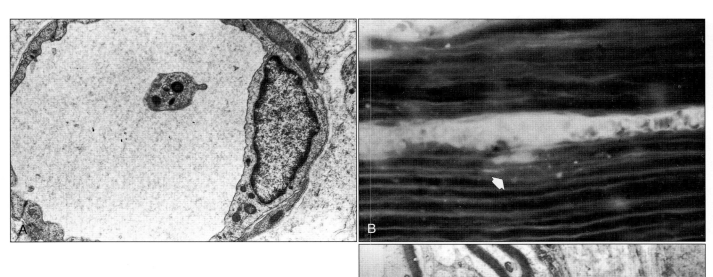

FIGURE 1-5 **(A)** Endoneurial microvessels have tight junctions. These intrafascicular microvessels are one of the sites of the blood–nerve barrier; the other is the perineurium. **(B)** Intrafascicular capillary in nerve whose blood supply was injected with a vital dye at the site at which the perineurium had been interrupted. Interruption of the perineurium can lead to leakage of serum from capillaries, as indicated by the extravascular dye in this study *(arrow)*. **(C)** Electron micrograph showing perineurium *(arrow);* myelinated and unmyelinated axons and a Schwann cell are seen to the left.

basement lamellae of the Schwann cells (Fig. 1-6).[10,90] Thus, the connective tissue component of nerve exists even at this microscopic level.

Axons contain certain organelles including mitochondria, neurofilaments, endoplasmic reticulum, microtubules, and dense particles.[44] Axons originate from their cell bodies which are in the spinal cord, dorsal root ganglia, and autonomic ganglia. Most of the "mother" neuron's cytoplasm is included in the volume of the axon since it is very long compared to the size of the neuron.[36,143] There is axoplasmic flow from the neuron to the axon's end stations and thus a proximal to distal gradient in endoneurial pressure.

In healthy nerve, there tend to be two sizes of fibers, large and small. The larger fibers are concerned with conduction of afferent as well as efferent messages connected with muscles, as well as afferent messages connected with touch, pressure, and some painful sensations. Smaller fibers conduct efferent messages concerned with autonomic function and afferent messages for temperature perception and most painful sensations.

Schwann cells are placed along the longitudinal extent of the axon.[115] In the case of larger fibers, the membrane of each Schwann cell wraps concentrically around a segment of axon, providing a lipoprotein coating or covering of myelin.[17] There is less envelopment of the axon as the edge of one Schwann cell approaches that of another. This is known as the "node of Ranvier."[105] Processes from adjacent Schwann cells interdigitate with each other at these nodal areas. The node of Ranvier permits ionic exchanges between the axoplasm of a nerve fiber and the intercellular space. This exchange, in turn, permits salutatory conduction of a nerve action

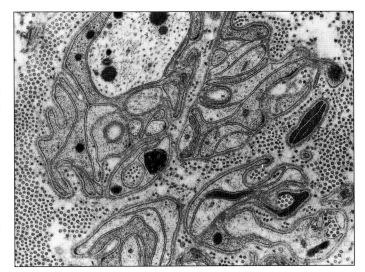

FIGURE 1-6 This electron micrograph shows unmyelinated fibers surrounded by basal lamina or endoneurium and by collagen fibrils.

potential impulse which travels from one node to the next. There is a basal lamina around each Schwann cell and its contents. The ability to form such a basal lamina differentiates the Schwann cell from other intraneural cells such as fibroblasts or mast cells.[10,22] Small and less myelinated fibers are enveloped by the membrane of a Schwann cell, but by no lipoprotein sheath or less of one than

5

in the larger and better myelinated fibers.[21,93] These fibers do not have the structural capacity for salutatory conduction, and impulses transmit along axon alone, making for slower conduction than seen in larger fibers. Thus, a wave of depolarization spreads continuously along such axons.

A Schwann cell not only provides myelin and some guidance structure in terms of a basal membrane, but is most likely the source of an as yet unidentified trophic or growth factor(s)[27,28,34,43,138] Such trophic factors may originate from Schwann cells proximal to the injury site as well as distal to it.[32,52,74,84] There is also evidence for neurotrophic interactions between regenerating axons and distal inputs such as muscles even in the adult animal.[24] In any case, the growth cone, which is the tip of an advancing neurite or regenerating axon, seems to depend on Schwann cell contact for elongation as well as guidance.[2,3,139,140] The local environment provides some adhesiveness and access to components such as laminin and fibronectin.[9,30,54] These, as well as other factors, provide an optimal setting for the fiber's growth cone and, therefore, the advance of the neurite.[29,31,112,146] Thus, the local environment at the injury and regenerative site remains extremely important, and this is so not only for the welfare of the growth cone, but also the Schwann cell.[10,138]

NEURONS AND AXOPLASM TRANSPORT

During peripheral nerve neurite regeneration, ribonucleic acid (RNA) at a neuronal level increases to presumably provide amino acids for the replenishment of axoplasm.[6,11,33,36] This increase in neuronal RNA persists until the regenerative process is finished.[40,41] Cytoskeletal proteins such as tubulin and neurofilament protein provide the building blocks for axonal regrowth.[14,15,116] Actin and probably myosin nourish the growth cone at the very tip of the advancing neurite.[137] The synthesized microtubules and neurofilaments form a network extending to the tip of the advancing neurite.[33]

Axoplasm contains proteins and cytoskeletal elements including microtubules and neurofilaments.[16,33] Axoplasm is continuously made and sustained by axonal transport mechanisms.[78] There is a continuous bidirectional fast transport system for axoplasm in nerve which has both anterograde and retrograde components. The slow component tends to carry more proteins and thus building blocks for growth than do the fast components. Slow transport at a rate of 1–2 mm per day moves the proteins for the neuron to the advancing neurite tip, but the local environment at the injury site may also provide important proteins for construction of the neurite tip.[18,96] Anterograde fast axonal transport of amino acids and proteins increases in response to injury, but only provides some of the less major and thus smaller building blocks.[95] Retrograde fast axonal transport, which accelerates during the early phase of regeneration, may provide varying concentrations of trophic or signal protein to the neuron, but this remains to be conclusively proven.[103] Again, the local environment may provide a more immediate signal to the spatially close growth cone.[69,137]

PERIPHERAL NERVE DEGENERATION AND REGENERATION

If the axon(s) are divided by injury, Wallerian degeneration occurs. This is a process that takes several weeks to be complete and includes the gradual dissolution of axoplasm and myelin distal to an injury and their gradual phagocytosis. The distal basal lamina

persists and Schwann cells proliferate in anticipation of axonal regrowth.

With serious injury to nerve, the important connective tissue layers as well as their enclosed nerve fibers are injured. The connective tissue response to most injuries is a proliferative one.[44,55,131] This leads to a disorganized connective tissue which can thwart effective axonal regrowth (Fig. 1-7).[59,133] Despite this, peripheral neurite regeneration is much more effective than that of axons or neurites in the CNS.[73] Peripheral nerve has a basal lamina provided by the Schwann cells and surrounding its axons while the CNS does not. The basal lamina, although destroyed at the injury site, survives proximal and distal to it (Fig. 1-8).[60,89] In the distal stump of an injured nerve, the lamina surrounds deposits of degenerating myelin and axoplasmic debris, which are gradually phagocytized.[7,101,141] The Schwann cells proliferate close to the growth cones and elongating neurites to form bands of Büngner.[104] As the neurites grow distally, the basal lamina tends to resist the expanding force of the growing neurite and to channel its advance within the sheath to reach the "guidance system of the distal stump" (Fig. 1-9). Trophic factors which may exist in both the central and the peripheral nervous system do help attract the new neurite. A proximal stump, separated by a distance from the distal stump, preferentially grows towards it rather than to non-neural tissue.[3,81] The relatively structured tubular system of a nerve undergoing Wallerian degeneration and then regeneration helps also to direct axonal regrowth (Figs 1-10 to 1-12).[104,117,130,144]

By comparison, in the CNS, where there is no basal laminar system, effective axonal regeneration may be poor because the expanding pressure of the neurite's terminal club is less restrained. This leads to rupture, loss of axoplasm, and release of lysosomal enzymes which can further damage the local environment.[140] Despite the relatively favorable circumstances for peripheral nerve regeneration, the growing neurite in higher-phylum animals such as primates can be readily blocked or deflected. The nerve fiber is forced to change pathways and/or divide many times by the disorganized proliferation of both endoneurial and interfascicular epineurial connective tissues in response to injury (Fig. 1-13).[104,117,131] This can result in distal stump axons of fine caliber and of relatively poor myelination. Of even greater consequence, axons may not regain their former sites of innervation or come close enough to them to mature and become functional. The factors responsible for such fibroblast proliferation and subsequent collagen alignment after injury are poorly understood (Fig. 1-14).[69,83,102,131] Unfortunately, practical methods to ameliorate such changes biochemically are not as yet available.[26,91,132]

Some triggers or modulators of fibroblastic activity are known.[46] Recent neurochemical work with human neuromas indicate that two cytokines secreted by macrophages, TNF and IL-1, increase dramatically after nerve injury.[83] These cytokines produce NGF which facilitates axonal regeneration but they also activate MAP and SAPK in the human neuroma fibroblasts. These activate protein kinesis then accelerate fibroblast proliferation.

Adequate regeneration of a nerve fiber takes time, both for the fiber to reach a distal innervational site and for the fiber to mature. Thus, a series of "delays" exist, even when axonal regeneration is quite successful (Table 1-1).

NEURAL BLOOD SUPPLY

Fortunately, blood supply to nerve is a rich one.[1,98] It is predominantly longitudinal with proximal input at the level of the roots or

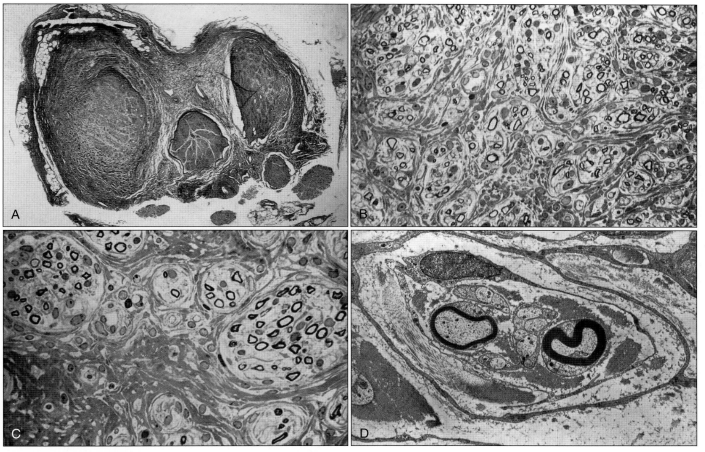

FIGURE 1-7 **(A)** Cross-section of an injured nerve showing intrafascicular as well as extrafascicular scar. **(B)** Small, fine, regenerated axons are mixed in with endoneurial scar in this low-power, Masson stained, microscopic cross-section. **(C)** Another area from the same cross-section shows several areas of relatively heavy scar mixed in with clusters of relatively small, regenerating axons. **(D)** Electron micrographic preparation showing fibroblasts and scar around regenerating axons.

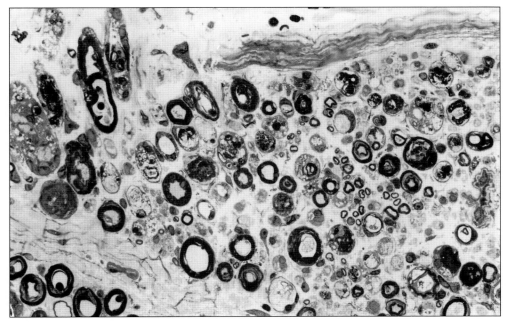

FIGURE 1-8 This photomicrograph shows areas of degenerating axons distal to a partial laceration to nerve.

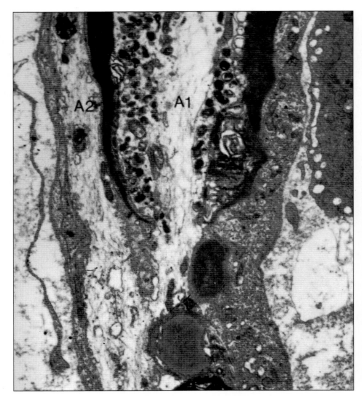

FIGURE 1-9 Process of axonal sprouting occurs in the proximal stump. A1 is the terminal sprout, and A2 is a collateral sprout. These sprouts are retained in the original basement lamella of the nerve fiber, and the regenerative unit thus formed crosses the suture line to reinnervate the distal stump or graft.

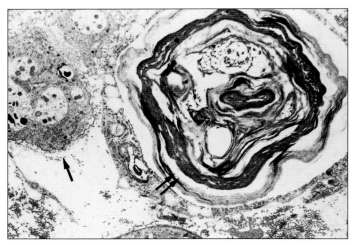

FIGURE 1-10 A regenerative unit *(singe arrow)* invades the distal stump next to a fiber undergoing Wallerian degeneration *(double arrow).*

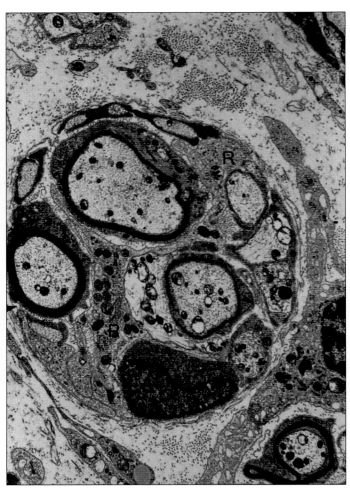

FIGURE 1-11 Axons of the regenerative unit start to myelinate as the regenerating fibers come into contact with the Schwann cells of the distal stump.

Table 1-1 Axonal growth characteristics
Initial delay while regenerating axons make up the area of retrograde degeneration.
Injury site delay while axons traverse injury site.
Distal delay as axons grow down the distal stump.
Terminal delay as axons both mature and reinnervate distal innervational sites.

spinal nerves and distal input connected with both the motor and sensory branches.[13] Vessels travel a course predominantly in the epineurium and interfascicular epineurium, but are also located within the fascicles themselves.[80] There is a collateral blood supply which feeds into the extensive epineurial longitudinal system via the mesoneurium (Fig. 1-15).[122] The mesoneurium as a layer is anatomically controversial although in the living subject it can usually be demonstrated as a fine, transparent membrane attaching nerve to adjacent soft tissue structures. These collateral vessels can be sacrificed during mobilization of a nerve without loss of function or decreased ability for the injured nerve to regenerate.[66] Longitudinal and intraneural vessels supply enough nourishment to maintain functional integrity and/or ability to regenerate.[8] Nonetheless, changes in blood flow to nerve can occur with different types of injuries.[97] In addition, the blood–nerve barrier can be disturbed in an animal such as a rat not only by various injuries but also by toxins.[63]

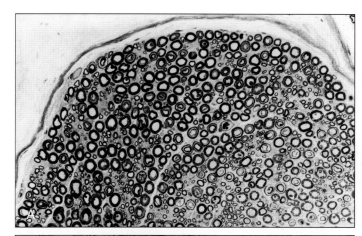

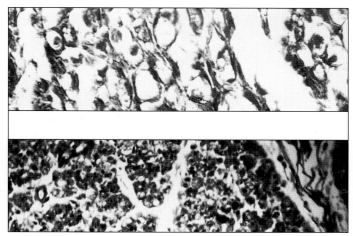

FIGURE 1-13 Degenerative changes in distal stumps of nerves studied at different time intervals. The top photograph shows degenerative axonal and myelin debris but with relatively open tubular system at 3 weeks after injury. The bottom photograph shows a distal cross-section 3 months after more proximal injury. Endoneurial fibroblasts have proliferated, and the tubular system has been somewhat closed down by connective tissue. Despite this distal stump change, axons that eventually become functional can grow distally, depending on the local injury milieu more proximally. (Masson stain ×40.)

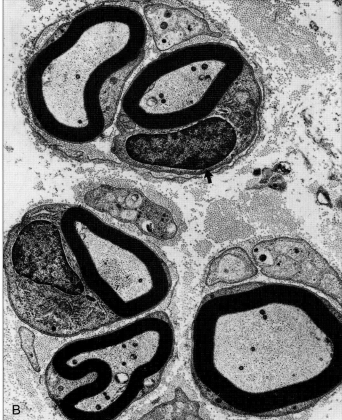

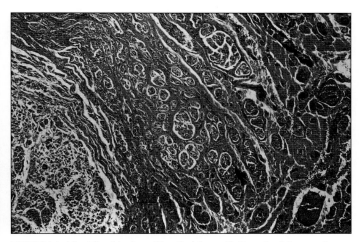

FIGURE 1-14 Fibroblast proliferation in graft. Despite this, small axons are seen at both intrafascicular and extrafascicular sites. (Masson stain ×35.)

FIGURE 1-12 **(A)** With regeneration, fibers in the distal stump mature until a normal pattern of myelinated and unmyelinated fibers is seen. **(B)** Each Schwann cell *(arrow)* is associated with a single large axon in the case of a myelinated fiber or with multiple small axons which remain either unmyelinated or poorly myelinated.

FASCICULAR STRUCTURE

Not as favorable for the surgeon as nerve's blood supply is the next anatomical fact, which is that fascicular structure changes position along the longitudinal course of the nerve every few centimeters (Fig. 1-16).[130] This makes fascicular matching between proximal and distal stumps, where there has been loss of neural substance, difficult. Fascicles also trade fibers or sometimes bundles of such with neighboring fascicles as they travel down the course of the

nerve.[90] This changing reorganization appears random, but that is not the case, because the process eventually provides the proper mix of afferent and efferent fibers for each branch. In addition, the more centrally placed fascicles, especially in the proximal segment of a nerve, contain fibers serving a variety of distal functions. As the nerve approaches the more distal extremity, there is greater differentiation of function into specific fascicles which then become predominantly motor or sensory. These fascicular positional changes and fascicular trade-offs are more dramatic in the proximal portions of a given nerve than distally.[85] Nonetheless, a fascicle may be a 9 o'clock position at one level and, within a few centimeters, be at a 12 o'clock or even a 2 o'clock position.[126]

The final unit of function within a fascicle is the nerve fiber, composed of the axon and its attendant Schwann cells. The

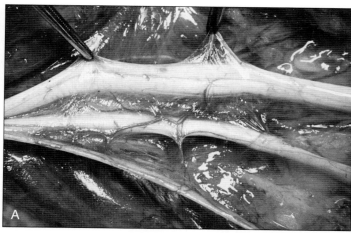

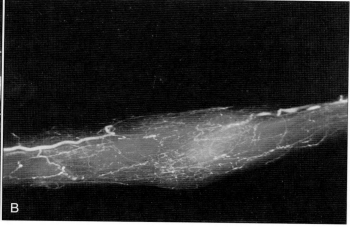

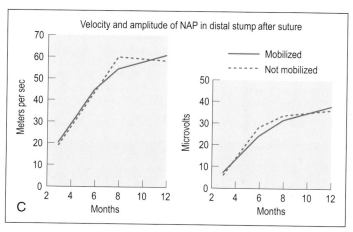

FIGURE 1-15 **(A)** Blood supply in the primate sciatic complex. Forceps are on the presumed mesoneurium. The longitudinal nature of the epineurial vessels is evident. Collateral vessels can be seen at several levels and reaching nerve via the mesoneurium. Tibial nerve is at the top, peroneal nerve is intermediate, and sural nerve is below. (From Kline D, Hackett E, Davis G, Myers B: Effect of mobilization on the blood supply and regeneration of injured nerves. J Surg Res 12:254–266, 1972.) **(B)** Primate sciatic nerve injured by severance and then sutured together. Animal was perfused with contrast to demonstrate reconstitution of microvessels, especially at the injury site. **(C)** These two graphs depict distal stump nerve action potential (NAP) velocity and amplitude in primate nerves that were severed and sutured. Nerve on one side was mobilized from sciatic notch to calf levels before repair, whereas that on the other side was not mobilized. NAP velocities and amplitudes were relatively similar at each time interval up to 12 months after repair, whether or not nerve was mobilized. (Adapted by Gilliatt RM (personal communication) from Kline D, Hackett E, Davis G, Myers B: Effects of mobilization on the blood supply and regeneration of injured nerves. J Surg Res, 1972.)

endoneurium surrounding the nerve fibers reacts to injury just as do the other connective tissue layers of the nerve. These nerve fibers and their fibrous coverings cannot be seen either by the naked eye or under the operating microscope; therefore, the structure that forms the subunit of various micro-operative procedures is the fascicle (Fig. 1-17).

OPERATIVE CONSIDERATIONS

Microdissection of nerve at a fascicular level is difficult although not impossible.[131,132] Grossly, or even under the operating microscope, fascicular structure can appear to be intact, and yet there may be severe axonal loss. Furthermore, the related endoneurial changes may be of such a nature as to prevent successful regeneration unless repair is instituted. This is particularly so with some contusive and many stretch injuries, where despite even gross fascicular continuity, intrafascicular change is often neurotemetic. Variability in this intrafascicular pathology also makes intraoperative electrophysiologic assessment of an injury in continuity imperative (Fig. 1-18).[64,65,92] Thus, electrical stimulation as well as stimulation and recording of nerve action potentials (NAPs) are, in our as well as other people's view, necessary intraoperative steps with most serious lesions in continuity.[68,145]

Microscopic operative technique is generally used to dissect fascicles within a nerve, and it should be stressed that such a dissection is along structural lines alone. A major assumption made by some clinicians during such procedures is that if the fascicle is grossly intact, the nerve fibers contained within that structure are likely to be normal or have the potential to become so. Although this may be true under some circumstances, it is far from universal. This is because intrafascicular neurotemetic changes can and often do occur despite maintenance of gross continuity of a fascicle. This is particularly so when stretching forces are the primary mechanism of injury or when nerve has been injured by injection.[69] Unfortunately, stretch is the leading cause or mechanism of serious nerve injury requiring operation; therefore, fascicular continuity by no means assures recovery unless the potential for such is shown by intraoperative electrical testing.[145]

BASIC RESPONSES TO INJURY

THE NEURON'S RESPONSE

The cell body, which is located in the anterior horn of the spinal cord, the posterior root ganglion, or in an autonomic ganglion, undergoes chromatolysis when an axon is interrupted.[116] Histologically, the neuronal swelling is accompanied by displacement of the Nissl substance to the periphery of the cell.[11] Thus, enlargement of a neuron after its axon is injured is usually regenerative rather than degenerative in nature.[6,20,75] Exceptions are found in severe proximal injury to neural elements, particularly the brachial plexus or the lumbosacral plexus, which can result in retrograde damage

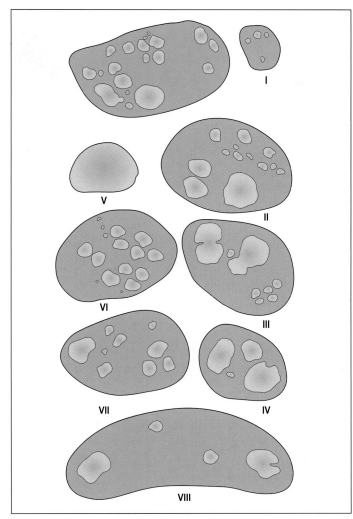

FIGURE 1-16 Change in fascicular pattern in radial nerve running from arm level (I) to forearm level (VIII). V represents the superficial sensory radial nerve, and VI and VII are the proximal and distal posterior interosseous nerves. (From Sunderland S: The intraneural topography of the radial, median, and ulnar nerves. Brain 68:243–299, 1945.)

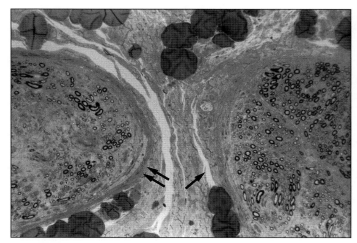

FIGURE 1-17 Elbow-level cross-section of radial nerve in a patient with preganglionic injury of C7 and C8 spinal nerves. The superficial sensory radial part of the nerve, which is made up of sensory axons, is preserved to the right *(single arrow)* whereas most of the motor fascicle, seen to the left, is degenerated *(double arrow)*. (Toluidine blue ×368.)

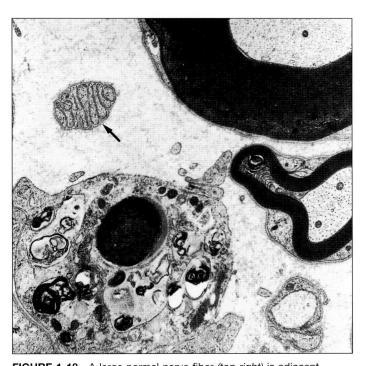

FIGURE 1-18 A large normal nerve fiber *(top right)* is adjacent to a smaller axon with a thinner myelin coating. At the lower left, a macrophage is digesting myelin debris. Above this is a band of Büngner *(arrow)* composed of a stack of Schwann cell profiles within a single basement lamella. Nerve fiber injury can be of a different degree within a single fascicle, and nerve fascicle injury can be of a different degree within a single peripheral nerve. The surgeon must be familiar with these concepts during evaluation of nerve lesions in continuity.

to the neuron serious enough to be incompatible with its survival.[53]

When neuronal chromatolysis is regenerative in nature, the cytoplasm increases in volume, primarily due to an increase in ribonucleic acid (RNA) and associated enzymes.[40] RNA changes from large particles to submicroscopic particles, and this change results in an apparent loss of Nissl substance. From 4 days after injury until a peak is reached at 20 days, the amount of RNA increases as does it metabolic rate.[37] RNA appears necessary for the reconstruction of axons, and it provides the polypeptides and proteins necessary for replenishment of axoplasm (Fig. 1-19). Its role as the central ingredient in regeneration has, however, been questioned by some. The argument has been advanced that the increase occurs only if regeneration is already proceeding successfully.[41,57] The RNA may serve only as a marker for regeneration rather than heralding it. In any case, it has been clearly shown that increased RNA volume and activity persist until axon regeneration and maturation cease. The closer the injury is to the spinal cord, the more hypertrophic are the neuronal changes, while with distal lesions, the

changes are less marked. Since a proximal injury requires a lengthier regeneration of the axon than a distal one, it is almost as if the neuron were able to anticipate the job ahead.

Methods for tracing axon connections back to the CNS have led to a number of interesting observations.[72] In a healthy axon-

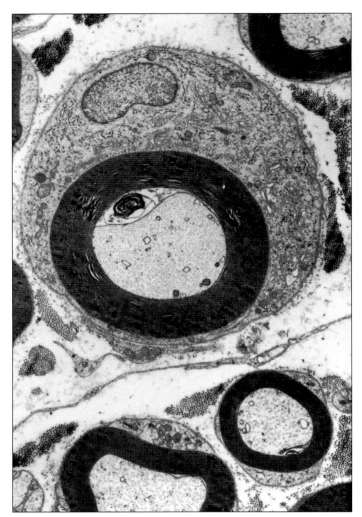

FIGURE 1-19 Axon is continuous with the nerve cell body in the spinal cord or posterior root ganglion. All protein synthesis occurs in the cell body and is transported down the axon. Surrounding the axon is the reduplicated surface membrane of the attendant Schwann cell – the myelin. By contrast, the cytoplasm of the Schwann cell is packed with organelles. A basement lamella coats the surface of the Schwann cell, and this forms a continuous structure along the length of the nerve fiber, made up of the continuous axon and a chain of discontinuous Schwann cells.

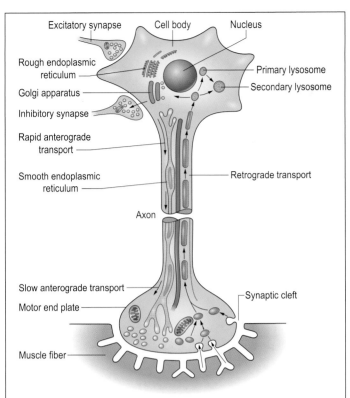

FIGURE 1-20 Diagram of a cell body with its supported axon and distal innervational site. The drawing shows some of the intraneuronal structures and the smooth endoplasmic reticulum, tubular structure, and microfilaments at the nerve level. Sites of metabolic exchange are noted. (Adapted from Lundborg G, Ed: Nerve Injury and Repair. Edinburgh, Churchill Livingstone, 1988.)

to-neuron relationship, metabolic building blocks for axoplasm are circulated from the nerve body down the axon and back up again (Fig. 1-20). As specified earlier, the axoplasmic flow of these metabolites may be supplemented along the axon's course by local exchange of both metabolites and waste products. Thus, some of the building blocks necessary for survival of the axon may be provided by the axon's local environment rather than by the neuron itself.[51,69]

Neurotrophic factor availability affects neuronal survival and these can originate from CNS glia, other neurons or non-neuronal sources, especially Schwann cells in the periphery.[107,147] Neurotrophins such as nerve growth factor (NGF), brain-derived nerve growth factor (BDNF), neurotrophin-3 (NT-3,) and NT-4/5 are transported to the cell body and help it to survive.[87] Prevention of regeneration to a distal stump leads to a greater apoptosis of sensory neurons than motor ones, possibly due to trophic factors from glia

and other neurons.[44,87] On the other hand, motor neurons can survive a year or more without axonal regeneration to the distal stump.[106]

Molecular genetic changes in neurons undergoing change due to axonal regeneration have also received relatively recent attention.[63] There are early neuronal increases in C-FOS, jun BV, and c jun m RNA. These changes can vary according to the nature of the injury. Significant changes in C-FOS protein content exist when nerve root avulsion is compared to more distal nerve injury.[149] The immediate early genes (IEGs) are activated by unknown mechanisms and appear to be blocked by administration of various growth factors.[63]

Despite a number of neuronal metabolic alterations in neuronal function, neurophysiological markers such as resting-potential and after potential spikes do not change.[19,39] There is, however, a disturbance in the neuron's central synaptic function.[38] Longer latency and increased temporal dispersion of the reflex discharge evoked by the afferent stimulation of the neuron occur. Degenerative changes in synaptic vesicles have also been demonstrated by electron microscopy and may relate to interference in synaptic function.[109]

Experimental work suggests some expansion of the sensory neuronal field in response to distal axotomy and subsequent regeneration.[51,62] Neighboring neurons whose axons were not sectioned were found to branch to feed the neuronal zone whose distal axons were sectioned.[57,142] There is also some experimental evidence that the motor neuronal zone subtending a nerve's injury can increase in size or expand in terms of level.[23,25,50] How effective such expansion is in terms of useful regeneration remains to be shown but has been recorded, even in the primate.[70,114] With increased interest in nerve transfers for stretch injuries to plexus with nerve root avulsion(s) functional magnetic resonance imaging (MRI) studies have shown some transfer of activity from the donor neuronal site to that recipient site.[88]

If the axon is freshly re-resected proximal to a previous transection site, new regenerative activity on the part of the neuron results and a new thrust of axoplasm occurs.[42] This has led to the suggestion that a possible way of accelerating axonal growth is by creating a conditioning lesion or a second axotomy several weeks after the initial injury.[86] This presumes that regeneration by means of a repair, which is delayed for several weeks, will be augmented by the primed and thus already increased metabolic activity of the neurons that was provided by the original injury. It is unclear at this time whether a second axotomy forces a completely new turnover of RNA to occur or whether it changes the peak activity already achieved by the first axotomy. In any case, such conditioning may play a role in the usual surgical procedure to repair nerve. An important step in neural repair, either by direct apposition or grafts after any interval of time, is to trim or resect not only the distal stump but also the proximal one back to healthy tissue.[5] Thus, a second axotomy is universal once repair is undertaken for a serious nerve lesion. Only the interval between the two axotomies may vary.

AXONAL RESPONSE TO INJURY

For clinical purposes, there are three basic ways in which nerve fibers can respond to trauma (Fig. 1-21), and this has been nicely delineated by Seddon[118] and enlarged upon by Sunderland.[127] It must, however, be kept in mind that the thousands of axons making up each nerve are not only of variable size and disposition, but also have different needs nutritionally as well as for oxygenation. As a result, many nerve injuries are composed of mixed elements of neurapraxia, axonotmesis, and neurotmesis.

Neurapraxia

With neurapraxia, there is a block in conduction of the impulse down the nerve fiber, and recovery takes place without Wallerian degeneration. This is probably a biochemical lesion due to a concussion or shock-like injury to the fiber.[117,130] In the case of the whole nerve, neurapraxia is brought about by compression or by relatively mild, blunt blows, including some low-velocity missile injuries close to the nerve. Thus, injury where there is the potential for compression or stretch can produce some element of neurapraxia (Fig. 1-22).[110] Peroneal paralysis due to a prolonged cross-legged position and radial or Saturday night paralysis due to compression of the radial nerve in axilla or outer arm are common examples of neurapraxic injures. Stimulation proximal to such an injury fails to produce muscle function distally while stimulation distal to the injury does. If the entire cross-section of the nerve is affected, a NAP will not transmit across the lesion but can be generated by stimulating and recording either proximal or distal to it.

Segmental demyelination of some fibers may occur, and others may actually undergo axonotmesis, producing occasional fibrillations in muscle seen by electromyography performed several weeks later. The overwhelming picture is, however, one of normal axons

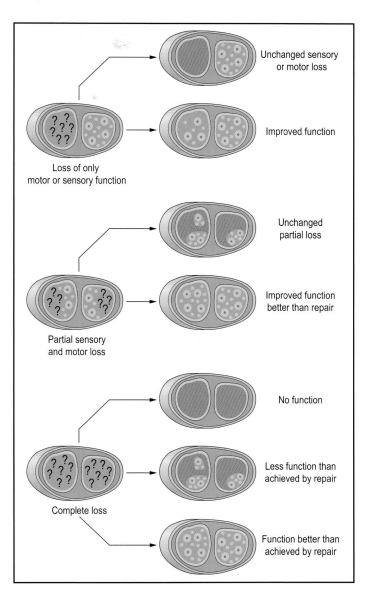

FIGURE 1-21 Various outcomes are shown for the three major types of injury to nerve. With loss of only motor or sensory function, the outcome can include either unchanged sensory or motor loss or improved function in both spheres. With time, the result with partial sensory and motor loss may be either unchanged partial loss or function that improves to a level better than repair would have given. With complete loss, there may be no functional return with time, less function than is achieved by repair, or better function than a repair might bring.

without Wallerian degeneration.[35,48] Such injury selectively affects the larger fibers serving muscle contraction as well as touch and position sense, while fine fibers subserving pain and sweating are spared.[125] Thus, these injuries often have an element of pain. Since connective tissue elements as well as most of the microscopic anatomy of the axon and its coverings are preserved, recovery is assured, but may require several days, or on occasion, even up to 5–6 weeks to occur.

Axonotmesis

By comparison, axonotmesis involves loss of the relative continuity of the axon and its covering of myelin, but preservation of the

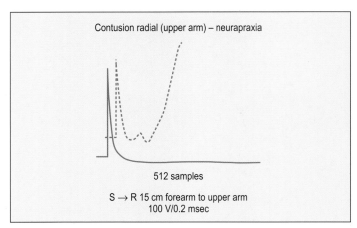

Contusion radial (upper arm) – neurapraxia

512 samples

S → R 15 cm forearm to upper arm
100 V/0.2 msec

FIGURE 1-22 Recording made noninvasively at the skin level distal to an area of contusion 5 days after the onset of a complete radial palsy. Summated trace is above and single trace below. The summated trace shows a nerve action potential (NAP) after the stimulus artifact, and this is followed by the take-off of an evoked muscle action potential (MAP). Ability to stimulate both an NAP and an MAP by stimulation distal to the lesion provides evidence of the presence of neurapraxic lesion.

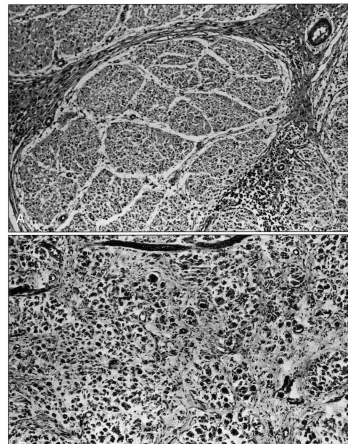

FIGURE 1-23 **(A)** Scarred distal stump with fine axons only. **(B)** Area of a distal stump with more adequate axonal regeneration than seen in **A**. Although the interval between injury and the making of these cross-sections was the same, the mechanism of the injury was different. Nerve injury in **B** was more axonotmetic than in **A**.

connective tissue framework of the nerve.[94] Due to loss of axonal continuity, Wallerian degeneration occurs. Electromyography 2–3 weeks later will show fibrillations and denervational potentials in musculature distal to the injury site.[47] Loss in both motor and sensory spheres is more complete with axonotmesis than with neurapraxia, and recovery only occurs through regeneration of the axons, a process requiring time (Fig. 1-23). Axonotmesis is usually the result of a more severe crush or contusion injury than that producing neurapraxia. After the elapse of 2–3 days, stimulation either proximal or distal to such a lesion does not produce muscle contraction. An NAP cannot be evoked across such a lesion or by recording from more distal nerve.

There is usually an element of retrograde proximal degeneration of the axon, and when regeneration occurs, this loss must first be overcome.[4] The regenerative fibers must cross the injury site and next regenerate down the distal stump. In the human, spanning of the injury site as well as axonal regeneration through the proximal or retrograde area of degeneration may require several weeks. Then, the neurite tip progresses down the distal stump only at an average rate of a millimeter per day. This rate may be faster if the injury is closer to the central nervous system such as with an injury to a plexus trunk or slower at a more distal site such as the wrist or hand. Thus, proximal lesions may grow distally as fast as 2–3 mm per day and distal lesions as slowly as 0.5 mm per day.[111]

Once sufficient numbers (4000 or 5000) of regenerating fibers penetrate the injury site, there will be restoration of an NAP recorded across it, but its amplitude will be small and conduction velocity greatly reduced.[64] Such a distal stump response can be recorded long before a muscle action potential can be evoked or decreases in denervational change can be recorded from muscle distal to the lesion.[65] Thus, there is a substantial period of time where regeneration can be satisfactory, and yet there is no more peripheral, clinical, or electrical evidence of such. As regeneration proceeds down the distal stump, this progress can be followed by NAP recordings. There is then a further delay once axons reach distal inputs while the latter are reconstructed and their axons

mature. At some point after axons reach muscle and before voluntary contraction can occur, stimulation of the regenerating nerve can produce muscle function. This finding may antedate clinical recovery by a number of weeks.[92] Regeneration with axonotmetic injury is superior to that of neurotmesis, even when such injures are corrected by surgical repair. With axonotmesis, the basement membrane system is relatively intact, and regenerating axon clusters are guided by Schwann cells and bands of Büngner enclosed within a relatively preserved distal endoneurium.

Neurotmesis

More severe contusion, stretch, or laceration produces neurotmesis, and not only axons but investing connective tissues lose their continuity. An obvious example of neurotmetic injury to nerve is one that transects it because both axonal and connective tissue continuity is lost. Many neophytes do not appreciate that most neurotmetic injuries do not, however, produce gross loss of continuity of the nerve, but rather, internal disruption of the architecture of the nerve sufficient to involve perineurium and endoneurium as well as axons and their coverings.

Denervational changes recorded by electromyogram (EMG) are the same as those seen with axonotmetic injury.[47] However, rever-

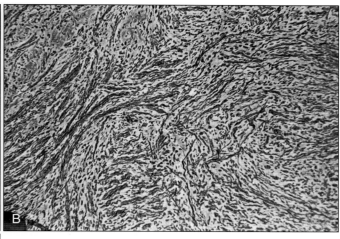

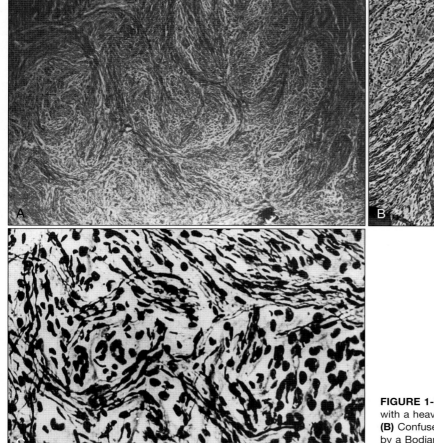

FIGURE 1-24 **(A)** Neurotmetic or Sunderland grade IV injury with a heavy proliferation of connective tissue. Masson stain. **(B)** Confused, disorganized axons from an injury site stained by a Bodian technique. **(C)** Confused and disorganized axons from another injury site.

sal of these changes and recovery are unlikely to occur because regenerating axons become mixed in a swirl of regenerating fibroblasts and collagen, producing a disorganized repair site or neuroma (Fig. 1-24). Thus, stimulation either above or distal to a neurotmetic segment of injury does not produce function nor are NAPs recorded across or distal to the lesion.[68] Furthermore, these abnormalities persist and do not improve as with neurapraxic and axonotmetic injuries. Although axons often reach the distal stump in great numbers in neurotmetic injuries, they often fail to find their pre-injury pathways (Fig. 1-25).[144] Most importantly, because of endoneurial proliferation and contraction of distal nerve sheaths, they may fail to regain sufficient axonal diameter and myelination to produce functional regeneration, even if they do reach proper destinations.

Biochemical and channel marking studies of human neuroma tissue has begun and some interesting observations have been made. For example, Gap 43, important in the early period of axonal regeneration, decreases with time.[49] In addition, Ankyrin G plays some role in changes in sodium channels in injured fibers, especially those associated with painful neuromas.[71]

Sunderland's grade I or first-degree injury corresponds to a neurapraxic injury (Fig. 1-26). Grade II injuries involve loss of axon continuity with preservation of endoneurium as well as fascicular structure and corresponds with an almost pure axonotmetic injury. Grade III is a mixed axonotmetic–neurotmetic injury with loss of both axons and endoneurium, but most of the perineurial and thus

some of the external fascicular structure is maintained. Grade IV injury involves loss of axons, endoneurium, and perineurium, and thus absence of fascicular structure with continuity maintained only by epineurium. This is a predominant neurotmetic injury. Grade V injury involves a transected nerve, and thus is neurotmetic by definition. Mackinnon has proposed a grade VI injury which is partial laceration of the nerve along with a partial segment in continuity and having a mix of axonotmetic and neurotmetic damage.[85]

With transection and repair, toughness or tensile strength at the injury or repair site reaches a maximum in 3–4 weeks.[76,136] In many partial lesions there is a spectrum of injury to fibers. If preservation of function or partial recovery of function returns by 6 weeks, the injury that permitted some axons to suffer only neurapraxia will usually have involved the remaining axonal population in axonotmesis, thus permitting their regeneration. With no evidence of reversal of neurapraxia at 6 weeks, the existing proportion of axonal involvement by axonotmesis versus neurotmesis remains undetermined. Predominance of injury type can be determined relatively early after injury only by combining operative inspection with intraoperative electrophysiological testing.[64,68,92]

DISTAL AXONS AND THEIR CONNECTIONS

Depending on the time it takes for axons to reach a distal innervational site, the endoneurial pathways will be expanded or decreased

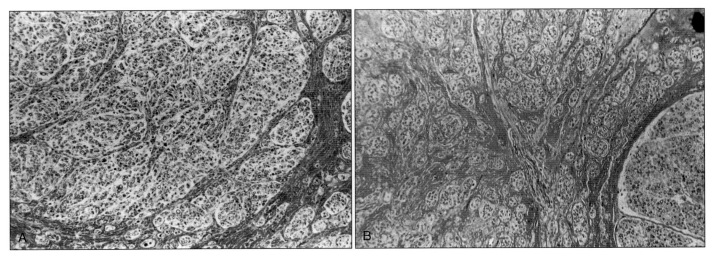

FIGURE 1-25 **(A)** Poor reinnervation of distal stump of nerve. The fibers are small, and those to the right are in an extrafascicular position. **(B)** Distal cross-section through graft site. Some axons are within the graft at lower right, but many are in extrafascicular tissue.

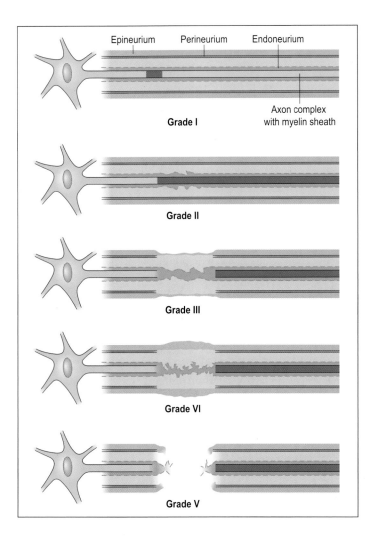

Epineurium   Perineurium   Endoneurium

Axon complex
with myelin sheath

Grade I

Grade II

Grade III

Grade VI

Grade V

FIGURE 1-26 This drawing exhibits diagrammatically the five types of injury as described by Sunderland. Grade I is a neurapraxic injury with a block in conduction without Wallerian degeneration. Grade II is a pure axonotmetic injury with maintenance of the connective tissue framework and, thus, the potential for excellent regeneration. Grade III is a more severe lesion which usually has a mixture of axonotmetic and neurotmetic axons. Grade IV is a neurotmetic lesion in continuity in which endoneurial and perineurial connective tissue layers as well as axons are disrupted. Grade V is a transecting injury with, by definition, interruption of all connective tissue layers. (Adapted from Kline D, Hudson A: Acute injuries of peripheral nerves. In: Youmans J, Ed: Neurological Surgery, 3rd edn. Philadelphia, WB Saunders, 1990:2423–2510.)

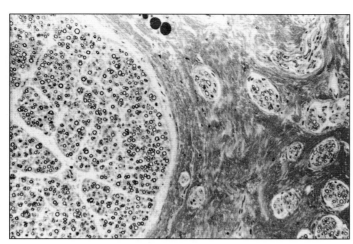

FIGURE 1-27 Fascicle of a distal stump on the left has been well innervated by axons which are maturing and regaining myelin thickness. Several regenerative units have missed the distal fascicle at the suture line and have grown into the extrafascicular epineurial tissues, forming a suture line neuroma to the right.

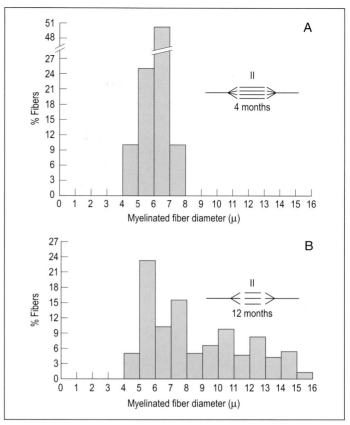

FIGURE 1-28 Composite graphs of myelinated axonal counts stratified by fiber size made 1 cm distal to a graft 2.54 cm in length at 4 months **(A)** and at 12 months **(B).** The majority of fibers are small and intermediate in size at 4 months. At 12 months, there are more large fibers, but even after this period, their numbers are relatively small.

in diameter. Usually, more than one fiber grows down a tube, but only those reaching a distal receptor and reinnervating it go on to mature and take on myelin, while others either degenerate or fail to mature (Fig. 1-27).[113]

Regenerating axons may not function effectively even after reaching distal end-organs unless they arrive close to their original site.[148] Regenerating fibers can induce some, but unfortunately not complete, change in end-organs not innervated by them prior to injury.[121] Cutaneous fibers do not cross certain boundaries even for sensory reinnervation, and they are certainly not effective in reinnervating motor sites. In addition, even regeneration of ulnar or median motor fibers into the fine hand muscles seldom produces even near-normal muscle function.[58,131] The ability of the central nervous system to relate to new end-organ contact on the part of the axon is limited in both the sensory and the motor spheres, but does occur, although usually with less than optimal results.[124] This is readily illustrated by the synkinesis seen with facial nerve regeneration, particularly that associated with hypoglossal-facial or accessory-facial anastomosis (Fig. 1-28).[114]

When denervated, the structure of muscle begins to change histologically by the third week after injury. The muscle fibers kink, and their cross-striations decrease.[129] Atrophy or shrinkage of the muscle mass may be evident clinically within a few weeks and will persist unless reinnervation occurs.[107] With continued denervation, particularly if this is accompanied by a lack of activity and movement, fibrosis replaces the muscle[108] so that by 2 years after denervation, the muscle can be totally replaced by scar tissue and/or fat.[56] For this reason, intervals of denervation beyond 2 years begin to impose major limitations on the motor function that can follow subsequent reinnervation, even by the most skillfully executed repair.

CONCLUSION

Based on the issues discussed in this chapter, the surgeon will appreciate that merely looking at and palpating a nerve at operation does not give the surgeon enough information so that the surgeon can decide whether to perform a neurolysis or resect the lesion and

effect repair. Function of the nerve must be assessed during operation by various electrophysiological techniques such as stimulation, and stimulation and recording of nerve action potentials. In the majority of instances, these electrophysiological techniques are applied to the nerve trunk as a whole, and individual fascicular function is usually not measured during the course of standard peripheral nerve operations. Nonetheless, if necessary, fascicular function can be assessed in the same fashion. Thus, optimal appreciation of function and structure during the course of peripheral nerve surgery is gained by using electrophysiological techniques as well as micro-operative techniques in a complementary fashion. Surgeons who treat disorders of peripheral nerves should be fully conversant with techniques that assess not only structure but also physiologic function intraoperatively. A combined anatomic and physiologic approach to nerve injuries provides the major emphasis of this book's hypothesis, and thus is re-emphasized throughout.

REFERENCES

1. Adams WE: Blood supply of nerves. J Anat 76:323–341, 1942.
2. Aguayo A, Attiwell M, Trecarten J, et al.: Abnormal myelination in transplanted Trembler mouse Schwann cells. Nature 265:73–75, 1977.
3. Aguayo A and Bray G: Cell interactions studied in the peripheral nerve of experimental animals. In: Dyck P, Thomas P, Lambert E,

et al. Eds: Peripheral Neuropathy. Philadelphia, W B Saunders, 1984.

4. Aitken JT and Thomas PK: Retrograde changes in fiber size following nerve section. J Anat 96:121–129, 1962.

5. Aldskoquis H, Arvidsson J, and Grant G: Axotomy – induced changes in primary sensory neurons. In: Scott E, Ed: Diversity, Development, and Plasticity. Oxford Univ. Press, New York, 1992.

6. Aleksavdrovskaya OV: Degeneration and regeneration of peripheral nerves in double injury. Tr Mosk Vet Akad 10:174–188, 1956.

7. Asbury A: The histogenesis of phagocytes during Wallerian degeneration procedures. Sixth International Congress of Neuropathology. Paris, Masson & Cie, 1970.

8. Bacsich P and Wyburn GM: The vascular pattern of peripheral nerve during repair after experimental crush. J Anat 79:9–14, 1945.

9. Bailey S, Eichler M, Villadiego A, et al.: The influence of fibronectin and laminin during Schwann cell migration and peripheral nerve regeneration through silicon chambers. J Neurocytology 122:176–184, 1993.

10. Baron-Van Evercooren A, Gansmuller A, Gumpel M, et al.: Schwann cell differentiation in vitro: Extracellular matrix deposition and interaction. Dev Neurosci 8:182–196, 1986.

11. Barr ML and Hamilton JD: A quantitative study of certain morphological changes in spinal motor neurons during axon reaction. J Comp Neurol 89:93–121, 1948.

12. Behrman I and Ackland R: Experimental study of the regenerative potential of perineurium at a site of nerve transection. J Neurosurg 54:79–83, 1981.

13. Bentley, FH and Schlapp W: Experiments on blood supply of nerves. J Physiol (London) 102:62–71, 1943.

14. Bisby M: Changes in composition of labeled protein transported in motor axons during their regeneration. J Neurobiol 11:435–455, 1980.

15. Bisby M: Regeneration of peripheral nervous system axon. In: Waxman S, Kocsis J, Stysp J, Eds: The Axon: Structure, Function, and Pathophysiology, Oxford University Press, New York, 1995.

16. Bisby MA: Synthesis of cytoskeletal proteins by axotomized and regenerating motoneurons. In: Reier PJ, Bunge RP, and Seil FJ, Eds: Current Issues in Neural Regeneration. New York, Alan R. Liss, 1988.

17. Bischoff A and Thomas PK: Microscopic anatomy of myelinated nerve fibers. In: Dyck PJ, Thomas PK, and Lambert EH, Eds: Peripheral Neuropathy. Philadelphia, WB Saunders, 1975:104–130.

18. Black MM and Lasek RJ: Slow components of axonal transport: Two cytoskeletal networks. J Cell Biol 86:616–623, 1980.

19. Bradley K, Brock LG, and McIntyre AK: Effects of axon section on motoneuron function. Proc Univ Otago Med Sch 33:14–16, 1955.

20. Brattgard SO, Edstrom JE, and Hyden H: The productive capacity of the neuron in retrograde reaction. Exp Cell Res 5(Suppl.):185, 1958.

21. Bray G and Aguyagoi AJ: Regeneration of peripheral unmyelinated nerves. Fate of the axonal sprouts which develop after injury. J Anat 117:3:517–529, 1974.

22. Bray GM, Raminsky M, and Aguayo AJ: Interactions between axons and their sheath cells. Ann Rev Neurosci 4:127–162, 1981.

23. Brushart TM, Henry EW, and Mesulam MM: Reorganization of muscle afferent projections accompanies peripheral nerve regeneration. Neuroscience 6:2053–2061, 1981.

24. Brushart TM and Mesulam MM: Alteration in connections between muscle and anterior horn motor neurons after peripheral nerve repair. Science 208:603–605, 1980.

25. Brushart TM and Seiler WA IV: Selective innervation of distal motor stumps by peripheral motor axons. Exp Neurol 97:289–300, 1987.

26. Bucko C, Joynt R, and Grabb W: Peripheral nerve regeneration in primates during D-penicillamine induced lathrism. Plast Reconstr Surg 67:23–28, 1981.

27. Bunge M, Williams A, Wood P, et al.: Comparison of nerve cell plus Schwann cell cultures with particular emphasis on basal lamina and collagen formation. J Cell Biol 84:184–193, 1980.

28. Bunge RP and Bunge MB: Tissue culture in the study of peripheral nerve pathology. In: Dyck PJ, Thomas PK, and Lambert EH, Eds: Peripheral Neuropathy. Philadelphia, WB Saunders, 1975:391–409.

29. Chang S, Rathjen FG, and Raper JA: Extension of neuritis on axons is impaired by antibodies against specific neural cell surface glycoproteins. J Cell Biol 104:355–362, 1987.

30. Cunningham BA, Hemperly JJ, Murray BA, et al.: Neural cell adhesion molecule: Structure, immunoglobulin-like domains, cell surface modulation, and alternative RNA splicing. Science 236:799–806, 1987.

31. Daniloff JK, Levi G, Grumet M, et al.: Altered expression of neuronal cell adhesion molecules induced by nerve injury and repair. J Cell Biol 103:020–945, 1986.

32. Davis A: The neurotrophic hypothesis: Where does it stand? Philosop Transect Royal Soc 351B:389–394, 1996.

33. Davison PF: Microtubules and neurofilaments: Possible implications in axoplasmic transport. Advances Biochem Psychopharmacol 2:168, 1970.

34. Dekker A, Gispen WH, and de Wied D: Axonal regeneration, growth factors and neuropeptides. Life Sci 41:1667–1678, 1987.

35. Denny-Brown D and Brenner C: Lesion in peripheral nerve resulting from compression by spring clip. Arch Neurol Psychiat 52:120, 1944.

36. Ducker T, Kempe L, Hayes G: The metabolic background for peripheral nerve surgery. J Neurosurg 30:270–280, 1969.

37. Ducker TB, Kaufmann FC: Metabolic factors in the surgery of peripheral nerves. Clin Neurosurg 24:406–424, 1977.

38. Eccles JC, Kryjevic K, and Miledi R: Delayed effects of peripheral severance of afferent nerve fibers on efficacy of their central synapses. J Physiol 145:204–220, 1959.

39. Eccles JC, Libet B, and Young R: The behavior of chromatolysed motoneurons studied by intracellular recording. J Physiol 143:11–40, 1958.

40. Edstrom JE: Ribonucleic acid changes in motoneurons of frog during axon regeneration. J Neurochem 5:43–49, 1959.

41. Engh CA and Schofield BH: A review of the central response to peripheral nerve injury and its significance in nerve regeneration. J Neurosurg 37:198–203, 1972.

42. Forman D, McQuarrie I, Laborre F, et al.: Time course of the conditioning lesion effect on axonal regeneration. Brain Res 182:180–185, 1980.

43. Friedlander DR, Grumet M, and Edelman GM: Nerve growth factor enhances expression of neuron-glia cell adhesion molecule in PC12 cells. J Cell Biol 102:413–419, 1986.

44. Fu S, Gordon T: The cellular and molecular basis of peripheral nerve regeneration. Mol Neurobiol 14(1–2):67–116, 1997.

45. Gerhart D, Drewes L: Glucose transporters at the blood–nerve barrier are associated with perineurial cells and endoneurial microvessels. Brain Res 508:46–50, 1990.

46. Germinez-Gallego G, Cuevas P: Fibroblast growth factors, proteins with a broad spectrum of activity. Neurologic Res 16:313–316, 1994.

47. Gilliatt R: Physical injury to peripheral nerves, physiological and electrodiagnostic aspects. Mayo Clin Proc 56:3641–3370, 1981.

48. Gilliatt RW, Ochoa J, Ridge P, et al.: Cause of nerve damage in acute compression. Trans Amer Neurol Assn 99:71–574, 1974.

49. Gilmer-Hill H, Jiang J, Ma S, et al.: Intraxonal GAP 43 in neuromas decreases over time after traumatic injury. Neurosurgery 51(5):1229–1237, 2002

50. Gorio A, Marini P, and Zanoni R: Muscle reinnervation. III. Motoneuron sprouting capacity, enhancement by exogenous gangliosides. Neuroscience 8:417–429, 1983.

51. Gorio A, Millesi H, and Mingrino S, Eds: Post Traumatic Peripheral Nerve Regeneration: Experimental Basis and Clinical Implications. New York, Raven Press, 1981.

52. Grafstein B: Cellular mechanisms for recovery from nervous system injury. Surg Neurol 13:363–365, 1980.

53. Grafstein B and McQuarrie I: Role of the nerve cell body in axonal regeneration. In: Cotman CW, Ed: Neural Plasticity. New York, Raven Press, 1978.

54. Gunderson RW: Response of sensory neurites and growth cones to patterned substrata of laminin and fibronectin in vitro. Dev Biol 121:423–432, 1987.

55. Guth L: Regeneration in the mammalian peripheral nervous system. Physiol Rev 36:441–478, 1956.

56. Guttmann E and Young JZ: Reinnervation of muscle after various periods of atrophy. J Anat 78:15–43, 1944.

57. Horch KW: Central responses of cutaneous neurons to peripheral nerve crush in the cat. Brain Res 151:581–586, 1978.

58. Hubbard JI, Ed: The Peripheral Nervous System. New York and London, Plenum Press, 1974.

59. Huber CG: Experimental observations on peripheral nerve repair. In: Medical Department, United States Army, Surgery in World War I: Vol. XI, Part I: Neurosurgery. Washington DC, US Government Printing Office, 1927.

60. Hudson A, Morris J, and Weddell G: An electron microscope study of regeneration in sutured rat sciatic nerves. Surg Forum 21:451–453, 1970.

61. Hudson A and Kline D: Progression of partial experimental injury to peripheral nerve. Part 2: Light and electron microscopic studies. J Neurosurg 42:15–22, 1975.

62. Jackson PC, Diamond J: Regenerating axons reclaim sensory targets from collateral nerve sprouts. Science 214:926–928, 1981.

63. Jacques L, Kline D: Responses of peripheral nerve to physical injury, Pt. 3 Ch. 36 In: Neurosurgery: The Scientific Basis of Clinical Practice, 3rd edn. Crockard A, Haywood R, Hoff J, Eds: London, Blackwell Scientific, 1998.

64. Kline G and DeJonge BR: Evoked potentials to evaluate peripheral nerve injuries. Surg Gynecol Obstet 127:1239–1250, 1968.

65. Kline DG, Hackett ER, and May P: Evaluation of nerve injures by evoked potentials and electromyography. J Neurosurg 31:128–136, 1969.

66. Kline DG, Hackett E, Davis G, et al.: Effects of mobilization on the blood supply and regeneration of injured nerves. J Surg Res 12:254–266, 1972.

67. Kline DG, Hudson AR, Hackett ER, et al.: Progression of partial experimental injury to peripheral nerve. Part 1: Periodic measurements of muscle contraction strength. J Neurosurg 42:1–14, 1975.

68. Kline DG: Physiological and clinical factors contributing to timing of nerve repair. Clin Neurosurg 24:425–455, 1977.

69. Kline DG and Hudson AR: Selected recent advances in peripheral nerve injury research. Surg Neurol 24:371–376, 1985.

70. Kline DG, Donner T, Happel L, et al.: Intraforaminal repair of brachial plexus: Experimental study in primates. J Neurosurg 76(3):459–470, 1992.

71. Kretschmer T, England J, Happel L, et al.: Ankyrin G and voltage gated sodium channels colocalizes in human neuroma. Key proteins of membrane remodeling after axonal injury. Neurosci Letters 323:151–155, 2002.

72. Kristensson K and Olsson Y: Retrograde transport of horseradish-peroxidase in transected axons. 3. Entry into injured axons and subsequent localization in perikaryon. Brain Res 126:154–159, 1977.

73. Lehman R and Hayes G: Degeneration and regeneration in peripheral nerve. Brain 90:285–296, 1967.

74. Levi-Montalcini R: The nerve growth factor 35 years later. Science 237:11545–1162, 1987.

75. Lieberman AR: The axon reaction: A review of principal features of perikaryal responses to axon injury. Int Rev Neurobiol 14:49–124, 1971.

76. Liu CT, Benda CF, and Lewey FH: Tensile strength of human nerves. Arch Neurol Psychiatry 59:322–336, 1948.

77. Low FN: The perineurium and connective tissue of peripheral nerve. In: Landon DN, Ed: The Peripheral Nerve. New York; John Wiley and Sons, 1976:159–187.

78. Lubinska L: Axoplasmic streaming in regenerating and normal nerve fibers. Mechanisms of Neural Regeneration. Progr Brain Res 13:1–71, 1964.

79. Lundborg G: Intraneural microcirculation and peripheral nerve barriers: Technique for evaluation – clinical implications. In: Omer GE and Spinner M, Eds: Management of Peripheral Nerve Problems. Philadelphia, WB Saunders, 1980.

80. Lundborg G: Structure and function of the intraneural microvessels as related to trauma, edema formation, and nerve function. J Bone Joint Surg 57A:938–948, 1975.

81. Lundborg G, Dahlin LB, Danielson N, et al.: Nerve regeneration across an extended gap: A neurobiological view of nerve repair and possible neuronotropic factors. J Hand Surg 7:580–587, 1982.

82. Lundborg G and Rydevik B: Effects of stretching the tibial nerve of the rabbit. A preliminary study of the intraneural circulation and the barrier function of the perineurium. J Bone Joint Surg 55B:390–401, 1973.

83. Lu G, Beuerman R, Zhao S, et al.: Tumor necrosis factor-alpha and interleukin-1 induce activation of MAP kinase and SAP kinase in human neuroma fibroblasts. Neurochem Int 30:401–410, 1997.

84. Mackinnon SE, Dellon AL, Lundborg G, et al.: A study of neurotropism in a primate model. J Hand Surg 11A:888–894, 1986.

85. Mackinnon SE, Dellon AL, Hudson AR, et al.: Alteration of neuroma formation produced by manipulation of neural environment in primates. Plast Reconstr Surg 76:345–352, 1985.

86. Malassy M, Bakker D, Dekker A, et al.: Functional magnetic resonance imaging and control over biceps muscle after intercostals-musculocutaneous nerve transfer. J Neurosurg 98:261–268, 2003.

87. McQuarrie I: Acceleration of axonal regeneration of rat somatic motor neurons by using a conditioning lesion. In: Gorio A, Millesi H, and Mingrino S, Eds: Post Traumatic Peripheral Nerve Regeneration. New York, Raven Press, 1981:49–58.

88. Meyer M, Matsuoka I, Wetmore C, et al.: Enhanced synthesis of brain derived neurotrophic factor in the lesioned peripheral nerve: different mechanisms are responsible for regulation of BDNF, NGF and MRNA. J Cell Biol 119:45–54, 1992.

89. Morris JH, Hudson AR, and Weddell G: A study of degeneration and regeneration in the divided rat sciatic nerve based on electron microscopy. Z Zellforsch 124:76–203, 1972.

90. Myers R: Anatomy and microanatomy of peripheral nerve. Neurosurg Clinics N Am (Burchiel K, Ed) 2(1):1–20, 1991.

91. Nachemson A, Lundberg G, Myrhage R, et al.: Nerve regeneration after pharmacologic suppression of the scar reaction of the suture site. An experimental study of the effects of estrogen-progesterone, methyl prednisolone acetate and cis-hydroxyproline in rat sciatic nerve. J Scand Plast Reconstr Surg 19:255–261, 1985.

92. Nulsen F, Lewey F: Intraneural bipolar stimulation: A new aid in assessment of nerve injuries. Science 106:301–303, 1947.

93. Ochoa J: Microscopic anatomy of unmyelinated nerve fibers. In: Dyck PJ, Thomas PK, and Lambert EH, Eds: Peripheral Neuropathy. Philadelphia, WB Saunders, 1975:113–150.

94. Ochoa J, Fowler TJ, and Gilliatt RW: Anatomical changes in peripheral nerves compressed by a pneumatic tourniquet. J Anat 113:433–455, 1972.

95. Ochs S: Axoplasmic transport-energy metabolism and mechanism. In: Hubbard J, Ed: The Peripheral Nervous System. New York, Plenum Press, 1974:47–67.

96. Ochs S: Axoplasmic transport – a basis for neural pathology. In: Dyck PJ, Thomas PK, and Lambert EH, Eds: Peripheral Neuropathy. Philadelphia, WB Saunders, 1975:213–230.

97. Ogata K and Naito M: Blood flow of perioneal nerve: Effects of dissection, stretching and compression. J Hand Surg (Br) 11:10–14, 1986.

98. Olsson Y: Vascular permeability in the peripheral nervous system. In: Dyck PJ, Thomas PK, and Lambert EH, Eds: Peripheral Neuropathy, 1st Edn, Vol. 1. Philadelphia, WB Saunders, 1965:131–150.

99. Olsson Y and Reese T: Permeability of vasa nervorum and perineurium in mouse sciatic nerve studied by fluorescence and electron microscopy. J Neuropath Exp Neurol 30:105, 1971.

100. Peale E, Luciano K, and Spitznos M: Freeze-fracture aspects of the perineurial sheath of rabbit sciatic nerve. J Neurocytol 54:385–392, 1976.

101. Pellegrino RG, Rithie JM, and Spencer PS: The role of Schwann cell division in the clearance of nodal axolemma following nerve section in the cat. J Physiol (Lond) 334:68, 1982.

102. Pleasure D, Bova F, Lane J, et al.: Regeneration after nerve transaction. Effect of inhibition of collagen synthesis. Exp Neurol 45:72–79, 1974.

103. Pleasure D: Axoplasmic transport. In: Sumner A, Ed: The Physiology of Peripheral Nerve Disease. Philadelphia, WB Saunders, 1980:221–237.

104. Ramon Y, Cajal S: Degeneration and Regeneration of the Nervous System. Trans May RM. New York, Oxford University Press, 1928.

105. Ranvier M: Leçons sur l'Histologie du Systeme Nerveux. Paris, F. Savy, 1878.

106. Rich K, Disch S, Elchlier M: The influence of regeneration and nerve growth factor on neuronal cell body reaction to injury. J Neurocytol 18:567–569, 1989.

107. Richardson PM: Neurotrophic factors in regeneration. Curr Opin Neurobiol 111:401–406, 1991.

108. Richter H and Ketelsen U: Impairment of motor recovery after late nerve suture: Experimental study in the rabbit. II: Morphological findings. Neurosurgery 10:75–85, 1982.

109. Robertis E: Submicroscopic morphology and function of the synapse. Exp Cell Res 5(Suppl):347–369, 1958.

110. Rudge P, Ochoa J, and Gilliatt RW: Acute peripheral nerve compression in the baboon. J Neurol Sci 23:403–420, 1974.

111. Rydevik B and Lundborg G: Permeability of intraneural microvessels and perineurium following acute, graded experimental nerve compression. Scand J Plast Reconstr Surg 11:179–187, 1977.

112. Salonen V, Peltonen J, Roytta M, et al.: Laminin in traumatized nerve: Basement membrane changes during degeneration and regeneration. J Neurocytol 16:713–720, 1987.

113. Sanders FK and Young JZ: The influence of peripheral connections on the diameter of regenerating nerve fibers. J Exp Biol 22:203–212, 1946.

114. Schemm GW: The pattern of cortical localization following cranial nerve cross anastomosis. J Neurosurg 18:593–596, 1961.

115. Schwann T: Microscopic Researches into the Accordance in the Structure and Growth of Animals and Plants. Trans. Smith H. London, Sydenham Society, 1847.

116. Sears TA: Structural changes in motoneurons following axotomy. J Exp Biol 132:93–109, 1987.

117. Seddon H: Degeneration and regeneration. In: Seddon H: Surgical Disorders of the Peripheral Nerves. Edinburgh, E & S Livingston, 1972:9–31.

118. Seddon H: Three types of nerve injury. Brain 66:237–288, 1943.

119. Shantaveerappa TR and Bourne GH: The "perineurial epithelium," a metabolically active continuous protoplasmic cell barrier surrounding peripheral nerve fasciculi. J Anat 96:527–536, 1962.

120. Shantaveerappa TR and Bourne GH: Perineurial epithelium: A new concept of its role in the integrity of the peripheral nervous system. Science 154:1464–1467, 1966.

121. Simpson SA and Young JS: Regeneration of fiber diameter after cross-unions of visceral and somatic nerves. J Anat 79:48, 1945.

122. Smith JW: Factors influencing nerve repair. II: Collateral circulation of peripheral nerves. Arch Surg 93:433–437, 1966.

123. Spencer PS, Weinberg HJ, and Paine CS: The perineurial window – a new model of focal demyelination and remyelination. Brain Res 965:923–929, 1975.

124. Sperry RW: The problem of central nervous reorganization after nerve regeneration and muscle transposition. Q Rev Biol 20:311, 1945.

125. Strain R and Olson W: Selective damage of large diameter peripheral nerve fibers by compression: An application of Laplace's Law. Exp Neurol 47:68–80, 1975.

126. Sunderland S: The intraneural topography of the radial, median, and ulnar nerves. Brain 68:243–299, 1945.

127. Sunderland S: A classification of peripheral nerve injuries producing loss of function. Brain 74:491, 1951.

128. Sunderland S and Bradley K: The cross-sectional area of peripheral nerve trunks devoted to nerve fibers. Brain 72:428–439, 1949.

129. Sunderland S and Ray LJ: Denervation changes in muscle. J Neurol Neurosurg Psychiatry 13:159–177, 1950.

130. Sunderland S: Nerve and Nerve Injuries. Baltimore, Williams & Wilkins, 1968.

131. Sunderland S: Nerve Injuries and Their Repair: A Critical Appraisal. Edinburgh, Churchill Livingston, 1991.

132. Terzis J, Sun O, Thomas P: Historical and basic science review. Past, present and future of nerve repair. Reconstr Microsurg 13:215–225, 1997.

133. Thomas PK and Jones DG: The cellular response to nerve injury, 3. The effect of repeated crush injuries. J Anat 106:463–470, 1970.

134. Thomas PK and Jones DG: The cellular response to nerve injury. 2. Regeneration of the perineurium after nerve section. J Anat 101:45–55, 1967.

135. Thomas PK and Olsson Y: Microscopic anatomy and function of the connective tissue components of peripheral nerve. In: Dyck PJ, Thomas PK, Lambert EH, et al., Eds: Peripheral Neuropathy, 2nd edn, Vol. 1. Philadelphia, WB Saunders, 1984:97–120.

136. Toby E, Meyer B, Shwappach J, et al.: Changes in the structural properties of peripheral nerves after transaction. J Hand Surg 21A:1086–1090, 1996.

137. Uzman B, Snyder S, and Villegas G: Status of peripheral nerve regeneration. In: Neural Regeneration and Transplantation. New York, Alan R. Liss, 1989.

138. Varon R and Bunge R: Tropic mechanisms in the peripheral nervous system. Ann Rev Neurosci 1:327–361, 1978.

139. Varon S and Adler R: Trophic and specifying factors directed to neuronal cells. Adv Cell Neurobiol 2:115–163, 1981.

140. Veraa R and Grafstein B: Cellular mechanisms for recovery from nervous system injury. A conference report. Exp Neurol 71:6–75, 1981.

141. Waller A: Experiments on the section of the glossopharyngeal and hypoglossal nerves of the frog. Phil Trans Roy Soc (London), 140:423–429, 1850.

142. Weddell G, Guttman L, and Guttman E: The local extension of nerve fibers into denervated areas of skin. J Neurol Psychiatry 4:206, 1941.

143. Weiss P: Neuronal dynamics and neuroplastic flow. In: Schmidt F, Ed: The Neurosciences (2nd Study Program). New York, The Rockefeller Press, 1970:840–850.

144. Weiss P: Technology of nerve regeneration. A review. J Neurosurg 1:400–450, 1944.

145. Williams HB, Terzis JK: Single fascicular recordings: An intraoperative diagnostic tool for the management of peripheral nerve lesions. Plast Reconstr Surg 57:562–569, 1976.

146. Yamada KM, Spooner BS, and Wessells NK: Ultrastructure and function of the growth cones and axons of cultured nerve cells. J Cell Biol 49:614–635, 1971.

147. Yono Q, Elliott J, Snider W. Brain derived neurotrophic factor rescues spinal motor neurons from axotomy induced cell death. Nature 360:753–755, 1992.

148. Zalewski A: Effects of neuromuscular reinnervation on denervated skeletal muscle by axons of motor, sensory, and sympathetic neurons. Am J Physiol 219:1675–1679, 1970.

149. Zhao S, Pang Y, Beuerman R, et al.: Expression of C-FOS protein in the spinal cord after brachial plexus injury: comparison of root avulsion and distal nerve transaction. Neurosurgery 42(6):1357–1362, 1998.

2

Mechanisms and pathology of injury

Rajiv Midha

OVERVIEW

- The clinician managing nerve injuries must understand the diversity of surgical lesions affecting nerves and how these differing mechanisms shape outcome.
- The bluntly transected nerve, which invariably entails a contusive injury to a length of nerve, does not do well with acute repair, but the sharply and neatly transected nerve does.
- Lesions in continuity caused by gunshot wounds, contusion, or stretch may or may not need surgery and are usually operated on after some delay.
- Progressive loss of function for nerve injuries in continuity is an important exception, where an acute operation to decompress the nerve may be in order.
- Some lesions, usually as a result of severe stretch forces, are so extensive or proximal, that little can be offered by direct nerve surgery.
- The behavior of an acutely compressed nerve differs from that of nerve more chronically entrapped.
- Electrical, thermal, and irradiation injuries share similarities to those resulting from ischemic damage to a limb in having an extensive length of nerve injury that is often not amenable to nerve repair.
- Injection injuries are often focal, and if not improving spontaneously should be explored and reconstructed depending on the intraoperative electrical studies.
- Iatrogenic injuries should be managed with exactly the same timing considerations as non-iatrogenic injuries, depending on the presumed injury mechanism.
- As the differences in injury response according to mechanisms are understood, a more rational approach for timing and selection of operation can be developed.

TRANSECTION

Soft tissue lacerations have the potential to transect nerves but sever the nerve sharply in only 30% of cases (Fig. 2-1).[19] These acute, sharp nerve injuries are favorable lesions to repair early. The remainder of soft tissue lacerations are more likely to leave the nerve in continuity but cause intraneural damage of variable severity, as these are from contusive and stretching mechanisms.[101] Knives, glass, propeller and fan blades, chain saws, auto metal,

surgical instruments, and other relatively sharp objects can partially or totally transect nerve, or they can bruise and stretch it without severance of the nerve (Figs 2-2 and 2-3).

Almost 15% of nerve injuries associated with a potentially transecting mechanism actually leave the nerve in *partial* continuity.[48] Loss of function results from a variable amount of neurotmesis, axonotmesis, and neurapraxia,[88] but the nerve or a portion of it is still in continuity. With time, this bruised and stretched segment of nerve thickens, and, depending on the severity of internal disruption, it may become a neuroma in continuity. This can be found even though functional loss distal to the soft tissue laceration is complete.

If a nerve is partially transected, the injury to those fibers cut is by definition neurotmetic or Sunderland grade V. On the other hand, those fibers not directly transected can have a variable degree of injury and be Sunderland grade II, III, or IV.[100] Functional loss can vary from mild and incomplete to severe and total. In addition, ability to recover is quite variable, as is the time required for recovery.[42] Serial electrical studies on partially lacerated and initially quantified functional loss in primates indicate some extension of loss within the first few hours.[53] This is presumably a result of loss of the perineurial barrier surrounding the various non-transected fascicles, with concomitant intrafascicular as well as extrafascicular swelling (Fig. 2-4).[43] Some of the progressive portion of the loss reverses through regeneration, but much does not. In the human, the partially transected portion of a nerve seldom regenerates well enough spontaneously to restore function. Functional recovery in some of these cases can be attributed to reversal of neurapraxia or regeneration in the bruised and stretched portion of the nerve rather than in the transected portion.

The physical appearance of a totally transected nerve varies acutely and with time and is related to the sharpness of the laceration. With sharp transection, the epineurium is cleanly cut, and there is minimal contusive change or hemorrhage in either stump. With time, even following sharp division, the stumps retract and become enveloped in scar. The amount of proximal and distal neuroma formed on either stump is much less compared with that formed in a more contusive or blunt transaction (Fig. 2-5).

Blunt transection is associated with a ragged tear of the epineurium acutely and an irregular, longitudinal extent of damage to a segment of the nerve. Bruising and hemorrhage can extend for several centimeters up or down either stump. With time, sizable proximal and distal neuromas develop. Retraction and proliferative scars around the stumps are often more severe than those seen with sharp transection.[18]

If the object penetrating the limb takes an oblique course through the soft tissues, the actual site of injury to the nerve may be at a distance from the entrance site (Fig. 2-6). Any laceration serious enough to damage a nerve can also cut or bruise muscle, tendons, or vessels, and function of these structures also requires evaluation and sometimes repair.[65] The sequence of such diverse repairs is addressed further in Chapter 6.

Operative iatrogenic transection may be sharp, as with scalpel injury, or blunt and rending, as with severe stretch during excessive retraction or manipulation of the limb or wound site. Nerve can also be inadvertently divided during surgery by electrocautery or by laser.

LESIONS (NEUROMAS) IN CONTINUITY

Most severe nerve injuries do not transect or distract nerve, but leave it in gross continuity. Depending on the series reported and the referral and practice pattern of the clinician, this figure can vary between 60% and 70% of serious nerve injuries.[73] If initial loss is partial in the distal distribution of such an injury, improvement is more likely to occur, but this is not always the case. Even with incomplete loss, predictability of outcome is limited. Prognosis is especially uncertain in cases of complete functional loss distal to a lesion in continuity (Table 2-1). In this circumstance, good recovery may occur spontaneously with time, or recovery may be partial and less than that which a good repair would achieve, or, surprisingly often, very little significant spontaneous return of function may occur. This variability makes prediction of outcome with lesions in continuity very difficult.[48,51]

Lesions in continuity can be either focal or diffuse, and may even have skipped areas of damage, depending on the mechanism of injury. In most cases, the entire cross-section of the nerve has a similar extent of internal damage.[47] In some cases, however, one or more fascicles may be partially or completely spared, with clinical examination showing partial neurological deficits. In a few cases, all or a portion of the fibers are concussed and have a temporary neurapraxic injury, resulting in a reversible deficit. In other cases, there is a spectrum of fiber injury types ranging from neurapraxic block in conduction to axonotmesis and neurotmesis.[90] Unfortunately, in these mixed grades of injury, axonotmesis and neurotmesis predominate.[87] Effective spontaneous regeneration depends on minimal connective tissue damage. With greater internal damage, an increasing degree of intrafascicular fibrosis results, frustrating regenerating axons and leading to their aberrant regrowth, despite

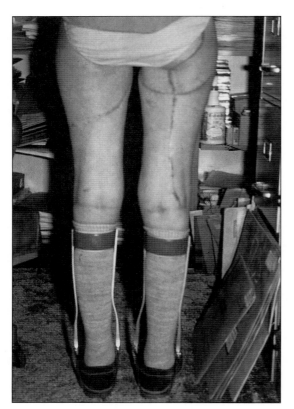

FIGURE 2-1 Healed lacerations and surgical scars in a teenager with bilateral sciatic transections from glass. Left side was repaired primarily by the referring surgeon. When the proximal stump on the right side could not be found beneath the transverse laceration, the patient was sent for a secondary repair. The proximal stump had retracted to the level of the buttock and a substantial longitudinal exposure of the sciatic nerve was needed to gain length for an end–end repair.

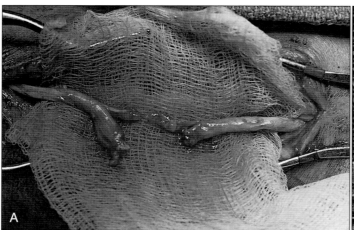
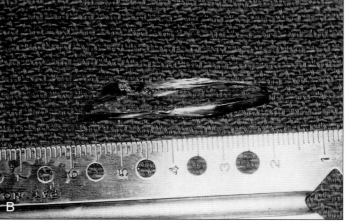

FIGURE 2-2 **(A)** Ulnar nerve severed somewhat obliquely by glass and exposed for repair several weeks later. Note the slightly bulbous but minimally neuromatous proximal and distal stumps. **(B)** A shard of glass responsible for a lacerative injury to nerve.

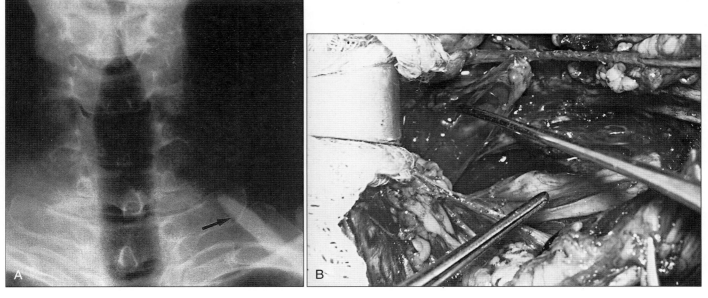

FIGURE 2-3 **(A)** Shard of glass *(arrow)* in neck and partially beneath the clavicle in a patient who sustained multiple head and neck lacerations from flying glass in a factory explosion. **(B)** Large piece of glass being extracted from beneath the left clavicle. This was lying just on top of the lower trunk, which it had contused but not lacerated.

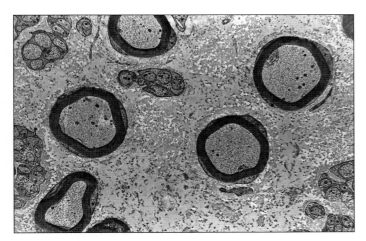

FIGURE 2-4 Electron micrograph showing area adjacent to partial non-human primate nerve injury site at which the perineurium had been disrupted. Axons demonstrate decreased myelin thickness and increased distance between them, suggesting endoneurial edema.

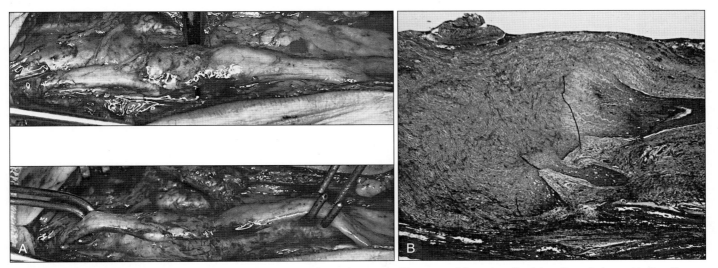

FIGURE 2-5 **(A)** Relatively sharp laceration to median nerve transecting most of it, exposed 5 weeks after injury *(top photograph)*. Despite some physical continuity, there was no conducted nerve action potential. **(B)** Large neuroma caused by a blunt transecting injury. Axons from the fasciculi to the right have attempted to grow to the left but are greatly disorganized and mixed with relatively heavy scar tissue. (Masson stain ×40.)

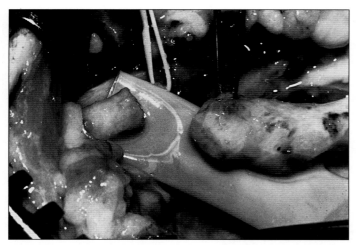

FIGURE 2-6 C5 spinal nerve lacerated by a knife at its junction with the upper trunk. The entry wound was just above clavicle in the posterolateral neck and reached C5 in an oblique fashion.

gross continuity of the nerve itself. The resulting neuroma in continuity contains a meshwork of connective tissue entwined with fine-caliber, poorly myelinated axons. Depending on the degree of internal disruption, spontaneous recovery may or may not occur. Unfortunately, with many stretch-contusive injuries, injury to perineurial and endoneurial layers is severe, considerable connective tissue proliferation occurs, and effective axonal regeneration is minimal.[87]

With the typical lesion in continuity, the nerve is acutely swollen, with extravasation of serum or blood, necrosis of axons with loss of their myelin coverings, and some disruption of the connective tissue elements.[87,118] Wallerian degeneration occurs, and axonal and myelin debris is phagocytozed from both the injury site and more distal nerve.[112] The Schwann cells, basal lamina, and distal connective tissue elements survive, and are well positioned and conducive for axonal outgrowth.[67] Unfortunately, the endoneurial and perineurial elements at the injury site rapidly proliferate and lay down poorly structured collagen, interfering with organized and properly directed axonal regeneration.[95] Because there is some retrograde damage proximal to the injury site with most nerve injuries, clusters of regenerating axons must first traverse this area of loss.[74] These regenerating axons next encounter poorly restructured collagen at the injury site, leading to further disorganization in their orientation.[49] Axons branch many times as they traverse the site of injury. Such axonal branching in the human may occur several hundred times.[117] Other axons may be deflected into peripheral connective tissue layers at the injury site as well as distally. As a result, axons reaching the distal stump are thin, poorly myelinated, and therefore less likely to reach prior distal end-organs than with a more axonotmetic injury. Many serious lesions in continuity are therefore not capable of regeneration of a quality to lead to recovery of useful distal function.[101]

If connective tissue disorganization is severe, regenerating axons, although penetrating the injury site by the thousands, are poor in caliber and misdirected.[118] On the other hand, if connective tissue involvement is mild with relative preservation of not only perineurial tissues but a proportion of the endoneurial pathways across the injury site, axons regenerate well, regenerative units reach distal structures after minimal branching, and individual axons come close to prior innervational inputs and eventually regain an adequate degree of caliber and myelination. This is the type of

Table 2-1 Management of neuroma in continuity
Partial injuries (incomplete loss with significant distal sparing)
Most cases improve with conservative treatment. Follow with serial clinical examination, supplemented with electrophysiological assessment

Operation may still be required:
    Expanding masses (hematoma, AV fistula, pseudoaneurysm) with clinical worsening;
    Lesion near entrapment site (example, peroneal nerve at lateral knee);
    Distal loss is partial, but major (in an important component of the nerve), and no further recovery occurs;
    Neuropathic pain, not amenable to pharmacotherapy and physiotherapy.

Complete injuries

Relatively focal lesions caused by fracture, GSW, iatrogenic insult:
    Follow by clinical and EMG studies for 2–3 months;
    Explore if no clinical or electrical improvement;
    Use intraoperative stimulation and NAPs to decide for or against resection.

Relatively lengthy lesion in continuity caused by stretch/contusion:
    Follow by clinical and EMG studies for 4–5 months;
    If no significant clinical or electrical improvement, explore;
    Use intraoperative stimulation and NAPs to decide for or against resection and graft repair;
    May need special studies (myelography, MRI, sensory and motor evoked potentials) to decide suitability for repair of a proximal spinal nerve.

spontaneous regeneration that can lead to restoration of useful function.

Predicting which lesion in continuity will recover adequate distal function spontaneously is difficult. The knowledge of the mechanism of injury can be somewhat helpful. Less severe compressive or contusive injury, a very mild stretch injury, or, surprisingly some gunshot wounds (GSWs) are more likely to spare some internal connective tissue architecture and permit a structured axonal regenerative response. The patient presenting with brachial plexitis usually recovers function over a period of time, but there are also exceptions with this disorder of unknown cause.[75,108] Those injuries resulting from the more contusive and stretching forces associated with high-speed land, water, and air accidents are less likely to regenerate in a fashion leading to useful distal function. Despite these generalizations, it is difficult to predict outcome, and most lesions in continuity have an uncertain future.[48] Most lesions in continuity are therefore clinically followed and re-evaluated at intervals for several months before surgical exploration, intraoperative recordings, and repair are undertaken (Table 2-1).[73]

A nerve that has been sutured or repaired by grafts also becomes a lesion or neuroma in continuity.[117] The size, firmness, and histologic appearance of such a lesion depends on the interval since repair, the thoroughness of resection of damaged tissue before suture, the accuracy with which the stumps and their fascicular structures were opposed, and the degree of tension on the repair site.[104] Variable proportions of the suture neuroma in continuity are derived from epineurial and interfascicular epineurial connective tissue proliferation, but the scar that usually thwarts successful regeneration is derived from the endoneurial fibroblasts.[76] Even with an excellent repair, the new lesion in continuity produced by the suture or grafts shows swirls of connective tissue and a variable number of misdirected axons. Some axons reach more distal fascicular structure, but others are misdirected at the repair site scar into extrafascicular sites. Even with a poor repair, however, a large number of axons may reach the distal stump of the nerve, because the neuronal thrust for regeneration of axons is great. Depending on the number of times they must divide to reach this level and the scar at the repair site, axons may or may not take on enough caliber to be functional. Even if the fibers are successful in reaching distal innervational sites and maturing at the level of the distal stump, they remain slender and relatively poorly myelinated for many years at the repair site.[117,118] With a poor repair, connective tissue proliferation is great. Axons are forced by the scar to divide many more times to traverse this barrier, distal extrafascicular placement is more likely, and maturity of fibers at the repair site and also more distally is less complete than with a more meticulous repair.

An important factor affecting recovery of function is whether regenerating fibers reach or come close to previously innervated sites for sensation and motor function. Poor specificity of regeneration with misdirection of axons into inappropriate end-organs plays an important role in reducing the outcome of nerve repair.[8]

NEUROPHYSIOLOGY OF LESIONS IN CONTINUITY

Because most lesions or neuromas in continuity have lost axonal continuity, the process of Wallerian degeneration occurs. This takes a finite amount of time so that stimulation distal to the injury site can produce muscular contraction for 1–3 days even though the patient cannot contract those muscles voluntarily. In the experimental setting, early-regenerating fine fibers can be stimulated and recorded from across a lesion in continuity. This requires direct stimulation and recording from the nerve. To record such nerve action potentials (NAPs) in the early days after injury, summation is necessary, as is a computer to average, integrate, and take the small potentials generated off the slope of the trace descending from the stimulus artifact peak. This is interesting but not clinically predictive because almost all lesions in continuity have such fine fibers penetrating the injury site. This type of early regenerative response is not predictive of a functionally useful degree of regeneration that takes several weeks or months to occur.

Intraoperative recording can produce reliable information about regeneration by 6–8 weeks after injury in relatively focal lesions in continuity caused by fractures and some contusions and GSWs.[51,105] Less focal lesions require more time for adequate regeneration to occur through the lesion in continuity and to be picked up by even direct operative NAP recording. Several thousand fibers greater than 6 μm in diameter are required to produce such an NAP.[52] In an adequately regenerating lesion in continuity, such a response can be traced through the injury site and into the distal stump. Amplification used is similar to that provided by an oscilloscope with a differential amplifier, and a computer is not necessary to integrate or summate such responses.[40,107]

With further time, adequate regeneration is heralded by reversal of distal denervational change in muscle and presence of nascent or early reinnervation potentials.[35] Insertional activity and eventually a muscle action potential (MAP) can be evoked on electromyography (EMG).[44] In addition, at some time before recovery of voluntary function, stimulation of the successfully re-growing nerve is able to produce muscular contraction. These more distally related regenerative changes take many months to occur, particularly in sciatic injuries, in proximal arm-level radial, median, and ulnar injuries, and in most brachial plexus injuries. Conduction velocity determinations, which are usually dependent on recording from distal reinnervational sites, remain slow, and this may be true for many months. Conduction across the injury site also remains slow for years and sometimes forever because, despite more distal axonal maturation, fiber diameter and myelination remain poor at the injury site. Velocity values assess large fibers only, whereas NAP amplitude and the area beneath the NAP curve give a rough estimate of the fiber spectrum involved. There are relative variables such as interelectrode distance, electrode contact, wound temperature, and moisture, and these factors must be assessed before final interpretation of NAP amplitudes is completed.[24,107]

STRETCH, TRACTION, AND CONTUSION

Blunt forces imparted to nerve remain by far the most common mechanisms underlying nerve injury.[31] The majority of serious injuries to nerve in patients are therefore caused by stretch, traction, and contusion. Normally, the nerve can withstand moderate stretch forces, given its elastin and collagen-rich perineurial layer which endow tensile strength, and its excellent ability to glide during physiologic motion (aided by the undulating course of nerve fibers in a longitudinal direction).[102] However, even 8% stretch leads to a disturbance in intraneural circulation and blood–nerve barrier function,[64] while stretch beyond 10–20%, especially if applied acutely, results in structural failure.[59] Such forces can therefore occasionally distract a nerve, pulling it totally apart, or more commonly leave it in continuity, but with considerable internal damage. If distracted by substantial forces, the nerve is frayed, and both stumps are damaged over many centimeters. Retraction and scar about both stumps are severe. If nerve is left in continuity, as is more likely, the degree of intraneural damage is variable and may, on occasion, present as a spectrum of fiber change including neurapraxia, axonotmesis, and neurotmesis.

Mechanisms responsible for a relatively mild degree of stretch may be associated with forces producing fractures or those related to lesser degrees of surgical retraction (Fig. 2-7).[91] More commonly, traction forces are sufficient to tear apart intraneural connective tissue structure as well as disconnect axons (Fig. 2-8).[97] Such lesions are Sunderland grade IV and are neurotmetic despite physical continuity of the nerve.[41] Less frequently, such forces result in a more axonotmetic or Sunderland grade II or III lesion which may have the potential for effective regeneration because of less connective tissue destruction.[100] A stretch mechanism is also responsible for segments of damage to nerve displaced by high-velocity missiles, especially with GSWs.[81]

Brachial plexus injury is a common disorder resulting from a stretch mechanism. Stretch or traction injuries to the plexus most commonly result from extremes of movement at the shoulder joint, with or without actual dislocation or fracture of the humerus or the clavicle. With blunt or traction forces, scapular, rib, or cervical spine fractures, or any combination of these, can also occur.[71,77] While a clavicular fracture attests to the disruptive force applied to the shoulder joint, rarely does the fracture itself produce a focal

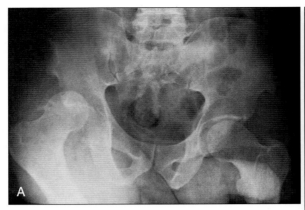

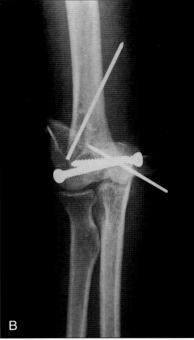

FIGURE 2-7 **(A)** Right hip dislocation resulted in a sciatic nerve injury. **(B)** Distal humeral fracture associated with ulnar nerve injury.

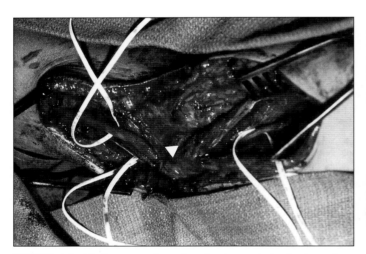

FIGURE 2-8 Median nerve *(arrowhead)* entrapped at a fracture site.

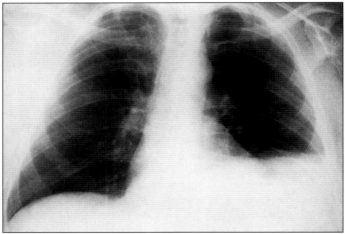

FIGURE 2-9 Elevation of left hemi-diaphragm from phrenic nerve injury associated with a severe stretch injury to the brachial plexus. This finding implies very proximal damage, likely preganglionic, to the C5 spinal nerve.

injury to the underlying plexus.[103] Either upper or lower elements of the plexus may suffer the predominant injury, or, with severe traction forces, all elements may be involved in addition to phrenic nerve and even subclavian vessels (Fig. 2-9). All grades of damage are possible. Spinal nerves and roots can be avulsed from the spinal cord or more laterally from truncal or more distal outflows. The stretched elements may be left in continuity and have a mixture of neurapraxia and axonotmesis. A combination of neurapraxia, axonotmesis, and neurotmesis may coexist but unfortunately these mixed grades of injuries are more commonly severe in degree, having significant neurotmetic components. Most traction injuries do not avulse or pull apart the plexus elements. Instead, the elements are left in some continuity but have a severe degree of internal disruption, essentially a Sunderland grade IV injury. Each plexus element may have a different grade of damage within the same injury site. In such cases, the lesion is not focal but extends over 5–6 cm or more of nerve.

The effect of stretch on peripheral nerve is similar throughout the body, but specific anatomic relationships contribute to characteristic patterns of injury in the case of brachial plexus stretch.[101] The attachment of the rootlets to the spinal cord is best appreciated by examination of an anatomic specimen. A surgeon can observe the delicate rootlets during spinal operations, and the radiologist can demonstrate these structures effectively by the use of water-soluble contrast material, provided sufficient concentration is maintained in the cervical area (Fig. 2-10).[10] Cervical myelography, followed by thin-section computerized tomography (CT), remains the best nonoperative method of demonstrating avulsions. Magnetic resonance imaging (MRI) is, nonetheless, becoming increasingly sensitive in delineating the actual root and rootlets themselves (Fig. 2-11), and may someday replace CT myelography.[17,22,38]

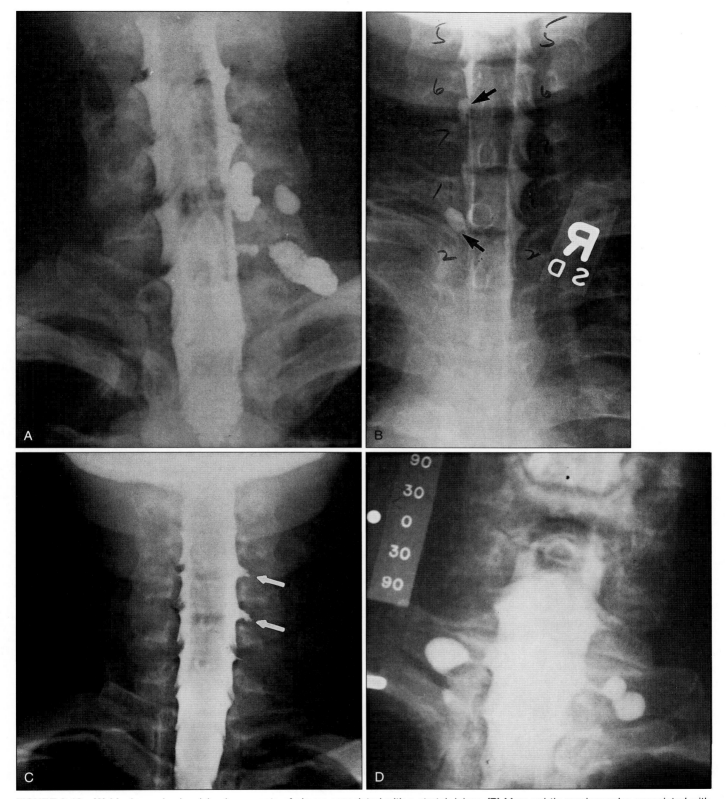

FIGURE 2-10 **(A)** Meningoceles involving lower roots of plexus associated with a stretch injury. **(B)** More subtle meningoceles associated with the left C7 and T1 spinal nerves *(arrows)*. **(C)** Small meningoceles *(arrows)* associated with the C5 and C6 spinal nerves. **(D)** Tarlov cysts involving the T1 roots bilaterally.

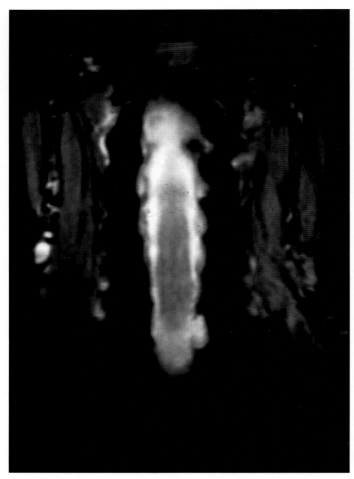

FIGURE 2-11 An excellent MRI sequence showing a meningocele negating the need for a CT myelogram. Although desirable, such detail cannot always be obtained by MRI sequences. CT myelography remains the gold standard.

Traction along the axis of the brachial plexus can literally tear their roots out of the spinal cord. Subsequent observation at open operation during a dorsal root entry zone procedure for pain reveals the absence of any dorsal proximal stumps and the presence of brownish staining of the pia in a line with unaffected rootlets above and below the primary lesion, as well as some cord atrophy on that side.[10,86] Similar observations, aided by endoscopes, have been made in surgery to repair avulsed nerve roots to the spinal cord.[9] Avulsion of rootlets subtended by a single spinal nerve does not imply avulsion of all the rootlets of the brachial plexus; likewise, rootlet avulsion may coexist with brachial plexus injuries more peripherally placed and affecting other elements of the plexus.

After the roots penetrate dura, they become spinal nerves. The spinal nerves run in the gutters of the foramina in the vertebrae for which they are named. At this intraforaminal level, the nerves are relatively tethered by mesoneurial-like connections to the gutters.[6] The spinal nerves then angle inferiorly to appear between the scalenus anticus and scalenus medius muscles and thus gain the posterior triangle of the neck. Spinal nerves are often injured in a characteristic fashion just as they run off the lip of the gutter of the transverse process. Forces here may distract spinal nerve from trunk, producing a rupture. Alternatively, they may produce severe intraneural damage resulting in lengthy lesions in continuity that involve not only spinal nerves and trunks but may extend into the divisions and rarely even into the more distal infraclavicular elements. A common finding with severe stretch injuries is to see cords pulled away from more proximal elements of the plexus such as roots and trunks. Unfortunately, under these circumstances, intraneural damage on these proximal elements often extends close to, if not all the way to, the spinal theca or cord.[101]

The clavicle, padded by the subclavius muscle, has an important relation to the plexus, but common clavicular fracture rarely involves the brachial plexus. However, the entire plexus may be tethered at this point, and abduction and adduction of the arm at operation may show acute angulation of the plexal elements below the clavicle if they cannot move freely in a normal fashion. Callus from a healing clavicular fracture may, on occasion, impinge directly on the plexus, where it may cause a brachial plexus palsy by compression, or prolong or aggravate underlying nerve injury.

Birth palsies from difficult deliveries are less common now because of improved obstetrical training and practice, but they still occur.[57,92,93] The most common is Erb's palsy, involving the upper and middle trunk, which is usually caused by forcible depression of the shoulder and arm during delivery of the infant.[33] Klumpke paralysis involves damage to the lower trunk, roots, or spinal nerves and occurs in circumstances where the arm remains caught in the pelvis and is held hyperabducted while traction is applied to the body. Like stretch injuries to plexus in adults, the outcome of obstetrical plexus palsies is variable, but unlike the adult injuries, which are usually caused by greater forces, those associated with delivery have a greater chance for spontaneous recovery.[21]

In addition to the brachial plexus, nerve elements that are prone to extensive and severe damage include the lumbosacral plexus from severe fractures and dislocations in the pelvis, sciatic nerve with hip dislocation, peroneal nerve with knee dislocation, and the axillary nerve with shoulder dislocation (Fig. 2-11).[31,54] Lumbosacral plexus stretch injuries are often lengthy lesions in continuity with distraction of lumbosacral roots, as suggested by pseudomeningoceles on myelography. Distal intraneural damage to the lumbar or sacral plexus can occur in association with some extensive pelvic fractures or, more rarely, with severe hyperextension of the thigh.

The peroneal nerve can be stretched in association with a variety of knee injuries and sometimes with fracture or avulsion of the fibular head.[115] Peroneal components of the sciatic nerve at the level of the sciatic notch and buttocks can be stretched with hip dislocation or fracture.[54] Relatively more focal stretch and contusive injuries with somewhat better prognosis result from simple fractures adjacent to nerves.[89,94] An illustrative example is the radial nerve palsy following a mid-humeral fracture, which exhibits a tendency to recover spontaneously in 70–80% of patients.[80,89]

The important point with stretch injuries is that, although some may improve, many do not and require operative reconstruction (Table 2-1). However, there may be no satisfactory operations on nerves for some of the most severe stretch injuries. If the major injury is neurotmetic, it can involve such a long segment of the nerve that the only operative method for replacing the resulting extensive neuroma is use of lengthy grafts. The results of repair with such lengthy grafts are often poor, and these are especially prone to fail at the proximal levels where many stretch injuries begin.

GUNSHOT WOUNDS TO NERVE

A frequent source of contusion and stretch injury to nerve is a GSW (Fig. 2-12). In some parts of the world, this is a common

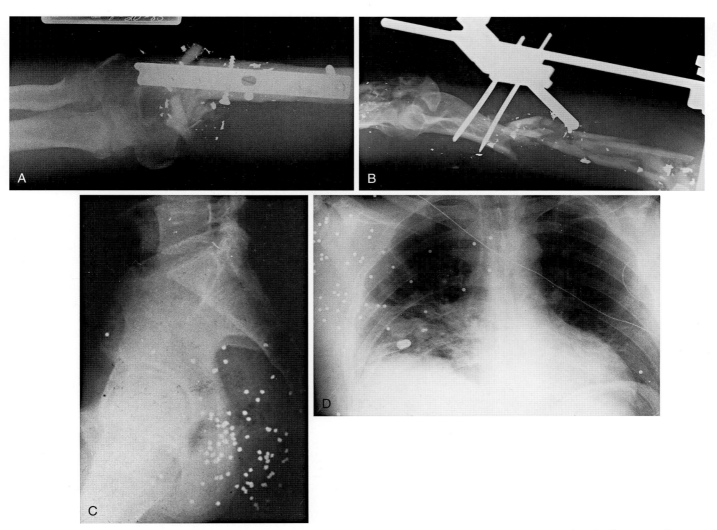

FIGURE 2-12 Various gunshot wounds (GSWs) involving nerves. **(A)** Severe GSW-fractured humerus (shown plated) and adjacent median nerve. **(B)** A forearm fracture managed with external fixation was caused by GSW that also injured both median and ulnar nerves. **(C)** Shotgun injury to buttock involved the sciatic nerve. **(D)** Shotgun injury involving right chest and infraclavicular plexus.

source of nerve injury even in a peacetime, civilian setting.[50] Most such injuries are not caused by direct hit of the nerve by the missile or its fragments; indeed in only approximately 15% of cases is there physical, albeit blunt, partial or complete transaction of the nerve.[81] In a few other cases, particularly shotgun blasts, pellets can become embedded in nerve, even though the nerve remains in gross continuity. Equally rarely, missile fragments may strike bone, fracturing it and driving bone fragments into the nerve, secondarily lacerating the nerve.

In the majority of cases, nerve injured by GSW is left in physical continuity.[50] Such lesions have a variable degree of intraneural derangement. This is because most (85%) of missile trajectories do not strike the nerve, providing a near miss, but can nevertheless injure the nerve with as much severity as a direct hit.[99] As the missile approaches nerve, the latter explodes away from its trajectory and then implodes back as the missile passes by.[84] These dual acute stretching forces, as well as contusive forces, can result in a neurapraxic block in conduction, axonotmesis, neurotmesis, or a mixture of two or even three of these injury grades. All too frequently, the contusive and stretching forces associated with GSW pull apart not only axons but also their connective tissue investments and even intraneural vasculature. Such damage extends over

a length of the nerve. Acutely, it produces a swollen, somewhat hemorrhagic neural segment. With time, as connective tissue proliferates and regenerative sprouts divide many times, a neuroma in continuity is produced. This lesion may or may not have the potential for useful regeneration, depending on the proportion of axonotmetic to neurotmetic changes.

If missiles transect or partially lacerate nerve, the lesion is a blunt and not a sharp injury. Acutely, the nerve end tends to be shredded and irregular, with hemorrhagic, contusive changes in both stumps.[114] Subsequently, a bulbous proximal neuroma and less-swollen distal neuroma form, as with other blunt transecting mechanisms such as auto metal, fan blades, propellers, and chain saws. Embedded shell fragments or spicules of bone may be associated with localized edema or hemorrhage. With time, intraneural connective tissue elements may proliferate around these foreign objects.

Because it takes time to determine the extent of tissue change, whether nerve is transected or stretched but left in continuity, delay in exploration and repair is usually indicated.[51] Associated vascular, osseous, pulmonary, or abdominal wounds may require more acute surgical intervention. Acute hematoma, traumatic aneurysm, arteriovenous fistula, and neural injury close to areas of potential entrapment may also require relatively early operation (Table 2-1). Some pain syndromes such as true causalgia are palliated by early sympathetic blocks and, in many cases, will respond to sympathectomy. On occasion, shell fragments embedded in nerve or intraneural pellets produce a severe dysesthetic pain. Manipulation of the nerve associated with their relatively early removal can sometimes help such pain.

An excellent example of the role of an associated injury is provided by vascular injury. Pseudoaneurysm is usually secondary to a relatively small hole or laceration in a major artery caused by a penetrating missile or a knife or other sharp instrument (Fig. 2-13). Blood under pressure dissects into and around the wall of the vessel. This produces an expanding mass which can compress adjacent nerves. This is especially true with pseudoaneurysms of the axillary, femoral, and popliteal arteries, sites at which vessels are in close juxtaposition to nerves. An axillary artery aneurysm, for example, may compress lateral, posterior, or medial cord and their peripheral outflow, since plexus elements are incorporated in the wall of the false aneurysm. Such compression, as well as stretching, often further compounds partial or incomplete injury to these

elements, leading to a progressive loss of function.[46] Few lesions produce clinical progression of peripheral nerve loss after the first few hours have passed. Pseudoaneurysm, arteriovenous fistula, and hematomas are the exceptions. Hence, progression of neurological deficit (and in some cases, a progressively severe pain syndrome) mandates an aggressive search for the cause of the compressive etiology, followed by urgent surgical exploration and decompression to prevent permanent loss of function.

ISCHEMIA AND COMPRESSION

ISCHEMIA

Peripheral nerve, like other neural tissues, is critically dependent on blood flow. Because it is rarely possible to compress a nerve segment without simultaneously affecting its blood supply, the relative roles of ischemia and physical deformation in compression lesions remain unsettled.[15] More recent evidence suggests that although ischemia may be primarily responsible for a mild type of rapidly reversible nerve lesion, direct mechanical distortion is the

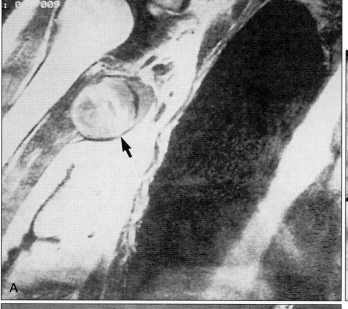

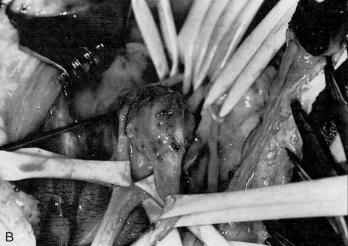

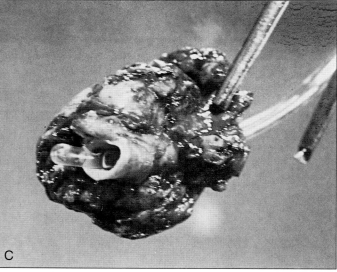

FIGURE 2-13 **(A)** Magnetic resonance scan of an axillary pseudoaneurysm *(arrow)* caused by a penetrating wound. **(B)** Exposure of pseudoaneurysm, which had compressed the lateral and medial cord, contributions to median nerve. **(C)** Another pseudoaneurysm which required resection of a segment of axillary artery for repair. Note that the artery was patent. Preoperative angiogram was normal.

major factor underlying more severe, long-lasting forms of pressure palsy such as Saturday night palsy or tourniquet paralysis.[113] Nevertheless, it is likely that in most compressive lesions, including chronic entrapment neuropathies, localized ischemia at the site of deformation plays some role.[20,116] Ischemia can produce a wide range of nerve fiber lesions and, if severe and prolonged, results in widespread axonal loss and Wallerian degeneration.[63]

In less severe degrees of ischemia, reduction in nerve fiber density is characteristically the result of early dropout of large myelinated fibers.[60] Although damage to a nutrient artery may lead to ischemic injury of a peripheral nerve, pure, isolated ischemic neurogenic lesions are uncommon in humans. An example is occasionally provided by a midforearm-level injury or by some vascular diseases affecting median nerve with its dominant median artery. Here, necrosis of the distal stump of the nerve may occur. More commonly, nerve trunks are involved along with other soft tissue structures of the limbs such as muscle and major vessels, with the severity of the nerve injury depending on the degree and duration of ischemia and compression. Studies on limb ischemia suggest that there is a critical period of approximately 8 hours, after which irreversible nerve injury ensues.[61]

The vascular anatomy of peripheral nerves, with rich anastomoses between longitudinal vessels in the epineurium, perineurium, and endoneurium and the regional segmental supply, allows the surgeon to mobilize long segments of nerve without producing ischemia. Nevertheless, extensive intraneural dissection by an inexperienced surgeon can jeopardize the microcirculation and result in ischemic damage.[62] Evidence also suggests that a transected nerve or one under tension is more sensitive to ischemia.[96] The surgeon should therefore minimize interruption of both regional and segmental longitudinal vascular supply, in addition to avoiding tension at the suture site.

COMPRESSION

The sequential pathology of nerve fiber injury is rather stereotyped and occurs regardless of the compressive agent (Fig. 2-14).[1] An exception to this rule appears to be the nerve fiber pathology that results from more minor forms of compression.[37] Compression of nerve fibers appears to produce myelinated nerve fiber changes that are peculiar to this mechanism.[2,78] These include alterations in paranodal myelination, axonal thinning, and segmental demyelination.[25–27,85] Wallerian degeneration results from more severe degrees of compression.

The degree of recovery after compression or ischemic injury may be accurately predicted in some clinical situations. The characteristic Saturday night palsy results from compression of the radial nerve against the humerus. Total radial nerve palsy often results, but there is return of motor and sensory function in the majority of cases without any need for surgical intervention. Most palsies associated with unconsciousness due to anesthesia and poor positioning or pressure during operation as well as those related to improper application of plaster casts carry a good prognosis for spontaneous recovery.[65] There are, however, important exceptions. Sometimes the compression or crushing injury has been severe enough or prolonged enough to cause damage that is irreversible unless operative repair is done (Fig. 2-15). The brachial plexus and the ulnar, sciatic, and peroneal nerves are most commonly affected by these more severe compressive etiologies.[82] Restoration of function after acute compression and ischemic injury may be less certain in some other circumstances. It may be difficult, for example, to

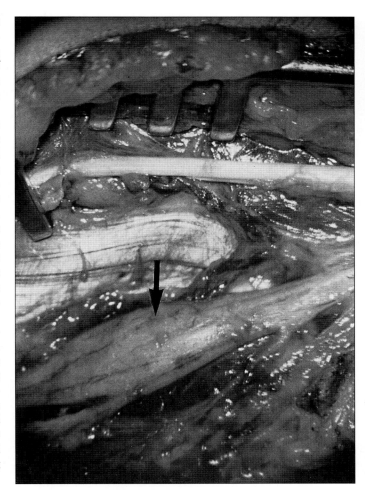

FIGURE 2-14 Enlargement of posterior interosseous nerve *(arrow)* just proximal to entrapment site at arcade of Frohse.

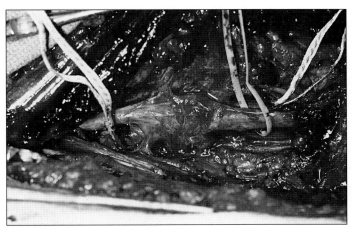

FIGURE 2-15 Crush injury to lateral cord of brachial plexus.

predict the degree of recovery that follows evacuation of hematomas or relief of aneurysmal compression of such structures as the brachial plexus and the femoral or sciatic nerves.[34] Although infrequent, there are also circumstances in which two levels of compression may exist.[110] The patient with cervical spondylolysis or relatively mild disc disease affecting a root or spinal nerve may be more likely to become symptomatic with an otherwise mild degree of compression of the median nerve at the wrist or ulnar nerve at the elbow. In these circumstances, multiple factors exist that affect the outcome of peripheral nerve surgery, including the identity and level of the nerve involved, the age of the patient, the extent of the pre-compression injury to nerve, and the timing of the corrective surgery.

Severe crushing injury, skeletal fracture with vascular compromise, and anticoagulant administration, resulting in hemorrhage, can lead to increased pressure within a fascial compartment. As a consequence of this, severe compression and ischemic damage to peripheral nerves as well as other soft tissues can result. A closed compartment syndrome with impending ischemic paralysis requires immediate decompression with properly placed and usually extensive, longitudinal fasciotomies.[98] Delay in treatment results in ischemic infarction of muscle, nerve, and other tissues, leading to contractures and other crippling deformities.

COMPARTMENT SYNDROMES

Volkmann contracture is a serious example of ischemic compression. Paralysis can follow manipulation with or without casting and immobilization of a closed fracture near the elbow that is associated with severe muscle swelling and hemorrhage into the anterior compartment of the forearm.[36] This type of ischemic injury is most frequently associated with supracondylar fracture of the humerus and dislocation of the elbow and can occur even before manipulation or casting is done. Actual infarction of the volar forearm musculature can occur. Blunt but contusive injury to the forearm, such as from a pool cue or baseball bat, can also result in enough swelling to compress nerves secondarily even though arterial injury or spasm may not be present. Two patients seen by us had been injured by pool cue blows to the forearm, and swelling led to both radial and median nerve palsies even though there was no fracture of the radius or ulna.

In the usual Volkmann case, there is injury to the brachial artery along with diffuse segmental damage to the median nerve and volar forearm muscles. The large median and sometimes radial nerve fibers serving motor and proprioceptive function are more severely involved than the smaller pain fibers. The EMG may aid in diagnosis by showing temporary but repetitive and spontaneous motor discharges from muscles most distal to the injury site.[44] Swelling of the forearm resulting in a painful paresthetic hand must alert the physician to an impending compartment syndrome long before more obvious signs of vascular compromise are apparent.

Ischemia of sufficient magnitude to produce Volkmann's contracture results in severe endoneurial scarring over so long a segment of the median nerve as to make spontaneous regeneration unlikely (Fig. 2-16). Bunnell believed that Volkmann's contracture was sufficiently explained by closed-space compression of the brachial vessel between the fracture and the lacertus fibrosus at the level of the elbow.[101] In any case, spasm of the artery results in ischemia and sometimes in actual infarction of soft tissues of the volar forearm compartment.

Section and repair of the damaged segment of the brachial artery may be necessary.[87] Anticoagulation alone may not suffice and may even be deleterious. We have seen one patient whose syndrome progressed shortly after heparinization, probably because of hemorrhage into an already ischemic musculature.

In addition to the median nerve, the radial and even occasionally the ulnar nerve may be involved because of a severely swollen elbow and forearm, particularly if the contracture was initially

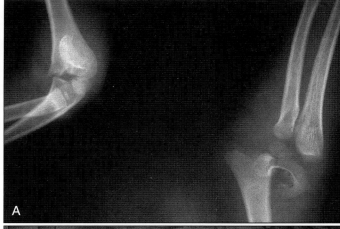

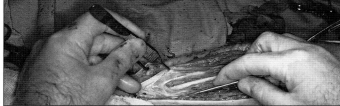

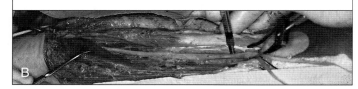

FIGURE 2-16 **(A)** Distal humeral fracture dislocation that resulted in brachial artery damage and Volkmann's ischemia. **(B)** Long-standing Volkmann's contracture caused by an intra-arterial morphine injection. The top photograph shows the fatty replaced pronator muscle, being grasped by forceps and pulled away from the pale-appearing median nerve. In the lower photograph, a lengthy segment of the abnormal median nerve (having sustained compressive and ischemic damage) is exposed.

associated with multiple contusive injuries at these levels. Immediate fasciotomy is in order because remedial operation for the more severe degrees of Volkmann's contracture, although possible, is disappointing.[109] Compression of the median nerve must be relieved by operation, especially in the region of the pronator teres and flexor digitorum sublimis muscles. Closed-space swelling of this type can be aggravated by a tight-fitting cast or by fixation of the elbow in acute flexion. Emergency treatment is necessary at the first signs of ischemia if irreversible neural damage and contractures of the extremity are to be prevented.

A related condition is the anterior compartment syndrome involving the leg, which results in a progressive peroneal palsy or foot drop. A fracture or fractures of the tibia and fibula may or may not be a concomitant finding, but soft tissue swelling is always present. Urgent extensive fasciotomy is indicated, just as with Volkmann's contracture. Tissue pressure can be readily measured by placing a needle in the swollen limb and attaching it to a saline-filled tube and manometer. If the difference between arterial pressure measured by cuff and tissue pressure measured by manometer is less than 40 mmHg, ischemic infarction is likely to occur.

In summary, extension of neural injury by compression and ischemia is a serious possibility if enough soft tissue swelling or an aneurysm, fistula, hematoma, or arterial insufficiency occurs in a relatively closed or confined neurovascular compartment. These lesions are particularly apt to occur with perforating wounds that involve arteries and with fractures but can also be caused by blunt or contusive trauma. Neural damage usually is preventable by expeditious decompression, but it becomes irreversible if severe ischemia involves a long segment of nerve persists for too long a period of time.

ELECTRICAL INJURY

Electrical injury by passage of a large current through a peripheral nerve usually results from accidental contact of the extremity with a high-tension wire.[16] If the individual does not succumb to respiratory or cardiac arrest, diffuse nerve and muscle damage results.[3] Pathologic reports of peripheral nerve damage caused by this mechanism are sparse, and guidelines for treatment are controversial.[23] Conservative management of the nerve injury itself and early orthopedic reconstruction of the extremity seem to be best.[39] Prognosis with most low-voltage injuries is excellent, but quite variable for high-voltage injuries.[39] Operative experience with seven such cases involving one or more peripheral nerves indicates that only a few of these lesions improve spontaneously with time. Resection of a lengthy segment of damaged nerve and repair by grafts is usually necessary and outcomes have not been good. Histologically, the segment of the nerve is virtually replaced, first with necrosis and then with connective tissue reaction, including a severe degree of both perineurial and endoneurial scar tissue. Fascicular outline may be preserved, but intrafascicular damage and fibrosis can be severe enough to prevent any but fine axon regeneration. The accompanying severe skin burns and necrosis of bone and other soft tissues frequently thwart reconstructive efforts.[58] The muscle in the extremity often is extensively coagulated, leading to severe contractures which further decreases the likelihood of useful reinnervation.

THERMAL INJURY

Although not a common mechanism of peripheral nerve injury, thermal injury by flame, steam, or hot elements can result in neural damage ranging from a transient neurapraxia to severe neurotmesis with extensive necrosis of nerve as well as adjacent tissues. In patients with circumferential burns, neural damage may be related to delayed constrictive fibrosis, resulting in a tourniquet effect. Patients with severe burns involving nerve present with complete motor and sensory loss. The clinical examination is often difficult because of associated soft tissue injuries, extensive skin loss, and often a massively swollen extremity. The degree of tissue necrosis, the extent of bacterial contamination, and the need for an adequate soft tissue bed make immediate reconstruction of nerve rarely feasible. Proper attention to the wound with repeated escharectomy, if indicated, increases the success of secondary repairs. In thermal injury, whether by direct effect or secondary to constrictive fibrosis, long lengths of nerves are often involved, necessitating nerve grafts. The prognosis for functional recovery is poor in such cases, especially if there is also extensive involvement of muscle and other soft tissues.

Serious surface burns caused by thermal agents can lead to coagulation necrosis of underlying nerves. Like electrical injuries, the more serious burns can affect a length of nerve. Experience with four patients who required graft replacement of both median

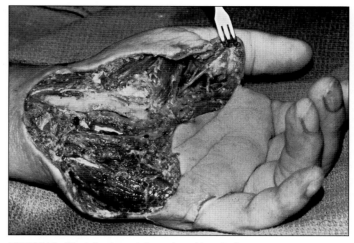

FIGURE 2-17 Infection of the palm of hand after carpal tunnel release. Despite the infection severity, median and ulnar nerve function was not significantly impaired.

and ulnar nerves at the wrist demonstrated the difficulty in providing useful recovery. Although all four had undergone prior skin grafts or other soft tissue transfers to provide coverage, tendon grafts were also necessary in two of these patients. In one of these cases, burn involved the palmar surface of the hand, and severe contractures were present despite extensive prior soft tissue operations. Infection can complicate any soft tissue wound involving nerve (Fig. 2-17). It is more likely to do so if the injury mechanism has produced necrosis of soft tissue, and thus it is often seen with thermal and electrical burns and some compartment syndromes. The nerve's epineurial and interfascicular connective tissue layers usually resist invasion unless they are extensively injured. In exceptional cases, infection can lead to an extensive segment of intraneural necrosis and a lengthy lesion that is difficult to repair with any success.

INJECTION INJURY

Injection injury, a surprisingly common category of neural injury, deserves special attention.

PATHOGENESIS

Injection injury is caused by a needle placed into or close to nerve, and damage results from neurotoxic chemicals in the agent injected. The extent of damage varies, depending not only on the agent injected but whether the needle and therefore the toxic agent were placed in or close to nerve. There are cases in which some or all of the injury relates to the damage done by the needle placement itself. Experimentally, damage from injection seems to require placement of the agent either within the epineurium or, for more serious damage, at an intraneural locus, either intrafascicular or in the connective tissue layers between the fascicles.[29] In the human, however, about 10% of patients subsequently found to have an injection injury have a delay of hours or even days before the onset of symptoms.[72] This suggests either a purely epineurial locus for deposition of the agent in these cases, placement of medication close to nerve, or in a tissue plane from which the agent can gravitate to and bathe the nerve.

The pathology of injection injuries also varies depending on the injection site and the agent injected.[7] The principal pathogenetic

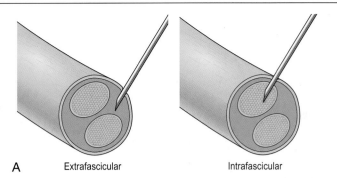

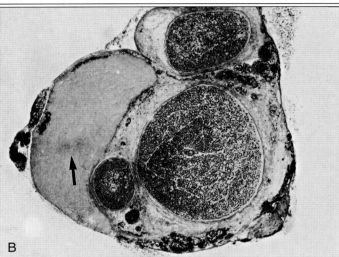

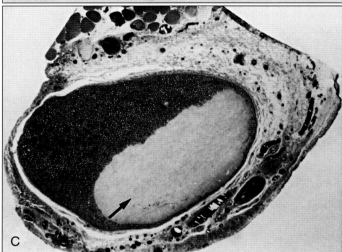

FIGURE 2-18 **(A)** The two intraneural sites for injection injuries. **(B)** Nerve injected at an extrafascicular site. **(C)** An intrafascicular injection *(arrow)* of collagen in a primate nerve.

mechanism, however, is necrosis.[55] With intraneural injection, there is acute edema and inflammatory changes, often with necrosis, which affects connective tissue elements, axons, and myelin (Fig. 2-18).[66] With time, connective tissue proliferation may occur, producing intraneural scar, thwarting effective axonal regeneration.[83] The blood–nerve barrier at both the perineurial and endoneurial capillary levels are severely disrupted,[30] a finding that may occur despite preservation of the fascicular outline. After the first few days, the injected segment is no longer swollen and may with further time appear shrunken or even as a segment of nerve with normal diameter. On gross inspection with or without magnification, the nerve usually appears to have excellent physical continuity. Even intraneural dissection may reveal good fascicular continuity despite intrafascicular damage that is quite neurotmetic. Some agents injected into epineurium or adjacent to nerve produce more proliferation of inflammatory tissue and scar than at an intraneural locus, but the necrosis at the latter locus is especially damaging and difficult for the regenerative process to overcome spontaneously.

CLINICAL FEATURES

In the usual clinical setting, needle placement results in an electric-like shock down the extremity, followed by or concomitant with a severe radicular burning pain and paresthesias as the agent is injected. Acute symptoms are variously described but are usually severe. Pain associated with the injection is described as searing, burning, electrical, or numbing, and with serious injection injury the sensation usually travels down the limb and in the distribution of the nerve injected.[79] With delayed onset, which seems to occur in about 10% of patients with injection injuries, the symptoms are less dramatic but nonetheless bothersome.[72] These include a burning pain, paresthesias, and radiation of a deep discomfort down the limbs and in the distribution of the less directly involved nerve.

Initial loss may be complete or incomplete in the distribution of the injected nerve. There can be a variable degree of sensory and motor loss. Sometimes, fiber dropout is mild, and although the lesion is painful, sensory or motor loss may be minimal. Occasionally, the absence of reflexes and conductive abnormalities in the distribution of the injured nerve are the only clinical findings. More often, clinical loss is more dramatic and more severe, including complete sensory or motor loss or both, accompanied by denervational changes on EMG. Initial loss may improve with time, but will often persist with the more severe injection injuries. Many of the latter injuries do not regenerate adequately or at all despite maintenance of physical continuity. If clinical loss remains complete or severe, it will not improve unless corrected by surgical intervention.

INJECTION SITES

The most common neural injection sites are the sciatic nerve at the buttock level and the radial nerve in the lateral upper arm.[72,111] Nonetheless, beside sciatic and radial nerves, we have seen injection injuries involving almost every other major nerve in the body (Fig. 2-19). Included have been injection injuries to femoral and lateral femoral cutaneous nerves as well as ulnar and median nerves at wrist, elbow, and upper arm levels. Although quite unusual, injection injuries of musculocutaneous and antebrachial cutaneous nerves and even portions of the brachial plexus have been seen. The most common site is sciatic at the buttock or proximal thigh level.[11] Classically, this is most likely to occur if the injection is not made in the upper outer quadrant of the buttock.[13,14] However, from the histories given, even this may not always be a safe site. If the patient is lying on one side or bent over while standing, the relation of the presumed upper outer buttock quadrant to the sciatic nerve can change. Another factor making sciatic injection more likely to cause injury is a thinly constructed buttock, which is more likely in a cachectic, chronically ill patient or a constitutionally thin individual.

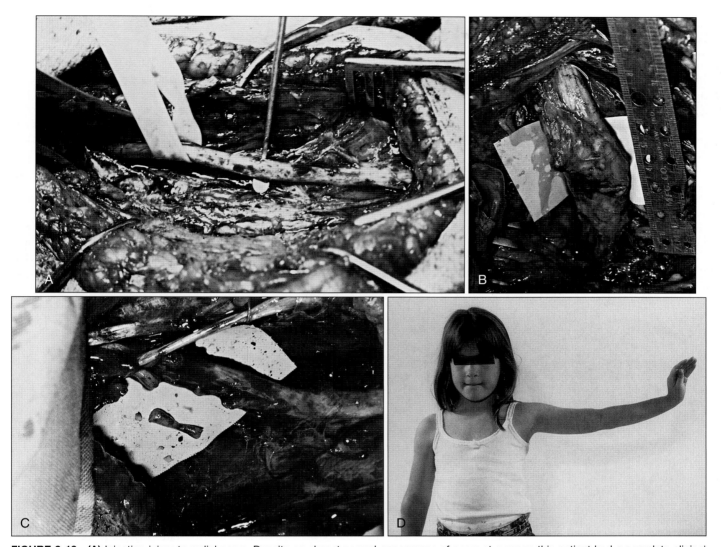

FIGURE 2-19 **(A)** Injection injury to radial nerve. Despite an almost normal appearance of nerve at surgery, this patient had a complete clinical loss and absence of NAPs on exploration 4.5 months post-injury. **(B)** Severe, granulomatous injection injury involving sciatic nerve at a buttock level. **(C)** Injection injury resulting in partial loss of function undergoing a split repair. **(D)** Recovery of radial function following repair of a radial injection injury.

The length of the needle used and the angle at which the needle penetrates soft tissues are factors, as is the force with which the injection is given. If the hub of the needle inverts skin and underlying soft tissue with enough force during injection, the tip of the needle can penetrate to a level deeper than surmised. This may be compounded if the needle penetrates soft tissue at an angle headed toward nerve rather than at a right angle to a horizontal plane through the body. Other factors, such as movement of the patient as the injection is being made, can sometimes play a role. If the patient shrugs or jerks up the shoulder, perhaps in anticipation of the pain connected with the event, or ability to see the approaching needle, an injection intended for the deltoid can injure the radial nerve. In part because of this, injection injury of radial nerve at the midhumeral level is the second most frequent site of injection injury. Infusions or needles intended for veins can also be inadvertently placed in nerves. This is more likely to occur to median or ulnar nerve, the former either at the wrist or elbow and the latter at the wrist. Infusion complications have, however, also been seen involving the brachial plexus, the femoral nerve, and the posterior tibial nerve at the ankle.

MANAGEMENT

The sciatic nerve lies in a trough beneath the piriformis muscle and posterior to the gemellus, quadratus, and obturator internus muscles, between the bony boundaries of the ischial tuberosity and the greater trochanter. Drugs not injected directly into the nerve may pool in this trough and bathe the nerve to produce neuritis. Intraneural damage is similar to the changes seen with antibiotic injection into the brain. Although the deficit in neural function usually is caused by intraneural neuritis and scar tissue rather than extraneural scarring, some authors believe that external neurolysis for this complication can reverse loss of function.[69] We do not agree with this; however, a lesion with partial loss of function and severe pain not responding to analgesics may be helped by internal neurolysis on a delayed basis. An occasional patient may have a true causalgia after injection, and they may benefit from sympathectomy, especially if recurrent sympathetic blocks have provided temporary relief. The pain in most of these patients can be managed effectively with tricyclic antidepressants (such as Nortriptyline) or newer anticonvulsant agents (Gabapentin), as these have demonstrated good benefit for neuropathic pain states.[45,70]

Sedatives and narcotics as well as antibiotics and steroids can cause injection neuropathy. If the complication is noticed immediately, 50–100 ml of normal saline can be placed in the region of the injection site in the hope of diluting the drug and avoiding permanent neuropathy. Open operative irrigation might be even more logical, but because such patients are not usually seen acutely, experience with either approach is lacking. If the nerve deficit is partial, expectant treatment is best, provided pain is not a severe problem, but if the deficit is complete after several months of observation, exploration becomes warranted. In this regard, if an injection injury to the sciatic nerve spares either the peroneal or tibial division but is complete in the other division, it is a complete lesion of one division, and this division may need resection and repair if function is to be regained.[54]

Our policy with injection injuries has been to expose the nerve that shows little or no function after 8–16 weeks and attempt to evoke an NAP through the injury.[72] If no response is recorded, the lesion must be resected. With sciatic palsies, one division may require resection and the other only neurolysis. The gross appearance of the nerve lesion is deceiving in many of these injection injuries. Segments that appear to inspection and palpation to be minimally injured may have such extensive axonal and endoneurial disruption as to preclude useful functional regeneration. In these cases, only resection and repair can provide hope for recovery. As a result, a severe palsy secondary to injection injury usually should be followed for only 2–4 months. If there is then no significant recovery, electrically or clinically, the nerve should be explored so that direct stimulation and evoked NAP studies can be made.

The final point to be emphasized is that neuropathy from drug injections must be prevented by proper education of nurses and ancillary personnel as well as physicians.

IRRADIATION INJURY

An iatrogenic cause of nerve damage much less common than injection is irradiation.[12,106] This usually affects the brachial plexus but can also occur at the level of the pelvic plexus.[32] Extensive scar formation in surrounding soft tissues and severe intraneural changes, consisting of myelin loss, axonal degeneration and extensive endoneurial fibrosis, often result.[68] Management of these difficult cases is addressed in subsequent chapters.

IATROGENIC INJURY

Unfortunately, iatrogenic damage to nerve remains a common etiology of nerve injury.[56] An earlier section addressed injection injuries, a not infrequent iatrogenic injury mechanism. Accidental injury to a peripheral nerve creates a situation that is distressing to both the physician and the patient. It is essential that the patient be managed with great care so that the situation is not subsequently aggravated by inappropriate actions.[4,5]

In the majority of iatrogenic cases we have seen, the originating physician was unaware that the nerve had been accidentally injured. The nerve may have been injured by inappropriate retractor pressure or more directly by cautery, incision, or suture (Fig. 2-20).

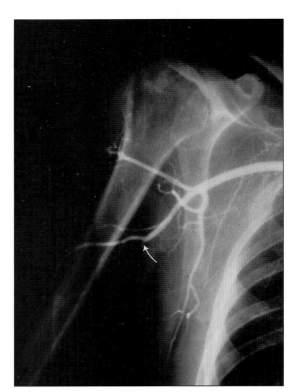

FIGURE 2-20 Axillary artery injury *(arrow)* following transaxillary first rib resection, also complicated by a severe injury to the medial cord.

Nerves may be injured by pressure while they are immobilized in the operating room or subsequently by plaster casts. Inappropriate operative management of peripheral nerves may also result in inadvertent complete or partial nerve injury.

DIAGNOSIS

Even though such injuries are iatrogenic in origin, the injury mechanisms involved are similar to non-iatrogenic injuries. Necessary in diagnosis is a thorough history, followed by a detailed motor and sensory clinical examination, and then supplemented by electrophysiologic studies. It is of great importance to undertake a careful, detailed, and sequential history from the patient and seek collateral forms of information from family members, medical notes and records, and any other ancillary investigations done. The true diagnosis may not be apparent for a few days if the patient is immobilized postoperatively or is suffering from postoperative pain and is under sedation. For example, it is not unusual for sciatic or femoral nerve palsy complicating hip surgery to be diagnosed days after the operation (Fig. 2-21). The local discomfort after a cervical lymph node biopsy may confuse the patient, but the symptoms resulting from trapezius palsy attendant on accessory nerve injury are usually reported by the patient within a few weeks of operation.

Record keeping should be of the highest order. It is totally inappropriate to re-dictate the original operative note after an iatrogenic injury is discovered postoperatively. Similarly, the chart should be carefully guarded so that it or portions of it are not lost. Any alteration or loss of records is liable to be interpreted as evidence of lack of honesty by the surgeon, even if this is not the case. Notes should be appropriate to the problem. Lengthy treatises concerning irrelevant issues, although accurate in themselves, may be subsequently interpreted as attempts to confuse rather than

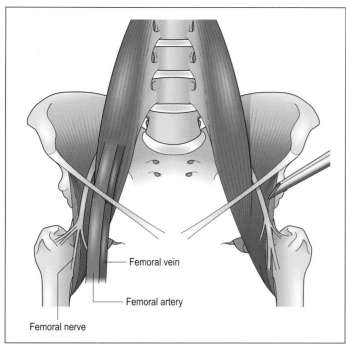

FIGURE 2-21 Damage to femoral nerve during the course of a hip joint repair in this illustrated case resulted from a blow to the nerve by a periosteal elevator that slipped on the anterior surface of the ileum.

- Femoral vein
- Femoral artery
- Femoral nerve

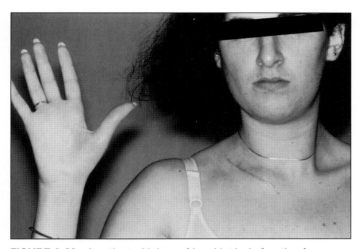

FIGURE 2-22 A patient with loss of hand intrinsic function from iatrogenic plexopathy caused by damage to the lower trunk during attempted supraclavicular sympathectomy for presumed reflex sympathetic dystrophy.

illuminate the clinical problem. It is most appropriate to consult an expert on nerve who records on the chart that such a consultation has occurred. The detailed results of the consult should be maintained in the patient's hospital and office records.

MANAGEMENT

The presumed mechanism of injury determines management. If the nerve damage arises and progresses following traction, limb lengthening, or application of plaster cast which may be causing external pressure, then discontinuation of the offending apparatus is clearly indicated.[28] If a sharp cut is made in a nerve and it is

recognized at the time of operation, the appropriate management is to reconstitute the nerve using standard microsuturing technique at the same operation. This allows end-to-end apposition. There is no requirement to trim the stumps, and retraction of nerve stumps will not have occurred. If there is a strong probability that blunt transection has occurred at operation, then it may be appropriate to reoperate several weeks after the iatrogenic injury, just as with non-iatrogenic blunt lacerations.

In the majority of instances, the assumption is made that a lesion in continuity is present. The patient is therefore managed appropriately for 3–4 months while evidence of spontaneous regeneration is sought by repeated clinical examinations supplemented by electrical studies. Patients may require appropriate splints and other orthotic devices as well as physical therapy during this time of waiting (Fig. 2-22).

Concern about legal consequences of iatrogenic injury may alter a physician's usual pattern of practice. The attending physician must be extremely vigilant that alteration of normal practice does not compromise the end result. We strongly advise that patients are managed using the usual clinical guidelines for each type of injury, whether it be sharp transection or a focal or lengthy lesion in continuity. Moreover, the timing of exploration should be the same, and not altered or extended because of the "false hope" that the nerve may spontaneously recover. As in every nerve injury case, every effort must be made to reduce the final disability by appropriate care of the limb after the second (nerve reconstructive) operation.

REFERENCES

1. Aguayo A: Neuropathy due to compression and entrapment. In: Dyek PJ, Thomas PK, Lambert EH, Eds: Peripheral Neuropathy. Philadelphia: WB Saunders, 1975:688–713.
2. Aguayo A, Nair CP, and Midgley R: Experimental progressive compression neuropathy in the rabbit. Histologic and electrophysiologic studies. Arch Neurol 24:358–364, 1971.
3. Aita JA: Neurologic manifestations of electrical injury. Nebr State Med J 50:530–533, 1965.
4. Birch R, Bonney G, Dowell J, et al.: Iatrogenic injuries of peripheral nerves. J Bone Joint Surg [Br] 73:280–282, 1991.
5. Birch R, Bonney G, and Wynn Parry C: Iatropathic Injuries. In: Birch R, Ed: Surgical Disorders of Peripheral Nerve. Edinburgh, Churchill Livingstone, 1998.
6. Bowden REM, Abdullah S, and Gooding MR: Anatomy of the cervical spine, membranes, spinal cord, nerve roots, and brachial plexus. In: Wilkinson MF, Eds: Brain. Cervical spondylosis and other disorders of the cervical spine. Philadelphia, WB Saunders, 1967.
7. Broadbent TR, Odom GL, and Woodhall B: Peripheral nerve injuries from administration of penicillin. Report of four clinical cases. JAMA 140:1008–1010, 1949.
8. Brushart TME: The mechanical and humoral control of specificity in nerve repair. In: Gelberman RH, Ed: Operative Nerve Repair and Reconstruction. Philadelphia, JB Lippincott, 1991:215–230.
9. Carlstedt T, Anand P, and Hallin R, et al.: Spinal nerve root repair and reimplantation of avulsed ventral roots into the spinal cord after brachial plexus injury. J Neurosurg 93:237–247, 2000.
10. Carvalho GA, Nikkhah G, and Matthies C, et al.: Diagnosis of root avulsions in traumatic brachial plexus injuries: value of computerized tomography, myelography and magnetic resonance imaging. J Neurosurg 86:69–76, 1997.
11. Clark K, Williams PEJ, and Willis W, et al.: Injection injury of the sciatic nerve. Clin Neurosurg 17:111–125, 1970.

12. Clodius L, Uhlschmid G, and Hess K: Irradiation plexitis of the brachial plexus. Clin Plast Surg 11:161–165, 1984.

13. Combes MA, Clark WK: Sciatic nerve injury following intragluteal injection: pathogenesis and prevention. Am J Dis Child 199:579, 1960.

14. Combes MA, Clark WK, and Gregory CF, et al.: Sciatic nerve injury in infants: recognition and prevention of impairment resulting from intragluteal injections. JAMA 173:1330–1339, 1960.

15. Denny-Brown D and Brenner C: Paralysis of nerve induced by direct pressure and tourniquet. Arch Neurol Psychiat 51:1–26, 1944.

16. Di Vincenti FC, Moncrief JA, and Pruitt BA: Electrical injuries: a review of 65 cases. J Trauma 9:497–507, 1969.

17. Doi K, Otsuka K, and Okamoto Y, et al.: Cervical nerve root avulsion in brachial plexus injuries: magnetic resonance imaging classification and comparison with myelography and computerized tomography myelography. J Neurosurg 96:277–284, 2002.

18. Ducker TB: Pathophysiology of peripheral nerve trauma. In: Omer GE and Spinner M, Eds: Management of Peripheral Nerve Problems. Philadelphia, WB Saunders, 1980.

19. Ducker TB and Garrison WB: Surgical aspects of peripheral nerve trauma. Curr Probl Surg 1:62, 1974.

20. Eames RA and Lange LS: Clinical and pathological study of ischaemic neuropathy. J Neurol NeurosurgPsychiatry 30:215–226, 1967.

21. Eng GD, Binder H, and Getson P, et al.: Obstetrical brachial plexus palsy (OBPP) outcome with conservative management. Muscle Nerve 19:884–891, 1996.

22. Filler AG, Kliot M, and Howe FA, et al.: Application of magnetic resonance neurography in the evaluation of patients with peripheral nerve pathology. J Neurosurg 85:299–309, 1996.

23. Fischer H: Pathological effects and sequelae of electrical accidents. Electrical burns (secondary accidents, renal manifestations, sequelae). J Occup Med 7:564–571, 1965.

24. Friedman WA: The electrophysiology of peripheral nerve injuries. Neurosurg Clin N Am 2:43–56, 1991.

25. Fullerton PM and Gilliatt R: Pressure neuropathy in the hind foot of the guinea-pig. J Neurol Neurosurg Psychiatry 30:18–25, 1967.

26. Fullerton PM and Gilliatt RW: Median and ulnar neuropathy in the guinea-pig. J Neurol Neurosurg Psychiatry 30:393–402, 1967.

27. Fullerton PM, Gilliatt RW, and Lascelles RG, et al.: The relation between fibre diameter and internodal length in chronic neuropathy. Proc Physiol Soc 19–20:26P–28P, 1965.

28. Galardi G, Comi G, and Lozza L, et al.: Peripheral nerve damage during limb lengthening. Neurophysiology in five cases of bilateral tibial lengthening. J Bone Joint Surg [Br] 72:121–124, 1990.

29. Gentili F, Hudson AR, and Hunter D: Clinical and experimental aspects of injection injuries of peripheral nerves. Can J Neurol Sci 7:143–151, 1980.

30. Gentili F, Hudson AR, and Hunter D, et al.: Nerve injection injury with local anesthetic agents: a light and electron microscopic, fluorescent microscopic, and horseradish peroxidase study. Neurosurgery 6:263–272, 1980.

31. Gentili F, Hudson AR, and Midha R: Peripheral nerve injuries: types, causes, and grading. In: Wilkins RH, Rengachary SS, Eds: Neurosurgery, 2nd edn, vol. 3. New York, McGraw-Hill, 1996:3105–3114.

32. Gilbert H and Kagen AR: Radiation Damage to the Nervous System. New York, Raven Press, 1980.

33. Gilbert A and Whitaker I: Obstetrical brachial plexus lesions. J Hand Surg [Br] 16:489–491, 1991.

34. Gilden DH and Eisner J: Lumbar plexopathy caused by disseminated intravascular coagulation. JAMA 237:2846–2847, 1977.

35. Gilliatt R: Physical injury to peripheral nerves, physiological and electrodiagnostic aspects. Mayo Clin Proc 56:361–370, 1981.

36. Goldner JL and Goldner RD: Volkmann's ischemia and ischemic contractures. In: Jupiter JB, Ed: Flynn's Hand Surgery. Baltimore, Williams & Wilkins, 1991.

37. Granit R, Leksell L, and Skoglund CR: Fiber interactions in injured or compressed region of nerve. Brain 67:125–140, 1944.

38. Grant GA, Goodkin R, and Kliot M: Evaluation and surgical management of peripheral nerve problems. Neurosurgery 44:825–839, 1999.

39. Grube BJ, Heimbach DM, and Engrav LH, et al.: Neurologic consequences of electrical burns. J Trauma 30:254–258, 1990.

40. Happel LT and Kline DG: Nerve lesions in continuity. In: Gelberman RH, Ed: Operative Nerve Repair and Reconstruction. Philadelphia, JB Lipincott, 1991:601–616.

41. Highet J: Effects of stretch on peripheral nerve. Br J Surg 30:355–369, 1942.

42. Hudson AR and Hunter D: Timing of peripheral nerve repair: important local neuropathologic factors. Clin Neurosurg 24:392–405, 1977.

43. Hudson AR, Hunter D, and Kline DG, et al.: Progression of partial experimental injury to peripheral nerve II: light and electron microscopic studies. J Neurosurg 42:15–22, 1975.

44. Kimura J: Electrodiagnosis. In: Diseases of Nerve and Muscles: Principles and Practice. Philadelphia, FA Davis, 1983:505.

45. Kingery WS: A critical review of controlled clinical trials for peripheral neuropathic pain and complex regional pain syndromes. Pain 73:123–139, 1997.

46. Kline DG: Peripheral nerve injury observed or incurred during vascular operations. Semin Vasc Surg 41:20–25, 1991.

47. Kline DG and Hudson AR: Acute injuries of peripheral nerves. In: Youmans J, Ed: Neurological Surgery. Philadelphia, WB Saunders, 1990.

48. Kline DG: Physiological and clinical factors contributing to the timing of nerve repair. Clin Neurosurg 24:425–455, 1977.

49. Kline DG: Macroscopic and microscopic concomitants of nerve repair. Clin Neurosurg 26:582–606, 1979.

50. Kline DG: Civilian gunshot wounds to the brachial plexus. J Neurosurg 70:166–174, 1989.

51. Kline DG and Hackett ER: Reappraisal of timing for exploration of civilian peripheral nerve injuries. Surgery 78:54–65, 1975.

52. Kline DG and Happel LT: A quarter century's experience with intraoperative nerve action potential recording. Can J Neurol Sci 20:3–10, 1993.

53. Kline DG, Hudson AR, and Hackett ER, et al.: Progression of partial experimental injury to peripheral nerve I: Periodic measurements of muscle contraction strength. J Neurosurg 42:1–14, 1975.

54. Kline DG, Kim D, and Midha R, et al.: Management and results of sciatic nerve injuries: a 24-year experience [see comments]. J Neurosurg 89:13–23, 1998.

55. Kolb LC and Gray SJ: Peripheral neuritis as a complication of penicillin therapy. JAMA 132:323–326, 1946.

56. Kretschmer T, Antoniadis G, and Braun V, et al.: Evaluation of iatrogenic lesions in 722 surgically treated cases of peripheral nerve trauma. J Neurosurg 94:905–912, 2001.

57. Levine MG, Holroyde J, and Woods JR Jr., et al.: Birth trauma: incidence and predisposing factors. Obstet Gynecol 63:792–795, 1984.

58. Lewis GK: Trauma resulting from electricity. J Int Coll Surg 28:724–738, 1957.

59. Liu CT, Benda CE, and Lewey FH: Tensile strength of human nerves: Experimental physiological and histological study. Arch Neurol Psychiat 59:322–336, 1948.

60. Lundborg G: Intraneural microcirculation and peripheral nerve barriers. Techniques for evaluation – clinical implications. In: Omer

GE and Spinner M, Eds: Management of Peripheral Nerve Problems. Philadelphia, WB Saunders, 1980.

61. Lundborg G: Ischemic nerve injury. Experimental studies on intraneural microvascular pathophysiology and nerve function in a limb subjected to temporary circulatory arrest. Scand J Plast Reconstr Surg Suppl 6:3–113, 1970.

62. Lundborg G: Structure and function of the intraneural microvessels as related to trauma, edema formation and nerve function. J Bone Joint Surg [Am] 57:938–948, 1975.

63. Lundborg G: Nerve regeneration. In: Lundborg G, Ed. Nerve Injury and Repair. London, Churchill Livingstone, 1988:149–195.

64. Lundborg G and Rydevik B: Effects of stretching the tibial nerve of the rabbit. A preliminary study of the intraneural circulation and the barrier function of the perineurium. J Bone Joint Surg 55B:390–401, 1973.

65. Mackinnon SE and Dellon AL: Surgery of the Peripheral Nerve. New York, Thieme Medical Publishers, 1988.

66. Mackinnon SE, Hudson AR, and Gentili F, et al.: Peripheral nerve injection injury with steroid agents. Plast Reconstr Surg 69:482, 1982.

67. Martini R: Expression and functional roles of neural cell surface molecules and extracellular matrix components during development and regeneration of peripheral nerves. J Neurocytol 23:1–28, 1994.

68. Match KM: Radiation-induced brachial plexus paralysis. Arch Surg 110:384–391, 1975.

69. Matson DD: Early neurolysis in the treatment of injury of the peripheral nerves due to faulty injection of antibiotics. N Engl J Med 242:973–975, 1950.

70. Merren MD: Gabapentin for treatment of pain and tremor: a large case series. South Med J 91:739–744, 1998.

71. Midha R: Epidemiology of brachial plexus injuries in a multitrauma population. Neurosurgery 40:1182–1189, 1997.

72. Midha R, Guha A, and Gentili F, et al: Peripheral nerve injection injury. In: Omer GE, Spinner M, and Van Beek AL, Eds: Management of Peripheral Nerve Problems, 2nd edn. Philadelphia, WB Saunders, 1999:406–413.

73. Midha R and Kline DG: Evaluation of the neuroma in continuity. In: Omer GE, Spinner M, and Van Beek AL, Eds: Management of Peripheral Nerve Problems, 2nd edn. Philadelphia, WB Saunders, 1998:319–327.

74. Morris JH, Hudson AR, and Weddel G: A study of degeneration and regeneration in the divided rat sciatic nerve based on electron microscopy. II. The development of the regenerating unit. Z Zellforsch Mikrosk Anat 124:103–130, 1972.

75. Mumentholer M: Brachial plexus neuropathies. In: Dyck PJ, Thomas PK, and Lambert EH, et al., Eds: Peripheral Neuropathy. Philadelphia, WB Saunders, 1984:1383–1394.

76. Nath RK, Mackinnon SE, and Jensen JN, et al.: Spatial pattern of type 1 collagen expression in injured peripheral nerve. J Neurosurg 86:870, 1997.

77. Noble J, Munro CA, and Prasad VSSV, et al.: Analysis of upper and lower extremity peripheral nerve injuries in a population of patients with multiple injuries. J Trauma 45:116–122, 1998.

78. Ochoa J and Marotte LR: The nature of the nerve lesion caused by chronic entrapment in the guinea-pig. J Neurol Sci 19:491–495, 1973.

79. Ochs G: Painful dysesthesias following peripheral nerve injury. A clinical and electrophysiological study. Brain Res 496:228–240, 1989.

80. Omer GE: Results of untreated peripheral nerve injuries. Clin Orthopaed Rel Res 163:15–19, 1982.

81. Omer GE: Nerve injuries associated with gunshot wounds of the extremities. In: Gelberman RH, Ed: Operative Nerve Repair and Reconstruction. Philadelphia, JB Lippincott, 1991:655–670.

82. Parks BJ: Postoperative peripheral neuropathies. Surgery 74:348–357, 1973.

83. Pizzolato P and Mannheimei W: Histopathologic Effects of Local Anesthetic Drugs and Related Substances. Springfield, Charles C Thomas, 1961.

84. Puckett WO, Grundfest H, and McElroy W, et al.: Damage to peripheral nerves due to high velocity missiles without direct hit. Neurosurg 3:294–299, 1946.

85. Rudge P, Ochoa J, and Gilliatt RW: Acute peripheral nerve compression in the baboon. J Neurol Sci 23:403–420, 1974.

86. Samii M: Dorsal root entry zone coagulation for control of intractable pain due to brachial plexus injury. In: Samii M, Ed: Peripheral Nerve Lesions. Berlin: Springer-Verlag, 1990.

87. Seddon H: Peripheral nerve injuries. London, Her Majesty's Stationary Office. Medical research council special report series, 1954.

88. Seddon HJ: Three types of nerve injury. Brain 66:238–288, 1943.

89. Seddon HJ: Nerve lesions complicating certain closed bone injuries. JAMA 135:691–694, 1947.

90. Seddon HJ: Surgical Disorders of the Peripheral Nerves. Baltimore, Williams & Wilkins, 1972.

91. Seletz E: Surgery of Peripheral Nerves. Springfield: Charles C Thomas, 1951:119–137.

92. Sever J: Obstetric paralysis: Report of eleven hundred cases. JAMA 85:1862–1870, 1925.

93. Sever JW: Obstetric paralysis: Its etiology, pathology, clinical aspects and treatment. Am J Dis Child 12:541, 1916.

94. Siegel DB and Gelberman RH: Peripheral nerve injuries associated with fractures and dislocations. In: Gelberman RH, Ed: Operative Nerve Repair and Reconstruction. Philadelphia, JB Lippincott, 1991:619–633.

95. Siironen J, Sandberg M, and Vuorinen V, et al: Expression of type I and III collagens and fibronectin after transection of rat sciatic nerve. Lab Invest 67:80–87, 1992.

96. Smith JW: Factors influencing nerve repair. II. Collateral circulation of peripheral nerves. Arch Surg 93:433–437, 1966.

97. Speed JS and Knight RA: Peripheral nerve injuries. In: Campbell's Operative Orthopaedics, vol 1. St Louis: CV Mosby, 1956:947–1014.

98. Spinner M: Injuries to the major branches of peripheral nerves of the Forearm. 2nd edn. Philadelphia, WB Saunders, 1978.

99. Spurling RG and Woodhall B: Medical Department, United States Army, Surgery in World War II: Neurosurgery, vol 2. Washington DC, US Government Printing Office, 1959.

100. Sunderland S: A classification of peripheral nerve injuries producing loss of function. Brain 74:491–516, 1951.

101. Sunderland S: Nerve and Nerve Injuries, 1st edn. Baltimore: Williams & Wilkins, 1968.

102. Sunderland S: Nerve and Nerve Injuries, 2nd edn. Edinburgh, Churchill-Livingstone, 1978.

103. Sunderland S: Nerve Injuries and their Repair. A Critical Appraisal. Melbourne, Churchill Livingstone, 1991.

104. Tarlov IM: How long should an extremity be immobilized after nerve suture? Ann Surg 126:336–376, 1947.

105. Terzis JK, Dykes RW, and Hakstian RW: Electrophysiological recordings in peripheral nerve surgery: a review. J Hand Surg [Am] 1:52–66, 1976.

106. Thomas JE and Colby MY Jr.: Radiation-induced or metastatic brachial plexopathy? A diagnostic dilemma. JAMA 222:1392–1395, 1972.

107. Tiel RL, Happel LT, and Kline DG: Nerve action potential recording method and equipment. Neurosurgery 39:103–109, 1996.

108. Tsairis P, Dyck PJ, and Muldner DW: Natural history of brachial plexus neuropathy. Arch Neurol 27:297–306, 1972.

109. Tsuge K: Treatment of established Volkmann's contracture. J Bone Joint Surg [Am] 57:925–929, 1975.

110. Upton AR and McComas AJ: The double crush in nerve-entrapment syndromes. Lancet 2:359–361, 1973.

111. Villarejo FJ and Pascual AM: Injection injury of the sciatic nerve (370 cases). Child's Nerv Syst 9:229–232, 1993.

112. Waller A: Experiments on the section of the glossopharyngeal and hypoglossal nerves of the frog, and observations of the alterations produced thereby in the structure of their primitive fibres. Phil Trans Roy Soc (Lond) 140:423–429, 1850.

113. Weisi H and Osborne GV: The pathological changes in rat nerves subject to moderate compression. J Bone Joint Surg 468:297–306, 1964.

114. Whitcomb BB: Techniques of peripheral nerve repair. In: Spurling RG, Ed: Medical Department, United States Army, Surgery in World War II: Neurosurgery, vol 2, part 2: Peripheral Nerve Injuries. Washington DC, US Government Printing Office, 1959.

115. White JC: The result of traction injuries to the common peroneal nerve. J Bone Joint Surg 408:346–351, 1968.

116. Williams IR, Jefferson D, and Gilliatt RW: Acute nerve compression during limb ischaemia – an experimental study. J Neurol Sci 46:199–207, 1980.

117. Woodhall B, Nulsen F, and White J, et al.: Neurosurgical Implications, Peripheral Nerve Regeneration. Washington, DC. Veterans Administration Monograph, 1957:569–638.

118. Zachary RB and Roaf R: Lesions in continuity. In: Seddon H, Ed: Peripheral Nerve Injuries. London, Her Majesty's Stationary Office, 1954.

3

Clinical and electrical evaluation

David G. Kline

OVERVIEW

- There are no substitutes for an accurate, detailed history and a thorough physical examination.
- Ability to accurately test muscle as well as sensory function is paramount.
- Development of a routine for testing upper and lower limb function is helpful.
- Even the limb which is in a cast can be tested as can the limb of an unconscious or uncooperative patient.
- The Tinel's sign is more valuable when absent than present.
- Injury to nerve results in retrograde as well as injury site and distal stump and distal innervational site changes so time required for recovery must take into account all of these delays.
- Electromyogram (EMG) testing involves muscle sampling for electrical activity, not just conductive studies.
- The three phases of EMG muscle testing, needle insertion, activity in muscle at rest, and the muscle action potential seen with contraction, need to be understood.
- Presence of nascent units suggests but does not guarantee subsequent useful muscle function.
- Denervational changes can persist despite useful muscle contraction.
- The EMG is a sampling method.
- Myelogram followed by computed tomography (CT) scan cuts remain valuable for plexus stretch-avulsive injuries.
- Magnetic resonance imaging (MRI) is most valuable for tumors involving plexus or nerve although future development of MRI will undoubtedly make it more valuable for nerve injuries and entrapments.
- Plain X-rays are still valuable when fractures are complicated by nerve injury.
- Angiography is especially important for pseudoaneurysms, A-V fistula, prior history of vascular trauma, and some tumors.

HISTORY

A monograph or even whole book could in itself be written on this topic and will not for purposes of this text be done. However, a few points require emphasis. Any good clinical examination begins with the history. From this, the time of the injury or onset of the condition and its potential mechanism(s) can usually be gleaned. Detail becomes important. Besides the patient's memory of events, review of available records of the patient's plight can be important as can review of the outcomes of electrical and radiologic studies done. Especially important is review of prior operative notes if those procedures involved the nerve and/or lesion in question. The latter review should, however, never substitute for re-taking the history orally from the patient or if need be loved ones or other caregivers. It is important to find out whether the patient feels his or her function has changed since the injury or onset of the difficultly and, if so, in what way. Along with the past medical history and a review of systems a history of drug use as well as social habits is important. For new patients Dr. Tiel and I ask them or family to fill out a history form which we can go over with them after the oral history is taken and the physical examination done.

CLINICAL AND ELECTRICAL EVALUATION

Important clinical questions associated with nerve lesions revolve around nerve involved, level of the injury, and severity of the injury.[36] It is especially important to determine how complete the loss is distal to the level of the injury since incomplete loss may improve with time while complete loss often does not.[32,83] To do this well requires intimate knowledge of the anatomical distribution of the nerve in question.[26] In addition, one needs to know how to test the muscles and sensory distribution(s) usually innervated by the nerve.[1,46,53] It is also important to know the trick or substitutive motions used by patients to provide movement despite paralysis, as well as the areas of skin where nerves have sensory as well as autonomic overlap.[17,22] Experience in examining the limb with paralysis is paramount.[22,39,70] Knowledge of innervational anatomy and variation in patterns is useless unless complemented by the ability to examine the limb in a comprehensive fashion.[31,63] Practice in examination is the key since, with time and patience on the part of the examiner, documentation of the severity of the loss becomes easier. Such clinical evaluation is especially useful if one learns to grade the severity of the injury not only for the important individual motor and sensory sites, but for the nerve as a whole. Others have attempted to standardize some of the nomenclature concerned with nerve, but unfortunately, there is not as yet a clearly acceptable set of criteria for grading clinical function.[17,54,64,70] As a result, the next chapter will be devoted to methods of grading and changes we have found useful in these methods.

EVALUATION IN THE EMERGENCY SETTING

There are few surgeons of experience who have not discovered paralysis denoting peripheral nerve injury some time after suturing a lacerated wound or treating a fracture of an extremity by open or closed methods. This oversight applies even more to inexperienced individuals such as senor medical students or interns working in busy emergency rooms. The question then arises as to whether the paralysis was present at the time of admission or whether it arose from what the patient or someone else thought was poor treatment. It should be an ironclad rule that an examination for a peripheral nerve injury be made and recorded for every patient suffering from a severe closed injury, fracture/dislocation, or lacerating wound of an extremity, whether the patient is conscious or unconscious. Most of the necessary acute observations and tests for distal motor function are quite simple. In addition, absence of a median or ulnar nerve injury can even be established in an unconscious patient merely by the direct observation of presence of sweating on the forefinger or little finger, or wrinkling of the skin of these digits after immersion in water.

Before one can exclude a lesion of a peripheral nerve, one must be certain that the most distal portion of that nerve is functioning.[26,32] Strong extension of the wrist does not preclude an injury to the posterior interosseous branch of the radial. This nerve innervates finger and thumb extensors after some but not all extensors to the wrist have received branches. Furthermore, flexing of the fingers does not preclude a distal median nerve paralysis. A lesion of the median nerve at the wrist can still give an opponens pollicis and abductor pollicis brevis paralysis, and, more importantly, anesthesia of the palmar surface of the thumb and first two or three fingers. A test worth remembering, then, must be one that establishes clearly the presence or absence of the most distal function of the nerve being tested. For the upper limb, one method of grossly reviewing innervation consists of asking the patient to make a five-fingered cone with the tips of the fingers and then extending the thumb (Fig. 3-1).[53,64] The intact ulnar nerve bunches the fingers into a cone by the action of the intrinsic hand muscles, the opponens pollicis muscle innervated by the median nerve opposes the palmar surface of the thumb to the pads of the terminal phalanges, and the radial nerve extends the thumb. The test is a good one, but the disadvantage is that a patient with an acute injury of an extremity may not move the fingers because of pain or fear of causing pain by movement. The test, moreover, is difficult to carry out with the arm in a cast extending to the metacarpophalangeal junctions. Nevertheless, if the test can be well executed, one can be quite certain that there is not a severe lesion of the median, ulnar, or radial nerves. If the great toe can be extended, the peroneal portion of the sciatic nerve is not divided; if the great toe can be actively flexed, the same may be said for the tibial portion of this nerve; and if the great toe can be extended and flexed, there cannot be a complete lesion of the sciatic nerve.

Kenneth Livingston has reported a simple method for the testing of the most commonly injured nerves of the upper extremity.[69,86] In testing the median nerve, perception of pinprick over the palmar surface of the distal phalanx of the index finger is observed. If there is good sensation there, complete interruption of the median nerve

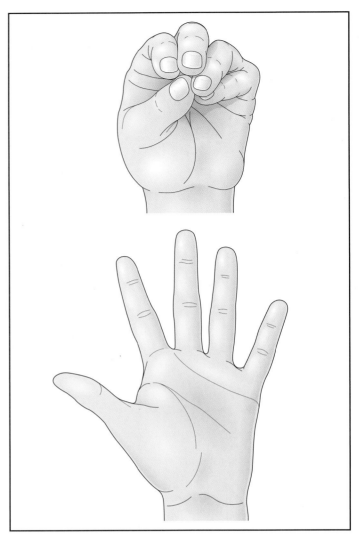

FIGURE 3-1 A rapid and relatively simple test of the distal function of median, ulnar, and radial nerves. Fingers and thumb are brought together by opponens pollicis (median) and opponens digiti quinti minimi (ulnar) as well as finger flexors (median and ulnar). Fingers are then opened up and extended by radial-innervated extensor muscles. This is called the cone test.

is excluded. For the ulnar nerve, the palmar surface of the distal phalanx of the little finger is tested for sensation. In testing the radial nerve, the ability to extend the distal phalange of the thumb with force rules out a serious lesion of that nerve. Sensory tests of the radial nerve are, as a rule, not sufficiently diagnostic. There can be objections to the use of sensory examinations in testing median and ulnar nerve function since they do not exclude hysterical or malingered anesthesia. In children, because of fear and lack of cooperation, both sensory and motor examinations may be impossible to carry out. The answers then as to function in that setting lie with careful and often repetitive observation of the limb as the child uses it to play and/or feed.

AUTONOMIC FUNCTION

Although careful sensory and motor evaluation is the key to the diagnosis of nerve lesions, a surprising amount of information can be gained from assessing autonomic function. Sweating results

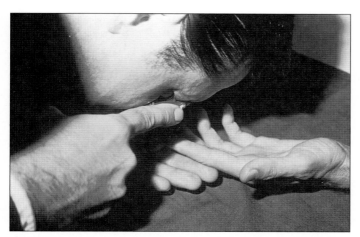

FIGURE 3-2 The cholinergic unmyelinated fibers that innervate sweat glands run in a peripheral nerve. Therefore, sweating is abolished in the peripheral nerve distribution of a transected nerve. This results in a very characteristic dryness and change in resistance when the fingers of the examiner slide over the affected area. Return of sweating to a previously denervated area is an early sign of nerve regeneration. The ophthalmoscope is a source of both illumination and magnification, and beads of sweat can be seen glistening on the dermal ridges. Unfortunately, return of sweating, like a positive Tinel sign, does not guarantee a successful result.

from stimulation of the sympathetic components of a peripheral nerve. The sympathetic fibers run in the peripheral nerve and not, to any significant extent, along vessels. The area of skin to which these sympathetic components are distributed thus corresponds to the sensory distribution of a peripheral nerve. After division of a nerve, the region where sweating is lost will therefore correspond with the area of anesthesia. Loss of sweating can be demonstrated by complicated methods such as Minor's starch-iodine method or quinizarine, or by the use of paper impregnated with an iron solution that changes color when moisture comes in contact with it.[3] These methods are not always available, but sweating or its absence can be observed directly with the ±20 lens of the ophthalmoscope or some other source of light.[30] This illuminates the highly refractile droplets of sweat under magnification as they appear on the papillary ridges of the finger.

The ophthalmoscope lens gives a magnification of only approximately 5 times, but this is sufficient to demonstrate the individual droplets as they appear at the mouths of the sweat ducts on the papillary ridges. This observation is most easily made in somewhat subdued surrounding light (Fig. 3-2). The droplets appear as highly refractile, rounded points of light. One may at first mistake sebaceous material for sweat. There are no sebaceous glands on the palmar surfaces of the hands, but sebaceous material commonly appears there from contact with the face or backs of the hands. The sebum is seen through the ophthalmoscope as a fine, scale-like, silver substance. With a little practice or by removing the sebum with ether, it can be readily differentiated from sweat. The secretion of the sebaceous glands is the end product of cellular disruption, and in contradistinction to the secretion of sweat glands, is not under control of the sympathetic nervous system.

Palpation of a denervated area may reveal a characteristic dry sensation, and there is limited resistance to the examiner's fingers gliding over the skin. If sweating can be demonstrated in the autonomous zones of the median and ulnar nerves, there cannot be

a complete lesion of either of these nerves, and surgical exploration in the near future, at least, is contraindicated.

When sweating occurs in normal individuals, it is, in general, symmetrical in intensity. The absence of sweating is only of significance, therefore, if it is unilateral. If sweat particles are seen in the autonomous zone of the ulnar nerve, complete division of that nerve cannot be present. The absence of sweat here, however, is only of importance if there is visible sweating in the corresponding area of the other hand. In another sense, the presence of sweating in the distribution of the nerve being tested is of more real value when evident than when absent.

Return of sweating may antedate sensory or motor return by weeks to months, but a return of sweating does not necessarily mean that sensory or motor function will follow. The regeneration of a few unmyelinated autonomic fibers does not, unfortunately, guarantee regeneration of the larger motor or sensory fibers. A test that is probably related to the presence or absence of autonomic function is the O'Rian wrinkle test.[62] Normally innervated fingers, immersed in tepid water, will wrinkle after 5–10 minutes. With denervation, the fingers will no longer wrinkle, while with reinnervation wrinkles will once again be seen.

Autonomic dysfunction resulting in discoloration of the skin and changes in skin temperature, in addition to changes in sweating pattern, is usually associated with pain such as true causalgia or reflex sympathetic dystrophy, and is discussed in succeeding chapters.

SENSORY FUNCTION

Sensory testing is important, but can be difficult and at times misleading. One must be certain that observations are made in autonomous zones where the likelihood of overlapping innervation from adjacent uninjured nerves is minimal. The autonomous zone for the median nerve (Fig. 3-3) includes the distal and volar surface of the forefinger and volar surface of the distal thumb. Autonomous sensory zones for the ulnar nerve (Fig. 3-3) include the volar and dorsal surfaces of the distal digit of the little finger. The radial nerve does not have a reliable autonomous zone, but if there is any sensory loss at all, it will usually be found over the region of the anatomical snuffbox.[61] Autonomous zones for the tibial nerve include the heel and a portion of the sole of the foot (Fig. 3-4), while a less autonomous zone for the peroneal nerve exists over the dorsum of the foot, especially just proximal to the big toe and the second toe.

Sensory return in nonautonomous areas usually precedes motor return. Sensory return in an autonomous area is usually a later development that follows the earliest motor return. In the case of median nerve injury, sensory recovery can be the primary concern from the standpoint of practical function (Fig. 3-5). The arrival of new sensory axons in the hand proximal to the autonomous zone at the fingertips can be recognized by sensory displacement.[46] With initial testing, the patient localizes the stimulus to another point within the median sensory area that is removed from the actual stimulus site. This does not occur due to overlapping innervation by neighboring nerves or with recovery from neurapraxia. Sensory displacement indicates that a regenerating axon has strayed into a sensory receptor that is remote from the one that the brain is accustomed to having it supply.

Two-point discrimination in the normal adult finger pad should span 3–5 mm. This can be tested simply with a bent paper clip or a pair of calipers. Values for return of good two-point discrimina-

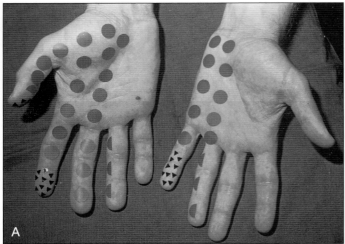

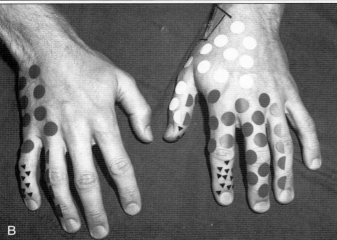

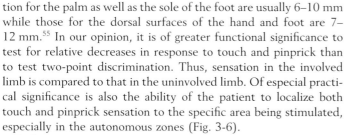

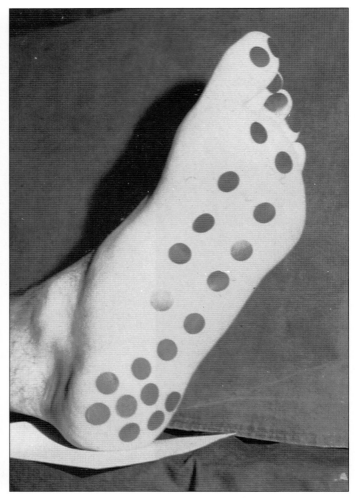

FIGURE 3-3 **(A)** Usual sensory zones of the hand for median (hand to the left in the photograph) and ulnar (hand to the right in the photograph) nerves. Small triangles indicate autonomous zones where loss can be due only to median or ulnar nerve loss. Conversely, recovery in an autonomous zone means that nerve has regenerated and reversal is not caused by overlap from an adjacent nerve.
(B) White circles on the dorsum of the hand to the right indicate the usual sensory territory of the radial nerve. Boxed area on the wrist indicates the "anatomical snuffbox," the area in which radial sensory loss, if present, will be found. Dark circles on the hand to the right in the photograph outline the usual median distribution; those on the hand to the left indicate their usual ulnar distribution. Small triangles indicate the dorsal surface autonomous zones for median and ulnar nerves, respectively.

FIGURE 3-4 The sensory examination of the sole of the foot must be performed with care because the peripheral nerve supply is complex. The calcaneal branches of the posterior tibial nerve are given off before the tarsal tunnel in many cases, so the heel may escape sensory disturbance in true tarsal tunnel syndrome in which compression is closer to the sole of the foot. The sensory distributions of the medial and lateral plantar nerves in the foot are roughly analogous to those of the median and ulnar nerves in the hand. However, the sural nerve clearly supplies the outer border of the foot. The femoral nerve contributes the saphenous branch, which usually supplies a strip of sensation to skin as far as the medial malleolus and instep. The circles on the heel of the foot indicate the usual autonomous zone for the tibial nerve.

tion for the palm as well as the sole of the foot are usually 6–10 mm while those for the dorsal surfaces of the hand and foot are 7–12 mm.[55] In our opinion, it is of greater functional significance to test for relative decreases in response to touch and pinprick than to test two-point discrimination. Thus, sensation in the involved limb is compared to that in the uninvolved limb. Of especial practical significance is also the ability of the patient to localize both touch and pinprick sensation to the specific area being stimulated, especially in the autonomous zones (Fig. 3-6).

Definite sensory recovery in autonomous zones, even with sensory displacement, can provide early evidence of regeneration in distal lesions of major sensory nerves such as the median and tibial nerves. On the other hand, sensory recovery usually occurs relatively late and can be very misleading as an indicator of eventual

useful motor recovery, particularly in the case of radial and peroneal nerves (Fig. 3-7).

For the majority of serious nerve lesions, and especially those proximal to the wrist or knee levels, sensation can be tested for relative perception and localization by having the patient close his eyes, stroking his fingers or foot areas bilaterally, and asking the patient to compare responses. Response to pinprick can be tested in the same comparative fashion. At the same time, the patient's ability to localize both touch and pinprick can be tested. Sensory responses can be graded for each nerve tested (see Chapter 4).

The area of sensory supply of a peripheral nerve should not be confused with the area of sensory supply of a segmental spinal nerve (dermatomal pattern). On occasion, the maps of the dermatomal and peripheral nerve distribution will overlap (Fig. 3-8).

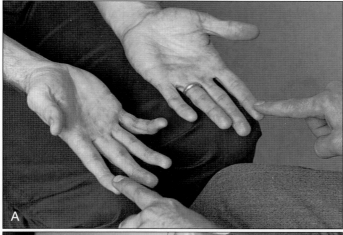

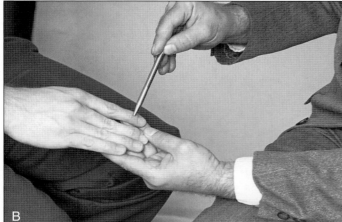

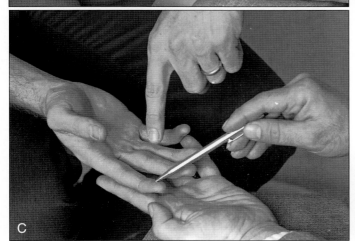

FIGURE 3-5 **(A)** In testing touch in median autonomous zones, the examiner modulates touch bilaterally on the volar surfaces of the forefingers, using his own forefingers as the stimuli. **(B)** Autonomous zone on dorsum of forefinger is tested for localization by touching it with a pen while the patient's eyes are closed. **(C)** Testing for localization on the volar surface of the forefinger. With eyes closed, the patient is able to point out accurately the area being stimulated.

FIGURE 3-7 Patient's radial sensory area in the region of the anatomic snuffbox is tested for localization by using the tip of the pen. There may not, however, be sensory loss even in this area despite a complete radial injury.

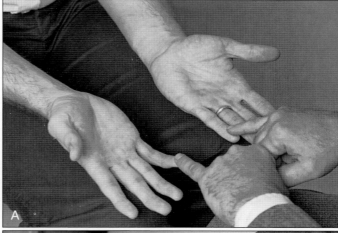

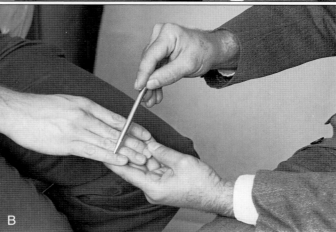

FIGURE 3-6 **(A)** In this photograph, the patient's response to touch is being compared by modulating touch, using the examiner's own little fingers on the patient's little fingers. **(B)** Here, ability to localize the pressure from the examiner's pen in an autonomous zone of the ulnar nerve is being assessed.

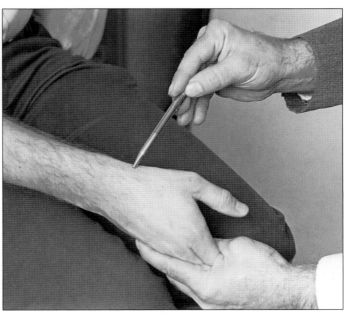

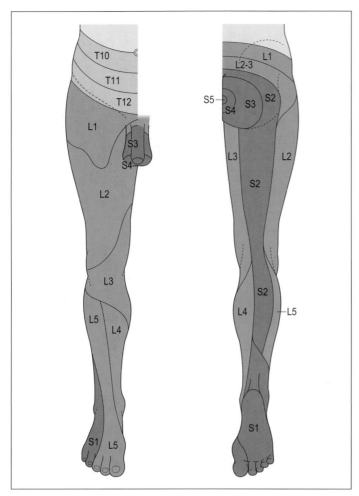

FIGURE 3-8 A dermatome is the area of skin supplied by a single spinal nerve. Patterns vary from patient to patient, but usually the inner aspect of the leg is supplied by L4, the outer leg by L5, and the lateral aspect of the foot by S1. The map of peripheral nerve distribution differs from that for nerve roots or spinal nerves. It is imperative that the differential diagnosis between spinal and peripheral conditions be made with care. Loss in the dermatome for L5 may mimic a peroneal nerve sensory loss; both L5 radicular pathology and peroneal nerve palsy can give rise to a foot drop. Likewise, radicular pathology involving the L2 root could be confused with meralgia paresthetica. The lower dorsal or thoracic dermatomes and those of the sacral roots are close posteriorly and yet separate anteriorly. These dermatomes are usually tested to assess the level of a spinal cord injury. (By comparison, sensory testing in the groin and area of the genitalia is used to assess ilioinguinal and genitofemoral nerve pathology.) A perianal target-like area of sensory loss is a reliable indicator of sacral root pathology. For completeness' sake, the surgeon should review the peripheral pathways subtending both perianal and perivaginal sensation, as well as the peripheral supply of the rectal sphincters. The clinician must be a master of both the lower and upper limbs. In most cases, the history can guide the examiner as to which of these two maps to consult in a given patient. Both authors have several examples of patients who underwent spinal surgery (often on the basis of a slightly abnormal scanning study or myelogram) even though the pathology was at a peripheral nerve level.

The information required for accurate clinical diagnosis can be determined by using simple stimuli applied with cotton wool, a pin and paperclip, or the examiner's touch. The examiner should not be deterred by absence of very specialized methods of sensory study as those techniques add little to the examination conducted by an experienced as well as thorough clinician. Special techniques, e.g. the use of laser beams, are used by those studying pain or the physiology of sensation, but are not necessary for practical diagnostic accuracy at the bedside.

The spinal nerve is derived from a single spinal segment and supplies a specific skin area of the embryo. The limb bud grows and drags the dermatomes to the periphery, leaving a gap in the body sequence, with a sudden jump from cervical 4 to the thoracic 2 levels. The peripheral nerve surgeon should be aware of the map for peripheral nerve distribution and areas of confusion which may arise when one attempts to differentiate a radicular from a peripheral nerve lesion. On sensory examination of the shoulder, it may be difficult to distinguish a C5 from an axillary nerve injury. The C6 dermatome may be confused with the median nerve sensory distribution so that a C5–6 disc may be removed instead of releasing the carpal tunnel. Sensory loss in the C8–T1 distribution may be confused with ulnar nerve pathology, and the surgeon must appreciate the peripheral sensory distribution of ulnar nerve, medial antebrachial cutaneous, and medial cutaneous nerves of the arm, so as to avoid confusion between radicular and peripheral nerve pathology.

MOTOR FUNCTION

There is no substitute for a thorough motor examination where major nerve injury is suspected. To do this well requires patience and perseverance as well as some experience. Each major peripheral nerve innervates a cascade of muscles. Once the physician learns these patterns and gains experience in testing them, his or her abilities to localize spinal cord and spine-related nerve root problems, as well as neuropathies, will be increased greatly. A good beginning is provided by the "MRC Handbook on Peripheral Nerve Examination," as well as a number of other texts.[1,53,64,69] Study of these and similar texts will also give the examiner an idea of the more common anomalies in innervation.[14,45,50]

Black and white photographs of various tests for muscle function are interspersed, not only in this chapter (Figs 3-9 to 3-18), but also in other chapters dealing with individual nerves and in the appendix as well.

A common error in clinical examination is to assume injury at a specific level and neglect examination of muscles innervated above this level (Fig. 3-11).[39,52] Another frequent error is failure to examine muscles innervated by other nerves in the limb. Muscles in the distribution of noninjured nerve(s) can sometimes substitute for loss and make the injury appear partial or even nonexistent. For example, the examiner can mistake abduction of the fingers, a function supplied by the ulnar nerve, for radial-innervated finger extension (Fig. 3-12A). The reverse can be true for ulnar palsy where extension of the fingers by radial-innervated extensor communis may provide some abduction (Fig. 3-12B). The classic example of substitutive movement is illustrated by a wrist-level median palsy where opponens pollicis is paralyzed. Extensor pollicis, which is radial-innervated, pulls the thumb away from the palm, ulnar-innervated adductor pollicis displaces the thumb toward and across the palm, and flexor pollicis longus, which is innervated above the wrist by

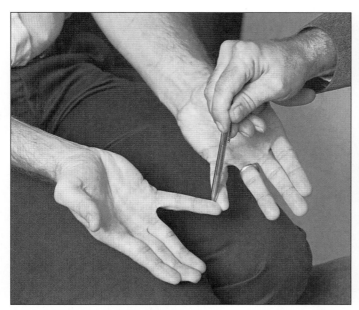

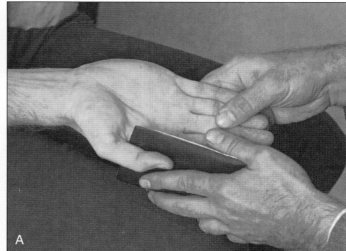

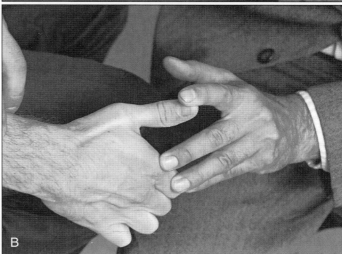

FIGURE 3-9 The abductor of the small finger is supplied by short twigs derived from the ulnar nerve in Guyon's canal, whereas the flexor of the terminal phalanx of the small finger is supplied by the ulnar nerve in the proximal forearm. Thus, abductor digiti minimi and flexor profundus to the ring finger are useful muscles to test to determine the level of injury to the ulnar nerve. The examiner is asking the subject to resist the passage of the pencil between the little fingers. The slightly atrophied hypothenar eminence of the patient's right hand gave way, demonstrating impairment of ulnar input on that side.

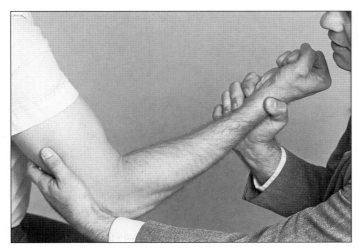

FIGURE 3-11 Triceps is primarily supplied by C7 through the middle trunk, the latter's posterior division, and the posterior cord to radial nerve. The initial branches to the three heads of this muscle arise in the axilla, and injuries to the radial nerve at a lateral humeral level, such as Saturday night palsy, are not accompanied by paralysis of triceps. Testing of this proximal muscle is therefore critical in determining the level of radial nerve injury. The examiner is resisting the patient's attempt to extend the elbow while inspecting and palpating the triceps. Loss of triceps function is not nearly as important to the patient as loss of elbow flexion because gravity extends the previously flexed elbow.

FIGURE 3-10 **(A)** The adductor of the thumb is supplied by the terminal branch of the ulnar nerve. Having passed around the hook of the hamate, the ulnar nerve crosses the hand to supply the intrinsic muscles and terminates in the adductor pollicis. This muscle is useful to test in assessing the ulnar nerve function, because its power is reduced by a lesion at any level along the course of the nerve. The patient is asked to maintain the card as the examiner attempts to pull the card away. The subject is instructed to keep the thumb straight. Because the ulnar-supplied adductor is weak, the card starts slipping out, so the patient responds by using his median-supplied flexor pollicis longus to supplement his effort (the Froment sign). **(B)** The extensor surfaces of the three bones of the thumb each have a tendon attached. All three of the muscles for these tendons are supplied by the posterior interosseous nerve (PIN) in the proximal forearm. The median-nerve-innervated muscles flex and oppose the thumb, but the function of the three PIN-supplied muscles is to retrieve the thumb from the flexed position, allowing subsequent grasping motions. In this photograph, the patient is attempting to extend the thumb against resistance, and the long (EPL) tendon is compared with thumb extension in the contralateral limb.

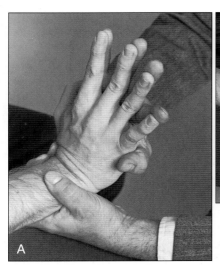

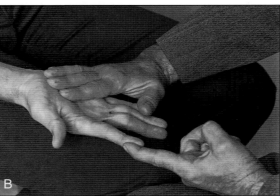

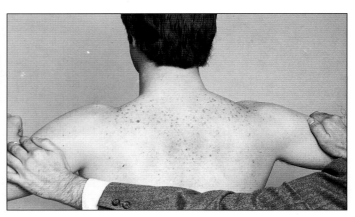

FIGURE 3-12 Testing interossei.
(A) The examiner places his fingers against the patient's, extending his wrist. He asks the patient to spread or abduct the fingers and then bring them back together or adduct them. In this fashion, the examiner takes away any ability for the patient to use the radial-innervated extensors to simulate a true abduction motion of the fingers.
(B) The first dorsal interosseous is being tested by asking the patient to abduct the forefinger against the examiner's forefinger, which is placed above the plane of the palm so that interosseous and not extensor communis to forefinger is tested.

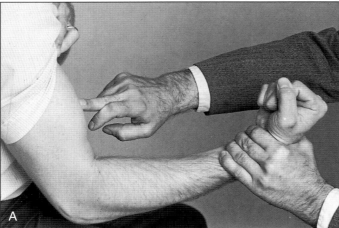

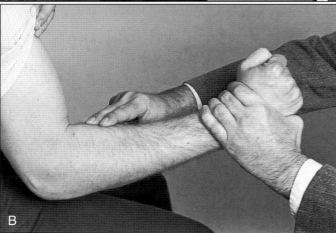

FIGURE 3-14 This patient is resisting the examiner's attempt to adduct or push the shoulders down and to the patient's side. The function of trapezius (cranial nerve XI) and deltoid (spinal nerve C5 through the upper trunk, the latter's posterior division, the posterior cord, and the axillary nerve) can be seen, palpated, and compared.

the median, pulls the tip of the thumb towards opposing fingers, completing the thumb's opposition-like motion.

The patient with a complete radial palsy can sometimes provide some dorsiflexion of the wrist by flexing the fingers and making a fist. Extensor tendons shortened by the palsy will then force the hand backward, even though they are not innervated.

Substitution can mislead the examiner. For example, despite complete biceps/brachialis palsy, the forearm can be readily flexed on the upper arm by the brachioradialis supplied by the radial nerve (Fig. 3-13). This further highlights the need for a thorough examination of all the major muscles in a limb where nerve injury is suspected.

In some patients with paralysis of the deltoid, a good deal of abduction can be gained by use of the supraspinatus to initiate abduction, and then use of the long head of the biceps to provide forward abduction (Figs 3-14 to 3-16). These substitutes for deltoid can be aided by scapular rotation as well as elevation of the shoulder by the levator scapuli and trapezius. This misleading set of circumstances can be obviated by the examiner passively elevating the patient's limb to the horizontal. He should then grasp the patient's deltoid with the other hand and ask the patient to sustain the abduction. Minor degrees of deltoid contraction can thus be readily

FIGURE 3-13 **(A)** Biceps is primarily supplied by the sixth cervical nerve through the upper trunk, the latter's anterior division, the lateral cord, and the musculocutaneous nerve. This muscle is both a powerful flexor of the elbow and supinator of the forearm.
(B) Brachioradialis is primarily supplied by C6 through the upper trunk, the latter's posterior division, the posterior cord, and the radial nerve. It is a modest flexor of the elbow but can hypertrophy in cases of biceps paralysis so as to flex the elbow more strongly. The examiner is testing elbow flexion against resistance in full supination (biceps) and with wrist partially pronated (brachioradialis). Biceps examination is key to the diagnosis of proximal upper element plexus injury or musculocutaneous nerve injury. Brachioradialis function is key to assessing progress after radial nerve injury.

appreciated. Gravity can also supplement or replace in part muscles providing function such as forearm extension, knee flexion, and plantar flexion. Testing of muscles serving these functions has to take this into account. Evaluation for completeness of injury, or conversely, return of function, can be difficult for injuries involving neural input to either the shoulder or to the fine muscles of the hand. In these areas especially, experience is the only effective teacher.

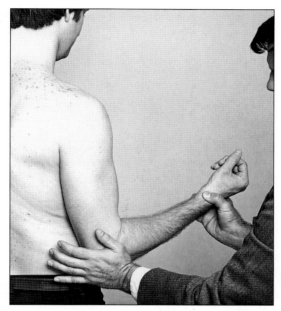

FIGURE 3-15 Internal and external rotation of the shoulder is checked against resistance. External rotation is accomplished by the infraspinatus supplied by the suprascapular nerve with input primarily from C5. Every effort should be made to regain external shoulder rotation during surgery on upper plexus elements, in addition to providing outflow for elbow flexion and shoulder abduction. Internal rotation is primarily accomplished by the pectoralis major, which has a very widespread innervation from the roots of the brachial plexus through the lateral and medial pectoral nerves (named for their cords of origin).

In some cases, anomalous innervation can also trick the examiner into believing he is dealing with either a partial or a complete lesion of the nerve. Some knowledge of the common anomalies helps avoid these misperceptions.[22,31,56,61,63,66]

With penetrating injuries, loss of function can be due to tendon transection, but usually when this is the case, the soft tissue injury will be much too distal to account for loss of function on a neural basis alone. Thus, the patient who has a wrist-level laceration, and inability to flex the distal phalanx of the thumb or forefinger, has such loss due to transection of the flexor pollicis longus or the flexor profundus and not due to median nerve laceration. Finally, "just as no man is an island unto himself," few serious injuries of an extremity involve only nerve without muscle, tendon, vascular or bone injuries. Thus, evidence of these as well as nerve injury should be sought (Fig. 3-17).[64,67]

SIMULATED MUSCLE WEAKNESS

As one attempts to grade muscle strength, lack of effort (LOE) on the part of the patient can usually be detected by an experienced examiner. LOE may result because motion is painful to the patient or because of lack of confidence to move the involved limb, or sometimes because of a need for secondary gain. One can be suspicious of LOE if the patient does not fully contract nearby muscles that are not at all related to the nerve injury in question. Thus, one can suspect LOE if the patient does not give full effort to wrist extension (radial nerve) or to flexion of the tip of the thumb (median nerve) when loss of hand intrinsics is suspected due to an elbow-level ulnar injury. A similar example for the lower extremity would be lack of full plantar flexion, foot inversion, and toe flexion in a patient with a fibular-level peroneal nerve lesion. One always has to be careful not to overlook a partial or mild palsy associated with a severe one, but then well-selected electrical tests will usually provide evidence of the former as well as document the latter.

Another sign of LOE is a tendency for the tested function to have a "staccato or give-and-take" contraction of the muscle concerned. An example of this behavioral aberration is sometimes seen when the flexor profundus of the forefinger is tested in a patient with a median palsy. The patient may provide only slight flexion,

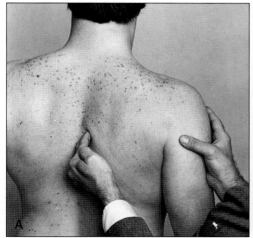 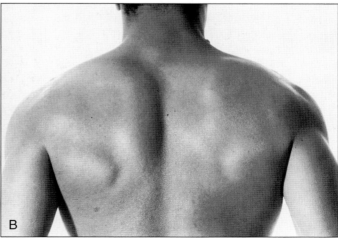

FIGURE 3-16 **(A)** Rhomboids on the patient's right side are palpated by the examiner's finger. The patient was asked to brace his shoulders backwards as if "at attention." **(B)** This patient's right rhomboid was paralyzed as a result of a stab wound. The nerve to rhomboids was cut as it departed the C5 spinal nerve. In brachial plexus stretch cases, paralysis of rhomboid or electrophysiologic evidence of denervation in that muscle indicates a very proximal C5 lesion.

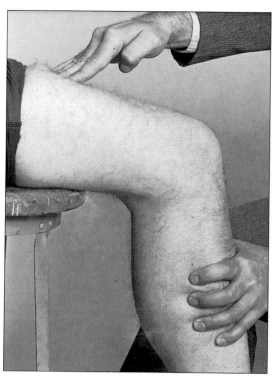

FIGURE 3-17 The usually massive quadriceps is supplied by the femoral nerve, which has both an extraperitoneal intra-abdominal course in the pelvis and a branching appearance in the right proximal thigh. The examiner is palpating the anterior thigh and also inspecting the lateral aspect of the thigh so as not be misled by any concomitant contraction of tensor fascia lata (supplied by superior gluteal nerve). The obturator nerve is tested by attempting to force the knees apart against an adducting motion of the thighs by the patient. This nerve has the same spinal nerve origin (L2, L3, L4) as the femoral. The presence of hip adduction in the absence of knee extension implies that the spinal nerves are intact and that the lesion is therefore in the femoral nerve itself. Femoral palsy due to injury may be accompanied by serious vascular and/or abdominal injury.

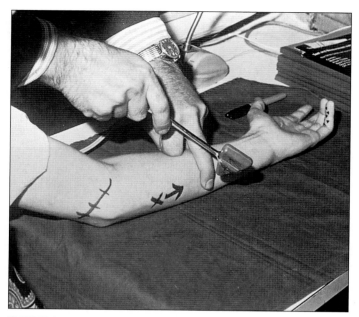

FIGURE 3-18 Attention to detail is important to both elicit and interpret a Tinel sign. The level of a left ulnar nerve injury is shown by the dotted line proximal to the elbow. Sharp percussion of the nerve at site "X" on a previous visit had elicited paresthesias, and the examiner is now attempting to elicit them at a more distal site on a subsequent visit. An advancing Tinel sign indicates that at least some fine fibers are growing down the nerve but does not guarantee a good clinical result. The absence of advance, however, indicates a poor chance of recovery. Note that the nerve is not percussed at the point of injury. Any focal nerve injury will respond with local paresthesias if directly percussed.

then extension, then a little more flexion, then once again, extension. This provides a back-and-forth or "give-and-take" type of motion rather than a sustained attempt at contraction that the examiner is asking for. This type of contraction could be due to severe paresis, but is more than likely due either to lack of concentration on the patient's part or LOE. Sometimes, with repeated exhortation on the part of the examiner, the patient will correct the aberration and provide a sustained and more complete contraction of the muscle in question.

A more obvious sign of LOE is "give-away-weakness" where the patient starts out with good contraction of a muscle, and then, in the midst of contracting that muscle, its strength seem to rather suddenly "give away" or fade. There is a muscle that can be tested without the patient's voluntary input and that is the latissimus dorsi. A patient claiming total paralysis of the arm and who has, in spite of that, excellent contraction of this muscle upon coughing has psychologic problems.

TINEL'S SIGN

Presence of a Tinel's sign provides some evidence favoring axonal regeneration. If paresthesias are obtained by distal nerve percussion, some continuity of sensory axons from the point percussed

through the lesion to the central nervous system is suggested. If the response moves distally with time, and particularly if progression down the extremity is associated with diminished paresthesias in response to tapping over the injury site, evidence for continued sensory fiber regeneration down the distal stump is present (Fig. 3-18). A positive Tinel's sign implies only fine-fiber regeneration, however, and tells the examiner nothing about the quantity or eventual quality of the new fibers. Over 50% of the World War Two soldiers who ultimately required resection and suture of nerve injuries had earlier shown an advancing Tinel's sign. Henderson studied a large group of patients with nerve injuries in a concentration camp where operation was not permitted.[23] He found the Tinel's sign to be useful as long as it advanced rapidly along the distal stump and was not confined to the injury alone. Even so, the majority of the patients who had a Tinel's advancing down the limb and distal to the lesion had not regained significant useful function on follow-up after the war.

On the other hand, if no Tinel's response is obtained, and sufficient time has elapsed for fine-fiber regeneration to occur (4–6 weeks), the absence of a Tinel's sign distal to a lesion is such strong evidence against regeneration as to constitute a significant negative finding.[40,69] In other words, a positive Tinel's sign is comparable to the finding of paresthesias on electrical stimulation of the distal nerve. Such a finding has no quantitative significance. On the other hand, an absent sensory response on tapping distal to the injury after an appropriate time lapse strongly suggests total neural interruption or extremely poor axonal regrowth to the level of the nerve being tapped.

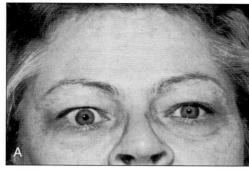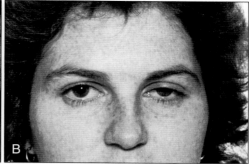

FIGURE 3-19 The examiner should automatically look for a Horner syndrome while taking the patient's history, particularly if there is any complaint of hand weakness. **(A)** This patient's small left pupil is obvious, but if there is any doubt, the lights should be dimmed – the normal contralateral pupil will then dilate, making the inequality of pupil size more obvious. This patient suffered from a breast carcinoma with invasion of C8 and T1 spinal nerves. **(B)** The difference in size of the palpebral fissure may be obvious initially, and this lady's ptosis accompanied an avulsion injury of C8 and T1 spinal nerves. The physical sign signals a proximal injury to the spinal nerve in this setting and is hence an unwelcome sign usually observed immediately when the patient enters the examining room. The ptosis rarely interferes with vision and frequently becomes much less severe with the passage of a few weeks. The relatively small pupil, however, remains.

OTHER FINDINGS ASSOCIATED WITH NERVE LESIONS

Because of autonomic fiber loss, skin in the distribution of the injured nerve and sometimes beyond it will feel dry and cool. Loss of sympathetic input to skin, sweat glands, and vasodilatory fibers to small skin arterioles presumably lead to these changes. With time, the skin can seem shiny in appearance and texture as it becomes less coarse or wrinkled. Of interest, if a digit with sensory and autonomic loss is immersed in water for several minutes, it will fail to wrinkle like a normally innervated finger or toe. More chronic deinnervation will make the skin appear shiny or glossy.

Proximal involvement of the C8 and/or T1 spinal nerves may also produce a Horner's syndrome which is due to loss of sympathetic fiber input to both the iris and the levator palpebrae superioris (Fig. 3-19).

Patients will frequently report a tendency for the denervated portion of an extremity to bruise easily. Skin and underlying soft tissues not only seem to bruise more readily than normal tissues, but also to heal more slowly. Thus, soft tissue hemorrhage seems to take longer to mobilize, and skin lacerations or scratches take longer to heal than usual. Of interest is the osteoporosis and actual shrinkage of bone architecture that can occur, especially to the fingers, with a long-standing palsy. Thus, denervated digits tend to narrow in diameter and taper down at their tips. This may be accompanied by what appears to be excessive and abnormal nail growth, the latter not only elongating more rapidly than normal, but also becoming thickened and at times ridged and/or discolored. Some patients, especially children or those with dementia as well as median or ulnar injury, will repetitively either suck or chew on their anesthetic fingers (Fig. 3-20). Occasionally, such individuals will even autocannibalize their fingers or hand. Skin and nail changes from such behavior should be obvious, but may be overlooked or not appreciated unless the nature of the responsible neuropathy is appreciated.

It is to be stressed that all or any of these changes can occur without the patient having either reflex sympathetic dystrophy (RSD) or causalgia.[18] Nonetheless, with these sympathetically related disorders, the onset of such findings may be accelerated as well as accentuated.[47,48,73] For example, the patient with RSD affecting the hand will frequently not trim his nails because this

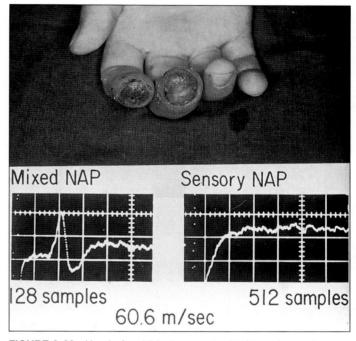

FIGURE 3-20 Hand of a child who sustained a laceration to the wrist and presented with a mutilated forefinger and long finger caused by sucking and chewing on them. The noninvasive, positive tracing to the left was recorded by stimulating median nerve at wrist and recording over the course of the median at the elbow. The flat trace to the right was obtained by stimulating over forefinger digital nerves and recording over median nerve just above the wrist.

activity is too painful for him. As a result, such a patient can present with long, often curved, "talon-like nails" such as an eagle or other bird of prey might have. Early in the course of the disorder, hyperhidrosis and vasoconstriction predominate.[18,48] The "sine qua non" for both of these disorders is a burning-like pain and a hand or foot that cannot be manipulated, even when the patient's attention is distracted from the examination.

The limb with disuse atrophy, or one immobilized too long by a cast or rigid splint, usually has severe distal changes affecting skin and other soft tissue as well as bone.[8,9] The easy tendency of the shiny, fragile skin and tapered fingers to bruise or slough can be reduced somewhat, but not eliminated by early vigorous and repetitive physical therapy.

Unusual sensory symptoms can occur with nerve lesions and/or their regrowth. These feelings are not always painful and may consist of tingling or a sharpened awareness of touch. For example, even itchiness of the palm, as well as fingers of the hand, can be associated with carpal tunnel syndrome.

TIME AND DISTANCE IN AXONAL REGENERATION

The time-honored rule of thumb for the rate of regeneration is 1 mm per day or 1 inch per month.[45,64] It is evident that the rate is faster at more proximal levels of the nerve and slower at more distal levels. However, it should be pointed out that this rule of thumb is applicable primarily to new fibers once they have reached the distal stump, and does not take into account the time necessary to traverse injury or repair sites, or the time necessary to mature and form meaningful distal connections. Thus, the overall rate of significant regrowth is much slower than is generally appreciated.[39,71] As a result, the regenerative process extends and continues over a greater period of time than is generally recognized or acknowledged.

There are several steps in the process (Fig. 3-21):

1. There is a variable extent of retrograde degenerative change after injury. The more blunt or stretching the force is, the lengthier this zone of injury is. New neurites must first overcome this defect, which may be a few millimeters or up to several centimeters proximal to the site of primary impact.
2. Axons must penetrate the original injury or repair site. Progress here is especially slow and requires much more time than studies in the rat or lower animals suggest.[39,40] This is especially so when grafts have to be interposed between stumps of a nerve to make up a gap. Here, axons traversing the graft repair site may require weeks of growth rather than days.
3. Once the new axons have reached the distal stump, they grow at 1 mm per day for the average nerve at mid-limb level. Rate of growth down the distal stump tends to be faster for lesions of proximal limb and much slower for those in distal limb. Rate may also be slow if substantial endoneurial proliferation has had time to occur before axons reach the distal stump.
4. Upon reaching distal target sites, further time, which can be several weeks or even a month, may be necessary before axonal-to-end-plate motor functions are reconstituted or significant sensory reinput occurs.
5. Fiber maturation with recovery of axonal volume and myelin thickness takes longer.

Thus, the regenerative process for a proximal plexus element or a long nerve such as the sciatic nerve may take 5–6 years for completion. Total time for maximal recovery for a median nerve injured at the wrist may be only 2–3 years, while the same nerve injured at the elbow level may not complete the process for 4 years or so.

Therefore, predictions of recovery based on measurements between the lesion or repair site and muscle(s) expected to be reinnervated, and application of the millimeter-per-day or inch-per-month rule must be tempered by the above additional factors.[38,40]

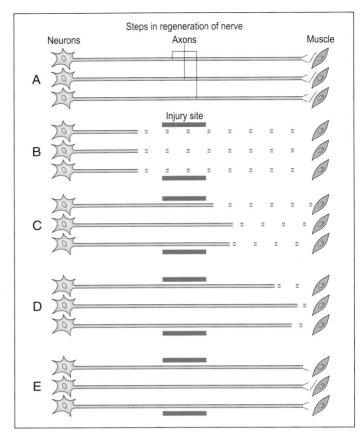

FIGURE 3-21 **(A)** The top drawing shows neurons, their axonal extensions, and their distal input, in this case to muscle. **(B)** After an injury that parts axons, there is a segment of retrograde degeneration and, over the ensuing weeks, Wallerian degeneration of the distal nerve. **(C)** Over a period of several weeks, axons of variable number and size traverse the injury site, reach the distal stump, and begin to descend in it. There is no spontaneous clinical function, nerve cannot be stimulated to produce distal function, and electromyography (EMG) shows a severe denervational pattern. Two to three months after injury, a nerve action potential (NAP) may be recordable by stimulating proximally and recording distally. Months may be required for axons to proceed on down the distal stump. **(D)** Axons begin to reach end inputs, but not enough time has passed or reconstruction occurred to permit spontaneous function. EMG may show some reversal of denervational change and signs of reinnervation such as nascent potentials. **(E)** More of the motor end plates have been reconstructed, and reinnervational changes by EMG are more pronounced. Time between D and E varies but may be weeks to a month or two.

It is also important to discuss when the time for useful recovery by spontaneous regeneration has passed post injury. Nerve repair may have little to offer beyond such a time.[22,25,27,38] If 24 or more months of total muscle denervation have elapsed, many muscles do not recover sufficient function even after regaining neural fiber input.[8,45] Atrophy can be so advanced and/or muscle actually replaced by fibrotic change and even fat, that the arrival of very healthy axons is like "sowing good seed on fallow ground."[44,71] This is less likely to be the case for relatively large, bulky muscles such as the biceps/brachialis or gastrocnemius-soleus than for those smaller muscles such as thenar and hypothenar intrinsics, or interossei and lumbricales. An exception referable to size appears to be the facial muscles, which may benefit from late reinnervation by facial nerve repair or by neurotization or nerve transfer procedures.

Other exceptions to the "24 month rule" may occur in a few lesions in continuity that have maintained or restored some distal continuity, even though it is not enough to produce useful distal function.[37,38,82] Sometimes, presence of distal fibers may keep enough of the distal stump and end-input architecture preserved or accessible so that very late repair after resection of the original lesion can, on occasion, produce function.

Implications of these observations referable to management are important.[25,60,78] This is because distance from injury site to the functional unit desired for reinnervation tempers the timing for surgical repair. Thus, the longer the distance, the earlier surgical intervention should be considered.[15] This is especially so with brachial plexus and proximal sciatic lesions. Relatively early timing for exploration and, if indicated, repair, also plays a role in upper arm median, ulnar, and some radial injuries.

In some cases, the distance between the injury site and the function desired is such that early or late repair, or even on occasion, spontaneous regeneration, will achieve little.[21,27] This is especially so for proximal ulnar lesions or their origins such as C8, T1, lower trunk, or medial cord. These proximal elements supply ulnar nerve and thus input to the very small and very distal intrinsic hand muscles. Unfortunately, lesions of the proximal peroneal division of the sciatic nerve have similar limitations in time. Peroneal-innervated muscles have a complex innervational as well as firing pattern for function. Input for these relatively lengthy muscles most likely occurs at multiple levels in a specific pattern. This complex input must be reinstituted to achieve recovery of useful dorsiflexion of the foot and/or toes. This is a difficult regenerative task even when circumstances are ideal.

Sensory and autonomic recovery is not subject to as severe limitations in time as is motor function.[64,71] This is an important consideration favoring median nerve repair at an axillary level even though it may contribute little to recovery of median-innervated hand function.[79] Repair of the tibial division of the sciatic nerve may be useful even at a buttock level despite the great distance and time involved for regrowth from such a proximal level. Some recovery of at least protective sensation on the sole of the foot usually results, even from graft repairs at this level. In addition, some degree of planter flexion usually results even though inversion of the foot and toe flexion may be poor.

ELECTROPHYSIOLOGICAL TESTING

Electrical tests are not only invaluable in working up and documenting recovery in the patient with injury, but are also important for entrapments, and at times, for nerve tumors.[26,40] Electrical tests need to be well selected as well as thorough, and should be done by individuals well versed in these techniques as well as interested in patients suffering from surgical nerve lesions as well as medical neuropathies. Although a thorough EMG will help localize the level of the lesion and the nerve involved, this should never substitute for a thorough physical examination, but rather should complement it.[5,6] Specific electrophysiologic findings will be emphasized in subsequent chapters. From the point of view of the surgeon, the following initial observations may be of value.

ELECTROMYOGRAPHY

Acutely and for the first few days after injury, nerve distal to the injury site can be stimulated to produce distal muscle function. This is so even though axons have lost their continuity proximal to the stimulating site. Response to stimulation persists because Wallerian degeneration takes time to proceed down the distal stump of a nerve. After 48–72 hours, the distal stump will no longer respond to stimulation, but sampling of muscle will show no denervational change. Such change takes several more weeks to come about. At 2–3 weeks, the electromyographer can help the clinician by documenting the extent of deinnervation as well as its distribution (Fig. 3-22).[5] With time and upon repeat EMG study, denervational changes may reverse or there may be nascent activity indicating reinnervation, especially in proximal muscles. Unfortunately, such physiologic evidence of fiber return to muscle does not promise effective function, but at the least it does indicate some nerve fiber regrowth to those sites where it is recorded.[34,43,76] EMG should, however, never substitute for clinical examination because even a muscle with extensive deinnervation by EMG may still contract if a portion of its input has been spared or has recovered.[40,69] Conversely, a few fibers may penetrate an injury site and reverse denervational change in a portion of a muscle, and yet

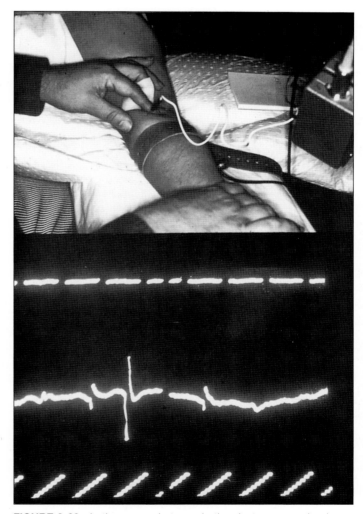

FIGURE 3-22 In the upper photograph, the electromyographer is recording from the pronator muscle in a patient who had sustained a more proximal gunshot wound involving the median nerve 4 months previously. The lower photograph shows recorded fibrillations and a denervational potential. A similar pattern was seen in other muscles sampled, including flexor superficialis, flexor profundus, and flexor pollicis longus, indicating a complete median lesion.

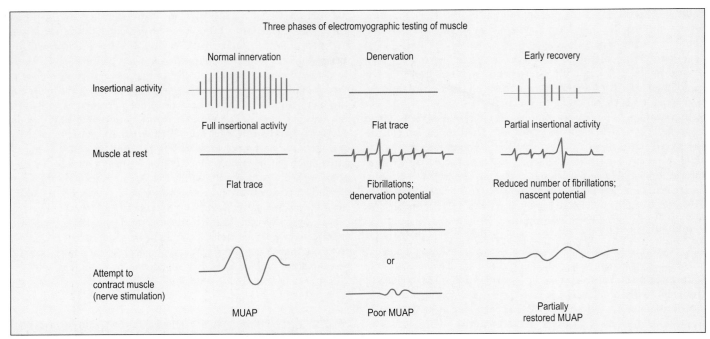

FIGURE 3-23 The three phases usually used on electromyography (EMG) recording from muscle with a needle, coaxially placed in muscle. Traces on EMG with normal innervation, denervation, and early recovery of innervation. The test further delineates these findings. MUAP, evoked muscle action potential.

sufficient regrowth through the remainder of the injury site may not subsequently occur, and thus, distal function can remain poor.

There are three phases or steps to performing an EMG (Fig. 3-23). The first phase is a brief burst of electrical or insertional activity in response to a needle being placed into muscle. The second phase occurs with the needle in muscle and the muscle at rest. The trace should remain flat in a healthy, well-innervated muscle. The third phase is the electrical response when the patient attempts to contract muscle, or the electromyographer stimulates nerve supplying it. With good innervation, this produces a muscle action potential or MUAP. The patient should be able to recruit or increase the firing of these MUAPs.

With serious denervation, there is loss or severe reduction in insertional activity. With the muscle at rest, instead of a flat trace, spontaneous firing of rapid biphasic, low-amplitude sharp waves or fibrillations occur. On attempted muscle contraction, there is no evoked MUAP or a poorly formed one, and recruitment is poor. With reinnervation, these changes begin to reverse, especially in muscle closest to the injury site. The intensity or frequency of fibrillations and denervational potential will decrease. There may also be nascent potentials which are broader based and higher in amplitude than fibrillations. Insertional activity will be partially restored, and some restoration of an MUAP will with time become evident, especially when nerve going to that muscle is stimulated. Eventually, even ability to recruit will begin to occur.

EMG can only suggest reinnervation once axons have regrown all the way to muscle.[19,35] Thus, a nerve can be regenerating well beyond an injury and on down the distal stump for months before reversal of denervationed changes or regenerative changes will be noted by EMG.[37,70] In these earlier weeks to months, only nerve action potential (NAP) recording will indicate regeneration.[37,38,74,77]

Usually, we will obtain a baseline EMG on any serious nerve lesion at 3 weeks or so post injury, and repeat this after 1–2 months in those lesions suspected to be in continuity. In addition, such lesions are monitored by physical examination as well as EMG for a period to determine if surgery is necessary. Occasionally, it may be of value to obtain an EMG earlier than 3 weeks to document existence of a preexisting injury or condition. This may be particularly helpful in a postoperative anesthetic or positioning palsy where existence of denervational changes a few days or at a week or so after operation may suggest a preexisting condition.

EMG results must be weighted carefully, taking into account the individual nerve, the level of the injury, time required for regrowth to the proximal muscles, and the clinical findings, especially those on motor examination.[5,40,76] Unfortunately, finding a decrease in denervation activity and even nascent activity does not mean eventual regeneration that will be functionally significant.[35,40,43] It favors this but does not guarantee it.[71] Conversely, denervational activity can persist for some time even when muscle is observed to contract, so clinical muscle testing remains paramount. Following repair, EMG can only be expected to be predictive and then only at a time when axons can be expected to have reached muscle based on an estimated rate of regeneration.[46] Thus, in an adult with a buttock-level sciatic nerve repair that is regenerating well, a decrease in denervation and/or reinnervational activity may not begin to occur for a year.[38,71] On the other hand, EMG signs of regeneration may occur by 3 months in brachioradialis muscle when there has been a midhumeral-level radial lesion that is axonotemetic.

The other facet of electromyographic testing involves conduction studies on nerves (Fig. 3-24). These tests are of greatest value for suspected entrapment(s) of nerve. They are of less predictive value for the seriously injured nerve since conduction may remain slow even years after restoration of clinical function. Because of distances involved, conduction studies done for elbow-level ulnar

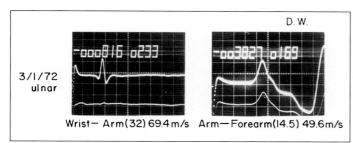

FIGURE 3-24 Noninvasively recorded nerve action potentials on whole ulnar nerve in a patient with an elbow-level entrapment. Response from stimulus over ulnar nerve at the wrist was recorded from distal upper arm *(left tracing)*. Conduction is normal over this length because the more normal conduction on distal nerve is averaged with that which is abnormal across the elbow. Right tracing was recorded distal to the elbow-level lesion. Top trace in each inset is a summated recording; bottom trace is a single nonsummated trace. Wrist to arm recording (to the left) was over a 32 cm distance with conduction at 69.4 meters per second, whereas that to the right was over a 14.5 cm distance and conducted at 49.6 meters per second.

entrapment may be normal in patients with clinical findings for such, and who with intraoperative testing over shorter distances have very abnormal velocities and reduced amplitudes.

NERVE STIMULATION

Nerve stimulation below the level of a neurapraxic injury will produce motor function while stimulation proximal to the injury will not. In addition, simple stimulation of a nerve that is regenerating can evoke muscle contraction(s) several weeks before the patient can do so voluntarily, providing axons have reached muscle (Fig. 3-25).[59] This simple observation may be a useful prognosticator of good clinical recovery and suggest further conservative management. Of course, stimulation of a nerve that has undergone Wallerian degeneration will fail to give muscle contraction. Thus, results of nerve stimulation can be a valuable observation in the early weeks after injury. After that, however, regeneration may be progressing down the distal stump quite well and yet not have reached muscle, so that stimulation could not be expected to make it contract.[40] On the other hand, there is a delay of weeks to several months after new fibers reach muscle before they mature enough and reinnervate enough motor units for voluntary contraction to occur.[70,78] Stimulation can produce muscle contraction at some point in time between when fibers first begin to reinnervate muscle and recovery of voluntary function occurs.

Simple nerve stimulation is especially helpful in early recognition of adequate peroneal recovery, and this can sometimes obviate need for operation.[71] With milder degrees of peroneal injury, stimulation at the head of fibula 4 or 5 months post injury may produce eversion (peroneus) or even foot dorsiflexion (anterior tibialis). The same could be said for an adequately recovering radial nerve injured at a midhumeral level. Under these circumstances, distal radial nerve stimulation may produce brachioradialis contraction 2–6 weeks before this is observable clinically. Depending on the injury mechanism and the extent of radial injury, this may be somewhere between 2.5 and 3.5 months post injury.

Care must be taken not to interpret muscle contraction in response to stimulation of adjacent uninjured nerves or contraction of muscles proximal to the injury site as contraction from muscles below or distal to the lesion.

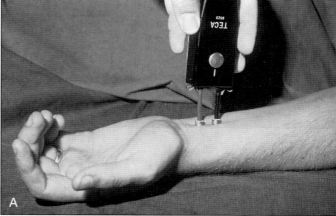

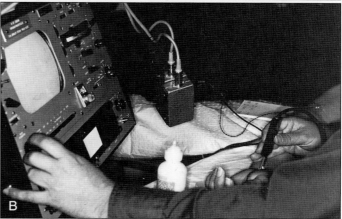

FIGURE 3-25 **(A)** Skin-level nerve stimulation by handheld electrode. Stimuli were delivered to the median nerve proximal to the wrist-level lesion to see if thenar intrinsics, and especially abductor pollicis brevis, would contract. **(B)** Electromyographer is varying stimulus voltage amplitude and duration to determine a threshold for distal muscle contraction in response to median stimulation.

Nerve action potential (NAP) recording across the lesion will provide earlier and also more reliable information about regeneration that stimulation alone, but for most nerves and injury sites requires operative exposure of the nerve (Fig. 3-26).[37,77]

SENSORY CONDUCTION STUDIES

Sensory nerve action potential (sNAP) studies are of a major use for brachial plexus stretch injuries.[7,34,42] They can sometimes differentiate preganglionic from postganglionic site(s) of injury. Lesions at a root or spinal nerve level restricted to the preganglionic region and not extending through the dorsal root ganglion or into the postganglionic area produce complete distal sensory loss, but also preserve distal sensory conduction. Injury of preganglionic fibers between the dorsal root ganglion and the spinal cord does not cause degeneration of the distal postganglionic fibers. Unfortunately, if the lesion is both pre- and postganglionic, the trace will be flat; thus, a negative study is not as helpful diagnostically as a positive one.[34,35,37] Sensory studies can be done by stimulating the hand in the C6 (thumb and index finger), C6–7 (index and long finger), and C8–T1 (little and ring finger) areas and recording from median, radial, and/or ulnar nerves more proximally. If the area stimulated is anesthetic to touch, then recording an sNAP indicates a preganglionic injury in the distribution of one or more roots.

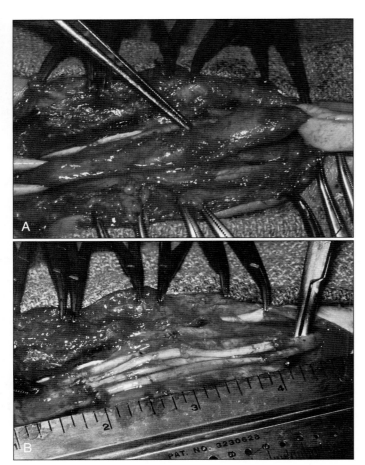

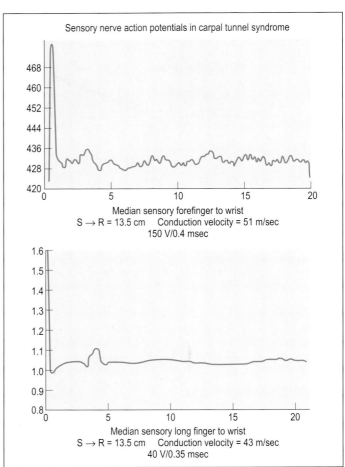

FIGURE 3-26 **(A)** Forearm-level lesion in continuity to the median nerve. Proximal and elbow level is to the right, and distal and hand level is to the left. There was no distal muscle contraction when either the proximal or distal stump was stimulated. **(B)** This lesion also did not transmit a nerve action potential and required a graft repair. Grafts were approximately 6 cm in length.

FIGURE 3-27 Noninvasively recorded sensory potentials in a patient recovering from carpal tunnel syndrome after carpal tunnel release. Amplification necessary to record forefinger to wrist response *(top graph)* was much greater than that required for response from long finger to wrist *(bottom graph)* even though velocity was greater. Conduction velocity is in meters per second (m/sec) and stimulus intensity is in volts and milliseconds (V/msec).

Distal sensory distributions of roots overlap. Even at a finger level, it can be difficult to be certain which root(s) have preganglionic injury.[35] Thus, stimulation of an anesthetic forefinger or even thumb can produce an sNAP if either C6 or C7 (or C6 as well as C7) are damaged at a preganglionic level. This makes it difficult to be certain that C6 has preganglionic injury. Some electromyographers feel that an sNAP recorded from the forearm cutaneous branch (brachial cutaneous) of the musculocutaneous nerve when there is volar forearm hypoesthesia strongly suggests preganglionic injury of C6. For C5, there are no specific stimulation or recording sites for noninvasive sNAP studies.[40] Thus, it is difficult to evaluate the upper spinal nerves or roots with this technique, and yet these are the very ones that one would like to know the most about. On the other hand, sNAP studies may provide useful information about the lower roots, especially C8 and T1.

Such sensory studies have replaced axon-response testing by histamine injection.[7] With preganglionic injury, injection of histamine into an anesthetic area of skin will produce a wheal much like normally innervated skin. Sensory conduction studies are also of great value for some entrapments. For example, sNAPs across the wrist will be abnormal relatively early in patients with carpal tunnel syndrome (CTS) (Fig. 3-27). On the other hand, sensory radial responses will be normal in a patient with posterior interosseous nerve (PIN) entrapment.

SOMATOSENSORY STUDIES

These tests involve peripheral stimulation and more central spinal cord or cortical recordings.[68,72] Recording sites include those over the spine (spinal cord-evoked potential [SEP]) and over cerebral cortex at a scalp level (evoked cortical responses [ECR]).[81] Somatosensory studies are primarily used in plexus injuries, and like sensory conduction studies (sNAPs), can be helpful in differentiating preganglionic from postganglionic lesions.[29,41] Recording an SEP or ECR requires only a few hundred intact fibers between point stimulated and that recorded from, so a positive response insures only minimal continuity of spinal nerve or root.[84] Thus, a negative study may be more important than a positive one. If done in the early months after severe plexus injury, and if distal sites are used for stimulation, as is the usual case, information provided about regeneration is minimal. One cannot have expected fibers to have grown enough to reach most of the distal sites used for stimulation. This requires many more months or even years after injury and/or repair. On the other hand, intraoperative somatosensory studies, particularly when spinal nerves or roots are directly stimulated close to or in their foramens, can be very valuable.[37,49]

Table 3-1 Evidence favoring complete injury with deinnervation

Complete sensory and sweating loss, especially in autonomous zones.
No voluntary muscle function on full effort.
No motor responses on stimulation of nerve below lesion site.
No electrical activity on EMG needle insertion, fibrillatious and deinnervation potentials, no muscle action potentials on voluntary effort. (Samples must be thorough.)
No nerve action potential (NAP) past lesion, provided enough time for regeneration has elapsed.

Table 3-2 Evidence favoring partial injury or functional regeneration

Preservation of the recovery of sensation or sweating in autonomous zones of nerve concerned.
Voluntary muscle function, especially against resistance in injured nerve's motor distribution.
Motor response on stimulation of nerve (must be discrete for nerve stimulation).
Ability to evoke and record nerve action potentials (NAPs) across and distal to injury site.

For a given nerve injury, a combination of electrophysiologic tests is often necessary to provide an optimal level of information about denervation and regeneration (Fig. 3-28). This is especially so with brachial plexus lesions where multiple electrical tests can provide a thorough work-up of the variety of lesions seen.

A combination of clinical and electrical tests can be used to determine whether or not loss due to injury is complete and how complete deinnervation is (Tables 3-1 and 3-2). Such a determination is of great importance since loss in the distribution of a nerve, which is complete, does not usually recover spontaneously. On the other hand, loss which is partial to begin with or which has improved either clinically or electrically is usually associated with spontaneous recovery.

RADIOLOGIC STUDIES

X-RAYS

Fractures can be associated with nerve injury, so radiographs of the traumatized limb with palsy are usually indicated (Fig. 3-29).[49] Midhumeral fractures are associated with radial nerve injuries. Incidence of serious radial palsy increases if humeral fracture is comminuted and/or compound and/or operation is necessary for fixation. Ulna or radius fractures, especially if comminuted, can be associated with a combined median and ulnar nerve injury, and, on occasion, posterior interosseous palsy. Unfortunately, hip dislocation or fracture has an incidence of sciatic palsy associated with it as do operations to restore hip function. More distal fractures of the femur can involve either or both the tibial and peroneal divi-

sions of the sciatic nerve. At times, though, a midshaft fracture of the femur can be related to a more proximal stretch injury to the sciatic nerve at a buttock level. One of the difficult lessons to learn is that the level of the nerve lesion does not always relate to the level of the fracture. Thus, more precise localization still hinges on good clinical and electrodiagnostic evaluation.

Cervical spine fractures can be associated with severe proximal and thus irreparable stretch injuries to the plexus, especially at the root or spinal nerve level of the involved vertebra.[2,4] Fractures of the humerus, clavicle, scapula, and/or ribs when present may provide rough estimates of the forces brought to bear on the neck, shoulder, and arm, as well as brachial plexus, but do not always help to localize the level or document the extent of injury.[42] Plexus damage is usually more proximal than such fractures would indicate and is usually at a root or spinal nerve level.[60,65] Occasionally, excessive callus formation from a fracture of the clavicle, mid-level humerus, elbow, hip, or head of fibula will entrap nerve or complicate partial neural injury at these levels.

MYELOGRAPHY

This radiologic study is still an important test for supraclavicular brachial plexus injuries as well as lumbosacral stretch injuries.[12,42,57,65] It is true that the myelogram can be falsely negative, so meningoceles can be absent at levels where damage to the spinal nerve and root has extended to the spinal cord.[2,15,24,33,51,58] It is also true that meningoceles can be present on roots that function normally or have the potential for recovery, and thus the study can be a false-positive one.[24,49,58] More commonly, in our experience, a meningocele means that either the root is avulsed or, although in gross continuity, has severe internal damage extending to a very proximal level.[40] In either case, the root at this level is usually not reparable. Thus, presence of a meningocele usually means there was enough force to produce an arachnoidal tear and that if the root is not functioning, damage has extended proximally.[71] Such a finding suggests but does not prove that other roots without a meningocele also have been damaged proximally.[71,80] Fortunately, this is not always the case. A number of our patients with meningoceles at some (usually lower levels) but not all levels have had successful repair of one or more spinal nerves at an upper level.

Other myelographic findings of importance with stretch injuries include subdural or extradural extravasation of contrast, evidence of cord swelling acutely, or, after a few weeks, spinal cord atrophy.[11,70,85] To date, the MRI with or without contrast does not substitute for a well-done myelogram using concentrated water-soluble contrast with good anteroposterior as well as lateral and oblique views followed by a computerized axial tomography (CAT) scan. CAT scan transverse cuts after placement of subarachnoid contrast by myelography will show the anterior as well as posterior roots as linear defects in the contrast when there is not preganglionic injury.[12] At the present time, MRI at most centers also has difficulty visualizing enough or all of the roots and spinal nerves to exclude proximal damage.[28,71]

Tumor involving plexus root(s) can also be partially evaluated by myelogram, which may show deformity of one or more root sleeves and/or compression or deformity of the lateral contrast column.[11]

CAT SCAN AND MRI

A CAT scan with metrizamide can miss one or more meningoceles because the cuts may not be fine enough to cover the entire course

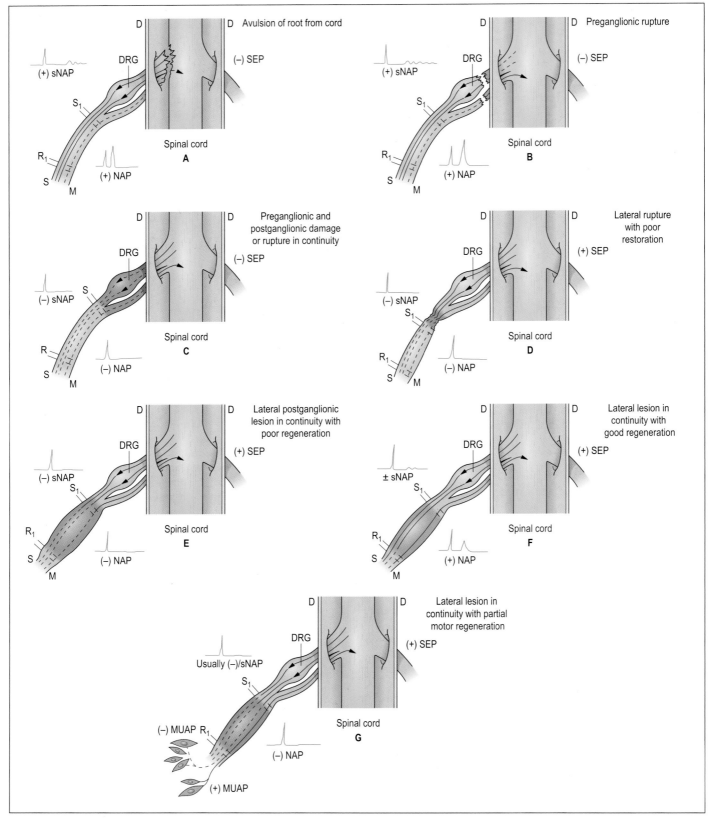

FIGURE 3-28 Variations in spinal nerve injury caused by stretch and their usual electrophysiologic findings. Injuries are progressively depicted from medial or proximal sites to more lateral or distal sites. Parts E, F, and G depict several sets of findings that are not uncommon with stretch injury to the plexus but not as widely known as A, B, C, and D. In G, a few hundred fibers have regenerated or were spared to distal muscle. Thus, the muscle has some contraction when the plexus element is stimulated but does not have an NAP because it does not have 4000 or more fibers greater in size than 5 microns. D, dura mater; DRG, dorsal root ganglion; M, muscle; MUAP, muscle action potential recorded by electromyography; NAP, nerve action potential; R_1, recording electrode; S_1, stimulating electrode; SEP, somatosensory-evoked potential recorded after stimulation of spinal nerve near spine; sNAP, sensory nerve action potential.

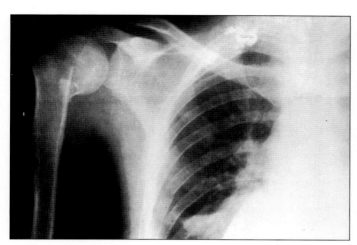

FIGURE 3-29 Shoulder radiograph showing fractured humeral neck associated with a stretch injury to the brachial plexus.

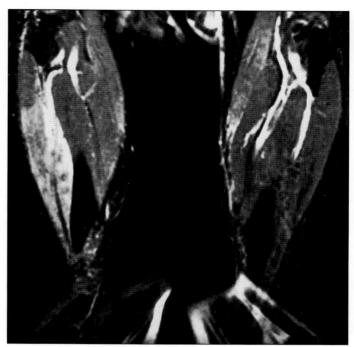

FIGURE 3-30 Magnetic resonance image of anterior and posterior compartment muscle in a patient with a severe peroneal palsy caused by a large intraneural ganglion cyst. T2 phase shows a "whitish-like density" of muscle characteristic of denervation.

of the nerve root, but usually are very useful for stretch injuries. CAT scans, of course, are valuable for tumors, as is the MRI scan.[2,16] Nonetheless, either study confined to the cervical spine can miss tumors of the plexus in lateral neck or shoulder. In an injury setting, MRI can show a nerve root,[20] but it seldom provides enough detail for all roots to preclude the need for a myelogram.[49] As the technology involved with MRI studies develops further, there will be the potential for the MRI to show all of each root and to compare the involved with the uninvolved side. MRI can also confirm degeneration of a nerve, but is not discriminating enough as yet to document regeneration into a previously degenerated site(s).[13] MRI has been shown by studies published in *The Lancet* to depict denervated muscle which will appear "whitish or dense" (Fig. 3-30). Such MRI changes seen within a few days after axonal loss have occurred and provide the earliest objective sign of such.[75] These changes on MRI gradually reverse as muscle is renervated. On the other hand, the MRI's forte in the nerve field is in depicting tumor(s) impinging on or arising from nerve(s), particularly those of the brachial plexus or pelvic plexus where inspection and palpation may not delineate the size and extent of the mass let alone its relationship to adjacent structures.[16]

ANGIOGRAPHY

The use of arteriography and venography will be discussed in some detail in the sections dealing with gunshot wounds and other penetrating wounds, and stretch/contusions to the brachial plexus as well as thoracic outlet syndrome. In some centers, it is probably overused when injury is blunt, but not done enough when there have been penetrating injuries or a suspected compartment syndrome. Occasionally, angiography will be useful for certain tumors involving nerves or plexus and for an entrapment such as that involving axillary nerve where arm abduction of the circumflex artery accompanying nerve will show occlusion.[10]

In most instances, the working clinical diagnosis will be obvious after the history and physical examination are recorded and selected electrical and radiographic studies are obtained. Occasionally, difficulty may be experienced. For example, both principle authors have seen C5–6 discectomies performed in patients with median nerve pathology and L4–5 discectomies performed in patients with peroneal nerve palsies.

SUMMARY

With a little practice, even the busy physician can learn much about nerve function by careful physical examination of the limb. This is also the case in the acute or emergent setting where, even when the patient's cooperation is lacking, much can be observed. Despite the importance of the sensory and autonomic territories for the median, ulnar, and tibial nerves, motor function and its accurate evaluation is of even greater importance for most major nerves. Substitute and trick movements need to be recognized, and lack of function due to tendinous and/or bony injury differentiated from neural loss. It is not only important to identify the nerve involved and the injury level in the limb, but also to ascertain whether loss, especially that to the motor system, is complete or incomplete, and, to determine the distribution and severity of such loss.

Although this text is not intended to replace a more thorough exposition of electrophysiologic evaluation of nerve and muscle, a selected exposure to electromyography (EMG), conductive studies, nerve action potential (NAP) recording, and somatosensory studies is important. It is most important to understand how such studies can evaluate a lesion and also appreciate some of their limitations. In a similar vein, the immense contributions of various radiologic studies to the field of nerve injury not only need to be understood, but in some cases, weighted appropriately to realize their limitations as well as their advantages.

REFERENCES

1. Aids to Investigation of Peripheral Nerve Injuries, Medical Research Council, Nerve Injuries Committee: MRC War Memorandum No. 7,

London, His Majesty's Stationary Office, 1943. London, Balliere Tindall, 1986.

2. Armington W, Harnsberger H, Osborn A, et al.: Radiographic evaluation of brachial plexopathy. Am J Neurorad 8:361–367, 1987.

3. Aschan W and Moberg E: Ninhydrin fiber printing test used to map out partial lesions to nerves of hand. Acta Chir Scand 123:365–370, 1962.

4. Bateman JE: The Shoulder and Neck, 2nd edn. Philadelphia, WB Saunders, 1978:565–616.

5. Bauwens P: Electrodiagnostic definition of the site and nature of peripheral nerve lesions. Ann Phys Med 5:149–152, 1960.

6. Birch R, Bonney G, and Wynn-Parry C: Surgical Disorders of the Peripheral Nerves. Edinburgh, Churchill Livingstone, 1998.

7. Bonney G: The value of axon responses in determining the site of lesion in traction injuries of the brachial plexus. Brain 77:588–609, 1954.

8. Brown P: Factors influencing the success of surgical repair of peripheral nerves. Surg Clin N Am 52:1137–1155, 1972.

9. Bunnell S: Active splinting of the hand. J Bone Joint Surg 28:732–736, 1946.

10. Cahill BR: Quadrilateral space syndrome. In: Omer GE Jr. and Spinner M, Eds: Management of Peripheral Nerve Problems. Philadelphia, Saunders, 1980:602–606.

11. Campbell JB: Peripheral nerve repair. Clin Neurosurg 17:77–98, 1970.

12. Carvalho GA, Nikkah G, Matthies C, et al.: Diagnosis of root avulsions in traumatic brachial plexus injuries: Value of computerized tomography, myelography, and magnetic resonance imaging. J Neurosurg 86:69–76, 1997.

13. Dailey AT, Tsuruda JS, Filler AG, et al.: Magnetic resonance neurography for peripheral nerve degeneration and regeneration. Lancet 350:1221–1222, 1997.

14. Dawson D, Hallett M, and Millender L: Entrapment Neuropathies, 2nd edn. Little Brown, Boston, 1990.

15. Drake CG: Diagnosis and treatment of lesions of the brachial plexus and adjacent structures. Clin Neurosurg 11:110–127, 1964.

16. Filler AG, Kliot M, Howe F, et al.: Application of magnetic resonance neurography in the evaluation of patients with peripheral nerve pathology. J Neurosurg 85:299–309, 1996.

17. Gelberman RH: Operative Nerve Repair and Reconstruction. Philadelphia, JB Lippincott, 1991.

18. Goldner JL: Pain: Extremities and spine – evaluation and differential diagnosis. In: Omer GE Jr. and Spinner M, Eds: Management of Peripheral Nerve Problems, 1st edn.. Philadelphia, Saunders, 1980:602–606.

19. Grundfest H, Oester YT, and Beebe GW: Electrical evidence of regeneration. In: Peripheral Nerve Regeneration. Veteran Administration Monograph. Washington, DC, US Government Printing Office, 1957:203–240.

20. Gupta RK, Mehta VS, and Banerji AK: MRI evaluation of brachial plexus injuries. Neuroradiology 31:377, 1989.

21. Guttmann E and Young JZ: Reinnervation of muscle after various periods of atrophy. J Anat 78:15–43, 1944.

22. Haymaker W and Woodhall B: Peripheral Nerve Injuries: Principles of Diagnosis, 2nd edn. Philadelphia, WB Saunders, 1953.

23. Henderson WR: Clinical assessment of peripheral nerve injuries. Tinel's test. Lancet 2:801–804, 1948.

24. Heon M: Myelogram: A questionable aid in diagnosis and prognosis of brachial plexus components in traction injuries. Conn Med 22:260–262, 1965.

25. Hubbard J: The quality of nerve regeneration. Factors independent of the most skillful repair. Surg Clin N Am 52:1099–1108, 1972.

26. Hudson A, Berry H, and Mayfield F: Chronic injuries of peripheral nerves by entrapment. In: Youmans J, Ed: Neurological Surgery: A Comprehensive Reference Guide to the Diagnosis and Management of Neurosurgical Problems, 2nd edn. Philadelphia, Saunders, 1982.

27. Hudson AR and Hunter D: Timing of peripheral nerve repair: Important local neuropathologic factors. Clin Neurosurg 24:391–405, 1977.

28. Iyer RB, Fenstermacher MJ, and Libshitz HI: Imaging of the treated brachial plexus. AJR Am J Roentgenol 167:225–229, 1996.

29. Jones SJ: Diagnostic use of peripheral and spinal somatosensory evoked potentials in traction lesions of the brachial plexus. Clin Plast Surg 11:167–172, 1984.

30. Kahn EA: Direct observation of sweating in peripheral nerve lesions. Surg Gynecol Obstet 92:22–26, 1951.

31. Kaplan EB and Spinner MB: Normal and anomalous innervation patterns in the upper extremity. In: Omer G, Spinner M, Eds: Management of Peripheral Nerve Problems. Philadelphia, WB Saunders, 1980.

32. Kempe L: Operative Neurosurgery, vol. 2. New York, Springer, 1970.

33. Kewalramani L and Taylor R: Brachial plexus root avulsion: Role of myelography. J Trauma 15:603–608, 1975.

34. Kimura J: Electrodiagnosis in Diseases of Nerves and Muscles: Principles and Practices. Philadelphia, FA Davis, 1983.

35. Kimura J: Electrodiagnosis in Diseases of Nerve and Muscles: Principles and Practice. 2nd edn. Philadelphia, FA Davis, 1989.

36. Kline DG: Macroscopic and microscopic concomitants of nerve repair. Clin Neurosurg 26:582–606, 1979.

37. Kline DG: Evaluating the neuroma in continuity. In: Omer GE and Spinner M, Eds: Management of Peripheral Nerve Problems. Philadelphia, WB Saunders, 1980. (See also Midha R, Kline D: 2nd edn. 1998.)

38. Kline DG: Operative experience with major lower extremity nerve lesions, including the lumbosacral plexus and the sciatic nerve. In: Omer GE Jr. and Spinner M, Eds: Management of Peripheral Nerve Problems, 1st edn. Philadelphia, Saunders, 1980:607–625.

39. Kline D: Diagnostic approach to individual nerve injuries. In: Wilkins R, Rengachary S, Eds: Neurosurgery. New York, McGraw Hill, 1985.

40. Kline DG and Hudson AR: Acute injuries of peripheral nerves. In: Youmans J, Ed: Neurological Surgery, 3rd edn. Philadelphia, WB Saunders, 1990.

41. Landi A, Copeland SA, Wynn-Parry CB, et al.: The role of somatosensory evoked potentials and nerve conduction studies in the surgical management of brachial plexus injuries. J Bone Joint Surg 62B:9–22, 1980.

42. Leffert RD: Clinical diagnosis, testing, and electromyographic study in brachial plexus traction injuries. Clin Ortho Relat Res 237:24–31, 1988.

43. Licht S, Ed: Electrodiagnosis and Electromyography. New Haven, Conn, E. Licht, 1961.

44. Liu CT and Lewey FH: The effect of surging currents of low frequency in man on atrophy of denervated muscles. J Nerv Ment Dis 105:571–581, 1947.

45. Lundborg G: Nerve Injury and Repair. Edinburgh, Churchill Livingston, 1988.

46. Mackinnon S and Dellon A: Surgery of the Peripheral Nerve. New York, Thieme, 1988.

47. Mayfield FH: Causalgia. Springfield, IL, Charles C Thomas, 1951.

48. Mayfield F: Reflex dystrophies of the hand. In: Flynn JE Ed: Hand Surgery. Baltimore, Williamson & Wilkins, 1966:1095 (see also 738–750).

49. McGillicuddy J: Clinical decision-making in brachial plexus injuries. Neurosurg Clin N Am 2:137–150, 1991.

50. McQuarrie I: Clinical signs of Peripheral Nerve Regeneration. In: Wilkins R and Rengachary S, Eds: Neurosurgery. New York, McGraw Hill, 1985.

51. McQuarrie I: Peripheral nerve surgery – today and looking ahead. Clin Plastic Surg 13:255–268, 1986.

52. McQuarrie I and Idzikowski C: Injuries to peripheral nerves. In: Miller T and Rowlands B, Eds: Physiologic Basis of Modern Surgical Care. St. Louis, CV Mosby, 1988:802–815.

53. Medical Research Council, Nerve Injuries Committee: Aids to Investigation of Peripheral Nerve Injuries. MRC War Memorandum No. 7, London, His Majesty's Stationery Office, 1943.

54. Millesi H and Terzis JK: Nomenclature in peripheral nerve surgery. Clin Plast Surg 11:3–8, 1984.

55. Moberg E: Objective methods for determining the functional value of sensibility in the hand. J Bone Joint Surg 40B:454–475, 1958.

56. Murphey F, Kirklin J, and Finlaysan AI: Anomalous innervation of the intrinsic muscles of the hand. Surg Gynecol Obstet 83:15–23, 1946.

57. Murphey F, Hartung W, and Kirklin JW: Myelographic demonstration of avulsing injury of brachial plexus. Am J Roentgenol 58:102–105, 1947.

58. Narakas A: The surgical treatment of traumatic brachial plexus injuries. Int Surg 65:521–527, 1980.

59. Nulsen FE and Lewey FH: Intraneural bipolar stimulation: A new aid in the assessment of nerve injuries. Science 106:301–304, 1947.

60. Omer G: The evaluation of clinical results following peripheral nerve suture. In: Omer G and Spinner M, Eds: Management of Peripheral Nerve Problems. Philadelphia, WB Saunders, 1980:431–438.

61. Omer GE and Spinner M: Peripheral nerve testing and suture techniques. Amercian Academy of Orthopaedic Surgeons Instructional Course Lectures, Vol. 24. St. Louis, CV Mosby, 1975:122–143.

62. O'Rian S: New and simple test of nerve function in the hand. Br Med J 3:615, 1973.

63. Prutkin L: Normal and anomalous innervation patterns in the lower extremities. In: Omer G and Spinner M, Eds: Management of Peripheral Nerve Problems. Philadelphia, WB Saunders, 1980.

64. Seddon HJ: Surgical Disorders of the Peripheral Nerves. Baltimore, Williams & Wilkins, 1972.

65. Simard J and Sypert G: Closed traction avulsion injuries of the brachial plexus. Contemp Neurosurg 50:1–6, 1983.

66. Spinner M: The anterior interosseous-nerve syndrome with special attention to its variations. J Bone Joint Surg 52A:84, 1970.

67. Spurling RG and Woodhall B, Eds: Medical Department, United States Army, Surgery in World War II: Neurosurgery, vol. II. Washington DC, US Government Printing Office, 1959.

68. Sugioka H, Tsuyama N, and Hara T, et al.: Investigation of brachial plexus injuries by intraoperative cortical somatosensory evoked potentials. Arch Orthop Trauma Surg 99:143–151, 1982.

69. Sunderland S: Nerve and Nerve Injuries, 1st edn. Baltimore, Williams & Wilkins, 1968.

70. Sunderland S: Nerves and Nerve Injuries, 2nd edn. Edinburgh and London, Churchill Livingstone, 1978.

71. Sunderland S: Nerve Injuries and their Repair: A Critical Reappraisal. Edinburgh, Churchill Livingstone, 1991.

72. Syneck V and Cowan J: Somatosensory evoked potentials in patients with supraclavicular brachial plexus injuries. Neurology 32:1347–1352, 1982.

73. Ulmer JL and Mayfield FH: Causalgia: A study of 75 cases. Surg Gynecol Obstet 83:789–796, 1946.

74. Van Beek A, Hubble B, and Kinkead L: Clinical use of nerve stimulation and recording. Plast Reconstr Surg 71:225–232, 1983.

75. West GA, Haynor DR, Goodkin R, et al.: Magnetic resonance imaging signal changes in denervated muscles after peripheral nerve injury. Neurosurgery 35:1077–1086, 1994.

76. Wilbourn A: Electrodiagnosis of plexopathies. Neurol Clin 3:511–529, 1985.

77. Williams H and Terzis J: Single fascicular recordings: An intraoperative diagnostic tool for the management of peripheral nerve lesions. Plast Reconstr Surg 57:562–569, 1976.

78. Woodhall B, Nulsen FE, White JC, et al.: Neurosurgical implications. In: Peripheral Nerve Regeneration. Veterans Administration Monograph. Washington, DC, US Government Printing Office, 1957:569–638.

79. Wynn-Parry CB: Rehabilitation of the Hand. London, Butterworth, 1966.

80. Yeoman P: Cervical myelography in traction injuries of the brachial plexus. J Bone Joint Surg 50B:253–257, 1968.

81. Yiannikas C, Chahani BT, and Young RR: The investigation of traumatic lesions of the brachial plexus by electromyography and short latency somatosensory potentials evoked by stimulation of multiple peripheral nerves. J Neurol Neurosurg Psychiatry 46:1014–1022, 1983.

82. Zachary RB and Roaf R: Lesions in continuity. In: Seddon HJ, Ed: Peripheral Nerve Injuries. London, Her Majesty's Stationery Office, Med. Res. Council Spec. Report Series No., 282, 1954.

83. Zalis A, Rodriquez A, Oester Y, et al.: Evaluation of nerve regeneration by means of evoked potentials. J Bone Joint Surg 54A:1246–1253, 1972.

84. Zhao OS, Kim DH, Kline DG, et al.: Somatosensory evoked potential induced by stimulating a variable number of nerve fibers in the rat. Muscle Nerve 16:1220–1227, 1993.

85. Zorub D, Nashold BS Jr, and Cook WA Jr: Avulsion of the brachial plexus, I. A review with implications on the therapy of intractable pain. Surg Neurol 2:347–353, 1974.

86. Livingston WK: Evidence of active invasion of denervated areas by sensory fibers from neighboring nerves. J Neurosurg 4:140–144, 1947.

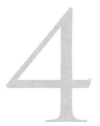

Grading results

David G. Kline

OVERVIEW

■ To evaluate nerve loss and recovery requires a system that is relatively simple but detailed enough to provide useful information.

■ The MRC system is such a system for individual muscles but was originally designed for grading loss with polio where slight muscle function has greater prognostic significance than it does for most nerve injuries.

■ The LSUHSC system grades contraction against gravity as a 2 and thus a 3 is contraction against gravity and mild pressure, and a grade 4 contraction against gravity and moderate pressure.

■ Equally important is grading of a whole nerve or plexus element's function. The American system, taking into account recovery of proximal muscles versus distal ones, was expanded for this purpose.

■ Since different nerves and plexus elements have different patterns of recovery, we have made some attempt to individualize the whole nerve grading system.

■ Same examples of outcomes using the LSUHSC grading system are included.

■ Still needed are better systems to evaluate the usefulness of any recovery gained in terms of acts of daily living and employment.

One of the central themes of this book is the use of data concerning results of management. Difficulties in obtaining such data have on several occasions, delayed publication of the first and second editions of the book. Nevertheless, a useful system for grading loss and recovery of sensory and motor function has always been paramount. Moreover, a system is needed not only for grading individual muscle and sensory responses but for evaluating function in the distribution of an entire nerve or plexus element. Most nerves and plexus elements innervate one or more proximal muscles, a group of more distal muscles, and also a distal sensory field of variable functional importance. There are a number of useful publications that have used or reported on various grading systems.[1–8,12–26] Discussion of the reasons for selection of the grading systems in use, however, has been difficult to find. In this book, the grading system used to evaluate recovery – the LSUHSC (LSUMC) system – is based on earlier British and American systems but includes some important changes.[9–11]

Both the British Medical Research Council (MRC) and the American systems for grading loss or return of motor function after nerve injury and repair were originally based on grading systems developed to evaluate paralysis associated with poliomyelitis (Tables 4-1 to 4-3). In the polio patient, retention or return of a very small amount of function held important prognostic and often therapeutic value. Grades 1, 2, and 3 in those systems took the muscle function only to the point of overcoming gravity, and function after that point received limited gradation. With nerve injury, small amounts of recovery are also important, but so is a gradual gradation after recovery of contraction against gravity. As a result, these systems were modified to create contraction against gravity and mild resistance. The LSUMC modified system also provides a grade 4 for contraction against moderate resistance and, finally, a grade 5 for contraction against maximal resistance (Table 4-4; Fig. 4-1). Sensory grades were also changed to accommodate a more practical and readily carried out examination, concentrating on ability to localize various stimuli.

For grading whole nerve function, we began with the MRC system, which takes into account proximal as well as distal muscle function. A similar but altered scheme was devised (Table 4-5), again expanding grades between 2 and 5. The designation of independent and synergetic movements, used for grade 4 in the MRC system and grade 5 in the American system, was eliminated even though this was a potentially valuable observation. Instead, grade 4 for whole nerve was made to include contraction of proximal and distal muscles against gravity and some resistance. It was determined that full recovery of function was unlikely with most serious injuries to major nerves, so grade 5 includes contraction of proximal and distal muscles against gravity and moderate rather than full resistance. These changes in the British and American systems for grading whole nerve function resulted in the system shown in Table 4-5.

GRADING UPPER AND LOWER EXTREMITY NERVE INJURIES

A severe high or proximal injury to radial nerve results in loss of triceps, brachioradialis, supinator, extensor carpi ulnaris (ECU) and radialis (ECR), extensor communis (EC), and extensor pollicis longus (EPL) function (Fig. 4-2). Sensory loss on the dorsum of the hand and over the anatomic snuffbox area is variable. For

Table 4-1 Muscle power grading (British system)

Grade	Description
0–None	No palpable muscle contraction
1–Trace	Palpable muscle contraction detectable by examiner
2–Poor	Active joint motion present with gravity eliminated
3–Fair	Muscle can move joint through full range of motion against gravity
4–Good	Full range of motion against gravity and some resistance
5–Normal	Full range of motion with a maximum force that is normal for the muscle

Table 4-2 Grading of entire nerve (British MRC system)

M5	Complete recovery
M4	All synergistic and independent movements are possible
M3	All important muscles contract against resistance
M2	Return of perceptible contraction in both proximal and distal muscles
M1	Return of perceptible contraction in proximal muscles
M0	No contraction in any muscle

Source: Seddon H: Peripheral Nerve Injuries. Medical Research Council Special Report Series No. 282 London, Her Majesty's Stationary Office 1954.

Table 4-3 Grading of entire nerve (American system)

M6	Complete recovery
M5	Some synergistic and isolated movements possible
M4	All important muscles have sufficient power to act against resistance
M3	Proximal muscles act against gravity; perceptible contraction in intrinsic muscles
M2	Proximal muscles act against gravity; no return of power in intrinsic muscles
M1	Return of perceptible contraction in the proximal muscles
M0	No contraction

Source: Woodhall B and Beebe G, Eds: Peripheral nerve regeneration: A follow-up study of 3656 WWII injuries. VA Medical Monograph, US Government Printing Office, Washington, DC, 1956.

Table 4-4 Louisiana State University Medical Center grading system for motor and sensory function

Individual muscle grades

Grade	Evaluation	Description
0	Absent	No contraction
1	Poor	Trace contraction
2	Fair	Movement against gravity only
3	Moderate	Movement against gravity and some (mild) resistance
4	Good	Movement against moderate resistance
5	Excellent	Movement against maximal resistance

Sensory grades

Grade	Evaluation	Description
0	Absent	No response to touch, pin, or pressure
1	Bad	Testing gives hyperesthesia or paresthesia; deep pain recovery in autonomous zones
2	Poor	Sensory response sufficient for grip and slow protection; sensory stimuli mislocalized with over-response
3	Moderate	Response to touch and pin in autonomous zones; sensation mislocalized and not normal with some over-response
4	Good	Response to touch and pin in autonomous zones; response localized but sensation not normal; no over-response
5	Excellent	Near normal response to touch and pin in entire field including autonomous zones

grading purposes, proximal muscles for a proximal radial lesion would be triceps and brachioradialis, and distal muscles would be ECR, ECU, EC, and EPL (Fig. 4-2). Sensory loss is less important and more variable with a radial lesion than with a median or ulnar lesion. Therefore, sensory grading is not included when function for the whole radial nerve is graded.

For a proximal radial lesion, the grading scale is as follows:

0 = Absent radial motor function.
1 = Some contraction of triceps; if brachioradialis contracts, it does so against gravity only.
2 = Triceps and brachioradialis contract against force, but there is little or no supination and no wrist extension.
3 = Triceps and brachioradialis contract against force; supination and wrist extension against at least gravity. There may be a trace of finger or thumb extension, or this may be absent.
4 = Triceps and brachioradialis contract against force; supination and wrist extension are present against force. There is usually a trace or better finger and thumb extension.
5 = Good triceps and brachioradialis function as well as supination and wrist extension; finger and thumb extension against at least gravity and some resistance.

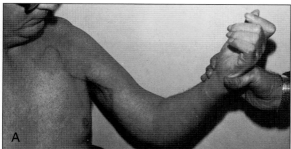

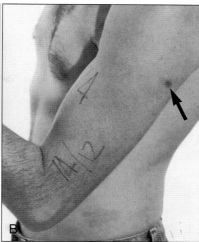

FIGURE 4-1 (A) Grading biceps in a patient who sustained lateral cord to musculocutaneous nerve and lateral cord to median nerve injuries as a result of stretch/contusion.
(B) Recovery of biceps 14 months after a gunshot wound *(arrow shows entry site)* and 12 months after a suture repair of the musculocutaneous nerve.

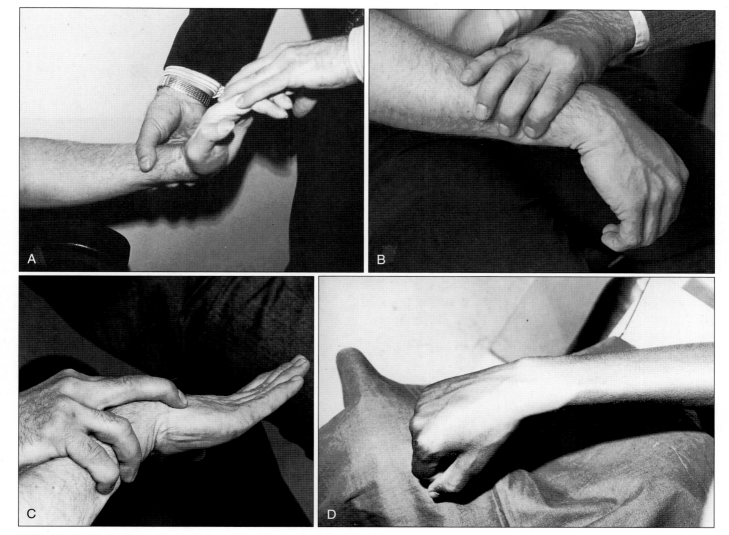

FIGURE 4-2 (A) Grading wrist extension in a patient with a posterior cord to radial nerve lesion. (B) Trace contraction of wrist extension. (C) Extension of wrist against gravity and some pressure. (D) Partial extension of wrist despite total radial palsy. Extensor tendons had shortened owing to denervation, and when this patient made a fist, the wrist cocked back.

Table 4-5 Louisiana State University Medical Center criteria for grading whole nerve injury

Grade	Evaluation	Description
0	Absent	No muscle contraction, absent sensation
1	Poor	Proximal muscles contract but not against gravity; sensory grade 1 or 0
2	Fair	Proximal muscles contract against gravity; distal muscles do not contract; sensory grade if applicable is usually 2 or lower
3	Moderate	Proximal muscles contract against gravity and some resistance; some distal muscles contract against at least gravity; sensory grade is usually 3
4	Good	All proximal and some distal muscles contract against gravity and some resistance; sensory grade is 3 or better
5	Excellent	All muscles contract against moderate resistance; sensory grade is 4 or better

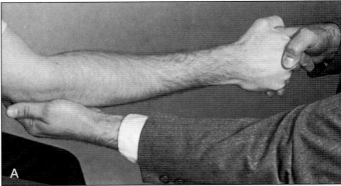

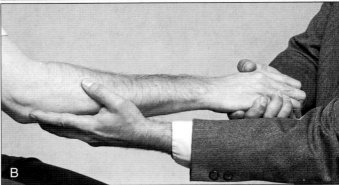

FIGURE 4-3 Steps in grading pronator. Hand and forearm are partially pronated in **(A)** and fully pronated against resistance in **(B)**.

Construction of a grading paradigm for a more distal radial lesion involving posterior interosseous nerve (PIN) would include the following criteria:

0 = No ECU, EC, or EPL muscle function.
1 = Either trace function or contraction against gravity only for ECU; absent EC and EPL muscle function.
2 = Recovery of ECU function; absent or trace only of EC or EPL muscle function or both.
3 = Recovery of ECU, some EC, weak or absent EPL muscle function.
4 = Recovery of moderate strength of EC and EPL; full strength in ECU muscle function.
5 = Recovery of full strength of EPL, EC, and ECU muscle function.

For grading of the more common midarm radial lesion, such as that caused by a fracture at a midhumeral level, the brachioradialis, supinator, and ECR are the proximal muscles, and the ECU, EC, and EPL are the distal muscles. By comparison, for a posterior cord lesion, the proximal muscles would be latissimus dorsi, deltoid, and triceps, and the more distal muscles would be brachiaoradialis, supinator, and ECR.

Such a template is easier for a femoral nerve lesion and somewhat more complex for a median or ulnar nerve lesion. For a proximal pelvic-level femoral lesion:

0 = Absence of iliacus as well as quadriceps muscle function.
1 = Contraction of iliacus against gravity but not pressure.
2 = Contraction of iliacus against gravity and some pressure; usually a trace of quadriceps function is present.
3 = Good iliacus contraction, and quadriceps contracts against gravity.
4 = Good iliacus function, and contraction of quadriceps against gravity plus some force.
5 = Contraction of both iliacus and quadriceps against considerable force.

By comparison, grading a proximal median lesion would include more detail because of its important distal sensory as well as motor input (Fig. 4-3). For a proximal median lesion:

0 = No median-innervated pronation or wrist or finger or thumb flexion, no thenar intrinsic function (abductor pollicis brevis and opponens pollicis); absent to poor median sensation.
1 = Pronation present but quite weak, median-innervated wrist and finger flexors contract, but not against gravity; sensory grade, if present, is 1.
2 = Pronation and wrist and finger flexion against gravity; more distal muscles either do not contract or have muscles function only; sensory grade is 2 or lower.
3 = Pronation as well as wrist and finger flexion against gravity and some resistance; some distal muscles such as flexor pollicis longus an even thenar intrinsics contract against gravity; sensory grade is usually 3.
4 = Pronators, wrist and finger flexors, flexor pollicis longus muscles, and even thenar intrinsics contract against some resistance; sensory grade is 3 or better.
5 = All median-innervated muscles contract against considerable force; sensory grade is 4 or better.

A similar system can be devised for the ulnar nerve, which also has a sensory field. A grading system for portions of the brachial plexus that eventually go to either the median or ulnar nerve also has design similarities to that used for the median nerve.

Grading systems for the sciatic nerve once again depend on both proximal and distal muscles but also work best if the tibial half of that nerve's function is evaluated separately from the peroneal half. For proximal tibial lesions:

0 = No gastrocnemius-soleus function, no inversion, no toe flexion, little or no sensation on the plantar surface of the foot.

1 = Trace gastrocnemius but no other tibial muscle function; trace to poor plantar sensation.

2 = Gastrocnemius contracts against gravity only; plantar surface usually has a sensory grade of 2 or less.

3 = Gastrocnemius-soleus contracts against gravity and some force; trace or better inversion; plantar sensory grade of 3 or better.

4 = Gastrocnemius contracts against moderate resistance, inversion grades 3 or better, either a trace or no toe flexion; sensation grades 4 or better.

5 = Gastrocnemius has full function, inversion grades 4 or better, toe flexion present; plantar sensation grades 4 or better.

For a proximal peroneal division lesion, grading includes a thigh muscle but excludes a less important sensory field:

0 = No or little short head of biceps function, no peronei, no anterior tibialis (AT), no extensor hallucis longus (EHL) or EC function.

1 = Short head of biceps contracts, no distal peroneal-innervated motor function.

2 = Short head of biceps contracts, peronei contract against gravity or better; no AT or more distal motor function.

3 = Short head of biceps contracts, peronei grade 3 or better; AT contracts, peronei grade 3 or better; AT contracts against gravity, but function of EHL and EC for toes is usually absent.

4 = Short head of biceps and peronei contract, as does AT, which is great 3 or better; EHL and EC may have trace function.

5 = Short head of biceps and peronei contract, AT grades 4 or better, and EHL and EC contract against at least gravity.

GRADING C5–C6 OR UPPER TRUNK LESIONS

Loss in this distribution involves supraspinatus, infraspinatus, deltoid, latissimus dorsi, bicep/brachialis, brachioradialis, and supinator muscle (Fig. 4-4). Although deltoid is more proximal than biceps/brachialis or brachioradialis, it often recovers later than these muscles because it requires a very complex innervation to work even against gravity. Infraspinatus seldom recovers after severe proximal plexus injury. These variations are reflected in the following grading scale:

0 = No function in the C5–C6 or upper trunk distribution.

1 = Some supraspinatus contraction, trace of biceps/brachialis, no deltoid.

2 = Supraspinatus contraction, but no deltoid contraction or trace only; contraction of biceps against gravity only.

3 = Supraspinatus contraction, trace only deltoid, contraction of biceps/brachialis or brachioradialis against gravity and some force.

4 = Supraspinatus contraction is against gravity or more, deltoid contracts against gravity or more, biceps/brachialis or brachioradialis contracts against moderate resistance; infraspinatus may or may not contract.

5 = Good recovery of supraspinatus function; deltoid contracts against gravity and at least mild resistance; biceps/brachialis or brachioradialis against great resistance; some recovery of supination; infraspinatus may or may not contract.

GRADING C5, C6, AND C7 LESIONS OR UPPER PLUS MIDDLE TRUNK LESIONS

Loss in this distribution includes supraspinatus, infraspinatus, supinator, deltoid, latissimus dorsi, biceps/brachialis, brachioradialis, and usually latissimus dorsi and triceps loss (Fig. 4-5). There is often some weakness in pronation. There may or may not be weakness or loss of wrist extension and finger and thumb extension. Less frequent is weakness in wrist and finger flexion. There may also be some sensory loss in the median distribution. It has to be recognized, though, that input from C7 is quite variable from patient to patient. The grading system is as follows:

0 = No function in the C5, C6, and C7 distribution.

1 = Some supraspinatus contraction, trace contraction of biceps/brachialis, but absent deltoid function and also no function in the more distal C7-innervated muscles.

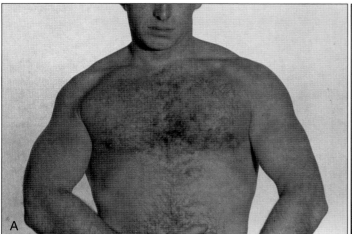
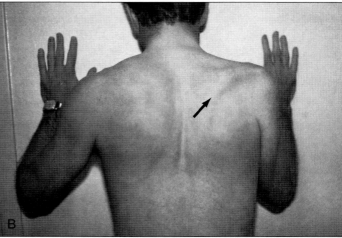

FIGURE 4-4 **(A)** Absence of the patient's right deltoid in an otherwise muscular young man. The only abduction of the arm was provided by supraspinatus, so deltoid (and thus axillary) function was 0. **(B)** In this patient, there was loss of not only deltoid but supraspinatus and infraspinatus function. Note the muscular atrophy on either side of the scapula's spinous process *(arrow)*. Supraspinatus function was trace only, as was that of deltoid; infraspinatus function was absent (0). This gave an overall grade for C5 function of 1.

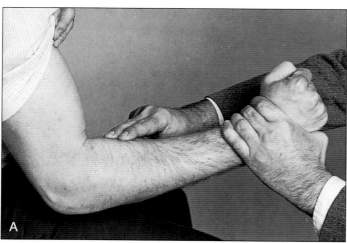
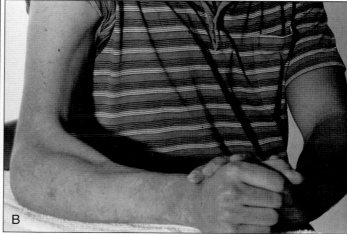

FIGURE 4-5 Grading brachioradialis. **(A)** Muscle contraction is palpated, and resistance is applied by the examiner as the patient flexes forearm that is partially pronated. **(B)** In this patient, biceps function was absent, but brachioradialis contracted against gravity and mild pressure (grade 3).

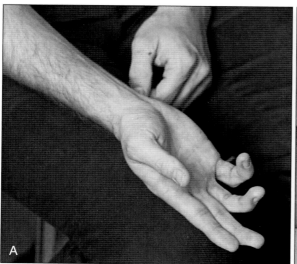
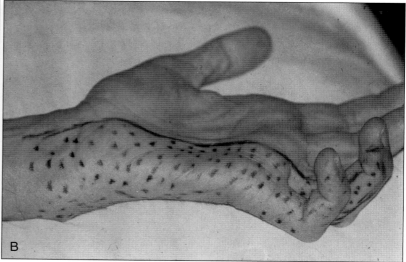

FIGURE 4-6 **(A)** Clawing associated with loss of function of lumbrical to little and ring fingers in an ulnar palsy. After flexor carpi ulnaris is tested, flexor profundus function in the little and ring fingers is assessed. Then, the hand intrinsic muscles are examined. **(B)** In this case of severe ulnar palsy caused by an elbow-level injury, loss was complete below the level of the flexor carpi ulnaris. Only a trace of abductor digiti minimi and opponens digiti minimi function was present (grade 1). Typical sensory loss with a proximal ulnar injury is evident.

2 = Supraspinatus contraction, trace contraction of deltoid, and contraction of biceps/brachialis against gravity only; no function of triceps or other distal C6- or C7-innervated muscles.

3 = Supraspinatus contraction; deltoid contracts against gravity, biceps/brachioradialis or brachioradialis against gravity and some resistance, triceps trace or better.

4 = Supraspinatus contraction, deltoid contracts against gravity or better, biceps/brachialis or brachioradialis against gravity and at least moderate resistance, and triceps against gravity; some true supination, some return of wrist, finger and thumb extension or flexion if these functions were absent before operation.

5 = Supraspinatus contraction, deltoid against some resistance, biceps/brachioradialis and brachioradialis against moderate or more resistance, some supination, triceps against gravity,

and some resistance and some contraction of wrist, finger, and thumb extensors or flexors if they were absent preoperatively.

GRADING C8–T1 LESIONS

Complete loss in this distribution always includes hand intrinsic muscle loss. This includes muscles in the ulnar distribution, which are hypothenars, interossei, lumbricals, and adductor pollicis (Fig. 4-6). There is also weakness of flexor pollicis brevis and sensory loss in the ulnar distribution. In the median distribution, function of thenar intrinsics, including abductor pollicis brevis and opponens pollicis, is lost; flexor pollicis brevis function is also lost because both distal median and ulnar outflows supply this muscle with dual innervation. There may or may not be further loss, including decreased extension of the fingers, which is sometimes worse in

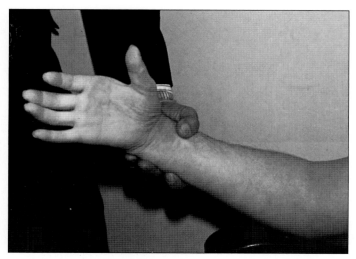

FIGURE 4-7 Interossei in this patient could contract, but not against resistance. This gave overall grade 2 function.

little and ring fingers than in forefinger and long finger, but occasionally occurs the other way around. In other patients, the flexor profundus muscles may be weak, and again the distribution of this loss varies from patient to patient, so that in some it affects fingers on the ulnar side of the hand more than on the radial side, and in other cases the other way around. On occasion, even wrist and finger extensors or totally paralyzed. Shoulder, upper arm, and usually forearm muscle functions are excellent, but the hand is severely affected (Fig. 4-7). The grading system is as follows:

0 = No function in C8–T1 distribution.
1 = Some but usually poor (grade 2 or less) sensation in ulnar distribution of hand; some recovery of finger extensor or finger flexor function if that had been absent previously (grade 2).
2 = Finger extensors or flexors functional if function was lost before (grade 3); ulnar sensation is grade 3 or better; hypothenars contract and are grade 2 or better; function of other intrinsics is trace or absent.
3 = Ulnar sensation is grade 3 or better; finger extensors or flexors, if function was lost before, grade 3 or better; hypothenar muscles grade 3 or better; most other hand intrinsics contract against gravity only.
4 = Ulnar sensation grade 3 or better; finger extensors or flexors, if function was lost before, grade 3 or better; hypothenars grade 3 or better; most other intrinsics contract against gravity and some resistance.
5 = Ulnar sensation grade 4 or 5; return of any lost finger extension or flexion; all intrinsics contract against at least moderate pressure or resistance.

GRADING C5–T1 LOSS

Complete loss of function in this distribution produces a flail arm. In the usual injury, rhomboids and serratus anterior still contract because of very proximal origin from spinal nerve branches to these muscles. Diaphragm usually functions, and there is a variable amount of paraspinal denervation. There is no other function preserved in the arm with a complete lesion in this distribution, so

shoulder movement, other than that provided by trapezius, is absent, as is elbow, wrist, and finger motion. Sensory loss is complete in median and ulnar distributions of the hand and even in the radial distribution on the back of the hand. Usually, there is no significant sensory perception below the elbow. Because of widespread autonomic loss, there is absence of sweating on all fingers. The grading scale is as follows:

0 = No sensory or motor function in the arm.
1 = Supraspinatus contracts against gravity; trace contraction of biceps/brachialis or brachioradialis.
2 = Supraspinatus contracts against gravity and some pressure; biceps/brachialis or brachioradialis contract against gravity.
3 = Supraspinatus is good, bicep/brachialis or brachioradialis contract against gravity, and some pressure; contraction of deltoid usually trace to against gravity; there may be a trace of triceps function.
4 = In addition to findings for grade 3 above, triceps contracts at least against gravity; deltoid contracts at least against gravity; there may be a trace of wrist and/or finger function.
5 = In addition to recovery of shoulder and arm muscle contraction against gravity and at least some resistance, there is either wrist flexion or extension, and there is some finger flexion.

GRADING LATERAL CORD LOSS

Loss in this distribution includes biceps/brachialis loss and sensory loss in the median distribution. Pronation is weak or absent, and wrist and finger flexion, including thumb flexion, may be weak. The grading system is a follows:

0 = No motor or sensory function.
1 = Trace of biceps/brachialis function with or without slight return of some sensation in median distribution (sensory grade 1).
2 = Biceps/brachialis contract against gravity; sensation in the median distribution is grade 1 or higher.
3 = Biceps/brachialis contract against gravity and some pressure; sensation is grade 2 or higher; any wrist or finger flexion weakness has improved.
4 = Biceps/brachialis contract against gravity and moderate pressure; sensation is grade 3 or higher.
5 = Biceps/brachialis contract against gravity and considerable pressure; sensation grades 3 or higher.

GRADING MEDIAL CORD LOSS

In addition to severe hand intrinsic muscle function loss and ulnar distribution sensory loss, there is a variable amount of forearm-level, median-innervated motor loss. This usually involves wrist and finger flexion weakness (see Fig. 4-7). Grading is as follows:

0 = No sensory or motor function.
1 = Return of wrist and finger flexion if absent or paretic previously.
2 = Some sensation in ulnar distribution (grade 2); weak (trace) hypothenar function.
3 = Return of contraction of hypothenars against gravity and some pressure; sensation in ulnar distribution grades 3; trace

or better function of interossei, lumbricales, and adductor pollicis.

4 = Hypothenars contract against gravity and mild pressure, as do interossei and lumbricales.

5 = Return of motor function of hypothenars, interossei, and lumbricales to grade 4 or better. Thenar intrinsics and adductor pollicis contract against at least gravity. Ulnar sensation is grade 4 or better.

GRADING POSTERIOR CORD LOSS

Posterior cord has as an initial branch, the thoracodorsal innervating latissimus dorsi and subscapularis branches. Its major outflow, though, is to all the radial-innervated muscles including triceps through extensor communis. The other major branch or nerve goes to the axillary nerve innervating the deltoid. Despite its proximity to posterior cord, recovery of deltoid, if it occurs, is relatively delayed. Grading is as follows:

0 = No motor function for deltoid or radial-innervated muscles.

1 = Some triceps contraction.

2 = Triceps contraction, latissimus contraction, trace of deltoid contraction.

3 = Grade 3 triceps and brachioradialis contraction, deltoid grade 2 or better, usually wrist extension a trace or better.

4 = Wrist extension is grade 3 or better, in addition to grade 3 or better triceps, and brachioradialis, deltoid contraction is grade 2 or better

5 = Recovery of deltoid to grade 3 or better as well as triceps, brachioradialis, and wrist extension to grade 3 or better; usually some finger extension is present.

OUTCOMES STUDIES

The use of grading systems can be illustrated by looking at a group of median nerve lesions at the level of the arm.

Table 4-6 lists outcomes in 51 patients comparing those not in continuity (12) to those in continuity (29) and tumors (10). A whole nerve grade of 3 or better was viewed as good and successful so those cases achieving that level are placed after the "slash" (/). For example, 2 of 3 cases having primary repair by suture achieved a grade 3 or better result. Most of the injuries having loss of continuity were due to lacerations.

Table 4-7 lists patients evaluated and operated on at the arm level by category of injury or lesion and also provides their postoperative grades. The grading system used for arm-level median lesions is found on page 68.

Lacerations, gunshot wounds, and tumors provided the majority of the cases. Even though lesions were at an arm level, outcomes were good. Grade 3 level equals return of pronation, wrist flexion, and some finger flexion by flexor superficialis as well as restoration of enough sensation in the median distribution to be at least protective. Fourteen patients achieved a grade 4 recovery because of return of flexor profundus as well as flexor pollicis longus and a sensory grade 4 by the LSUHSC grading system. Few patients gained a grade 5 level, since this required recovery of excellent sensation as well as median-innervated intrinsic muscles.

Table 4-6 Operations on median nerve at arm level (51)
Not in continuity (12)
Primary repair   Suture 3/2*

Secondary repair
  Graft 8/5
  Suture 1/1

In continuity (29)
  Positive NAP (17/16)
  Negative NAP
    Graft 7/5
    Suture 5/5

Tumors – 9 of 10 removed with grade 3 or better function.

( ) Number of cases.

*Number of cases/number improving to grade 3 or better.

Table 4-7 Results of operation on 51 arm level median palsies function grade (postoperative)

Etiologies	Total cases	5	4	3	2	1	0	Nonoperative*
Laceration†	15	1	6	4	4	0	0	3
Gunshot†	12	2	6	3	1	0	0	10
Fracture†	5	0	1	3	1	0	0	0
Contusion†	4	0	1	3	0	0	0	1
Compression	4	2	0	1	1	0	0	3
Injection	1	0	1	0	0	0	0	2
Tumor	10	6	2	1	1	0	0	2
Total	51	11	17	15	8	0	0	21

*18 of 21 patients in the nonoperative category reached a grade of 3 or better.

†Prior operations included vascular repair (16), fracture repair (4), fasciotomy (1), and prior operation on nerve itself (5).

Table 4-8 Pain grades

Grade	Description
P4 (100%)	Severe enough to prevent all activity and causes distress
P3 (75%)	Prevents some activity
P2 (50%)	Interferes with activity
P1 (25%)	Annoying

Source: Omer GE and Spinner M, Eds: Management of Peripheral Nerve Problems. Philadelphia, WB Saunders, 1980:434.

Throughout the text similar tables showing outcomes will be found. In some instances such as the section on median, radial, combined upper extremity, and femoral nerve, intervals between injury and operation on the nerve are also provided.

GRADING PAIN

Some interesting attempts have been made to grade pain (Table 4-8). Various investigators have devised questionnaires and body diagrams for patients on which patients are requested to describe their pain. Attempts have also been made to quantify or grade such systems. All investigators agree, however, that grading of pain is very difficult to achieve in a satisfactory fashion. For purposes of this text, we have tried to describe the pain pattern whenever possible rather than attempting to grade this response or outcome.

SUMMARY

If results of management are to be used to formulate future therapy, they must not only be graded for motor and important sensory function but individualized for different anatomic levels. There are always potential criticisms of a grading system. The MRC system is such a system for individual muscles but was originally designed for grading loss with polio where slight muscle function has greater prognostic significance than it does for most nerve injuries. Grading such small amounts of function, although sometimes important for nerve injures, pales in comparison to grading contraction against gravity and against mild, moderate, and great resistance. For this reason, the Louisiana State University Medical Center system goes for 0 = no function, to 1 = trace, to 2 = contraction against gravity, to 3 = contraction against gravity and contraction against considerable or full resistance.

It is also important to be able to grade a whole nerve's function level by level. For the results reported in this text, this has been done by comparatively grading function for the proximal or closest muscles to the level of a given nerve's injury and for those in the nerve's more distal distribution. Individual grading tables have thus been developed for most major nerves at their more important levels.

The system is presented only to be enlarged upon, changed, or redirected. Clearly, the older British and American systems, although valuable, do not provide quite as much information as that proposed here. Conversely, the LSUHSC grading system presented has not addressed itself to the limb for activities of daily living or employment, although the case summaries provided in later chapters provide some insight in this regard.

REFERENCES

1. Bateman JE: Results and assessment of disability in iatrogenic nerve injuries. In: Bateman JE: Trauma to Nerves in Limbs. Philadelphia, WB Saunders, 1962:285–305.
2. Bowsen RE and Napier JR: The assessment of hand function after peripheral nerve injuries. J Bone Joint Surg 43B:481, 1961.
3. Daniels L and Worthingham C: Muscle Testing, 3rd edn. Philadelphia, WB Saunders, 1972.
4. Dellon AL: Results of nerve repair in the hand. In: Dellon AL: Evaluation of Sensibility and Re-education of Sensation in the Hand. Baltimore, Williams and Wilkins, 1981:193–201.
5. Evarts CM: Examination of the musculoskeletal patient. In: Evarts CM, Ed: Surgery of the Musculoskeletal System. New York, Churchill Livingston, 1983:9–17.
6. Groff RA and Houtz SJ: Recovery and regeneration. In: Manual of Diagnosis and Management of Peripheral Nerve Injuries. Philadelphia, JB Lippincott, 1945:33–35.
7. Haymaker W and Woodhall B: Peripheral Nerve Injuries, Principles of Diagnosis, 2nd edn. Philadelphia, WB Saunders, 1953.
8. Highet WB: Grading of motor and sensory recovery in nerve injuries. Report to the Medical Research Council. London, Her Majesty's Stationery Office, 1954.
9. Kline DG and Hurst J: Prediction of recovery from peripheral nerve injury. Neurol Neurosurg Updated Series 5:2–8, 1984.
10. Kline DG and Judice D: Operative management of selected brachial plexus lesions. J Neurosurg 58:631, 1983.
11. Kline DG and Nulsen F: Acute injuries of peripheral nerves. In: Youmans J, Ed: Neurological Surgery, 2nd edn. Philadelphia, WB Saunders, 1981.
12. Mannerfelt L: Motor function testing. In: Omer GE and Spinner M, Eds: Management of Peripheral Nerve Problems. Philadelphia, WB Saunders, 1980:16–29.
13. Mannerfelt L: Studies on the hand in ulnar nerve paralysis. Acta Orthop Scand Supple 87:1–176, 1966.
14. McNamara MJ, Garrett WE, Seaber AV, et al.: Neurorrhaphy, nerve grafting and neurotization: A functional comparison of nerve reconstruction techniques. J Hand Surg 12A:35A–360, 1987.
15. Medical Research Council: Aids to the Examination of the Peripheral Nervous System. Memorandum No. 45. London, Her Majesty's Stationery Office, 1976.
16. Miller RG: Injury to peripheral motor nerves. AAEE Mimeograph No. 28. Muscle Nerve 10:698–710, 1987.
17. Millesi H: Brachial plexus injuries – management and results. Clin Plast Surg 1:115–120, 1984.
18. Mumenthaler M and Schliak H: Lasionen peripherer Nerven, Diagnostik und Therapie. Stuttgart, George Thieme Verlag, 1977.
19. Omer G: Results of untreated peripheral nerve injuries. Clin Orthop Rel Res 163:15–19, 1982.
20. Omer G: The evaluation of clinical results following peripheral nerve suture. In: Omer G and Spinner M, Eds: Management of Peripheral Nerve Problems. Philadelphia, WB Saunders, 1980.
21. Pollock LJ and Davis L: The results of peripheral nerve surgery. In: Peripheral Nerve Injuries. New York, Paul B Hoeber, 1933: 545–561.
22. Seddon HJ: Results of repair of nerves. In: Seddon HJ: Surgical Disorders of the Peripheral Nerves. Baltimore, Williams & Wilkins, 1972:299–315.
23. Spinner M: Factors affecting return of function following nerve injury. In: Spinner M: Injuries to the Major Branches of Peripheral Nerves of the Forearm, 2nd edn. Philadelphia, WB Saunders, 1978:42–51.
24. Sunderland S: Nerves and Nerve Injuries. Baltimore, Williams & Wilkins, 1968.

25. Tinel J: Prognosis and treatment of peripheral nerve lesions. In: Joll CA, Ed: Nerve Wounds. London, Bailliere, Tindall and Cox, 1917:297–299.

26. Woodhall B and Beebe GW, Eds: Peripheral nerve regeneration: A follow-up study of 3656 World War II injuries. Washington, DC, US Government Printing Office, 1956:115–201.

5

Nerve action potential recordings

David G. Kline

OVERVIEW

- The majority of serious nerve injuries requiring operation leave the nerve in gross continuity.
- Judging the potential for a lesion in continuity to regenerate adequately is difficult by inspection, palpation, and even by internal neurolysis and simple stimulation, especially in the early months after injury.
- Use of both stimulation and recording across a lesion in continuity, or what is termed nerve action potential (NAP) recording, provides a measure of the severity of the lesion as well as its potential for recovery.
- Proper electrodes, use of adequate recording equipment, and attention to the details involved in such an electrophysiologic technique are important for optimal results.
- Recordings made proximal to a lesion or from known intact nerves or elements can be used to check the equipment.
- Recordings done over a 30-year period have been matched with histology of resected specimens where traces have been flat and outcomes where NAPs are present. Such data confirm the importance of NAP recordings for such injuries
- NAP recordings can also be used to locate or verify the site(s) of entrapments and to help in the excision of tumors, especially those that are intraneural.
- One can seldom discern the contents of a book by only viewing its cover. Nerve lesions in continuity need to be tested to decide whether they should be resected or not.

Evaluation of lesions in continuity is extremely challenging since preoperative studies, at least in the early months post injury, cannot prove the need for resection and repair, and even intraoperative inspection can be misleading (Fig. 5-1).[2,12,14,19,48,49] Whenever possible, we have tried to evaluate lesions in continuity by stimulation and recording studies of the whole injured peripheral nerve by nerve action potential (NAP) or compound nerve action potential (cNAP) studies. Where such studies have led to resection of a lesion in continuity, the resected segment has been evaluated histologically. Excellent correlation between negative NAP recordings and neurotemetic lesions has been demonstrated in many hundreds of resected nerve specimens. The intraoperative electrical studies have also been correlated with the preoperative severity and clinical course of the patient.[24–26,29] A number of laboratory studies in

primates have also been done.[27,28] NAP studies in those controlled experiments could be correlated with the histology at the recording site. In the primate, an NAP could be recorded distal to a successfully regenerating injury or repair site many weeks to months before there was electromyogram (EMG) evidence of recovery. The presence of an NAP usually related to the presence of 4000 to 5000 nerve fibers 5 microns or greater in diameter with some degree of early myelination. Similar clinical studies using NAP recording have also been subsequently repeated and reported by a number of other investigators.[1,9,20–22,31,34,36,42,43,45,50] The usefulness of the technique (Table 5-1) has also been further substantiated by more recent editorials and papers.[10,32,33,38,44]

Since NAP recordings and results will frequently be referred to in subsequent chapters, review of some of the related important basic considerations as well as instrumentation involved is in order. What follows is partially abstracted from recent as well as older publications on this topic.[17,18] Results with recording for various categories of lesions will be found in the chapter on Grading and in the tables in other chapters on specific nerves (Table 5-2).

BASIC CONSIDERATIONS FOR NAP RECORDING

In healthy nerve, stimulation of a nerve fiber membrane produces a conducted impulse or NAP when stimulus intensity exceeds the fiber's threshold.[8,18] Various axons which respond to lower-intensity stimuli do so because of their membrane properties.[46] The medium-sized fibers have the lowest threshold, the large fibers have the intermediate threshold, and finally the fine or small fibers have the highest threshold.[6,7] NAP amplitude can vary depending on the intensity of the stimulus applied to the whole nerve and, therefore, the number of fibers stimulated.[13,18] If the stimulus is supramaximal in intensity, then NAP amplitude and its integral (area covered by the NAP) will be maximal (Figs 5-2, 5-3).[23,39]

Threshold for stimulation and therefore ability to evoke an NAP depends on both the duration of applied current and the intensity of the stimulus. If the duration is decreased too much, then the intensity must be increased to reach threshold. An injured but regenerating nerve has a spectrum or range of various-sized fibers

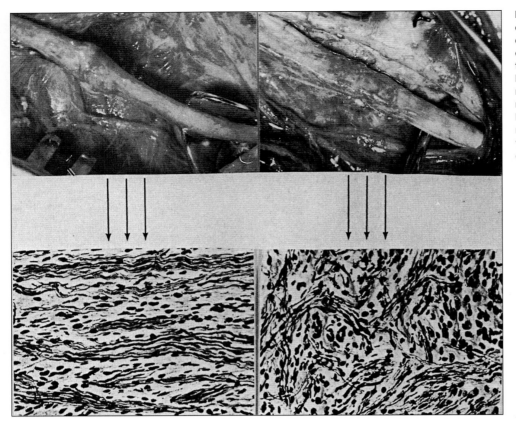

FIGURE 5-1 The usual problem encountered in evaluating a lesion in continuity intraoperatively without electrical recordings. The lesion at the top left appeared irregular and felt firm, but had a very structured and relatively mature axonal pattern at the regenerative site *(bottom left)*. The lesion at the top right appeared relatively non-neuromatous but had a very disorganized regenerative pattern composed of fine axons *(bottom right)*.

Table 5-1 Rationale for NAP recording
Sixty percent or more of nerve injuries have some degree of continuity.
If exploration is determined by failure of anticipated recovery, repair, if needed, will be too late.
Operative inspection and palpitation of a neuroma in continuity can be misleading.
Operative stimulation and recording (NAPs) can provide early information about significant recovery by 8 weeks post injury.
To transmit an NAP through an area of injury requires at least 4000 axons greater than 5 μ in diameter at the recording site.
Presence of an NAP recorded distal to a lesion in continuity in the early months post injury promises recovery without resection and repair.
In an occasional case, one portion of the cross-section of the nerve will be more severely injured than the remainder, and, despite an NAP recorded distal to the injury, will require a split repair.

Table 5-2 Timing for NAP recording
Two to four months for relatively focal contusions due to fractures and gunshot wounds and lacerations in continuity.
Four to five months for stretch injuries, especially those involving plexus.
At any time for partial injuries, entrapments, and other compressive lesions and tumors
In the acute setting, can be used to identify an area of conductive block, although lesion may be due to neurapraxia, axonotmesis, and/or neurotmesis.

reaching the distal stump.[15] This spectrum of fiber sizes alters with the interval after injury and/or repair.[30,40] Small axons, including regenerating fibers, have a much higher threshold and may require substantially greater stimulation to cause an NAP.[17,46] In some abnormal fibers, even maximal intensity of stimuli may not evoke a response without also increasing stimulus duration. This fact is useful for clinical recording because the relatively short stimulus used to reduce stimulus artifact as seen on the oscilloscope screen is also less likely to stimulate small, fine fibers. This helps, because the surgeon needs to evaluate the status of medium-sized or larger fibers between the site stimulated and that recorded from.[18,25] In this fashion, NAP recording can assess regeneration where fiber populations and numbers are different from healthy nerve.[5,16]

Nerve fibers embedded in scar or within tumor will require higher currents for stimulation since both the capacitance and resistance of such tissue tend to shunt stimuli away from the neural tissue.[17] Connective tissue surrounding nerve can also shunt current away from electrodes used for recording. Thus, recording from a regenerating nerve may require not only more intense stimuli to evoke a response, but also higher amplification and very low background noise level for adequate recordings. Surrounding tissues can also reduce NAP amplitude and distort its form. Computer averag-

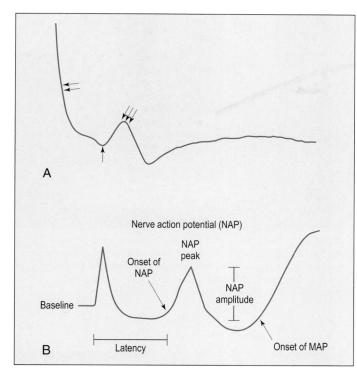

FIGURE 5-2 **(A)** Healthy nerve action potential (NAP) recorded from median nerve. NAP onset is marked by arrow. Downsweep of stimulus artifact is marked by double arrow and peak of NAP amplitude by triple arrow. **(B)** Drawing to show the important features of an evoked NAP. In this instance, the onset of a muscle action potential, or MAP, is also shown. The size of the stimulus artifact will vary according to stimulus intensity.

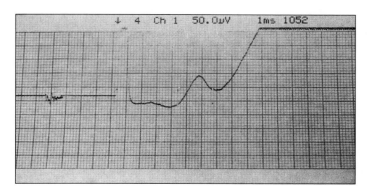

FIGURE 5-3 Nerve action potential recorded distal to an injured upper trunk of the plexus, indicating regeneration across the lesion. This plexus element underwent neurolysis rather than resection and repair. Amplitude is set on 50 μV and timebase on 1 millisecond per division.

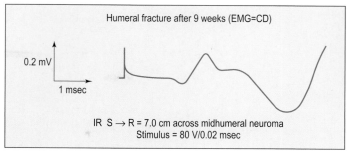

FIGURE 5-4 Recording made across neuroma involving radial nerve in humeral groove secondary to fracture 9 weeks previously. Loss was complete below triceps clinically and by electromyography (EMG). CD, complete denervation; IR, invasive recording; R, recording, S, stimulus. The NAP indicates excellent early regeneration, and as a result only a neurolysis was done. Overall radial recovery was grade 4/5 by 3 years postoperatively.

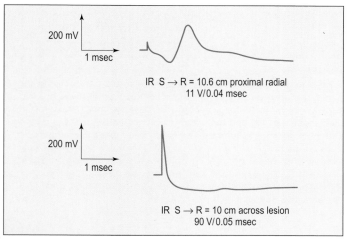

FIGURE 5-5 Operative nerve action potential (NAP) recordings proximal to a radial lesion *(top trace)* and across it *(bottom trace)*. Only a tiny NAP is seen in the lower trace. Lesion was resected and was largely neurotmetic or Sunderland grade IV histologically. Stimulus parameters were 11.0 V at 0.04 msec for proximal trace and 90 V at 0.05 msec for lower trace. IR, invasive recording; S → R, stimulus to recording (distance).

ing may improve noise level and help make the evoked response look better or larger, but does not reflect the activity required for intraoperative decision-making as accurately as a single trace (Fig. 5-4).[17,43]

In a myelinated axon, impulse conduction occurs when a region of active membrane, usually involving several nodes of Ranvier, excites adjacent nodes. Thus, distance between nodes and the number of nodes responding determine the axon's conduction velocity.[3,4,7] Another factor in determining velocity is the time required to reproduce the action potential at each node.[39] Distribu-

tion of conduction velocities amongst myelinated axons is related to both fiber diameters and distances between nodes.[11] The axonal diameter affects the flow of electrical current down the length of an axon and helps determine how many nodes of Ranvier act as a unit.[46] Distribution studies of conduction velocities provide a relationship between NAP, tracing shape and axon composition in the whole nerve.[7]

The presence of a compound nerve action potential or NAP indicates viable axons (Figs 5-5, 5-6). At the recording site in primates, an NAP seems to require at least 4000 moderate or larger-sized fibers with some degree of myelination.[27,28] When this requirement is met in vivo, direct recording does not require excessive amplification or summation. Recording an NAP distal to an injury site correlates with a satisfactory clinical outcome due to spontaneous regeneration.[24] Resection and repair of such a lesion would usually give a less satisfactory outcome. By comparison, though, resection of a non-conducting lesion is necessary since spontaneous recovery will be poor or non-existent without repair.[26]

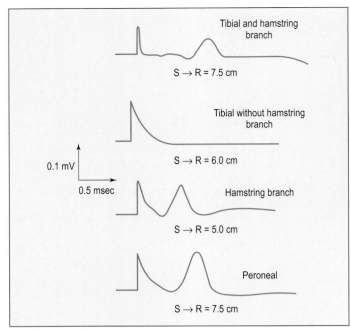

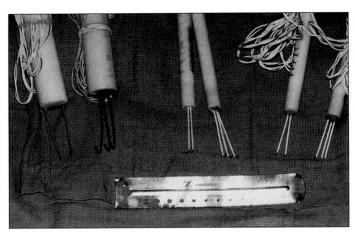

FIGURE 5-6 Recordings made operatively in a patient with lesions in continuity involving both divisions of the sciatic nerve. Recording made from the tibial and hamstring branches together was positive *(top)*. When the hamstring branch was dissected away, tracing from tibial alone was flat and that from the hamstring branch was positive. Thus, the tibial nerve had a neurotmetic injury while the hamstring branch was viable. Nerve action potential recorded from peroneal nerve is seen at the bottom. This patient had a graft repair of the tibial division and only a neurolysis of the peroneal division. Stimulus artifacts in this series of traces have the same amplitude since stimulus intensity was relatively constant.

FIGURE 5-7 Electrodes used for intraoperative nerve action potential recordings. Maxi-electrodes are to the left, mini-electrodes are in the center, and micro-electrodes are to the right. Bipolar recording electrodes are to the left in each pair, and tripolar stimulating electrodes are to the right in each pair.

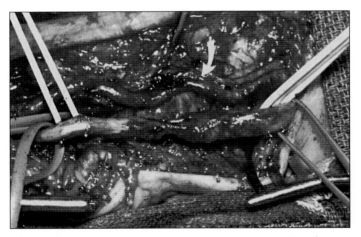

FIGURE 5-8 Recording from ulnar nerve injury in the region of Guyon's canal. Tripolar stimulating electrodes are to the right and bipolar recording electrodes are to the left. There was no transmission in this complete lesion, so a resection and repair were necessary. Ulnar artery has been mobilized away from the ulnar nerve and is seen at the top *(arrow)*.

ELECTRODES USED FOR NAP STIMULATION AND RECORDING

Electrodes are made of either a noble metal such as platinum or medical-grade stainless steel in order to minimize electrolysis associated with metal in contact with the nerve during stimulation. Eighteen-gauge wire is bent like a shepherd's crook on one end so that nerve can be suspended in the crook and gently lifted away from other tissues. The other ends of the wires are placed through the center of a drilled-out Delrin or Teflon rod and soldered to leads for attachment to instrumentation used for stimulating and recording.[17] The drilled-out center of the rod is then sealed with a surgical epoxy cement. When materials are carefully selected, the electrodes can withstand autoclaving, gas sterilization, and water absorption (Fig. 5-7; Table 5-3).

The ends of the two active electrodes used for stimulation are separated by at least 3 mm (Fig. 5-8). Electrode tips are separated by a longer distance of 5–7 mm for stimulation of big nerves such as sciatic or some brachial plexus elements since a larger volume of tissue is involved (Fig. 5-9). If electrode tips are spaced too closely, not all fibers will be stimulated. Stimulation of a nerve both in continuity and in situ differs from the classic physiologic recording in vitro with one or both nerve ends killed. As a result, some small but important alterations in electrode configuration are necessary.

If two stimulating electrode tips are used, there is not only a current generated in the gap between the two but it also flowing

Table 5-3 Intraoperative NAP recording

Stimulus	Setting
Duration	0.05–0.1 msec
Intensity	1.0–125 volts
Frequency	1–2 per second
Recording amplification	20–5 mv per division
Time frame	0.5–2.0 msec per division
Frequency filters	1–3 Hz

msec, milliseconds; mv, millivolts; Hz, Hertz.

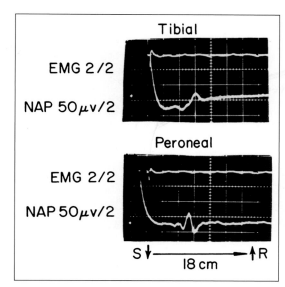

FIGURE 5-9 Nerve action potential (NAP) and evoked electromyographic (EMG) recordings made on tibial and peroneal nerves after evacuation of an old popliteal blood clot and neurolysis of nerves involved by scar. Despite presence of an NAP (lower trace on each graph), no muscle action potential could be recorded from gastrocnemius or from peronei. It was concluded that the NAPs, which conducted at 30 m/sec, were regenerative but that not enough fibers had yet reached musculature to produce an evoked muscle action potential.

away from the electrodes through nerve as well as through other body tissues and back again to nerve. This shock is almost instantaneous but still tends to give a large stimulus artifact. When stimulating and recording montages are relatively close, as they have to be in some clinical situations, the "after-slope" of this stimulus artifact can obscure the evoked NAP. One way to minimize this is to use three tips for the stimulating electrode.[16,26] The outermost two tips are a common anode and are connected one to the other while the middle tip is the cathode. Application of a potential difference between the outermost and innermost active electrodes still produces two currents but neither involves the whole nerve, and thus the stimulus artifact is reduced. The tripolar stimulation electrode also limits the spread of the stimulation current along a longitudinal course in the nerve, making for a more precise and somewhat isolated site of stimulation. Generally, the fidelity of recordings from larger nerves will be optimal if larger-caliber electrodes are used and better for smaller nerve if finer-caliber electrodes are used.

Recording electrode configuration is also important. The electrodes are bipolar and each wire or tip at the recording site is separated by 4–5 mm so that one electrode is recording from an active and the other from a relatively inactive portion of the nerve. The bipolar electrode's recording tips should be separated by as much as a centimeter for relatively large nerves such as the sciatic, femoral, or proximal median. If these two recording tips are too close together on the nerve, amplitude of the evoked NAP can be reduced, or the NAP can be eliminated altogether. When the distance between stimulating and recording electrode montages is large, there is also a need to separate the two recording electrode tips by a greater distance than when recordings are made over a short distance. There is a larger length of active nerve due to greater temporal dispersion in conduction when recordings are made over a long distance. The time of arrival of responses at the recording

site is thus quite variable. This temporal dispersion is due to differences in conduction velocities amongst different-sized myelinated axons.

Distance between stimulating and recording electrode sets is also important. If they are too close, the stimulus artifact will still be extensive despite use of a tripolar stimulating electrode.

Fine electroencephalogram (EEG) needles can also be placed in nerve to both stimulate and record NAPs.[21] When done carefully, this is not damaging even to intact nerve. Needle recordings are especially useful when the surgical exposure of nerve is limited or at a deep level. Usually, two needles are placed in the nerve or element to be evaluated several millimeters apart for stimulation proximally, and then two needles separated by several millimeters more distally.

Lead-in and lead-out wires from the stimulating and recording electrodes should be separated by several inches if possible, otherwise capacitance between the wires can further increase stimulus artifact and also produce other electrical noise.[41] Shielding is usually used for lead-out wires since isolation needs to be maximized. Electrode-to-wire connections and integrity of the wire can be readily checked by use of an amp meter.

Grounding can be provided by attaching the lead-out from a Bovie pad affixed to the patient's skin to the grounding portion of the recording machine. The electrosurgical unit is turned off to provide safe grounding and to reduce unwanted electrical noise. Operating room equipment, which is either battery-operated or motor-driven, such as body and fluid warmers, TCD machines and fluorescent lights should be turned off, or better yet, should be disconnected by having their plugs removed from nearby wall sockets. This reduces the possibility of 60 cycle interference. A single wave isolated from a 60 cycle recording may be misinterpreted as a positive NAP by an inexperienced observer.

STIMULATING AND RECORDING EQUIPMENT

Most electromyographic (EMG) machines manufactured within the last 20 years or so will have the necessary built-in stimulating and recording parameters for satisfactory NAP recording.[17,28] In recent years, we have found it convenient to use the TECA, model TD 20 which is self-contained and provides some degree of flexibility (Fig. 5-10).[25,26] We also have access to a larger Nicolet Spirit Machine which can be programmed for a variety of operative electrophysiological studies. Dr. Robert L. Tiel uses a very compact machine, an XLTEK Neuromax C1004, for his NAP recordings.[41] One can also construct a system using a Grass model stimulator (S-44) with a stimulus isolation unit (SIU-6) to provide stimulation.[29] Recording can be done using an oscilloscope with a differential amplifier, as is available for the Tektronix 7000 series. A trigger wire can be led from the stimulator to the oscilloscope so that a trace will be prompted with each stimulus delivered to the stimulating electrode(s) (Table 5-4).

Whether a compact EMG machine such as the TECA TD 20 or a larger system is used, attention must be paid to both the high- and low-frequency filters. The low-frequency filter setting is usually placed in the 5–10 Hz range or lower and the high-frequency setting at 2500 Hz or higher. These settings tend to decrease stimulus artifact and noise without filtering out the evoked NAP response. If over filtered, the stimulus artifact will be greater and the amplitude as well as the integral of the NAP less. If a 60 Hz notch filter is built into the recording instrument, it is usually better not to use

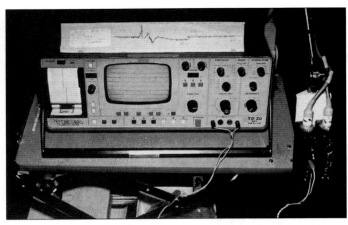

FIGURE 5-10 TECA TD 20 electromyography instrument used for stimulation and recording. Stimulating electrodes are led out of the stimulating portion of the instrument at the bottom and recording electrodes into differential amplifier to the right of the photograph. Tracing propped on top of the instrument is of a nerve action potential recorded at a site distal to a stretch injury involving an axillary nerve.

Table 5-4 Intraoperative NAP recording steps

If possible, place both stimulating and recording electrodes proximal to the injury site, separated by 3–4 cm and record a proximal NAP. An adjacent, less-involved element or nerve can be tested to check the equipment when proximal nerve is not available.

Keeping stimulus duration brief, gradually increase stimulus intensity until NAP is evoked. Gradually increase amplification. Try different low- and high-frequency filters to optimize the evoked response.

Move distal recording electrodes into or onto the injury site to see if an NAP response is maintained.

Amplification setting may have to be increased further and/or filters further adjusted.

Move recording electrodes distal to the injury site to see if an NAP response can be evoked to that level and if so, how far down the distal stump it can be recorded.

Observe muscle(s) distal to stimulation site(s) for contraction.

---

it for NAP recording. The filter device itself can generate a wave resembling an NAP.

TECHNIQUE FOR STIMULATING AND RECORDING NAPS

Short-duration stimuli are used both to decrease stimulus artifact and to decrease stimulation of fine fibers which may or may not mature with further time and lead to useful function. Typical settings range between 0.05 to 0.1 msec in duration. This requires increased voltage for adequate stimulation. While healthy nerves may require voltages between 3 and 15 V, regenerating nerve may need 100 V or more. Frequency of stimulation should be kept at

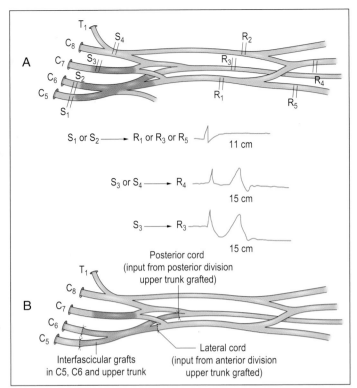

FIGURE 5-11 Use of nerve action potential (NAP) recording to sort out a stretch injury involving right C5, C6, and C7 spinal nerves and their more distal outflows as viewed from the side. In this case, recordings proximal to the injury sites were not possible. Stimulation of C5 and C6 and recording from upper trunk divisions as well as lateral and posterior cords gave no NAPs. Stimulation of C7 to middle trunk, and posterior cord gave an NAP, as did stimulation and recording from the lower plexus elements. A graft repair extending from proximal C5 and C6 to lateral and posterior cords was carried out. It would have been difficult to make the correct intraoperative decisions regarding resection without the use of NAP recordings.

2 per second or less to prevent damage to nerve with these short-duration, high-voltage stimuli.

NAPs are recorded with the oscilloscope set between 50 μV and 5 mV per division on the oscilloscope face. The time base is set at 0.5–2 msec per division. We usually begin by recording the NAP proximal to the injury site by both stimulating and recording above it (Fig. 5-11).[24] If electrodes as well as stimulating and recording equipment are working, and 3–4 or more centimeters of nerve can be exposed proximal to the lesion in continuity, an NAP response should be recordable. Alternatively, NAPs are recorded from an adjacent, healthy nerve or plexus element. These maneuvers ensure that the entire system is functioning properly. If the recordings are suboptimal, all equipment is checked in a systematic way before any attempt is made to record from the injured nerve. Recording electrodes are then moved onto the lesion site and beyond to see if an NAP can be recorded and, if so, how far distal to the injury site (Fig. 5-12). If a proximal segment of the injured nerve is not available for a baseline recording, then an adjacent uninvolved nerve may be used to check the electrodes and the stimulation and recording settings. These settings can then be used as a starting point to stimulate and record from the injured nerve (Fig. 5-13). Intensity of stimulation and, if need be, duration can be increased as well as amplification used for recording. There are cases, particu-

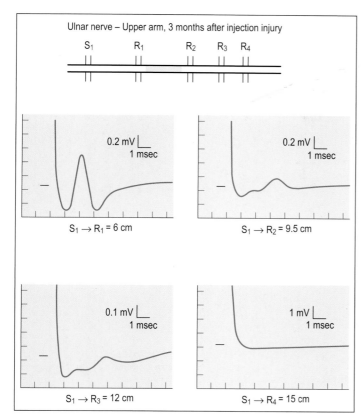

FIGURE 5-12 Operative nerve action potential (NAP) studies on an injection injury of the ulnar nerve at 3 months after injury. S_1 to R_1 is a recording proximal to the lesion. S_1 to R_2 is a recording across the lesion, and S_1 to R_3 and S_1 to R_4 are recordings made more distally. This nerve was regenerating well despite complete loss of function clinically, and electrically, more distally. Therefore, only neurolysis was performed and the lesion was not resected. (From Kline D: Microsurgery of peripheral nerves: Selection for and timing of operation. In: Bunke H and Furnas D, Eds: Symposium on Clinical Frontiers in Reconstructive Microsurgery. St. Louis, CV Mosby, 1984:341–349.)

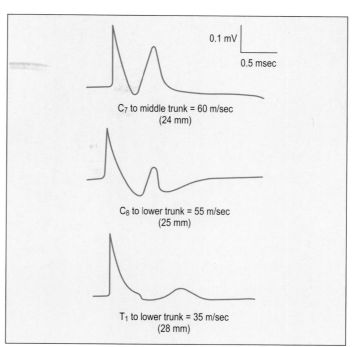

FIGURE 5-13 Operative nerve action potential recordings from a patient suspected of thoracic outlet syndrome. T1 to lower trunk trace is reduced in amplitude, has a broad base, and is relatively slow at 35 m/sec. This indicates an irritative and/or compressive lesion involving T1 to lower trunk. A neurolysis of the lower elements of the plexus was done. C7 to middle trunk recordings were normal by comparison.

larly when severe plexus stretch injuries are studied intraoperatively, where one cannot record from nerve proximal to injury site or even from other uninvolved or less involved nerves.[26] One must then be content with stimulating at the lesion site or even distal to it and recording below or distally.

Response of distal muscle to stimulation of nerve proximal to a lesion is also noted since contraction usually indicates good regeneration not only through the lesion but to that muscle.[35,37] Since the limb must therefore be available for inspection and palpation throughout the operation, appropriate draping at the start of the operation is essential. In general, however, in the early months post injury, such obvious evidence of sparing or recovery will usually not be present unless the lesion was partial to begin with.

The objective in operative recording is to measure an NAP distal to the lesion. In the initial 9 months after injury, the NAP's amplitude and conduction velocity are not as important as the simple presence or absence of a response. Presence of an NAP indicates axons of sufficient number, caliber, and maturation to presage useful recovery of function for at least a portion of the injured cross-section of nerve. Absence of an NAP indicates that recovery will not occur without resection and repair. An NAP recorded a year or more after injury across a lesion in continuity with severe

clinical loss should have moderately good amplitude and conduction great than 30 m/sec.

In some cases, an NAP is present but visual inspection of the conducting segment suggests that one portion of the lesion's cross-section is more severely involved than another. Then, the lesion can be split into groups of fascicles, and these fascicular groups or individual fascicles can be tested separately.[41,42,47] Usually, some fascicles conduct and others do not. This leads to a split repair, in which a portion of the nerve is repaired by direct suture or graft and a portion by neurolysis alone.

As stimulation and recording begin, the stimulus intensity (voltage) is gradually increased, and the amplification for recording is also increased until an NAP is seen. Different filter settings can also be tried. The stimulating electrodes are usually placed proximally since that stimulation site ensures activation of a maximal number of fibers.[40,41] If a stimulus site proximal to an injured but regenerating nerve is accessible, more normal fibers can be stimulated proximally than distally.[16,18] This decreases the need for a high-intensity stimulus and, as a result, decreases the stimulus artifact recorded distally. Stimulating and recording electrode tips are used to lift and hold the nerve away from other tissues or tissue fluids (Figs 5-14 to 5-16).

More distal evoked muscle action potentials (MAPs) can be picked up by the recording electrodes placed on nerve. These responses, however, are quite delayed compared to NAPs. Their calculated velocities are slow, usually less than 20 m/sec. They are also larger in amplitude than NAPs and more likely to be polyphasic and to have a broader base than an NAP.

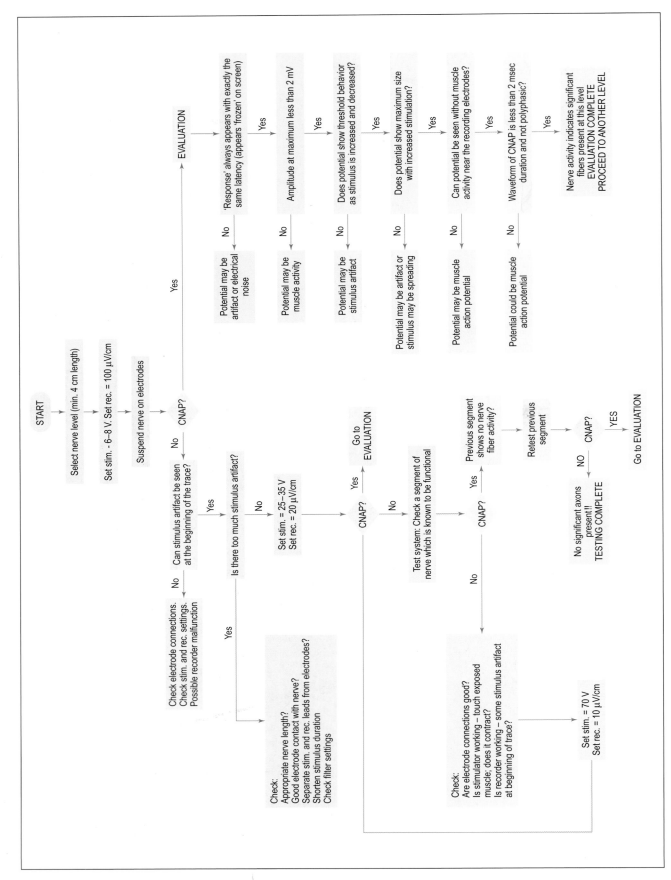

FIGURE 5-14 Algorithm for use with evaluation of nerve action potential results.

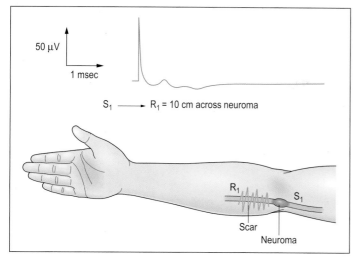

FIGURE 5-15 Ulnar neuroma caused by fracture and contusion at the level of the elbow. Despite complete clinical loss below flexor carpi ulnaris and complete denervation as confirmed by electromyography, a nerve action potential could be recorded to a point 6 cm distal to the neuroma. As a result, a neurolysis, transposition, and submuscular burial were done.

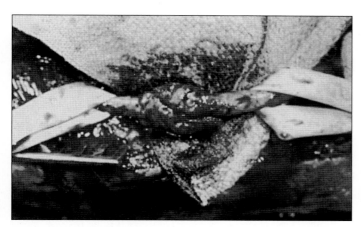

FIGURE 5-16 Large ulnar lesion in continuity caused by contusion associated with a fracture, which conducted a nerve action potential, much to our surprise. The patient recovered a great deal of function after neurolysis and transposition beneath pronator teres and flexor carpi ulnaris.

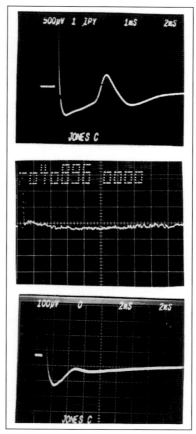

FIGURE 5-17 A series of electrical traces recorded from an injured median nerve at a forearm level with complete loss distal to the injury. Top trace was an operative trace made proximal to the injury site. Bottom trace was recorded operatively across the injury site at 3.5 months, indicating early but adequate regeneration through the lesion. Middle trace was an attempt to evoke a response across the lesion noninvasively and at a skin level. However, even with summation, the small potential seen in the bottom trace could not be recorded noninvasively. This nerve did well with only a neurolysis.

NAP trace may be flat, much as with a lesion present lateral to the dorsal root ganglion (Table 5-5).

OTHER PRECAUTIONS

If an extremity is operated on under tourniquet and the latter is inflated for 60 minutes or longer, the tourniquet should be left down for 20 or more minutes before NAP recording is tried. Ischemia as well as low wound temperature can block successful recordings.[17,40] In several earlier cases done under tourniquet, NAP traces were flat and yet regeneration as shown by either histologic study of resected segment or subsequent clinical course was adequate.[25] One also has to be careful of local anesthetic use that may also temporarily block conduction. Since the block can persist for many hours, absence of an NAP may not under theses circumstances indicate resection. On the other hand, muscle paralysis by curare-like drugs does not interfere with NAP recording. Discussion with the anesthetist preoperatively will result in anesthetic technique in which neuromuscular blockade used in induction will have worn off by the time the surgeon has dissected the area of injury. The surgeon is thus able to stimulate normal and/or injured

PREGANGLIONIC PLEXUS LESIONS

With a plexus lesion, where spinal nerves or roots are injured at a preganglionic level but are intact postganglionically, rapidly conducting (60–80 m/sec) and relatively large-amplitude NAPs can be recorded (Fig. 5-17). This is due to the fact that the large and well-myelinated sensory fibers have been spared Wallerian degeneration and, when stimulated, conduct a rapid and large response. These responses differ from slower, lower-amplitude regenerative NAPs and may even be faster and larger than those seen when recording from an intact plexus element.[13,26] If there is doubt, the proximal part of the spinal nerve can be stimulated and an attempt made to record somatosensory evoked potentials via cutaneous electrodes placed previously over the upper and posterior cervical spine area. With preganglionic injury, these evoked responses will be absent. If there are both pre- and postganglionic lesions, the

Table 5-5 Results* of NAP recordings for injuries 1967–2001

Nerve	No. patients	+ NAP neurolysis	+ NAP split repair	– NAP suture or graft
Accessory	55	19/19+	1/1	35/25
Axillary	99	30/29	2/2	67/40
Median	125	73/69	3/3	49/39
Radial	119	64/63	2/2	53/46
Ulnar	126	85/80	5/5	36/24
Multiple nerves	53	62/55	5/5	64/42
Plexus lacerations	20	26/24	2/2	31/24
Plexus GSW	118	128/120	2/2	163/92
Plexus stretch	481	319/280	27/23	1007/502
Tibial divisions	352	219/199	5/5	128/99
Peroneal divisions	347	219/159	3/3	125/54
Tibial	70	39/33	2/2	29/24
Peroneal	241	95/81	3/3	143/60
Femoral	89	44/44	0/0	45/40
Total	2295	1422/1255 (94.7%)	62/58 (94%)	1975/1101 (56%)

*Grade 3 or better recovery on the LSUHSC grading scale.

+Number of nerves or elements studied/number gaining a grade or better level of recovery.

nerve, observe the effect of appropriate muscle contraction, and then elicit NAPs from nerves which give no response to direct stimulation. Once the NAP recording phase of the operation is concluded, the anesthetist can use whatever anesthetic technique he or she prefers.

Noninvasive recording of whole or NAPs is possible for some nerve lesions, but has a definite incidence of false-negative traces, as subsequently shown by intraoperative NAP studies. Such recordings are more readily achieved with nerves distal in the extremity and close to skin such as median or ulnar close to the wrist. Occasionally, stimulation of a nerve close to but uninvolved by the injury will produce a false-positive study, so patients have to be carefully selected for such a noninvasive approach.

CONCLUSION

The majority of serious injuries affecting nerve leave it in continuity. Some lesions recover enough function in the early months after injury to make operative intervention unnecessary; some do not, and then the operative decision whether to resect the lesion or not can be difficult. Inspection and palpation can be misleading, and simple stimulation may provide contraction in muscles with relatively early innervation distal to the lesion; however, with serious injuries to most major nerves, stimulation cannot be expected to do so for many months. Furthermore, an occasional lesion with an injury site that has primarily poor regenerative potential will permit a few hundred axons to reach a distal muscle site and thus respond to stimulation. By comparison, an adequately regenerating nerve

will have thousands of axons extending through the injury site and into the distal stump by 2–3 months post injury, and yet will not have enough distal muscular input to reverse denervational changes seen by EMG or for the nerve to respond to simple stimulation. Where injury involves an element of stretch, even finding fascicular continuity by internal neurolysis can be misleading because intrafascicular injury can be neurotemetic rather than axonotemetic.

One way to measure regeneration into the distal nerve is to both stimulate and record across the injury site. This is NAP recording. These studies have been performed on almost all of the lesions in continuity reported in this text. Since presence or absence of an operative NAP has helped direct the operative management in this series, the rationale for this operative approach, the techniques and equipment used for such recordings, and the overall results with a variety of lesions in various nerves are summarized in this chapter. Emphasized is whether or not a response is present rather than its configuration, latency, or velocity.

If an NAP was present in this series, the lesion usually had an external neurolysis if unassociated with pain or an internal neurolysis if severe and neuritic pain was a problem. Some lesions in continuity having an NAP had more obvious severe injury to one portion of the nerve than to another. In these cases, the nerve was split into groups of fascicles and differentially evaluated by NAP recordings. A split repair was then usually done.

Those lesions in continuity not transmitting an NAP 2 or more months post injury were resected and proven to be neurotemetic or Sunderland grade IV histologically. NAP recording was also used as an investigative tool for entrapments such as those involving ulnar, posterior interosseous, or peroneal nerves or plexus elements in presumed thoracic outlet cases as well as in tumors arising from or involving nerve(s).

REFERENCES

1. Calder H, Mast J, and Johnstone C: Intraoperative evoked potential monitoring in acetabular surgery. Clin Orthop 205:160–167, 1994.
2. Carter G, Robinson L, Chang V, et al.: Electrodiagnostic evaluation of traumatic nerve injuries. Hand Clin 16(1):1–12, 2000.
3. Collins W, O'Leary J, Hunt W, et al.: An electrophysiological study of nerve regeneration in the cat. J Neurosurg 12:39–46, 1955.
4. Cragg BG and Thomas PK: Changes in conduction velocity and fiber size proximal to peripheral nerve lesions. J Physiol 157:315–327, 1961.
5. Cragg BG and Thomas PK: The conduction velocity of regenerated peripheral nerve fibers. J Physiol (London) 171:164–175, 1964.
6. Dawson GD: The relative excitability and conduction velocity of sensory and motor nerve fibers in man. J Physiol (London) 131:436–451, 1956.
7. Dorfman L et al.: Conduction Velocity Distributions: A Population Approach to Electrophysiology of Nerve. New York, WR Liss, 1981.
8. Erlanger J and Gasser H: Electrical Signs of Nervous Activity. Philadelphia, University of Pennsylvania Press, 1937.
9. Freidman W: The electrophysiology of peripheral nerve injuries. Neorosurg Clin N Am 2:1:43–56, 1992.
10. Gabriel E, Villavicencio A, and Friedman A: Evaluation and surgical repair of brachial plexus injuries. Sem Neurosurg 12(1):29–48, 2001.
11. Galbrath J and Meyers R: Impulse conduction. In: Gelberman R.H., Ed: Operative Nerve Repair and Reconstruction. Philadelphia, JB Lippincott, 1991:19–45.
12. Gilliatt R: Physical injury to peripheral nerves: Physiologic and electrodiagnostic aspects. Mayo Clin Proc 56:361–370, 1981.
13. Gilliatt RW and Sears TA: Sensory nerve action potentials in patients with peripheral nerve lesions. J Neurol Neurosurg Psych 21:109–118, 1958.
14. Grundfest H, Oester YT, and Beebe GW: Electrical evidence of regeneration. In: Woodhall B, Beebe GW, Eds: Peripheral Nerve Regeneration. Washington, DC, US Government Printing Office, 1956.
15. Gutman E and Sanders F: Recovery of fiber numbers and diameters in the regeneration of peripheral nerves. J Physiol 101:489, 1943.
16. Hallin RG, Wiesenfeld Z, and Lungregord H: Neurophysiological studies of peripheral nerve functions after neural regeneration following nerve suture in man. Int Rehabil Med 3:187–192, 1981.
17. Happel L and Kline D: Nerve lesions in continuity. In: Gelberman R, Ed: Operative Nerve Repair and Reconstruction. Philadelphia, JB Lippincott, 1991.
18. Happel L and Kline D: Intraoperative neurophysiology of the peripheral nervous system In: Deletis V, Shils J, Eds: Neurophysiology in Neurosurgery. New York, Academic Press, Elsevier Sci, 2002:269–194.
19. Hodgkin A and Huxley A: Currents carried by sodium and potassium ions through the membrane of the giant axon of Loglio. J Physiol 116:449, 1952.
20. Hudson A and Hunter D: Timing of peripheral nerve repair: important local neuropathologic factors. Clin Neurosurg 24:392–405, 1977.
21. Hudson AR and Trammer B: Brachial plexus injuries. In: Wilkins R, Rengachary S, Eds: Neurosurgery. New York, McGraw Hill, 1985.
22. Kaplan B, Freidman W, and Gravenstein D: Intraoperative electrophysiology in treatment of peripheral nerve injuries. J Fla Med Assoc 71:400–403, 1984.
23. Kimura J: Electrodiagnosis in Diseases of Nerve and Muscle: Principles and Practice. Philadelphia, FA Davis, 1983.
24. Kline DG and Hackett ER: Reappraisal of timing for exploration of civilian peripheral nerve injuries. Surgery 78:54–65, 1975.
25. Kline DG and Hackett ER: The neuroma-in-continuity: A management problem. In: Wilkins RH and Rengachary S, Eds: Neurosurgery. New York, McGraw-Hill, 1984. See also Midha R, Kline D: Evaluation of neuroma in continuity. In: Omer G, Spinner M, and Van Beek A, Eds: Management of Peripheral Nerve Problems. Philadelphia, WB Saunders, 1998.
26. Kline DG, Hackett ER, and Happel L: Review of surgical lesions of the brachial plexus. Arch Neurology 43:170–181, 1985.
27. Kline DG and DeJonge BR: Evoked potentials to evaluate peripheral nerve injuries. Surg Gynecol Obstet 127:1239–1250, 1968.
28. Kline DG, Hackett ER, and May PR: Evaluation of nerve injuries by evoked potentials and electromyography. J Neurosurg 31:128–136, 1969.
29. Kline DG and Nulsen FE: The neuroma-incontinuity: Its preoperative and operative management. Surg Clin N Am 52:1189–1209, 1972.
30. Lyons W and Woodhall B: Atlas of Peripheral Nerve Injuries. Philadelphia, WB Saunders, 1949.
31. McGillicuddy J: Clinical decision-making in brachial plexus injuries. Neorosurg Clin N Am 2:1:137–150, 1992.
32. Midha R and MacKay M: Principles of nerve regeneration and surgical repair. Sem Neurosurg (N Af ed) 12(1):81–92, 2001.
33. Nath N: Preface to Seminars in Neurosurgery 12(1):3, 2001.
34. Nelson KR: Use of peripheral nerve action potentials for intraoperative monitoring. Neurol Clin 6:917–933, 1988.
35. Nulsen FE and Lewey FH: Intraneural bipolar stimulation: A new aid in the assessment of nerve injuries. Science 106:301, 1947.
36. Oberle J, Antoniadis G, Ruth S, et al.: Value of nerve action potentials in surgical management of traumatic nerve lesions. Neurosurgery 41(6):1337–1344, 1997.
37. Seddon HJ: Surgical Disorders of the Peripheral Nerves. Baltimore, Williams & Wilkins, 1972.
38. Spinner M: Peripheral nerve problems – past, present, and future In: Management of Peripheral Nerve Problems, 2nd Edn. WB Saunders, 1998.
39. Sumner A: The Physiology of Peripheral Nerve Disease. Philadelphia, WB. Saunders, 1980.
40. Sunderland S: Nerves and Nerve Injuries, 2nd edn. Edinburgh, Churchill-Livingstone, 1978.
41. Tiel R, Happel L, and Kline D: Nerve action potential recording method and equipment. Neurosurgery 39(1):103–109, 1996.
42. Terzis J and Dykes R: Electorphysiological recordings in peripheral nerve surgery: A review. J Hand Surg 1:52–66, 1976.
43. Van Beek A: Intraoperative nerve stimulation and recording techniques In: Management of Peripheral Nerve Problems, 2nd Edn. WB Saunders, 1998.
44. Van Beek A, Hubble B, and Kinkead L: Clinical use of nerve stimulation and recording. Plast Reconst Surg 71:225–232, 1983.
45. Vanderark G, Meyer G, Kline D, et al.: Peripheral nerve injuries studied by evoked potential recordings. Mil Med 135(2):90–94, 1970.
46. Waxman SG: Physiology and Pathobiology of Axons. New York, Raven Press, 1978.
47. Williams HB and Terzis JK: Single fascicular recordings: An intraoperative diagnostic tool for the management of peripheral nerve lesions. Plast Reconstr Surg 57:562–569, 1976.
48. Woodhall B, Nulsen F, White Jet al.: Neurosurgical implications. In: Peripheral Nerve Regeneration. Washington, DC, V.A. Monograph, US Government Printing Office, 1957.
49. Zachary R and Roaf R: Lesions in continuity. In: Seddon H, Ed: Peripheral Nerve Injuries. Her Majesty's Stationery Office, Med. Res. Council Spec. Report, Series No. 282, 1954.
50. Zalis A, Rodriguez A, Oester Y, et al.: Evaluation of nerve regeneration by means of evoked potentials. J Bone Joint Surg 54A:1246–1253, 1972.

Operative care and techniques

Robert J. Spinner

OVERVIEW

- Thorough physical examination and adequate electrodiagnostic and radiologic studies are necessary prerequisites.
- Mastery of the anatomy needed for exposure and repair is a necessity.
- Exposure of the nerve proximal and distal to the injury site and a thorough external neurolysis of lesions in continuity or if there has been nerve transection is important.
- Operative nerve action potential recordings across lesions in continuity permit a relatively early decision for or against resection.
- Where repair is necessary, an end-to-end epineurial-level suture is preferred provided tension is minimal and such can be provided by mobilization, nerve transfer, and/or mild flexion of elbow, knee, or hip
- If the gap for repair is large, and end-to-end repair is not possible without moderate tension at the repair site, then autologous grafts are needed.
- Grafts are placed using interfascicular repair and donors such as sural, antebrachial cutaneous, or superficial sensory nerves.
- Internal neurolysis is done for nerve lesions transmitting an NAP and having neuritic pain not managed well by pharmacology. Other indications for internal neurolysis are asymmetric lesions where one portion of the cross-section is functional and one part is not. Differential NAP recordings can then lead to a split repair.
- Postoperative wound care that is meticulous, instruction of the patient and family, and postoperative outpatient follow-up are all important.
- Provision of exercises to maintain range of motion (ROM) and to strengthen the limb is needed, as eventually are orders for physical and occupational therapy.
- Postoperatively, patients and their families will appreciate a realistic assessment of potential outcomes and an estimated timetable for any recovery of function.

PREOPERATIVE EVALUATION, CARE, AND COUNSELING

The preoperative assessment of patients with nerve-related problems should be conducted in a systematic, logical approach. Evaluation should include a comprehensive history and physical examination, typically supplemented by electrodiagnostic and imaging studies. The decision to operate is a joint decision by the patient and the surgeon but the type of procedure, and the timing of intervention are based on a surgeon's knowledge and experience. Timely referral is necessary if, and when, the initial physician does not feel comfortable treating or operating on a patient. Sequential examinations may be necessary to determine if delayed surgery is indicated or not, depending on the presence of clinical and/or electrical signs of recovery.

Whether or not surgery is being considered in the near or distant future, physicians should address early on the patients' rehabilitative needs as well as any pain and psychological issues. Physical therapy is an important and necessary part of a treatment plan to maintain passive and active range of motion in affected and neighboring joints and strengthen muscles that are functioning. Injured nerves do not recover by being put to rest. Immobilized joints stiffen rapidly. A potentially successful operation on nerve(s) can be markedly compromised when joint contractures develop. Range of motion (ROM) exercises must be performed frequently and repetitively. Provision of physical therapy once a day during the workweek does not suffice to keep a paralyzed limb sufficiently mobile. The patient and his or her family must be shown how to provide ROM not only to joints subtended by the paralysis but also to those above and below. Such home ROM must be done many times a day. All too often, a patient presents with a stiff and painful shoulder, elbow, or wrist whose neuropathy originated only weeks earlier. A similar scenario can affect the lower extremity. Hip, knee, or ankle stiffness can readily occur if non-weight-bearing has been (wrongly) advised after nerve injury. There are, admittedly, clinical settings in which concomitant bony, vascular, or tendinous injury requires a period of immobilization. Even in these settings, though, structured therapy directed toward shoulder, fingers, hip, or foot helps to maintain the limb as optimally as possible. From the outset, the patient must assume responsibility for the denervated limb. A passive attitude, in which the patient assumes that the physical therapist will do the work, is associated with bad clinical outcomes.

Neuropathic pain may be severe and may be even more of an issue than the new neurologic deficit. Neuropathic pain should be treated aggressively, as it impedes both a patient's desire to perform physical therapy and his or her psychology and overall well-being.

While many physicians feel comfortable initiating a program consisting of pharmacologic agents and physical therapy in patients with mild pain, a multidisciplinary pain center may be helpful in dealing with more severe or refractory pain syndromes. In these cases, specialists in pain management can titrate one or more medications, or utilize other modalities in an attempt to control patients' pain more effectively.

The patient's psychological state during both the preoperative and postoperative period is of the utmost importance. This factor alone may be the single most important determinant of overall outcome. Depression and anxiety are common after significant nerve injury. These emotional responses result from many factors: physical limitations, pain, cosmetic concerns, and economic hardships. They should be explored with the patient and managed appropriately. A depressed patient who does not initially obey the surgeon's instructions and who subsequently fails to participate in a vigorous home physical therapy program may also complain bitterly of dysesthesias and pain. Such a psychological state can defeat the results that could have been realized after successful surgery. Conversely, a patient who optimizes residual and returning function rather than complaining of the deficit is more likely to regain a useful, functioning limb, even if perfection is not achieved.

The surgeon has many counseling responsibilities. First, he or she must educate the patient and the family about the nature of the nerve-related problem, the indications for surgery, the advantages and disadvantages of surgery and specific techniques, possible complications and realistic outcomes to expect with operative or non-operative intervention in terms of restoring or improving function, form and pain. Preoperatively, the surgeon should try to provide a description of the possible procedures (with planned incisions) to be done, such as neurolysis, suture, nerve grafting, and split repair, and nerve transfer, and give the patient some idea of results with each. Postoperatively, the surgeon has a feel for the procedure's possible success and can usually provide a more accurate estimate of expected recovery or lack thereof. A more precise prognosis hinges on the operative findings. Unfortunately, recovery of significant function rarely can be promised, and because of the severity of the lesion (e.g. the nerve involved, or concomitant injuries), or timing of intervention, failure can result. The patient and the patient's family must be made to understand that the operation may not work (Table 6-1). The fact that restoration of useful function after major injuries often takes years rather than weeks or months to occur must be emphasized. Patients are usually unaware of these time frames and may expect immediate postoperative recovery. Despite advance preparations, some patients still awaken from their operation disappointed that their limb movement has not been magically restored and with the belated realization that they face a lengthy period of waiting and hard work on their part to optimize any recovery that may occur. There must also be a commitment to long-term self-care of the limb and completion of a certain number of follow-up visits. In our practice, we have developed pamphlets describing some of these issues in relatively simple language for patient use.

OPERATIONS

SCHEDULING

The timing of surgery depends on many factors, but especially the type of injury (e.g. laceration, blunt transection, stretch/contusion, compression, etc.) and the timing of presentation. The duration of

Table 6-1 Preoperative care

Initial wound or injury care for soft tissue damage of anteries, tendons, bones, chest, abdomen, etc.
Appropriate radiographs and, on occasion, scanning studies.
Early clinical grading of both motor and sensory function.
Baseline electromyogram at 2–3 weeks.
Institution of early range of motion and, it possible, strengthening exercises of spared or potentially injured functional units.
Several visits for clinical examination and electromyographic evaluation if delayed surgery is indicated.
Realistic appraisal of possible outcomes for the patient and the patient's family.
Preoperative clearance by medical and anesthesia services; preoperative antibiotic administration.

surgery varies considerably. A brachial plexus procedure may be concluded in 3–12 hours, depending on the pathology revealed and the reconstruction attempted. On occasion, operations may be performed in two stages, with a total duration well in excess of 12 hours. If bone, vessel, or tendon work is required, this is best accomplished before nerve surgery, either at the same or in a separate (previous) operation. In this way, nothing in subsequent procedures will disturb a delicate nerve repair.

Preoperative clearance should be obtained by medical and anesthesia services.

THE OPERATIVE TEAM

The surgeon and his or her team should be well rested and prepared for the surgery. To do this well, the operator should have a detailed and profound knowledge of the immediate and surrounding anatomy of the site of nerve injury. Electrophysiologists or technicians should be available to assist in the performance of nerve action potential (NAP) or other nerve recordings (e.g. electromyography, somatosensory evoked potentials, and motor evoked potentials). Usually, a single surgical assistant suffices, but segments of complex operations may necessitate additional help, and appropriate individuals should be available to harvest sural nerves and close multiple operative wounds simultaneously. The operating room nurse is an important member of the team. It helps if the scrub nurse is interested in and has some knowledge of the basic anatomy, physiology, and pathology of nerve injuries and tumors. The scrub nurse should be in charge of the sterilization, packaging, and subsequent arrangement of the various surgical instruments, as well as the electrodes and other equipment needed for operative recordings. The anesthesiologist should be familiar with the specifics of peripheral nerve surgery – such as avoiding paralytic agents when surgeons are dissecting around nerves or performing certain intraoperative recordings, and maintaining patient immobility at the conclusion of the procedure, while dressings and casts are being applied. Pathologists should be available to review histologic sections; the scheduled pathologist should have reviewed any slides obtained from any previous biopsy before the new specimens are examined. Biopsies may be of single fascicles, and the pathologist must be comfortable handling small specimens. On occasion, a vascular surgeon should be on standby, should an arterial injury occur during a difficult re-exploration of an infraclavicular exposure after a previous arterial repair was done.

POSITIONING

The patient should be positioned so as to avoid pressure palsies. Limbs must be available for inspection during surgery. Broad exposure is helpful. Both legs must be available for potential sural nerve donation and access to the chest is necessary for intercostal nerve harvesting. Limbs may need to be moved during surgery, and draping should accommodate this. Drapes at the root of limbs should not be so snug as to cause a venous tourniquet effect. Surface electrodes for somatosensory evoked potential recording should be checked immediately before skin preparation to ensure they have not moved during patient positioning.

If an operating microscope is to be used later in the procedure, it helps to position and sometimes drape it before the procedure begins. Trial positioning of the microscope should ensure that, if the instrument is subsequently used, both surgeon and assistant can work in comfort for prolonged periods without cervical or lumbar strain. The lens and eyepiece can be partially focused and positioned for the surgeon and the surgeon's assistant. In addition, this "dry run" will help place the scrub nurse and the instrument table(s). A display monitor for the microscope should be prepared, as it allows all personnel in the operating room the opportunity to visualize this delicate part of the procedure well.

INSTRUMENTATION

There is no set position for the instrument tray; adaptation and innovation are necessary according to potential access required for graft donation, positioning of the surgeon and assistant, and location of the anesthetic equipment. The operating technician or instrument nurse should have comfortable access during potentially prolonged operations.

We prefer a variety of scalpels including a long-handled plastic knife holder with a No. 15 blade and long-handled Metzenbaum scissors for most dissections (Fig. 6-1). Cushing or similar forceps are used for much of the dissection, and ophthalmic forceps are used for fascicular work. Penrose drains and fine plastic loops (Vasaloops) are helpful for neural retraction. A variety of hemostats, Moynihans, and self-retaining retractors are necessary, as is an assortment of microinstruments, including several types of bipolar forceps, microscissors, and microforceps. Instruments are conveniently separated into macro- and micro-sets. Especially useful for initial placement of drains around nerves is a Jacobsen with a curved but blunt tip, or what we term a "click-a-clack."

Variable-caliber, pressure-controlled suction tubes are needed during the macro- and microstages of the operation. Large-caliber, high-pressure suction tubes tend to injure the sites of nerve surgery. A cell saver may be helpful for large operations or those in which blood loss is predicted to be high. Provision of both the Bovie and a good bipolar coagulator is necessary.

INITIAL (MACRO) EXPOSURE

The initial approach, such as skin incision and soft tissue dissection to reach nerves, in most nerve operations may be performed with

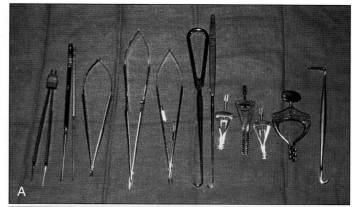
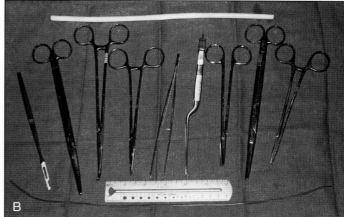

FIGURE 6-1 Display on operating table of some of the instruments more commonly used during peripheral nerve surgery. **(A)** Fine bipolar forceps, microscissors, and right-angled dissector for passing drains beneath nerves (curved Jacobsen or "click-a-clack"), vein retractors, and a variety of small Alm and mastoid retractors as well as a small plastic rake. **(B)** No. 15 scalpel blade on a long-handled knife, a long variety of Metzenbaum scissors, Moynihans, a Cushing-Gerald forceps with teeth, bayonet-shaped bipolar forceps with relatively broad tips, other Metzenbaum scissors, and a needle-nosed suture holder. A Penrose drain (top), and a rule and a plastic loop (bottom).

or without magnification, depending on the surgeon's preference. During the initial exposure, cutaneous nerves should be identified and protected whenever possible. Dissection of nerve and attendant scar, as well as preservation of adjacent structures, is aided by the use of loupes or microscope. Exposure should be generous. Normal nerve above and below the injury should also be exposed to allow identification of discrete nerve elements with injury, particularly in plexus cases. The surgeon must control bleeding from vessels above and below the site of injury. The surgeon should operate with confidence and reasonable speed during exposure of the area, based on a sound knowledge of key anatomic landmarks and structures (Fig. 6-2). Use of a microscope too early in the dissection will unnecessarily prolong it. The pace of progress subsequently slows when painstaking dissection of complex injuries and attendant scar is required. Great care must be exercised in placing self-retaining retractors so that adjacent structures are not injured during prolonged surgery.

CLOSURE

It is best to close all wounds except the main access wound before nerve grafting. This ensures minimal disturbances after the nerve

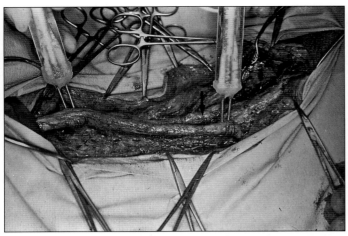

FIGURE 6-2 Exposure and neurolysis of contused sciatic complex. Sciatic nerve and its tibial and peroneal branches have been exposed completely with a 360-degree dissection around each element. Electrodes to the left are around the whole sciatic nerve and those to the right are hooked around the peroneal nerve, while the black arrow points to the tibial nerve.

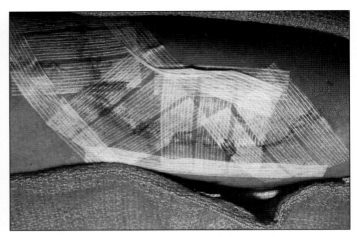

FIGURE 6-3 Steri-Strips applied to wound closed subcutaneously after exploration of the radial nerve at the level of the elbow.

repair has been made. Careless application of sponges during closure can cause grafts to adhere to gauze so that suture lines are disrupted. Careless removal of self-retaining retractors can disrupt suture lines. Tight fascial closure around repaired nerve(s) should not be attempted so as to avoid the potential for extrinsic compression. Skin closure should be meticulous because scars tend to spread badly if care is not given to this end stage of the operation (Fig. 6-3). Suction drains should be placed well away from graft sites. Suction bulbs should be deflated prior to their removal, and drains should be removed carefully so as not to damage the nerves repaired. Vigorous cleaning of skin near the site of nerve repair must be avoided, and a senior member of the team should supervise application of dressings, slings, or casts. The tired operating team must maintain vigilance during the closure phase, or all the good work may be undone in a single, careless moment.

OPERATIONS COMMONLY DONE

EXTERNAL NEUROLYSIS

This procedure is the cornerstone for almost all peripheral nerve surgery. Neurolysis is done before intraoperative electrical recordings, and is necessary before suture or graft repair. External neurolysis involves cleaning the nerve of investing tissues, including scar. As used in this text, neurolysis means freeing up the nerve in a full, circumferential fashion, over some length. For the injured nerve, this includes resection of epineurial scar tissue. Simple exposure or unroofing of a nerve, such as might be done by section of the transverse carpal ligament in an uncomplicated case of carpal tunnel syndrome, does not constitute external neurolysis.

External neurolysis is usually done by freeing up more normal nerve proximal and distal to the site of scarring and alternatively working toward the injured site, in a circumferential fashion around the nerve. This can usually be done with a No. 15 scalpel blade on a long-handled plastic knife holder or sometimes more readily by a pair of Metzenbaum scissors. This portion of the dissection can be helped by gently displacing the nerve to one side or the other by use of a 4 × 4 inch moistened sponge or by gentle traction on adjacent tissues with Gerald forceps.

Nerve proximal and distal to the injury site can be encircled with Penrose drains (Fig. 6-4). These drains can be used to elevate and shift the nerve to ensure dissection along its epineural surface. Finer loops such as Vasaloops can be used on smaller nerves or branches of larger nerves, but if used on a larger nerve, they unduly constrict it. At times, epineurial bands or constrictive circles of mesoneurium can be observed. These should be sharply lysed without injuring underlying nerve. Exposure of more healthy nerve proximal to the injury site is a luxury not available to the surgeon for many supraclavicular plexus injuries or with lesions of the sciatic nerve close to the sciatic notch. In those settings, exposure of more distal elements or nerve along with dissection proximally helps, as does careful attention to surrounding anatomic details or landmarks.

Resection of epineurial scar may require use of fine dissection scissors or microscissors, but sometimes it can be done by scalpel blade (Fig. 6-5). As much fascicular tissue is spared as possible. Bleeding points at an epineurial or subepineurial level are coagulated using fine-tipped bipolar forceps while the surgical assistant irrigates the area with saline.

NERVE ACTION POTENTIAL RECORDINGS

External neurolysis is the first step in preparation of performing intraoperative electrical evaluation of any lesion in continuity. There are those who believe that close microscopic inspection of the nerve after external neurolysis or use of internal neurolysis and attempts to trace fascicles through the injury site are the only operative observations necessary in order to make decisions about the need for complete or partial resection. In contrast, we favor use of intraoperative stimulation and recording studies to evaluate such lesions.

After external neurolysis has been completed, stimulating and recording electrodes are placed on the nerve, proximal to the level of the lesion if possible. Stimulation should produce a recordable NAP above or proximal to the lesion. The recording electrodes are then moved into the region of the injury, and changes in the evoked NAP are noted. Recording electrodes are then moved distally to see if a response is transmitted beyond the lesion in continuity. If there is an NAP, the time interval since injury is 9 months or less, and severe pain in the distribution of the nerve or element is not a problem, then one can be content with the external neurolysis

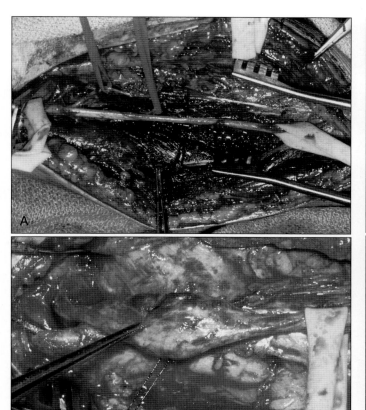

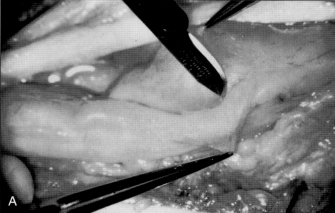

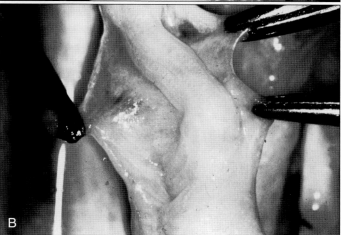

FIGURE 6-4 **(A)** Complete external neurolysis and 360-degree circumferential exposure of a stretch injury site. Penrose drains encircle the proximal nerve to the left and distal nerve to the right. **(B)** Exposure of a more severe lesion in continuity. Penrose drain encircles the distal nerve to the right.

FIGURE 6-5 **(A)** Resection of epineurial scar. **(B)** Epineurium and scar teased away from main nerve trunk. Forceps grasp the epineurium, which has been dissected away from the fascicles.

alone and be confident of recovery of function. If, on the other hand, there is no NAP transmitted across the lesion, resection and repair are usually indicated.

INTERNAL NEUROLYSIS

Internal neurolysis involves the careful splitting of nerve into its individual fascicles or bundles of fascicles. Internal neurolysis requires magnification and, usually, use of microinstruments as well. It is more easily accomplished on nerves in the distal portion of the extremity than proximally, where there are more fascicular interconnections. An indication for internal neurolysis is an injury that is more severe to one portion of a nerve than another and which, despite presence of a transmitted NAP across the lesion, requires a split or partial repair. Another indication is pain of a severe, neuritic nature for which conservative pharmacologic management has failed and in which the pain pattern is associated with partial or no major anatomic dysfunction. Both of these situations can sometimes be helped by internal neurolysis, but there may be a price paid in terms of further decrease of function, even if the procedure is carefully done.

Fascicles or groups of fascicles are isolated over a length by sharp dissection and elevated by Vasaloops or fine drains (Fig. 6-6). It usually helps to split apart the fascicles proximal and distal to the injury site, and then to trace them through the region of injury. Sometimes, maintenance of a group or groups of fascicles is pref-

erential to splitting the nerve apart fascicle by fascicle, and this is left to the judgment of the individual surgeon, based on the fascicular pattern of that particular nerve at that level (Fig. 6-7). Fascicular groups or individual fascicles should then be cleaned of interfascicular epineurium or scar. It is then important to test each fascicle or group of fascicles by NAP recordings, for it is pointless to leave behind functionless and non-repaired tissue. The remaining bundles or fascicles are thoroughly irrigated with sterile saline, and bleeding points are coagulated with the bipolar forceps. Occasionally, interfascicular repair without interposition of grafts is indicated, and then an internal neurolysis of each stump (if the lesion is caused by transection) or of whole nerve (if the lesion is blunt) is performed (Fig. 6-8). Refer to the split repair section later in this chapter for further discussion.

END-TO-END SUTURE REPAIR

If a nerve has been transected or if a short nerve gap exists following the resection of a lesion in continuity, a surgeon can sometimes achieve an end-to-end epineurial repair. If transection is present, dissection should proceed whenever possible from more normal proximal and distal nerves toward their stumps. Sharp dissection is usually necessary to free stumps from adjacent and scarred soft tissues. Stumps are then trimmed back to healthy epineurium and fascicular structure. Structure of the proximal stumps is readily

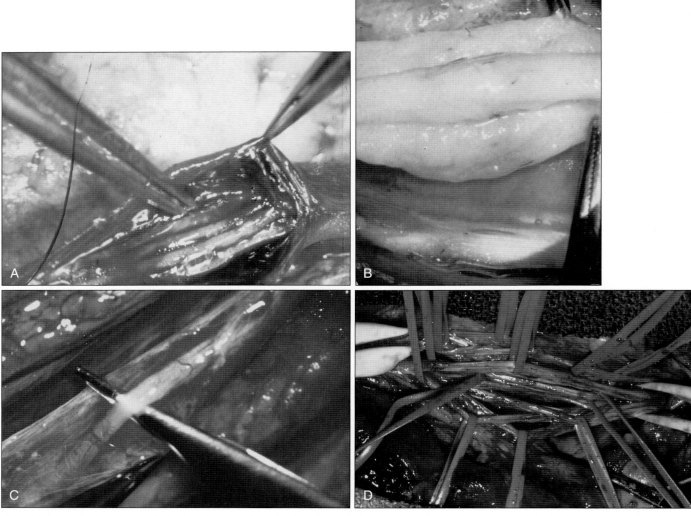

FIGURE 6-6 **(A)** Internal neurolysis showing a portion of epineurium retracted by forceps. **(B)** Exposed fascicles before separation by sharp dissection. **(C)** Dissection of a single fascicle shown beneath fine Metzenbaum scissors. **(D)** Extensive internal neurolysis of a sciatic nerve lesion. Fascicles were split apart both by sharp dissection with a scalpel and by use of fine Metzenbaum scissors and microscissors.

evident because the freshened fascicles pout from beneath the trimmed epineurium (Fig. 6-9). Depending on the time interval between the occurrence of the nerve injury and the operation for repair, distal stump fascicles may be surrounded by a variable amount of scar. The distal stump is resected back to a discernible fascicular pattern and one which is relatively soft to palpation by the gloved finger or by a double-ended dissector or with the handle of the scalpel. It helps to section these stumps after placing them on a piece of sterile tongue blade or similar firm surface or using a Miter box. We prefer a fresh scalpel blade mounted on a scalpel handle so that the orientation of the cuts can be readily controlled, and so that nerve at the site of section is not unduly squashed or squeezed. Nerve beyond the stump can be steadied by the gloved thumb and index finger or can be held on top of the cutting surface by fine-toothed forceps grasping the epineurium.

Blood from either sectioned stump is irrigated away. Sometimes, such bleeding, if caused by oozing from multiple small vessels, can be diminished by placing a piece of muscle or Gelfoam beneath a cotton paddy and against the stump. This is held in place for a few minutes to tamponade the bleeding source. If bleeding is arterial, the bleeding point in the stump may have to be searched out and coagulated by the fine-tipped bipolars. Under these circumstances, it helps if the surgeon's assistant irrigates away the blood as the bleeding vessel is sought out.

After bleeding is controlled and the stumps are as fresh as possible, the suture repair is carried out (Fig. 6-10). Prior to this, the stumps are mobilized, usually both proximally and distally, to perform the repair with mild tension only. Transposition and limb positioning may further help minimize a nerve gap. The length may vary from nerve to nerve at different sites with these techniques. Transposition of the ulnar nerve anterior to the elbow or of the radial nerve beneath the biceps/brachialis muscles for an arm-level radial nerve repair, or performance of a partial fibulectomy for a peroneal repair are useful procedures to gain nerve length. In addition, flexion of the elbow for most nerve repairs of the arm and flexion at the knee helps gain length for most sciatic nerve repairs.

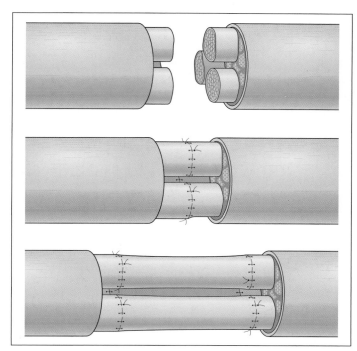

FIGURE 6-7 Groups of fascicles have been dissected out in a nerve with a nerve gap *(top)*. This nerve may be repaired by fascicular repair *(center)* or by a grouped interfascicular repair *(bottom)*.

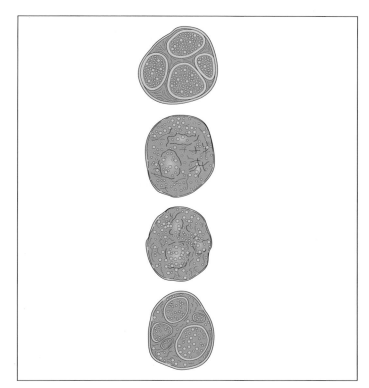

FIGURE 6-8 Usual histologic result of an interfascicular repair without grafts. More normal fascicular pattern is present at top. Proximal to distal extent of scar mixed with axons *(middle two drawings)* tends to be longer than in an end-to-end repair. Many axons have reached the distal stump fascicles *(bottom)*, but some are at extrafascicular loci. (Adapted from Hudson A, Hunter D, Kline D, Bratton B: Histological studies of experimental interfascicular graft repairs. J Neurosurg 51:333–340, 1979.)

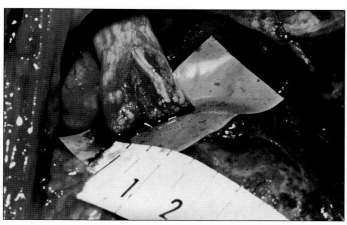

FIGURE 6-9 Several large groups of fascicles trimmed back to healthy tissue are evident on this freshly prepared proximal stump.

These limbs may need to be immobilized for several weeks in order to prevent tension on the repair before mobilization is allowed. However, we believe that the short period of immobilization is worthwhile, especially when a direct nerve repair can be accomplished (without tension) rather than an interpositional graft repair. We do not believe that a minor amount of tension with an end-to-end repair is bad or deleterious, but certainly that tension which could lead to distraction is to be avoided. Usually, the gap after resection of a neuroma or of a lesion in continuity is too lengthy to allow direct repair, so grafts are often used for repair. In general, if there is debate about the integrity or possibility of distraction of an end-to-end repair, it is better to resort to grafts. If a completed end-to-end repair distracts with slight movement of the limb despite mobilization of the nerve stumps and provision of some joint flexion, it is better to take down the repair and replace it with grafts than to risk distraction in the postoperative period.

Repair is done by first placing two lateral sutures at the 3-o'clock and 9-o'clock positions (Figs 6-11, 6-12). Sites for these sutures may be close to longitudinally oriented vessels at an epineurial level or in relationship to major fascicles or bundles seen on the face of both stumps. This helps the surgeon to align the fascicular structure as much as possible. As the surgeon and the assistant tie these laterally placed sutures, it is helpful to make the first tie a surgeon's knot, especially if there is any tension on the repair. After the lateral sutures are tied, their ends are clamped with a fine hemostat and the lateral edges are spread somewhat so that there is a clear delineation of the proximal and distal intervening epineurial edges. These are approximated by interrupted sutures to appose the two stumps rather than "accordion" them together. The lateral sutures are then rotated to expose the back side of the repair site. This side is then closed by a number of finely spaced sutures. Epineurium should be reapposed within reason, but this should not be overdone. Thus, the number of epineurial sutures placed should permit accurate coaptation and no more. Excess suture will result in additional scarring. Some prefer to reinforce any suture repair with fibrin glue. Other workers use only a few sutures to oppose nerve stumps and use fibrin glue circumferentially for the repair.

The caliber of the suture used varies with the size of the nerve to be sutured and the degree of tension predicted for the repair site. As the suture needle traverses the epineurium, a little of the deeper structure is usually included so that fascicular coaptation is

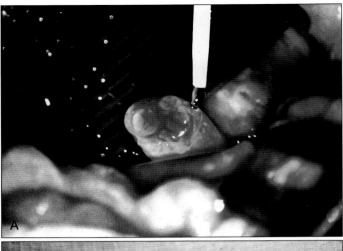

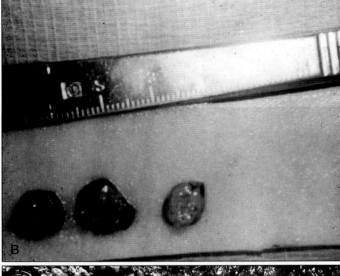

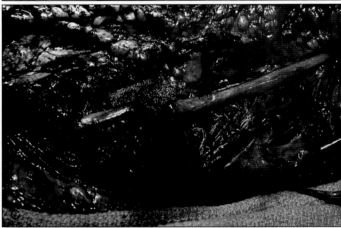

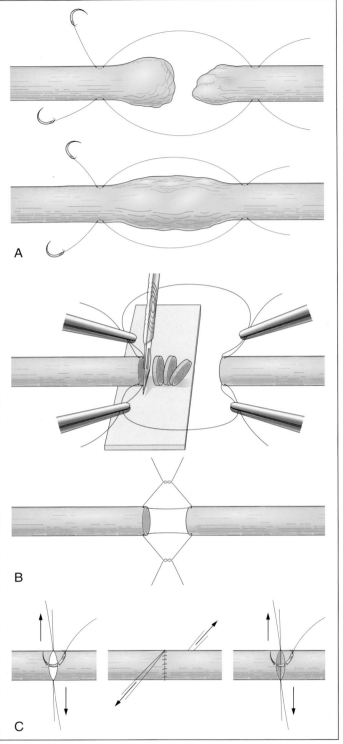

FIGURE 6-10 **(A)** Sectioning back to healthy-appearing fascicular structure. The freshly sectioned end is being irrigated with heparanized saline. **(B)** Segments or sections of scarred nerve removed from a lesion in continuity. Note the absence of a healthy fascicular pattern as seen in **A**. **(C)** Freshly trimmed nerve stumps after resection of an injection injury involving arm-level radial nerve. An end-to-end repair was then done.

FIGURE 6-11 **(A)** Pre-placement of lateral sutures on both a transected nerve *(top)* and a lesion in continuity *(bottom)*. **(B)** Sectioning back to healthy proximal stump tissue and pulling together the pre-placed lateral sutures. **(C)** Placement of epineurial sutures on uppermost epineurial borders, rotation of the nerve using lateral sutures, and placement of apposing epineurial sutures.

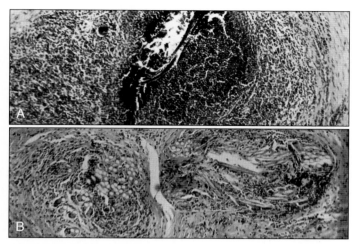

FIGURE 6-12 Histologic comparison of two different types of suture used to repair nerve. The top photograph **(A)** shows a heavy inflammatory response to silk, whereas the lower photograph **(B)** shows less response to Mersilene. Sections were taken 6 weeks after sutures were placed (H & E, ×40).

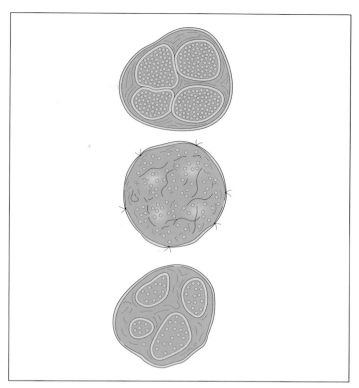

FIGURE 6-13 Usual histologic picture of an epineurial or end-to-end repair several months after operation. Normal proximal stump morphology is seen at the top. Axons mixed with scar are seen in the middle at the center of the repair site, and some restoration of distal stump fascicular structure is seen at the bottom. (Adapted from Hudson A, Hunter D, Kline D, Bratton B: Histological studies of experimental interfascicular graft repairs. J Neurosurg 51:333–340, 1979.)

maintained. Most polyfascicular nerves are repaired when possible by an epineurial end-to-end technique. We have repaired some oligofascicular nerves using fascicular suture. The latter becomes more useful for some distal median and ulnar repairs in which mixed motor–sensory fascicles can sometimes be defined well.

Sometimes, there is disparity between the stump sizes, usually with the proximal being greater in caliber than the distal stump. If this is the case, sutures can be placed at the 12-o'clock and 6-o'clock positions after the lateral sutures are tied. Then, a suture is placed midway between each of these sutures, and this is repeated again until the epineurium is reapposed circumferentially in a symmetric fashion. After the epineurium is closed, the repair site is gently grasped by the moistened tips of the gloved thumb and index finger. The suture site is then rolled back and forth between the fingertips several times to align the stumps and their fascicular structure as well as possible, and to make sure the sutures are securely tied and that distraction with slight movement does not occur.

Two important points demand special emphasis. The leading cause for failure of repair is inadequate resection of injured nerve back to healthy tissue. The second leading cause is distraction of the repair site at some time postoperatively. Both of these complications can be avoided if individual lesions are well selected for end-to-end repair. Nonetheless, graft repair should be used if gaps are long or tension is great; in these cases, inadequate resection and subsequent distraction of the repair are risks. If a gap is small (a few centimeters or less in length), end-to-end suture works well and, in our experience, gives better results than grafts (Fig. 6-13). If a gap is larger and cannot be readily made up by mobilization or mild positioning of the extremity without significant tension on the repair site, then grafts are in order and should give results superior to suture.

NERVE GRAFTING

We prefer to narrow the inter-stump gap somewhat before placement of grafts. After a lengthy lesion in continuity is resected, both stumps are mobilized and the limb is immobilized in mild flexion. We do not believe that there is an advantage to attempting to

minimize gap lengths further with positioning of the limb in flexion, when relatively long interposed grafts are already necessary; in these cases, we prefer early protected motion at the neighboring joints. After grafts have been decided on, epineurium from each stump is trimmed, and then each stump end is split into multiple bundles or fingers of fasciculi (Fig. 6-14). This is usually done by microscissors after visualizing the fascicular pattern on each stump. Sometimes, the nerve end is placed on a firm surface such as a tongue blade and split into quarters or fifths lengthwise by use of a scalpel. Similarly disposed ends or tails are then created on the opposite stump. Interfascicular epineurial tissue or scar is then trimmed from between the fasciculi or groups of fasciculi.

The gap is then measured, and the number of grafts necessary to close it is calculated. Individual graft length, which should be a little longer than the gap to account for retraction and shrinkage, is then multiplied times the number of grafts needed. This gives the length of donor nerve to be harvested. The majority of grafts are fashioned from the sural nerve. Cutaneous nerves of the forearm or arm (medial antebrachial or brachial cutaneous nerve, superficial radial nerve, etc.) can be used if these potential donor nerves are uninvolved by injury themselves.

Sural grafts are usually harvested through a mildly curvilinear incision on the posterolateral calf and leg. Others have described harvesting the nerve through several short incisions along the leg, sometimes aided by a tendon stripper or an endoscope. The sural nerve can be most reliably located lateral to the Achilles tendon and an inch or so above the lateral malleolus. It usually lies beneath

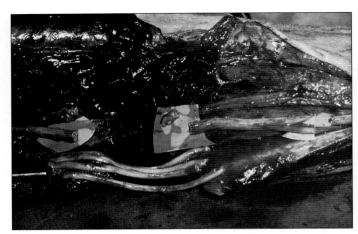

FIGURE 6-14 Preparing a plexus lesion involving multiple elements for graft repair. Grouped interfascicular grafts are about to be sewn in place at the bottom of the photograph; at the top, elements have been sectioned back to healthy tissue. Note that the grafts are somewhat longer than the gap to be bridged.

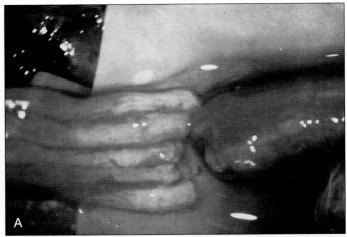

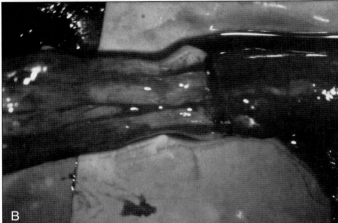

FIGURE 6-15 **(A)** Grafts have been led out of groups of proximal stump fascicles to the left (out of picture). They lie next to the distal stump, which is ready to be split into groups of fascicles to receive the grafts. **(B)** Grafts have been sewn to groups of fascicles on the right without tension. Only a few sutures are necessary to coapt each graft to each group of fascicles.

the lesser saphenous vein. A segment of nerve can be readily dissected free, elevated by a Vesseloops, and then traced proximally. If significantly large branches are encountered, they are traced back down the limb distally and, if necessary, used as graft material too. Any large proximal branches can be traced beneath gastrocnemius/soleus fascia to their origin from peroneal divisions of the sciatic nerve or sometimes peroneal and tibial nerves themselves. Care should be taken not to cause a traction injury to the sural nerve during harvesting. This may damage the sural nerve itself or even the peroneal, tibial, or sciatic nerves. The sural nerve is then sectioned proximally and distally after the desired length is dissected free. The bipolar forceps tip is usually used to attempt to seal shut the ends of the proximal fascicles. Whether this is done or not, it is important to leave the proximal stump buried beneath muscle, especially if shorter grafts are harvested farther down the leg. If only a short segment is needed, it is probably better to take a longer length of sural nerve than necessary. This ensures that the proximal sural end lies beneath some muscle or fascia rather than remaining relatively exposed farther down the limb in the subcutaneous tissue.

The medial brachial or antebrachial cutaneous nerve can be harvested from the medial arm. If used for distal plexus or proximal nerve injuries, these nerves can be located as they originate from the medial cord. They can then be located distally and dissected free from brachial vessels and other soft tissues. As with sural nerve harvest, the fascicles of the proximal ends are coagulated by the bipolar forceps after removal of a segment of nerve. Typically the medial brachial cutaneous nerve is very small, while the medial antebrachial cutaneous nerve is of a better size.

The superficial radial nerve is a relatively large-caliber nerve that can be harvested through a dorsoradial incision along the forearm. The nerve can be easily identified just above the wrist level where it runs in the subcutaneous tissue and traced proximally. Additional length of donor nerve can be obtained by dissecting this sensory branch away from the radial nerve to a point above the elbow.

After donor nerve has been harvested, it is handled gently, kept moist in isotonic saline, and then moved to the graft site. Excessive mesoneurial or other tissue is removed from the nerve by sharp dissection. Donor nerve is then divided into segments about 10% longer than the gap to be closed. Grafts are sewn in place to proxi-

mal and distal fascicular groups of the stumps by two lateral sutures (Fig. 6-15). Because donor graft caliber is usually smaller than what it is sewn to, the lateral sutures are used to spread or "fishmouth" the end of the graft segment to cover as much of the fascicular structure as possible (Fig. 6-16). Sometimes, a third or even a fourth suture is used. In some settings, such as placement of intraforaminal-level spinal nerve grafts, only one suture can be accurately placed, usually running through the center of the proximal stump of the spinal nerve as well as the center of the end of the donor nerve. Usually, 7-0 or 8-0 nylon or Prolene suture is used. Finer suture is more difficult to handle even with magnification, and a larger-caliber suture takes up too much of the intraneural space. Fibrin glue can also be used to hold together approximated nerve stump and grafts.

Depending on the setting, all of the grafts can be sutured first proximally and then distally, or each graft can be sewn in one at a time. The former approach is especially useful when one needs to sew grafts in difficult locations, such as close to the clavicle. The clavicle can be mobilized by the surgeon and retracted by the assistant so that one set of graft ends can be sewn in, and then traction on the clavicle relaxed or retracted in the opposite direction as the other set of ends is sutured in place.

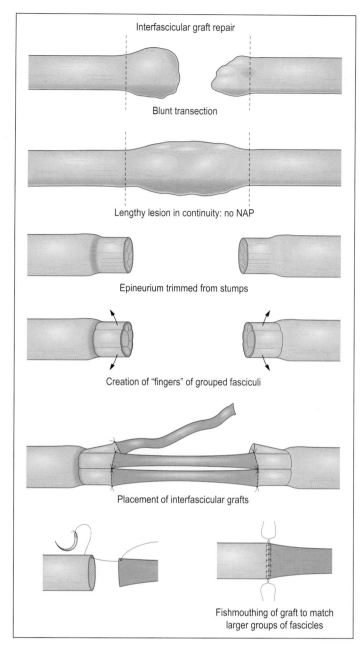

FIGURE 6-16 Drawing of steps necessary for the usual interfascicular graft repair done either for a blunt transection with retraction of neuromatous stumps or for a lengthy lesion in continuity requiring resection. Epineurium is trimmed from both stumps after they have been sectioned back to healthy tissue. Groups of "fingers" of fasciculi are fashioned and then bridged with graft. Note how the end of each graft has been spread or "fishmouthed" to cover stump fascicular structure.

It is important to reinspect the graft coaptations at the completion of the repair because graft ends can be easily distracted as other grafts are being sutured in place (Fig. 6-17). The graft site is then irrigated and bleeding points are coagulated with the bipolar forceps. As with end-to-end repair, it is important to place the grafts in a bed as free of scar tissue as possible.

At the present time, several groups are using entubulation techniques to reconstruct small nerve gaps or instead of an end-to-end suture. Preliminary clinical studies suggest that useful reinnervation can be obtained for gaps <3 cm in length. The primary uses of nerve

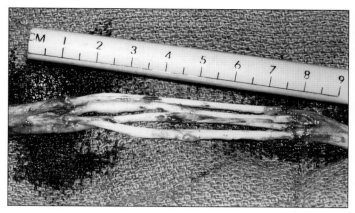

FIGURE 6-17 A completed grouped interfascicular repair using 4 sural grafts 7 cm in length. (From Dubuisson A, Kline D: Indications for peripheral nerve and brachial plexus surgery. Neurol Clin North Am 10:935–951, 1992, with permission).

conduits thus far have been in small nerves such as digital nerves as well as in mixed nerves such as the median or ulnar nerves at the wrist level. Some surgeons are reporting other uses such as in spinal accessory nerve repair or even in more proximal-level major peripheral nerve reconstruction. The obvious benefit would be decreased donor morbidity by avoiding nerve graft harvesting. Nonresorbable materials such as Silastic have been used for many years, but often have to be removed at a secondary operation. Autologous tissues fashioned into tubes and newer biodegradable substances are currently available on the market and are being advocated by some for short gaps. Much research will continue in this field, especially with different types of tubes in which various growth factors can be placed in the tube and delivered to the repair site.

There has been much experimental and some clinical interest in vascularized nerve grafts, but, to date, the potential advantages and reported results do not seem to warrant this more extensive procedure for routine uses. There may be some potential benefit to a vascularized nerve graft when an extremely long gap exists or when there is an avascular bed.

After placement of grafts, we usually place the upper limb in a sling, particularly for brachial plexus cases. We do limit shoulder abduction of the shoulder for about 3 weeks but still encourage circular motions and partial shoulder abduction until then. Figure 6-18 shows the usual histologic appearance several months after repair.

SPLIT REPAIR

When a portion of the cross-section of an injury site is more severely involved than the rest, the nerve can be split into fascicles or bundles of fascicles by internal neurolysis (Fig. 6-19). Testing of the individual components often leads to resection of some and relative sparing of others. After clearing those to be left behind of extrinsic scar, those resected are repaired, usually by inlaying one or more grafts between their stumps. This is termed split repair. As with end-to-end or whole nerve graft repair, it is important to resect the damaged segments back to healthy tissue and to gain as relaxed a repair as possible.

If nerve is partially transected and repaired acutely, split repair usually entails simple end-to-end suture of the transected portion. If a small gap exists, a slight undulation in the relatively uninjured portion of the nerve is acceptable with either acute or more delayed

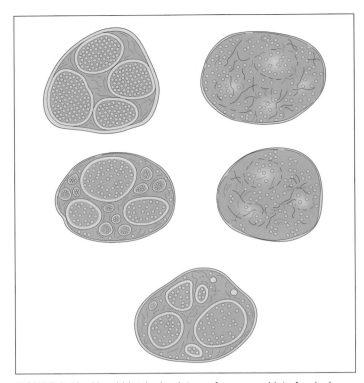

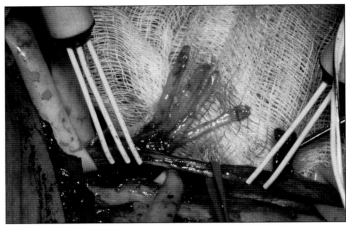

FIGURE 6-19 Stimulation (to the left) and recording (to the right) from a portion of nerve to be retained without repair because of detection of a nerve action potential (NAP) conducted across this segment of nerve. Grafts have been sewn into fascicular groups to the left and will next be sutured into those on the right of the photograph. This portion of the injury did not conduct an NAP. (From Dubuisson A, Kline D: Indications for peripheral nerve and brachial plexus surgery. Neurol Clin North Am 10:935–951, 1992, with permission).

FIGURE 6-18 Usual histologic picture of a grouped interfascicular repair using multiple grafts several months after repair. More normal fascicular pattern is seen at top left. Site of scar, axons, and disorganization are seen at interface between proximal stump and proximal grafts *(top right)*. At the mid-segment of the grafts, some of their fascicular structure is still evident, with regenerated axons within but also external to fascicles *(middle left)*. In the more distal portion of the grafted segment, more disorganization is evident, especially close to and at the level of the coaptation of the graft to the distal stump's groups of fascicles *(middle right)*. At the bottom center is the distal stump morphology; regenerated axons are both intrafascicular and extrafascicular. (Adapted from Hudson A, Hunter D, Kline D, Bratton B: Histological studies of experimental interfascicular graft repairs. J Neurosurg 51:333–340, 1979.)

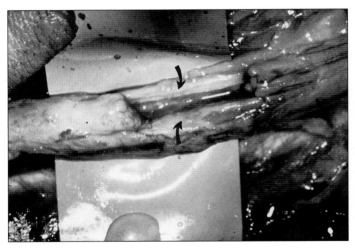

FIGURE 6-20 Preparation for split or partial repair by grafts. End to the right of the photograph has been split into bundles for receipt of grafts; the portion of the fascicular structure to the left remains to be split. Retained portions of the nerve are indicated by arrows.

repair. On the other hand, if a good deal of undulation results, or if there is the potential for kinking to develop, it is better to lay in grafts to fill the gap (Fig. 6-20). Split repairs usually have a favorable outcome, especially if the portion spared repair is proved to be either intact, only partially injured, or regenerating by intraoperative electrophysiologic evaluation.

NERVE TRANSFER (NEUROTIZATION)

Nerve transfer (neurotization) is the substitution of a functioning but expendable nerve or part of nerve to a nonfunctioning nerve. There are a variety of potential nerve transfers, including extraplexal sources (such as C3 and C4 spinal nerves or descending cervical plexus, spinal accessory nerve, intercostal nerves, phrenic nerve, hypoglossal nerve, and contralateral C7) and intraplexal sources (such as the thoracodorsal nerve, pectoral or triceps branches and ulnar or median nerve fascicles). Nerve transfers may be performed to supply motor or sensory function.

Nerve transfers are indicated for preganglionic injuries (where nerve grafting would not be possible). For example, intercostal nerves may be transferred to the biceps branch (or to the musculocutaneous nerve) as part of a reconstructive strategy to allow elbow flexion in a patient with a C6 avulsion. Another possibility would be to transfer a fascicle of the ulnar nerve (Oberlin's procedure) to the biceps branch in the same clinical scenario (assuming the ulnar nerve was functioning, such as in a patient with a C5–6 brachial plexus lesion). Because of the recently reported successful outcomes with distal nerve transfers, such as Oberlin's transfer, many surgeons are using nerve transfers preferentially instead of nerve grafting in situations of postganglionic injury (i.e. where nerve grafting could be performed). The rationale behind using nerve transfers is that they often allow additional reconstructive options in cases of severe brachial injury. Some surgeons would also suggest that nerve transfers allow more reliable recovery than nerve grafting in postganglionic injury, but this remains controversial.

Other surgeons are using a nerve transfer to power free functioning muscle transfer (e.g. free gracilis transfer; see Chapter 16 for full description of this procedure). This procedure consists of moving a muscle with a neurovascular pedicle, and reattaching the muscle and reconnecting the nerve and vessels in another location so that the transferred muscle can subserve another function (such as elbow flexion). Free functioning muscle transfer is an effective procedure, especially in late cases (e.g. after 1 year), where nerve procedures (such as nerve grafting or nerve transfers) by themselves are not effective.

Surgeons must carefully weigh the advantages and disadvantages as well as the risks and benefits of performing a specific nerve transfer. Every nerve that is selected for a nerve transfer has a function, and its sacrifice will result in *some* potential loss. Obviously, certain nerve transfers that are being used by some surgeons across the world have a higher risk of downgrading function than others (e.g. phrenic nerve and contralateral C7). See Chapter 16 for a full description on nerve transfers for brachial plexus injury.

OTHER PROCEDURES

Peripheral nerve surgeons must be aware of other procedures to muscle/tendon (e.g. transfers), bone (e.g. osteotomy, amputation, etc.) or joint (e.g. fusion) that may be helpful to a patient, even if the procedure itself is not part of his or her operative armamentarium (see Chapter 20 for further details about these procedures and their indications). These procedures should always be considered when patients present too late for typical nerve-related surgery or when previous reconstructive attempts have failed.

RESECTION OF PAINFUL NEUROMAS

Some injuries to nerves lead to the formation of painful neuromas. If these involve relatively unimportant sensory nerves or branches of mixed motor–sensory nerves, the neuroma can be resected without repair. Examples include medial or lateral antebrachial cutaneous nerves, dorsal cutaneous branch of the ulnar, palmar sensory branches of the median or ulnar, superficial sensory branch of the radial (SSR), and sural and saphenous portions of the sciatic and femoral complexes. It is important under these circumstances to resect not only the neuroma but, if in continuity, portions of the nerve both distal and proximal to it. It is also necessary to remove surrounding scar and any branches from adjacent, less injured nerves. The latter can contribute to the neuroma or at least be a partial generator of painful impulses, as pointed out by Mackinnon and Dellon (Surgery of the Peripheral Nerve, New York, G. Thieme, 1988), and need resection. This is more likely to be a problem with SSR and saphenous nerve neuromas than with others.

Treatment of the freshly sectioned proximal end of nerve associated with a neuroma remains controversial. An ideal treatment to ensure against recurrence is lacking. Any injury to nerve, even fresh and sharp section of it, leads to neuroma and may eventually result in a painful neuroma. At this time, we prefer to place the freshly sectioned nerve as deep in soft tissues as possible, preferably deep to muscle. We do not suture the end to muscle, turn the nerve back on itself, curve or angulate it proximally, ligate it, bury it in bone, or inject it with sclerosing materials. We prefer to attempt to seal shut the ends of the fascicles in the proximal stump by coagulation with the fine tips of the bipolar forceps. This is done under magnification and only in the proximal stump. The situation may be helped by resecting 6 cm or more of nerve to discourage regrowth, restoration of continuity, and a resultant neuroma, which may again be painful.

POSTOPERATIVE CARE

This phase of care differs somewhat from nerve to nerve, for upper and lower limbs, and for plexus and non-plexus operations (Table 6-2). Nonetheless, some common features require special emphasis. The tensile strength of nerves, whether repaired end-to-end or by grafts, appears to be maximal by 3 weeks postoperatively. Some care in not overstretching, abducting, or extending the limb is necessary in the early weeks, but not later on. It is true that if an end-to-end repair is done under some tension, then extension of the limb even after 3 weeks postoperatively should be done gradually. A physical therapist who is aware of the implications of working out a limb after neural repair is of invaluable help. Often, a parent or other loved one can, if carefully instructed, help the patients themselves to do this. Again, nerves do not heal by being placed at rest, nor do joints regain mobility without motion. Structured therapy is of help, but the patient and his or her family must help by moving the paralyzed or paretic limb many times a day.

Wound care is the same as that for other soft tissue operations with a few exceptions. Limbs should be checked frequently for excessive swelling, bleeding and vascular insufficiency, evolving neurologic deficit, or new neuropathic pain. Collections of blood or serum in and around the repair site should be minimized by careful and patient intraoperative hemostasis. If they arise postoperatively, then it is best to aspirate or surgically evacuate sizable collections (even those not causing compression); if untreated, they may lead to severe scarring about the repair sites.

Although intact nerve is relatively resistant to invasion by infection, the same may not be true of injured or surgically manipulated nerve with altered blood-to-nerve barriers. A soft tissue infection in a limb after nerve has been operated on, with or without repair, requires aggressive treatment with antibiotics and sometimes incision, debridement, and drainage. All of our patients who have

---

Table 6-2 Postoperative care

Check limbs and dressings frequently for excessive swelling or bleeding and vascular insufficiency.
Institute early and aggressive pulmonary care; chest radiograph especially for brachial plexus dissections.
Keep immobilization of the limb as minimal as possible.
Institute early range of motion, especially of joints well proximal and distal to the operative site.
Daily wound care; early mildly compressive dressings followed by noncompressive coverage by dressings.
Removal of drain, if used.
Frank discussion with the patient and family about operative findings, repairs done, possible outcomes, expected course of rehabilitation, and pain patterns that may occur.
Discharge instructions regarding wound care, need for physician follow-up, expected postoperative visits, and use of medications.

undergone lengthy procedures receive perioperative intravenous antibiotics followed by a course of oral antibiotics.

Dressings are usually changed daily postoperatively until the patient is discharged. Dressings are applied in such a fashion as to provide mild compression of the wound site and more distal limb. If the patient is discharged after a few days, he or she is usually sent home with a dressing on. The patient is urged to keep the wound dry and either to return for inspection and removal of sutures or staples in 7–10 days, or, if coming from a distance, to see his or her local physician at about the same time. If the skin was closed in a subcuticular fashion, then Steri-Strips should be soaked off the wound edges 8–10 days after operation. Usually, patients are instructed to keep the arm or leg elevated for a portion of each day for several weeks or more postoperatively. This should not be done, however, by neglecting frequent movement of the involved limb. In addition to receiving an antibiotic, the patient is usually sent home with one or more medications for pain. If potentially addictive drugs are prescribed for a week or two postoperatively, then it may also be necessary to provide an analgesic of lesser potency and with less potential for addiction so that the patient can switch over to the lesser drug after a period of time.

It is necessary to explain to the patient and to family and friends at the hospital what was done, what to expect, when the patient is to return for follow-up, and, if possible, what the realistic outlook is for recovery or improvement, especially in function. Provision of some timetable in this regard is helpful. We usually try to provide the patient with a rough drawing of the operative findings. We inform patients that they may experience some painful shocks and dysesthesia several weeks or more after surgery, even though they might not have been present immediately postoperatively while the patient was in the hospital. Dysesthesia or pain associated with regeneration is more painful to some patients than to others, and the nature and meaning of this should be explained to the patient. We summarize special instructions for wound care, limb movement, return visit for wound check by us or another physician, and a tentative idea of future postoperative visits (i.e. 6 months, 1 year, 3 years, 5 years, etc.).

COMPLICATIONS OR LIMITS TO OPERATIONS

Specific complications for specific nerves are discussed at the end of each appropriate chapter. Each type of operation on a particular nerve at a specific level has some limit to its ability to aid return of function. Some estimate of these limits can be given preoperatively and then refined further for the patient and family postoperatively. Failure to improve or limited improvement, as such, is not necessarily a complication. Nonetheless, it should always be pointed out as a possibility to the patient.

The second major possible negative outcome is that function of a partially injured nerve may be further decreased as a result of the operation. This is certainly the case if a lesion in continuity with partial distal retention of function is associated with severe pain and the lesion is resected or a repair of the entire cross-section of the nerve is done. Further loss can also occur following external neurolysis or especially internal neurolysis of a partially injured nerve. The surgeon needs to warn the patient of these possibilities, even though their likelihood is small when the operator is experienced.

New loss in the distribution of a nearby or related nerve, branch, or element can also occur, even if the dissection seemed careful

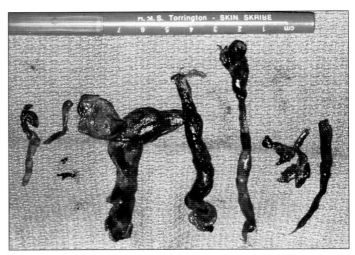

FIGURE 6-21 Clots removed from pulmonary arterial tree. Acute pulmonary embolectomy was necessary 3 days postoperatively in this patient.

and retraction or other manipulation was not excessive. Good visualization of structures related to the injured nerve or element is paramount if new or further loss is to be avoided. Such loss may be minimized by dissecting out related structures, mobilizing them to a variable degree away from the injury site, and protecting them maximally. Be mindful that iatrogenic injuries do occur, even with experienced surgeons, but frequently can be avoided if they have a good understanding of the regional anatomy. Be careful and remain humble.

Pain that was not present preoperatively can result either at the site of injury or at the donor site of a nerve graft, or milder pain can sometimes be increased by operation. These distressing changes can also occur despite good technique and should be pointed out to the patient. If a partially injured nerve or adjacent element is stretched, bruised, compressed, or complicated by clot in a potentially tight space, or if a potential and related area of entrapment is not removed or is incompletely released, increased neuritic pain as well as further loss of function is even more possible.

Wound complications such as hematoma, seroma, or wound infection can occur. Exposures are often necessarily large, and wounds are exposed for a lengthy period. This can lead to infection unless care of soft tissues is as meticulous as possible and postoperative wound care is also carefully maintained.

Pulmonary complications can always occur, especially if general anesthesia is necessary (Fig. 6-21). Complications include atelectasis, pneumonia, pulmonary embolus, and even acute respiratory distress syndrome. Careful attention must be given to good pulmonary toilet and maintenance of good pulmonary function postoperatively, especially after lengthy nerve operations with the patient under general anesthesia. Pleural effusion, pneumo- or hemothorax, and diaphragmatic paralysis are more likely with brachial plexus or thoracic outlet procedures and abdominal complications with pelvic plexus procedures.

USE OF GROSS ANATOMY DURING OPERATION

The peripheral nerve surgeon must be intimately familiar with the gross anatomic features pertaining to the site of injury and the injured nerves. Performing clinical examination and interpreting electrodiagnostic testing or imaging studies are exercises in applied anatomy, and it is from the clinical data that the site and completeness of nerve injury are estimated. At operation, the surgeon must be familiar with all structures in the operative field as well as those beyond the periphery of vision. He or she must have a working knowledge of both the normal and variant anatomy. Frequently, the surgeon seeks areas of normal anatomy from which to commence the dissection, because the site of peripheral nerve injury may be significantly distorted by scarring.

BONES OR OSTEOLOGY

The surgeon should first study the bones, preferably with the individual bones at hand. After knowledge of the elementary skeletal features is mastered, the soft tissues can be added until the complete anatomic picture is assembled.

Upper limb

The transverse processes of the cervical vertebrae should be studied with care. At operation, the surgeon can palpate the anterior tubercles of the transverse processes. These tubercles mark the lateral extremity of the gutters of the transverse processes, which support the spinal nerves. Scalenus anticus is attached to the anterior tubercles and scalenus medius to the posterior tubercles, so that the spinal nerves gain access to the posterior triangle of the neck by running between these muscles. It is appropriate also to realize the anatomy of the vertebral artery within the cervical vertebrae, because bony dissection within the foramen brings the operator close to that structure.

The bones of the pectoral girdle and shoulder joint should be examined with care. The clavicle is grooved on its undersurface by the subclavius muscle, which is always seen in brachial plexus dissections. With the clavicle in hand, the surgeon should review the attachment of pectoralis major and deltoid in an anatomy textbook. Division of a portion of the lateral clavicular attachment of pectoralis major is necessary to gain access to the upper medial cord and its divisions of origin. The reciprocal attachments of trapezius and deltoid to the clavicle are usually undisturbed during routine plexus surgery, but, on occasion, exposure of the suprascapular nerve proximal to the transverse scapular ligament may be improved by dividing clavicular fibers of trapezius close to the bone.

The scapula should be examined with care, noting the points of attachment of levator scapulae, rhomboids, serratus anterior, trapezius, deltoid, and the short scapular muscles. Careful study allows the surgeon to gain an appreciation of the combined muscle functions that result in rotation of the scapula in the later phases of shoulder abduction. An understanding of mechanisms involved in winging of the scapula, which is so characteristic of both trapezius palsy and serratus anterior palsy but also a rhomboid paralysis, is also gained by studying the exact points of attachment of these muscles to the shoulder blade. In trapezius palsy, the levator scapulae has to take over the suspensory function. An appreciation of the attachment of that muscle to the scapula permits the surgeon to understand the function of the muscle in an injury to cranial nerve XI. The examiner cannot be deceived into thinking that the trapezius fibers are contracting when, in fact, levator scapulae is being examined. The rhomboid muscle is often assessed as a clinical indicator of proximal C5 spinal nerve injury. The attachment of this muscle to the scapula should be noted in an appropriate atlas.

The scapula should be examined both individually and while articulated to the clavicle so that the clinician can note the exact position of the scapular notch and transverse scapular ligament. In the articulated skeleton, the angle formed between the scapula and clavicle becomes more acute the more laterally the surgeon dissects the suprascapular nerve from its takeoff at the upper trunk, and the space becomes more and more confined. The attachment of the external rotators of the shoulder joint should be traced on the bone. Often, the surgeon hopes to regain elbow flexion in upper plexus surgery, but reinnervation of the external rotators is of significant importance; failure to achieve external rotation in addition to elbow flexion, limits the functionality to a patient attempting to utilize the reinnervated elbow flexion in activities of daily living.

The very small size of the glenoid should be appreciated. The upper point of attachment of the deltoid should be delineated on the articulated scapula and clavicle. If this muscle is paralyzed from either a C5 spinal nerve, upper trunk, or axillary nerve injury, the head of the humerus slides down on the small articular surface, causing the characteristic clinical picture of subluxation of the shoulder joint. On the anterior aspect of the scapula, the coracoid process provides an extremely useful landmark and reference point during axillary or infraclavicular dissection. Note the point of attachment of pectoralis minor, biceps, and coracobrachialis. No matter how extensive the scarring is in the axilla, the coracoid can always be palpated, thus providing an anatomic landmark for the surgeon and a reference point for the neural and vascular structures contained in the axilla.

The surgeon should hold the humerus and examine the points of attachment of supraspinatus and deltoid. The C5-innervated muscles abduct the shoulder joint, and the subsequent combined action of trapezius and serratus anterior rotates the scapula to achieve the full range of scapular abduction. The exact point of attachment of pectoralis major to the humerus should also be noted. The tendon on this great muscle is usually partially and sometimes totally divided close to the humerus during the axillary exposure. While examining this region, the surgeon should note the point of attachment of latissimus dorsi. The shining tendon of this great back muscle is a constant companion during posterior axillary dissection, and the relation of this tendon to the quadrangular and triangular spaces is well appreciated by examining its point of insertion into the humerus. The surgeon should trace the humeral attachments of triceps so that the passage of the radial nerve and its relation to the spiral groove are clearly understood. Farther distally, the bony attachments of brachioradialis and extensor carpi radialis longus should be examined with care; these muscles are important in the differential diagnosis of radial nerve and posterior interosseous nerve palsy. The point of origin of the common forearm flexors and the pronator teres should also be observed; this anatomy may be important in ulnar nerve transpositions at the elbow or developing the internervous plane for median nerve dissections in the proximal forearm and distal arm.

The two forearm bones should be examined on an articulated skeleton. A detailed study of the insertion of the biceps tendon reveals why that muscle is a powerful supinator of the forearm. It is essential to understand the bony attachments of the two heads of flexor carpi ulnaris if the surgeon is to develop a complete understanding of the anatomy related to the ulnar nerve at the elbow joint. Similarly, the two points of origin of the supinator muscle should be carefully defined so that a subsequent understanding of the course of the posterior interosseous nerve is facilitated. One must also look carefully for the bony markings of the point of attachment of the superficial flexors of the forearm. An understanding of the anatomy of the upper portion of this muscle is essential for dissection of the median nerve distal to pronator teres. Note also the detailed points of origin of the median- and ulnar-innervated deep flexor musculature; testing of these muscles forms the basis of the clinical diagnosis of median and ulnar nerve lesions.

Next, examine an articulated hand. The four points of attachment of the transverse carpal ligament should be identified with care. Each of these four points can be palpated in the living hand. The pisiform bone is analogous to the patella in that it is a sesamoid bone. Note with care the relation of the ulnar nerve to this bone and the subsequent path of the deep motor branch around the hook of the hamate. The lateral points of attachment of the transverse carpal ligament, the scaphoid, and the trapezium should be identified, and the clinician should then understand the distal extent of the transverse carpal ligament, whose complete division in carpal tunnel surgery is so important. At this stage, it is appropriate to visualize the complex curvatures of the articular surfaces of the scaphoid and trapezium. These surfaces allow for rotation of the thumb and hence the clinical movement of opposition as opposed to pure flexion.

Lower limb

The bones of the lower limb should also be examined, in both the disarticulated and the articulated states. The anterior surface of the sacrum should be reviewed, drawing out the points of attachment of the piriformis muscle. The surgeon can then get a firm appreciation of the manner in which the descending trunk formed from L4 and L5 spinal nerve crosses in front of the sacroiliac joint to join the sacral spinal nerves at the origination of the lumbosacral plexus. These neural elements escape the pelvis as the sciatic nerve and gluteal branches. The sciatic courses below or through piriformis and is usually next observed by the surgeon in the buttock en route to the thigh. The surgeon should next examine the outer surface of the pelvic ring and trace in detail the attachments of the gluteal musculature. Note particularly the relation of the uppermost extent of the sciatic notch to the posterior iliac crest. In fashioning appropriate incisions for sciatic notch surgery, all these points are of the utmost importance if appropriate exposure is to be obtained. The anterior superior iliac spine should be palpated to remind the observer of its relation to the lateral femoral cutaneous nerve of the thigh.

Next, examine the articulated hip joint. Although it is unnecessary for the peripheral nerve surgeon to master the intricate detail of the short muscles of the hip, the relation of both the sciatic nerve and the femoral nerve to the hip joint is very important. In the articulated skeleton, the bony attachments of the adductors should be examined at both the pelvic and femoral attachments. These muscles are supplied by the obturator nerve, which has the same roots of origin as the femoral nerve, a useful point of distinction between individual peripheral nerve and lumbar plexus injury. It is also important to identify and then trace the origins and insertions of the hamstring muscles, as these are frequently examined in assessing proximal sciatic nerve function. In particular, note the course of biceps femoris, because this muscle is often dissected during mid-thigh sciatic exposure.

The articulated knee joint should be examined from behind. The point of insertion of biceps femoris into the head of the fibula can be readily seen. This bony prominence can be palpated intraopera-

tively and serves as a guide to the adjacent peroneal nerve as it winds around the neck of the fibula; its terminal branches continue on into the anterior and lateral compartments of the leg.

The medial and lateral malleoli should be clearly identified. The former serves as a guide to the tibial nerve as it leaves the leg to enter the foot, and the latter leads to the sural nerve, which is frequently used as a source of grafts.

The peripheral nerve surgeon need not master all the details of the small bones of the foot, but several points are of importance. The bony origin of extensor digitorum brevis should be delineated, because this muscle is frequently used in electrophysiologic studies. Points of attachment of the peroneus tendons and those of the anterior and posterior tibial muscles should also be studied, because these groups are often used in assessing the nerves of the lower limb.

MUSCLES

The clinician must have a complete understanding of the function of the major muscles, because weakness or paralysis is the basis of clinical diagnosis of peripheral nerve lesions. In addition, incisions to expose peripheral nerves are fashioned so that the dissection is made on the surface or edge of muscles or between muscles, but occasionally, muscle fibers have to be split to gain an appropriate exposure.

The posterior and somewhat lateral border of sternocleidomastoid is frequently dissected during an initial supraclavicular exposure of the brachial plexus. The clavicular origin is often divided to allow greater exposure of the lower plexus elements. The surgeon should immediately recognize the branches of the cervical plexus as they wind around the posterior border of sternocleidomastoid. These cervical plexus branches serve as a good indicator that the dissection is sufficiently extended superiorly to allow detailed dissection of the underlying C5 spinal nerve, and these nerves (and the great auricular nerve) also serve as a preliminary guide during dissection of the accessory nerve in the posterior triangle of the neck. The omohyoid is a readily recognized feature in the early stages of plexus exposure, but the plexus is still obscured by the supraclavicular fat pad. Palpation of the characteristic anterior rounded surface of scalenus anticus through this fat rapidly orients the surgeon to the proximal outflow of the brachial plexus. This muscle should be studied in exquisite detail. Mastery of all the relationships of this muscle serves to elucidate the three-dimensional anatomic relationships at the root of the neck.

The function and appearance of the majority of the muscles in the upper limb can be learned by quiet periods of contemplation in the dissecting room and by studying the appropriate texts. It is well, however, to review in detail the function of the extrinsic and intrinsic muscles of the hand, as these structures are keys to the understanding of median, ulnar, and radial nerve injuries of the upper limb.

The appearance of the psoas muscle during a retroperitoneal approach should also be reviewed. This muscle is the guide to the dissection of the femoral nerve and its spinal nerves of origin. The anatomy of the inguinal ligament should be viewed in the dissecting room so that the surgeon clearly understands the relation of the femoral artery and the femoral nerve to that structure. On the posterior aspect of the pelvis, the peripheral attachments of gluteus maximus should be studied with care, and the relationship of the inferior border of gluteus maximus, the buttock crease, and the sciatic nerve should be reviewed. These are all points of importance during proximal exposure of the sciatic nerve. At this time, it is also appropriate to review the appearance, bony attachments, and relation of the iliotibial tract or tensor fasciae latae. In patients with femoral nerve palsies, the action of this muscle can confuse the uninitiated so that tensing of the investing fascia could be misinterpreted as evidence of quadriceps function.

It is well to become thoroughly familiar with the insertional sites and appearances of the muscles around the popliteal fossa. These structures should be viewed from the posterior aspect, because it is from this aspect that the surgeon will be operating on the tibial and peroneal nerves. In the leg, the details of the relation between the peroneal nerve and the peronei muscles should be viewed by examining a dissected specimen. The surgeon should also examine the posterior aspect of the (lower) leg so as to fully understand the plane of approach for extended exposure of the tibial nerve in its course toward the ankle. The short muscles of the foot should be reviewed to the extent that the surgeon is clearly able to dissect the medial and lateral plantar nerves in their proximal portion during tibial nerve surgery through the region of the tarsal tunnel and the plantar tunnels.

VESSELS

The peripheral nerve surgeon not only must know vascular anatomy but must also be capable of dealing with vascular pathology during nerve dissections. The anatomy of the subclavian artery should be thoroughly understood and the point of origin of the vertebral arteries mastered. These vessels must be protected during surgery on the stellate ganglion and upper thoracic sympathetic trunk. A more lateral exposure of the plexus is greatly aided by either resection or division of a portion of scalenus anticus after the phrenic nerve has been identified, mobilized, and protected. This exposure allows the surgeon to divide the thyrocervical artery and other small branches. This permits mobilization of the subclavian artery superiorly and inferiorly, offering full access to the first thoracic and eighth cervical spinal nerves and the lower trunk of the brachial plexus. In supraclavicular plexus dissections, branches of the transverse cervical artery are usually secured and divided to allow detailed access to the nerve structures. In the axilla, the surgeon needs to study the course of the axillary artery. Such study pays dividends when a tedious dissection through a scarred infraclavicular plexus is undertaken. The origin of the median nerve embraces the artery, and following the medial motor head of the median nerve proximally leads the surgeon to the medial cord, which may be tucked out of sight behind the posteromedial border of the artery. Initial dissection of the posterior cord is usually lateral to the artery in the upper axilla and may be medial to the artery in the lower axilla. If the artery is drawn medially, the circumflex humeral vessels are revealed, and these serve as an excellent guide to the quadrangular space if the surgeon is having difficulty in locating the axillary nerve. Palpation of the brachial artery in the arm is a rapid guide to the exposure of the median nerve. In the distal forearm, the ulnar artery is very closely applied to the ulnar nerve.

In cases of combined nerve and vascular injury, it is appropriate for the surgeon to study the collateral circulation with care so that these vessels are not interrupted during subsequent peripheral nerve surgery. For example, it may be imperative to preserve the circumflex humeral vessels or to preserve the radial collateral artery running behind the humerus in the event of obstruction to the main blood supply.

In dissections at the root of the neck, the internal jugular vein is usually seen. The angle between the major draining veins of the upper limbs and the internal jugular vein should be approached with care, because numerous lymph channels, in addition to the major named lymphatic trunks, may be injured in this dissection. Previous injury may cause scarring and attachment of the internal jugular vein to the deep surface of sternocleidomastoid. This large and important draining vein in the neck should be treated with caution throughout the dissection. The cephalic vein delineates the groove between deltoid and pectoralis major (deltopectoral interval), and this vein is often divided during axillary exposure. As a general statement, veins that obscure the nerves under dissection are usually divided, but if the patient's venous return has previously been compromised by injury, the surgeon may have to preserve as many venous structures as possible.

Arteriovenous malformations may accompany peripheral nerve injury, and traumatic pseudoaneurysm formation is one of the causes of subsequent deterioration of peripheral nerve function after injury. When dissecting in the root of the neck or the axilla, the surgeon must always be prepared to manage such arterial or venous injuries appropriately. A particular note of caution is issued with regard to previous procedures done to repair vessels, particularly by grafts. The surgeon should ascertain before nerve surgery whether such grafts have been placed in a normal or extra-anatomic position and also have some idea of their length. Imaging studies may be particularly helpful.

NERVES

The clinician must be familiar enough with the course of nerves so that their relation to the skin at that level can be easily defined. Part of the clinical examination involves palpation or percussion of the nerve along its course. In most instances, the nerve or element of origin must also be examined for function. This type of preoperative inspection aids the placement of a proper skin incision and also helps direct the deeper portion of the dissection. Masses arising in nerve can be moved from side to side but not axially; this point is useful in their identification by the clinician. Palpation of a mass in a peripheral nerve often results in paresthesia in the appropriate distribution.

The branches of the cervical plexus form a useful landmark during dissection for accessory nerve injury and during the dissection of the C5 spinal nerve. The phrenic nerve, attached to the front of scalenus anticus by the prevertebral fascia, is a useful guide and leads the surgeon up to the C5 spinal nerve, thus establishing the plane of outflow of the spinal nerves. The junction of C5 and C6 to form the upper trunk is usually a characteristic landmark, and the suprascapular nerve leaving the upper trunk usually indicates the take-off of anterior and posterior divisions. The position of the sixth spinal nerve having been established, it is usually fairly easy to display the seventh spinal nerve, which continues as the middle trunk. This, of course, requires a deeper dissection with removal of the overlying scalene anterior muscle. There may on occasion be difficulty in identifying the lower trunk; it may be tucked behind the subclavian artery.

In the axilla, the median nerve is usually readily found in the distal portion of the dissection. If this nerve is followed superiorly to its lateral sensory head, the musculocutaneous nerve can be found, and if the medial head is followed, the ulnar and medial antebrachial and brachial cutaneous nerves are usually readily identified. The posterior cord appears as a flattened, tape-like structure in the upper axilla and is usually readily identified, but in the lower portion of the dissection, it may be easy to confuse the more rounded distal posterior cord with the distal medial cord. In the arm, the inexperienced surgeon may confuse the medial antebrachial cutaneous nerve with the median nerve, but the former is a much smaller nerve than the latter. In the forearm, the SSR is usually readily identified, and tracing this proximally leads the surgeon to the larger posterior interosseous nerve. The median and ulnar nerves at the wrist are usually quite characteristic in their appearance, but contusion and hemorrhage may cause confusion. We have had to reoperate on patients in whom median and ulnar nerves had been sewn to tendons at this level or more proximally in the forearm (Fig. 6-22).

The appearance of the femoral nerve in the retroperitoneal space is quite characteristic, and the nerve should not be confused with a psoas tendon. In the thigh, the main trunk of the femoral nerve lies in a separate fascial compartment from the femoral artery and divides rapidly into numerous branches in a very characteristic fashion.

In the buttock, the large sciatic nerve should be defined with ease, but care is required during that dissection with the superior and inferior gluteal nerves as well as the posterior cutaneous nerve of thigh and proximally placed hamstring branches. The characteristic appearance of the sciatic nerve and its two divisions should guide the dissector proximally to allow identification of the other nerves mentioned. Divergence of the tibial and peroneal components of the sciatic nerve in the lower thigh is quite characteristic, but the exact level of this divergence is not constant. Sural nerve often has contributions from peroneal and tibial nerves.

The appearance of the peroneal nerve deep to the investing fascia and just proximal to the neck of the fibula is quite characteristic. Nonetheless, the surgeon must be certain to identify the rounded tendon of insertion of biceps femoris, which on occasion may mimic the peroneal nerve in appearance. At the level of the ankle, the tibial nerve is in close proximity to vessels and surrounding tendons, and the characteristic point of branching into medial and lateral plantar nerves is another familiar landmark. In the leg, the

sural nerve can be readily differentiated from its attendant lesser saphenous vein, and in similar fashion, the saphenous nerve can be distinguished from adjacent greater saphenous vein.

Inexperienced surgeons should repeatedly visit the dissection room. Review of prosected specimens helps the surgeon review the entire anatomy surrounding the proposed site of operation. Then in the more limited exposure experienced in the operating room, the surgeon will be much more comfortable in establishing the relation between the structures viewed through a surgical incision. It must be remembered, however, that dissection to display specific points in an anatomy museum in itself alters the relation among those structures. What may appear as a very straightforward pattern in a dissected anatomy specimen may be much less obvious when the surgeon deals with individual variations in anatomy as well as distortion of relations by the scar of injury or tumoral displacement.

The standard anatomy texts that should be consulted include those that display dissections in as lifelike and non-diagrammatic form as is possible. The differential coloring of tissues in these texts aids comprehension but may give a misleading impression of simplicity which is rapidly dispelled when the surgeon confronts reality in the operating room. There is, however, no substitute for gaining experience by assisting experienced surgeons who are totally familiar with the anatomy of the peripheral nerves. At the same time, the student learns technical maneuvers that enable the operator to dissect with dexterity and without causing undue damage to tissues. Finally, in this age of sophisticated imaging and electrodiagnosis, it is worth repeating that interpretation of not only the extremely important clinical findings but also the imaging and electrophysiologic studies is all based on a thorough mastery of human anatomy.

SUMMARY

Operative intervention should only be contemplated after a thoughtful, comprehensive, and timely preoperative evaluation has been performed. A successful operation is based on the surgeon's understanding of the indications and contraindications of various procedures and the advantages and disadvantages of a given procedure in any circumstance. A surgeon must possess an intimate knowledge of the anatomy of the involved limb, shoulder, neck, or pelvis. Exposure must be generous and, whenever possible, should include more normal proximal and distal nerve so that the injury site is worked out by dissecting from normal to abnormal. An appreciation of related structures such as vessels, tendons, and other nerves is necessary, as well as is skill in dissecting those out and retracting them gently in order to preserve them. Great attention must be given to hemostasis and the gentlest handling of tissues. There is not only a spectrum but a flow of procedures or repair strategies. External neurolysis is first performed. Nerve action potential recording can then assess lesions in continuity. Depending on the preoperative assessment and intraoperative findings, the following procedures may be performed: external neurolysis alone (when a nerve action potential is obtained across a lesion); internal neurolysis for selected circumstances such as severe neuritic pain or split repair; epineurial end-to-end repair following transection injury or when a short nerve gap exists after resection of a neuroma; interfascicular graft repair following ruptures or when a longer nerve gap exists after resection; or nerve transfer (neurotization) for preganglionic injury. Peripheral nerve surgeons must be aware of other procedures that exist for muscle/

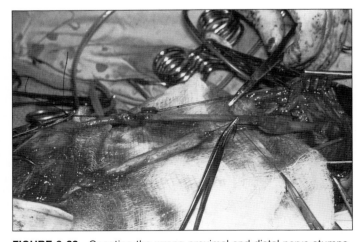

FIGURE 6-22 Coapting the wrong proximal and distal nerve stumps or suturing nerve to tendon or vessel may complicate repair but can be avoided. The proximal stump of a nerve (to the right) was mistakenly sewn to a severed portion of tendon (to the left). Distal stump of the nerve was found at a distance from the tendon and is being drawn toward the proximal neuroma by a suture held with a hemostat.

tendon (e.g. transfers), bone (e.g. osteotomies) or joint (e.g. fusions or arthrodeses) that may be helpful to a patient, even if these procedures themselves are not part of his or her operative armamentarium. A rational and well-reasoned program for preoperative and postoperative care as well as careful instruction of the patient and family is equally important. A reasoned and well-balanced prognosis and outline of expectations and limits of recovery must be shared with the patient and family.

Specific operative approaches are covered in some detail under each major nerve or neural complex. Nonetheless, some general comments were in order and have been presented in this chapter.

7

Radial nerve

Daniel H. Kim

OVERVIEW

- The radial nerve has major contributions from the C6–C8 nerve roots and is the major outflow of the posterior cord distal to the origin of the subscapular, thoracodorsal, and axillary nerves.

- The motor input occurs at an arm and forearm level and is more important than the radial nerve's sensory function. Muscles supplied by the radial nerve include the triceps, anconeus, brachioradialis, extensor carpi radialis longus (ECRL), and extensor carpi radialis brevis (ECRB). The continuation of the radial nerve, the posterior interosseous nerve (PIN) supplies the extensor carpi ulnaris (ECU), supinator, extensor digitorum communis, extensor digiti minimi, abductor pollicis longus, extensor pollicis longus and brevis, and the extensor indicis muscles. Hand intrinsic muscles are not supplied by the radial nerve, as occurs with the median and ulnar nerves.

- In the Louisiana State University Health Sciences Center (LSUHSC) series presented in this chapter, most serious radial injuries were associated with fractures, lacerations, contusions, and gunshot wounds, but a number of injection injuries and entrapments also required surgery. The value of neurolysis based on intraoperative nerve action potential stimulation and recording and of end-to-end suture anastomosis repair and graft repair can be obtained from the tables.

- Dissection of the radial nerve at an arm level can be challenging because the nerve is deep to the triceps in the posterior arm and deep to the axillary then brachial artery and other nerves in the axilla and medial arm.

- Recovery, either spontaneously or with a good repair, is excellent and is superior to that of other major nerves, with the exception of the musculocutaneous or the tibial nerves. Results with repair of the PIN can be excellent as can recovery after release of PIN entrapment. Restoration of finger and thumb extension, however, often does not come close to the excellent function achieved in the more proximal radial-innervated muscles, and as a result tendon transfers to restore finger and thumb extension remain important. The tables provide data on treatment and outcomes according to the level of nerve involved and mechanism of injury and lesion. The data for this chapter on the radial nerve evolved from experience with 295 cases, 205 of which underwent surgery.

APPLIED ANATOMY

The radial nerve is the major outflow of the posterior cord after the originations of the upper and lower subscapular nerves and the thoracodorsal and axillary nerves from this cord. The posterior cord is formed from divisions derived from the upper, middle, and lower trunks of the brachial plexus and there is thus an anatomic potential for a widespread radicular origin of nerve fibers contained in this cord. Specifically for the radial nerve, the radicular origins include the C5–C8 spinal roots.

The posterior cord is so named because of its relation to the axillary artery, but it is important to remember that the posterior cord, as well as the medial and lateral cords, each bears that strict relation to the artery only for the short distance in which the artery is covered by the pectoralis minor muscle.

Posterior cord branches and the muscles which they innervate include the upper and lower subscapular nerves, which together supply the subscapularis muscle, and the lower subscapularis nerve supplies the teres major. The thoracodorsal nerve innervates the latissimus dorsi muscle and the axillary nerve, the deltoid muscle. The radial nerve supplies the triceps, anconeus, brachioradialis, extensor carpi radialis longus (ECRL) and extensor carpi radialis brevis (ECRB) muscles. The posterior interosseous nerve (PIN), a continuation of the radial nerve, innervates the extensor carpi ulnaris (ECU), supinator, extensor digitorum communis, extensor digiti minimi, abductor pollicis longus, extensor pollicis longus and brevis, and the extensor indicis muscles (Figs 7-1, 7-2).

The triceps branches leave the dorsal aspect of the radial nerve close to its origin from the posterior cord, are variable in number, and run obliquely to supply one or more of the three heads of the triceps muscle. The surgeon must remember to guard these branches while delineating the radial nerve and dissecting through dense scar encompassing it in the distal axilla. Important branches to the triceps muscle, which have arisen either more proximally or at the axillary level of dissection may be encased within the scar tissue.

The radial nerve can be approached from either the medial or lateral aspect of the axillary or brachial artery during axillary dissection. Usually, there is little difficulty in defining the radial nerve from the medial side of the artery in the inferior axilla, and dissection through the fat behind the artery rapidly reveals the characteristic tapelike nerve that is one of the largest branches of the plexus.

The axillary nerve as it relates to the radial nerve is best approached by a lateral exposure of the artery at the level of the coracoid process. This is most easily accomplished by freeing up and displacing medially the axillary artery and its accompanying axillary veins. An anatomical reference point for the radial nerve here is the point of origin of the axillary nerve at approximately the level of the coracoid process. This bony protuberance is easily palpable and is the site of the lateral attachment of the pectoralis minor muscle.

The circumflex humeral vessels are blood vessels associated with the radial nerve which tether the axillary artery and veins as they run to the level of the quadrangular space. The quadrangular space is formed by the teres major and minor muscles, the humerus and the long head of the triceps muscle (Fig. 7-3).

Between the quadrangular space and the level of the coracoid process, the axillary nerve is defined behind the axillary artery, and concomitantly, the origin of the radial nerve is noted and dissected out. At this level, the nerve is found just medial to the profundus branch of the axillary artery.[51] It is usually easiest to define the radial nerve in the inferior axilla and to dissect upward, taking precautions already described if there is scar tissue superficial to the subscapularis muscle.

The circumflex humeral vessels mentioned may become crucial anastomotic branches if there has been an accompanying vascular injury. The surgeon should operate with extreme care if previous vein grafts have been inserted after an axillary artery injury, since the damaged vessels may be densely adherent to the posteriorly located radial nerve. The profunda brachial, also called the deep brachial artery, a branch of the axillary artery, accompanies the radial nerve as it leaves the axilla. The latissimus dorsi tendon's "shining silver surface" defines the lower border of the posterior axilla and is an operative landmark (Fig. 7-4). The quadrangular space and, downward, the triangular space are identified by sliding a finger upward and over the teres major muscle. In the normal situation, the dissection of the radial nerve at the lower axilla is very easy, but direct injury or severe scarring may require the identification of these basic anatomical landmarks before any detailed dissection of the nerve.

The ulnar nerve is of a smaller caliber and has a rounder configuration than the radial nerve in most patients. The medial cutaneous nerve of the forearm is considerably smaller than the ulnar nerve to which it may be closely related. The ulnar nerve is initially a nerve of the flexor compartment of the arm, and it remains a close associate of the axillary artery, whereas the radial nerve deviates progressively farther posteriorly as the artery travels distally. The

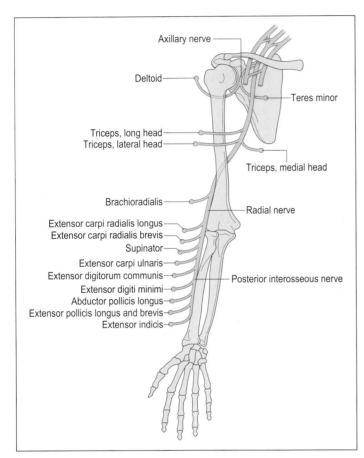

Axillary nerve
Deltoid
Teres minor
Triceps, long head
Triceps, lateral head
Triceps, medial head
Brachioradialis
Radial nerve
Extensor carpi radialis longus
Extensor carpi radialis brevis
Supinator
Extensor carpi ulnaris
Extensor digitorum communis
Posterior interosseous nerve
Extensor digiti minimi
Abductor pollicis longus
Extensor pollicis longus and brevis
Extensor indicis

FIGURE 7-1 This figure shows the muscles supplied by the radial nerve and its continuation, the posterior interosseous nerve.

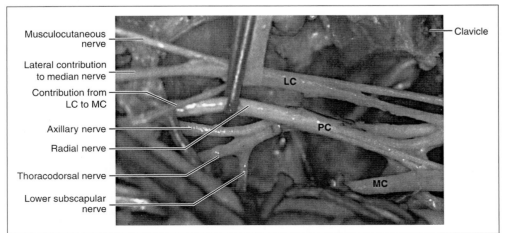

Musculocutaneous nerve
Lateral contribution to median nerve
Contribution from LC to MC
Axillary nerve
Radial nerve
Thoracodorsal nerve
Lower subscapular nerve
Clavicle
LC
PC
MC

FIGURE 7-2 Note the divisions forming the posterior cord on the right of which the radial nerve is seen as the main outflow. The relationships of the axillary and thoracodorsal nerves may vary and a characteristic pattern is shown in this dissection. Note the point of origin of the musculocutaneous nerve. To demonstrate the posterior cord and its branches, when dissecting at the back of the axillary nerve, the surgeon must be careful not to forcefully retract the musculocutaneous nerve. LC, lateral cord. PC, posterior cord. MC, medial cord.

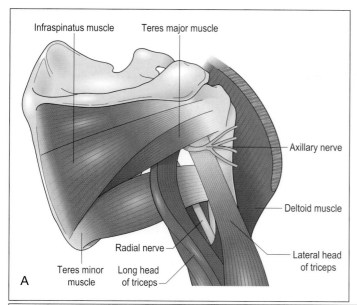

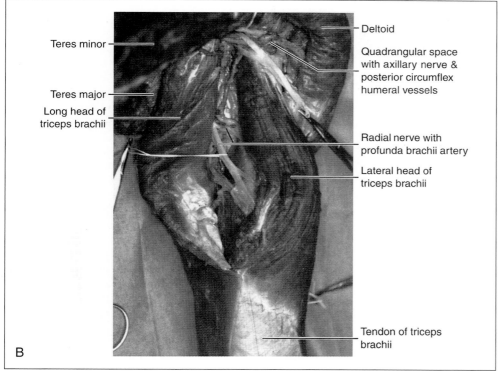

FIGURE 7-3 **(A)** This drawing shows a posterior view of the anatomy of the arm-level radial nerve. The intermuscular septum has been sectioned and the lateral and long heads are retracted. The radial nerve is seen winding around the posterior humerus to reach the humeral groove. Superiorly, the deltoid has been sectioned and is shown turned laterally; the axillary nerve and its relationship to the teres major and teres minor can then be seen. **(B)** This is a right arm cadaveric dissection showing the posterior view of the triangular space with the exiting radial nerve.

motor branch of the radial nerve to the medial head of the triceps may lie close to the ulnar nerve. With experience, the surgeon can distinguish these nerves from the much larger radial nerve, but the uninitiated may identify nerves incorrectly during dissection medially and posteriorly to the distal axillary artery through dense scar tissue. The operator must remember that the radial nerve is destined for the extensor compartment of the arm and in the process enters the medial aspect of the spiral groove. The surgeon will then be able to focus on the target by palpating the humerus and the axillary and brachial arteries and demonstrating the latissimus dorsi tendon's "shining silver surface" and the long head of the triceps muscle. It is not an easy procedure to identify the radial nerve deep to the fascia and posterior to the palpable brachial artery and then

to trace the nerve lying on the long head of the triceps muscle to the proximal end of the spiral groove.

THE RADIAL NERVE IN THE ARM

The radial nerve winds around from the medial to the lateral side of the arm directly applied to the humerus and then pierces the lateral intermuscular septum, at which point it is both relatively fixed and exposed. In the spiral groove, the nerve is covered by the lateral head of triceps muscle and, at this point, the nerve is reduced to four or five fascicles, which is the least number in its entire course. In the spiral groove further muscular branches are given off to the medial and lateral heads of the triceps muscle. The

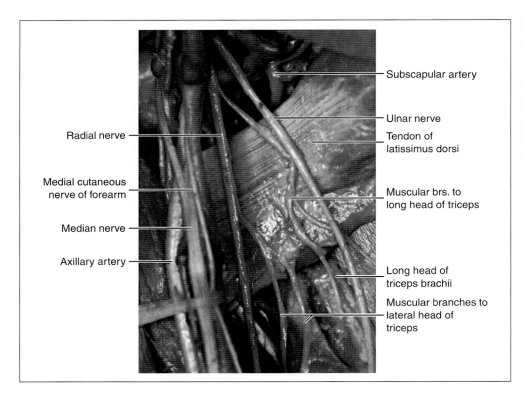

Radial nerve

Medial cutaneous
nerve of forearm

Median nerve

Axillary artery

Subscapular artery

Ulnar nerve

Tendon of
latissimus dorsi

Muscular brs. to
long head of triceps

Long head of
triceps brachii

Muscular branches to
lateral head of
triceps

FIGURE 7-4 This dissection of the posterior axillary region shows the relationship of the radial nerve to the latissimus dorsi tendon and the very proximal outflow of triceps branches. The tissues have been dissected to illustrate these key surgical facts but in the natural state the ulnar nerve and the medial head of the median nerve are closely applied at this level of the axilla.

triceps muscle has a peculiar nomenclature applied to it and this is one of the factors that may cause confusion regarding the anatomy of the radial nerve in the arm. Viewed from behind, the lateral head of the triceps muscle is appropriately named, and its humeral attachment is to the lateral border of the spiral groove. The head medial to the lateral head is, unfortunately, called the long head. The so-called medial head is more deeply placed, but appropriately borders the medial lip of the spiral groove.[12]

The usual Saturday night palsy that is caused by compression of the nerve in the spiral groove does not have triceps palsy as a feature. This suggests that the proximally placed motor branches to the triceps are more important to triceps motor function than those branches in the spiral groove.

The anconeus muscle's nerve supply is given off in the spiral groove. This small muscle is of little importance during the clinical examination, but an electrode can be placed within its substance to check for early denervation. In the presence of radial nerve palsy, denervation of the anceoneus signals that the injury to the radial nerve is proximal to the outflow of this branch.

In the distal lateral arm, the radial nerve is identified in the trough found by separating the brachialis muscle from brachioradialis muscle. The radial nerve gives a branch to the brachioradialis 2–3 cm proximal to the elbow and 7–8 cm distal to the humeral groove. The brachialis is one of the few muscles of the body that receives a twin nerve supply from both the radial and the musculocutaneous nerves; thus, a patient suffering from a radial nerve injury very seldom exhibits brachialis muscle weakness. Conversely, a patient suffering from a musculocutaneous nerve injury very seldom exhibits any significant flexion power based on only a radial nerve supply to the brachialis muscle. These unimportant radial nerve branches to the brachialis arise from the medial aspect of the nerve.

An anatomic feature of considerable clinical significance relates to the point of branching of the motor supply to brachioradialis

and ECRL muscles. Both of these muscles are usually supplied by several nerve branches issuing from lateral side of the main radial nerve in the distal arm proximal to the elbow. Thus, close to the elbow joint, radial branches supply a portion of brachioradialis, brachialis, and sometimes ECRL muscles, and also the radio-humeral joint and the annular ligament of the joint.

THE RADIAL NERVE AT THE ELBOW AND IN THE PROXIMAL FOREARM

The radial nerve spirals around the humerus, pierces the lateral intermuscular septum, and then enters the antecubital fossa (Fig. 7-5). The nerve gains the flexor compartment of the arm underneath the brachioradialis and ECRL muscles. The major division of the nerve into its direct forearm continuation, the superficial sensory radial nerve (SSRN), and the posteriorly inclined posterior interosseous nerve (PIN), a predominantly motor nerve, becomes readily apparent if the brachioradialis muscle is gently retracted laterally and the radial nerve tented up on a sling.

SUPERFICIAL SENSORY RADIAL NERVE

The superficial sensory radial nerve (SSRN) can be easily demonstrated in the antecubital fossa and as it courses distally in the forearm under the edge of the brachioradialis muscle lateral to the radial artery (Fig. 7-6). It is readily available as a nerve graft in this superficial position. The fascicles destined for the SSRN can be split off the anterior part of the distal radial nerve by dissecting from below upward for approximately 4 cm under the operating microscope or loupes, while the fascicles destined for the PIN are placed more posteriorly at this level. At the junction of the middle and distal third of the forearm, the sensory nerve once again enters the extensor aspect of the limb and winds around the radius deep to the brachioradialis tendon. The nerve pierces the deep fascia

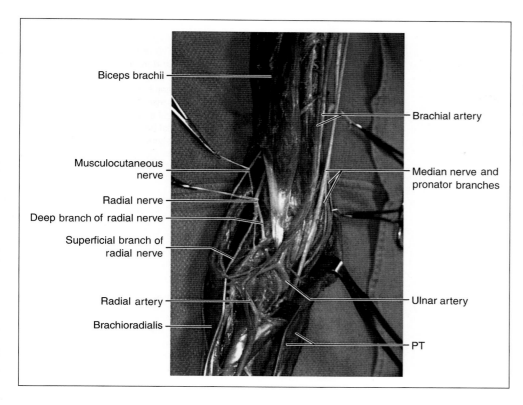

Biceps brachii

Brachial artery

Musculocutaneous nerve

Median nerve and pronator branches

Radial nerve

Deep branch of radial nerve

Superficial branch of radial nerve

Radial artery

Ulnar artery

Brachioradialis

PT

FIGURE 7-5 It is important to find the correct interval between the brachialis and brachioradialis muscles, so that the nerve can be displayed, as shown in this cadaveric dissection. The superficial sensory radial nerve is easily found and can be traced back to the main radial nerve and also to the point of origin of the posterior interosseous nerve.

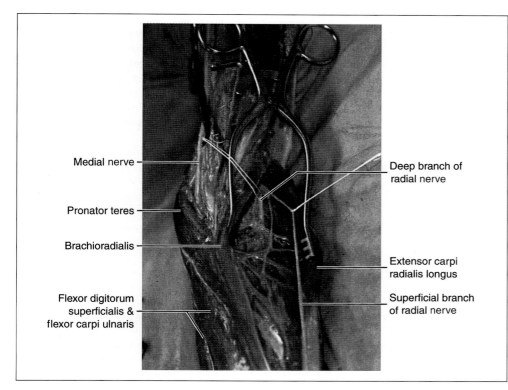

Medial nerve

Pronator teres

Brachioradialis

Flexor digitorum superficialis & flexor carpi ulnaris

Deep branch of radial nerve

Extensor carpi radialis longus

Superficial branch of radial nerve

FIGURE 7-6 The superficial sensory radial nerve is easily found under the medial margin of the brachioradialis and can be "tented up" with a Vasoloop as shown. This displays the origin of the posterior interosseous nerve (deep branch of radial), which runs toward the arcade of Frohse, to gain the interval between the superficial and deep heads of the supinator muscle. In this dissected specimen, the brachioradialis muscle has been displaced medially. In the operating room the same exposure can be obtained by displacing the brachioradialis muscle laterally.

and breaks into four or five branches. These branches run across the anatomical snuffbox superficial to the thumb extensor tendons and are posterior to the wrist joint and to the scaphoid bone. These terminal distal branches are well described in anatomy texts, but from a functional point of view, they supply an extremely variable area of skin on the dorsum of the hand. The SSRN traditionally supplies the radial dorsum of the hand, the thenar web space, a variable portion of the dorsal surface of the thumb and index finger and the radial side of the middle finger.

POSTERIOR INTEROSSEOUS NERVE

The remaining motor fibers of the radial nerve in the distal arm are diverted into the PIN at the level of the forearm (Fig. 7-7). This

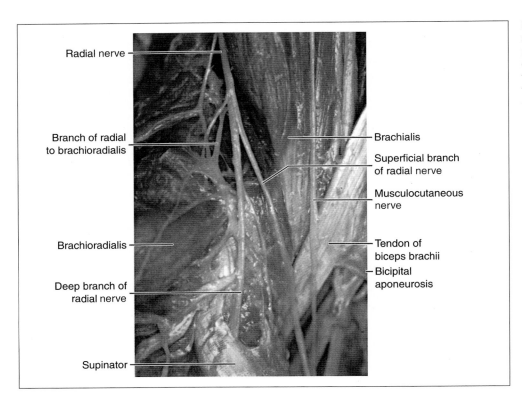

Radial nerve

Branch of radial
to brachioradialis

Brachioradialis

Deep branch of
radial nerve

Supinator

Brachialis

Superficial branch
of radial nerve

Musculocutaneous
nerve

Tendon of
biceps brachii

Bicipital
aponeurosis

FIGURE 7-7 This dissection of the right arcade of Frohse shows the posterior interosseous (PIN) running deep to the tendinous upper margin of the superficial head of the supinator then winding around to the extensor compartment of the forearm. Intraoperatively, the PIN in this region is usually surrounded by small arteries and veins, each of which is carefully controlled to keep the dissection clean and the various planes displayed.

nerve supplies all the extensor muscles of the back of the forearm, with the exception of the ECRL, which is usually supplied by the main radial nerve, but can be supplied by a branch from the SSRN. Although some texts state that the point of divergence of the main motor and main sensory continuations of the nerve is at the level of the epicondyle, our data are in keeping with the data reported by Sunderland. In Sunderland's study of 14 of 20 specimens, the point of divergence was between 1 and 2 cm distal to the epicondyle.[58]

Having left the main radial nerve, the PIN is destined to leave the flexor compartment of the forearm and to enter the extensor compartment. It achieves this by spiraling around the radius between the superficial and deep heads of the supinator muscle as it inclines backward and downward. The PIN is surrounded by small arteries and veins, which the surgeon must appreciate, i.e. a "leash" of blood vessels usually crosses the nerve transversely and must be coagulated and sectioned to fully expose the PIN. These vessels are easily seen with the naked eye; however, their anatomical relationship to the nerve is more exactly defined with the aid of operating loupes.

The supinator and the important ECU muscles are supplied by the PIN before that nerve is lost from view between the two heads of the supinator muscle. The branches to the ECRL and ECRB muscles may be partially hidden by the small vessels in this area and ECRL branches may arise from the proximal SSRN, distal whole radial nerve, or, less frequently, the proximal PIN. These variations are not unlike those noted at the point of origin of the radial and axillary nerves. The surgeon should define the specific anatomy with care because some of the motor branches here are of smaller caliber.

The anatomy of the heads of the supinator muscle is key to understanding the remaining course of the PIN (Figs 7-8, 7-9). This muscle has a superficial head originating from the lateral epicondyle of the humerus and a deep head with its origin from the ulna, and both heads insert into the radius. The nerve runs between the superficial and deep heads of the supinator and the PIN's course runs at almost right angles to the upper border of superficial head of the supinator. The PIN runs beneath the proximal edge of the volar or superficial supinator, which is sometimes fibrous and sometimes muscular.

In either case, the volar supinator forms an arch or arcade superficial to the PIN known as the arcade of Frohse. The PIN is therefore almost as closely related to bone as the radial nerve is to the humerus, and may be directly apposed to the radius in some cases.

THE RADIAL NERVE IN THE MIDFOREARM LEVEL

After traveling under the distal border of the supinator muscle, deep to the superficial layer of extensor muscles, the PIN immediately breaks up into short branches, which supply the extensor musculature, including the ECU and extensor digitorum, and two long branches, which innervate the extensor indicis, extensor pollicis longus and brevis, and the abductor pollicis longus muscles. Each of the three bones of the thumb receives one or more tendons on its dorsal surface. These tendons include those of the (1) extensor pollicis longus to the distal phalanx, (2) the extensor pollicis brevis, (3) the median-innervated abductor pollicis brevis to the proximal phalanx, and (4) the abductor pollicis longus to the metacarpal bone. With the exception of the median-innervated abductor pollicis brevis, the remaining three muscles are supplied by the PIN branches and are, therefore, affected in both radial and PIN lesions.

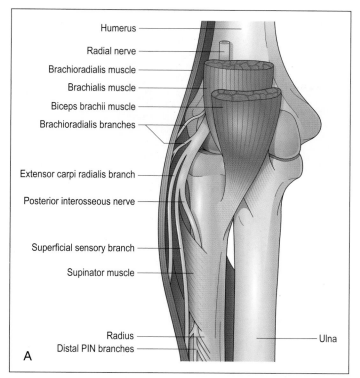

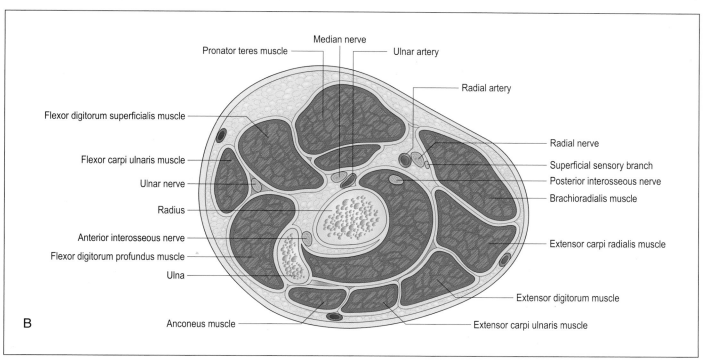

FIGURE 7-8 **(A)** The supinator is shown in this drawing (note the origin of the ulnar head; the superficial head is derived from the distal humerus). The radial nerve, after supplying branches to the brachioradialis and the extensor carpi radialis muscles, runs across the front of the elbow joint under the brachioradialis. The superficial sensory radial nerve (SSRN) continues in that line. The PIN, the motor continuation of the radial nerve, runs posteriorly between the two heads of the supinator. The nerve then winds around the radius to reach the extensor compartment of the forearm. **(B)** This is a cross-section of the forearm. The posterior interosseous nerve (PIN) is shown between the two heads of the supinator. The SSRN is found by retracting the medial edge of the brachioradialis. As the PIN winds around the radius, it lies further posterior to the radius and can be exposed by dissecting into the interval between the extensor digitorum communis and the ECRB muscles.

Of lesser importance is the fact that the abductor pollicis longus may act as a weak wrist flexor and abductor pollicis brevis may weakly extend the distal interphalangeal joint of the thumb in the absence of function of the extensor pollicis longus.

CLINICAL PRESENTATION & EXAMINATION

The radial nerve is the nerve of the extensor compartments of the arm and forearm. From the clinician's viewpoint, its prime function is that of motor control, but it is a mixed motor and sensory nerve. The clinical features of this major upper limb nerve are conveniently considered at the axillary, arm, forearm and hand levels.

UPPER ARM

A key clinical point in assessing the level of nerve injury in a patient with suspected radial nerve pathology is whether that patient's latissimus dorsi muscle innervated by the thoracodorsal nerve and

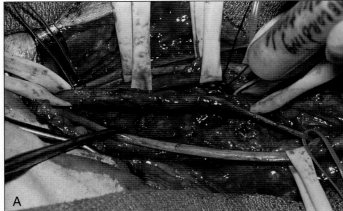

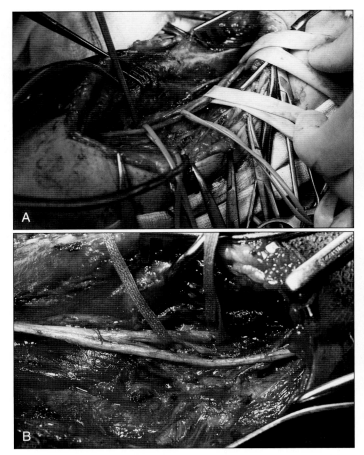

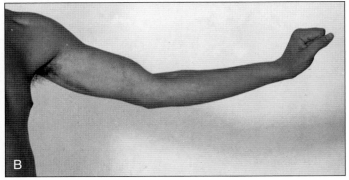

FIGURE 7-9 **(A)** The exposure of the left superficial sensory radial nerve (SSRN), encircled by two Vasoloops, and the more medial posterior interosseous nerve (PIN) is shown. The instrument points to the course of the PIN beneath the volar supinator. **(B)** The exposure of the right PIN (encircled by tapes) and the SSRN branch of the radial nerve is seen here. The extensor carpi ulnaris muscle branch can be seen arising from the proximal PIN. A portion of the volar supinator has been opened to provide this exposure.

FIGURE 7-10 **(A)** Contusion and stretch injury from a gunshot wound affecting the posterior cord to the radial segment. The initial triceps branch is encircled by a Vasoloop and the more medial axillary nerve by two Penrose drains. The proximal ulnar nerve is retracted by a vein retractor inferiorly and a Penrose drain distally. Stimulation and recording over the posterior cord to radial segment gave a nerve action potential at 5 months despite complete radial loss, so only a neurolysis was done. **(B)** There was recovery of wrist extension and some finger extension after several years.

the axillary-innervated deltoid muscle are functioning. If both of these muscles are clinically active, then the lesion spares the posterior cord, which supplies the branches to these intact muscles, and is in the radial nerve itself.

If a patient presents with an isolated deltoid and triceps palsy in the presence of normal wrist extension, there is only one anatomical site where the injury could have occurred, and that is in the axilla at a point where the axillary nerve and the main nerve supply to triceps are closely related to one another. Most surgeons are surprised to find how proximal the point is at which the medial and long heads of the triceps muscle are supplied. The triceps is the major extensor muscle affecting the elbow and, as such, its function is usually aided by gravity. It serves as the main antagonist of the elbow flexors, which are situated in front of the humerus, and the triceps can be readily observed and palpated as the individual attempts to extend the elbow. The triceps is best tested with the shoulder partially abducted and the elbow partially flexed to avoid the effects of gravity. If the patient is seated, the patient is asked to extend the elbow so that the forearm is parallel to the floor. If there is a question of triceps function, gravity can also be eliminated by placing the patient in a supine position and asking the patient to push up with the forearm.

Outflow to the triceps muscle from the posterior cord originates primarily from the C7 root through the middle trunk and its posterior division, and also from C6 and sometimes even the C8 root. Its reflex, however, is predominately a C7 one. Few radial nerve injuries involve triceps loss, because the origin of the triceps is very proximal (Fig. 7-10). The exception is provided by cord-to-nerve-level stretch injuries and some gunshot wounds (GSWs) which involved the cord-to-nerve level. One form of radial nerve compression is Saturday night palsy caused by prolonged radial nerve compression at the axillary level as a result of draping the arm over the back of a chair and may in some cases result in a high enough radial palsy to include triceps loss.

Humeral fractures or operative manipulation for their repair may result in isolated injury to the triceps branches (Fig. 7-11). Secondary repair of this complication is difficult owing to the branches being torn out of muscle or injured over their entire length. Other than an occasional and unusual penetrating injury, the mechanism for an isolated triceps loss from nerve injury is usually a stretch injury causing combined deltoid and triceps palsies. Sometimes, an actual avulsion occurs, not only of the axillary nerve as it runs into the quadrilateral space, but of the triceps branches, which are

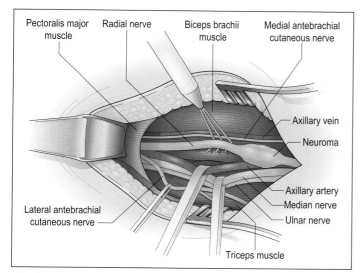

FIGURE 7-11 This is a drawing of the radial nerve exposed in the medial upper arm prior to its winding around the humerus to reach the lateral arm. A lesion in continuity is shown with a stimulating electrode placed proximally on the radial nerve. Recording electrodes were placed on the lateral arm exposure of the radial nerve (not shown) to attempt to obtain a response across the spiral groove. The spiral groove is a frequent site of radial nerve damage, especially with humeral fractures.

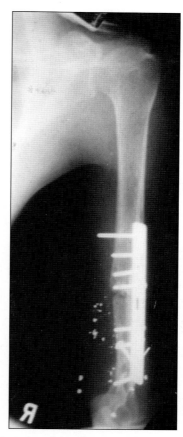

FIGURE 7-12 A shotgun injury fractured the humerus and resulted in a complete radial palsy with sparing of the triceps muscle function. A radial lesion in continuity was resected at 4 months after injury, since there was no intraoperative nerve action potential recorded across the injury. Graft repair resulted in a grade 3–4 recovery when the patient was evaluated at 3 years postoperatively. Exploration of such a nerve injury at the time of acute fracture fixation usually shows a swollen, angry-appearing nerve. There is no way to assess the potential for recovery in such a lesion in continuity at that time.

pulled away from the muscle itself. Effective repair of this extensive injury is difficult, in our experience.

MIDHUMERAL LEVEL

Injury to the radial nerve at a midarm level owing to humeral fracture is the most common mechanism for radial injury[21,24] (Figs 7-12, 7-13) and approximately 20% of such fractures have an associated radial palsy.[3,41] The incidence increases with oblique fractures, compound or complex fractures, and those requiring open surgical manipulation for reduction.[1,14] The nerve may also be injured during subsequent removal of hardware associated with the fracture repair.[18] Other mechanisms of injury at this level include GSW, contusion, simple compression or stretch without fracture, injection injury, tumor and, rarely, entrapment.

The hallmarks of injury at this level are loss of the brachioradialis and more distal radial-innervated functions with sparing of triceps function.[42,47] The patient with a radial nerve injury at the midarm level retains significant triceps function because of the high origin of triceps motor branches. The brachioradialis is the first target muscle downstream, and is tested on repeated clinical examinations as the clinician documents the presence or absence of regeneration. Patients with complete radial nerve palsies at the mid-upper arm level exhibit the characteristic wrist drop and finger drop resulting from lack of function of all the muscles on the extensor aspect of the forearm. This includes muscles supplied by the PIN as well as a paralysis of the ECRL, which receives a branch either directly from the radial nerve or from SSRN.

DISTAL ARM

The radial nerve can be injured at the distal arm level by accidental drug injection, distal humeral fracture (Fig. 7-14), direct contusion, or GSW,[24,28] although it is relatively protected because it lies beneath and between the brachialis and triceps muscles in the lower third of the arm. Again, the brachioradialis is the key proximal muscle involved, and this muscle is best tested by asking the patient to flex the forearm with the latter placed halfway between pronation and supination. The resultant bulge of the muscle belly is felt on the radial side of the proximal volar forearm. In addition to the brachioradialis, the biceps muscle also contracts under these circumstances. The brachioradialis flexes the elbow joint and supplements the biceps muscle functions. Inspection and palpation can separate the effects of the brachioradialis muscle in gaining flexion of the forearm. This can be a very important substitute in a patient suffering from musculocutaneous nerve injury.

ELBOW LEVEL

The ECRL and ECRB are the next muscles downstream supplied by the radial nerve. Branches to these two muscles originate either from the whole radial nerve before it divides into PIN and SSRN or from the latter itself. These muscles extend the wrist in a radial direction and are important for certain functions such as the use of a hammer. An elbow-level radial nerve injury causes loss of

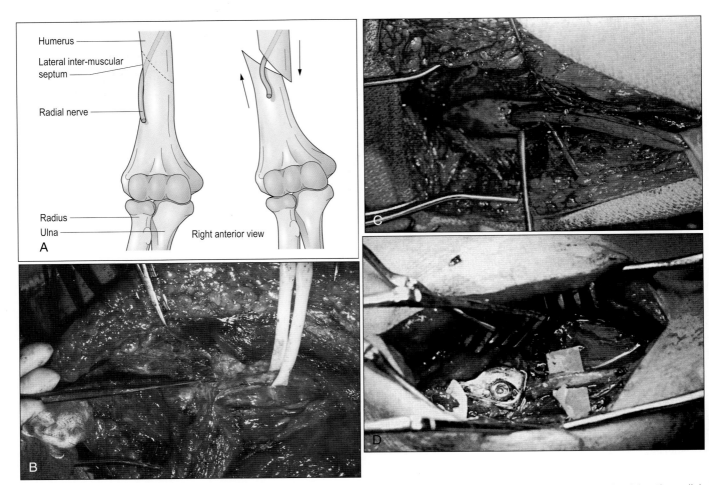

FIGURE 7-13 **(A)** The drawing shows the usual level and fracture mechanism for a radial nerve injury. **(B)** Scar and callus involving the radial nerve is seen intraoperatively at a midhumeral level. **(C)** The radial nerve is shown caught in the middle of a healed fracture. **(D)** The radial nerve is entrapped by plate and screws used to stabilize a humeral fracture. Resection and repair of each lesion seen in **B, C,** and **D** was necessary.

function of ECRL and ECRB muscles. A PIN injury or entrapment results in sparing of ECRL and ECRB function, but there is an absence of the PIN-supplied ECU extension in an ulnar direction. As a result, the hand deviates in a radial direction on attempted dorsiflexion of the wrist.

Elbow-level lesions involving the whole radial nerve are caused by penetrating wounds in this area and, less frequently, by fractures or dislocations of the elbow, by cysts or tumors in this region, or, occasionally, by Volkmann ischemic contractures.[43] The latter are usually caused by supracondylar humeral fractures and dislocations of the elbow.[32] Brachial arterial contusion or stretch results in ischemia of forearm musculature and even of the forearm nerves themselves. In summary, functional loss with elbow-level lesions of the radial nerve includes all muscles innervated by the radial nerve, except the triceps, brachioradialis, and, sometimes, ECR.

POSTERIOR INTEROSSEOUS NERVE

Posterior interosseous nerve involvement seriously affects the function of more distal muscles, but spares some supination provided by the biceps muscle. The most common involvement of PIN is by spontaneous entrapment;[23,27,33,52] however, the PIN can be damaged or compressed by penetrating or contusive soft tissue wounds, fractures of the radius or ulna, tumors originating from bone or soft tissue, or operations to repair fractures in this area.[5,9,55,57] The patient may present with dysfunction of all muscles innervated by PIN or, initially, with only paralysis of extension of one or more fingers at the metacarpophalangeal joints (Fig. 7-15). Subsequent paralysis of other PIN-innervated muscles usually occurs. Thus, extension of the wrist is weak, especially in an ulnar direction from weakness of the ECU, and the patient cannot extend the fingers at the metacarpophalangeal joints from weakness of the extensor digitorum and cannot extend the thumb due to weakness of the extensor pollicis brevis and longus muscles. Entrapment is usually caused by a fibrous edge of the proximal portion of the superficial head of the supinator or infrequently by a scarred vascular complex or connective tissue band just before the entry of the PIN between the two heads of the supinator.[45,53]

This region is complex anatomically and includes the arcade of Frohse. Spinner has also described entrapment of the PIN by the edge of ECRB with pronation.[52] Chronic irritation can lead to an entrapment-like syndrome perhaps related to stressful supination and pronation; a small number of isolated cases have been reported in swimmers, Frisbee and tennis players, violinists, and music conductors. These disorders should not be confused with "tennis elbow," which is related to lateral elbow pain with repeti-

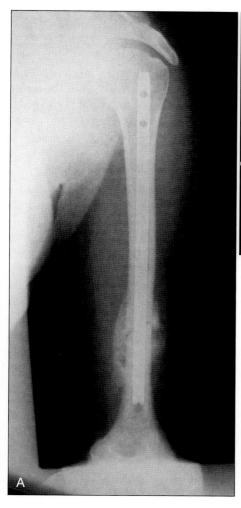

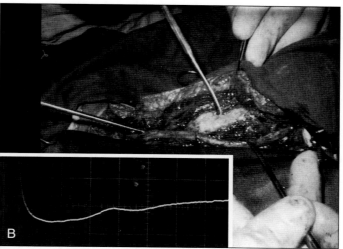

FIGURE 7-14 **(A)** A radiograph is seen of a distal humeral fracture associated with a radial palsy. The latter did not improve over a 4-month period, so exploration and nerve action potential (NAP) recordings were done. **(B)** The nerve was adherent to callus at the distal lateral arm level, but transmitted a positive NAP, which is shown in the insert of Fig. 7.14B. As a result, only a neurolysis was performed. The subsequent recovery was excellent.

tive pronation/supination. Impingement on the PIN is not part of that problem, which is usually caused by epicondylitis, instead.[13]

The "radial tunnel syndrome" has been characterized by some authors as pain and tenderness in the region of the forearm brachioradialis muscle, especially on deep palpation with wrist flexion or dorsiflexion, or on pronation or supination against pressure.[29,35] Implied is irritation of the PIN, but without any measurable clinical or electromyographic loss of function in that nerve's distribution. The exact nature of this disorder, however, remains unclear.

PIN branches to the supinator muscle usually leave the nerve proximal to its entry between the two heads of the supinator muscle.[54] The supinator muscle is a supplement to the powerful biceps in the action of supination. Supination should be tested with the elbow extended to reduce the substitutive effect of the biceps, which is an effective supinator if the elbow is flexed. The patient is asked to turn the hand palm up from a pronated or palm-down position.

The ECU branch has a variable origin but usually arises from the PIN in the region of the arcade of Frohse.[52] This muscle extends the wrist in an ulnar direction, as opposed to the ECR, which extends it in a radial direction. The ECU has a more proximal nerve input from either the SSRN or the whole radial nerve before it divides into the PIN and SSRN.

Wrist dorsiflexion can sometimes be simulated by flexing the fingers to make a fist despite the absence of the ECU and ECR

muscles, especially if the extensor communis muscle is somewhat fibrotic and shortened because of either direct injury or chronic paralysis. Wrist extension is accomplished by the action of numerous tendons, of which the ECRB is the most powerful. This movement brings the hand into the "position of function" and takes up the slack of the long flexors to the digits so that a powerful grip can be sustained by those tendons. The ECRL and ECRB muscles, however, can extend the wrist with moderate power, albeit with a clear radial drift. Thus, a radial nerve palsy presents with a total wrist drop, but a patient suffering from PIN palsy exhibits wrist extension, though weak and asymmetrical (Figs 7-15, 7-16). After leaving the cover of the volar supinator, the PIN reaches the dorsal expansion of the forearm and branches in a "peslike" fashion to supply the extensor communis muscle of the forefinger, long, ring, and little fingers.

The long extensors of the forearm extend the fingers at the metacarpophalangeal joints. Both radial- and PIN-palsied patients exhibit finger drop at the knuckle joint.[15] In a hand without paralysis, the interphalangeal joints are extended by the function of the intrinsic musculature of the hand supplemented by long extensor tendon activity. This may give rise to some confusion in the clinician's mind, when a patient with a wrist drop may yet be able to extend the fingers. This confusion is easily removed by passively extending the patient's wrist and then asking the patient to straighten the fingers at the metacarpophalangeal joints. A patient with paralyzed long extensors is unable to extend the metacarpophalangeal joints, even though the digits can be extended reasonably well with the metacarpophalangeal joints flexed by using the lumbricales.

Another method for testing the extensor communis and extensor pollicis longus is to place the patient's hand palm down on a flat surface and then ask the patient to lift each finger and thumb individually against resistance applied by the examiner.[17] In this position, the examiner can also test the extensor indicis of the forefinger and the extensor digiti minimi of the little finger. Another test of finger extension is to have the patient make a fist and then extend each finger individually without holding the other fingers back with the thumb.

Most important is the method of testing the extensor pollicis longus function, because the abductor pollicis longus and brevis muscles can simulate this function well. The examiner places the patient's forearm in a position that is halfway pronated, with the ulnar side of the hand on a flat surface.[62] The patient is then instructed to pull the thumb away from the forefinger in a parallel direction against resistance.

MID-DORSAL FOREARM

At the level of the dorsal or extensor surface of the forearm, mechanisms of injury include laceration and, less frequently, GSW, fracture, and tumor.[2,6] The pattern of loss in the extension of the fingers and thumb is quite variable, depending on which branches are disrupted or contused.[52] Injuries are often associated with some degree of direct muscle damage, and this makes successful repair especially difficult.

SUPERFICIAL SENSORY RADIAL NERVE

The superficial sensory radial nerve (SSRN) may be readily injured between the elbow and the wrist, but with penetrating injury at the upper forearm level, the SSRN is often spared, although the PIN is much more vulnerable. The sensory territory of the radial nerve encompasses the dorsum of the hand and some of the wrist. The area of loss on the dorsum of the hand may be small, even with complete radial nerve injury (Fig. 7-17),[46] because of overlap from the median and ulnar nerves, the antebrachial cutaneous

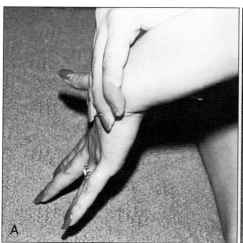
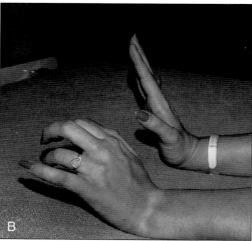

FIGURE 7-15 (A) In posterior interosseous nerve (PIN) palsy, wrist extension is poor because of weakness of the extensor carpi ulnaris muscle, and finger and thumb extension is poor or absent altogether because of weakness of the extensor communis and extensor pollicis longus muscles. (B) In early and less severe PIN-entrapment, the degree of finger extension weakness varies from digit to digit. In this case, finger extension was absent for the ring finger, the forefinger and the thumb, and quite weak for the little and long fingers.

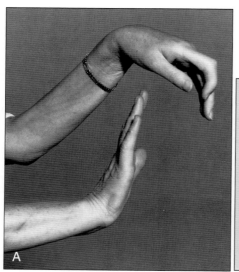
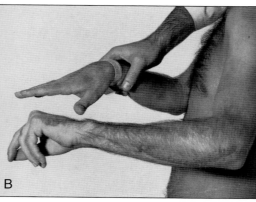

FIGURE 7-16 These figures compare the clinical presentation of a radial and a posterior interosseous nerve (PIN) palsy. (A) A complete radial palsy involves the patient's left arm compared with the normal function of the right arm. (B) A PIN palsy involves this patient's left arm. The patient can only partially extend the wrist, and finger and thumb extension is poor.

nerve, or the forearm branch of the musculocutaneous nerve. The closest the radial nerve has to an autonomous zone for sensation is the anatomical snuffbox region, which is located between the abductor pollicis and extensor pollicis longus muscles.

Superficial sensory nerve damage is often associated with a painful paresthesia, which may have a burning nature, making contact with the dorsum of the hand especially uncomfortable. Sensory loss in a radial distribution unassociated with pain or paresthesias does not interfere with hand function.

SUBSTITUTE OR TRICK MOVEMENTS

In testing for radial palsy, the examiner must be aware of a number of possible trick or substitute movements that can mimic radial-innervated function. Even though the extensor communis muscle is paralyzed, the interosseous muscles can appear to extend the fingers as they are abducted. True extensor function can be tested by placing the hand on a flat surface and asking the patient to extend the fingers above the surface one by one. With extensor communis muscle paralysis, the examiner may be fooled into thinking the ulnar-innervated interossei muscles are also weak, because with finger drop or fingers in a downward flexed position at the metacarpophalangeal joint, the interosseous muscles, which abduct and adduct fingers, do not perform well. This can be minimized by testing for abduction and adduction with the fingers on a flat surface or forcing the fingers into a hyperextended position, thus substituting for extensor communis muscle function, and having the patient abduct and adduct the fingers against those of the examiner. It must be re-emphasized that wrist extension by radial-innervated muscles can also be mimicked by a movement in which the fingers are flexed and the wrist is forced into a degree of extension. This occurs when the extensor tendons have been shortened as a result of paralysis or direct injury to muscle or tendons.

Supinator muscle function can also be mimicked by biceps/brachialis muscle contractions, particularly if the elbow is flexed or at least not fully extended, because the partial insertion of the biceps muscle into the proximal ulna tends to pull the forearm,

and thus the hand, into a palm-up position. Biceps/brachialis muscle function can be mistaken for brachioradialis muscle function and vice versa, particularly if the forearm is not partially pronated when brachioradialis function is tested. Gravity alone can substitute for triceps function, but palpation of the triceps during extension of the forearm should confirm this muscle's participation.

ELECTROPHYSIOLOGICAL STUDIES

Even though radial nerve function is important for a useful hand, the radial nerve differs from the median and ulnar nerves since there are no radial-innervated hand intrinsic muscles. Electrical studies therefore concentrate on the triceps, the one arm muscle innervated by the nerve, and, in addition, the proximal and mid-forearm muscles, i.e. the brachioradialis, ECR, ECU, supinator, extensor communis, and extensor pollicis longus muscles are evaluated.

Proximal injury to the upper arm is detected by denervational changes in the triceps and in the more distal muscles. If posterior cord involvement has resulted in radial distribution loss, then, in addition to triceps changes, there are denervational changes in the deltoid, latissimus dorsi muscles, and sometimes the subscapularis muscle. Not all of the triceps muscle may show such changes, because this muscle has three parts and a number of triceps branches leave the posterior cord close to the origination of the radial nerve.[48]

Midhumeral-level injury is documented by electrical change in the brachioradialis and more distally innervated muscles, but absence in the triceps. Of importance is the time required for reversal of denervational changes in the brachioradialis.[41] The brachioradialis muscle receives proximal input in the distal third of the arm and other input from branches at the level of the elbow and even somewhat more distally. The common axonotmetic injury associated with midhumeral-level damage secondary to fracture may require 3–4 months for enough axons of sufficient caliber and myelination to reach the brachioradialis muscle and adequate motor end-plate reconstruction to occur so that the number of fibrillations and denervational potentials decrease in this muscle. Other signs of re-innervation include nascent potentials and the return of evoked muscle action potentials on stimulation of the more proximal radial nerve. Somewhat antedating this reversal in electromyographic denervational changes is the contraction of the brachioradialis muscle in response to stimulation of the radial nerve in the lower lateral arm.[37] A stimulus site is usually found several inches above the elbow, where the nerve is located usually between, although somewhat deep to, the biceps/brachialis and triceps muscles. An attempt can also be made to stimulate the radial nerve in the humeral groove as it winds around the humerus to travel from a medial to a lateral position in the mid-upper arm. After the brachioradialis muscle begins to recover, the ECR muscle usually shows electrical signs of recovery a few months later.[60] This recovery is then followed by recovery in the ECU muscle. Unfortunately, electrical and clinical recovery in the extensors communis, pollicis longus, indicis proprius, and digiti minimi is less certain, and if recovery does occur, it is delayed for another 6–9 months.[4] This is so even though more proximal muscles have recovered good function.

An interesting observation can sometimes be made by placing a needle in the anconeus, an almost vestigial muscle overlying the

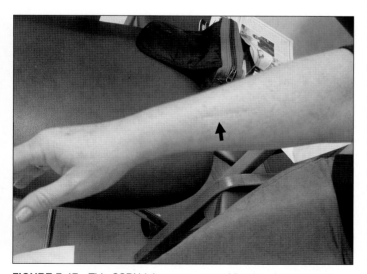

FIGURE 7-17 This SSRN injury was caused by the placement of fixation pins to stabilize the forearm *(arrow)*.

lateral olecranon of the ulna. Reversal of denervational changes in that muscle may antedate similar changes in the ECR and ECU muscles and, occasionally, in the brachioradialis muscle by some weeks.

With elbow-level lesions, the ECR and ECU muscles may recover electrical loss relatively quickly. Unfortunately, with some penetrating injuries, these muscles may have sustained a severe enough branch injury that they do not recover. Return of wrist extension under these circumstances may be dependent on recovery of more distal extensor communis and pollicis longus muscles. Electrical assessment for recovery should include these muscles, because the ECR and especially the ECU muscles may remain deinnervated under some circumstances.

The supinator muscle is a difficult one to evaluate, but fortunately the electrodiagnostic concomitants of a volar forearm PIN palsy are as striking as its clinical counterparts. Sensory conduction from the SSRN is spared or, at worst, mildly reduced in velocity. If a needle is placed by a skilled electrodiagnostician, the supinator muscle shows only partial denervational changes, the ECR muscle is spared, and the ECU, extensor communis, and extensor pollicis longus muscles exhibit changes. With supinator-level entrapment, the onset of denervational changes in these muscles may be delayed beyond the usual 3 weeks, but motor conduction velocities to the same muscles are prolonged early in the course of the entrapment.[11] To stimulate the PIN without surgical exposure, needle electrodes are usually necessary. The whole radial nerve can be stimulated at the elbow or above with recordings from the extensor indicis, extensor pollicis longus, or extensor communis muscles. Recovery of more normal conduction velocities may take many months to occur, even after a technically successful decompression of PIN.

With dorsal forearm lesions to the branches of the radial nerve, the results of electrodiagnosis are variable since the distribution of loss may not be uniform: some portions of the extensor pollicis longus and especially the extensor communis muscles have loss, and other portions do not. Such findings highlight the difficulties of surgical repair at this level, to be discussed.

SURGICAL EXPOSURE

MEDIAL ARM

The exposure of the radial nerve between its origin from the posterior cord to the medial border of the spiral groove is straightforward, but the surgeon must pay attention to certain details to avoid injury to other peripheral nerves.

In the usual case, as described earlier, the thoracodorsal nerve is a branch of the posterior cord, but occasionally it may be a branch of the axillary nerve, and, rarely, a branch of the radial nerve. Thoracodorsal fascicles are discrete, so they can be split back to the level of the posterior cord and appropriately excluded from repair.

The operator must be careful not to damage branches to the triceps, and this accident is less likely to occur if the surgical dissection proceeds in a proximal to distal direction.[22] Like the thoracodorsal nerve, the triceps branches can usually be split back and away from the posterior cord and proximal radial nerve. The triceps branches can have a very proximal take-off from the radial nerve or the posterior cord junction with the radial nerve. The latissimus dorsi muscle's "shining silver tendon" and fascia is a familiar landmark on the posterior wall of the axilla. The axillary nerve leaves

the axilla by running through the quadrangular space whose lower border is the tendon of the latissimus dorsi. The axillary nerve can also be split away from the posterior cord over quite a distance, but it is difficult to follow proximally through divisional and trunk levels, although the posterior division of the upper trunk is its usual origin. Although the median and ulnar nerves are nerves of the flexor compartment of the arm and the radial nerve is in the extensor compartment, these nerves are closely related throughout their proximal course, and prolonged retraction of median and ulnar nerves should be avoided during the dissection of the radial nerve itself.

The radial nerve runs across the latissimus dorsi and takes an oblique course toward the medial aspect of the arm, where it lies on the volar surface of the triceps, behind the medial intramuscular septum.

As the dissection nears the elbow, a number of vessels, including the radial collateral artery, may be encountered. The radial collateral artery may be an important component of the vascular anastomosis around the elbow joint, particularly if prior injury has resulted in occlusion of the brachial artery.[25] In this circumstance, the artery should be carefully guarded during dissection of the radial nerve.

The proximal radial nerve can also be approached posteriorly and this alternative exposure is well described by Henry.[20] The patient is positioned prone with the operative arm at the side. An incision is made curving medially beneath the lower border of the deltoid and then extended inferiorly between the long and lateral heads of the triceps (Figs 7-18 to 7-20). The latter are palpable because there is a slight depression between them. The fascia is then split, taking care to stay in the midline. The radial nerve, including its triceps branches, is exposed and can be traced through the spiral groove to the junction of the middle and lower thirds of the forearm. This approach is excellent as long as more distal nerve does not need to be exposed to gain length or to harvest forearm-level SSRN for use as a graft.

IN THE SPIRAL GROOVE

The radial nerve can be exposed on both the medial and lateral aspects of the arm. By operating alternatively from these two aspects of the arm, the segment of the nerve immediately behind the humerus can be exposed without injuring the triceps musculature (Fig. 7-21).[25] If irreparable injury to the radial nerve immediately behind the humerus is evident grossly or by intraoperative evoked nerve action potential (NAP) studies, the radial nerve is sectioned through to areas of normal fascicular pattern both proximal and distal to the injury (Fig. 7-22). As with other nerve lesions

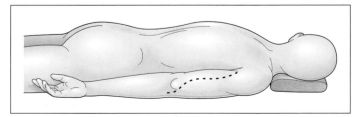

FIGURE 7-18 This is the incision for the posterior approach to the radial nerve with the patient prone. This approach provides some exposure of the radial nerve proximal to, through, and below the humeral groove.

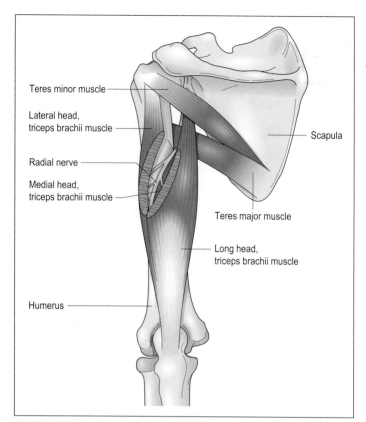

FIGURE 7-19 This drawing illustrates the junction of the lateral and long heads of the triceps seen posteriorly, which is an important landmark for the posterior approach to the radial nerve. By splitting these two heads, the nerve is seen in its direct relationship with the posterior aspect of the humerus.

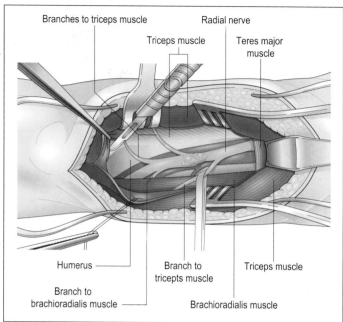

FIGURE 7-20 This illustration shows the triceps muscle split to expose the midarm-level radial nerve as seen from a posterior approach. The Army-Navy retractor to the right is displacing the deltoid muscle proximally.

requiring resection, it is very important to section back to healthy non-neuromatous tissue before attempting repair.[31] The operator then has a proximal stump on the medial aspect of the humerus and a distal stump on the lateral aspect of the arm.

Transposition of the distal stump beneath the biceps/brachialis muscles and anterior to the humerus permits the repair to be done on the medial side of the upper arm and regains some length, especially if the elbow is partially flexed.[36,48] This can be done by burrowing through muscle with a large hemostat or Kocher anterior to the humerus, pulling a silk suture through, gently tying the suture to the distal stump and very gently pulling it through the tunnel thus created. Depending on the length of resection, restoration of continuity may also be accomplished by passing grafts anterior to the humerus. The latter maneuver permits some shortening of the distance between the proximal and distal stumps, but in practical terms it is usually difficult to accomplish this with grafts less than 5 cm in length in adult patients.

LATERAL ARM

On leaving the spiral groove, the radial nerve moves from the extensor compartment and enters the flexor compartment of the arm by passing through the lateral intramuscular septum. The nerve in the lateral arm can be difficult to locate and usually requires a skin incision and deeper dissection extending from the arm, across

the elbow, to the forearm. Important for this dissection is the identification of the brachioradialis and brachialis muscles. The surgeon then places one thumb on the brachialis and the other thumb on the brachioradialis.[49] Pushing these two muscles apart reveals the radial nerve deep in the created valley (Fig. 7-23). If this does not demonstrate the radial nerve, it can be readily located deep to the brachioradialis muscle at the elbow and proximal forearm level and traced proximally into the arm.[25]

ANTECUBITAL FOSSA

The nerve is dissected out between the brachialis and brachioradialis muscles. At this level, it lies somewhat beneath the latter muscle, which needs to be retracted laterally to expose the nerve.[49] The nerve should be gently "tented forward" on a Penrose drain to reveal the branches to the brachioradialis and ECRL muscles, as well as its major divisions into the SSRN and PIN. The point at which the PIN leaves the SSRN is variable but easily demonstrated by gently retracting the more proximal radial nerve upward with a Penrose drain. It is essential that the surgeon has an adequate view of this region, and this is accomplished by extending the skin incision distally over the brachioradialis muscle and, if needed, onto the dorsal forearm. More distal exposure of the SSRN is an easy matter as overlying deep fascia is sectioned and the brachioradialis muscle is retracted. This nerve is handled with care because it may be useful as a donor graft. Fascicles of the SSRN nerve can be dissected back into the main radial nerve trunk with relative ease, and this may be an important maneuver to insure that subsequent regeneration of the main radial nerve is directed solely into the PIN. This is especially important if the intent of surgery is to restore the important muscles innervated by the PIN.

121

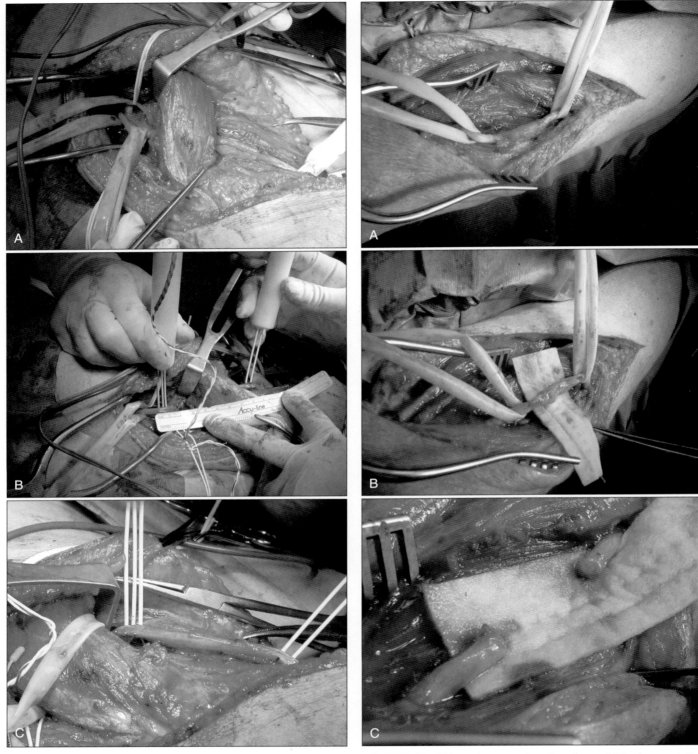

FIGURE 7-21 The right arm-level radial nerve had a focal neuroma in continuity. **(A)** The patient was placed supine and the nerve was exposed proximally (to the left of the triceps muscle and encircled with a Penrose drain) and distally. **(B)** A recording was made across the radial nerve under the triceps muscle and **(C)** distal to the triceps muscle. There was significant scar, which decreased the nerve action potential recording and a neurolysis was performed.

FIGURE 7-22 This patient was placed supine and this shows a left forearm elbow-level radial nerve injury. **(A)** The upper and lower retractor teeth are displacing the medial and lateral heads of the triceps muscle, respectively, as shown in this intraoperative photograph. **(B)** The radial nerve was carefully isolated as shown. **(C)** Nerve action potentials were not recordable across the lesion and a neuroma was resected. A graft repair was performed.

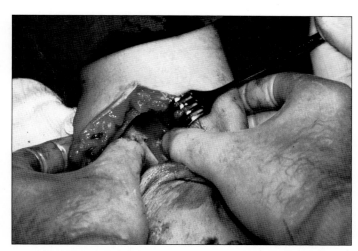

FIGURE 7-23 This shows a method of exposing the radial nerve at the level of the elbow. The operator's left thumb is retracting against the brachioradialis muscle and the right thumb against the biceps/brachialis muscles: the nerve is found deep in the groove between these muscles.

POSTERIOR INTEROSSEOUS NERVE

The exposure of the radial nerve on the medial and lateral aspects of the arm and in the antecubital fossa is relatively straightforward; however, dissection of the PIN can be difficult, particularly if there is a great deal of scarring and adjacent soft tissue injury.[19] The PIN leaves the main radial nerve to reach the interval between the superficial and deep heads of the supinator. The nerve then passes between the two heads of that muscle and winds around the lateral aspect of the proximal radius to reach the extensor aspect of the forearm. As the PIN reaches the dorsal forearm, it branches to supply most of the extensor musculature. The key to understanding this anatomy is an appreciation of the detailed structure of the supinator muscle.[63] This muscle has humeral and ulnar heads of origin and a single point of insertion onto the radius.

Numerous small vessels surround the PIN as it approaches the upper border of the superficial head of the supinator in the forearm. These vessels form leashes both volar and posterior to the nerve and can bleed vigorously if entered without preparation. These vessels must be coagulated with bipolar forceps discretely to avoid injuring the PIN itself and the branches running from that nerve to the supinator muscle. The arcade of Frohse is usually well defined and is often of a tendinous nature (Figs 7-24, 7-25). By dividing the superficial head of the supinator, the surgeon can expose the PIN as it winds around the forearm into the extensor compartment. At this point, the operator usually has difficulty with the exposure and should switch the approach to that placed on the dorsum of the forearm. This may be accomplished though either a separate or the same skin incision (Fig. 7-26).

A surgical instrument passed from the flexor aspect of the proximal exposure along the course of the distal PIN but superficial to it can serve as a useful landmark after the dorsal forearm approach is initiated. The surgical instrument can then be palpated and used as a guide as the operator splits the superficial extensor layer on the posterior aspect of the forearm, thus displaying the distal heads of the supinator muscle. Here, the PIN is running at right angles to the supinator muscle fibers.

Division of the superficial head of the supinator is then finished, taking care that the cut does not injure the numerous fine branches innervating the various extensor muscles. Repair of the PIN itself is usually a reasonably simple matter after the approach anatomy is mastered, but repair of the fine distal branches may be quite difficult.[38] Not only are the branches small, but they are usually enmeshed in heavy scar tissue.

SUPERFICIAL SENSORY RADIAL NERVE

Exposure of the SSRN is straightforward in the proximal forearm (Fig. 7-27). An appropriately placed longitudinal incision defines the nerve, which may be a useful donor for graft repair of injuries of either the radial nerve or PIN. After it arises from the main radial nerve, the SSRN courses beneath the brachioradialis muscle, but above or superficial to the ECRL muscle. The SSRN supplies the skin over the radial side of the dorsum of the wrist and hand and branches terminate on the dorsal surface of the radial three-and-a-half digits. Particular attention should be given to the relationships between the wrist-level branches of the SSRN, the brachioradialis tendon, and the three tendons destined for the proximal and distal phalanx of the thumb. In this area, there is frequent overlap with terminal branches of the lateral antebrachial cutaneous nerve of the forearm or the distal lateral branch of the musculocutaneous nerve.[33] This needs to be appreciated if the operation is intended to resolve painful neuromas. These branches can contribute to the neuroma, and pain can recur unless the neuroma is removed along with these involved branches.

RESULTS

The outcome of surgical repair of the radial nerve with or without tendon transfer is considered excellent by most authors in the field.[24,26,36,64] The radial nerve is felt to be the most favorable major nerve in the body in terms of return of function, either spontaneously or after repair.[7,40,44] This is also reflected in our personal series.

Those patients referred for possible surgery and selected for conservative management almost invariably recovered to a grade 4 or 5. Even those requiring operative exploration fared extremely well. This is not surprising in cases in which intraoperative NAP studies indicated significant regeneration through a lesion in continuity and, as a result, only neurolysis rather than resection and repair was done. Significant recovery also occurred with repair, whether by end-to-end suture anastomosis or by grafts. Such good results can be related to several factors. All muscles receiving motor input from the radial nerve receive it relatively proximal in the limb compared with the median- and especially the ulnar-innervated muscles. Thus, the terminal muscles innervated by the radial nerve are in the middle third of the forearm and not in the hand. Furthermore, although the radial nerve has a significant sensory outflow, this destination is to the dorsal aspect of the forearm and hand sensory areas, which are relatively less important than other sensory areas. Imperfect recovery of sensation in these areas does not affect use of the limb and hand as much as it would in the median or even the ulnar distributions.

Despite favorable results with the proper management of radial nerve injuries, recovery of the extensor communis and especially the extensor pollicis longus muscles is difficult to obtain.[50] This is especially so with upper arm lesions, in which recovery of the brachioradialis muscle, improved supination, and some wrist extension

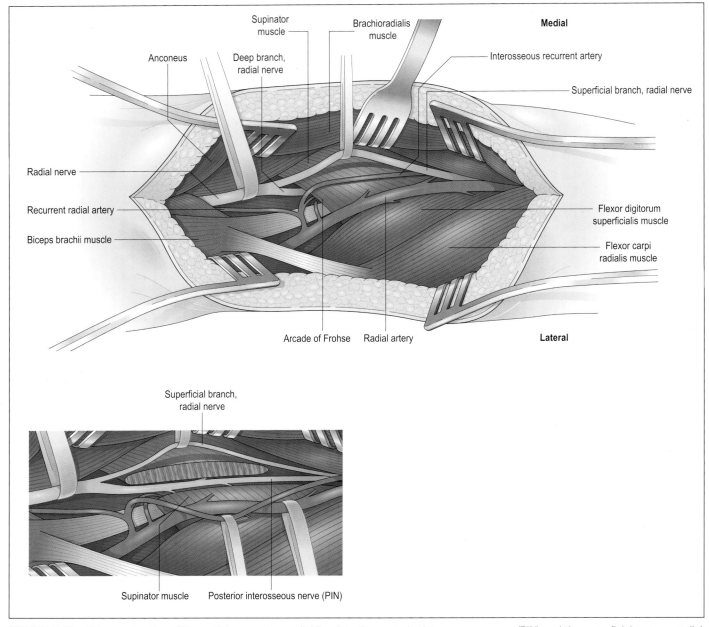

FIGURE 7-24 This is a drawing of the radial nerve shown dividing into the posterior interosseous nerve (PIN) and the superficial sensory radial nerve with the associated radial artery and branches. The PIN runs beneath the arcade of Frohse. The inset shows sectioning of the volar supinator. Within the supinator canal, branches of the more dorsal supinator muscle are seen; distally, early branches to extensor of the fingers and thumb are visible.

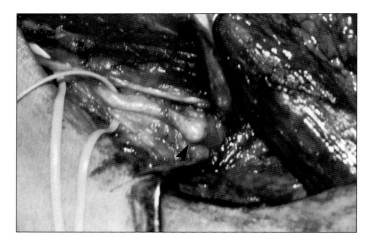

FIGURE 7-25 A neuroma of the posterior interosseous nerve is seen *(arrowhead)* located just proximal to the arcade of Frohse.

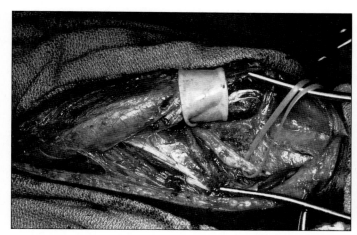

FIGURE 7-26 Exposure of distal posterior interosseous nerve (PIN) on the dorsum of the forearm and take-off point (at the level of the plastic loop) of the extensor communis, pollicis longus, and indicis branches. The more distal supinator has been divided to expose the distal PIN; the exposed brachioradialis muscle is retracted superiorly by a Penrose drain.

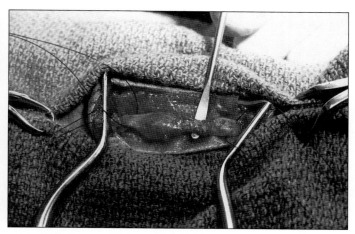

FIGURE 7-28 An SSRN injury in continuity with a more proximal bulbous enlargement to the left is seen in this intraoperative photograph. This lesion was resected along with the nerve well proximal and distal to the injury site. The proximal end was left buried beneath the brachioradialis muscle after sealing the exposed fasciculi with the bipolar coagulator.

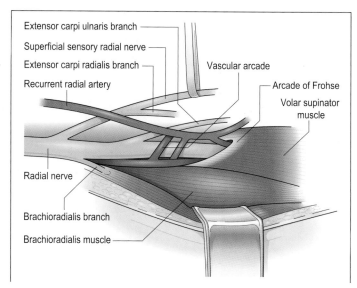

FIGURE 7-27 This is a drawing of the anatomy of the radial to superficial sensory radial nerve and posterior interosseous nerve complexes viewed from a volar approach at a proximal forearm level. (From Cravens G and Kline D: Posterior interosseous palsies. Neurosurgery 27:397–402, 1990.)

usually provided by ECR muscle is expected. In these lesions, recovery of extension of fingers and thumb and even ECU is less certain.[39] Fortunately, use of a portion of the flexor carpi ulnaris (FCU) or flexor superficialis as a tendon transfer to the extensor expansion of the digits is an excellent substitute under these circumstances.[10] If it is properly done, good finger and even some degree of thumb extension can be gained.[61] Because results are good, some feel that tendon transfer rather than neural repair is the primarily indicated procedure.[16,59] We do not agree with this, preferring to reserve tendon transfer for cases in which neural regeneration is unlikely or does not occur. On the other hand, even if a transfer is done before neural regeneration is completed, we have not seen it complicate the result. Although we do not hesitate

to recommend tendon transfer if appropriate, we do not advocate early transfer unless it is estimated that the chances for successful neural recovery are quite poor.

Less encouraging are those repairs attempted at the distal terminus of the PIN, where identification and reconstruction of branches on the dorsum of the forearm are difficult. Very proximal lesions involving radial outflow at the posterior cord or upper radial nerve levels and dorsal forearm injuries involving the extensor communis and pollicis longus branches both share in the difficulty of obtaining recovery of digit extension and the more likely need for tendon transfer.[56]

Equally frustrating can be the treatment of SSRN neuromas, which at times can resist any form of management (Fig. 7-28).[33] We prefer sharp section, bipolar coagulation of the individual fascicles under magnification, and then placement of the proximal nerve in healthy soft tissue free of scar, rather than burying the nerve in bone, wrapping it in Silastic, or capping it. If repair of the SSRN is elected to minimize neuroma formation and recurrence of pain and paresthesias, it must be meticulous. Unfortunately, similar symptoms can occur as a result of the inevitable neuroma in continuity that occurs with either end-to-end suture anastomosis or graft repairs.

Patients likely to have a prolonged wrist drop and inability to extend the fingers and thumb should be fitted with a dynamic dorsiflexion splint.[8] This splint holds the wrist in a mildly extended position and is fitted with an outrigger with rubber bands and finger pads. This permits the patient to flex against an extensor-like resistance and tends to maintain the optimal length of the extensor communis and pollicis longus muscles.

FURTHER ANALYSIS OF RESULTS IN THE RADIAL NERVE SERIES

The mechanisms of injuries or lesions involving the radial nerve are seen in Table 7-1. Included in the series are a relatively large number of fractures, lacerations, blunt contusions, and GSWs. Although not usually injury related, there were also a large number of entrapments, mostly affecting PIN, and tumors, usually involv-

Table 7-1 Radial nerve – mechanisms of injury

Mechanism	Operative cases	Nonoperative cases
Fracture	53	32
Laceration	44	3
Blunt contusion or Volkmann volar compartment syndrome	29	21
Tumor	25	6
Entrapment	22	10
Gunshot wound	16	6
Injection	9	3
Prior suture or neurolysis	7	3
Dislocation	0	2
Sleep compression	0	4
Totals	205	90

Table 7-2 Radial nerve injuries by level*

Level	Operative cases	Nonoperative cases
Arm	83	37
Posterior interosseous nerve	37	12
Elbow	30	15
Radial sensory	21	14
Dorsal forearm	9	2
Total	180	80

*Excludes tumors or those injuries involving several levels.

Table 7-3 Arm-level radial nerve: operative findings, operations, and results in 83 injuries*

Operative finding	NAP	Operation	Result
Transection		Primary suture	5/4
Transection		Secondary suture	8/6
Transection		Secondary grafts	5/3
In continuity lesion	+	Neurolysis	22/21
In continuity lesion	−	Suture	14/13
In continuity lesion	−	Grafts	29/26

*Number of nerves operated/number of nerves reaching ≥ grade 3 result. Cases having poor follow-up (<1 year) were graded as <3. NAP, nerve action potential.

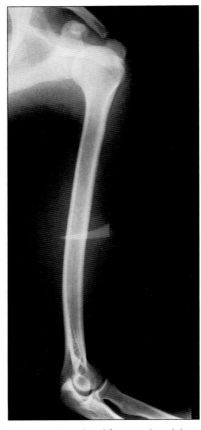

FIGURE 7-29 A penetrating shard from a glass injury seen in this plain film of the humerus caused a midhumeral-level transected radial nerve. This was repaired within 24 hours of the injury. Retained glass fragments can usually be visualized by appropriate soft tissue radiographs regardless of the lead content of the glass.

ing the upper arm-level radial nerve. Only 90 of the radial lesions evaluated did not require surgery.

As can be seen in Table 7-2, the largest category was that of lesions involving the arm-level radial nerve, followed by those involving the PIN and the elbow-level radial nerve. Radial nerve sensory lesions and dorsal forearm radial branch lesions were less frequent, especially those requiring operation.

AT THE ARM LEVEL

Table 7-3 shows the number of radial nerves having surgical intervention which were transected and the number in continuity, operations performed, and results by a whole nerve grading system. Eighteen arm-level radial nerves, which underwent surgery, were found to be transected, while 65 were in continuity. Knife and glass wounds were responsible for most transections; a few were caused by fan and propeller blade injuries, GSWs, and compound fractures of the humerus (Figs 7-29, 7-30). Of the five having primary end-

to-end suture anastomosis repair within 72 hours of injury, four recovered to a grade 3 or better level. Six of eight secondarily sutured nerves recovered adequately, as did three of five secondarily repaired by grafts.

A number of blunt contusive injuries to the radial nerve, two injection palsies, and four GSWs had recordable intraoperative

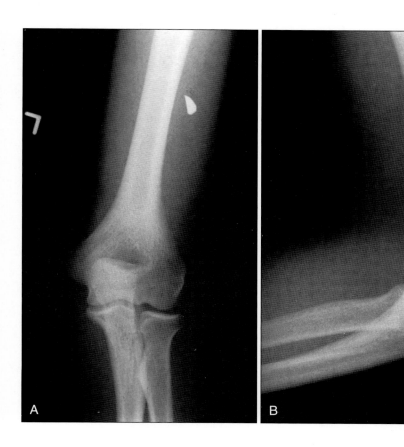

FIGURE 7-30 **(A)** Anteroposterior and **(B)** lateral plain X-rays of a missile embedded in the left arm. A patient gave the history of using an ax which struck a piece of metal embedded in a tree trunk. A resultant missile fragment penetrated the arm and was found embedded in the radial nerve as it lay in the humeral groove. This was repaired secondarily, a few weeks after the incident. Secondary repair of a nerve injured in this fashion probably gives a better result than an acute or primary repair, provided that good care is given to the soft tissue wound.

Table 7-4 Arm-level radial nerve: graded results by mechanism in 93 operative cases

Mechanism	No.	Grade				
		5	4	3	2	1
Fracture	36	8	16	8	3	1
Contusion	13	1	6	4	1	1
Laceration	12	4	5	2	1	0
Gunshot wound	10	1	5	3	1	0
Tumor	10	5	3	2	0	0
Injection	9	5	3	1	0	0
Compression	3	0	2	0	1	0
Totals	93	24	40	20	7	2

No., number of cases.

Table 7-5 Arm-level radial nerve: graded results by mechanism in 39 nonoperative cases

Mechanism	No.	Grade				
		5	4	3	2	1
Fracture	21	8	6	5	1	1
Contusion	7	2	4	1	0	0
Gunshot wound	5	4	0	1	0	0
Tumor	2	0	1	1	0	0
Dislocation	2	1	1	0	0	0
Laceration	2	2	0	0	0	0
Totals	39	17	12	8	1	1

No., number of cases.

NAPs across their lesions despite a total distal functional deficit. These lesions in continuity had neurolysis and did well. Where there was no NAP transmitted, despite gross continuity, and resection was necessary, end-to-end suture anastomosis repair led to acceptable recoveries in 13 of 14 cases and graft repair to good recoveries in 26 of 29 instances. For purposes of this table, if follow-up was not available, recovery was graded as 0.

Tables 7-4 and 7-5 show the grades achieved in the operative and nonoperative categories at this level according to the type of lesion. Striking is the large number of grade 3 or better results (82%) in those selected for operation. Despite this, it was difficult to restore a grade 5 finger and thumb extension, especially in the fracture, contusion, and GSW categories (Figs 7-31, 7-32). Here, lesions tended to be lengthier and more likely to require graft repair than the laceration and injection categories, in which, if repair was necessary, end-to-end suture anastomosis was more likely than graft repair. Despite the inability to restore full finger extension, most patients functioned well and did not wish tendon transfers to be done. The interval between the injury and/or the onset of symptoms and operation is shown in Table 7-6.

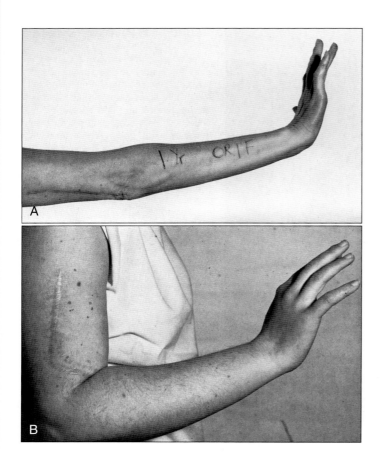

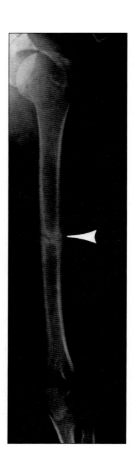

FIGURE 7-31 **(A)** Recovery of radial function in a patient with humeral fracture requiring open reduction and plating is shown. Wrist extension was normal by 1 year, but finger extension, although greatly improved, had not fully recovered at that time. **(B)** Recovery of radial function in another patient is seen 2.5 years after 13-cm grafts were placed at an axillary to arm level.

FIGURE 7-32 A healed midhumeral fracture is shown, which was *(arrowhead)* treated by closed reduction and associated with a radial palsy. This palsy reversed spontaneously with an almost complete recovery of what must have been an axonotmetic or Sunderland grade 2–3 lesion by 2 years after injury.

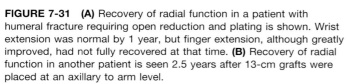

Table 7-6 Arm-level radial nerve: operative intervals (n = 93)

Mechanism	No.	Months											
		0	1	2	3	4	5	6	7	8	9	12	>12
Fracture	36	0	0	1	7	10	9	5	0	2	2	0	0
Contusion	13	0	0	0	1	5	3	3	1	0	0	0	0
Laceration	12	5	3	3	1	0	0	0	0	0	0	0	0
Gunshot wound	10	0	0	1	2	3	3	0	1	0	0	0	0
Tumor	10	0	1	2	0	1	1	2	1	0	0	0	2
Injection	9	0	0	0	1	3	0	3	2	0	0	0	0
Entrapment	3	0	0	0	0	0	0	1	1	0	1	0	0
Totals	93	5	4	7	12	22	16	14	6	2	3	0	2

No., number of cases.

The three entrapments were both spontaneous in onset and occurred at a midhumeral level in the area of the humeral groove.[30,34] In one case, a middle-aged man had a hobby of overhead softball pitching and may have had an element of chronic stretch as well as entrapment involving nerve at this level.

Five of the nine injection injuries to the radial nerve required resection and repair (Figs 7-33, 7-34). Results were good, although extension of fingers and thumb usually remained weak. One patient who had resection of a large neurofibroma along with nerve done elsewhere required a very proximal and lengthy graft repair with poor results. Results in those patients selected for conservative management were excellent, although functional loss was partial at

the start in almost one-third of these cases. In the other cases, spontaneous improvement clinically or by electromyography was evident by 3–4 months after injury. Also of interest were the two tumor patients who had tumor resection elsewhere, had partial deficit, and in both cases improved enough spontaneously so that operative repair was not needed.

CASE SUMMARIES – ARM LEVEL

CASE 1

A 27-year-old airline stewardess noted pain radiating down her arm to the back of her hand while serving food in flight. If her lateral upper arm knocked against a chair back or passenger, radicular pain was reproduced. She had no café au lait spots or other history of tumors and examination by an airline physician revealed a mass 3 cm in diameter below the deltoid and adjacent to the triceps, which could be moved from side to side but not up and down. There were no neurological deficits.

At operation, a discrete intraneural tumor was noted with fascicles spread around it like a basket (Fig. 7-35). By splitting the fascicles apart over the bulk of the tumor and by some interfascicular dissection proximally and distally, the tumor mass could be exposed. One fascicle entering and leaving the core of the tumor did not transmit an NAP. This feeding fascicle was sectioned, the fascicles dissected away from the capsule of the tumor, and the schwannoma was then removed "in toto."

Postoperatively, she had only a mild sensory deficit over the dorsum of the hand and no motor dysfunction. She has done well, with a 2.5 year period of follow-up.

COMMENT

A nerve tumor should always be considered as a possible etiology for any mass in an extremity. Both the patient's symptoms and physical findings suggested tumor involving the radial nerve. Schwannomas and most neurofibromas characteristically do not cause a neurological deficit and usually can be removed without causing any serious loss unless there has been prior biopsy or attempted removal.

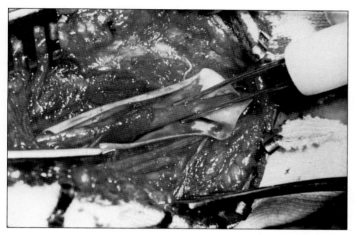

FIGURE 7-33 This is an intraoperative photograph of the result of a radial injection just below the lateral head of the triceps muscle. There was no brachioradialis muscle contraction in response to intraoperative stimulation either at or above the lesion 4 months after injury, so the lesion was resected and a repair was done. Stimulating electrodes are on the proximal stump of the nerve. (Photograph provided courtesy of Dr. Glenn Meyer of Milwaukee, Wisconsin.)

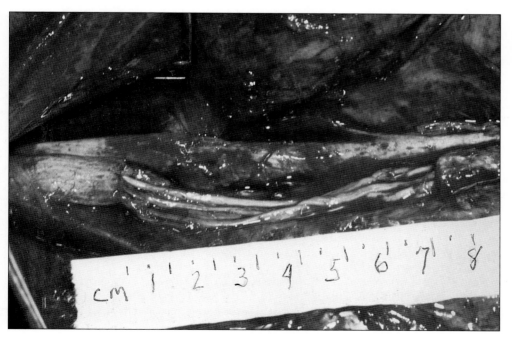

FIGURE 7-34 An intraoperative photograph showing a split repair of nerve injection injury using antebrachial cutaneous nerve grafts is shown.

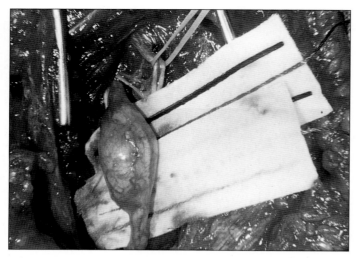

FIGURE 7-35 This is a typical neural sheath tumor involving the radial nerve at the lateral arm level. The lateral triceps muscle has been split to expose the lesion. A plastic loop is around several triceps branches.

CASE 2

A 19-year-old male received a morphine injection in his lateral arm below the deltoid muscle in preparation for a laminectomy. He felt an "electric shock" sensation travel down his arm to the back of his hand and had immediate wrist drop. Electromyography performed a week later showed absence of motor units in the brachioradialis and all of the more distal radial-innervated muscles. Radial sensory responses were recorded on several occasions and seemed to show a progressive decrease of the sensory NAP amplitudes and eventual loss. Examination a month later showed no function of the brachioradialis muscle, poor supination, and loss of wrist, finger, and thumb extension. Electromyography showed a severe denervational pattern with fibrillations as well as lack of motor units. Subsequent clinical and electrical follow-up at 2.5 months was the same, so the radial nerve was explored.

Exploration began in the lateral arm between the biceps and triceps muscles. A several-centimeter segment of nerve in the spiral groove was somewhat atrophic and was also invested in some scar tissue. Nerve action potential recording on the lateral arm segment distal to the lesion gave a very small potential. As a result, the radial nerve was exposed proximally by a separate incision and dissection in the high medial arm. The NAP recording from nerve proximal to the spiral groove gave a response of good amplitude conducting at 80 m/sec and recording across the spiral groove gave an NAP, but of much smaller amplitude, conducting at 30 m/sec. An internal neurolysis was done, and only a small amount of neural tissue and scar was resected. The histological study showed myxoid material surrounding degenerated nerve fibers and forming a perineurial halo. A few of the axonal bundles had myxoid material within their confines.

He has recovered grade 4–5 function even in finger and thumb extension. The follow-up has extended to 3.5 years.

COMMENT

Injection injuries are preventable, and all who give injections should be thoroughly trained to avoid these painful neuropathies. In this case, the NAP recording helped make the decision against resection.

CASE 3

A 20-year-old patient sustained a midarm humeral fracture. Loss of strength of muscles innervated by the radial nerve was immediate and complete below the triceps muscle. The fracture was treated in a closed fashion by cast placement, but clinical and electromyographic loss remained complete. As a result, the radial nerve was explored at 4.5 months after injury. This was done by exposing the distal arm-level nerve between the triceps and biceps muscles laterally. There was no NAP along this segment, so the more proximal radial nerve was exposed in the medial arm near the axilla. Stimulation there and recording from the lateral arm segment gave no NAP.

A lesion in continuity 3 cm in length centered at the humeral or spiral groove was resected. The distal nerve was then mobilized to a point below the elbow. Branches to the brachioradialis muscle were defined and protected. The distal nerve was then transposed by placing it beneath the biceps/brachialis and anterior to the distal humerus. With mild flexion of the elbow, enough length was gained to allow an end-to-end suture anastomosis on the medial side of the arm.

Wrist extension returned to a grade 5, and extension of fingers to a grade 3, but the extensor pollicis longus grade was only a trace. The follow-up extended to 3 years. The patient was able to use the limb quite well; therefore, tendon transfer was not necessary.

COMMENT

It is appropriate to wait a few months for results because the majority of radial nerve injuries associated with fracture recover spontaneously. If no brachioradialis function is present by 4 months, exploration should not be further delayed.

CASE 4

A 42-year-old woman sustained a 38-caliber GSW at the midarm level and the humerus was partially splintered, but not totally fractured. Loss of radial nerve function was complete clinically and electrically, and persisted for 4 months. A partially transected nerve was found. Four grafts of approximately 5 cm in length were placed. At 2 years postoperatively, the brachioradialis muscle function was grade 5, supination grade 4, and wrist and finger extension grade 3.

COMMENT

Frequently and surprising to some, GSWs are associated with lesions in continuity and not total division of the nerve. It is thus appropriate to wait 3 months to see if there is clinical recovery. In this case, none was found and, therefore, the patient was explored, revealing the pathology of a partially transected nerve. Figure 7-36 shows the results in another GSW case.

AT THE ELBOW LEVEL

Transections of the elbow-level radial nerve were caused by lacerations in nine cases and a gunshot wound and fracture in one case apiece. Primary repair of three sharp transections at this level was quite successful. All three had grade 3 or better outcomes. Of interest was the number of lesions in continuity having a positive intraoperative NAP and their good recovery with neurolysis. This was because six of nine distal humeral fractures not only had left nerve in continuity but also were regenerating and thus had the recordable intraoperative NAP. The one fracture-associated lesion requiring repair had lengthy grafts and only recovered to grade 2 (Table 7-7).

Both Volkmann volar compartment syndrome cases involving elbow-level radial nerve had recovery after early fasciotomy and neurolysis. Five of seven lesions in continuity requiring graft repair

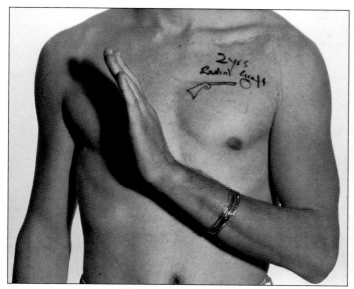

FIGURE 7-36 A radial gunshot wound in this young man was repaired by 4-cm grafts 2 years before. There was excellent return of wrist extension and some recovery of finger extension.

Table 7-7 Elbow-level radial nerve: operations and results in 37 injuries*

Operative finding	NAP	Operation	Result
Transection		Primary suture	3/3
Transection		Secondary suture	2/2
Transection		Secondary grafts	6/4
In continuity lesion	+	Neurolysis	17/17
In continuity lesion	–	Suture	2/2
In continuity lesion	–	Grafts	7/5

*Number of nerves operated/number of nerves reaching ≥ grade 3 result. Cases having poor follow-up (<1 year) were graded as <3. NAP, nerve action potential.

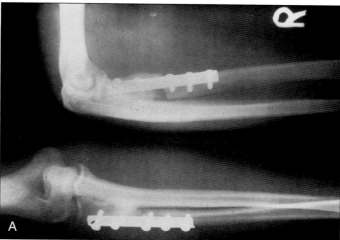
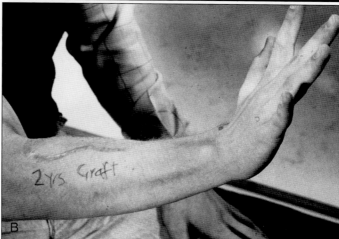

FIGURE 7-37 **(A)** This plain film shows a fracture of the radius which required plate and screw repair. An associated posterior interosseous nerve injury required graft repair 3 months later. **(B)** The patient recovered excellent wrist and some, but not complete, finger and thumb extension by 2 years after graft repair.

recovered to grade 3 or better (Fig. 7-37). See Tables 7-8 to 7-10 for more details on elbow-level lesions.

CASE SUMMARIES – ELBOW LEVEL

CASE 1

A 19-year-old male sustained a plate glass injury in which a shard of glass penetrated his lateral arm above the elbow. An acute exploration 8 hours after the injury showed a transected radial nerve. The nerve was neatly but somewhat obliquely transected.

After minimal trimming of both stumps, an end-to-end suture anastomosis repair was done using 6–0 nylon suture. He was fitted with a dynamic wrist and finger dorsiflexion splint with outrigger, rubber bands, and finger pads. With the help of this device and home exercises, he managed well.

At a clinic visit 1 year postoperatively, the brachioradialis and ECR muscles were grade 3 and supination was grade 2. There was only a trace of finger and

Table 7-8 Elbow-level radial nerve: graded results by mechanism in 35 operative cases

Mechanism	No.	Grade				
		5	4	3	2	1
Laceration	9	4	3	1	1	0
Fracture	9	2	5	1	1	1
Gunshot wound	6	1	4	1	0	0
Tumor	5	2	2	1	0	0
Contusion	4	0	2	1	1	0
Prior suture	2	0	1	0	1	0
Totals	35	9	17	5	4	0

No., number of cases.

131

thumb extension. By 3 years after operation, the brachioradialis muscle function had improved to grade 4 and wrist and finger extensors were grade 3–4. He no longer used the dorsiflexion splint and was managing his college classes and extracurricular activities, including baseball, without difficulty.

COMMENT

Sharp injuries due to laceration should be explored primarily, before stumps have an opportunity to retract. In this case, early surgery allowed end-to-end suture anastomosis repair.

CASE 2

This 8-year-old female lost her balance when she attempted to walk across the top of a swing set. While falling, she was impaled on a deer hook used to cure meat. She was rescued by her father, who found her hanging from the swing set with the hook embedded into her right elbow at the antecubital level. She required transfusions and acute repair of her brachial vein. She had a complete radial palsy below the branches to the brachioradialis. This included supination, wrist and finger extension, and sensation on the dorsum of the hand.

A transected radial nerve at the elbow level was repaired after trimming both stumps by end-to-end suture anastomosis using 6–0 nylon. This repair was done shortly after referral 4 months after the accident.

With the help of a tendon transfer 1 year later, a good result was gained. Wrist extensors by 3 years after neural repair were grade 4–5, the extensor communis muscles was grade 4, and extensor pollicis longus and supinator muscles were grade 3.

COMMENT

Repair for a complete loss of function associated with a penetrating wound of this nature could have occurred 2–4 weeks after injury. Tendon transfers can be tailored to specific residual defects if nerve suture is not entirely successful. Generally, we will wait several years after the initial nerve repair before recommending tendon transfer, unless the likelihood of recovery is very poor.

POSTERIOR INTEROSSEOUS NERVE LESIONS

The grading system used for evaluating PIN lesions is found in Table 7-11. Table 7-12 shows some of the details on 15 injured PINs, which underwent operation. Tables 7-13 and 7-14 show outcomes for operative and nonoperative cases by category. In cases in which there was complete preoperative loss, there were four transections caused by laceration and one associated with a fracture (Table 7-12). Of the lacerating injuries transecting PIN, one was repaired within 72 hours by suture and three by secondary suture. Despite a sharp mechanism for injury and complete preoperative loss, two were in gross physical continuity. Neither transmitted an NAP, and both required a repair, with eventual good results.

Each of the six fracture-associated PIN palsies had complete loss preoperatively (Fig. 7-37). In three cases, prior operative manipulation and plate and screw fixation of the fracture may have played a role in the origin of the PIN loss. One of these had three operations in an attempt to stabilize fractures of both the radius and ulna. In another case in which a fracture of the radius had been fixated, there was no continuity of the PIN. Grafts were necessary because a 6.3 cm gap resulted after stumps were trimmed to healthy tissue. The other four PIN palsies associated with fracture and operated on were in continuity. Two PIN lesions transmitted NAPs and had neurolysis, but two did not and required graft repairs. One patient had undergone prior neural operation.

Table 7-9 Elbow-level radial nerve: graded results by mechanism in 16 nonoperative cases

Mechanism	No.	Grade				
		5	4	3	2	1
Fracture	6	0	2	4	0	0
Contusion	4	3	1	0	0	0
Volkmann's volar contracture	2	0	0	1	1	0
Tumor	2	1	1	0	0	0
Gunshot wound	1	0	1	0	0	0
Prior suture	1	0	0	1	0	0
Totals	16	4	5	6	1	0

No., number of cases.

Table 7-10 Elbow-level radial nerve: operative intervals (n = 37)

Mechanism	No.	Months										
		0	1	2	3	4	5	6	7	8	9	12	>12
Laceration	9	3	3	1	1	0	1	0	0	0	0	0	0
Fracture	9	0	0	1	0	0	4	1	3	0	0	0	0
Gunshot wound	6	0	0	0	1	2	1	1	1	0	0	0	0
Tumor	6	0	0	0	1	0	1	2	0	1	1	0	0
Contusion	4	0	0	1	1	1	1	0	0	0	0	0	0
Prior suture	3	0	0	0	0	0	0	0	0	1	1	1	0
Totals	37	3	3	3	4	3	8	4	4	2	2	1	0

No., number of cases.

Excellent results were achieved by suture or grafts in both the laceration and fracture categories. Twenty-four PIN lesions transmitted NAPs. Despite good neural recovery, two had tendon transfers to help improve their function. Three contused PINS had recordable NAPs, underwent neurolysis, and have had substantial recovery (see Table 7-12).

Table 7-11 Grading of posterior interosseous nerve function

Grade	Description
0	No extensor carpi ulnaris (ECU), extensor communis (EC) or extensor pollicis longus (EPL)
1	Trace or against gravity only of ECU, but absent EC and EPL
2	Recovery of ECU but absent or trace only EC and EPL
3	Recovery of ECU and some EC but only weak or absent EPL
4	Recovery of moderate strength EC and EPL as well as full strength in ECU
5	Recovery of full strength in EPL and EC as well as in ECU

CASE SUMMARY – FOREARM-LEVEL POSTERIOR INTEROSSEOUS NERVE

CASE 1

This 25-year-old motorcyclist skidded off the road and struck a barbed wire fence. He sustained multiple ragged lacerations to the forearm, which were debrided, packed, and left open. The distal stump of a transected radial nerve was marked with a vascular clip and several weeks later the granulated areas were covered with skin grafts. The radial deficit was total from the supinator muscle and distally.

Unfortunately, repair of the radial nerve required grafts 8 cm in length. Grafts extended from main radial to the PIN just proximal to the arcade of Frohse, and the latter was sectioned. No attempt was made to repair SSRN, but one graft was led to a distal brachioradialis branch. Follow-up extended to 5 years. Wrist and finger extension including that to the thumb recovered to grade 3 level; supination remained absent and there was no sensory return.

COMMENT

Even in complex injury cases such as this, the radial nerve is worth repairing because of the known favorable outlook for this particular nerve.

POSTERIOR INTEROSSEOUS NERVE ENTRAPMENT

The PIN normally travels between the volar and dorsal levels of the supinator to reach the dorsum of the forearm. After exiting

Table 7-12 Posterior interosseous nerve injuries with complete preoperative loss (n = 15)

Nerve Injury	Operative findings	NAP	Operation	Result	F/up
Laceration	Transection		Secondary suture	4	2
Laceration	Transection		Secondary suture	4	1.5
Laceration	Transection		Secondary suture	4*	3
Laceration	Transection		Primary suture	5	3
Laceration	In continuity	–	Secondary suture	4	1.5
Laceration**	In continuity	–	Secondary suture	5	3.5
Radial fracture with plate/screw fixation	Transection		Grafts	4	2.3
Radial fracture	In continuity	+	Neurolysis	4	2
Radial fracture with elbow dislocation	In continuity	+	Neurolysis	4-5	2
Radial fracture with plate/screw fixation	In continuity	–	Grafts	4	2.5
Radial fracture with plate/screw fixation	In continuity	–	Grafts	3–4	2.5
Radial/ulnar fractures ***	In continuity	–	Grafts	3*	3.5
Contusion with brick	In continuity	+	Neurolysis	4	3
Contusion with pool cue	In continuity	+	Neurolysis	5	4.5
Contusion with stick	In continuity	+	Neurolysis	5	3.5

*A tendon transfer helped recovery.

**This case had a prior primary suture.

***This patient had three prior operations for stabilization of the fractures.

NAP, nerve action potential; F/up, follow-up in years.

Table 7-13 Posterior interosseous nerve entrapment results (n = 17)

Pre- to postoperative grade	No.
0 to 5	3
0 to 4	1
0 to 3	1
1 to 5	2
2 to 4	4
3 to 4	1
3 to 5	4

No., number of cases.

Table 7-14 Posterior interosseous nerve: graded results by injury mechanism in 40 operative cases

Mechanism	No.	Grade				
		5	4	3	2	1
Entrapment	19	10	7	2	0	0
Laceration	7	1	6	0	0	0
Fracture	7	0	5	2	0	0
Tumor	3	2	1	0	0	0
Contusion	3	1	2	0	0	0
Prior suture	1	1	0	0	0	0
Totals	40	15	21	4	0	0

No., number of cases.

between these two muscle heads, the PIN branches to supply extensors of the fingers and thumb. Compression usually occurs at the arcade of Frohse, which is the proximal portion of the volar supinator, and there may or may not be a fascial edge at this level.

This PIN entrapment syndrome is not rare if the examiner knows to look for it.[22] It may or may not be associated with proximal forearm pain, but it usually lacks the paresthesias and the sensory symptoms associated with most entrapments of other nerves. Instead, the patient presents with a painless decrease in extension of the fingers and thumb,[23] which may initially affect some fingers more than others. As the palsy progresses, there is weakness in the ECU amd extensor pollicis longus as well as the extensor communis muscles. Function of the ECR muscle and sensation in the distribution of the SSRN branch are maintained. With dorsiflexion of the wrist, the hand drifts in a radial direction and finger and thumb drop occur because of the weakness in extension of these digits. Table 7-11 shows the LSUHSC grading system used to evaluate loss and recovery in the PIN distribution.

Electromyography shows denervational changes in only the more severe PIN entrapments. Conductive studies can be done but require experience if they are to be done accurately on this segment of the radial nerve.

In our experience and that of others, loss of function may improve spontaneously in several months, especially if the onset was related to vigorous or repetitive wrist and forearm motion. If reversal of loss does not occur or if loss progresses, operative decompression is indicated. This is a favorable entrapment to treat surgically providing the decompression is thorough and includes division of the entire volar head of the supinator (Fig. 7-38).[11,63] A "leash" of blood vessels may encircle or cross over the nerve proximal to the muscular or fascial edge of the true arcade of Frohse, but this is seldom responsible for the entrapment.

Results with neurolysis of PIN and division of the volar supinator for PIN entrapments are excellent in well-selected patients. In two cases in our series, the entrapment was bilateral; in the remainder it was unilateral. PIN entrapment occurred with a male-to-female ratio of nine to five; the right-to-left sided ratio was the same. The mean age was 30 years and the length of follow-up averaged 3.4 years.

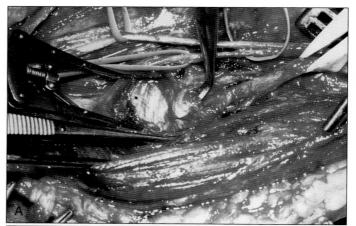
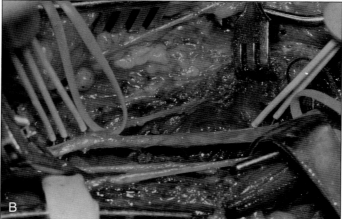

FIGURE 7-38 **(A)** The posterior interosseous nerve (PIN) is shown intraoperatively at the level of the arcade of Frohse. A double-ended dissector is beneath the somewhat fibrous edge of the volar head of the supinator. The superficial sensory radial nerve with the extensor carpi radialis branch arising from it is seen behind or deep to the instrument. **(B)** The volar supinator has been incised. The recording electrode is on the more distal PIN to the right of the photograph whereas the stimulating electrode is quite proximal on the PIN and to the left.

One-half of the PIN cases having surgery were caused by entrapment. Table 7-13 shows the grade assigned to each case before operation and the grade achieved after operation. Despite entrapment as a mechanism, loss was complete preoperatively in five of these patients and quite severe (grade 1 or 2) in another six. In each instance, intraoperative recordings showed an NAP across the entrapment site, which was either at the arcade of Frohse or beneath the supinator muscle. Conduction velocities were slowed, and NAP amplitudes were usually diminished. Fifteen of the entrapped nerves recovered to either grade 4 (six cases) or grade 5 (ten cases) level.

Tables 7-14 and 7-15 show the graded results in both the operated and unoperated categories. The three tumors involving PIN that had operations included a ganglion cyst, a lipoma, and a neurofibroma. Loss preoperatively was partial or, in the neurofibroma case, minimal. Fortunately, most neurological function was maintained; in the ganglion cyst case, pre- to postoperative function improved from grade 3 to grade 4. Tumors operated on previously and having neurological deficit included a patient with a neurofibroma in which function was a grade 2 and a schwannoma in which it was 4. Both improved remarkably with time. The six entrapments not having operations were seen within 2 months of onset and had improved by 5 months after occurrence. Despite severe loss related to sleep compression in two cases and fracture in seven instances, acceptable recovery occurred usually over a 6–7-month period.

Table 7-16 illustrates the tendency for PIN palsy, whether of spontaneous or traumatic origin, to preferentially have involved the right side, especially in females. The higher incidence of entrapments involving the right side versus the left side may be related to greater use of the right arm for repetitive motions.

DORSAL FOREARM BRANCH

As can be seen in Table 7-17, nine injuries at this level had surgery. Despite gaining some good results with transections repaired acutely by end-to-end suture anastomosis repair and secondarily by graft repair, two graft repairs failed. These dissections, especially if done secondarily, were difficult because it was a challenge to find distal branches to which to graft. This was especially so in two cases in which prior operation had failed.

Proximal lead-out could sometimes be located only by dissecting out PIN beneath the brachioradialis muscle and tracing it through and underneath the volar head of the supinator to its transection point, either at a branch level or at the distal PIN itself. The three patients with lesions in continuity who had operations were caused by contusion in two instances and fracture of the radius in one. Two other contusive injuries at a forearm level caused by blunt objects improved with time and did not need repair. An alternative to neural repair with injury at this level is tendon transfer, and one of the failed graft repairs subsequently had this done with good result.

Table 7-15 Posterior interosseous nerve: graded results by injury mechanism in 14 nonoperative cases

		Grade				
Mechanism	No.	5	4	3	2	1
Entrapment	6	5	1	0	0	0
Fracture	4	2	2	0	0	0
Sleep compression	2	0	2	0	0	0
Prior tumor resection	2	1	1	0	0	0
TOTALS	14	8	6	0	0	0

No., number of cases.

Table 7-17 Dorsal forearm branches: operations and results in 9 injuries

Operative finding	NAP	Operation	Result
Transection		Primary suture	2/2
Transection		Secondary grafts	4/2
In continuity lesion	+	Neurolysis	1/1
In continuity lesion	−	Neurolysis/grafts	1/1*
In continuity lesion	−	Graft	1/0**

*Initial neurolysis followed by later graft repair.

**Tendon transfer reversed most loss.

Table 7-16 Etiology and handedness of operated posterior interosseous nerve palsy (n = 34)

	Female		Male		Total	
	Right	Left	Right	Left	Right	Left
Laceration	1	0	3	2	4	2
Fractures*	2	1	3	0	5	1
Contusion/compression	1	0	0	2	1	2
Tumors	2	0	1	0	3	0
Entrapment	4	1	7	4	11	5
Totals	10	2	14	8	24	10

SUPERFICIAL SENSORY RADIAL NERVE LESIONS

Because the suture of a lacerated SSRN often results in a painful hyperesthesia on the dorsum of the hand as well as a tender, painful neuroma, we decided some years ago to excise such injured nerves. A similar approach has yielded even greater success with injured but painful sural and saphenous nerves. The sensory distributions of all three are not of great functional importance unless median, ulnar, or tibial sensory distributions are also absent. This approach has provided good relief in eight isolated SSRN lesions, but the other three have retained some symptoms. As pointed out by Mackinnon and Dellon,[33] it is important to excise the neuromas and tissues surrounding it as well as the nerve proximal to it. Fine branches from the lateral musculocutaneous or antebrachial cutaneous nerves can with time contribute to or be incorporated in the SSRN neuroma. This can occur whether these adjacent nerves are injured by the same forces injuring the SSRN or not. Excision has also been used for the persistently painful contusion-injured SSRN, because neurolysis in two earlier cases did not seem to work.

Twenty-one SSRN cases underwent operations. Thirteen cases have been managed conservatively, but not always successfully (Tables 7-18, 7-19). In those with persistent symptoms, neither patient nor insurer could always be convinced of the need for operation, especially because total relief of pain could not be promised.

Table 7-18 Superficial sensory radial neuroma: operative results (n = 21)

Nerve injury	Operation	Result*
Laceration	Neurolysis	0/0
Laceration	Excision	11/8
Contusion	Neurolysis	2/0
Contusion	Excision	6/6
Prior suture	Neurolysis	0/0
Prior suture	Excision	2/2

*Number of cases/number improved.

Table 7-19 Superficial sensory radial neuroma: nonoperative cases (n = 13)

Nerve injury	Result*
Compression	4/0
Prior suture	2/0
Contusion	6/1
Fracture	1/1

*Number of cases/number improved.

CASE SUMMARY – SUPERFICIAL SENSORY RADIAL NERVE

CASE 1

This 25-year-old male sheet metal worker was carrying a pile of iron sheets when the tape holding them together broke and he sustained a laceration of the volar mid-forearm area. Exploration with a tourniquet in place showed a partial laceration of muscles including brachioradialis, flexor carpi radialis, flexor pollicis longus, superficial flexor of the long finger, and palmaris longus tendon. A partial laceration of the SSRN branch of the radial nerve was noted. Muscle and tendon transections were repaired. Per the outside notes, the partially divided area of the SSRN was trimmed to healthy tissue, but the remaining nerve was left in continuity, and then the whole nerve in that area was placed beneath muscle.

When seen 1 year later, the patient was complaining of a dull aching pain with intermittent "electric shocks" along the radial side of the volar aspect of the forearm. There was hypoesthesia on the SSRN portion of the dorsum of the hand, including the dorsum of the thumb and the anatomic snuffbox region. Motor function of the hand was quite good, but there was some sensory decrease on the more volar forearm in the antebrachial cutaneous distribution. Tapping on the long volar forearm scar gave paresthesias down the radial side of the forearm. Skin-level NAP recordings showed a small-amplitude SSRN NAP conducting at 30 m/sec.

At exploration, neuromas in continuity were found on both the SSRN and one of the lateral antebrachial cutaneous nerve branches. The former transmitted only a small, slow NAP, and the latter did not conduct at all. A proximal and distal length of both nerves, including their lesions, were resected. Proximal fascicles were sealed by use of a fine-tipped bipolar forceps and placed beneath the brachioradialis muscle.

The patient did well postoperatively with good relief of pain. Unfortunately, he was lost to follow-up after 1.5 years.

COMMENT

Isolated SSRN neuromas can present difficult management problems because the patient frequently strikes the neuroma during day-to-day tasks.

POTENTIAL COMPLICATIONS

True complications with surgery on this nerve were infrequent in our series. Failure to recover more distal radial function in muscles such as the extensor communis or extensor pollicis longus is more of a recognized limitation of repair of this nerve than a true complication.

If proximal nerve is involved with heavy scar, it is possible to injure otherwise uninvolved triceps branches. This can occur as the nerve is laid out on the proximal and medial aspects of the arm or sometimes even in the region of the humeral groove. This occurred twice in this series, but fortunately some of this loss reversed with time. In the region of the elbow, brachioradialis branches can be inadvertently sectioned. Of potentially even more serious import is damage to the ECR branch, which can be inadvertently injured because of its variable origin from whole radial nerve or SSRN below the elbow.

Experience with reoperation on previously operated PIN entrapments or injuries suggests that frequently the entire volar head of the supinator has not been sectioned. This would seem to be indicated in the majority of cases at this level. Similarly, repair of an injured SSRN often does not relieve the pain and paresthesias associated with such injury, and resection of a length of this nerve seems preferable if pain is the dominant problem.

REFERENCES

1. Alnot JY and Le Reun D: Les lesions traumatiques du tronc nerf radial au bras. Rev Chir Orthop Reparatic Appar Mot 75:433–442, 1989.
2. Barton NJ: Radial nerve lesions. Hand 5:200–208, 1973.
3. Bateman JE: Trauma to Nerves in Limbs. Philadelphia, WB Saunders, 1962.
4. Bowden REM and Shell DA: The advance of functional recovery after radial nerve lesions in man. Brain 73:251–266, 1950.
5. Bowen TL and Stone KH: Posterior interosseous nerve paralysis caused by a ganglion at the elbow. Surgery 48B:774–776, 1966.
6. Boyd HB and Boals JC: The Monteggia lesion. A review of 159 cases. Clin Orthop 66:94–100, 1969.
7. Brown PW: Factors influencing the success of the surgical repair of peripheral nerves. Surg Clin North Am 52:1137–1155, 1972.
8. Bunnell S: Active splinting of the hand. J Bone Joint Surg 28:732–736, 1946.
9. Capener W: The vulnerability of the posterior interosseous nerve of the forearm. J Bone Joint Surg 48B:770–773, 1966.
10. Chuinard R, Boyes J, Start H, et al.: Tendon transfers for radial nerve palsy: Use of superficialis tendons for digit extension. J Hand Surg 3:560–570, 1978.
11. Cravens G and Kline D: Posterior interosseous palsies. Neurosurgery 27:397–402, 1990.
12. DiRosa F: Radial nerve: Anatomy and fascicular arrangement. In: Brunelli G, Ed: Textbook of Microsurgery, New York, Masson, 1988.
13. Emery SE and Gifford JF: One hundred years of tennis elbow. Contemp Orthop 12:53–58, 1986.
14. Garcia A and Maeck BH: Radial nerve injuries and fractures of the shaft of the humerus. Am J Surg 99:625–627, 1960.
15. Goldner JL: Function of the Hand Following Peripheral Nerve Injuries. Am Acad Orthop Surg Instruct, Course Lectures 10. Ann Arbor, MI, JW Edwards, 1953.
16. Griswold BA: Early tendon transfer for radial transection. Hand 8:134, 1976.
17. Guarantors of Brain: Aids to the Examination of the Peripheral Nervous System. London, Baillière Tindall, 1989.
18. Gurdjian ES, Hardy WG, Lindner DW, et al.: Nerve injuries in association with fractures and dislocations of long bones. Clin Orthop 27:147–151, 1963.
19. Hall HH, Mackinnon SE, and Gilbert RW: An approach to the posterior interosseous nerve. Plast Reconstr Surg 74:435–437, 1984.
20. Henry AK: Extensile Exposure: Applied to Limb Surgery. Baltimore, Williams & Wilkins, 1945.
21. Holstein A and Lewis GB: Fractures of the humerus with radial nerve paralysis. J Bone Joint Surg 45A:1382–1386, 1963.
22. Hudson AR and Mayfield FH: Chronic injuries of peripheral nerves by entrapment. In: Youmans JR, Ed: Neurological Surgery, 2nd edn, vol. 4. Philadelphia, WB Saunders, 1982.
23. Hustead AP, Mulder DW, and MacCarty CS. Nontraumatic progressive paralysis of the deep radial (posterior interosseous) nerve. Arch Neurol Psychiatry 69:269, 1958.
24. Jayendrahumar J: Radial nerve paralysis associated with fractures of the humerus. Clin Orthop 172:171–175, 1983.
25. Kempe L, Ed: Operative Neurosurgery, vol 2. New York, Springer-Verlag, 1970.
26. Kettlekamp DB and Alexander H: Clinical review of radial nerve injury. J Trauma 7:424–432, 1967.
27. Lichter RL: Tardy palsy of the posterior interosseous nerve with a Monteggia fracture. J Bone Joint Surg 57A:124–125, 1975.
28. Ling CMS and Loong SC: Injection injury of the radial nerve. Injury 8:60–62, 1976.
29. Lister GD, Belsole RB, and Kleinert HE: The radial tunnel syndrome. J Hand Surg 4:52–59, 1979.
30. Lotem M, Fried A, Levy M, et al.: Radial palsy following muscular effort: A nerve compression syndrome possibly related to a fibrous arch of the lateral head of the triceps. J Bone Joint Surg 53B:500–506, 1971.
31. Lyons WR and Woodhall, B: Atlas of Peripheral Nerve Injuries. Philadelphia, WB Saunders, 1949.
32. McGraw J: Neurological complications resulting from supracondylar fractures of the humerus in children. J Pediatr Orthop 6:647–650, 1986.
33. Mackinnon S and Dellon A: Surgery of the Peripheral Nerve. New York, Theime Medical Publishers, 1988.
34. Manske PR: Compression of the radial nerve by the triceps muscle: A case report. J Bone Joint Surg 59A:835–836, 1977.
35. Moss SH and Switzer HE: Radial tunnel syndrome. A spectrum of clinical presentations. J Hand Surg 8:414–419, 1983.
36. Nickolson OR and Seddon HJ: Nerve repair in civil practice. Br Med J 2:1065–1071, 1957.
37. Nulsen FE: The management of peripheral nerve injury producing hand dysfunction. In: Flynn JE, Ed: Hand Surgery. Baltimore, Williams & Wilkins, 1966.
38. Omer GE: Evaluation and reconstruction of forearm and hand after acute traumatic peripheral nerve injuries. J Bone Joint Surg 50A:1454–1460, 1968.
39. Omer GE: Injuries to the nerves of the upper extremities Bone Joint Surg 56A:1615–1624, 1974.
40. Omer GE: The results of untreated traumatic injuries. In: Omer G and Spinner M, Eds: Management of Peripheral Nerve Problems. Philadelphia, WB Saunders, 1980.
41. Packer JW, Foster RR, Garcia A, et al.: The humeral fracture with radial nerve palsy. Is exploration warranted? Clin Orthop 88:34–38, 1972.
42. Pollock FH, Drake D, Bovill E, et al.: Treatment of radial neuropathy associated with fracture of the humerus. J Bone Joint Surg 63A;239–243, 1981.
43. Reid RL: Radial nerve palsy. Hand Clin 4:179–182, 1988.
44. Sakellorides H: Follow-up of 172 peripheral nerve injuries in upper extremity in civilians. J Bone Joint Surg 44A:140–148, 1962.
45. Samu M: The arcade of Frohse and its relationship to posterior interosseous nerve paralysis: J Bone Joint Surg [Br] 50:809–812, 1968.
46. Savory WS: A case in which after the removal of several inches of the musculospiral nerve, the sensibility of that part of the skin of the hand which is supplied by it was retained. Lancet 2:142, 1868.
47. Seddon H: Nerve lesions complicating certain closed bone injuries. JAMA 135:691–194, 1947.
48. Seddon H: Surgical Disorders of the Peripheral Nerve, Baltimore, Williams & Wilkins, 1972.
49. Seletz E: Surgery of Peripheral Nerves. Springfield, Ill, Charles C. Thomas, 1951.
50. Shaw JL and Sakellorides H: Radial nerve paralysis associated with fractures of the humerus. J Bone Joint Surg 49A:899–902, 1967.
51. Sobotta JJ: Atlas of Human Anatomy, 9th English edn, 3 vols. Munich, Urban & Schwartzenberg, 1974.
52. Spinner M: Injuries to the Major Branches of Peripheral Nerves of the Forearm, 2nd Edn. Philadelphia, WB Saunders, 1978.
53. Spinner M: The arcade of Frohse and its relationship to posterior interosseous nerve paralysis. J Bone Joint Surg [Br] 50:809–812, 1968.
54. Spinner M, Freundlich BD, and Teicyer J: Posterior interosseous nerve palsy as complication of Monteggia fractures in children. Clin Orthop 58:141–145, 1968.
55. Stin F, Grabias S, and Deffer P: Nerve injuries complicating Monteggia lesions. J Bone Joint Surg 53A:1432–1436, 1971.
56. Steyers CM: Radial nerve results. In: Gelbermann R, Ed: Operative Nerve Repair and Reconstruction. Philadelphia, JB Lippincott, 1991.

57. Strachan JC and Ellis BW: Vulnerability of the posterior interosseous nerve during radial head resection. J Bone Joint Surg 53B:320–323, 1971.

58. Sunderland S: The intraneural topography of the radial, median, and ulnar nerves. Brain 68:243–299, 1945.

59. Sunderland S: Observations on injuries of the radial nerve due to gunshot wounds and other causes. Aust NZ J Surg 17:253, 1948.

60. Trojabarg W: Rate of recovery in motor and sensory fibers of the radial nerve: Clinical and electrophysiological aspects. J Neurol Neurosurg Psychiatry 33:625–630, 1978.

61. White WL: Restoration of function and balance of the wrist and hand by tendon transfers. Surg Clin North Am 40:427–459, 1960.

62. Woodhall B and Beebe WG: Peripheral Nerve Regeneration: A follow-up study of 3656 W W II injuries. VA Medical Monograph. Washington, DC, US Government Printing Office, 1956.

63. Young MC, Hudson AR, and Richards RR: Operative treatment of palsy of the posterior interosseous nerve of the forearm. J Bone Joint Surg 72A:8:1215–1219, 1990.

64. Zachary RB: Results of nerve suture. In: Seddon HJ, Ed: Peripheral Nerve Injuries. Medical Research Council No. 282. London, Her Majesty's Stationery Office, 1952.

8

Median nerve

Robert J. Spinner

SUMMARY

The median nerve carries important sensory as well as motor functions. Unlike the radial nerve, the median nerve does not innervate arm muscles, but it does provide important input to both forearm-level extrinsic and hand intrinsic muscles, especially to the thumb. Although the anatomic relationship of the median nerve is usually straightforward in the arm, it is complex at the elbow and proximal forearm, where the relationships of pronator teres and flexor digitorum superficialis muscles and the anterior interosseous nerve branch supplying other muscles are important. It is also at this level that the Martin-Gruber connection can occur, or more proximally, entrapment by a Struthers ligament.

Data analyzed for the median nerve included 250 patients with median nerve lesions. This included operative outcomes on 167 patients: 49 with arm-level involvement, 69 with elbow and forearm lesions, and 49 at the wrist level (exclusive of 376 cases of carpal tunnel syndrome). Analysis of arm-level data showed surprisingly good results not only for lacerations but also gunshot wounds and even some lesions associated with fracture and contusion. Grade 5 recoveries occurred mainly with partial lesions to begin with, or with complete lesions in which neurolysis was based on a positive nerve action potential (NAP) across the lesion. Major residual deficits involved intrinsic muscles such as thenar muscles, although lack of true opposition and abduction was usually substituted for nicely by ulnar- and radial-innervated thumb muscles. Elbow- and forearm-level median nerve lesions also fared well with proper management. Median nerve loss due to Volkmann's ischemia or electrical injury was difficult to reverse. Relief of neuritic pain was also not always possible, especially if iatrogenic injection injury was the mechanism. Wrist-level lesions involving the median nerve had similar restrictions in outcome of thenar-intrinsic function as lesions occurring more proximally in the limb, although overall grades for sensory return were higher. The clinical subset of carpal tunnel syndrome has been summarized with emphasis on failed carpal tunnel release, a type of case often referred to these authors for neurologic repair.

CLINICALLY AND SURGICAL RELEVANT ANATOMY

AXILLA

The median nerve originates at the axillary level from the lateral and medial cords, forming the characteristic "V" that in turn overlies the axillary to brachial artery junction. The lateral cord contribution to the median nerve is called the "sensory root" in that it provides critical sensory fibers to the hand. In addition, it supplies some function to the forearm and wrist. The medial cord contribution to the median nerve forms the "motor root" and supplies some of the intrinsic muscles of the hand.

The lateral cord to median nerve junction is usually easily seen during the initial brachial plexus exposure in the axilla, but the motor contribution from the medial cord may be posteromedial to the artery and only clearly seen when searched for and dissected away from the vessel. In a few cases, lateral or medial cord input to median nerve may pass posterior to the axillary artery. In others, the lateral cord may contribute some of its fibers destined for the median nerve by way of a proximal branch to the medial cord contribution to the median nerve. In almost a quarter of cases, lateral cord fibers destined for the median nerve can travel in more proximal musculocutaneous nerve, leaving it more distally to enter the median nerve which has already been partially constituted by input from the medial cord and that portion of the lateral cord not contributing to the musculocutaneous nerve.[40]

Fascicles destined to form the musculocutaneous nerve may not separate from the lateral cord, but may instead travel through the lateral head of the median nerve and leave it to achieve their destination on the medial edge of biceps and brachialis. In rare cases, the median nerve in the upper arm may be bifid as far as the elbow.[89] Of surgical importance is the fact that the course of the median nerve from its origin to most destinations is straight. As a result, not much length can be gained by mobilization. This makes some period of immobilization after repair of the median nerve mandatory if there is any tension on the repair.[90]

ARM

Injury to the portion of the median nerve in the arm may be complicated by damage to the brachial artery and vein, and even the ulnar nerve, caused by the median nerve's close proximity to these structures. Both motor and sensory loss involve the entire distribution of the nerve and are quite characteristic (Figs 8-1, 8-2). The radial nerve penetrates between the subscapularis muscle and the long head of the triceps, so it is deep as it descends to leave the medial upper arm to travel to the lateral side of the arm. As a result, the radial nerve is better protected and less likely to receive an injury concomitant with those involving the median and ulnar nerves and brachial vessels, even at a proximal arm level. Stretch injuries involving the cord to nerve level of the brachial plexus and very proximal penetrating injury to the arm are exceptions, in which the radial nerve may also be involved.

Median nerve injuries are often associated with ulnar nerve involvement. Such injuries are devastating. With the exception of extension of the wrist and extension of the fingers at the metacarpophalangeal joints only (radial and posterior interosseous nerve innervation), the hand is totally paralyzed.[99] Unless successful recovery is gained through regeneration, a severely clawed hand results. Such deformity involves all four fingers, resulting in a "main en griffe."[79]

Injuries to the median nerve along the medial aspect of the arm can be caused by glass, knife, or gunshot wounds, or they can be iatrogenic and associated with a vascular bypass procedure or construction of an arteriovenous fistula for renal dialysis.[47] Median nerve damage at this level is rarely associated with a fracture of the humerus (the radial nerve being more common).[8] Mechanisms of injury to the median nerve at a proximal level also include those secondary to angiography.[9] Damage results from direct penetration by a needle or catheter or, in some cases, from compression secondary to pseudoaneurysm of the axillary or brachial artery or a hematoma.

High median nerve palsy, with or without radial or ulnar nerve palsy, can be caused by compression or contusion of the nerve in the axilla or the proximal and medial arm (Fig. 8-3). Such a syndrome may be seen in stuporous people who hang an arm over a chair or park bench, or after one's sleeping partner rests his or her head for a prolonged period on the medial arm. More commonly, the patient lies in a lateral recumbent position and rests his or her own head on the lateral midhumeral area of the arm; this produces a radial nerve palsy below the triceps branches. Radial nerve palsy is also a much more common sequela of prolonged use of crutches than median nerve palsy, but crutch palsy can, on occasion, involve the median nerve with or without concomitant radial nerve involvement.

Loss, with proximal median nerve involvement, is total if the injury is severe enough to affect the entire cross-section of the nerve. In addition to median nerve distribution sensory loss, pronator function (both pronator teres and quadratus) is markedly reduced or lost, as is palmaris longus, flexor carpi radialis, flexor digitorum superficialis (to all fingers), as well as flexor digitorum

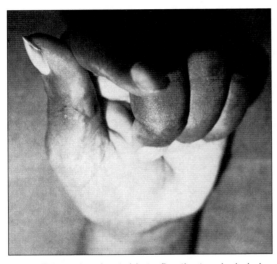

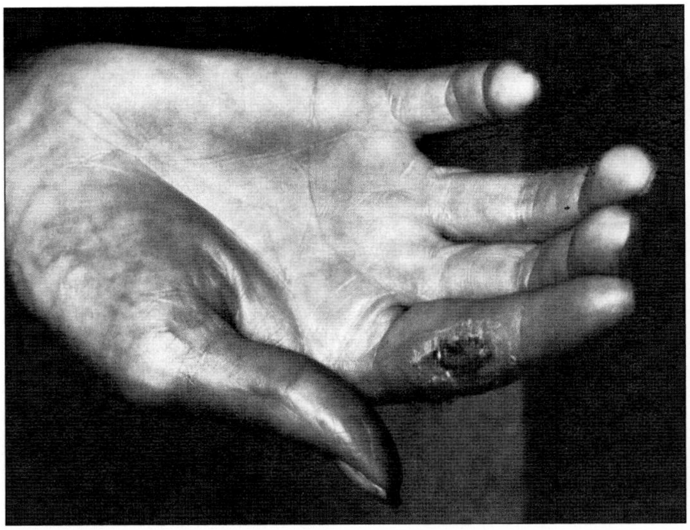

FIGURE 8-1 This patient is unable to flex the terminal phalanges of the thumb and index finger, suggesting a proximal median neuropathy. In a complete high median nerve lesion, the individual may display a typical "pope" or "prelate hand," in which the index finger can not be flexed at the distal or middle phalanges.

FIGURE 8-2 A burn to the anesthetic zone of index finger after proximal median nerve injury. Patients must guard and protect their anesthetic skin.

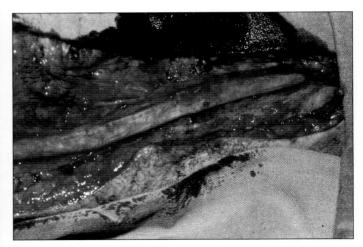

FIGURE 8-3 Contusion of median nerve at arm level, which did not transmit a nerve action potential at 6 months and required resection and repair. Note the absence of an obvious focal neuroma. You can't tell a book by its cover!

profundi function to the index and, in about half of cases, the middle finger. In addition, the flexor pollicis longus is paralyzed. Intrinsic muscles to the hand are also involved, including the thenar muscles and the median-innervated lumbricals. The pronator teres is the most proximal muscle innervated by the median nerve. Branches to the pronator teres, which is located in the forearm and elbow, usually arise at the level of the distal arm and innervate the muscle at the level of the flexor crease of the elbow or sometimes at the proximal forearm level. Very rarely, the pronator teres can be innervated by the musculocutaneous nerve, which can, even less frequently, innervate also the palmaris longus and flexor carpi radialis. The more distal pronator quadratus serves as a much weaker pronator than does the pronator teres; the pronator quadratus receives a branch from the anterior interosseous nerve in the mid forearm and travels along the interosseous membrane. Pronator teres is tested by having the patient extend the elbow. The patient's hand is then grasped by the examiner, and the patient is asked to rotate the hand from a palm-up, or supinated, position to a palm-down, or pronated, position (Fig. 8-4). Pronator quadratus function may be examined by resisting pronation with the elbow flexed.

After innervating the pronator teres and palmaris longus, the next important and proximal branches from the median nerve arise 2.5 cm or so below the elbow flexion crease and innervate the flexor digitorum superficialis.[89] The flexor digitorum superficialis results in flexion at the middle interphalangeal joint, while the flexor digitorum profundus results in flexion at the distal interphalangeal joint. In testing isolated flexor digitorum superficialis function, one must keep the other fingers fully extended. One can test the index and middle fingers in isolation. When testing the flexor digitorum superficialis function to the little and ring fingers, the index and middle fingers should be fully extended, and the little and ring fingers can be tested for flexion at the middle phalanges together. The flexor digitorum profundi should be tested in a slightly different manner. When testing the index and middle fingers, all other digits should be kept fully extended, and the finger being tested should be held in extension at the middle phalanx and only the distal interphalangeal joint be tested. The ulnar two digits are tested in combination by keeping the index and middle fingers extended and the ulnar two digits kept mildly flexed at the metacarpophalangeal joints; flexion at the distal interphalangeal joints can then be tested together.

Commonly, middle finger flexor digitorum profundus receives innervation from the median and ulnar nerve; this pattern of dual innervation often spares it from full loss of flexion in median palsy.[89] On the other hand, flexor digitorum profundus to the index finger is always median-innervated, making it a good marker muscle for the median nerve (Fig. 8-5).

In a patient with a high median nerve paralysis, wrist flexion is in an ulnar direction because the flexor carpi ulnaris is no longer balanced by flexor carpi radialis. Distal flexion of the thumb is lost, as is pure abduction of the thumb at right angles to the palm, and true opposition movement of the thumb is also not possible. With total paralysis of the flexor pollicis longus and some shortening of the tendon, the patient and examiner may yet believe that there is contraction at the distal interphalangeal joint of the thumb, after extending the thumb and suddenly relaxing it, because the shortened flexor tendon pulls the tip of the thumb into a partially flexed position. Lumbrical function to index and middle fingers is weak or absent unless all lumbricals are innervated by the ulnar nerve, a circumstance occurring approximately 15% of the time.

The palmaris longus receives its innervation at a proximal forearm level. Its loss is of little functional importance because this muscle serves only as a corrugator of palmar skin. Nonetheless, the palmaris longus may be an important muscle for the electromyographer to test because it receives relatively proximal input from the median nerve.[92,102] The palmaris longus tendon, which is more superficial and ulnar to the flexor carpi radialis, may be congenitally absent in approximately 10% of the population. As the median nerve passes beneath the palmaris longus, it is somewhat adherent to the undersurface of the flexor digitorum superficialis, which it supplies. The tendons of the flexor digitorum superficialis insert on the middle phalanx of each of the four fingers and thus flex the proximal and middle phalanges of the fingers toward the palm.

At the level of the upper arm, and usually at its midpoint, there may be a proximal Martin-Gruber anastomosis with fibers crossing between the median and ulnar nerves. This is an unusual variation, seen in less than 3% of dissections; the true Martin-Gruber anastomosis, which is at forearm level, occurs in at least 15% of the population.[40]

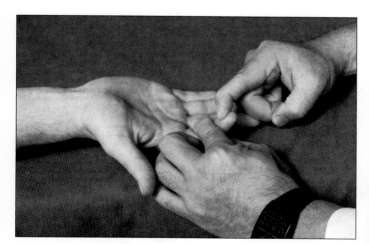

FIGURE 8-4 Testing flexor digitorum profundus to the index finger. The patient's middle phalanx is held fixed by the examiner's left index finger. The patient's middle, ring, and little fingers are kept in an extended position by the examiner's right middle and ring fingers. The patient is asked to flex or pull the distal phalanx toward the palm. Function is graded by the examiner applying counter-pressure with his right index finger.

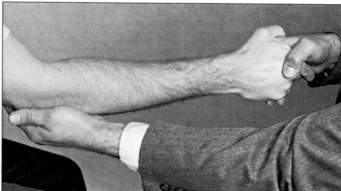

FIGURE 8-5 To test both pronator quadratus and pronator teres function, pronation is readily tested with the elbow flexed 90 degrees (demonstrated) and fully extended. The patient is asked to turn the palm of the hand downward against resistance.

Compression by Struthers ligament

The median nerve can be compressed beneath the ligament of Struthers in the distal arm (Fig. 8-6). This ligament is typically associated with a supracondylar spur or process, estimated to be present in 0.7–2.7% of the population. Of course, not all patients with such a spur or a ligament develop neurovascular compression. The ligament arises from the supracondylar process, which is located approximately 8 cm above the medial epicondyle on the medial side of the humerus. The ligament inserts into the medial epicondyle. The median nerve and brachial (or ulnar) artery pass beneath the ligament wherein these structures may be compressed. In addition, the ulnar nerve, which runs posterior to the ligament, may also be involved.

The diagnosis, although rare, must be considered in every patient with suspected carpal tunnel syndrome (CTS), especially those who failed CTS, or specifically when there is evidence of a proximal-level median nerve lesion. Surgeons should palpate for a spur, examine for a more proximal site of percussion tenderness and check an oblique X-ray of the distal humerus if considering this entity.

At operation, the ligament of Struthers should be released and the supracondylar spur, when present, resected. Surgical results have been quite good in the approximately 50 reported cases of high median nerve compression.

ELBOW/PROXIMAL FOREARM

At the elbow and proximal forearm level, mechanisms of injury to the median nerve are much the same as at the upper arm level. Distribution of loss may be the same, although function of pronator teres may be spared because its branches may leave the median nerve just proximal to this level. In addition to the usual categories of trauma, the median nerve can be injured at the level of the elbow by needles or catheter placement in the course of venipuncture or arterial catheterization.[93]

Pronator syndrome

The pronator syndrome is a controversial disorder described as compression of the median nerve where it passes between the superficial and deep heads of the pronator teres muscle. The nerve can be compressed by a hypertrophied pronator teres muscle and specifically its distal fascial edge, beneath which the main median nerve courses. The nerve may also be compressed more proximally by the bicipital aponeurosis (lacertus fibrosus) or more distally by the superficialis arch. The bicipital aponeurosis, which is an extension of the distal biceps tendon and inserts on the flexor fascia of the forearm, can also hypertrophy and occasionally cause compression of the median nerve at this level.

The pronator syndrome manifests itself primarily with vague forearm pain. Patients described with this syndrome may also have neurologic symptoms and signs related to median nerve involvement distal to the innervation of the pronator teres. Such loss is typically incomplete. Often, patients have many subjective complaints with few objective findings. Complete forms of high median nerve compression can occur, such as from an evolving hematoma beneath the bicipital aponeurosis.

Testing for the pronator syndrome is described at length elsewhere; it yields variable results.[35,66,82,87] Diagnosis is sometimes provided by electrical conduction studies if they are positive, but typically they are negative, and in this situation it does not exclude

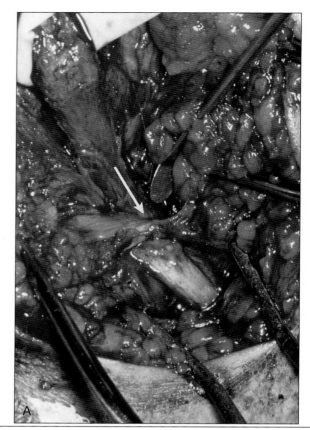

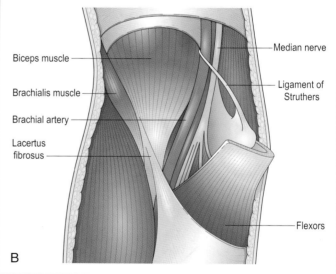

FIGURE 8-6 **(A)** Median nerve entrapped by a Struthers ligament *(arrow)* just proximal to the elbow. This teenager had prior unsuccessful CTRs bilaterally and had a contralateral Struthers ligament entrapping the median nerve at this level as well. **(B)** Drawing of the usual anatomy of a Struthers ligament running volar to both the brachial artery and median nerve.

the syndrome. Clinically, the physician questions specifically for a history of pain and looks for tenderness in the region of the proximal volar elbow, specifically in the area of the pronator teres, as well as symptoms of loss in the more distal median nerve distribution. Several tests have been advocated for the pronator syndrome which may help in establishing a diagnosis and localizing the level of the lesion. If pain is reproduced when the patient is asked to pronate the forearm against resistance and then extend the elbow, the site of pathology is the pronator teres. If pain occurs when the examiner tests the flexor digitorum superficialis of the middle finger, then the localization is at the flexor digitorum superficialis arch. If the patient's pain is reproduced with resistance to flexion of the elbow and supination of the forearm, then the bicipital aponeurosis is the offending structure.

Pronator syndrome should be suspected in patients with forearm pain and symptoms suggestive of median nerve compression. Carpal tunnel syndrome must be excluded. Electrodiagnostic studies are typically not diagnostic. Because of the difficulties diagnosing this clinical entity, when conservative measures fail, we believe that carpal tunnel release (CTR) should be considered, even before proximal median nerve decompression (unless electromyogram confirms a more proximal compression). If surgery for pronator syndrome is performed, all potential sites of compression should be specifically explored and decompressed: bicipital aponeurosis, pronator teres, and flexor digitorum superficialis arch. Double crush lesions although rare are possible, so complete decompression is recommended.

Martin-Gruber anastomosis

There are a number of variations of Martin-Gruber anastomosis.[82] Fibers destined for some of the ulnar-innervated hand intrinsics may travel in an elbow-level branch from the median to ulnar nerve or through the anterior interosseous nerve branch of the median nerve. Loss with injury to more proximal median or to anterior interosseous nerves may then be more serious than usual. Conversely, injury to the ulnar nerve proximal to the anastomosis gives less hand-intrinsic paralysis than usual. Ulnar fibers carried by the usual Martin-Gruber anastomosis eventually innervate the first dorsal interosseous, lumbricals, adductor pollicis, and the ulnar portion of the flexor pollicis brevis.

In another variation of the anastomosis, median nerve fibers destined for the thenar eminence cross over to the ulnar nerve in the proximal forearm (Fig. 8-7). These fibers then return to the thenar branch of the median nerve at a palmar level (Riche-Cannieu

anastomosis). If this forearm level of crossover occurs, loss with injury to the anterior interosseous nerve gives not only paralysis of flexor digitorum profundus to the index finger and flexor pollicis longus, but also weakness of thenar intrinsics.[89] Injury to the median nerve at a wrist level in such a limb would spare thenar intrinsics, but injury to the ulnar nerve would involve their loss as well as the usual ulnar-innervated intrinsic paralysis.

Forearm-level connections from the ulnar to median nerve are more unusual, but they do occur. In these cases, fibers destined for some ulnar intrinsics are carried in the median nerve to the hand. At the palmar level, these fibers branch to trade back to the ulnar nerve branches.

Ischemic contracture of Volkmann

A devastating complication of a supracondylar fracture or elbow dislocation caused by severe, blunt trauma is Volkmann ischemic contracture. Here, contusion or stretch of the brachial artery results in spasm of this vessel, secondary ischemia, and even resultant frank infarction of volar flexor compartment musculature. Under these circumstances, median nerve and sometimes radial (or posterior interosseous) and ulnar nerves receive not only ischemic damage but also compression secondary to ischemic infarction and swelling of the soft tissues of the volar compartment of the forearm. A less common but still observable set of circumstances occurs with acute swelling secondary to a large contusive blow to the forearm. This we have seen secondary to pool cue injuries to the forearm, and high-speed vehicular accidents in which the forearm is severely contused. Severe and prolonged compression of the forearm resulting from drug misuse and sleeping on the arm was responsible for several of our cases and has already been reported elsewhere in the literature.[72] Under these circumstances, even though there is no fracture, median nerve, and occasionally also the posterior interosseous nerve, can be acutely compressed by swollen tissue in the volar compartment.

In addition to a swollen, painful forearm, the patient with impending compartment syndrome has paresthesias, usually in the median distribution, but sometimes in the radial and ulnar distributions as well. These symptoms can progress in severity, and with time, there is dampening or loss of the radial pulse and ischemic symptoms and findings in the hand, especially at the fingertips (pallor). In addition to extensive damage to volar forearm musculature, the ensuing median sensory and motor neuropathy and, at times, radial and ulnar losses, make for a complex and difficult to reverse syndrome.[77] Various devices and techniques have been used to measure pressure in the anterior compartment more objectively. Early fasciotomy and neurolysis of the median and often the posterior interosseous nerve is necessary.[55] However, a good index of suspicion for the diagnosis and, as a result, early fasciotomy are preferable, in our experience.

Anterior interosseous nerve syndrome

The anterior interosseous nerve branch leaves the main trunk of the median nerve beneath the flexor digitorum superficialis muscle to travel in a somewhat oblique and radial direction. This nerve branches to supply not only the flexor digitorum profundus to the index and, at times, the middle fingers, but also the flexor pollicis longus and the pronator quadratus. Dysfunction of the flexor digitorum profundus and the flexor pollicis longus muscles results in the clinical manifestation of the anterior interosseous nerve syndrome. The paresis or paralysis of these finger flexors is demonstrated by a loss of the pinch mechanism between the index and

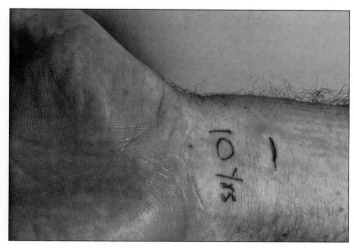

FIGURE 8-7 Thenar atrophy in a patient who had an unrepaired median laceration at the lower forearm level caused by a glass injury received 10 years before in which there was no Martin-Gruber anastomosis.

thumb and difficulty on the part of the patient in making an "O" with these two digits (Fig. 8-8). Function of the flexor digitorum profundus to the middle fingers is seldom totally lost because of either sharing of this digit's innervation through the ulnar nerve or a shared tendon origin with that of the ring finger. Patients may have the complete form or an incomplete form with weakness of only some of those muscles innervated by the anterior interosseous nerve. Characteristically, the syndrome lacks median sensory abnormality, so that the observer may mistake anterior interosseous nerve loss as tendon ruptures of the thumb and index finger.

The anterior interosseous nerve syndrome can occur spontaneously and be related to entrapment or follow penetration or, less frequently, contusive injury to the forearm.[69] Almost always, an individual with entrapment has the onset of the syndrome heralded by spontaneous pain in the proximal forearm as well as loss of dexterity in the use of the thumb and index fingers. If ulnar fibers travel in the anterior interosseous branch, then loss involves not only thumb and index pinch but more distal ulnar intrinsic muscles as well.[86]

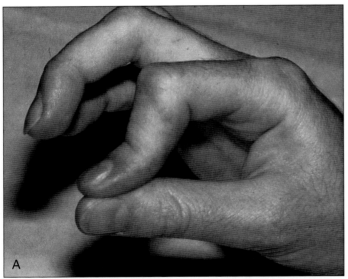

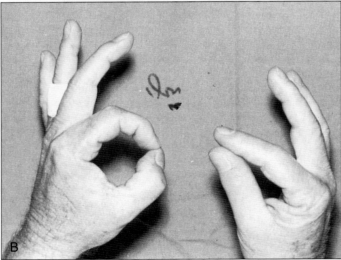

FIGURE 8-8 Anterior interosseous nerve palsy with loss of flexor digitorum profundus to index finger and flexor pollicis longus. The patient has poor pinch **(A)** and is unable to make an "O" with the index finger and thumb **(B)**.

On occasion, compression of the median nerve at the elbow level or even more proximally may selectively damage a fascicle destined for the anterior interosseous nerve and thus mimic a more distal lesion. This has been referred to as the "pseudo-anterior interosseous nerve" syndrome.[2,41,97] In addition, recently, intraepineurial constrictions have been noted within the median nerve, producing clinical pictures of anterior interosseous nerve syndrome.[34] Fascicle(s) at one or more levels may be affected. Some have recommended intraepineurial exploration of the median nerve if no pathology has been seen during an anterior interosseous nerve decompression, and derotation of any torsion if this is present.[34]

While spontaneous entrapments do occur producing anterior interosseous nerve syndrome, Parsonage-Turner syndrome (brachial neuritis or plexitis) also selectively targets the anterior interosseous nerve. Patients should be asked specifically about the onset of symptoms, the presence of antecedent pain, or sensory abnormalities elsewhere, and physicians should specifically examine clinically and electrically other muscles that are often sites of brachial plexitis (such as the serratus anterior, rhomboid, deltoid, supraspinatus) both on the affected side and also the contralateral side, as bilateral findings occur in approximately 10% of cases.

We favor a 6-month period of observation prior to performing surgical decompression in cases of "entrapment." Neurologic recovery follows decompression in many cases. Surgeons, however, may be taking credit for the relatively favorable natural history of Parsonage-Turner syndrome, a condition that typically would not need operative intervention. Tendon transfers can help those patients with poor return of function.

MID-FOREARM

At the middle or distal forearm area, the median nerve can be injured in association with a fracture involving the radius or ulna.[1] Loss includes flexor pollicis longus function, thenar intrinsic muscles, and lumbricals to index and sometime middle finger as well. Distal forearm injuries involving median nerve may also involve ulnar nerve, tendons, and important vessels.[14]

Other than the flexor pollicis longus branch, which usually leaves the median nerve trunk at the junction of the middle and distal third of the forearm, there are no motor branches from median nerve distal to the anterior interosseous nerve before the nerve reaches the palmar portion of the hand. An important sensory branch originating in the distal forearm is the palmar cutaneous branch, which leaves the radial side of the median nerve at a variable distance proximal to the wrist flexion crease. This branch supplies sensation over the dorsoradial aspect of the thenar prominence and the middle and distal phalanges of the thumb.

As pointed out earlier, the Martin-Gruber anastomosis is relatively common. Fibers destined for some of the distal median-innervated hand intrinsic muscle can leave the median nerve at the forearm level as a branch anastomosing with the ulnar nerve. They travel down the distal ulnar nerve to the distal third of the forearm, where a branch from the ulnar nerve may reanastomose with the distal median nerve. In many cases, fibers destined for the median nerve do not leave the ulnar nerve until the palmar level. Here, a branch leaving the deep ulnar nerve, termed the Riche-Cannieu anastomosis, provides fibers that travel back into the main median or, more commonly, to the recurrent thenar branch to innervate thenar musculature. Implications of these connections are extensive. Injury to median nerve at the distal forearm level can, in some patients, result in only median distribution sensory loss with little or no thenar muscular loss. In other patients, the reverse situation may apply. Ulnar nerve fibers destined for intrinsics and lumbricals of little and ring fingers travel in the median nerve for a distance down the forearm before reanastomosing with the ulnar nerve at the distal forearm or palmar levels.

The palmar cutaneous branch can be injured during the course of median nerve dissection at the wrist level or with blind scissoring of subcutaneous and wrist-level transverse carpal ligament fibers during the course of CTR. An occasional spontaneous laceration of the wrist, with or without main median nerve transection or damage, can involve this branch, as can contusive or crush injury at this level. Another mechanism producing injury to this branch is inadvertent damage or involvement during the course of tendon repair, tendon grafting, or tendon transfer procedures.

WRIST

At the wrist level, the median nerve is in close proximity to the palmaris longus tendon, and is located somewhat laterally to it or on its radial side. It is also volar or superior to the tendons of the flexor digitorum superficialis and profundus tendons.

Damage to the median nerve at the wrist level provides a common set of clinical circumstances. Because the nerve lies immediately volar to the flexor tendons, associated tendon injuries, particularly with sharp mechanisms, are common, as are injuries to the radial or ulnar arteries.[11] Loss is to all intrinsic muscles innervated by the nerve and also the median nerve sensory distribution, except for that of the palmar cutaneous branch, which again usually arises several centimeters proximal to the wrist crease. Although somewhat variable, the median cutaneous sensation is to the volar thenar eminence of the thumb and to the distal palm on the median side of the hand, the volar surface of the index, middle and radial portion of the ring fingers and the dorsal surfaces of the distal portions of these digits. Despite overlap with other nerves to the digits of the hand, there is an autonomous zone for the median nerve on the volar and dorsal surfaces of the distal phalanx of the index finger. Not uncommon is a partial injury, with either sensory loss accompanied by partial or complete motor sparing, or vice versa.

If injuries to the median at the wrist level are operated on acutely, the motor fascicle can be stimulated. If the patient is operated on later, while awake, the proximal face of the sensory fascicle can be stimulated.[26,98] More distally at the palmar level, the median nerve gives rise to a recurrent thenar branch to the abductor pollicis brevis, opponens pollicis, and flexor pollicis brevis, the last sharing its innervation with that of the deep branch of the ulnar nerve.

These anatomical and clinical considerations become very practical when dealing with the most common surgical neuropathy, which is entrapment of the median nerve beneath the transverse carpal ligament.

The median nerve can, on occasion, be bifid at the wrist level and proximal palm, and this can lead to confusion at the time of CTR. A smaller sensory branch may also leave the median nerve in the distal forearm, travel with it, and enter the palm along with the larger main median nerve. Some patients also have a palmar cutaneous branch that arises from the volar surface of the median and penetrates the transverse carpal ligament to supply the palm. This branch can be inadvertently injured during CTR, leading to a painful sensory neuroma.[56] At a variable level of the palm, the recurrent or thenar motor branch leaves the radial and somewhat dorsal side of the median nerve to supply the thenar muscles. Release of the flexor retinaculum must therefore be performed on

the ulnar side of the nerve to avoid injury to the thenar motor branch. Still, even with this technique, special care must always be taken, even during routine CTR, as variations of the recurrent branch exist, including an ulnar take-off from the median nerve, that may make it susceptible to iatrogenic injury.

The flexor pollicis brevis flexes the proximal phalanx of the thumb, and this function is aided by the flexor pollicis longus, which inserts on the more distal phalanx of the thumb. The abductor pollicis brevis pulls the thumb away from the palm at a right angel (Fig. 8-9). It can be tested by placing the dorsum of the hand on a flat surface and asking the patient to raise the thumb away from the palm at a right angle. One can palpate the thenar muscle mass and, in a healthy subject, can feel and see contraction of a portion of the abductor pollicis brevis as it is being tested. If the extensor pollicis mechanism is weak or paralyzed, as a result of radial nerve injury, it is difficult to test for abductor pollicis brevis function unless one provides some support along the dorsal aspect of the thumb. With the thumb supported in this fashion, the patient then attempts abduction against resistance. The abductor pollicis longus is innervated by the posterior interosseous nerve of the radial nerve and its tendon can be palpated in the anatomic snuff box.

The opponens pollicis pulls the thumb toward the palm in an oblique direction and permits the patient to touch the palmar surface of the thumb to the base of the little finger at the metacarpophalangeal joint level. The thumb rotates in opposition so that the thumb nail and small fingernail become parallel, in contrast to the position at rest, in which the nails are at right angles to each other. One can test the opponens pollicis by placing the examiner's index finger on top of the middle finger, placing both near the metacarpophalangeal joint of the patient's little finger, and asking the patient to use the thumb to press against the examiner's fingers as the examiner attempts to separate index and middle fingers (Fig. 8-10). With a healthy opponens pollicis, the examiner cannot separate the index finger away from the middle finger. It is best to ask the patient to refrain as much as possible from using the distal flexor mechanism of the thumb, which can substitute for a true

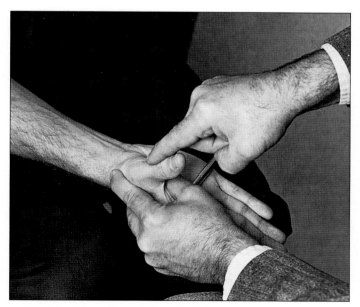

FIGURE 8-9 Abductor pollicis brevis is tested by having the patient abduct or pull the thumb up and away from the palm and at a right angle to it. Thenar contraction can be palpated at the same time.

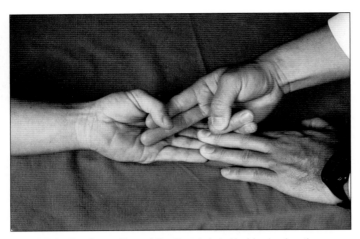

FIGURE 8-10 Opposition of the thumb is tested by having the patient press thumb down against the examiner's index and middle fingers. When there is full strength of opponens pollicis, the examiner will have trouble separating these two fingers.

opponens function. The opponens pollicis is one of the more difficult muscles in the body to test, because other thumb muscles can substitute for its function so readily.

In the presence of a distal or wrist-level median nerve palsy, the patient may still pull the thumb away from the palm, using extensor pollicis longus and brevis (radial-innervated) and adduct the thumb across the palm with the adductor pollicis (ulnar-innervated). The patient then uses the more proximal and thus intact median-innervated flexor pollicis longus to pull the tip of the thumb and thumb phalanges down toward the palmar surface, completing a simulated opponens pollicis or opposition-like maneuver.

PALM AND FINGERS

Median nerve injury at a palmar level can give variable findings, because there is some variation of the take-off of the digital branches and even of the thenar recurrent branch. Small branches or twigs leave the proximal digital nerves to supply lumbricals and, in the case of the ulnar nerve, interosseous muscles. The digital nerves then continue on to eventually supply sensation to the skin of the volar digits. Feeling is also provided for the volar and dorsal surfaces of the distal phalanx and the volar surface of the middle phalanx of the index finger. Sensation is also provided to a portion of the volar surface of the middle finger and sometimes to some of the ring finger along its radial aspect. Laceration to fingers or thumb is frequent and can involve the digital nerves. Crush and contusive injury can also be responsible for digital distribution sensory loss. As might be suspected under these circumstances, sensation is usually diminished or absent along the corresponding half of the palmar portion of the finger.

COMMENTS ON ELECTRODIAGNOSTIC STUDIES

Muscles innervated by the median nerve are all at or distal to the level of the elbow. Therefore, for arm injuries that are severe and complete, denervational change is present in all median-innervated muscles and at loci quite distal to the injury site. This means that reversal of such electrical changes, even in proximally innervated

muscles such as pronator teres, palmaris longus, flexor carpi radialis, and flexor digitorum superficialis takes a number of months. Sampling of the palmaris longus is difficult except for the experienced electromyographer, as is differentiating the flexor superficialis from pronator teres and the median-innervated portion of the flexor digitorum profundus from that portion innervated by the ulnar nerve. Nonetheless, the flexor digitorum profundus is a good diagnostic muscle because its ulnar half is innervated by that nerve and its radial half by the median nerve. Skillful medial placement of the needle electrode can assess the ulnar-innervated flexor digitorum profundus, whereas lateral placement assesses the median-innervated portion of the flexor digitorum profundus.

In checking for the anterior interosseous nerve syndrome, the median-innervated flexor digitorum profundus to the index finger is sampled along with the flexor pollicis longus, the next muscle downstream from the flexor digitorum profundus. Stimulation of the median nerve above the elbow and recording of muscle action potentials (MAPs) from the muscles provide a latency value that is increased if the anterior interosseous nerve branch is entrapped or partially injured. With more severe injury to the proximal median nerve or its anterior interosseous branch, denervational changes are also present in the flexor pollicis longus and the flexor profundus to the index finger. With mid-forearm-level injury to the median nerve, the flexor pollicis longus is the key muscle to needle in addition to thenar intrinsics such as the abductor pollicis brevis and opponens pollicis. These thenar intrinsic muscles should also be needled with evaluation of wrist-level injury to the median nerve.[92] Altered latencies for MAPs can also be recorded from these thenar muscles with entrapment of the median nerve at the wrist or with CTS.

Sensory conduction is more likely to be abnormal with early CTS than motor conduction. Sensory latencies are determined by stimulating digital nerves and recording a nerve action potential (NAP) from the wrist proximal to the flexor crease (orthodromic conduction) (Fig. 8-11). The latter site can also be used for stimulation of the median nerve so that needle recordings of MAPs from thenar intrinsic muscles can be accomplished or sensory NAPs can be recorded at skin level from more distal fingers (antidromic conduction). One of the difficulties in recording digital sensory potential in an antidromic fashion is that the recordings may be contaminated by MAPs arising from the thenar eminence, or more frequently, from lumbrical muscles.

Peripheral metabolic neuropathies have slowing of conduction as great as might be expected across the wrist with CTS, but conduction is also at least as slow more distally, such as from the palm to the digits. Electrical sampling of the thenar eminence musculature usually does not show denervation except in severe cases of CTS. On the other hand, if a MAP is recorded from thenar intrinsics after stimulation of median nerve at the wrist, then motor conduction across the carpal tunnel can be determined. In addition, forearm-level slowing of conduction is frequently seen in the more severe examples of CTS, indicating some retrograde degeneration of axons.

Pronator syndrome or compression of median nerve at the elbow level may be difficult to document electrically, especially in its early stages. If denervation is present, it can be found in proximal muscles as well as distal ones. Because the median nerve penetrates between the deep and superficial heads of pronator teres in 85% of cases, a tendinous band within the muscle may in a few cases constrict the nerve. This can result in slowing of conduction and a mild, partial median nerve syndrome distal to this level.

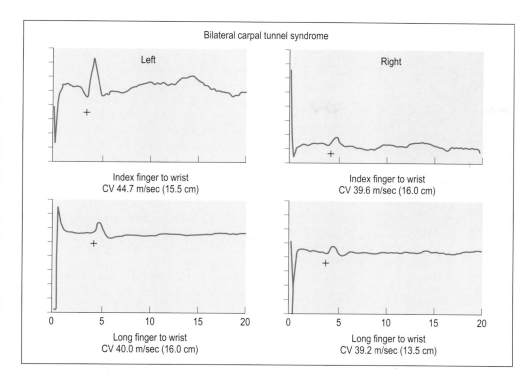

Bilateral carpal tunnel syndrome

Left

Right

Index finger to wrist
CV 44.7 m/sec (15.5 cm)

Index finger to wrist
CV 39.6 m/sec (16.0 cm)

Long finger to wrist
CV 40.0 m/sec (16.0 cm)

Long finger to wrist
CV 39.2 m/sec (13.5 cm)

FIGURE 8-11 Typical abnormal sensory conduction studies in a patient with bilateral CTS. Stimulation sites were digital nerves, and recording site was the wrist. Since the distance between stimulation and recording sites, and latency between stimulation and onset of evoked response, were known, conduction velocities could be calculated. CV, conduction velocity.

SURGICAL EXPOSURE OF THE MEDIAN NERVE

ARM

Exposure of the median nerve at this level can be, but is not always, straightforward. Incision is made superficial to the cleft between biceps/brachialis and triceps and over the course of the usually palpable brachial artery. As lateral and medial cord branches blend together to form median nerve, they do so directly over and often somewhat attached to the volar surface of the axillary to brachial artery junction. The nerve may be somewhat adherent to the artery at this level and must be carefully dissected away. The medial antebrachial cutaneous nerve is of a smaller caliber and is usually easily distinguished from the median nerve. The median nerve takes an almost straight course down the arm and toward the volar elbow but more distally tends to lie more lateral to brachial artery, although the nerve's mesoneurium tends to adhere the nerve to the vessel. By contrast, the ulnar nerve, after its origin from the medial cord, begins to take a slightly oblique course as it heads for the region of the olecranon on the posterior part of the elbow. On rare occasions, the median nerve at the arm level may send a branch to biceps brachii. Quite rare is a connection between the ulnar and median nerves at the level of the arm and comprising a proximal Martin-Gruber anastomosis. Whenever possible, these connections, if present, should be preserved during the dissection. As the median nerve approaches the elbow, it may give an early branch to the proximal pronator teres.

With injury and concomitant scar, it is important to skeletonize at least a portion of the artery so it can be protected as the median nerve is manipulated away from it and repaired. In a practical sense, adequate exposure and identification usually involve some exposure of not only the artery but also the ulnar nerve. Venous branches running to the brachial and eventually axillary vein often cross the median nerve at the arm level and may have to be ligated or coagulated to adequately expose median nerve and to gain length for operative electrical studies and repair. This can be done without compromise of important venous drainage because this drainage is located medially, inferiorly, and somewhat parallel to the artery and nerve rather than crossing the latter.

ELBOW AND FOREARM

The median nerve, along with the brachial artery, runs beneath the bicipital aponeurosis at the level of the elbow. After giving some branches to the pronator teres, the median nerve then goes deep to this muscle. Exposure at the elbow usually begins with an incision over the distal arm's brachial groove that runs slightly transversely in the elbow flexion crease and then extends distally, overlying the cleft between the brachioradialis and the pronator teres. The median nerve tends to lie beneath the lateral or radial edge of the pronator teres as it runs deep to this muscle and the flexor digitorum superficialis. There are many branches at the elbow level, and these can be dissected out to provide some mobility for the main nerve. These take an oblique course toward the pronator teres, palmaris longus, flexor carpi radialis, and flexor digitorum superficialis, and should be preserved when possible (Fig. 8-12).

Beneath the flexor digitorum superficialis, the median nerve divides into the anterior interosseous nerve and main median nerve. The anterior interosseous nerve supplies the median half of the flexor digitorum profundus, primarily to the index and to a variable extent of the middle finger. The anterior interosseous nerve branch also supplies the flexor pollicis longus in the mid to distal forearm and the pronator quadratus in the distal forearm. There can be some variation in the take-off of the anterior interosseous nerve or in the relationship of the tendinous origin of the deep head of the pronator teres crossing over the anterior interosseous nerve.

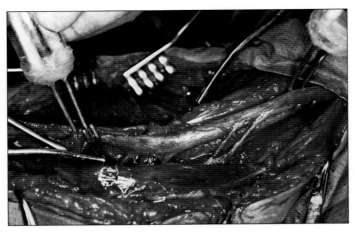

FIGURE 8-12 Anatomy of the median nerve at the level of the elbow. Arm is to the right and forearm is to the left. Lacertus fibrosus (bicipital aponeurosis) has been sectioned and pronator teres split away to expose this portion of the nerve. Pronator teres, flexor digitorum superficialis, and anterior interosseous nerve branches can be seen.

DISTAL FOREARM AND WRIST

The skin incision begins on the volar wrist and extends proximally on the forearm. It is made in an up-and-down fashion and just to the radial side of the palmaris longus. The nerve stays beneath muscle until it reaches the more distal forearm, where it nestles between multiple tendons. The wrist-level extension of the transverse carpal ligament is the antebrachial fascia that covers the nerve. This fascia must be opened to expose the nerve at the wrist. At this level, the median nerve lies somewhat deep to the palmaris longus and yet superficial to both the flexor digitorum superficialis and profundus tendons. As the nerve approaches the distal forearm, a branch leaves its dorsal surface to run to the pronator quadratus. Just above the wrist, the palmar cutaneous branch leaves the radial side of the nerve and can usually be dissected out and spared. Most of the surrounding tendons, especially those adjacent to or somewhat overlying the median nerve, can be mobilized and encircled with a Penrose drain to retract them from the nerve. Care must be taken in placing self-retaining retractors at this level because not only tendon but also nearby ulnar nerve and artery or radial artery can be easily damaged.

As the median nerve enters the palm of the hand, it runs under the transverse carpal ligament, which should be sectioned whenever the nerve is exposed and manipulated at the wrist or distal forearm levels. Soft tissue swelling can otherwise extend distally and lead to secondary entrapment at this level.

PALM AND HAND

Incisions for exposure for injuries and CTS are usually made in a palmar crease. Palmar skin is thick, but the amount of subcutaneous tissues varies from patient to patient. The underlying transverse carpal ligament usually has a grayish color and is especially thick at the heel of the palm. If there is an opportunity, we usually open the ligament first at the midpalmar level where it is not as thick, and then with scalpel or scissors, the ligament is opened more proximally and distally (Fig. 8-13). Even if the incision is not extended proximal to the wrist level, which we usually do not do

for routine CTR, subcutaneous tissue of the wrist is undermined from the level of the palmar incision. One blade of the Metzenbaum scissors is then slid on top of the median nerve and the other blade on top of transverse carpal ligament. Wrist-level ligament and antebrachial fascia of the distal forearm are then sectioned with the scissors. Usually, this is done on top of but toward the ulnar side of the median nerve to avoid cutting the palmar cutaneous branch. This branch usually arises from the radial side of the nerve several centimeters above the wrist crease. In the distal palmar space, the superficial palmar arch of vessels tends to lie superficial to the digital nerve branches and to cross them in a transverse fashion. The deep palmar arch is dorsal and thus deep to the digital nerve branches. These digital branches head toward the base of the middle and index finger. They give off small branches to underlying lumbricals and are sometimes accompanied by small arterial and venous branches from the palmar arcades of vessels.

Origin of the thenar recurrent branch is somewhat variable. This branch can run obliquely and forward from the nerve if it originates at a proximal palmar level, or, as is more usual, runs transversely if it arises from the median nerve at a mid-palmar level. In some instances, the thenar recurrent has a more distal origin and actually takes a backward course to go to thenar muscles. The branch can and often does divide before reaching musculature. Great care must be taken in dissecting along the radial side of the median nerve at a palmar level to preserve the recurrent thenar branch.

Serious injury involving the main median nerve before it branches at the palmar level may require internal neurolysis. One way to do this and preserve as much nerve as possible is to isolate digital and recurrent thenar branches first. These are then dissected proximally through the lesion in continuity. This results in an internal neurolysis of the nerve in which scar from not only epineurium but also interfascicular epineurium is removed.

Differential recording of NAPs can be done at a fascicular level or from a group of fascicles as well as from nerve as a whole. Grafts, if necessary, can extend from bundles or groups of fascicles proximally to digital and thenar recurrent branches distally.

Many routine operations, such as CTR, are performed using local or monitored anesthesia. A tourniquet may be utilized. These patients are operated on and return home on the same day. In the case of CTS, the transverse carpal ligament should be inspected before incision to exclude its penetration by a palmar cutaneous branch. This branch should be preserved to minimize palmar paresthesias and pain. In cases where tenosynovitis is present, we prefer to do an external neurolysis of the median nerve, clearing or freeing the nerve at least at the palmar level 360 degrees around. Inflammatory tenosynovium may be resected in select cases. We usually also resect a strip of traverse carpal ligament on either side to minimize reformation of the ligament. We do not close the ligament but we do close the subcutaneous tissue with No. 3 or 4 resorbable suture, and the skin, either with mattress or running subcuticular absorbable suture with Steri-Strips. Before closure, any oozing or bleeding points are sought out and coagulated with use of the bipolar forceps. A serious surgical complication at this level is a palmar hematoma of sufficient size to compress the median or ulnar nerves. As a result, meticulous hemostasis is very important. A mildly compressive dressing is applied using a soft, circular wrap of dressings. A boxing-glove-like dressing is fashioned, leaving the tips of the fingers and thumb exposed so the patient can be encouraged to move and use them relatively early postoperatively.

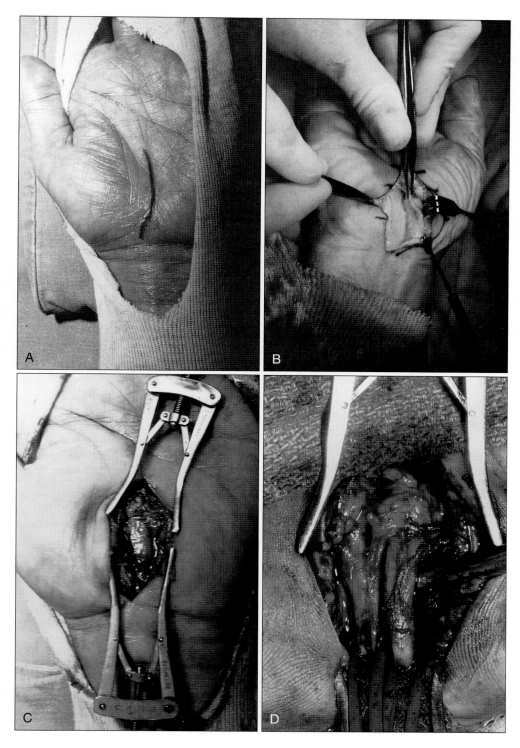

FIGURE 8-13 **(A)** Usual palmar incision for CTR. **(B)** Initial exposure after palmar skin incision has been made. Palmar aponeurosis has been divided. **(C)** The median nerve, in this case, is scarred and thickened after exposure through a palmar incision. **(D)** In another case, a bifid median nerve was exposed at the time of a CTR.

RESULTS

Results with a number of other series of median nerve injuries have been published and are worth careful study.[6,32,39,52,65,79–81] Some of these reports have been nicely reviewed by Cooney.[18] Many of these and other series have tended to be weighted toward more distal median injuries since they were reported by orthopedists, plastic surgeons, or those interested in hand surgery.[5,55,58,64,100] There are a few exceptions, but most of these summarizations are based on war wounds involving this nerve (Tables 8-1 to 8-

3).[68,70,74,99,101,102] Although a variety of tendon transfers is available for median nerve palsy, those done in these patients seemed much less effective than those done in other patients with radial or ulnar nerve palsies.[71,77]

The results of patients evaluated with median nerve injuries over a 30-year period of time was recently reported.[44] Of 250 adult patients with median nerve lesions, 83 patients recovered spontaneously. One hundred and sixty-seven patients underwent surgical exploration when they had not demonstrated clinical evidence of return of function and the majority of these operated patients went on to achieve satisfactory recoveries. The best results were seen in

Table 8-1 Median cases – series reported

Series	Median cases	Total no. of nerve cases
Alexander – Britain WW I	179	876
Burrow & Carter – Britain WW I	242	1406
Worster-Drought – Britain WW I	323	1008
Frazier – U.S. Army I	269	2390
Frazier/Silbert – U.S. Army I	88	378
Pollock/Davis – U.S. Army I	172	985
Tinel – French Army I	67	408
Foerester – Germany WW I	800	3907
Bristow – Britain WW II	451	2636
Woodhall/ Beebe – U.S. WW II	707	2276
Sunderland – Australia WW II	66	365

Table 8-2 Median nerve secondary suture repair results (Seddon)

Arm and elbow level	36% M3 S3+ or better recovery
Forearm level	25% M3 S3+ or better recovery
Wrist level	43.6% M3 S3+ or better recovery

Table 8-3 Median nerve repair results (Dellon)

High-level suture repair	30% M4 or better recovery
	17% S3+ or better recovery
Low-level suture repair	45% M4 or better recovery
	33.5% S3+ or better recovery
Combined high and low graft repair	33% M4 or better recovery
	26% S3+ or better recovery

M, motor grade; S, sensory grade.

patients who had lesions in continuity and present NAPs and in patients who were treated early with primary repair of transected nerves. However, surprisingly favorable results may be seen even when a surgeon performs neuroma resection and grafting based on absent NAPs. The grading system used, as well as the mechanisms of injury and outcomes in these patients are summarized in Tables 8-4 to 8-6. This series did not include operative results of 376 cases of CTS and 18 digital nerve injuries (both groups are summarized later in this chapter) as well as 68 median nerve tumors (47 nerve sheath and 21 benign nonneural sheath tumors, which are summarized in Chapter 23 and in a recent report[45]).

ARM-LEVEL LESIONS

Table 8-7 lists patients seen and evaluated and those operated on by mechanism leading to loss. Approximately two-thirds of patients were operated on within the first 3 months. Lacerations, followed by gunshot wounds, were responsible for the largest subtypes of injuries. In our series, median nerves injured at an arm level did surprisingly well in that a very large number of those operated on had restoration of enough sensation in the median nerve distribution to be at least protective. In addition, pronation by a means of pronator teres and some degree of wrist and finger flexion were recovered. This degree of return provided a grade of 3 using the LSUHSC system (Fig. 8-14). Forty-two of 49 patients achieved this level. While this group included 19 (of 20 patients) who required only external neurolysis because an NAP could be recorded, it also included 12/14 patients following suture or graft repair following neuroma resection, and 5/6 patients in whom primary or secondary end-to-end suture repair was done and 6/9 who had graft repair when the nerve was not in continuity. More than a dozen patients gained a grade of 4 owing to recovery of flexor pollicis longus and flexor profundus to the index finger as well as more proximal median-innervated muscles and at least S3 sensation. Few patients requiring proximal repair gained a grade 5, which required recovery of median-innervated thenar intrinsics as well as excellent sensory return (S4 or S5). Two that did were gunshot wounds in which, at operation, an NAP could be recorded across

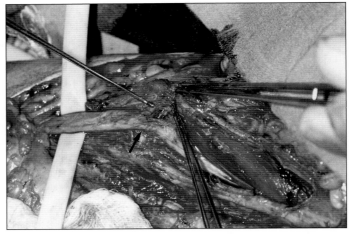

FIGURE 8-14 This median nerve was injured at a proximal level when a Swan-Ganz catheter was removed and a suture was placed in the nerve *(arrow)*. Exploration was timely and done 3.5 months later because of complete clinical and electrical loss. Resection was necessary, and over a 3.5-year period, the patient regained a sensory grade of 3 and motor grade of 3 to 4.

a lesion in continuity several months after wounding. Both cases had a neurolysis, and as predicted, recovered considerable function. Other gunshot wounds had no recordable NAPs through lesions in continuity and were resected and repaired by end-to-end suture in all but one case. Despite such a proximal level for repair, function returned to a grade 4 level in the vast majority of cases. Other cases recovering after operation to grade 4 or grade 4 to 5 levels included lacerations repaired either primarily or secondarily or those contused nerves needing only a neurolysis rather than resection because of the presence of an NAP.

Laceration

Four of the 17 lesions of proximal median nerve associated with a lacerating injury left the nerve in continuity, had an NAP on recording across an area of contusion, and recovered to a grade of either

Table 8-4 The LSUHSC grading system for motor and sensory function*

Grade	Evaluation	Description
Individual muscle grades		
0	Absent	No contraction
1	Poor	Trace of contraction
2	Fair	Movement against gravity only
3	Moderate	Movement against gravity & some (mild) resistance
4	Good	Movement against moderate resistance
5	Excellent	Movement against maximum resistance
Sensory grades		
0	Absent	No response to touch, pinprick, or pressure
1	Bad	Testing produces hypoesthesia or paresthesia; deep pain recovery in autonomous zones
2	Poor	Sensory response sufficient for grip & slow protection; sensory stimuli mislocalized with overresponse
3	Moderate	Response to touch & pinprick in autonomous zones; sensation to mislocalized & not normal with some overresponse
4	Good	Response to touch & pinprick in autonomous zones; response localized, but sensation not normal; no overresponse
5	Excellent	Near normal response to touch & pinprick in entire field including autonomous zones
Grading of proximal median nerve (MN) lesion†		
0	Absent	No MN-innervated pronation or wrist/finger/thumb flexion; no thenar intrinsic function (abductor pollicis brevis & opponens pollicis muscles); absent-to-poor MN sensation
1	Bad	Pronation present, but quite weak; MN-innervated wrist & finger flexors contract, but not against gravity; sensory grade, if present, is 1
2	Poor	Pronation as well as wrist & finger flexion against gravity; more distal muscles either do not contract or have trace function only; sensory grade is ≤2
3	Moderate	Pronation as well as wrist & finger flexion is against gravity & some resistance; some distal muscles such as flexor pollicis longus & even thenar intrinsics contract against gravity; sensory grade is usually 3
4	Good	Pronators, wrist & finger flexors, flexor pollicis longus muscles, & even thenar intrinsics contract against some resistance; sensory grade is ≥3
5	Excellent	All MN-innervated muscles contract against considerable force; sensory grade is ≥4.

*The LHUHS muscle grading system was used to evaluate preoperative loss and postoperative recovery of motor and sensory function. This system is based on earlier British and American systems, but includes some important changes.

†Grading a proximal MN lesion involves more detail because of its important distal sensory and motor input.

4 (three cases) or 5 (one case). Three primary suture repairs were done; two had a grade 3 or better result (one a grade 4 result, and one a grade 5). All three patients receiving secondary grafts regained a grade 3 or better result. Four of seven patients who had a graft repair of a transected nerve reached a grade 3 level or better (Figs 8-15, 8-16). Many of these patients had previous operations for vascular repair.

Gunshot wounds

Only 13 of 24 patients evaluated required operation as 11 demonstrated spontaneous improvement while under initial observation. There was only one failure in this group of 13 operated patients and that was an individual who required 10 cm (4 inch) grafts to replace a segment of proximal median nerve damaged by a shotgun blast. Fortunately, most proximal median nerve injuries caused by gunshot wounds that required resection were focal enough to be repaired by suture or, in one case, by split repair.

Fractures and stretch/contusions

Twelve of 13 lesions fared well with repair. All seven patients with fracture-related contusion required placement of grafts because of their lengthy up-and-down nature. One such repair, left unrepaired until 12 months after injury, not unexpectedly failed. Six patients with stretch injuries had lesions in continuity in which an NAP was

Table 8-5 Mechanisms of injury to the median nerve at various levels in 167 patients

Mechanism of injury	No. of cases				
	Arm	Elbow/forearm	AIN	Wrist	Total
Laceration	17	19	0	27	63
Gunshot wound	13	9	0	2	24
Fracture	7	4	0	3	14
Stretch or contusion	6	11	4	9	30
Compression	5	2	5	6	18
Injection	1	9	1	0	11
Volkmann ischemic contracture	0	2	0	0	2
Electrical	0	1	0	2	3
Arteriovenous fistula	0	1	0	0	1
Burn scar	0	0	1	0	1
Total	49	58	11	49	167

Table 8-6 Lesion categories and types of surgery performed in 167 patients with median nerve lesions

Lesion category & type of surgery	No. surgically treated	No. with grade ≥3 outcome (%)
Not in continuity		
1st suture repair	11	10 (91)
2nd suture repair	9	7 (78)
2nd graft repair	22	15 (68)
In continuity		
NAP present		
neurolysis	76	72 (95)
NAP absent		
suture repair	21	18 (86)
graft repair	28	21 (75)

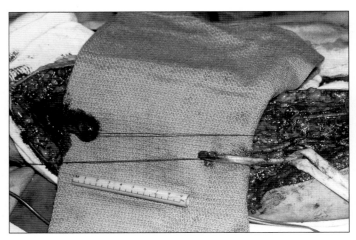

FIGURE 8-15 Long gap in the median nerve at the arm level caused by a blunt transection injury. Grafts required for repair had to be 10 cm long despite mobilization of both nerve ends and mild flexion of the elbow.

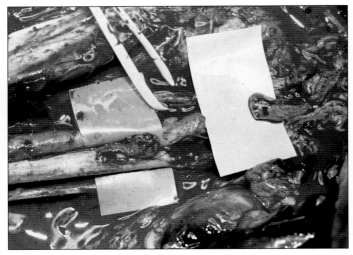

FIGURE 8-16 Preparation of a bluntly lacerated median nerve at an axillary level for repair.

Table 8-7 Outcomes in 49 patients who underwent surgery for median nerve lesions at the arm level

Factor	No. of cases evaluated	No. surgically treated	No. with grade ≥3 outcome
Mechanism of injury			
Laceration	21	17	13
Gunshot wound	24	13	12
Fracture	8	7	6
Stretch or contusion	8	6	6
Compression	8	5	4
Injection	1	1	1
Total	70	49	42
Lesion category & type of surgery			
Not in continuity			
1st suture repair		3	2
2nd suture repair		3	3
2nd graft repair		9	6
In continuity			
NAP present			
Neurolysis		20	19
NAP absent			
Suture repair		5	5
Graft repair		9	7

1st, primary; 2nd, secondary.

recorded. All six of these patients achieved a grade 3 or better result.

Compressive and injection injuries

Severe high median nerve palsy resulting from either compression by a crutch or a sleep palsy from placing arms over the back of a chair was usually managed conservatively, although a few cases required operation. Four of five patients obtained operative results of grade 3 or better with two obtaining grade 5 function. Those treated conservatively had partial loss to begin with or, in the early weeks after compression, showed significant improvement and had an eventual good result with spontaneous regeneration.

The one injection injury was caused by an attempted needling to draw blood from the medial upper arm. Loss, although present, was minimal. Neurolysis was done for pain, and fortunately this improved and eventually disappeared. Damage under these circumstances is usually more extensive and may require resection and repair. Such a lengthy injection injury to arm level median nerve is seen in Figure 8-17.

ARM-LEVEL LESION CASE SUMMARIES

CASE 1

This 19-year-old youth was shot in the right midarm with a 22-caliber pistol. Wound of entrance was on the medial arm and the exit site was posterolateral. There was no humeral fracture. Acutely, a repair of the brachial artery was done by use of a vein graft. Postoperatively, median loss was thought to be incomplete because of retention of some pronator and finger flexor function. Despite these

findings, electromyogram done at both 1 and 2 months after injury showed a severe denervational pattern.

The median nerve was exposed along the medial arm 9.5 weeks after injury. A lesion in continuity 2.6 cm in length was tested by NAP stimulation and recording. There was no distal muscle response on stimulation, and no NAP transmitted across the lesion, so it was resected. This was repaired by an end-to-end suture. Histologic studies showed the resected segment to be neurotmetic or a Sunderland grade 4 lesion.

By 3 years postoperatively, sensation in the median nerve distribution graded 4, as did motor function. The patient was able to use his arm to work as a carpenter.

COMMENT

Some gunshot wounds leaving nerves in continuity get better spontaneously, but if there is no substantial clinical improvement by 3 months or so, then exploration, is certainly indicated.

CASE 2

A 24-year-old man sustained a propeller laceration just below the axilla to the medial arm while water skiing. He also sustained a scapular fracture. He required acute repair of the proximal brachial artery, and then, 2 days later, he was returned to the operating room for primary suture of a divided and probably bluntly transected median nerve. Ulnar nerve, although badly injured, was found in continuity and left alone.

The patient was then referred because of persistent complete loss of median and ulnar function clinically and electrically. When explored by us at 6 months after injury, a suture neuroma of median nerve and a lesion in continuity of ulnar

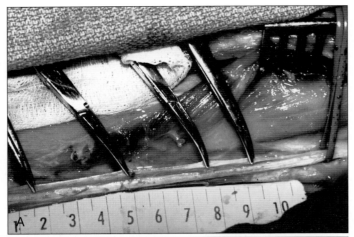

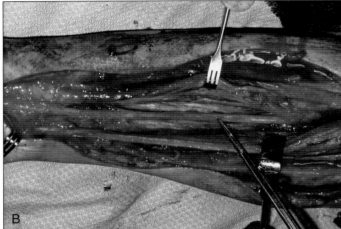

FIGURE 8-17 **(A)** Lengthy injection injury involving the median nerve in a physician as the result of an axillary level anesthetic block. **(B)** The ulnar nerve is being gently retracted to better expose the injured median nerve. This severe lesion in continuity required resection and a graft repair.

nerve were found. Neither nerve transmitted an NAP beyond their lesions. Both lesions in continuity were resected to healthier tissue. Stumps were then sutured end-to-end. Length was made up by mobilization of both stumps and transposition of the distal ulnar nerve to a submuscular position volar to the elbow.

Follow-up at 8 years showed partial median recovery with motor and sensory grades of 3. Ulnar nerve recovery was worse and graded only a 2 overall. The patient used the arm and hand to help his dominant right upper extremity, but only as a helper limb.

COMMENT
Perhaps a better initial management of this case would have been a delay of repair of the median for several weeks, because this was a blunt transection. At that time or later, the ulnar nerve could have been evaluated by NAP recordings, and more timely repair of this nerve could also have been done.

CASE 3
This 36-year-old man had renal failure resulting from glomerulonephritis. A Gore-tex shunt was placed from the brachial artery to vein for dialysis. Immediately postoperatively, he experienced arm pain radiating to the hand as well as painful paresthesias in the fingers and thumb. Both median and ulnar palsies were noted. The palsies appeared to progress in early months after placement of the shunt. Symptoms were initially thought to be caused by a relatively ische-

mic limb and possible nephritic neuropathy, but when seen 8 months later, it was apparent that both the symptoms and the clinical loss related to the proximal arm-level shunt site. Electromyography showed partial denervation in most median- and ulnar-innervated muscles, including those proximal in the limb, such as pronator teres, flexor digitorum superficialis, flexor carpi ulnaris, and flexor profundi. Conduction studies showed marked slowing along more distal median and ulnar nerve.

The shunt and nerves were approached through a medial upper arm incision between the biceps and triceps and extending up to the axillary area. Both median and ulnar nerves were found entrapped and compressed beneath a limb of the shunt. There was also relatively heavy scar at this point. Nerves were cleaned by working beneath the shunt. Small but definite NAPs could be recorded across both nerves. Postoperatively, the patient had almost immediate relief of the neuritic pain. Function gradually recovered even though the shunt was still used for dialysis. Median and ulnar nerve function each graded 4 overall. When the patient was seen in follow-up 3 years later, he was using his arm for most tasks.

COMMENT
Some patients who develop a peripheral neuropathy after arteriovenous shunt for dialysis have compression and entrapment as a cause rather than an ischemic or metabolic mechanism.

ELBOW AND FOREARM-LEVEL LESIONS

Lacerations
Lacerations to median nerve at elbow level were fairly frequent and comprised 19 of 58 cases operated on at this level (Table 8-8). Five had prior vascular operations for repair of brachial artery or vein. Some of these cases also had primary suture repair of the nerve elsewhere, and several of these required re-repair. The need for re-repair had no correlation with whether magnification had been used at the time of the original suture but did relate to how sharp the original transection had been.[63] In general, 17/19 patients recovered grade 3 or better function following surgery; in fact, the majority of these patients regained grade 4 or better function. The three primary repairs done by ourselves at the elbow level fared well, with recovery to grade 4 in all cases (Table 8-8). Secondary repairs of lacerations also had acceptable results. Four of six grafted nerves recovered grade 3 function or better, as did one of the two end-to-end sutures. The case report presented at the end of this section demonstrates the usual situation with laceration at this level.

Gunshot wounds
Gunshot wounds all produced lesions in continuity and required operation in 9 of 11 cases. Seven of the nine (77%) operated patients improved to grade 3 or better levels (Table 8-8). Not all, though, required neuroma resection and repair. Three had NAPs, indicating early and effective regeneration, were spared resection, and recovered nicely. Of these six remaining patients in whom NAPs were not obtained, four had acceptable results, but the other two did not, following graft repair or end-to end suture repair.

Fracture or contusions
Fracture or contusions to median nerve did well at this level unless they were complicated by Volkmann ischemic contracture. There were, unfortunately, four of these cases, two of which were not operated on for neural reconstruction because of late referral. The two operated on had neurolysis, one early (within 24 hours) and one late (at 4 months). Both patients had recovery of median nerve

Table 8-8 Outcomes in 58 patients who underwent surgery for median nerve lesions at the elbow and forearm levels

Factor	No. of cases evaluated	No. surgically treated	No. with grade ≥3 outcome
Mechanism of injury			
Laceration	26	19	17
Gunshot wound	11	9	7
Fracture	7	4	4
Stretch or contusion	14	11	10
Compression	6	2	2
Injection	19	9	8
Volkmann ischemic contracture	4	2	2
Arteriovenous fistula	2	1	1
Electrical	1	1	0
Total	90	58	51
Lesion category & type of surgery			
Not in continuity			
1st suture repair		3	3
2nd suture repair		2	1
2nd graft repair		6	4
In continuity			
NAP present			
Neurolysis		32	30
NAP absent			
Suture repair		4	3
Graft repair		11	8

function to grade 3 only. The other contused nerves usually had partial deficit to begin with, or they had demonstrable NAPs or muscle response to stimulation and did not have resection.

Injection injuries

Injection injuries to the median nerve at the elbow provided a relatively large category with 19 cases. Deficits were usually, but not always, partial; without exception, they were associated with severe pain. Injection injuries to elbow-level median nerve were usually caused by attempted venipuncture or catheterization of the brachial artery. In nine instances, operation was felt to be indicated because of severe pain and paresthesias (Table 8-8). Eight patients had neurolysis only, and one had a suture repair. Some amelioration of pain was gained as well as preservation of function in the cases having neurolysis. Pain was helped in the one case having resection and repair, but less than grade 3 functional result was obtained. Ten cases improved spontaneously and did not require operation (Table 8-8).

The single *electrical injury* at this level was a late referral, required grafts over a 7.6 cm distance, and had only a grade 2 result.

More than one-third of patients with elbow-level injury to the median nerve had prior operations done for associated injuries. Half of these operations involved previous attempts to repair the nerve. Still, more than half of these patients were operated on at 5 months or later.

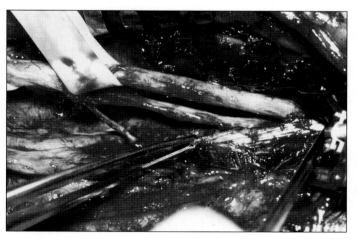

FIGURE 8-18 Fascial band compressing the anterior interosseous nerve branch of the median nerve at the junction of the upper and middle third of the forearm.

Fifteen patients were evaluated with anterior interosseous nerve lesions, and 11 underwent operation. Anterior interosseous nerve or division was entrapped in five cases and injured by injection in three cases, stretch in four, and burn scar in three. Four of the five patients with entrapments were significantly benefited by release and neurolysis of the nerve (Figs 8-18, 8-19; Table 8-9).

Table 8-9 Outcomes in 11 patients who underwent surgery for AIN lesions

Factor	No. of cases evaluated	No. surgically treated	No. with grade ≥3 outcome
Mechanism of injury			
Compression by bone or soft tissue	5	5	4
Injection	3	1	1
Stretch	4	4	3
Burn scar	3	1	1
Total	15	11	9
Lesion category & type of surgery			
Not in continuity			
1st suture repair		0	0
2nd suture repair		0	0
3rd suture repair		0	0
In continuity			
NAP present			
Neurolysis		8	7
NAP absent			
Suture repair		1	1
Graft repair		2	1

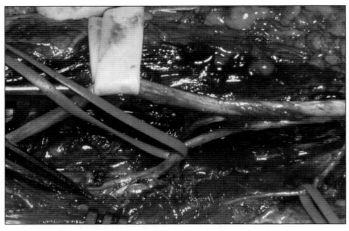

FIGURE 8-19 The anterior interosseous nerve branch is retracted by a Vasoloop, and the main median nerve is retracted by a Penrose drain.

ELBOW-LEVEL LESION CASE SUMMARIES

CASE 1

This 28-year-old woman lacerated her elbow on a plate glass window. She had soft tissue repair and primary suture repair of the median nerve in the antecubital fossa 4.5 hours after injury. She had a complete median nerve palsy below the pronator teres which persisted for 6 months. Electromyography at that time showed complete denervation with no evidence of reinnervation of palmaris longus or flexor digitorum superficialis.

The median nerve was explored at 6.5 months after injury (Fig. 8-20). A partially distracted suture repair was found, and it did not transmit an NAP or have muscle response on stimulation. Neuromas and intervening scar were resected and the nerve was re-repaired.

The patient has done well with recovery of acceptable median nerve function. Median-innervated finger flexion began to occur by 6 months postoperatively. Follow-up at 5.5 years gave median sensation a grade of 3 and motor a grade of 4 to 5. Thenar intrinsics and index lumbricals graded 3 to 4.

COMMENT

Even with a primary repair of a sharp injury, proper mobilization of the stumps and postoperative immobilization for several weeks may be necessary to avoid distraction and, at times, even disruption of a repair.

CASE 2

A 38-year-old man had open catheterization of the brachial artery for cardiac angiography. After this procedure, the patient had neuritic pain in the median nerve distribution. He described painful dysesthesias that extended down the forearm to the hand. Sympathetic blocks were tried elsewhere but gave only partial relief. Percussion or palpation over the healed incision used for angiography gave pain and some electric shock-like stimuli radiating to the hand. Electromyography showed only mild denervation change in median-innervated muscles, but conduction across the elbow was slowed.

Exploration at 3 months after injury showed a swollen and somewhat scarred median nerve segment beneath the lacertus fibrosus. NAP conduction across the lesion was 38.5 m/sec before and after external and partial internal neurolysis. Function was maintained, and, fortunately, pain was helped a good deal. Follow-up has extended to 4 years.

COMMENT

Severe, non-causalgic pain resulting from local nerve injury should usually be managed by direct operation on the nerve rather than by a more central procedure.

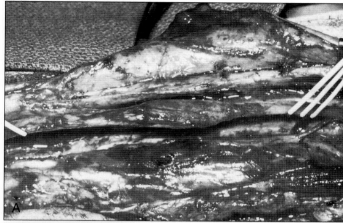

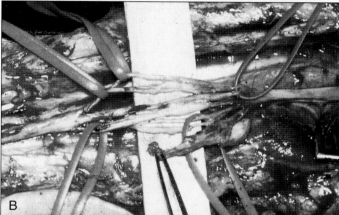

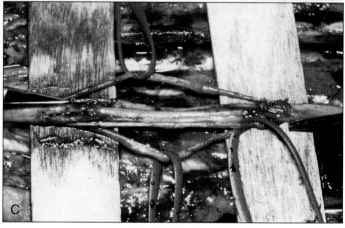

FIGURE 8-20 **(A)** Median nerve lesion in continuity at forearm level resulting from a contusive but partial laceration. Loss before operation was partial, and neuritic pain was a major problem. A nerve action potential (NAP) could be transmitted through the lesion. **(B)** Lesion was split into groups of fascicles; some transmitted NAPs, but most did not. Others, such as the one held by the forceps, were obviously neurotmetic. **(C)** A split repair was done. Three fascicular groups had a neurolysis, and four were replaced by grafts 3.2 cm (1.25 inches) in length.

CASE 3

This 23-year-old man had a water ski flip up and strike the medial surface of the arm above the elbow. Despite direct pressure to the wound, he lost a great deal of blood and required transfusions on reaching the hospital an hour later. The wound was explored, and a short segment of brachial artery was found

missing. Ends were trimmed, and an end-to-end arterial anastomosis was achieved. Lacerated and partially thrombosed veins were ligated. The distal end of the median nerve was found beneath pronator teres muscle and tagged with a suture. Postoperatively, there was a pulse to Doppler only, but over several days, a palpable pulse returned. Two months later, the wound was re-explored, but the nerve stumps were found widely apart, and because the surgeon did not feel comfortable attempting a graft repair the wound was closed.

The patient was subsequently referred for graft repair. He had a complete median palsy including loss of pronator both clinically and by electromyography. There was a diminished but present radial pulse and adequate vascular perfusion of the limb. At exploration 3.5 months after injury, the proximal end of the median with a neuroma was found above the elbow in the medial brachial groove and somewhat adherent to the underlying brachial artery. This was dissected off the vessel and trimmed back to healthy fascicular tissue. The tagged distal stump was found below the elbow and beneath the pronator teres. After trimming of this stump, a 10-cm gap existed. This was bridged with five grafts using both sural and antebrachial cutaneous nerves.

Follow-up has extended to 9 years. The patient uses the hand to turn valves in an oil refinery and has excellent wrist flexion and finger and thumb flexion. Thenar intrinsics remain quite weak, but he does not feel impeded by that. Sensory recovery is less complete, but grades 3 to 4. He still has some pins and needles feeling at the tip of the thumb and index finger. The overall grade for median nerve recovery is 4.

COMMENT

Even though this was a complex and lengthy proximal injury, repair gave at least protective median distribution sensation despite the use of long grafts.

CASE 4

A 39-year-old carpenter received a stab wound at the elbow level. Entry point was superior to the medial epicondyle, and the knife had been directed laterally and superiorly. Because the median nerve loss, although severe, was felt to be partial, he was managed with physical therapy and not referred for further evaluation. On examination 1 year after injury, pronator teres graded 3 to 4, flexor digitorum superficialis was quite weak, and flexor digitorum profundus to the index finger was absent. Flexor digitorum profundus to the middle finger was grade 4, probably because its innervation was shared with that to the ring finger. Flexor pollicis longus function was absent. There was a trace only of abductor pollicis brevis and opponens pollicis, and index and middle finger lumbricals were weak. Sensory grade in the median nerve distribution was 2 to 3. Electromyography showed a severe denervation pattern in the median distribution, with a few nascent units in the flexor digitorum superficialis and pronator teres but not elsewhere.

At exploration, a sizable neuroma in continuity was found at the level of the elbow. There was severe scarring just distal to the neuroma. The distal median nerve appeared atrophic. Stimulation proximal to the neuroma and recording distally showed a very small NAP. Because a year had elapsed and the response was small, the lesion was resected. Conduction velocity of this small NAP across the neuroma was relatively fast at 70 m/sec. This suggested that the original laceration had spared a small portion of the nerve. This was shown to be the case on histologic examination, at which a small fascicle was found to be spared. The rest of the neuroma consisted of fine fibers mixed with scar. There were only a few moderate-sized fibers.

An end-to-end suture was done after resection of the neuroma. Follow-up was at 14 years. The patient could make a fist but still could not curl his index finger entirely into the palm. He could, however, flex the tip of the thumb, and this function graded 3 to 4. Sensation in the median nerve distribution graded 4. Although he had some residual stiffness and pain in the fingers, he used the hand for work as a carpenter.

COMMENT

Even though a lesion may be partial or nearly complete but not complete, conservative management is not justified in the absence of appropriate improvement, and operation should not be unduly prolonged. See Figures 8-21 and 8-22 for additional examples.

Considerable judgment is required to manage cases with complete loss of function and minor degrees of recovery or cases with partial loss with little recovery. At operation, a decision may have to be made even after NAP recordings to sacrifice minor function so that an adequate repair can be done to provide a better end result.

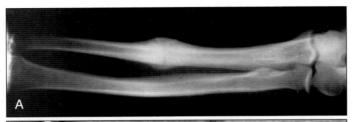

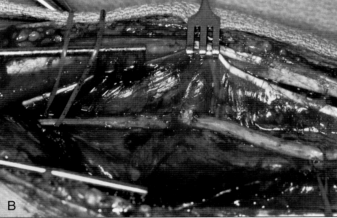

FIGURE 8-21 **(A)** Radius fracture involving the median nerve at a mid-forearm level. United fracture is seen on the lateral forearm radiograph. The distal median nerve loss was still complete at 5 months. The nerve was found entrapped in cicatrix at the fracture site. **(B)** Resection and end-to-end repair were required.

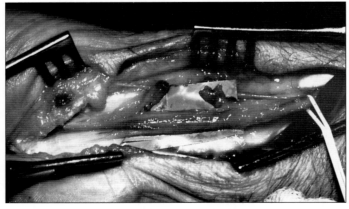

FIGURE 8-22 Distal forearm median injury from resection of a "ganglion" at the wrist level. The "ganglion" was in fact a median nerve schwannoma. Split repair of damaged fascicles by graft was performed; undamaged fascicles were retained.

FOREARM-LEVEL LESION CASE SUMMARIES

CASE 1

A 56-year-old man sustained a 22-caliber gunshot wound to the proximal forearm. The wound was debrided acutely and a sympathectomy was done for what was thought to be true causalgia. This gave only partial relief of his severe pain, which was primarily neuritic and not sympathetically mediated. Pronator teres and fingers flexors, including flexor profundus to index and flexor pollicis longus graded 3 to 4. Thenar intrinsic and median-innervated lumbrical functions were absent. Median distribution sensation graded 3 to 4. Electromyography suggested a lesion involving median nerve but distal to the anterior interosseous nerve branch.

Exploration at 5 months showed a lesion in continuity on the main median nerve distal to the anterior interosseous branch. An NAP could be transmitted across the lesion, but stimulation gave no distal muscle function. Only an external neurolysis was done.

The pain was helped a good deal. Follow-up at 10 years showed good use of the limb. Overall motor function graded 4 to 5; median nerve distribution sensation was quite acceptable and graded 4.

COMMENT

Sometimes, even external neurolysis may help neuritic pain, but this is by no means a universal outcome. Generally, severe pain from local nerve injury is best treated at least in the early months after trauma by direct repair of the nerve rather than by more central procedures.

CASE 2

This 14-year-old fell playing basketball and sustained a fracture of the radius and ulna. Weakness in finger and thumb flexion and hand intrinsics was noted, as well as sensory loss in the median nerve distribution. Fractures were treated by closed manipulation and then casted for 6 weeks. The patient then received intensive physical therapy, but a complete median palsy involving flexor pollicis longus and more distal thenar and lumbrical function was noted. Ulnar-innervated hand intrinsics worked but were weak, grading 3. Sensory loss was only in the median distribution.

Median and ulnar nerves were exposed at mid-forearm level 4.5 months after injury. Both nerves were bound down in cicatrix at the fracture site. Both nerves conducted an NAP before and after external neurolysis.

Follow-up after a 4.5-year period showed good recovery of motor and sensory functions, not only in the ulnar but also in the median nerve distributions. He uses the arm to compete as an amateur in golf tournaments.

COMMENT

All fractures involving a limb require a thorough neurologic examination. Not all blunt injuries to nerve can be managed expectantly.

CASE 3

This 33-year-old man sustained an extensive and complete to median nerve plate glass laceration to the mid-forearm. The soft tissue wound was repaired acutely, and a large gap found in the median nerve was not repaired. Clinical examination and electromyography showed complete loss, including that to flexor pollicis longus and more distal muscles. He maintained flexor digitorum superficialis and profundus function, and ulnar and radial function was normal. Unfortunately, referral for nerve repair was quite delayed. Three interfascicular grafts 7.6 cm in length were placed at 14 months after injury.

A Tinel sign advanced down the forearm to the wrist in the early months after repair, but overall grades were only 3 for both median sensory and distal motor evaluation at 6 years.

COMMENT

Even though injury is complex to non-neural tissues and requires extensive management, any significant neural injury should not be neglected too long. Ideally, this known transection to the median nerve should have been repaired either acutely or within a few weeks of the original injury once other soft tissues had healed.

CASE 4

A 21-year-old woman had a caesarean section and postoperatively received a venipuncture injury to the volar forearm involving the anterior interosseous nerve.

When seen a month after the incident, flexor digitorum profundus of the index fingers graded 3, and flexor pollicis longus was absent. Electromyography showed denervation in muscles in the anterior interosseous nerve distribution. By comparison, there was a healthy median sensory response conducting at 55 m/sec. It was elected to follow the patient for 3 months because there was partial function of the flexor digitorum profundus.

By 3 months after injury, flexor pollicis longus had returned and graded 2 to 3. Follow-up at 3 years showed a good pinch and excellent flexor pollicis longus as well as flexor digitorum profundus of the index finger.

COMMENT

A similar case in an older individual was operated on at 3 months after venipuncture injury because of severe pain, although anterior interosseous deficit was partial. A neurolysis was done, and anterior interosseous function improved to a grade of 4; however, pain, although diminished, was not completely eliminated. It is difficult to relieve pain caused by needled penetration of a nerve such as the median. Sometimes, external neurolysis helps even though the nerve appears, to gross inspection, to be quite normal. In other cases, neurolysis and its attendant manipulation of the nerve do not change the pain pattern.

CASE 5

A 37-year-old woman sustained a stress fracture of the right distal radius after lifting a heavy crate. The limb was immobilized, but when the cast was removed at 6 weeks after injury, there was inability to flex either the tip of the thumb or that of the index finger. There was no sensory loss. The elbow and proximal portion of the median nerve and anterior interosseous branch were surgically explored 8 weeks after injury. The median complex appeared normal, but only a very small NAP could be recorded from the anterior interosseous branch. A neurolysis was done. Recovery began 6 months later, and function was normal by 1.5 years. At last follow-up, 3.5 years later, function of the right hand was normal. The patient had developed, in the interim and spontaneously, decreased pinch of the opposite left thumb and index fingers, and these muscles graded 4 on examination. The patient, however, refused further investigation and subsequently has been lost to follow-up.

COMMENT

The anterior interosseous nerve syndrome is quite characteristic, and the clinical diagnosis should be made without difficulty. The subsequent spontaneous occurrence on the contralateral side can occur with almost all entrapments. However, beware of Parsonage-Turner syndrome masquerading as an isolated anterior interosseous nerve entrapment, especially when bilateral findings are present.

WRIST-LEVEL LESIONS

Lacerations to nerve predominated at this level (Table 8-10). Ten of the 27 laceration cases operated on had prior suture and were thought to be failing or to have failed. Most (8 of 10) required re-repair either by suture or grafts. Despite this, only two failed to gain a grade of 3 or better. Our impression was that at this distal level, aggressive management was necessary in order to optimize results, particularly if sensory loss was significant. Some of the remaining patients had neurolysis because nerves either were recovering after suture or were left in continuity despite laceration as a mechanism of injury. Despite a sharp mechanism for injury, some nerves were found to be contused rather than divided, and, because of NAPs transmitted across the lesion, had only neurolysis (Table 8-10). Painful paresthesias were also a problem in a few of these cases and were sometimes but not always helped by neurolysis.

Smaller numbers of patients had nerve contused by gunshot wound, fracture of the wrist, direct but blunt blows, stretch, or electrical injuries (Table 8-10). Results with neurolysis if an NAP was recorded were excellent, and repair by either end-to-end suture or grafts, also gave good results (Table 8-10). Even the two patients with electrical injury gained some degree of recovery (grade 3 to 4) by graft repair.

Associated ulnar nerve lesions and tendon injuries were not uncommon in the laceration category. This combination of injuries made total rehabilitation of the hand more difficult and down-graded the eventual results. The intervals between injury and operation were spread out between 0 and 12 months or more. While more than half of the wrist-level lesions were operated on during the first 6 months after injury, 10% were operated on after more than 12 months due to late referral. Those cases operated on acutely were transections caused by knives and had a primary end-to-end coaptation with excellent results (grade 4 or better). Outcomes were also good with delayed repair after either blunt transection or resection of lesions in continuity. In the entire series, only four of the 49 operated cases (8%) did not gain a grade 3 or better result.

The nonoperative category at this level also fared well. Approximately 90% of these patients achieved grade 3 or better function. Failures in conservative management were mainly caused by very late referral or refusal of operation. Patients with prior suture were sent for follow-up care and did well in four of six cases that were seen relatively early (less than 1 year after repair). If seen late, 18 months or more after prior suture, re-repair for motor return of thenar intrinsics was not thought to be worthwhile, especially if motor rather than sensory deficit was the major remaining deficit.

WRIST-LEVEL LESION CASE SUMMARIES

CASE 1

This 28-year-old man sustained a 22-caliber gunshot wound to the right distal forearm near the wrist. This was a through-and-through injury entering the volar forearm and wrist and exiting the dorsum of the forearm. There was no fracture, and the patient had a good radial pulse but a complete median palsy from the wrist more distally. The puncture wounds were dressed, and he received tetanus toxoid and was placed on antibiotics. The palsy did not resolve over a 3-month period. Electromyography confirmed a complete median nerve palsy with denervation in the abductor pollicis brevis and opponens pollicis. Sensory studies

Table 8-10 Outcomes in 49 patients who underwent surgery for median nerve lesions at the wrist level

Factor	No. of cases evaluated	No. surgically treated	No. with grade ≥3 outcome
Mechanism of injury			
Laceration	31	27	25
Gunshot wound	2	2	2
Fracture	12	3	3
Stretch or contusion	17	9	8
Compression	8	6	5
Electrical	4	2	2
Injection	1	0	0
Total	75	49	45
Lesion category & type of surgery			
Not in continuity			
1st suture repair		5	5
2nd suture repair		4	3
2nd graft repair		7	5
In continuity			
NAP present			
Neurolysis		16	16
NAP absent			
Suture repair		11	9
Graft repair		6	5

showed no evoked sensory NAPs after stimulation of digital nerve of the index finger and recording from the wrist.

On exploration at 3.5 months after wounding, there was no NAP evoked across a lesion in continuity at the wrist and stimulation gave no thenar intrinsic function. The lesion was resected, and an end-to-end suture repair was done. The resected segment was neurotmetic (Sunderland grade IV injury) on histologic study.

Sensation in the median distribution at 3.5 years postoperatively graded 4, whereas thenar intrinsic motor function graded only 3. He has been able to work as an electrician's helper.

COMMENT

Most of the time, gunshot wounds do not divide nerve but produce a lesion in continuity with a variable potential for recovery. Unfortunately, physical continuity does not guarantee useful recovery. Thus, in the absence of improvement in the early months after wounding, exploration and operative recordings are in order.

CASE 2

This 26-year-old man sustained a knife wound to the wrist and a wrist-level median palsy which was complete. At exploration 1 month later, the nerve was found to be partially transected yet still in continuity. There was no response to stimulation above or below the lesion. The partial transection was completed, and both ends were trimmed to healthy tissue. An end-to-end suture was done. Histologic examination of the resected segment showed several small but spared fascicles.

Follow-up extended to 3.5 years and indicated sensory recovery to a grade of 4; thenar intrinsics and lumbricals graded 3 to 4.

COMMENT

Not all penetrating, sharp injuries divide or transect nerve; some may only stretch or contuse nerve and not divide any portion of the nerve. In this case, most but not all of the nerve was divided. The remaining fascicles were, however, bruised and stretched, and this gave a complete deficit. In other cases, fascicle in continuity can be spared but, on testing, those in this case were not functional and therefore they were resected. NAP recording at 1 month could not be hoped to give evidence of functional regeneration, even if it were occurring. Simple stimulation in this case did show that the fascicles in continuity had been seriously injured.

CASE 3

This 4-year-old boy fell on a broken glass bottle and sustained a laceration of the distal forearm. Initial examination showed a loss of distal thumb flexion as well as blunting of sensation on the tips of the thumb and index finger and on some of the middle finger. It was impossible to test thenar intrinsics or lumbricals since the child was crying and uncooperative for most of the examination.

The wound was explored acutely, and both a divided flexor pollicis longus tendon and a transected median nerve were found. The nerve required minimal trimming of both stumps since epineurium had been neatly transected. Both the nerve and the tendon were repaired end-to-end. After closure of the forearm-to-wrist laceration, the wrist and palm were wrapped with circular gauze dressings with the fingertips and thumb tip exposed so they could be moved voluntarily and passively.

The child did well. By 1.5 years after injury, median nerve sensation graded 4 and thenar intrinsics almost 4. Electromyographic studies showed abundant thenar nascent changes, and sensory NAPs from index to above wrist could be obtained and conducted at 30 m/sec.

COMMENT

Clinical or electrical evaluation of children with nerve injury can be quite difficult. The surgeon must retain a high index of suspicion for serious injury, and examination may need to be repeated.

CASE 4

Another youngster, who was only 1 year of age, fell and lacerated her right wrist on a piece of metal. The soft tissue wound was cleaned out and sutured in an emergency room. The child tended to suck the fingers of this hand, and the mother brought the child back to the hospital because of ulcerated, eroded fingertips. This involved primarily the index and the middle fingers. Further examination by another neurosurgery service showed absent median sensation, yet there was no apparent atrophy of the thenar eminence, and abduction and opposition of the thumb appeared to be done with ease.

At exploration, a neuroma in continuity involved median nerve, but it was more severe on the volar than on the dorsal surface. Nerve transmitted an NAP, so an internal neurolysis was done, splitting the nerve into bundles, half of which transmitted and half of which did not. A split repair was done, using sural grafts to replace the presumed sensory portion of the nerve.

The metal fragment must have transected or badly stretched the sensory portion of the nerve, but spared, for the most part, the motor portion. Resolution of changes in the skin and nails and restoration of good sensory function occurred over the next 2 years.

COMMENT

In this case, despite apparent retention of median motor function, exploration and eventual repair were certainly indicated because of serious sensory loss in an area of great functional importance.

DIGITAL NERVES – PALMAR AND FINGER LEVELS

Most patients seen in consultation in this category were sent by us to a hand surgeon if repair was indicated, but 18 were managed by us.

Lacerating and contusive injuries were responsible for the majority of these lesions, but in four instances, injury was associated with CTR (Figs 8-23 to 8-25; Table 8-11). In eight instances, operation was not judged worthwhile, either because of incomplete loss predicted to improve or because the patient refused operation. Two patients with finger amputations and digital stump neuromas were helped by trimming the digital nerves back to a palmar level, coagulating the fascicles exposed with fine-tipped bipolars, and burying stumps as deeply in the palm as possible. There were three digital nerve repairs done at distal palmar or finger levels, and each had useful recovery of sensation to a grade 4 level. One of these patients had extensive tendon lacerations and a secondarily stiff hand, making for a delayed and incomplete recovery. Contusive injuries operated on usually had an extensive neurolysis without repair, but one patient with extensive palmar contusion did require a graft repair, with recovery of sensation to only grade 2 to 3.

Digital nerves inadvertently injured during CTR for CTS required neurolysis in two instances and repair in two others. Results were good for restoration of some useful sensory function (grade 3), but painful paresthesias and a tender palmar wound remained a problem in two of these patients. One patient had a hematoma of the palm caused by a duck knife wound. Sensory symptoms in the digits improved after the hematoma was evacuated. The palmar electrical

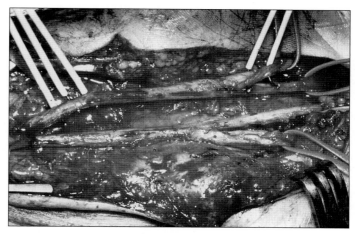

FIGURE 8-24 Direct injury to palmar median nerve. The nerve has been split into two major bundles. One large medial bundle is being stimulated, and recording is from thenar recurrent motor branch.

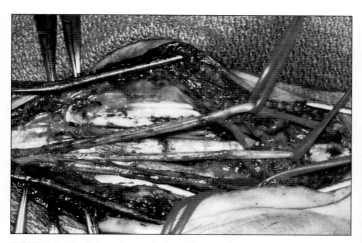

FIGURE 8-23 Internal neurolysis of the median nerve at a palmar level for very painful lesion in continuity caused by contusion. A nerve action potential transmitted to recurrent thenar and each digital sensory branch, so each group of fascicles was cleared of scar tissue and none was resected.

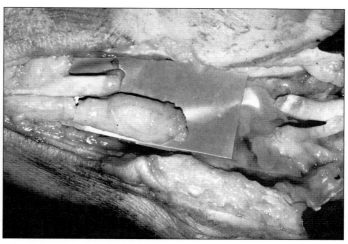

FIGURE 8-25 Preparation of palmar median nerve injury for grafts. Digital branches are to the right. Previous suture was with catgut and no splint was used. The neuroma is undergoing resection.

Table 8-11 Median nerve – digital nerve injuries – results (n = 18)

Mechanism	No. operated/significantly improved	
	Operated	Unoperated
Palmar or finger lacerations	4/3	3/2
Contusion / finger avulsion	1/1	4/3
Prior carpal tunnel release	4/3	0/0
Electrical	1/0	0/0
Missile	0/0	1/1
Total	10/9	8/6
Operations	No. operated/significantly improved	
Neurolysis	3	3
Suture	2	2
Graft	2	1
Evacuation of hematoma	1	1
Resection of digital nerve for neuroma	2	2

injury appeared to be helped somewhat by neurolysis of the median complex in that painful paresthesias in the fingers decreased.

DIGITAL NERVE CASE SUMMARY

This 36-year-old gardener and handyman was injured with an electric hedge clipper, sustaining a blunt laceration to his left index finger along its radial side at the level of the metacarpophalangeal joint. A primary end-to-end repair of a digital nerve was attempted elsewhere. Over the next few months, he developed severe hyperesthesia and pain referred to the tip of the index finger. There was extreme tenderness at the junction of the palm and index finger, and tapping there gave paresthesias radiating to the tip of the index finger.

At exploration 7 months after injury, there was a suture neuroma 2.5 cm in length, and it was apparent that there had been partial distraction of the repair site of the radial digital nerve. This was resected, and the gap was bridged by a 2.6 cm sural nerve graft. To date, the severe pain and hyperesthesia have been relieved, but sensory return on the tip of the index finger grades only 3 after 2.5 years of follow-up.

COMPLICATIONS

Dissection of the proximal median nerve can be associated with injury to the brachial artery, on which it lies. This occurred several times, but fortunately, the vessel could be directly repaired by one or more fine vascular sutures. It helps to encircle the vessel with tapes both proximal and distal to the epicenter of the nerve injury. Then, if hemorrhage occurs during the nerve dissection, the bleeding can be readily controlled and the vessel sutured. Retraction at this level can also compress proximal ulnar nerve, but we had no serious sequelae related to that.

At the elbow level and below, there is not only the risk of arterial or serious brachial venous injury, but also the risk of injury to the posterior interosseous and superficial sensory radial branches of the radial nerve. We were fortunate to be able to avoid any serious loss in those distributions, although sometimes a patient with operation on median at this level reported either a mild decrease in sensation on the dorsum of the hand or mild finger or thumb extension weakness.

Full exposure of midforearm-level median nerve includes splitting or dividing some of flexor digitorum superficialis, and some new or addition weakness in finger flexion may be present postoperatively. Thrombosis of the median artery has been reported at this level as a result of injury, or sometimes because of vasculitis, or less frequently, operation. We have not seen that occur as a result of an operation, but did do a neurolysis on a patient who had thrombosis of this vessel and severe neuropathy as a result of an unspecified vasculitis.

Complications of managing injury at the wrist included injury to nearby ulnar nerve and artery and section of thenar sensory branches or, in the palm, palmar sensory or recurrent motor branches.

Each of our wrist-level median injuries operated on by ourselves had prophylactic section of the transverse carpal ligament, but despite this, one patient who regenerated through a repair appeared to develop CTS several years later and required a neurolysis at the palmar level. Wound healing or infection was seldom a problem.

CARPAL TUNNEL SYNDROME

Carpal tunnel syndrome (CTS) is by far the most common entrapment neuropathy. Surgical results are extremely rewarding with expected improvement or resolution of symptoms in approximately 90% of cases. CTS results from compression of the median nerve at the level of the wrist or palm. The transverse carpal ligament, which is about the size of a postage stamp, extends in a somewhat quadrilateral fashion from the ulnar side of the wrist and the pisiform bone over to the base of the thumb. The median nerve passes beneath the transverse carpal ligament at the level of the wrist along with nine flexor tendons. Any condition that decreases the space within the carpal tunnel or increases the volume of its contents can result in the clinical manifestations of CTS. There may be a predisposition in some patients in whom the carpal canal has less volume than normal.[7] CTS is usually caused by hypertrophy of the ligament with secondary compressive or frictional injury to the median nerve (Figs 8-26, 8-27).[21,62] Pressure within the canal and presumably on the nerve is usually elevated in the symptomatic patient.[9,28] Injury to or inflammation of soft tissues can produce swelling in this region. As a result, secondary compression of an

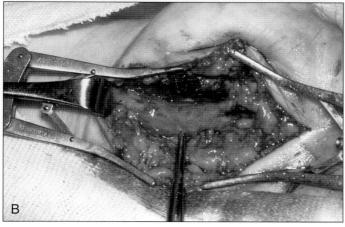

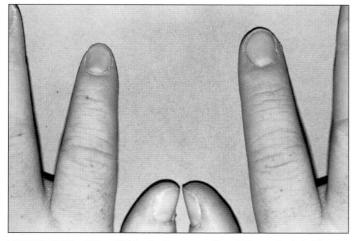

FIGURE 8-26 **(A)** Thinned and discolored segment of palmar-level median nerve (on background) caused by hypertrophied transverse carpal ligament. **(B)** Scarred and thickened segment of median nerve in a patient with long-standing CTS.

FIGURE 8-27 This child had a long-standing CTS on the left. Note the tapering of the left index finger compared with the right side.

already snug but previously uncompromised nerve in the carpal canal can also occur.

CTS has been associated with pregnancy, especially in the third trimester, rheumatoid arthritis, synovitis of the flexor tendons, prior trauma including acute fractures of the wrist (either a Colles' fracture or a reverse Colles' fracture), endocrinological conditions such as thyroid disorders or acromegaly, and a host of other less common diseases and injuries involving the wrist and wrist joints.[3,24,38,54,61] Its relationship to repetitive, cumulative activities remains controversial. The syndrome can also occur spontaneously, and actually this is its most frequent presentation.[10,88,94]

Onset of CTS is usually associated with numbness and paresthesias in the median nerve distribution, particularly at the tips of the fingers. Such symptoms can appear to spread to involve ulnar-innervated fingertips as well. The paresthesias frequently awaken the patient at night, and he or she gets up and attempts to "shake it off" or run cool or warm water over the hand to try and improve the symptoms. Wrist position, such as dorsiflexed when driving a car may reproduce symptoms. With time, the sensory symptoms become permanent, and weakness of the hand, particularly of the thenar intrinsic muscles innervated by the median nerve, is evident. Abduction and opposition of the thumb can be weak, as can lumbrical function, especially for the index and, less so, for the middle finger. Weakness may be described as "stiffness." Atrophy of the thenar eminence may also occur with long-standing and severe CTS. Usually, however, the patient comes to the physician complaining of only sensory symptoms and perhaps some mild clumsiness of the hand. Fine hand movement such as opening a bottle, turning a doorknob, or holding a pen or pencil between index and thumb can be affected. Patients may complain of wrist pain or pain in the forearm, arm, and even the shoulder. Such symptomatology is usually evident before atrophy occurs and in some patients is as bothersome as the sensory symptoms.[75]

Inability to localize stimuli in the median distribution, particularly in its autonomous zone, is a late finding with CTS, whereas blunting of sensation or hyperesthesia on stroking the volar tip of the index finger, middle finger, or thumb is an earlier finding. Comparison of blunt stimuli to sharp ones may be altered relatively early as well. Often, however, there is no sensory change to testing, even to two-point discrimination, despite the fact that the patient has many sensory complaints. Tapping on the wrist and sometimes the proximal palm gives paresthesias into the hand which may not always be restricted to the median nerve distribution. A Phalen sign, in which acute, sustained flexion or sometimes extension or dorsiflexion of the wrist gives median distribution paresthesias, is occasionally present, but it is frequently absent more than one would suspect, even with an acutely symptomatic CTS.[87] Even if the Phalen sign is negative, application of pressure by the examiner's thumb over the nerve at the wrist level as the wrist is either extended or flexed sometimes reproduces the patient's median distribution paresthesias.

Although CTR for CTS is one of the most straightforward and successful operations known, it can and does fail. Of course, the leading cause for failure or partial relief is that there can be other causes for paresthesias, numbness, or pain in the fingers and hand.[36,78] Most of these simulators are readily differentiated from CTS. Some of these causes include cervical disc and degenerative disease of the spine resulting in radiculopathy, cervical rib involving C7 to middle trunk, proximal median neuropathy, pronator or anterior interosseous nerve syndrome, or compression of the median nerve in the distal arm by a Struthers ligament[42,48,49,66,76,85] or other types of neuropathy (such as from diabetes) and various arthropathies of the wrist.

CTS can complicate or add to these primary diagnoses, and if so, CTR is still indicated. On the other hand, patients with CTS are often subjected to repeated periods of traction, steroid therapy, myelography, scalenotomy and first rib resection, and even psychotherapy before the transverse ligament is sectioned, frequently with relief of symptoms.

The diagnosis may be missed because the numbness and pain that would be expected to be confined to the distal sensory distribution of the median can involve the whole hand and can radiate up or down the arm.[12] On rare occasions, the presentation may be confined to thenar loss and atrophy caused by compression of the recurrent motor or thenar branch,[4] and the neurologist or surgeon has difficulty conceiving of CTS as the cause of the symptoms.

Although much has been written about the work-up of CTS, a few points are worth re-emphasis. The diagnosis of CTS is usually straightforward and can almost always be readily made by taking a careful history. Characteristic is a tingling pain mixed with numbness and associated paresthesias. The onset may be insidious or sudden, but discomfort is usually worse at night and often awakens the patent from an otherwise sound sleep. A Tinel sign on tapping or percussion is almost always present over the course of the nerve, particularly at the wrist and proximal palm. There may or may not be objective sensory decrease or median-innervated motor abductor pollicis brevis, opponens pollicis brevis, and index finger lumbrical weakness or thenar atrophy.

While the diagnosis can be made on clinical grounds alone, we routinely use electrodiagnostic studies to confirm the diagnosis, grade the degree of compression, and exclude other diagnoses. CTS can be present without electrical concomitants, but they are almost always there if searched for carefully, or there is an alternate explanation for their absence.[33,37,46] Intraoperative conduction changes are even more likely to be present than those recorded noninvasively. This is probably because the operative recordings can be made just across the involved portion of the nerve and thus over a shorter segment of median than is utilized by the usual less invasive studies.[23] Even though compound MAPs recorded from thenar muscles after stimulation at the wrist or above may be normal, those sensory NAPs recorded at wrist after stimulation of digital nerves at the fingers or, better yet, in the palm, usually have a slowed conduction across the carpal tunnel.[84]

A period of nonoperative therapy is appropriate, especially for patients with intermittent or mild symptoms. This may consist of nonsteroidal antiinflammatory agents, splinting and corticosteroid injection into the carpal canal, and work and activity modification, all of which have different successes.[31] Surgery has been shown to be an effective treatment for CTS, statistically significantly more so than nonoperative measures.[30]

RESULTS WITH CARPAL TUNNEL RELEASE THROUGH A PALMAR INCISION

Outcomes in a relatively small group of patients in whom follow-up was available are summarized in Table 8-12. The procedure was relatively successful in relieving or improving pain and paresthesias. Some reversal of sensory loss or motor loss was possible but less likely, particularly if such loss was severe or had been present for some time. The majority of the patients seemed pleased with their outcomes, but as can be seen in Table 8-12, three required a repeat CTR, five had some worsening of their symptoms, and a

Table 8-12 Results of carpal tunnel release by palmar incision – LSUHSC series (n = 376 CTRs in 340 patients*)

Prominent pain improved	246 of 282 (87%)
Prominent paresthesias improved	230 of 249 (92%)
Significant numbness improved	82 of 146 (56%)
Significant weakness improved	20 of 48 (42%)
Patients satisfied with results	303 of 340 (89%)
Major symptoms persisted	23 cases (6%)
Deficit increased	5 cases (1%)
Required repeat operation	3 cases (1%)
Complications	
Wound, hematoma	1 case
Superficial wound infection	3 cases
Addiction to narcotic	1 case
Reflex sympathetic dystrophy	1 case
Other diagnosis	2 cases

*Average follow-up period was 18.5 months.

few patients had complications which, fortunately, were usually mild.

We do not perform internal neurolysis and epineurotomy or tenosynovectomy routinely as these procedures have not been shown to be helpful in most series.[59] Internal neurolysis, however, was performed in patients with neuropathic pain, and tenosynovectomy was done when there was evidence of severe tenosynovitis. In patients with isolated or advanced cases of thenar atrophy, we performed neurolysis of the recurrent motor branch.

LIMITED OPEN, ENDOSCOPIC, AND PERCUTANEOUS TECHNIQUES

Various operative approaches and techniques have been advocated by surgeons over the years.[73] Outcomes from comparative trials have been summarized nicely.[88] While these limited techniques have advantages and advocates, at this time, we still prefer to perform our CTRs using the traditional method, namely open release of the transverse carpal ligament under direct visualization in an open manner.

A limited open technique often results in an issue of semantics about the length of a skin incision. Typically, a single incision is made in the mid-palm, but sometimes in the wrist crease. Occasionally, two small incisions may be made, one in the mid-palm, and the other at the wrist crease. The ability to inspect the carpal canal is more limited than with an open approach. The technique may be supplemented by use of various ligament knives for a relatively blinded release.

The most popular endoscopic techniques are the Agee (single) and Chow (dual) portal systems. The major advantages of these techniques are the smaller incision and the biomechanical and anatomic advantages afforded by the technique on minimizing the dissection and retention of the pulley effect on the flexor tendons.

These result in a quicker postoperative recovery (return of grip and pinch strength), earlier return to work, and decreased pillar pain. The disadvantages relate to a steep learning curve and a risk of incomplete release. The endoscopic technique may be slightly more expensive and is often more time consuming than an open approach. A recent meta-analysis has demonstrated a threefold risk of associated neurologic complication rate with the endoscopic technique.[91] The increased rate of neurologic injury has also been seen with other percutaneous techniques; not all comparisons, however, agree with such conclusions. Ultimately, the relatively small early benefits from endoscopic (and presumably percutaneous) techniques must be weighted against the inherent risk to neurovascular structures from limited visualization. Several studies have demonstrated no significant differences between patients treated with endoscopic and open techniques at 3–6 months postoperatively.

FAILED CARPAL TUNNEL RELEASE

Surgical CTR is an extremely successful operation for a very disabling condition, providing patients to be operated on are well selected.[19,25,67,75,95] Still, approximately 10–20% of patients may have persistent or develop recurrent symptoms, at least to some degree, or an occasional individual may develop increased symptoms or even new symptoms which differ from those present before surgery.[22,35,36,57] In some clinics, this has led to attempts at conservative, nonsurgical management.[27] These methods can work but require careful, repetitive follow-up, and the patient often comes to surgery anyway.[35,60] Results from secondary surgery range from 50% to 70% in most series. Failed CTS is typically due to errors of diagnosis or treatment.[15,16] Poor outcomes have been reported in those with worker's compensation or ongoing litigation, those who have had multiple previous operations, or who have symptoms outside of the median nerve distribution, or negative electrodiagnostic studies.

PERSISTENT SYMPTOMS AFTER CARPAL TUNNEL RELEASE

Persistent symptoms may be due to an underlying neuropathy or a more proximal site of compression. If the initial diagnosis was correct, persistent symptoms are often caused by incomplete division of the transverse carpal ligament, either in the distal palms or at the level of the wrist (Fig. 8-28).[43] There may be a proximal extension of the transverse carpal ligament or thickening of what some term the antebrachial fascia at the wrist level. A Tinel sign is usually present at the wrist or distal palm, even many months after the original surgery. New sensory/motor velocity studies may or may not be of help, because conductive abnormalities across the carpal tunnel may persist for many months and sometimes years after even the most successful CTR. The diagnosis of incomplete CTR may be suspected if the incision for the original CTR was placed over the wrist, suggesting the possibility of retention of distal palmar ligament. An inappropriately placed wrist or palmar incision or a very short wrist or distal palmar incision may suggest the possibility of persistent entrapment.[17] Less frequently, hypertrophic and sometimes inflamed synovium may have enveloped the nerve and may have been overlooked at surgery (Fig. 8-29).[50] Even less frequently, a ganglion cyst, lipoma, accessory lumbrical muscle, or other lesion may have intruded on the carpal tunnel and served as a precipitating or complicating feature of CTS. It is possible to

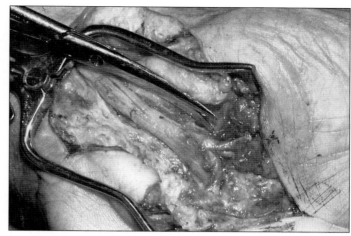

FIGURE 8-28 Median nerve in a patient with persistent CTS who did not have the distal portion of the transverse carpal ligament completely sectioned at previous operation.

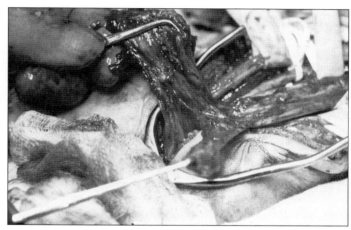

FIGURE 8-29 Tenosynovitis caused by tuberculosis resulted in compression of the median nerve at the level of the distal forearm and wrist with less involvement of the ulnar nerve. The patient presented with a palpable fullness at the wrist and symptoms suggestive of CTS. An extensive synovectomy was necessary, and then the patient was started on antitubercular drugs.

overlook such a lesion, especially if the surgeon's principal focus is release of the transverse carpal ligament and not careful inspection of the median nerve and its bed.

RECURRENT CARPAL TUNNEL SYNDROME

Although debated by some, we are convinced that the transverse ligament can reform with time. For that reason, we favor excision of a strip of ligament on either side of the transection at the time of the initial CTR. Nonetheless, reformation of the ligament is difficult to confirm without reoperation. Because such reconstitution does occur, it brings into question the efficacy of purposeful incomplete transverse ligament section or procedures to imbricate or reconstitute the ligament after section in an attempt to improve gripping power between the thumb and other fingers after CTR.[83]

Postoperative scar setting in and around the released nerve has been cited as a cause for recurrence. This is more likely to be a

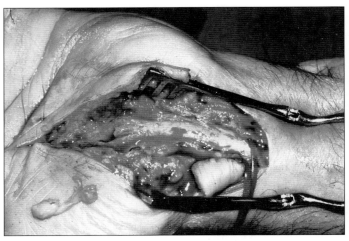

FIGURE 8-30 Injury to a sensory fascicle of the median nerve during previous CTR. The neuroma of the sensory fascicle has been resected and laid on the palmar skin.

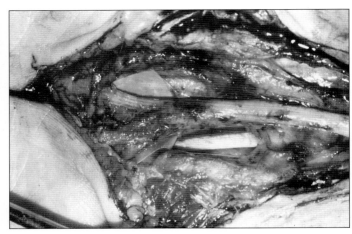

FIGURE 8-31 Injury to the palmar portion of the median nerve caused by prior CTR attempted through a transverse wrist incision.

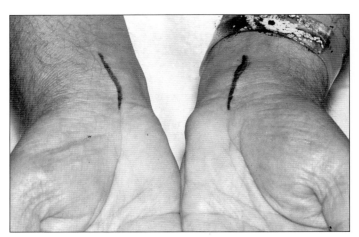

FIGURE 8-32 Failed bilateral CTR with approach made through longitudinal wrist incisions. Some thenar eminence atrophy is evident on the right.

factor if hemostasis at the time of the original surgery was less than adequate, if a palmar or wrist hematoma complicated the original surgery, or if wound healing was incomplete or poor as a result of infection or dehiscence of the wound.

INCREASED OR NEW SYMPTOMS AFTER CARPAL TUNNEL RELEASE

It is not unusual for numbness and paresthesias and even pain to increase after CTR (Fig. 8-30). Usually, such symptoms in an otherwise successful CTR are temporary. They are caused by an irritable nerve, perhaps one severely compressed but recently manipulated during CTR. If such symptoms do not resolve in a matter of weeks, or if they are very severe with or without new and significant sensory or motor loss, then there is the possibility that the nerve has been inadvertently injured during CTR. This is more obvious if there is new and significant deficit, but direct neural injury can sometimes be the source of severe pain without additional or new deficit. Sometimes this is caused by overenthusiastic manipulation of the nerve; other times, it results from inadvertent direct surgical injury to the nerve, and in other cases, it may be caused by ill-advised invasion of the nerve. At the present time, there is no indication for internal neurolysis on the vast majority of spontaneously and previously unoperated median nerves associated with CTS.[20,29,57] Inadvertent injury can and does occur, even in the hands of surgeons who are very experienced with this operation (Fig. 8-31). This is seldom related to anatomical variation of the nerve and its branches, although this is always a possibility.[51,96] The median nerve can be injured, as can the adjacent ulnar nerve during any procedure, including open and endoscopic techniques.[13,53]

If the pattern of loss and pain does not improve in the early months after CTR, then reoperation is in order. This is especially true if a prior operative incision appears to be badly placed (Fig. 8-32). Neurolysis of distal palmar branches may help but is often only the initial step in working out the extent of the direct neural injury. Internal neurolysis of the main median nerve at palmar and sometimes wrist level may be necessary. After internal neurolysis, intraoperative NAP recordings can identify or confirm the portion of the nerve that is damaged and help the surgeon decide whether

to resect and repair that segment or to be content with a neurolysis. The time necessary for recovery then depends on what type of repair is necessary, time interval between injury and repair, patient age, and all of the other usual factors that play a role in nerve regeneration. Restoration of function once lost does not follow the usual timetable for recovery after CTR.

Sometimes, a branch of the nerve can be severed or damaged during the course of CTR (Fig. 8-33). This may be the thenar, which provides median motor input to the thenar eminence and which, if damaged, produces thenar atrophy and weakness (Fig. 8-34).[53] This may or may not be reparable, depending on the relation of the injury to the input of this branch to muscle. A palmar-level digital nerve can also be injured and require repair, especially if its supply is to thumb and index finger. Digital nerves destined for middle finger, or less frequently, little finger may be resected if there is avulsion, neuroma, or severe damage over a length, because a hypoesthetic long or ring finger is preferable to one with severe hyperesthesia and hyperpathia.

Less obvious but of great diagnostic importance is damage to the palmar cutaneous branches. These injuries can be associated not only with numbness but with painful paresthesias, especially if a neuroma forms at the injury site. The palmar cutaneous nerve may

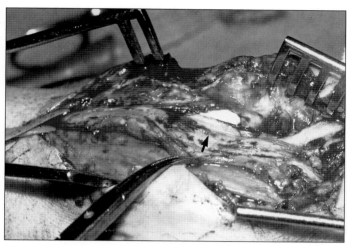

FIGURE 8-33 Severe palmar median injury *(arrow)* which required graft repair. A CTR had been attempted through a transverse wrist incision.

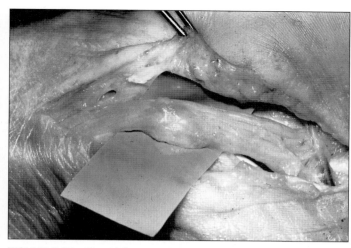

FIGURE 8-35 Direct injury to palmar median nerve despite direct inspection through a palmar incision. A portion of the nerve lesion required repair.

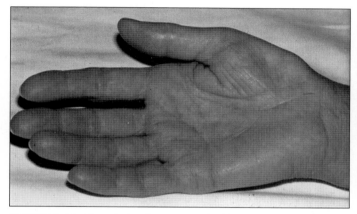

FIGURE 8-34 Thenar atrophy as a result of inadvertent section of the recurrent thenar branch during CTR. A retinaculotome had been used through a small wrist-level incision.

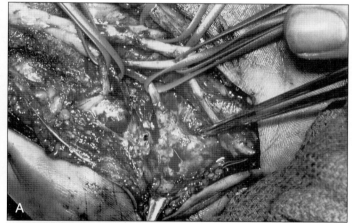

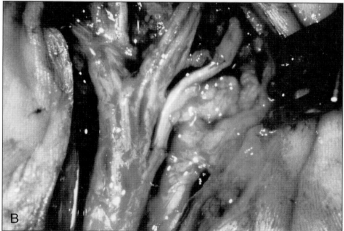

FIGURE 8-36 **(A)** Digital branch injury as a result of CTR. Neuroma and severe scar are evident at the tips of the forceps. Less involved thenar recurrent and other digital branches are encircled by Vasoloops. **(B)** Injury to a digital nerve was resected. A narrow sural nerve graft has been sewn in place with monofilament suture to replace the resected segment of digital nerve.

penetrate the transverse carpal ligament and thus be damaged even with a direct exposure and section of the ligament, and especially if a less open or a closed procedure is used. Unfortunately, even direct inspection of the nerve can lead to inadvertent branch or whole nerve injury (Fig. 8-35). The thenar sensory branch has a somewhat variable origin from the radial side of the distal median as it approaches the wrist. This branch can be damaged if scissors are used on top of the nerve at the wrist level to divide antebrachial fascia or ligament, especially if done subcutaneously from a palmar entry site. Resection of the injured branch and any attendant neuroma is usually preferable to attempted repair, because the latter invariably leads to some degree of neuroma formation, which in itself may become painful (Figs 8-36 to 8-38).

Occasionally, a patient sustains operative injury to the ulnar nerve or its superficial or deep palmar branches. Reoperation then depends on the severity of the loss and its attendant symptoms. Under these circumstances, it is often found that the transverse carpal ligament over the median nerve has also not been released fully at the time of the original surgery.

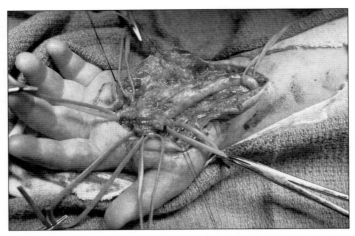

FIGURE 8-37 Contusive injury after CTR requires dissection of all branches of median nerve.

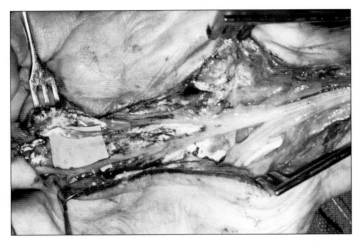

FIGURE 8-38 Distal injury to digital nerve branches.

MEDIAN NERVE ENTRAPMENT: CASE SUMMARY

This 15-year-old female had presented elsewhere with numbness and tingling in her thumbs and fingers at age 12. A bilateral CTR had been done. Symptoms quickly recurred and a repeat bilateral CTR was done 1 year later. However, after her symptoms persisted, she was seen by an orthopedist who ordered radiographs of her elbow, and bilateral medial, distal humeral spurs were found. A presumptive diagnosis of a Struthers ligament compression of the median nerve at the level of the elbow was made, and the patient was then referred for further work-up and possible surgery.

Electrical work-up at LSUHSC showed conductive slowing not only at the wrist but also at the elbow level for both median nerves. Both nerves were exposed at the elbow level and found to be compressed by a Struthers ligament running from the humerus to medial epicondyle (see Fig. 8-6). Compression was most severe on the left. Intraoperative NAP studies showed significant slowing of conduction across both nerves at the level of the Struthers ligaments. The ligaments were resected and an external neurolysis was done on the median nerves at that level. The median nerves at wrist and palmar level were also explored. They were, as might be expected, heavily scarred. An external neurolysis was done on both nerves. Intraoperative NAP studies confirmed significant slowing at this level as well. However, it was evident from this operation that these

changes were most likely secondary to the prior CTRs and that the primary problem was at the elbow level for both limbs.

Recovery has been slow but good, and 4 years later she uses both hands and arms normally.

COMMENT

Even though CTS is a common diagnosis, other disorders must be ruled out, particularly in individuals who are not middle-aged or older.

REFERENCES

1. Abbott L and Saunders J: Injuries of the median nerve in fractures of the lower end of the radius. Surg Gynecol Obstet 57:507–511, 1933.
2. Al-Qattan MM and Robertson GA. Pseudo-anterior interosseous nerve syndrome: a case report. J Hand Surg 18A:440–442, 1993.
3. Beard L, Kumar A, and Estep HL: Bilateral carpal tunnel syndrome caused by Grave's disease. Arch Intern Med 145:345–346, 1985.
4. Bennett JB and Crouch CC: Compression syndrome of the recurrent motor branch of the median nerve. J Hand Surg 7:407–409, 1982.
5. Birch R and Raji AR: Repair of median and ulnar nerves. Primary suture is best. J Bone Joint Surg 73B:154–157, 1991.
6. Birch R, Bonney G, and Wynn Parry CB: Surgical Disorders of the Peripheral Nerves. Edinburgh, Churchill Livingstone, 1998.
7. Bleeker M, Bohlman M, Moreland R, et al.: Carpal tunnel syndrome: Role of carpal canal size. Neurology 35:1599–1604, 1985.
8. Blom S and Dahlback L: Nerve injuries in dislocation of shoulder joint and factures of neck of humerus. A clinical and electromyographic study. Acta Chir Scand 136:461–466, 1970.
9. Boswick J and Stromberg W: Isolated injury of the median nerve above the elbow. J Bone Joint Surg Am 49A:481–487, 1967.
10. Brain WR, Wright AD, and Wilkinson M: Spontaneous compression of both median nerves in the carpal tunnel: Six cases treated surgically. Lancet 1:277–282, 1947.
11. Carroll R and Match R: Common errors in the management of wrist lacerations. J Trauma 14:553–558, 1974.
12. Cherington M: Proximal pain in carpal tunnel syndrome. Arch Surg 108:69, 1974.
13. Chow J: Endoscopic release of the carpal ligament: A new technique for carpal tunnel syndrome. Arthroscopy 5:19–24, 1989.
14. Chow J, Van Beek A, Bilos K, et al.: Anatomical basis for repair of ulnar and median nerves in the distal part of the forearm by group fascicular suture and nerve grafting. J Bone Joint Surg [Am] 68:273–280, 1986.
15. Cobb TK and Amadio PC: Reoperation for carpal tunnel syndrome. Hand Clin 12:313–323, 1996.
16. Cobb TK, Amadio PC, Leatherwood DF, et al.: Outcome of reoperation for carpal tunnel syndrome. J Hand Surg 21A:347–356, 1996.
17. Connolly W: Pitfalls in carpal tunnel decompression. Aust NZ J Surg 48:421–425, 1978.
18. Cooney WP: Median nerve repairs: The results of treatment. In: Gelberman RH, Ed: Operative Nerve Repair and Reconstruction. Philadelphia, JB Lippincott, 1991.
19. Cseuz KA, Thomas JE, Lambert EH, et al.: Long-term results of operation for carpal tunnel syndrome. Mayo Clin Proc 41:232–241, 1996.
20. Curtis RM and Eversmann WW Jr: Internal neurolysis as an adjunct to the treatment of the carpal tunnel syndrome. J Bone Joint Surg 55:733–740, 1973.
21. Dawson D, Hallett M, and Millender L: Entrapment Neuropathies, 2nd edn. Boston, Little, Brown, 1990.

22. Eason SY, Belsole RJ, and Greene TL: Carpal tunnel release: Analysis of suboptimal results. J Hand Surg 10B:365–369, 1985.

23. Eversmann WW Jr and Ritsick JA: Intraoperative changes in motor nerve conduction latency in carpal tunnel syndrome. J Hand Surg 3:77–81, 1978.

24. Freshwater F and Arons MS: The effect of various adjuncts on the surgical treatment of carpal tunnel syndrome secondary to chronic tenosynovitis. Plast Reconstr Surg 61:93–96, 1978.

25. Gainer JV and Nugent GR: Carpal tunnel syndrome: Report of 430 operations. South Med J 70:325–328, 1977.

26. Gaul J Jr: Electrical fascicle identification as an adjunct to nerve repair. J Hand Surg 8:289–296, 1983.

27. Gelberman RH, Aronson C, and Weisman MH: Carpal tunnel syndrome: Results of a prospective trial of steroid injection and splinting. J Bone Joint Surg 62A:1181–1184, 1980.

28. Gelberman RH, Hergenroeder PT, Hargens AR, et al.: The carpal tunnel syndrome: A study of carpal canal pressures. J Bone Joint Surg 63A:380–383, 1981.

29. Gelberman RH, Pfeiffer G, Galbraith R, et al.: Results of treatment of severe carpal tunnel syndrome without internal neurolysis of the median nerve. J Bone Joint Surg 69:896–903, 1987.

30. Gerritsen AA, de Vet HC, Scholten RJ, et al.: Splinting vs surgery in the treatment of carpal tunnel syndrome: a randomized controlled trial. JAMA 288:1245–1251, 2002.

31. Gerritsen AA, de Krom MC, Struijs MA, et al. Conservative treatment options for carpal tunnel syndrome: a systematic review of randomised controlled trials. J Neurol 249:272–280, 2002.

32. Haase J, Bjerve P, and Semesen K: Median and ulnar nerve transactions treated with microsurgical interfascicular cable grafting with autologous sural nerve. J Neurosurg 53:73–84, 1980.

33. Harris CM, Tanner E, Goldstein MN, et al.: The surgical treatment of the carpal tunnel syndrome correlated with preoperative nerve-conduction studies. J Bone Joint Surg 61A:93–98, 1979.

34. Haussmann P and Patel MR: Intraepineurial constriction of nerve fascicles in pronator syndrome and anterior interosseous nerve syndrome. Orthop Clin N Am 27:339–344, 1996.

35. Hudson A and Mayfield F: Chronic injuries of nerve by entrapment. In: Youmans J, Ed: Neurological Surgery, 2nd Ed. Philadelphia, WB Saunders, 1983.

36. Hudson A, Kline D, and Mackinnon S: Entrapment neuropathies. In: Horowitz N and Rizzoli H, Eds: Postoperative Complications of Extracranial Neurological Surgery. Baltimore, Williams & Wilkins, 1987.

37. Iyer V and Renichel GM: Normal median nerve proximal latency in carpal tunnel syndrome: A clue to coexisting Martin-Gruber anastomosis. J Neurol Neurosurg Psychiatry 39:449–452, 1976.

38. Jain VK, Cestero RVM, and Baum J: Carpal tunnel syndrome in patients undergoing maintenance hemodialysis. JAMA 242:2868–2869, 1979.

39. Kallio PK and Vastamaki M: An analysis of the results of late reconstruction of 132 median nerves. J Hand Surg 18B:97–105, 1993.

40. Kaplan E and Spinner M: Normal and anomalous innervation patterns in the upper extremity. In: Omer G and Spinner M, Eds: Management of Peripheral Nerve Problems. Philadelphia, WB Saunders, 1980.

41. Katirji MB: Pseudo-anterior interosseous nerve syndrome. Muscle Nerve 9:266–267, 1986.

42. Kelly MJ and Jackson BT: Compression of median nerve at elbow. Br Med J 2:283, 1976.

43. Kessler F: Complications of the management of carpal tunnel syndrome. Hand Clin 2:401–406, 1986.

44. Kim DH, Kam AC, Chandika P, et al.: Surgical management and outcomes in patients with median nerve lesions. J Neurosurg 95:584–594, 2001.

45. Kim DH, Murovic JA, Tiel RL, et al.: Operative outcomes of 546 Louisiana State University Health Sciences Center peripheral nerve tumors. Neurosurg Clin N Am 15:177–192, 2004.

46. Kimura J: The carpal tunnel syndrome. Localization of conduction abnormalities within the distal segment of the median nerve. Brain 102:619–635, 1979.

47. Kline DG and Hackett E: Reappraisal of timing for exploration of civilian nerve injuries. Surgery 78:54–63, 1978.

48. Laha RK, Dujovny M, and DeCastro SC: Entrapment of median nerve by supracondylar process of the humerus: Case report. J Neurosurg 46:252–255, 1977.

49. Lake PA: Anterior interosseous nerve syndrome. J Neurosurg 41:306–309, 1974.

50. Langloh RD and Linscheid RL: Recurrent and unrelieved carpal tunnel syndrome. Clin Orthop 83:41–47, 1972.

51. Lanz U: Anatomical variations of the median nerve in the carpal tunnel. J Hand Surg 2:44–53, 1977.

52. Larsen R and Posch J: Nerve injuries in the upper extremity. Arch Surg 77:469–475, 1975.

53. Louis D, Green T, and Noellert R: Complications of carpal tunnel surgery. J Neurosurg 62:352–356, 1985.

54. Low PA, McLeod JG, Turtle JR, et al.: Peripheral neuropathy in acromegaly. Brain 97:139–152, 1974.

55. Lundborg G: Nerve Injury and Repair. New York, Churchill Livingstone, 1988.

56. MacDonald RI, Lichtman DM, Hanlon JJ, et al.: Complications of surgical release for carpal tunnel syndrome. J Hand Surg 3:70–76, 1978.

57. Mackinnon S: Secondary carpal tunnel surgery. Neurosurg Clin N Am 2:75–91, 1991.

58. Mackinnon S and Dellon A: Surgery of the Peripheral Nerve. New York, Thieme Medical Publishers, 1988.

59. Mackinnon S, McCabe S, Murray J, et al.: Internal neurolysis fails to improve the results of primary carpal tunnel decompression. J Hand Surg 16:211–218, 1991.

60. Mahoney J, Lofchy N, Chow I, et al.: Carpal tunnel syndrome: A quality assurance evaluation of surgical treatment. R Coll Phys Surg Can Ann 25:20–23, 1992.

61. Massey EW: Carpal tunnel syndrome in pregnancy. Obstet Gynecol Surg 33:145, 1978.

62. McLellan DL and Swash M: Longitudinal sliding of median nerve during movements of the upper limb. J Neurol Neurosurg Psychiatry 39:566–570, 1976.

63. McManamny D: Comparison of microscope and loupe magnification: Assistance for the repair of median and ulnar nerves. Br J Plast Surg 36:367–372, 1983.

64. Michon J, Amend P, and Merle M: Microsurgical repair of peripheral nerve lesions: A study of 150 injuries of median and ulnar nerves. In: Samii M, Ed: Peripheral Nerve Lesions. Berlin, Springer-Verlag, 1990.

65. Millesi H, Meissl G, and Berger A: The interfascicular nerve grafting of the median and ulnar nerves. J Bone Joint Surg 54A:727–730, 1972.

66. Morris HH and Peters BH: Pronator syndrome: Clinical and electrophysiological features in seven cases. J Neurol Neurosurg Psychiatry 39:461–464, 1976.

67. Mumenthaler M: Clinical aspects of entrapment neuropathies. In: Samii M, Ed: Peripheral Nerve Lesions. Berlin, Springer-Verlag, 1990.

68. Nickolson OR and Seddon HJ: Nerve repair in civil practice. Br Med J 2:1065–1071, 1957.

69. O'Brien MD and Upton ARM: Anterior interosseous nerve syndrome. J Neurol Neurosurg Psychiatry 35:531–536, 1972.

70. Omer GE: Evaluation and reconstruction of forearm and hand after acute traumatic peripheral nerve injuries. J Bone Joint Surg 50A:1454–1460, 1968.

71. Omer GE: Tendon transfers for the reconstruction of the forearm and hand following peripheral nerve injuries. In: Omer GE and Spinner M, Eds: Management of Peripheral Nerve Problems. Philadelphia, WB Saunders, 1980.

72. Osborne A, Dorey L, and Hardey J: Volkmann's contracture associated with prolonged external pressure on the forearm. Arch Surg 104:794–799, 1972.

73. Paine K: The carpal tunnel syndrome. Can J Surg 6:446–449, 1963.

74. Platt H and Woods RS. Discussion on injuries of peripheral nerves. Proc Royal Soc Med 30:863–874, 1937.

75. Posch JL and Marcotte DR: Carpal tunnel syndrome: An analysis of 1201 cases. Orthop Rev 5:25–35, 1976.

76. Rask MR: Anterior interosseous nerve entrapment (Kiloh-Nevin syndrome). Clin Orthop 142:176–181, 1979.

77. Riordan DC: Tendon transplantations in median nerve and ulnar nerve paralysis. J Bone Joint Surg 35A:312–320, 1953.

78. Rosenbaum RB and Ochoa JL: Carpal Tunnel Syndrome and Other Disorders of the Median Nerve. 2nd edn. Woburn, Butterworth-Heinemann, 2002.

79. Sakellorides H: Follow-up of 172 peripheral nerve injuries in upper extremities in civilians. J Bone Joint Surg 44A:140–148, 1962.

80. Samii M: Use of microtechniques in peripheral nerve surgery – experience with over 300 cases. In: Handa H, Ed: Microneurosurgery. Tokyo, Igaku-Shoin, 1975.

81. Seddon H: Surgical Disorders of the Peripheral Nerves. Edinburgh, Churchill Livingstone, 1975.

82. Seigel D and Gelberman R: Median nerve: Applied anatomy and operative exposure. In: Gelberman RH, Ed: Operative Nerve Repair and Reconstruction. Philadelphia, JB Lippincott, 1991.

83. Serodge H and Serodge E: Pisi-triquetral pain syndrome after carpal tunnel release. J Hand Surg 14:858–873, 1989.

84. Simpson JA: Electrical signs in the diagnosis of carpal tunnel and related syndromes. J Neurol Neurosurg Psychiatry 19:275–280, 1956.

85. Smith R and Fisher R: Struthers ligament: A source of median nerve compression above the elbow. Case report. J Neurosurg 38:778–781, 1973.

86. Spinner M: The anterior interosseous nerve syndrome with special attention to its variations. J Bone Joint Surg 52A:84–89, 1970.

87. Spinner M: Injuries of the Major Branches of Peripheral Nerves of the Forearm. 2nd edn. Philadelphia. WB Saunders, 1978.

88. Sunderland S: The nerve lesion in the carpal tunnel syndrome. J Neurol Neurosurg Psychiatry 39:615–626, 1976.

89. Sunderland S and Ray L: Metrical and non-metrical features of the muscular branches of the median nerve. J Comp Neurol 85:191–200, 1946.

90. Tarlov IM: How long should an extremity be immobilized after nerve suture? Ann Surg 126:336–376, 1947.

91. Thoma A, Veltri K, Haines T, et al.: A meta-analysis of randomized controlled trials comparing endoscopic and open carpal tunnel decompression. Plast Reconstr Surg 114:1137–1146, 2004.

92. Thomas CK, Stein RB, Gordon T, et al.: Patterns of reinnervation and motor unit recruitment in human hand muscles after complete ulnar and median nerve section and resuture. J Neurol Neurosurg Psychiatry 50:259–268, 1987.

93. Tindall S: Painful neuromas. In: Wilkins R and Rengachary S, Eds: Neurosurgery. New York, McGraw-Hill, 1985.

94. Tindall SC: Chronic injuries of peripheral nerves by entrapment. In: Youmans J, Ed: Neurological Surgery, 3rd edn. Philadelphia, WB Saunders, 1990:2511–2542.

95. Tuckmann W, Richter H, and Strohr M: Compression Syndrome Peripherer Nerven. Berlin, Springer-Verlag, 1989.

96. Werschkul J: Anomalous course of the recurrent motor branch of the median nerve in a patient with carpal tunnel syndrome. J Neurosurg 47:113–114, 1977.

97. Wertsch JJ, Sanger JR, and Matloub HS. Pseudo-anterior interosseous nerve syndrome. Muscle Nerve 8:68–70, 1985.

98. Williams H and Jabaley M: The importance of internal anatomy of the peripheral nerves to nerve repair in forearm and hand. Hand Clin 2:689–707, 1986.

99. Woodhall B and Beebe G: Peripheral Nerve Regeneration: A review of 3,652 WW II Injuries. VA Monograph. Washington, DC, Government Printing Office, 1957.

100. Young V, Way R, and Weeks P: The results of nerve grafting in the wrist and hand. Ann Plast Surg 5:212–215, 1980.

101. Zachary RB and Holmes W: Primary sutures of nerves. Surg Gynecol Obstet 82:632–651, 1946.

102. Zachary R: Results of nerve suture. In: Seddon H, Ed: Peripheral Nerve Injuries. Medical Research Council Special Report Series No. 282. London, Her Majesty's Stationery Office, 1954.

9 Ulnar nerve

Daniel H. Kim

OVERVIEW

- The level of greatest importance for the ulnar nerve is the hand, where it innervates most of the intrinsic muscles. Complete ulnar loss at this level results in severe deficits and clawing of the little and sometimes ring fingers.

- The flexor carpi ulnaris (FCU) muscle receives ulnar nerve input at the arm level and just below the elbow, so it is frequently spared with distal arm- and elbow-level lesions and sometimes even more proximal arm-level injuries. Because the flexor digitorum profundus branch supplying the little finger leaves the ulnar nerve 2.5–5.0 cm below the elbow, flexion of the distal phalanx of the little finger is lost with complete ulnar lesions at or above the elbow. Flexion of the ring finger is not completely lost, however, because the tendinous slip is shared with the median-innervated flexor digitorum profundus to the long finger.

- The ulnar nerve can be transposed anterior to the elbow and deep to the pronator and FCU muscles. Unlike the median nerve in which it is difficult to make up lost nerve length, this maneuver gains 2.5–3.8 cm of length. Despite this advantage, results with repair of this nerve at almost any level are less than those achieved with median or radial nerve repair. Flexor digitorum profundus muscle strength can usually be regained, as can ulnar sensation, some degree of hypothenar function, and even some adductor pollicis function, providing a grade 3 recovery. Harder to regain are interosseous and lumbrical functions, except more frequently with lacerations or more focal injuries to the nerve at the level of the wrist, sometimes at the elbow level, and only seldom at the level of the arm. Tendon transfer to substitute for lumbrical muscle function loss helps the patient to extend the little and ring fingers.

- The series from Louisiana State University Health Sciences Center (LSUHSC) of 231 ulnar nerve injuries analyzed in this chapter supports the contention that ulnar nerve repair is worthwhile and should not be abandoned in favor of reconstructive procedures alone.

- Intraoperative recordings on entrapped elbow-level ulnar nerves indicated that the conductivity was most abnormal either within or just proximal to the olecranon groove and not at the level of the more distal cubital tunnel. There were only a few exceptions to this finding. Thus, the entrapment injury or irritative site appeared to be maximal within the olecranon notch segment of the nerve and not more distally at a forearm level.

- At LSUHSC, a modified Learmonth procedure with thorough neurolysis and then placement of the nerve deep to the pronator teres and FCU muscles was performed in 364 cases of elbow-level entrapped ulnar nerve. Only two cases had to be redone.

- A large number of simple ulnar decompressions, medial epicondylectomies, and subcutaneous transpositions done elsewhere have been sent to LSUHSC with pain, paresthesias, and sometimes progressive palsy. Some have been helped by reoperation and submuscular placement of the nerve. Simpler procedures for entrapment are effective much of the time, but are less so than a more formal submuscular transposition.

APPLIED ANATOMY

The ulnar nerve is important for coordinated hand function. In the arm and forearm, it innervates the flexor carpi ulnaris (FCU) and flexor digitorum profundus III and IV muscles and in the hand, the adductor pollicis, flexor pollicis brevis, lumbrical III and IV, hypothenar (the abductor, opponens and flexor digiti minimi muscles), and all dorsal and palmar interosseous muscles (Fig. 9-1). The ulnar nerve originates at an axillary level from the medial cord, which is medial to the axillary artery, hence the cord's name (Fig. 9-2). The medial cord gives a large motor branch to the median nerve, and then gives rise to the medial and lateral antebrachial cutaneous nerves and the ulnar nerve. Initially, the ulnar nerve travels posterior to the axillary artery, but then takes an oblique course away from the artery down the upper arm toward the olecranon notch. At the midarm level, the nerve passes either through or beneath the firm, fibrous intermuscular septum.

Almost 70% of limbs have an arcade of Struthers beneath which the nerve may pass just distal to the intermuscular septum. This arcade is formed by a thickening of the deep, investing fascia of the distal portion of the arm and muscle fibers from the medial head of the triceps. As one dissects proximally from the medial epicondyle, the ulnar nerve is often covered by these triceps fibers and some fascia.

In the distal arm (Fig. 9-3), the nerve is usually adherent to the proximal muscle belly of the FCU. Branches supplying this muscle proximal to the elbow usually arise from the dorsal surface of the

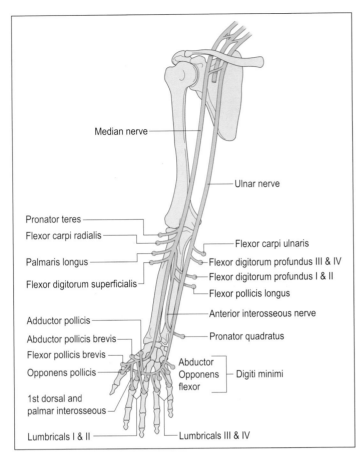

FIGURE 9-1 Muscles supplied by the ulnar nerve. Published with permission of MS Greenberg MD from the 6th edn. of his Handbook of Neurosurgery, 2006.

In the figure the following labels appear: Median nerve, Ulnar nerve, Pronator teres, Flexor carpi radialis, Flexor carpi ulnaris, Palmaris longus, Flexor digitorum profundus III & IV, Flexor digitorum profundus I & II, Flexor digitorum superficialis, Flexor pollicis longus, Anterior interosseous nerve, Adductor pollicis, Pronator quadratus, Abductor pollicis brevis, Flexor pollicis brevis, Opponens pollicis, Abductor Opponens flexor Digiti minimi, 1st dorsal and palmar interosseous, Lumbricals I & II, Lumbricals III & IV.

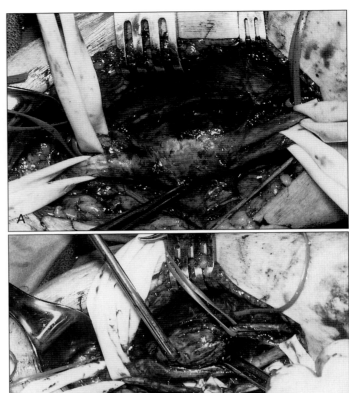

FIGURE 9-2 (A) An injury to the medial cord and the ulnar and proximal median nerves associated with an axillary angiogram. **(B)** A pseudoaneurysm of the axillary to brachial arterial junction, as well as direct injury to the ulnar and median nerves were each present. Both the ulnar and the median nerves required graft repair. After proximal and distal control of the artery, the aneurysm was evacuated, but an initial repair of a large, ragged hole in the artery was unsuccessful. A subsequent vascular graft repair by the vascular service was necessary.

nerve and tend to tether the nerve at this level. Both arteries and veins run parallel to the ulnar nerve in this region and are usually quite adherent to it.

Only 1% of the population has a Struthers ligament, which arises from a small, epicondylar-like process on the medial surface of the distal humerus. The ligament usually passes over the brachial artery and median nerve, and sometimes the ulnar nerve as well, on its way to insert on the medial epicondyle. In these few cases, the ulnar nerve can pass beneath this structure just proximal to the notch area.

As the nerve enters the olecranon notch, it tends to take on an ovoid rather than a round shape and is often adherent to the base of the notch. The nerve is covered by a raphe of connective tissue or fascia extending across the olecranon notch. Small neural articular branches may leave the inferior surface of the nerve and penetrate the joint space and small arteries and veins usually accompany the nerve into the notch and also lie on its floor.

In the distal portion of the olecranon notch, the nerve passes into a more constricted area bounded superficially by an aponeurotic arch extending to the medial epicondyle. Just distal to the notch, the nerve passes beneath the two heads of the FCU (Fig. 9-4), and distal to the notch, the nerve gives rise to relatively short branches that supply the FCU muscle. Occasionally, an anomalous, radial-innervated muscle, the anconeus epitrochlearis, arises from the medial border of the olecranon and adjacent triceps tendon and inserts into the medial epicondyle. If present, this muscle forms part of the cubital tunnel, reinforcing the aponeurosis of the two heads of origin of the FCU muscle.

Branches to the medial half of the flexor digitorum profundus muscle arise deep to the FCU muscle and the nerve and have a short course to this muscle. At this point, the nerve lies on the ulnar side of the flexor digitorum profundus muscle. If the surgeon's proximal phalanx of the little finger is placed into the olecranon groove and the tip is pointed toward the ulnar surface of the wrist, the course of the nerve in the proximal forearm is outlined.

In the more distal forearm, the ulnar nerve remains deep to the FCU muscle and medial to the flexor digitorum superficialis tendons. Throughout the distal forearm, the nerve is closely applied to the ulnar artery, which usually approaches the nerve at a midforearm level and lies on its radial side. The radial artery, the cohort of the ulnar artery, lies on the inner or ulnar side of the superficial sensory radial nerve.

At the proximal forearm level, there may be a Martin-Gruber anastomosis. Under these circumstances, the anterior interosseous branch of the median nerve gives rise to a branch that goes to the ulnar nerve.[63] This branch can take fibers, especially those destined

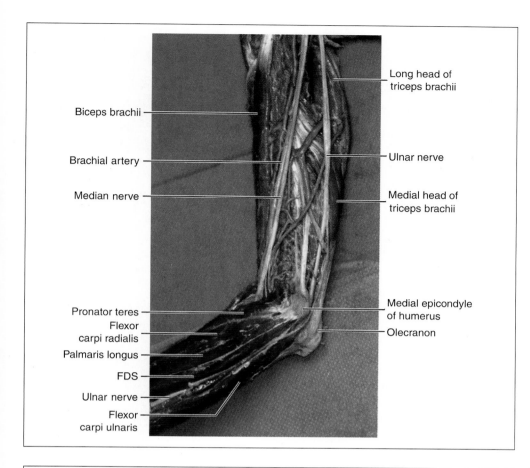

Biceps brachii

Brachial artery

Median nerve

Pronator teres
Flexor carpi radialis
Palmaris longus
FDS
Ulnar nerve
Flexor carpi ulnaris

Long head of triceps brachii

Ulnar nerve

Medial head of triceps brachii

Medial epicondyle of humerus
Olecranon

FIGURE 9-3 A view of the right medial arm shows the ulnar nerve at the distal arm, where it passes between the medial epicondyle and olecranon.

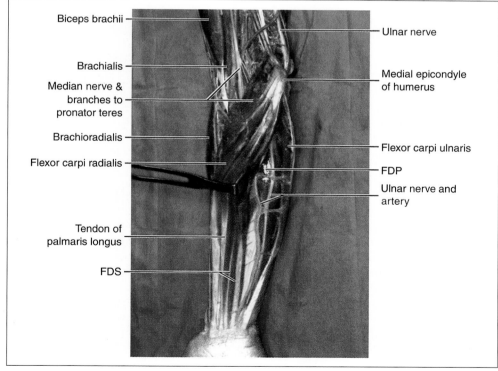

Biceps brachii

Brachialis

Median nerve & branches to pronator teres

Brachioradialis

Flexor carpi radialis

Tendon of palmaris longus

FDS

Ulnar nerve

Medial epicondyle of humerus

Flexor carpi ulnaris
FDP
Ulnar nerve and artery

FIGURE 9-4 The ulnar nerve is seen to enter the proximal volar forearm by passing between the two heads of the flexor carpi ulnaris.

for the abductor pollicis brevis and opponens pollicis, from the median nerve to the forearm-level ulnar nerve. These fibers then "trade back" to the distal median nerve at a wrist or palmar level (a Riche-Cannieu anastomosis). Ulnar motor fibers can also descend in the proximal median nerve and then return to the ulnar nerve at a forearm level through a branch from the anterior interosseous nerve.

The dorsal cutaneous nerve arises from the ulnar nerve, approximately 5–8 cm proximal to the wrist crease (Fig. 9-5) and this branch supplies sensation to the dorsum of the hand on the ulnar

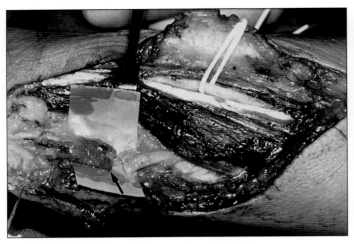

FIGURE 9-5 This is an operative photograph showing a transected dorsal cutaneous branch of the ulnar nerve. The surgeon has made a cut on one side of the neuroma *(arrow)*.

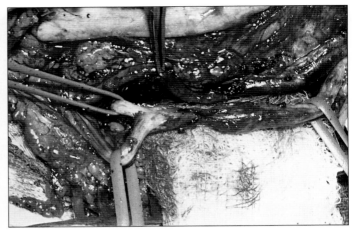

FIGURE 9-6 An ulnar injury at the palmar level in Guyon's canal, proximal to the superficial and deep ulnar branches. The injury was secondary to an attempted arthroscopic release of the transverse carpal ligament. No nerve action potential was transmitted across this lesion. After resection to healthier proximal and distal tissues, a graft repair was performed with four sural grafts 3.5 cm in length.

side and a portion of the dorsum of the little and ring fingers and ulnar half of the long finger. Sometimes it arises separately from the main ulnar nerve as far proximal as the olecranon notch and in rare cases can arise as far distally as Guyon's canal.

As the ulnar nerve passes through the wrist, it enters Guyon's canal or tunnel. The radial border of Guyon's canal is formed by the junction of the roof, which is the palmar carpal ligament including the palmaris brevis muscle, with the floor represented by the transverse carpal ligament, i.e. flexor retinaculum and origins of the thenar muscles.[49] The flexor retinaculum in turn attaches to the radial and anterior surfaces of the hook of the hamate. The radially located hamate and hook are more distally related to Guyon's canal than are the ulnar-sided pisiform bone and its FCU muscle insertion. The hamate and the pisiform bones are the most prominent landmarks in this region. The nerve is covered by an expansion of the FCU tendon and the antebrachial fascia. The more distal portion of the canal or tunnel is composed of pisohamate and pisometacarpal ligaments on either side, the opponens digiti minimi muscle deep or dorsally, and superficially there is overlying hypothenar fat and the palmar fibrous arch.[74]

As the ulnar nerve passes radial to the pisiform bone and superficial to the medial extension of the transverse carpal ligament, it quickly divides into the superficial and deep branches (Fig. 9-6). The superficial branch crosses the flexor digiti minimi muscle, gives a small branch to the palmaris brevis muscle, and then provides a variable and lengthy segment composed of digital sensory branches to the little and ring fingers. The deep branch passes backward and downward between the heads of the flexor and abductor digiti minimi muscles, winding around the hook of the hamate and running toward the thumb within the concavity of the palmar arch. The deep branch divides early to supply the remaining hypothenar muscles, which include the abductor, opponens, and flexor digiti minimi muscles. On occasion, a hypothenar branch may arise from the ulnar nerve proximal to the take-off of the superficial and deep branches. The principal deep branch travels toward the thumb and through the deep palmar space to further branch and supply all the interosseous muscles and lumbrical muscles for the ring and little fingers and the adductor pollicis and a portion of the flexor pollicis brevis muscles.

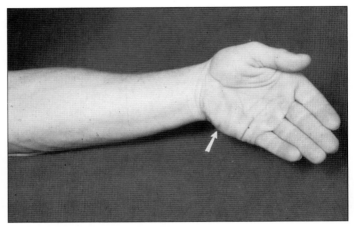

FIGURE 9-7 An alternative method to grading the strength of the flexor carpi ulnaris muscle is to have the patient flex and adduct the hand against applied pressure *(arrow)*.

CLINICAL PRESENTATION AND EXAMINATION

The most proximal muscle innervated by the ulnar nerve is the FCU. The FCU muscle is a major wrist flexor, particularly in an ulnar direction, and is supplied by branches both above and below the elbow. The clinician can readily grade the strength of this muscle by grasping the patient's hand in a handshake position and asking the patient to cock the wrist in a flexed, ulnarward direction (Fig. 9-7).

The flexor digitorum profundus muscle is not as straightforward in its examination, since this muscle has a two-nerve supply in the sense that usually the forefinger and the long finger are innervated by the median nerve and ring and little fingers by the ulnar nerve. The long finger profundus muscle shares a tendinous slip with the ring finger profundus muscle, so that even with a complete ulnar palsy, the function of the ring finger profundus muscle will appear intact unless the long finger is held extended as the ring finger profundus is tested. As a result, even complete ulnar nerve injury may cause only mild weakness of flexion of the distal phalanx of the ring finger. Distal flexion of the little finger will, however, usually be absent (Fig. 9-8). These subtle findings can be overlooked, especially when the ulnar nerve injury is severe, leading to extensive sensory and hand intrinsic muscle loss with clawing of the little and ring fingers (Fig. 9-9).

In terms of localizing the level of injury, the flexor digitorum profundus muscle is still important to evaluate. Preservation of its function in conjunction with distal hand intrinsic muscle loss usually indicates a more distal forearm or wrist-level lesion. An exception is ulnar entrapment at the elbow where hand intrinsic muscles tend to preferentially drop out with relative sparing of not only the FCU muscle, but also of the flexor digitorum profundus muscle.

The dorsal cutaneous nerve branch supplies sensation to the dorsum of the hand and a portion of the dorsum of the little and ring fingers and sometimes the ulnar half of the long finger. Injury which requires repair and is located proximal or distal to the origin of this branch may benefit from excision of this branch so that mainly motor fibers and the more important sensory fibers can be directed to the distal nerve (Figs 9-10, 9-11).[80] Injury proximal to this distal forearm-level branch from the ulnar nerve gives rather complete ulnar sensory loss. The latter includes loss on the dorsum of the hand and the dorsum of portions of the little and ulnar half of the ring fingers and the volar aspects of most of the little finger and the ulnar half of the ring finger. Loss may at times involve the dorsum of the ulnar half of the long finger as well. The autonomous zone for the ulnar nerve includes the volar aspects of the little finger's intermediate and distal phalanges, and the dorsal surface of its distal phalanx.[62] Loss in that distribution can only mean injury to the ulnar nerve proper or its more distal superficial sensory branch. Recovery in that distribution, if loss had been present previously, can only occur as the result of ulnar nerve regeneration and is not due to sprouting from adjacent nerves (Fig. 9-11).[55] On the other hand, injury to the ulnar nerve distal to the dorsal cutaneous branch spares sensation on the dorsum of the hand and fingers.

Hypothenar function is totally ulnar innervated. Abduction of the little finger by the abductor digiti minimi muscle is best tested by giving the patient a target against which to push that is volar to the horizontal plane of the hand, since the extensor digitorum communis tendon to the little finger can mimic abduction by an ulnarward movement as the digit is extended (Fig. 9-12). Opposition provided by the opponens digiti minimi muscle is not easy to test either, because the flexors can substitute for much of its function.[32] The examiner can cross his or her own fore- and long fingers and place them on the palm between the palmar crease and the heel of the palm. The patient, using the opponens digiti minimi muscle, should be able to reach this target and, by pressing down, be able to prevent the examiner from spreading his or her own forefinger away from the long finger. The other two ulnar-supplied hypothenar muscles, the flexor digiti minimi and palmaris brevis, are more difficult to isolate and to test with specificity than are the abductor digiti minimi and opponens digiti minimi muscles.[33]

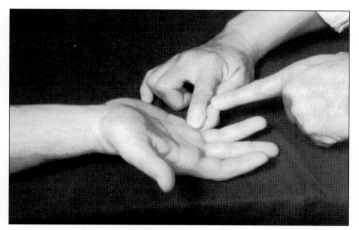

FIGURE 9-8 Testing the flexor profundus muscle of the little finger. The proximal phalanges are stabilized by one of the examiner's forefingers while the patient flexes the distal phalanx of the little finger against the examiner's other forefinger.

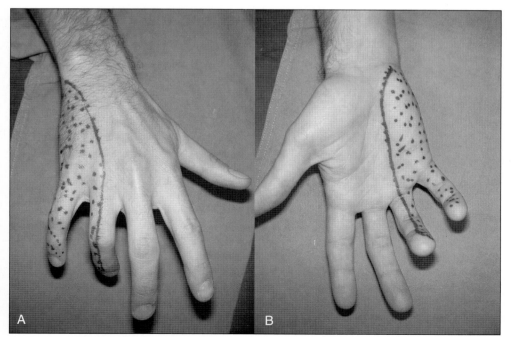

FIGURE 9-9 Ulnar sensory and motor loss, caused by an arm-level ulnar injury, with typical "clawing" of the ring and little fingers is seen in **(A)** and **(B).** The denervated ulnar intrinsic muscles fail to fix or hold the metacarpophalangeal joints, so the radial-innervated long extensors hyperextend the knuckle joints. Because the paralyzed intrinsic muscles fail to extend the interphalangeal joints, the median-innervated forearm flexors hyperflex the joints.

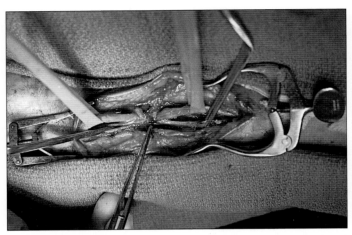

FIGURE 9-10 A distal forearm ulnar injury just proximal to the dorsal cutaneous branch is shown. The latter was dissected from the proximal stump and sacrificed so downflow to the distal stump excluded the distal dorsal cutaneous branch when the nerve was repaired. The level of the wrist is to the right of this photograph.

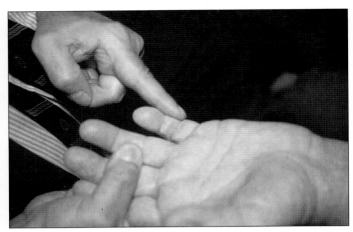

FIGURE 9-12 The patient abducts the little finger against resistance to exhibit strength of the abductor digiti minimi muscle.

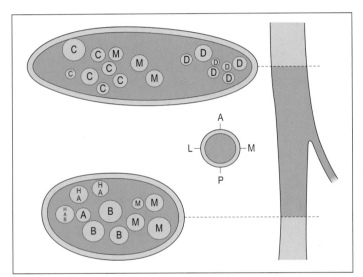

FIGURE 9-11 The ulnar fascicular pattern just proximal *(top diagram)* and then distal *(bottom diagram)* to the dorsal cutaneous branch. Repair of ulnar lesions at this level can be done by splitting away the dorsal cutaneous outflow from the more proximal nerve so that all of the proximal outflow goes to more distal downflow, which is associated with the important hand intrinsic muscles and sensation on the volar aspect of the little and ring fingers and hypothenar regions. (Circular diagram shows the orientation of nerve cross-sections: A, anterior; L, lateral; P, posterior; M, medial.) A, cutaneous fibers from ulnar side fifth finger; B, cutaneous fibers from the fourth interspace; C, combined superficial cutaneous fibers; D, dorsal cutaneous fibers; H, cutaneous fibers from the hypothenar eminence; M, deep muscular fibers. (From Sunderland S: Nerves and Nerve Injuries. Baltimore, Williams & Wilkins, 1968.)

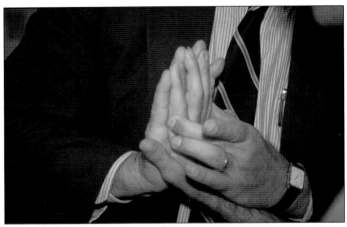

FIGURE 9-13 To test the interossei, the examiner places his or her palm, and the palmar surfaces of the fingers, and thumb against the palm and palmar surfaces of the patient's fingers and thumb with the patient's wrist in extension. The patient is asked to spread the fingers and then bring them back together.

The interosseous muscles are examined by having the patient place the hand and fingers palm down on a flat surface and asking him or her to spread and then bring the fingers back together. An even more reliable test of these muscles is for the examiner to place his or her palm and palmar surfaces of the fingers and thumb against the patient's palm and palmar surfaces of the fingers and thumb. This is done in such a way as to place the patient's wrist and fingers in hyperextension, thus removing the ability of the extensor muscles to mimic the function of the interosseous muscles (Fig. 9-13).

Ulnar-innervated lumbrical muscles are those of the little and ring fingers. Their loss can result in an "ulnar claw" of one or both of these fingers. This complication of ulnar nerve injury occurs because the function of the lumbrical muscles is to set the metacarpophalangeal joint, permitting the extensor digitorum communis muscle to extend the more distal digits. If this function is absent, the flexors are not opposed by an efficient extensor mechanism, and the fingers are pulled toward the palm. An "ulnar claw" is more likely to occur and to be more severe with distal lesions in which the flexor digitorum profundus function is intact and the fingers are pulled into more flexion. The lumbrical muscles can be tested individually by the examiner holding the first phalanx of the finger in a somewhat extended position and asking the patient to straighten or to extend the intermediate phalanx (Fig. 9-14).

The adductor pollicis muscle can be readily palpated and graded for strength by having the patient press the thumb against the side of the palm. With paralysis, a Froment's sign is present. This sign

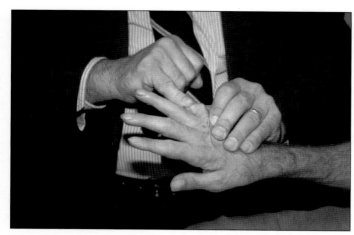

FIGURE 9-14 To examine the lumbrical muscles innervated by the ulnar nerve, the examiner holds the finger being examined in an extended position and asks the patient to straighten or extend the intermediate phalanx of the fourth, then fifth digits.

occurs when upon grasping a sheet of paper between the thumb and index finger, the distal phalanx of the thumb is flexed, rather than being kept straight, indicating abnormal function of the adductor pollicis and first dorsal interosseous muscles. In addition, the thumb is pulled toward and held against the side of the palm by the median-innervated flexor pollicis longus muscle, which substitutes for the adductor pollicis muscle. The flexor pollicis brevis muscle is innervated by both the ulnar and median nerves, and if the median supply to this muscle is intact, it is difficult to impossible to detect any weakness in this muscle, even with complete ulnar nerve loss.

ELECTROPHYSIOLOGICAL STUDIES

ELECTROMYOGRAPHY

Localization of the injury site is relatively straightforward for the ulnar nerve, but there are exceptions. As is the case for the median-innervated pronator teres muscle, the first discernible branches, in this case to the FCU, do not reach muscle until the distal level of the arm. As a result, injury which includes the FCU could be anywhere along the nerve's course in the proximal arm. Because the origin of the ulnar nerve is from the medial cord, loss caused by a severe injury at that level and mimicking ulnar injury includes denervational changes not only in ulnar-innervated hand intrinsic muscles, but also in those innervated by the median nerve in the thenar eminence.

The FCU muscle receives neural input from both above and below the elbow, but for electrophysiological testing, usually its two heads are sampled somewhat distal to the elbow. Denervational changes in the distribution of this muscle indicate a proximal ulnar lesion. The ulnar-innervated portion of the flexor digitorum profundus muscle is very important from an electrophysiological standpoint.[50] Denervational changes in the flexor digitorum profundus III and IV muscle with preservation of the FCU muscle indicates an injury or lesion at the elbow or distal arm level. Performing an electromyogram (EMG) of this muscle is not easy because the profundus is deep to the pronator teres and flexor superficialis muscles. In addition, the median-innervated flexor digitorum profundus I and II are close by, and it can be difficult to be certain

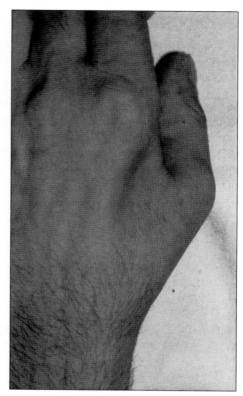

FIGURE 9-15 Atrophy of the first dorsal interosseous muscle in a patient with no sensory loss in the hand and normal long flexor activity in the medial two digits. An electromyogram showed severe denervation in this muscle and the adductor pollicis. The deep branch of the ulnar nerve was compressed by a ganglion cyst.

that the ulnar-innervated flexor digitorum profundus III and IV are being sampled.

As with upper arm-level injuries, precise electrical localization of forearm-level lesions is difficult.[36] After the flexor digitorum profundus III and IV, the next muscles innervated by the ulnar nerve are the hypothenar muscles in the hand. Sampling of the hypothenar eminence muscle mass, which is a prominent landmark, is straightforward. Nonetheless, if atrophy has occurred and the patient is unable to voluntarily contract these muscles, separation of the abductor digiti minimi muscle from the opponens digiti minimi muscle can be difficult if not impossible. Similarly, differentiating the palmar from dorsal interosseous muscles by needle examination can be difficult, also. Fortunately, these last two ulnar-innervated muscles share a relatively common neural input, so their differentiation is of little practical importance in terms of localization of injury. Nonetheless, the first dorsal interosseous muscle is a landmark muscle for an ulnar nerve electrophysiological work-up (Fig. 9-15).

The lumbrical muscles, although very important for hand function, are such small, deeply located slips of muscle that reliable sampling of their function is difficult. Near to the lumbrical muscles is the adductor pollicis muscle. With partial injuries or entrapments, the adductor pollicis muscle is often spared. Because the flexor pollicis brevis muscle has a dual innervation from both the ulnar and median nerves, sampling the flexor pollicis brevis for an ulnar nerve electrophysiological work-up is of limited value.

Variations in the ulnar and median innervation of the hand, such as the Martin-Gruber anastomosis, are more thoroughly discussed in Chapter 8.

CONDUCTION STUDIES

Ulnar nerve injury is the classical setting for use of the electrophysiological study to assess function by nerve conduction.[2]

Entrapment, whether in the olecranon notch or, less frequently, beneath the distal origins of the FCU muscle, can be assessed by stimulating the ulnar nerve above and below the elbow. The electrodiagnostician then records from the hypothenar muscles or first dorsal interosseous muscles and subtracts the two latencies. This results in the latency value for conduction across the elbow. Stimulation either above or below the elbow and recording quite distally from the hypothenar muscles has the drawback that conduction is over a relatively normal forearm level with both. As a result, milder conductive abnormalities across the elbow may not be documented. An alternative is to stimulate the nerve at one site well above the elbow and to record from both the FCU muscle above the elbow and the ulnar-innervated flexor digitorum profundus muscle below the elbow. Again, the latencies are subtracted to give the conduction across the elbow.

With elbow-level entrapment there is a relationship between the severity of the palsy and the amount of slowing across the notch. After transposition though, conduction velocity (CV) change does not always keep pace with clinical improvement. In early or mild cases, conduction not only between the elbow and the wrist, but even at the elbow, can be normal preoperatively. Distance over which latencies are recorded may play a role, especially if conduction is normal or only slightly abnormal, not only above but below or distal to the compression site.

For some proximal forearm-level lesions, conduction recordings from the flexor digitorum profundus muscle, instead of those from hand intrinsic muscles, can be used after stimulation of the nerve at the elbow. Differentiation of Guyon's canal entrapment of the deep branch of the ulnar nerve can also be made by comparing conduction from the proximal forearm to that across the wrist with the recording from the first dorsal interosseous muscle.

Wrist-level involvement of the whole nerve can be tested by sensory nerve action potential (sNAP) studies performed by either stimulating from the little finger digital sensory nerves and recording at the wrist or vice versa.[30] As with the median nerve, use of sNAP recordings can be helpful in assessing milder lesions, especially those located at a wrist or palmar level.

SURGICAL EXPOSURE

ARM LEVEL

Proximal exploration of the ulnar nerve in the arm is carried out using a medial incision centered in the groove between the biceps/brachialis and triceps muscles. The incision is over, but superficial to, the distal axillary and proximal brachial arteries. Depending on the level of the lesion, exposure of the medial cord, its branches to the antebrachial cutaneous nerves, the median nerve, as well as the ulnar nerve, may be necessary (Fig. 9-16). Although there may be variations in the anatomy at this level, the origin of the ulnar nerve from the medial cord is defined after the formation of the proximal median nerve and its inputs from the lateral and medial cords become apparent.[3,75] The ulnar nerve can then be traced distally and somewhat obliquely as it runs toward the olecranon notch, using sharp dissection and carefully dissecting the intermuscular septum at the midarm level. There are usually no ulnar branches of concern at the arm level until the nerve approaches

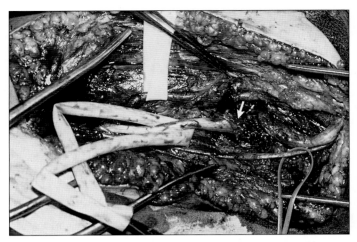

FIGURE 9-16 An ulnar nerve somewhat obliquely transected by glass at the proximal arm level is seen intraoperatively *(arrow)*. There has been only slight distraction of the stumps over a 5-week period. The Vasoloop is around an antebrachial cutaneous nerve, and the Penrose drain to the left surrounds the distal ulnar nerve stump. The Penrose at the top of the photograph encircles the brachial artery.

the elbow level, so dissection along the nerve at the midarm level is usually straightforward.

If the lesion is in the more distal arm, the ulnar nerve can be readily exposed just proximal to its entry point to or in the olecranon notch, and traced proximally. Any dissection in this area should also include sectioning of the intermuscular septum. In the distal arm, the nerve is often covered by a superior expansion of the triceps muscle fibers or fascia, and these need to be sectioned for adequate exposure.[42] The nerve at this level may be tethered to the underlying muscle by short branches to the proximal FCU muscle. It helps to dissect the nerve to an epineurial level and encircle it with Penrose drains at one or more distal arm levels. The drains are then used to shift the nerve as the surgeon clears these branches or dissects them back into the main nerve to gain length. At this level, the arteries and veins often join the mesoneurium and are closely applied to the nerve or epineurium itself. These vessels can be carefully stripped away from the nerve by the use of a Metzenbaum scissors for dissection and a bipolar coagulator to coagulate the collateral branches. The dissection of a distal arm lesion usually includes a distal elbow-level transposition of the ulnar nerve, so the lower level of the dissection should include clearing the nerve through the olecranon notch, opening the cubital tunnel, and splitting apart the two heads of the FCU muscle.

ELBOW AND FOREARM LEVEL

The incision begins on the medial distal arm, curves over the volar elbow lateral to the medial epicondylar region and then comes gently back down the medial proximal forearm. Dissection of the ulnar nerve through and beyond the olecranon notch region requires good lighting, some retraction, and the use of the bipolar coagulator (Fig. 9-17).[56] The overlying extension of the epicondylar fascia is sectioned and the nerve is carefully mobilized out of the olecranon notch using the bipolar coagulator to coagulate arteries and veins accompanying the nerve through this region. Because the nerve is often closely confined or is sometimes already entrapped at this level, the technique must be especially gentle. Small articular branches are usually sacrificed; however, the branches to the FCU

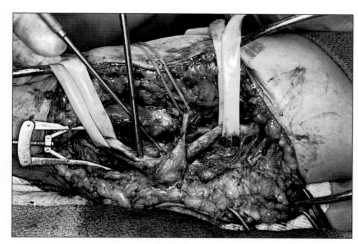

FIGURE 9-17 This is an intraoperative photograph of an ulnar injury in the olecranon notch region. This lesion required a split repair. The nerve was then transposed volar to the elbow and buried deep to the pronator teres and the flexor carpi ulnaris muscles.

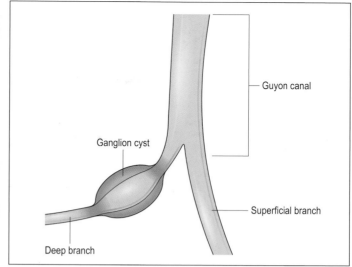

FIGURE 9-18 This drawing depicts compression by a ganglion cyst of the deep branch of the ulnar nerve just distal to Guyon's canal. Most of this patient's hand intrinsic muscle weakness reversed after removal of the cyst and decompression of this branch.

muscle are usually maintained, but freed over a length to aid mobilization of the ulnar nerve itself.[16,42] The nerve can then be traced below or distal to the olecranon notch by encircling it with a drain and dissecting around it while carefully sectioning the overlying FCU fascia and muscle. Care must be taken to preserve the ulnar flexor digitorum profundus III and IV branches, which usually originate from the lateral or radial side of the nerve, 2–4 cm distal to the olecranon notch. Flexor carpi ulnaris branches originating more superficially can be dissected back up and into the main trunk of the nerve to gain length or can be sectioned, if necessary. It is important to split the heads of the FCU muscle distal to the point at which the flexor digitorum profundus branches exit the ulnar nerve in order to adequately uncover the nerve. The muscle bellies of the FCU can be spread and held apart with a mastoid, or in more slender patients with an Alm retractor.

DISTAL FOREARM AND WRIST LEVEL

In the more distal forearm, the skin incision can parallel the superior edge of the FCU tendon. The tendon and originating muscle belly can be retracted medially after encircling them with one or more Penrose drains. The forearm portion of the nerve tends to lie beneath a line extending from the medial epicondyle to the palpable portion of the pisiform bone. For midforearm-level exposure of the ulnar nerve, some of the muscle belly of the FCU may have to be split as well. The nerve lies in the interval between the FCU and the flexor digitorum profundus muscles.[75] The dorsal cutaneous branch of the ulnar nerve arises from the posteromedial or ulnar aspect of the nerve and can usually be isolated and encircled with a plastic loop. Injury to the ulnar nerve at a distal forearm level often involves the adjacent and parallel ulnar artery, which usually adjoins the ulnar nerve at a midforearm level. This vessel may have to be isolated for subsequent repair or obliteration.[9] Most of the veins in this area can be coagulated as the nerve is elevated by drains and sharply cleared of investing tissue or scar.

Exposures at the wrist and palmar levels use a distal forearm incision on the radial side of the FCU muscle, curving gently on the radial side of the hypothenar eminence, and pointing toward the interval between the ring and little fingers. As the nerve approaches the wrist, it lies beneath or dorsal to the palmar carpal

ligament and volar to the transverse carpal ligament and the palmar surface of the flexor digitorum profundus tendons. The first is sectioned and the latter two usually preserved as a bed for the nerve. The ulnar artery remains on the lateral, i.e. radial, side of the nerve as the nerve passes on the radial side of the pisiform bone. In the more distal tunnel, the overlying fibrous arch of the palmar fascia should be incised for adequate exposure. The artery has usually branched, as has the nerve by this point, and vessels, as well as superficial and deep ulnar branches, are often intertwined. These relations should be established under magnification with the help of one or more Alm retractor(s) carefully placed to spread adjacent tissues. The superficial palmar branch, which exits the more distal tunnel along with an arterial branch, is first mobilized along with the more distal sensory branches. Then, the deep palmar or terminal branch of the ulnar nerve can be exposed, usually beneath and slightly lateral to or on the ulnar side of the deep or terminal branch of the artery (Fig. 9-18). As the nerve and vessel exit the distal ulnar tunnel, they pass around the hook of the hamate bone and deep to a fibrous arch, which is the site of origin of the hypothenar muscles. Dissection in the palmar area must be done in a measured and deliberate fashion and magnification, use of fine instruments, and the bipolar forceps are mandatory.

RESULTS

ARM LEVEL

In early literature, results reported for ulnar nerve repair were not encouraging,[1,65,70,71] and reports based on both world wars were especially dismal.[68,72,81,85,86] On the other hand, some more recent reports have been more optimistic.[8,37,48,60,61] Many recently published series have been relatively small and, more importantly, have consisted primarily of wrist-level injuries with few injuries included at an arm or elbow level.[77,78]

Associated injuries to tendons, bones, vessels, or other nerves can downgrade results, as can a fixed, clawed hand, even if

Table 9-1 The LSUHSC* muscle grading system for ulnar nerve injury

Grade	Evaluation	Description
0	Absent	No muscle contraction; absent sensation.
1	Poor	Proximal muscles such as FCU and FDP-V contract, but not against gravity; sensory grade is 1 or 0.
2	Fair	Proximal muscles (FCU and FDP-V) contract against gravity, distal intrinsic muscles do not contract; sensory grade, if applicable, is usually 2 or lower.
3	Moderate	Proximal muscles (FCU and FDP-V) contract against gravity and some resistance; some distal muscles, usually hypothenar muscles and occasionally lumbricals, contract against little resistance; sensory grade is usually 3.
4	Good	All proximal and some distal hand intrinsic muscles, such as interosseous and lumbricals to the little and ring finger muscles, contract against pressure with some resistance; sensory grade is 3 or better.
5	Excellent	All muscles, including hand intrinsics, contract against moderate resistance; sensory grade is 4 or better.

*LSUHSC, Louisiana State University Health Sciences Center; FCU, flexor carpi ulnaris muscle; FDP-V, flexor digitorum profundus muscle to little finger.

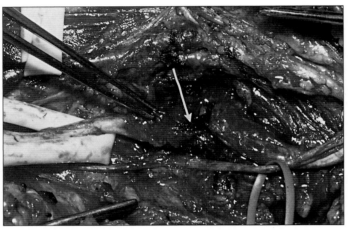

FIGURE 9-19 An old glass injury at the medial cord-to-ulnar nerve junction is shown *(arrow)*. The forceps are on a distal stump neuroma, and the Vasoloop is around an antebrachial cutaneous nerve. Since this injury was almost a year old and involved the very proximal ulnar nerve, results were poor even after 3 years of follow-up. The flexor carpi ulnaris muscle and the flexor digitorum profundus muscle to the ring finger were grade 4, and the flexor digitorum profundus muscle to the little finger was grade 3 to 4. Sensation in the ulnar nerve territory was grade 3. The hand intrinsic muscle function remained absent.

Table 9-2 Arm-level ulnar nerve mechanisms of injury (n = 62)

Mechanism of injury	Operative patients	Nonoperative patients
Laceration	18	5
Fracture	11	1
GSW	7	4
Stretch/contusion	6	5
Tumor/Infection*	5	0
Total	47	15

n, number; GSW, gunshot wound.

*Four tumors and 1 case of hidradenitis had operations without significant deficit.

successful repair returns nerve fibers to the hand intrinsic muscles.[39] Most of the ulnar nerve's input goes to the fine hand intrinsic muscles which are important for a useful hand and are difficult to reinnervate in a functional fashion (Fig. 9-19).

On the other hand, the flexor digitorum profundus muscle branches to the little and ring fingers and sensation in the ulnar distribution are less important for a useful hand than intrinsic muscle function.[56] Nonetheless, recovery of these motorsensory functions and some intrinsic function from the hypothenar and adductor pollicis muscles is possible, so the nerve should be repaired whenever indicated.

As pointed out by other authors in other series of patients and applicable to the LSUHSC patients, ulnar-injured extremities required maximal rehabilitation in terms of repetitive and sus-

tained physical and occupational therapy and home exercises.[81] Pre- and postoperative grades at each level were determined by the use of criteria included in Table 9-1.

Table 9-2 shows mechanisms of injuries or lesions involving the ulnar nerve at the arm level. Forty-seven of 62 lesions evaluated at this level were treated surgically.[43] There were five tumors (Fig. 9-20) and one case of hidradenitis, and preoperative loss was mild in these cases. Despite a large number of lacerations and puncture wounds affecting the high ulnar nerve, only eight of 18 patients having surgery had complete transection of the nerve; the remainder had partially transected nerve, or the injury had bruised and stretched it, giving lesions in continuity. Primary end-to-end suture anastomosis repair within 48 hours was possible in five transected cases and led to grade 3 recoveries in three (Table 9-3). Secondary end-to-end suture anastomosis repair and graft repair were less successful, with only one of three transections having eventual good results (Fig. 9-21). Split repair was performed for partial transection in three cases and all three patients had useful recoveries.

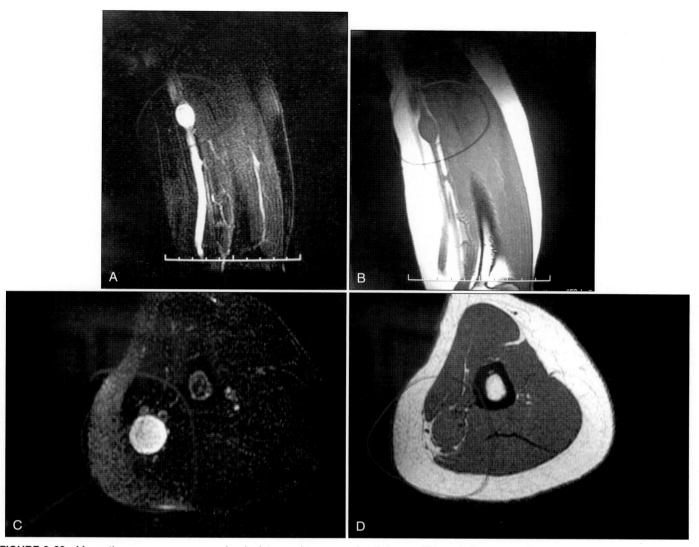

FIGURE 9-20 Magnetic resonance neurography depicts an ulnar nerve sheath tumor. This technique uses phased-array surface coils and fast T$_1$-spin echo pulse sequences on a standard 1.5-Tesla magnetic resonance imaging system.

There were 31 lesions in continuity having surgery (see Table 9-3). These included seven associated with lacerations. Most of the lesions were caused by relatively blunt lacerations from fans, propeller blades, or auto metal and the nerves were either partially lacerated or contused over a length. Seven lesions in continuity were associated with gunshot wounds (GSWs), six with blunt soft tissue contusions, and 11 with fractures (Fig. 9-22). In these cases, exploration was delayed for up to 4 months to determine whether early signs of spontaneous recovery would occur. This delay also permitted operative nerve action potential (NAP) studies to be done to prove or disprove the need for resection.[45]

Intraoperative recordings showed positive NAPs in 18 cases and 17 had neurolysis, with 15 (88%) of 17 having recoveries of grade 3 or better. One case associated with a lacerating injury had a split repair despite a positive NAP because one portion of the cross-section of nerve was more severely involved than the rest. In 13 cases without recordable NAPs across their lesions, four had suture repairs and six had graft repairs. Despite the absence of NAPs in three cases, only neurolysis was done due to the extensive length and proximal location of the lesion. Only one of these three cases had a significant recovery, and this was only to grade 3 level.

Three patients who underwent suture repairs and three patients who underwent graft repairs recovered to grade 3 or better level. Four of five schwannomas were totally resected with preservation of their preoperative functions, and the hidradenitis case in which the ulnar nerve required extensive neurolysis had the same result.

ARM-LEVEL CASE SUMMARIES

CASE 1

This 12-year-old boy fell through a plate glass window and sustained a laceration in the axilla. The soft tissue wound was repaired, but there was an ulnar nerve palsy. Examination 1 month later showed partial function of the FCU muscle, but a complete distal palsy. At exploration 1 week later, a lesion in continuity was found at a location near the nerve's point of emanation from the medial cord. The lesion conducted a small NAP. Because the loss was severe, it was postulated that only one or two fascicles going to the FCU muscle had been spared severance. The lesion was resected and an end-to-end suture anastomosis repair was done. The histology of the resected segment showed a neurotmetic lesion with the exception of two small, intact fascicles.

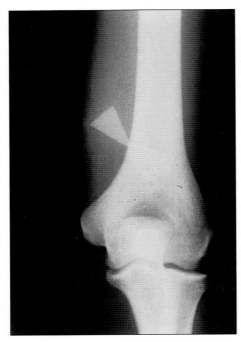

FIGURE 9-21 A radiograph shows a shard of glass that transected the ulnar nerve several inches above the elbow. This glass fragment was missed in the primary exploration, but found when the patient was examined because of total ulnar nerve palsy. The nerve was repaired secondarily a month later. The overlying triceps fibers, or arcade of Struthers, was divided to expose the nerve at this level.

Due to the patient's young age, he recovered function of the flexor digitorum profundus muscle by 1 year, and by 3.5 years his hand intrinsic muscles were grade 3 to 4, and sensation was grade 4.

COMMENT

This is a proximal ulnar nerve injury with a reasonable result, probably related to both the sharp mechanism of injury and the patient's age.

CASE 2

This 21-year-old male lacerated the medial surface of his distal arm on a piece of glass. A primary end-to-end suture anastomosis repair without transposition was done elsewhere. He presented 10 months later with severe pain and paresthesias in an ulnar nerve distribution. There was a tender mass 5 cm proximal to the tip of the elbow, and tapping in that location gave paresthesias down the ulnar side of the forearm. Motor loss was complete distal to the FCU muscle, and this included an absent flexor digitorum profundus to the little finger. Sensory loss was also complete and in the ulnar nerve distribution.

The area was explored 11 months after injury. A suture neuroma in continuity was found which did not transmit an NAP and this was resected. The 4 cm gap was shortened by transposition of the distal stump beneath the FCU and pronator teres muscles. This was carried out by dissecting the distal ulnar nerve through the olecranon notch area and below the elbow just distal to the flexor digitorum profundus muscle branches. A suture was placed in the epineurium and then a large, curved hemostat was used to create a tunnel beneath the FCU and the pronator teres muscles. By reaching through the tunnel from the arm to the forearm level with a long hemostat, the suture was grasped and the attached distal stump was drawn through the tunnel. Then, just proximal to the tunnel, an end-to-end suture anastomosis repair was accomplished without tension.

Follow-up after 2 years and 11 months found the flexor digitorum profundus muscle to the little finger to be grade 4, hypothenar muscles grade 3, interos-

Table 9-3 Arm-level ulnar nerve injuries (n = 42)

Operation*	No. of cases / no. recovered to ≥grade 3
Transection	
1° suture repair	5/3
2° suture repair	2/1
2° graft repair	1/0
2° split graft repair	3/3
Lesions in continuity	
Positive NAP	
Neurolysis	17/15
Split graft repair	1/1
Negative NAP	
Neurolysis	3/1
Suture repair	4/3
Graft repair	6/3

n, number; NAP, nerve action potential.

*Does not include tumors.

seous and lumbrical muscles to the little and ring fingers grade 2 to 3, and the adductor pollicis muscle was grade 3. Sensation in the ulnar nerve distribution was grade 4.

COMMENT

Serious injury to the ulnar nerve close to the elbow should usually include transposition as one of the surgical steps in its management.

CASE 3

This 11-year-old boy was waiting for his father to pick him up at a boys' boarding school on the coast. While waiting, he and several other boys made a small fire on the beach and placed a CO_2 canister, similar to those used to make cocktails, into the fire in an attempt to turn it into a rocket. The cartridge exploded, and a shard of metal sharply lacerated his proximal and medial arm. He was seen in a local hospital where the wound was probed for foreign bodies. No foreign bodies were found; however, it was noted that the ulnar nerve was almost completely divided, i.e. little was left in continuity. He was then brought to LSUHSC, where examination showed a complete ulnar nerve palsy with the exception of function of the FCU muscle (Fig. 9-23). Since the wound was sharp and caused by penetrating metal rather than a GSW, and because the nerve was known to be almost completely divided, a relatively acute repair was performed. At the operating table 1 day after injury, a relatively clean but partial division of the nerve was confirmed. This was converted to a complete division, a few millimeters of tissue were trimmed off the ends, and an end-to-end suture anastomosis repair was performed using 6–0 nylon.

Some FCU muscle function was still present postoperatively. By 4 months, this was found to be grade 4 and by 6 months, the flexor digitorum profundus muscle to the little finger had begun to recover. The hypothenar muscles began to contract by 1 year, and by 4 years postoperatively the intrinsic muscles were grade 3. Sensory return was grade 4. Youth and the relatively sharp nature of the injury helped, and the patient now uses the limb and the hand in an almost normal fashion. Some atrophy of hand intrinsic muscles, however, is present. His weakest muscle remains the lumbrical muscle to the little finger.

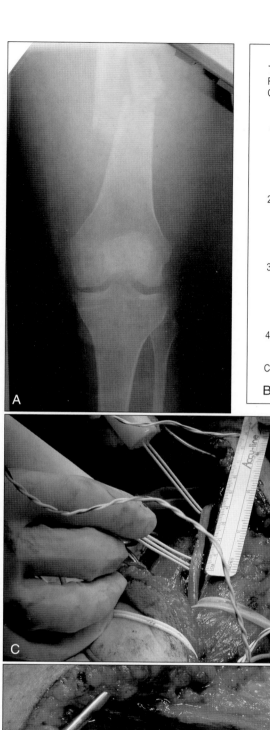

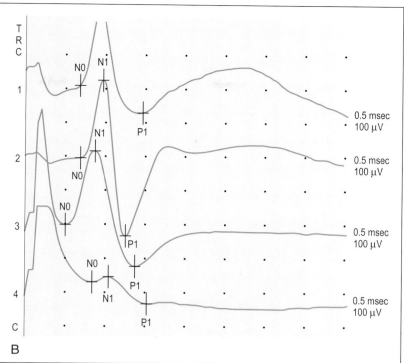

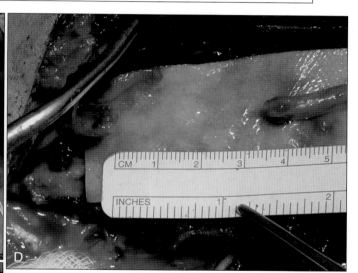

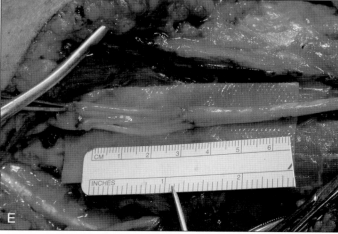

FIGURE 9-22 **(A)** Plain lateral X-ray of a humeral fracture, which resulted in an ulnar nerve injury. **(B)** Intraoperative nerve action potentials were positive proximal to the neuroma *(1, 2, 3)* and present, but small, into the proximal neuroma. Traces recorded beyond that point were flat. **(C)** Stimulating and recording electrodes are seen on the nerve proximal to the neuroma. **(D)** The neuroma was resected and **(E)** an intrafascicular graft repair was performed.

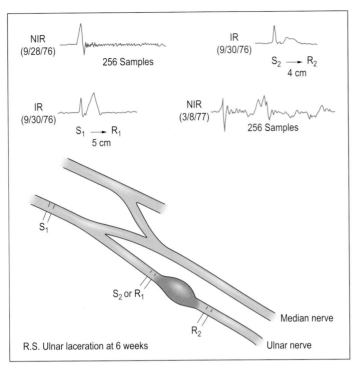

FIGURE 9-23 A partial ulnar lesion caused by an exploded fragment of a CO_2 canister. The flexor carpi ulnaris muscle was spared. Although noninvasive recording of the nerve action potential (NAP) showed no ulnar conduction, a small NAP was recordable across the lesion by invasive recording *(lower left recording)*. The lesion was resected and repaired end-to-end, and 5.5 months later a small NAP could be recorded noninvasively from the more distal ulnar nerve. Because the patient was only 12 years old at the time of injury, he even regained substantial recovery of the hand intrinsic muscles (grade 3) over a 6-year period of follow-up.

ELBOW AND FOREARM LEVELS

The mechanisms of injury were more varied at this level than in the upper arm, but contusions, lacerations and fracture-associated lesions still predominated (Table 9-4).[43] Unlike the arm-level major lesion, which was laceration, for the elbow and forearm levels it was stretch/contusion. Most of the contusions and fracture-associated injuries were either partial at the start or had a recordable NAP, and thus only underwent neurolysis and a transposition.

Lacerations including punctures was the second largest category of injuries to the elbow and forearm-level ulnar nerve, and 42 such cases had surgery. Thirty-one of 42 operative cases involved transections of the nerve (Table 9-5). Most were reparable by primary or secondary suture. Early end-to-end suture anastomosis was reserved for those severed by glass or a knife, and secondary end-to-end suture anastomosis was done for those more bluntly transected or, if sharply cut, those referred too late for primary repair (Fig. 9-24). The patient with resection without repair had undergone several prior unsuccessful repairs and had severe pain as the result of a lengthy and large neuroma in continuity. Resection of the neuroma, and some proximal and distal nerve, reduced pain such that a nonaddictive analgesic could be used. Lacerating injuries causing nerves to be contused and stretched, or partially lacerated, fell into the lesions in continuity group. Cases with NAPs transmitted across the lesion underwent neurolysis or split repairs. Those without NAPs required repair, usually by end-to-end suture

anastomosis or graft. Almost all operations at this level included transposition and submuscular placement.

A few patients with lesions had undergone earlier operation, but repair had failed in two cases, which resulted in re-operation. In both cases, acute repair of bluntly injured nerves had been attempted elsewhere.[47] In 13 lesions in continuity after resection, gaps were long enough to require a graft repair (Table 9-5; Fig. 9-25). One of five GSWs involving the ulnar nerve at this level required graft repair and subsequent transposition, whereas the others had only neurolysis or neurolysis and transposition (Fig. 9-26).

Table 9-4 Elbow- and forearm-level ulnar nerve mechanisms of injury (n = 272)

Mechanism of injury	Operative patients	Nonoperative patients
Stretch/contusion	41	26
Laceration	42	14
Fracture/dislocation	19	10
GSW	3	2
Injection	2	0
Volkmann's contracture	2	1
Electrical	1	1
Hematoma	0	1
Tumor	6	0
Total	115	154

n, number; GSW, gunshot wound.

Table 9-5 Forearm- and elbow-level ulnar nerve injury (n = 110)

Operation*	No. of cases / no. recovered to ≥grade 3
Transections	
1° suture repair	11/9
2° suture repair	12/8
2° graft repair	7/4
Resection	1/0
Lesions in continuity	
Positive NAP	
Neurolysis	57/54
Negative NAP	
Suture repair	13/10
Graft repair	7/5
Split graft repair	1/1

n, number.

*Does not include tumors.

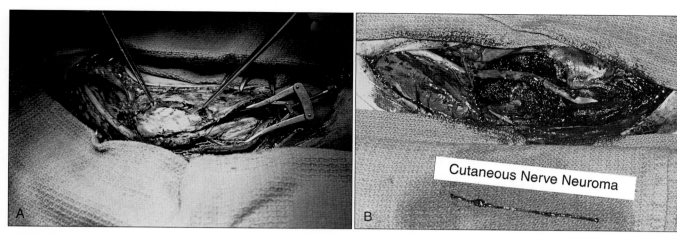

FIGURE 9-24 *(A)* Nerve has been cleared through the region of the olecranon notch by a complete external neurolysis. A trough has been made in the proximal forearm muscle by sectioning completely through pronator teres and the more volar portion of flexor carpi ulnaris. *(B)* Nerve has been placed in the muscle trough. Note that a neuroma and segment of antebrachial cutaneous nerve have been resected and are placed on the drape. This patient had prior neurolysis for olecranon notch-level entrapment and had injury to antebrachial cutaneous nerve.

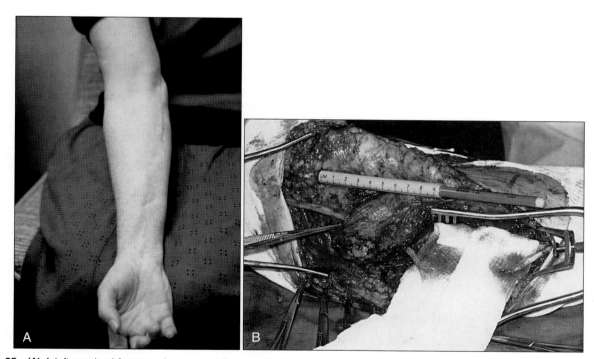

FIGURE 9-25 **(A)** A left proximal forearm ulnar nerve injury resulted from a blunt laceration. **(B)** At surgery this lengthy gap in the ulnar nerve at a proximal forearm level was partially shortened by transposing the proximal nerve beneath the pronator teres muscle. The ends of the ulnar nerve have been split into fascicular groups preparatory to the placement of sural grafts. The necessary grafts were 5.5 cm in length; without transposition, the required length would have been 10 cm.

Only one nerve injured by injection required repair, but others at 3.5 months after injection had recordable NAPs across a lesion in continuity. These cases underwent neurolysis, and over 1.5 years experienced acceptable recoveries.

A Volkmann's contracture case involved the median, radial, and ulnar nerves. Neurolysis was performed on all three nerves, and transposition of the ulnar nerve and fasciotomy were performed early, but the outcome was only fair.

Not unexpectedly, the electrical injury at the elbow involving ulnar nerve required repair at 4 months after injury. Graft repair was done, with only a grade 2 level attained. Burns by electricity tend to result in lengthy up-and-down lesions and are often associ-

ated with other severe soft tissue damage, making these lesions difficult to treat.[19,35,53]

With suture or graft repairs, 21 (68%) of 31 patients with lesions not in continuity achieved functional recoveries of grade 3 or better. Of 14 cases, 11 lesions (79%) in continuity without recordable NAPs but having repair showed grade 3 or greater improvement. The best results for lesions in continuity were those cases having positive NAPs. Of these, 59 (91%) out of 65 patients achieved grade 3 or better functional recoveries.

Recovery for most of the cases treated without operation was good. Several patients might have benefited from surgery, but were seen for the first time at LSUHSC a year or more after injury.

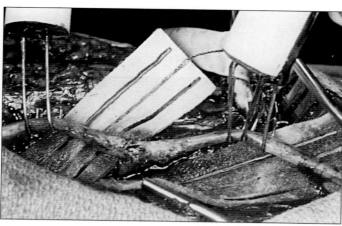

FIGURE 9-26 An ulnar nerve injured by a gunshot wound near the origin of the flexor digitorum profundus muscle branch is shown. The hand is to the left of the picture, and the shoulder is to the right. A nerve action potential could be recorded across this lesion at 5 months after injury, so it was not resected. Stimulating electrodes are to the right, and recording electrodes are to the left. After neurolysis, the nerve was transposed and buried deep to the proximal forearm muscles.

Lesions caused by mild compression, such as an operative complication, usually improved with time.[67] A few at the level of the elbow did, however, require transposition.

ELBOW- AND FOREARM-LEVEL CASE SUMMARIES

CASE 1

This 27-year-old man sustained a GSW to the right elbow from a .38-caliber pistol, resulting in an olecranon fracture. The wound was debrided acutely with removal of bone chips and, at the time of surgery, the ulnar nerve looked bruised. The nerve was unroofed where it lay in the olecranon notch and further distally as it ran beneath the two heads of the FCU muscle and the elbow was subsequently casted. After cast removal, it was evident that there was a complete ulnar nerve palsy below the FCU muscle accompanied by severe pain not only at the level of the elbow, but also radiating down the ulnar side of the forearm. There was an early claw deformity involving the little finger more than the ring finger. Electromyography showed complete denervation of the flexor digitorum profundus muscle to the little finger and of the hand intrinsic muscles. These clinical and electrical findings were still present when the patient was first seen at LSUHSC 3 months after injury. As a result, the nerve was explored 13 weeks after injury.

At surgery, the nerve was swollen and firm just before it entered the olecranon notch and throughout its course from within the notch to the forearm level. The nerve was encased in heavy scar and so an external neurolysis was performed as well as resection of part of the intermuscular septum and splitting of the two heads of the FCU muscle. There was a small but definite NAP recordable across the lesion, but not beyond a point 3.8 cm below the olecranon notch where the flexor digitorum profundus branches left the nerve. Thus, there was a conducted response and the conduction velocity was 32 m/sec. As a result, a transposition was done, and the nerve with its lesion in continuity was placed deep to the FCU and pronator teres muscles. Fascia and some muscle were then closed gently over the nerve.

Postoperatively, most of the patient's neuritic pain was gone, and after a 3.5-year period, the functional grades achieved were: ulnar sensation, grade 3 to 4; flexor digitorum profundus V, grade 4; flexor digitorum profundus IV, grade 5; hypothenar muscles, grade 3 to 4; interossei, grade 4; lumbrical V, grade 3; lumbrical IV, grade 4; and adductor pollicis, grade 4. He has had restoration of a fair grip in the right hand, though to only 60% of the left hand grip. As a bank clerk, he uses the hand for both writing and computer work.

COMMENT

Despite complete distal clinical and electrical loss, intraoperative evaluation indicated neurolysis and transposition, rather than resection. Fortunately, his neuritic pain improved as well as his function.

CASE 2

This 48-year-old man, a passenger in a vehicle involved in an auto accident, had his right elbow badly contused due to the car door being flung open and then closing on his limb. He had bruising and swelling of the elbow and a partial ulnar nerve palsy. The patient reported that a mild, initial hand weakness had progressed with time. He was first seen 4 months after the accident. The FCU muscle and flexor digitorum profundus muscle to the ring and little fingers functioned well. The hypothenar muscles were grade 2 and interossei, grade 1 to 2. The lumbrical muscle to the little finger was absent and that to the ring finger was grade 2 to 3. The adductor pollicis muscle function was much improved at grade 3 to 4. Sensation was poor, but loss was partial and was grade 3.

The patient underwent neurolysis, NAP stimulation and recording, and transposition at 5 months after injury. The nerve appeared tight in the region of the olecranon notch and was somewhat decreased in caliber at that level even after neurolysis. Nerve action potentials were found to conduct across this area, but only at 20 m/sec.

He eventually made a good recovery, with hand intrinsic muscles and sensation each reaching an overall grade of 4 by 3 years and 2 months, postoperatively.

COMMENT

Despite incomplete loss in the distribution of the ulnar nerve and a blunt injury, operation to provide a better environment for the nerve seemed indicated. This was especially so in this case, in which some progression of loss was suggested by the patient's history, even though there was no opportunity to document it.

WRIST LEVEL

Table 9-6 lists the mechanisms for injury at the wrist level. In the LSUHSC ulnar nerve injury series, the wrist or palm level had the smallest number compared with other levels.[43] The leading mechanism of injury was laceration, as it was at the other levels. There were 12 transected nerves, and six transections were sharp enough and seen acutely enough to have primary repair.[46] As at the arm level, the nerves having secondary repair had at least a grade 3 recovery, with one reaching a grade 4 level (Table 9-7). One neuroma caused by transection had been long-standing and the nerve was resected, rather than repaired. The other laceration-associated lesions left nerves in some degree of continuity: 12 had positive NAPs and 11 had neurolysis with recovery, and one had a split repair based on differential fascicular recordings.[82]

There were 10 digital nerve repairs with variable results, but usually with recovery of enough sensation to be protective. Five other patients had digital nerves with neuromas resected, with improvement in pain and hypersensitivity.

Both nerve injuries due to an electrical mechanism of injury and undergoing surgery required graft repair, and only one regained a grade 3 functional level. A third such lesion was managed conservatively because the loss was partial soon after injury. Five

Table 9-6 Wrist-level ulnar nerve mechanisms of injury (n = 80)

Mechanism of injury	Operative patients	Nonoperative patients
Laceration	16	3
Stretch/contusion	5	4
Fracture/dislocation	4	5
GSW	2	1
Electrical	2	1
Prior surgical injury	1	2
Tumor	2	0
Total	32	16

n, number; GSW, gunshot wound.

Table 9-7 Wrist-level ulnar nerve injury (n = 32)

Operation	No. of cases / no. recovered to ≥grade 3
Transections	
1° suture repair	6/4
2° suture repair	2/2
2° graft repair	1/1
Split graft repair	2/2
Resection	1/0
Lesions in continuity	
Positive NAP	
Neurolysis	11/11
Split graft repair	1/1
Negative NAP	
Suture repair	3/2
Graft repair	3/1

n, number.

*Does not include tumors.

contusions and two of four lesions associated with wrist fracture or dislocation not only had lesions in continuity, but had positive NAPs and, as a result, neurolysis with recovery.

The results of repair from other series are summarized in Tables 9-8 and 9-9.

OTHER CASE SUMMARIES

CASE 1

The arm of a 22-year-old male went through a plate glass window, and he required immediate repair of the brachial artery and biceps tendon. Nerve ends

Table 9-8 Ulnar nerve secondary suture repair (Seddon*)

Ulnar nerve level	M3 S3 or better recovery
Upper arm and elbow	20%
Forearm	25%
Wrist	44.5%

*British system.

M, motor grade; S, sensory grade.

Table 9-9 Ulnar nerve repair results (Dellon)

Location of repair	Recovery
High-level suture repair	≥17% M4 ≥20% S3+
Low-level suture repair	≥32% M4 ≥34.7% S3
Combined high and low Graft repair	≥43% M4 ≥21% S3
Digital nerve All-level suture repair All-level graft repair	≥59% S3 ≥29% S3

M, motor grade; S, sensory grade.

were tagged with tantalum clips, and the limb was casted. The patient had complete loss of both median and ulnar nerve functions. The only muscle partially spared was the pronator teres, which was grade 3. Two weeks later, the wound was explored at LSUHSC. The median and ulnar nerve stumps had retracted and, after trimming these, four antebrachial cutaneous nerve grafts were used to bridge the 6.4 cm gap in the median nerve, and the gap in the ulnar nerve was made up by transposition. As a result, an end-to-end suture anastomosis repair of that nerve could be done. The immediate postoperative period was uncomplicated.

At follow-up after 6 years, the patient could make a fist and could enclose his flexed fingers with his thumb. If he extended his fingers, the little finger tended to abduct. In the median nerve distribution, he had excellent pronation and function of the flexor digitorum superficialis, flexor digitorum profundus, and flexor pollicis longus muscles. The abductor pollicis brevis and opponens pollicis muscle strengths were grade 3 to 4 and median nerve sensation was grade 3. The overall median nerve grade was 4. In the ulnar distribution, he had excellent FCU muscle function. Flexor digitorum profundus and even hypothenar muscles were grade 4. The interosseous and lumbrical muscles were grade 3, while the abductor pollicis muscle was grade 3 to 4. Sensation was grade 3, and the overall ulnar nerve grade was 3 to 4. He could localize stimuli, but two-point discrimination remained poor. The patient would look at this hand when he used it for fine tasks, and he still had trouble picking up fine objects and buttoning clothes, but could use the hand to turn door knobs and could also turn the lid of a jar. As a grocery store owner, he was able to stock shelves and cut meat. He said he could use the hand to write with a pen or pencil if necessary, but his grip was somewhat different because he used more of his fingers to balance the grip of the thumb than before the accident.

COMMENT

If a decision is made not to repair a divided nerve at the time of acute operation, we recommend tacking the stump with an epineurial stitch to adjacent muscle or fascia. This prevents stump retraction. Placing a tantalum or other metallic clip(s) on a stump(s) is of no benefit.

CASE 2

A 42-year-old male electronics engineer had progressive numbness and weakness in the ulnar nerve distribution after using a hammer vigorously with the right hand. He subsequently developed a partial clawing of the right little and ring fingers. There was a Tinel sign at the wrist but no palpable mass. Ulnar-innervated hand intrinsic muscles were grade 2 to 3. The flexor digitorum profundus I and II muscle to the little finger was preserved. The sensory examination was normal. Conduction along the ulnar nerves was mildly slowed at both elbows, but was markedly slowed at the level of the right wrist.

At exploration several months after the onset of symptoms, a ganglion cyst 1.5 cm in diameter was found compressing the deep branch of the ulnar nerve. This branch was dissected off the lateral side of the cyst. After excision, the neck of the cyst was ligated and then oversewn with fascia. He has done well post-operatively, with gradual restoration of the ulnar-innervated hand intrinsic function.

COMMENT

Not all hand intrinsic loss is related to the more common elbow-level lesion since entrapment at the wrist can occur. In addition, complicating mass lesions such as this patient's ganglion cyst may play a role in entrapments. Absence of sensory loss in the presence of ulnar intrinsic muscle motor loss alerts the examiner to the wrist level as the site of the pathology. An EMG report of some or slight ulnar nerve slowing at the elbow should not outweigh the clinical findings indicating the wrist as the level of involvement.

COMPLICATIONS

The median nerve can be injured by retraction or non-gentle handling as the ulnar nerve is approached in the proximal arm. Fortunately, this complication was not experienced with any LSUHSC patients.

The potential complications associated with various transpositions or attempts to treat ulnar nerve entrapment at the elbow are legion. For the LSUHSC patients, a modified Learmonth transposition, placing the nerve deep to the pronator teres and FCU muscles, was almost always carried out. Despite dividing and then re-attaching a portion of these muscles, weakness in their distribution was seldom a problem. There were several patients, however, who had increased weakness in the flexor digitorum profundus muscle innervating the little or ring fingers. In addition, a patient with partial hand intrinsic muscle loss before manipulation of the nerve due to entrapment had some increased intrinsic loss postoperatively.

Complications at the forearm level included loss of the ulnar artery. This occurred in two LSUHSC patients, but had no serious consequences in terms of vascular insufficiency to the hand.

Decompression of an entrapped ulnar nerve through Guyon's canal can be incomplete and lead to failure to improve. In the relatively small LSUHSC series of cases at this level this complication was avoided.

A number of patients in the LSUHSC series of ulnar nerve injuries, as in other authors' series, required tendon transfer(s) to reduce the tendency for clawing.[4,54,69] When this had not been done

because of stiffness in little and ring fingers, progressive casting and, in a few instances, capsulotomies had to be done.[66]

ULNAR NERVE ENTRAPMENT AT THE ELBOW LEVEL

The most common ulnar nerve lesion is entrapment at the level of the elbow. The predominant involvement is within the olecranon notch, though compression can occur at several levels. The nerve is normally tightly constrained as it passes over the floor of this structure and spontaneous entrapment is usually associated with adhesions in the region of the olecranon notch. The aponeurotic arch overlying the notch and extending to the medial epicondyle can also thicken and compress the nerve. Flexion of the elbow moves the nerve through this tight area and may produce a frictional injury. In the less frequent and more distal cubital tunnel syndrome the nerve is compressed by the origins of the two heads of the FCU muscle.[1,23] Occasionally, the ulnar nerve rides up and out of the olecranon notch or groove as the arm is flexed. Rarely, the nerve is spontaneously compressed proximal to the notch by a Struthers ligament.

Entrapment is more likely to occur if there has been a prior elbow fracture or dislocation, but the majority of patients do not give this history.[28] Soft tissue contusion of the forearm and elbow without fracture can be a predisposing factor, as can diabetes mellitus, a history of alcoholism, rheumatoid arthritis, and tumor or ganglion arising at the level of the elbow. There may be a history of repetitive pressure on or trauma to the nerve. The patient may repetitively rest the elbow on a hard surface such as a desk, bar top, or car window ledge. One patient who developed unilateral entrapment was a telephone operator who rested her right elbow on a table as she held the phone to her ear. Another patient who had bilateral entrapment worked as a fitter for wedding dresses. She would rest both elbows on a low table as she reached up to pin or sew beads or sequins on a dress on a bride-to-be or mannequin.

SYMPTOMS

With ulnar nerve entrapment at the elbow level, patients commonly complain of paresthesias in an ulnar distribution, particularly in the little and, sometimes, the ring fingers. Often, the sensory syndrome is rather specific in that symptoms are present on the ulnar, but not radial side of the ring finger. Sensory fibers are usually affected before motor fibers. Paresthesias may be spontaneous or may be prompted by the use of the hand. In other cases, rather than spontaneous tingling or "electric shock" sensations, the patient may notice only hyperesthesias mixed with hypoesthesias of the little and ring fingers. This is followed by numbness in a similar distribution. With time, weakness in the hand intrinsic and hypothenar muscles may develop. The former may be initially manifested by spontaneous abduction of the little finger or a Wartenberg's sign caused by palmar interosseous muscle weakness. With time, atrophy of intrinsic muscles is evident. Occasionally, the entrapment presents first as weakness in the hand, and the patient has difficulty with fine movements. If the dominant hand is involved, holding a pen or pencil and writing are tedious. Turning a doorknob or unscrewing the lid of a jar or top of a bottle is difficult. In some cases, symptoms do not progress, and they may, on occasion, even regress if the elbow is rested or the patient avoids putting pressure on it.

PHYSICAL FINDINGS

Examination usually shows hypoesthesias mixed with hyperesthesias in the ulnar distribution of the hand. This is most likely on the volar and distal dorsal surfaces of the little finger. Usually, some degree of hand intrinsic muscle weakness is present, especially if the strength of the individual muscles of one hand is compared with that of the other. Intrinsic muscles showing the earliest weakness are the lumbrical muscle to the little finger and the abductor digiti minimi muscle. Weakness of the flexor digitorum profundus muscle supplying the little finger usually occurs later than weakness of the hand intrinsic muscles. Most striking under these circumstances is the appearance of the hand. There is shrinkage of the intrinsic muscles evident by inspection of the dorsum of the hand, as well as the palmar side along the hypothenar eminence. An ulnar claw deformity may develop later in the course of the entrapment owing to the lack of input of the lumbrical muscle(s) to the little and, sometimes, the ring finger.

Tenderness is usually present at the elbow, but of even greater importance is a Tinel sign at that level. Tapping over or proximal to the notch gives paresthesias in the distribution of the ulnar nerve, particularly into the little and, sometimes, the ring finger. The nerve may translocate out of the olecranon groove, which can be felt as the patient flexes and extends the elbow. Some, but not all patients with translocation of the nerve become symptomatic. Occasionally, this phenomenon is noted where there has been a prior neurolysis without transposition or a medial epicondylectomy or failed subcutaneous transposition.[11] The rate or progression of loss of function is extremely variable and unpredictable.

DIFFERENTIAL DIAGNOSES

The differential diagnoses include those disorders or traumatic episodes that involve the lower plexus elements. This includes lower cervical root radiculopathy caused by spurs or disc herniations. Thoracic outlet syndrome with lower spinal nerve compression could in part mimic ulnar neuropathy, but in those cases there is often loss not only of hand intrinsic muscles innervated by the ulnar nerve, but also of the thenar intrinsic muscles innervated by the median nerve. In addition, a Horner syndrome may alert the examiner to a more proximal or central pathology.

Amyotrophic lateral sclerosis (ALS) can begin with hand muscle loss on one side in one-third of cases. With time, however, the loss involves more of the arm and also the opposite arm and hand, but there is no sensory loss. As with spontaneous ulnar nerve entrapment, the peak period of presentation of ALS is between 40 and 60 years of age.

Another important neurological differential diagnosis is syringomyelia. Truncal or contralateral hand findings may suggest the diagnosis, although there is usually also dissociated sensory loss.

More distal lesions of Guyon's canal can mimic elbow-level entrapment, particularly if the deep branch is involved, because the maximal deficit is in the hand intrinsic muscles in entrapments at both levels. Spontaneous entrapment can be bilateral almost 20% of the time, although the contralateral side is often not symptomatic initially, and thus ulnar entrapment is usually unilateral on initial presentation. Symptoms are not always related to occupation but can be. Generally, cases have been categorized as follows:

Group I. Mild symptoms without motor involvement and minimal gross abnormality found at surgery. Most will recover fully even if symptoms were present for months to years.

Group II. Various sensory symptoms and mild to moderate atrophy of the hand intrinsic muscles. Almost 50% of patients experience reversal of muscle atrophy, including loss of intrinsic muscle function, after careful transposition.

Group III. Severe sensory and motor loss with hand intrinsic muscle wasting and reduced strength. Surgery may relieve or help pain and may increase sensation but, at best, only gives partial return of hand intrinsic muscle function.

In the usual case, the initial symptoms include intermittent hyper- and paresthesias in an ulnar distribution. These symptoms are often associated with elbow flexion. Sometimes, numbness is not noticed until it is pointed out to the patient at the time of examination. The patient may or may not notice lateral instability of the fingers in which the index finger slips sideways on gripping a knife or a pencil. There may be loss of stability of the little finger. During grasp, there may be loss of synchrony of digital flexion, and with intrinsic loss, coordination of the thumb and digits may be poor.

ELECTROPHYSIOLOGICAL STUDIES

An electrophysiological workup of ulnar nerve entrapment usually, but not always, confirms conductive slowing across the elbow.[7,20] Nonetheless, careful inspection and palpation of the limb and clinical testing of function remain paramount in the diagnosis of ulnar entrapment, just as with most nerve lesions.[15] This is especially so with ulnar entrapment at the elbow, because most electrophysiological conductive studies involve a segment of more normal nerve both proximal and often well distal to the area of compression in the olecranon notch, though with more severe entrapment, conduction for a variable length proximal and distal to the site of compression may be slowed as well.[31] Severe and especially sustained entrapment leads to denervational changes in the hand intrinsic muscles, including hypothenar, lumbrical and, especially, interosseous muscles,[40] while input to the adductor pollicis muscle is sometimes preserved. Conductive studies of the wrist-level ulnar nerve can usually exclude more distal entrapment in Guyon's canal (Fig. 9-27).

ULNAR NERVE ENTRAPMENT AT THE WRIST LEVEL

Three levels of entrapment can occur at the wrist level.[34]

SENSORY AND MOTOR BRANCH

Zone I consists of the ulnar nerve in the proximal aspect of Guyon's canal where it is proximal to its bifurcation into the deep branch and superficial branches.[29] This area is the most frequent site of spontaneous distal entrapment, and can be seen with wrist fractures and ganglion cysts.[5,58] There is ulnar sensory loss that does not include the dorsal cutaneous branch distribution, which supplies the dorsal hand; loss does include distal ulnar motor loss of the intrinsic muscles. Sensory conduction from the little and, sometimes, the ring finger is delayed across the wrist.

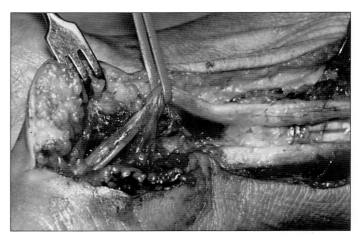

FIGURE 9-28   The ulnar nerve is shown in the region of Guyon's canyon. Both superficial and deep branches were entrapped at this level by an ulnar expansion of fascia while deep to nerve there was a thickened transverse carpal ligament.

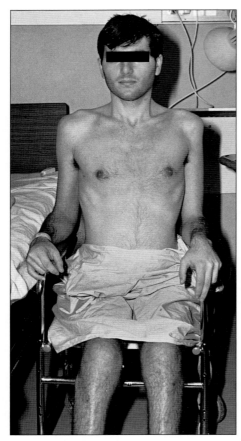

FIGURE 9-27   The paraplegic patient shown was referred with the suspected diagnosis of syringomyelia. Instead, compression and entrapment of both ulnar nerves at the level of the olecranon notch was found. The patient habitually rested his elbows on firm wheelchair arms.

DEEP MOTOR BRANCH

The deep motor branch comprises the zone II level of ulnar entrapment at the wrist level. Etiologies of entrapment here include repeated palmar trauma or pressure, ganglion, or carpal synovitis.[24,41] An unusual cause is hard labor or pressure of the palm against the handlebar during long-distance biking.[21,44] With trauma or pressure, the pisohamate ligament can thicken. On electrophysiological testing, conduction to the abductor digiti minimi muscle is usually normal, but that to the first dorsal interosseous is abnormal. Clinical loss and denervational changes occur in the palmar and dorsal interosseous, little and ring finger lumbrical, and adductor pollicis and deep head of the flexor pollicis brevis muscles.[73] Sensation is intact.

SUPERFICIAL BRANCH

Compression at the superficial branch level, or zone III, at the distal aspect of Guyon's canal gives pure sensory loss in a typical ulnar distribution that splits the ring finger. It is the least common entrapment at the wrist level. There is sparing of sensation in the superficial sensory distribution or dorsum of the hand.

OPERATIVE TECHNIQUES

ULNAR NERVE ENTRAPMENT AT THE ELBOW LEVEL

The arm is placed on an arm board. The elbow is positioned in extension with a folded towel under it and the hand is placed palm up. A mildly undulating skin incision is extended from the medial surface of the distal arm toward the medial volar surface of the elbow and then down along the proximal and medial side of the forearm (Fig. 9-28). Dissection is carried through the subcutaneous tissues, first at a forearm and then at an upper arm level. The antebrachial cutaneous nerves should be preserved and, if possible, mobilized toward the radial side of the forearm. The ulnar nerve can be easily located within the olecranon notch and then traced proximally into the distal arm and distally into the proximal forearm. At LSUHSC the nerve is usually identified first in the arm where it lies adherent to the superior muscle fibers of the FCU.

The ulnar nerve is covered 70% of the time by an arcade of Struthers which is composed of fibers originating from the medial posterior aspect of the medial intermuscular septum and medial border of the humerus to the fascia of the medial head of the triceps and coracobrachialis.[79] This arcade is a rare cause of entrapment in and of itself.

At this level, the ulnar nerve is also often adherent to the dorsal belly of the triceps and must be sharply dissected away. Major branches to the proximal FCU muscle should be preserved whenever possible. If needed, branches can be dissected back and split away from the main trunk of the ulnar nerve so they are lengthened in preparation for transposition.

There may also be major collateral vascular input to the nerve at this level, which should be dissected out and preserved if possible. Dissection is carried proximally enough to identify the point at which the nerve comes under the intermuscular septum.[76] The septum is sectioned or, more frequently, a segment resected so that the course of the nerve in the distal upper arm is free after transposition (Fig. 9-29). The nerve is then encircled with a Penrose drain. Dissection can then proceed by following the nerve distally and unroofing the olecranon notch. The nerve is encircled distally

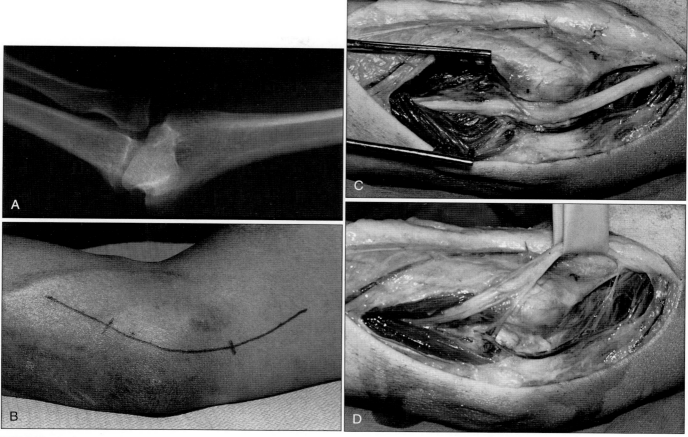

FIGURE 9-29 **(A)** A fracture dislocation of the elbow associated with a subsequent onset of tardy ulnar palsy is seen. **(B)** This is the usual type of incision to expose an entrapped ulnar nerve. **(C)** This is the ulnar nerve in the olecranon notch: proximal is to the right and distal to the left where the two heads of the flexor carpi ulnaris muscle have been split. **(D)** The nerve has been temporarily moved volar to the elbow so that the line of incision in the volar musculature can be ascertained.

with a Penrose drain and dissected in a circumferential fashion as it runs in the proximal forearm.

An alternative for distal exposure is to place the proximal phalanx of the surgeon's little finger in the notch and to point the tip of the surgeon's little finger towards the FCU muscle insertion at the wrist. This gives the approximate course of the ulnar nerve in the proximal forearm, where it lies deep to the two heads of the FCU muscle, but above the flexor digitorum superficialis muscle (Fig. 9-30). A longitudinal incision can then be made through fascia, and the fibers of the FCU muscle are split to expose the deeper forearm portion of the ulnar nerve. Smaller branches to the FCU muscle may be encountered just distal to the notch and these can either be dissected back into the main ulnar nerve to lengthen them for transposition, or they can be sacrificed by sectioning.

At approximately 2.5–5 cm distal to the olecranon notch, ulnar nerve branches to the ulnar half of the flexor digitorum profundus muscle arise. These take off from the radial and somewhat dorsal surface of the ulnar nerve and run a relatively short course to the flexor digitorum profundus muscle. It is very important to preserve this muscular input. After the ulnar nerve has been cleared to approximately 8 cm below the olecranon notch, it can be encircled with another Penrose drain.

Dissection is then carried into the olecranon notch alternatively from the upper arm and forearm levels. Bipolar forceps coagulation should be used in the olecranon notch because both arteries and veins accompany the nerve and are deep to it, lying on the floor of the notch, and these vessels bleed frequently. Usually, small neural branches to the elbow joint can be cut and thus sacrificed. After the nerve is free circumferentially, it is ready for transposition. The radial side of the pronator teres muscle is dissected distally and some of the lacertus fibrosis is sectioned to mobilize the proximal pronator muscle. A trough is made in an oblique and slightly curved fashion all the way through the pronator and proximal portion of the FCU muscles leaving a cuff of muscles and fascia along the distal medial epicondyle. The detached distal muscle mass is then gently elevated and slightly undermined, as is that portion left attached to the medial epicondyle.

The ulnar nerve is then placed in the muscle trough, and some fascia and superficial pronator muscle is reattached to the cuff of muscle and fascia on the medial epicondyle with 1–0 suture (Fig. 9-31). The FCU muscle is also reattached to the cuff of muscle along the distal portion of the medial epicondyle. The forearm FCU muscle is then closed over the nerve, but not before carefully grasping the nerve proximally and distally with gloved fingers

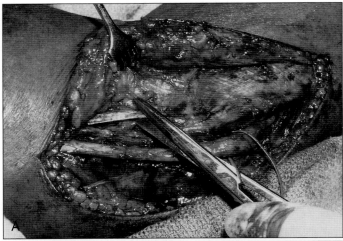

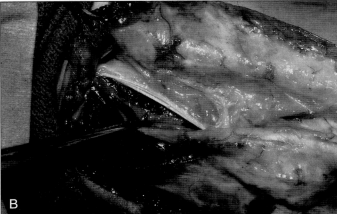

FIGURE 9-30 **(A)** Sectioning the intermuscular septum before transposition of the ulnar nerve is carried out as shown. An alternative step is to actually resect a segment of this fibrous tissue. **(B)** The operation is shown here being repeated on a subcutaneously transposed ulnar nerve, where the intermuscular septum had not been divided.

making sure it moves freely by gently tugging back and forth beneath the already partially closed volar musculature. The longitudinal split in the more distal FCU is closed only superficially so as not to compress the underlying nerve. Other soft tissues and the skin are usually closed subcutaneously without a drain.

If there has been a previous operation, this elbow incision is used, but is usually extended somewhat proximally and distally into the arm and forearm, respectively. This was especially necessary if a short elbow-level incision was used for a medial epicondylectomy or a neurolysis without transposition at elbow level. Because of the prior operation and usually subcutaneous position of the previously transposed nerve, a good deal of scar tissue is usually encountered. It is thus helpful to extend the proximal exposure far enough to find healthier nerve and then to trace the nerve throughout the scar and previously placed tacking sutures using sharp dissection with a No. 15 blade on a long, thin scalpel handle. In some cases, it is necessary to locate the distal forearm level ulnar nerve and work back toward and through the elbow level scar as well.

As has been reported by others, at LSUHSC some entrapment cases that had prior surgery were felt to be candidates for reoperation (Fig. 9-32).[6,57] There were a variety of findings common to these cases.

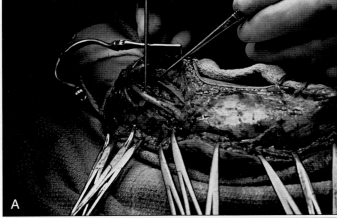

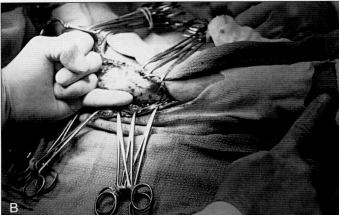

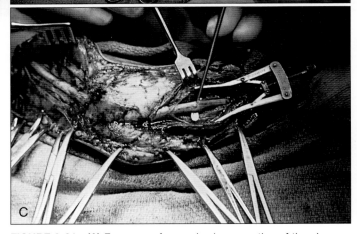

FIGURE 9-31 **(A)** Exposure of a proximal-arm portion of the ulnar nerve prior to transposition is seen. **(B)** A method of determining the forearm course of the ulnar nerve is illustrated. The base of the surgeon's ring finger rests in the olecranon notch and points toward his right forefinger, which is placed over the wrist portion of the ulna. A line projected between the two outlines the course of the nerve. **(C)** The ulnar nerve is exposed both above and below the olecranon notch. The spatula is beneath the distal or forearm-level nerve.

1. Extraneural scar over a length of the nerve was universal. Thus, great care must be taken in dissecting out the ulnar nerve.
2. Some cases had epineural thickening, intraneural scar, or even a neuroma, most likely related to injury from the prior operation(s). Several patients had sustained damage to the antebrachial cutaneous nerves or branches, and this appeared

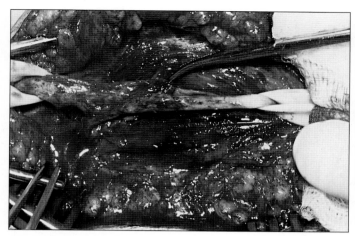

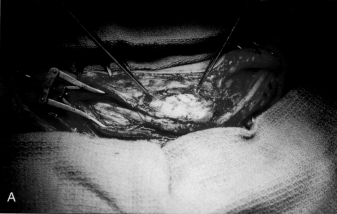

FIGURE 9-32 The appearance of an ulnar nerve is seen after two attempts to treat it surgically for entrapment. The first operation was a simple decompression through the olecranon notch and the cubital tunnel, whereas the second was a subcutaneous transposition volar to the elbow. When seen by one of the authors, the patient had an ulnar neuropathy with motor grades averaging 3 to 4 and sensation at grade 4. The patient had painful paresthesias in the ulnar nerve distribution and an exquisitely tender elbow with a Tinel sign over that portion of the nerve. An external neurolysis was performed and the nerve was buried deep to the pronator teres and flexor carpi ulnaris muscles. Over 1 year, the patient's pain has improved greatly, and motor grades are 4 with a sensory grade of 4+.

to be responsible for some of their persistent symptoms (Fig. 9-33).[17]

3. There was angulation or kinking of the nerve as it passed over the volar pronator teres muscle or more commonly as it left this subcutaneous site to penetrate between the two heads of the FCU muscle. In other cases, because of slippage or initial incomplete transposition, the nerve was found to be passing on top of the medial epicondyle. In some cases, the nerve was kinked or angulated at two separate levels. Usually, the intraoperative NAP recording showed marked conductive delays at either or both of these sites of angulation.

4. If prior medial epicondylectomy had been tried and had failed, the nerve was found to be partially volar, but still passing over the medial prominence of the epicondylar region. Because of a presumed limited neurolysis, angulation or kinking either proximally or distally was sometimes found (Fig. 9-34).

5. Several transpositions with submuscular burial done elsewhere had to be redone in this series. In two of these cases, the muscle trough had been incompletely created, the more medial FCU muscle was not divided or was incompletely divided, and the forearm-level nerve was severely angulated. In several other patients undergoing reoperations, it was apparent that the nerve had been placed in the pronator teres muscle rather than below it, and this may have led to persistent symptoms, as suggested by Dellon's experimental studies.[18]

DOCUMENTATION OF THE ULNAR ENTRAPMENT SITE

For study purposes, each of the ulnar nerves in the LSUHSC series of ulnar entrapments, whether having had surgery or not, had intraoperative NAP recordings made from the nerve both proximal to the olecranon notch and across the notch *before* the nerve was released at that level. After these recordings were made and the

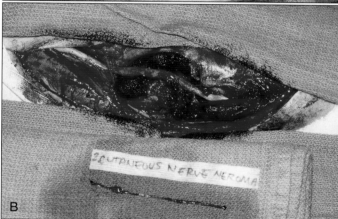

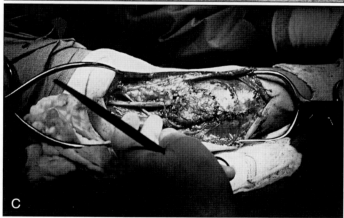

FIGURE 9-33 **(A)** This nerve has been cleared through the region of the olecranon notch by a complete external neurolysis. A trough has been made in the proximal forearm muscle by sectioning completely through the pronator teres and the more volar portion of the flexor carpi ulnaris muscles. **(B)** The nerve has been placed in the muscle trough. Note that a neuroma and segment of the antebrachial cutaneous nerve have been resected and are placed on the drape. This patient had undergone prior neurolysis for olecranon notch-level entrapment and experienced injury to the antebrachial cutaneous nerve. **(C)** The transposed nerve with closure of the pronator teres and flexor carpi ulnaris muscles over it. The proximal nerve is to the left and distal to the right in these figures.

nerve was freed entirely from the notch, NAP inching studies were done to see where the abnormality in conduction velocity (CV) and NAP amplitude were first evident, and where they were maximal. Results in cases without previous operations indicated the following observations:

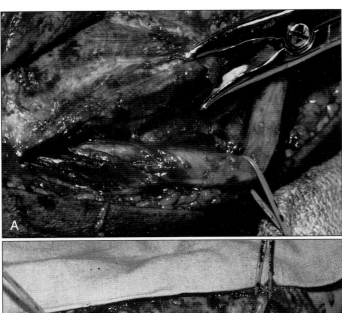

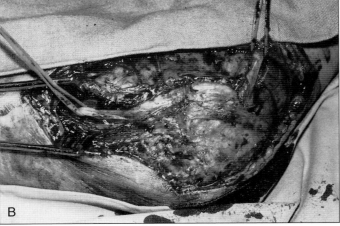

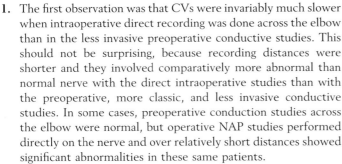

FIGURE 9-34 **(A)** The Ehni procedure is shown here. The ulnar nerve has been mobilized, and the medial epicondyle has been cleared of some of the pronator and flexor carpi ulnaris muscle origins. A Leksell rongeur was used to remove some of the medial epicondyle. **(B)** A scarred and somewhat angulated ulnar nerve that had been placed subcutaneously is seen. The nerve was subsequently cleared of scar and placed below the forearm musculature.

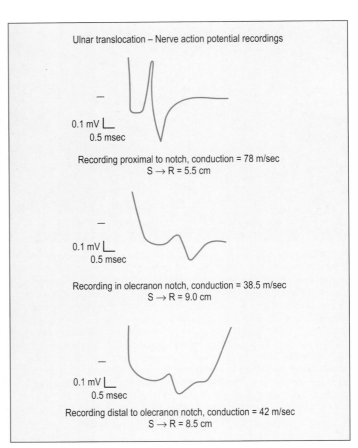

Ulnar translocation – Nerve action potential recordings

0.1 mV
0.5 msec

Recording proximal to notch, conduction = 78 m/sec
S → R = 5.5 cm

0.1 mV
0.5 msec

Recording in olecranon notch, conduction = 38.5 m/sec
S → R = 9.0 cm

0.1 mV
0.5 msec

Recording distal to olecranon notch, conduction = 42 m/sec
S → R = 8.5 cm

FIGURE 9-35 Intraoperative nerve action potential (NAP) recordings from a patient with mild but significant ulnar neuropathy and translocation of the nerve over the medial epicondyle on flexion and extension. The top tracing shows the recording proximal to the olecranon notch. The middle tracing shows an NAP recorded with an electrode on the nerve just proximal to the notch (where the amplitude is decreased and the velocity is slowed). The bottom tracing also shows a relatively small NAP amplitude and slowed response when the recording electrode was placed about 1 cm beyond the notch area.

1. The first observation was that CVs were invariably much slower when intraoperative direct recording was done across the elbow than in the less invasive preoperative conductive studies. This should not be surprising, because recording distances were shorter and they involved comparatively more abnormal than normal nerve with the direct intraoperative studies than with the preoperative, more classic, and less invasive conductive studies. In some cases, preoperative conduction studies across the elbow were normal, but operative NAP studies performed directly on the nerve and over relatively short distances showed significant abnormalities in these same patients.

2. Although amplitudes of NAPs across the olecranon notch sometimes increased immediately after neurolysis of the nerve, CV seldom did acutely (Fig. 9-35). In a few cases, amplitude decreased, presumably because of manipulation of the nerve in the region of the notch.

3. Although the CV was often slowed at the arm level in the ulnar nerve involved by a more distal entrapment, CV changes were usually maximal either just proximal to the notch or within the notch segment of the nerve itself.

4. The NAP amplitude was usually maintained in the upper arm, but began to dampen as the nerve approached the olecranon notch or was in the notch itself (Fig. 9-36).

5. It was rare for either CV or NAP amplitudes to be maintained through the notch area. In other words, the entrapment, injury, or irritative site appeared to be maximal within the olecranon notch segment of the nerve and not more distal beneath the two heads of the FCU muscle or what has been termed the "cubital tunnel."

These observations usually correlated well with the physical appearance of that portion of the ulnar nerve in the olecranon notch or groove. Sometimes, the nerve was swollen, injected, and "angry" in appearance in the notch area, but usually it had a compressed, narrowed, and/or scarred appearance.[10] In many of the cases, electrophysiological and, sometimes, gross pathological abnormalities began somewhat proximal to the olecranon portion of the nerve; in most others, changes were more severe in the "notch" portion of the nerve. There were only a few cases in which recordings were maximally abnormal just distal to the olecranon notch or in the

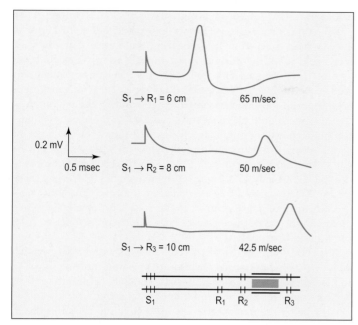

FIGURE 9-36 Typical nerve action potential recordings made operatively in a patient with ulnar entrapment neuropathy. In the top trace, S_1 to R_1 was recorded well proximal to the entrapment site; S_1 to R_2 was recorded just proximal to the olecranon notch and began to show slowing of conduction. A recording made more distally (S_1 to R_3) was also slowed.

area of the "cubital tunnel." These observations to date support the concept that most elbow-level entrapments originate in the olecranon notch or groove and not at a more distal site.

RESULTS

The following outcomes were accumulated with the help of Dr. John Reeves.

Ulnar nerve entrapment at the elbow level

The grading system used to evaluate the ulnar entrapments is found in Table 9-10 and is the scale used at LSUHSC. The system does not match or compare proximal with distal recovery, but instead concentrates on hand intrinsic motor and sensory function. These two modalities are the most seriously affected by most elbow-level ulnar entrapments. Most group I patients, as described in the prior section on differential diagnoses were grade 5 preoperatively, whereas group II usually were grade 4 preoperatively. Severe cases or group III patients were grade 3 or less preoperatively. Evaluated in that fashion, 15 patients in the series having surgery and 1.5 years or longer follow-up were in group I, 134 were in group II, and 311 were in group III.[43]

Among the 460 cases of ulnar entrapment undergoing operations for ulnar nerve entrapments, the incidence of bilaterality of the lesions studied was 65 (14%). One hundred and forty-seven patients had prior unsuccessful ulnar neurolysis and/or subcutaneous transpositions elsewhere in an attempt to stabilize or reverse the palsy. The patients who had undergone previous operations underwent repeat neurolysis and submuscular transposition. In a few patients, spontaneous cases were related to operative positioning or inadvertent compression during the course of an operation, but in most, a clear-cut cause was lacking (Fig. 9-37).

Table 9-10 Grading for ulnar entrapments

Grade	Description
0	No hand intrinsic muscle function; sensation grade is 0 to 1.
1	No hand intrinsic muscle function; sensation grade is 1 to 3.
2	Hand intrinsic muscle function is a trace (grade 1) or contract to antigravity (grade 2); sensation grade is 2 to 4.
3	Hand intrinsic muscle function is a grade 3; sensation grade ≥3.
4	Hand intrinsic muscle function is a grade 4; sensation grade is 4 or 5.
5	Hand intrinsic muscle function is a grade 5; sensation grade is 4 or 5.

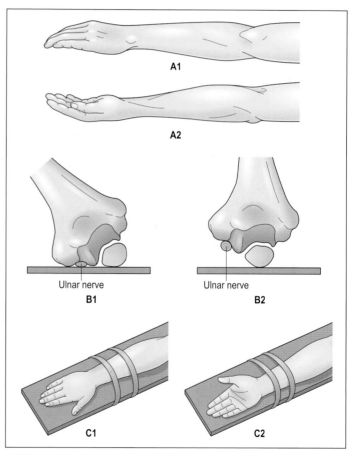

FIGURE 9-37 If the arm is extended and the elbow is held down on a firm surface such as an arm board, it is better to place the hand palm up, rather than palm down. The palm-up position is less likely to lead to compression of the ulnar nerve in the region of the olecranon notch.

The proper procedure to use for surgical management of ulnar entrapment remains most controversial, and there are advocates of each of the many different operational procedures. Operations include neurolysis without transposition, release of only the "cubital tunnel," neurolysis and transposition of the nerve to a subcutaneous site, medial epicondylectomy or the Ehni procedure, transposition to an intramuscular site and, finally, neurolysis with transposition to a submuscular site.[12,22,27,59,64,83,84] The last approach, originally described by Learmonth and refined by Leffert and Dellon and others, was used at LSUHSC for operative management of entrapments severe enough not to respond to conservative treatment.[13,51,52]

Tables 9-11 and 9-12 depict results in terms of grade stabilization or change after operation in fresh cases and in those having previous surgery elsewhere and requiring repeat operation. Follow-up for patients reported in these tables was a minimum of 1.5 years.

In the patients with fresh operations, with no prior surgery, and who had 1.5 years or more follow-up, 340 (93%) of 364 cases had an improvement in their level of motor function, and usually sensory function, postoperatively. There were 14 patients (4%) who had severe preoperative loss, i.e. were grade 1, 78 (21%) of patients were grade 2, 154 (42%) grade 3, 107 (29%) grade 4, and 11 (3%) were grade 5. At follow-up 212 (58%) improved one

Table 9-11 Pre- and postoperative grades for ulnar nerve entrapments undergoing initial operations* (n = 364 cases)

Postoperative grades	Preoperative grades				
	1	2	3	4	5
1					
2		1	2		
3		1	32	2	1
4		9	23	81	8	1
5		3	21	71	98	10

*Motor function improved one grade in 212 patients (58%), two grades in 95 patients (26%), and three or four grades in 33 patients (9%). No change in function was observed in 22 patients (6%) and function worsened in two patients (0.5%). (Table adapted from J Neurosurg 98:1001, 2003, with permission from the Journal of Neurosurgery.)

Table 9-12 Pre- and postoperative grades for ulnar nerve entrapments status – post prior operations* (n = 96 cases)

Postoperative grades	Preoperative grades				
	1	2	3	4	5
1	2				
2	1	2	1		
3	3	9	10		
4	1	4	23	12	
5	0	0	9	15	4

*Motor function improved one grade in 48 patients (50%), two grades in 16 patients (17%), and three grades in 1 patient (1%). No change in function was observed in 30 patients (31%) and function worsened in one patient (1%). (Table adapted from J Neurosurg 98:1001, 2003, with permission from the Journal of Neurosurgery.)

grade, 95 (26%) improved two grades and 33 (9%) improved by either three or four grades. Twenty-four patients did not improve. Twenty-two remained unchanged; 10 of those were at an excellent level (grade 5) at the start, and another eight were at grade 4 level. Two patients dropped one grade postoperatively: one patient was grade 5 and the other was grade 4 before surgery. This may have been caused by manipulation of the nerve during the operation.

It was more difficult to improve function in those patients who had undergone prior operations. Table 9-12 shows the course of 96 patients with 1.5 or more years of follow-up who had undergone one or more prior operations. Of the 96 patients, 50% improved one grade, but only 17% improved by two grades and 1% by three grades. Thirty (31%) of 96 cases had no improvement. Only one-seventh of these were grade 5 at the start. Fortunately, only one patient in this reoperative category had a decrease in function from the preoperative grade.

A special subset in the category of patients with prior operation were those who presented with severe pain and some neuropathy. In the first LSUHSC series of 368 cases of ulnar nerve entrapment, both severe pain and severe neuropathy (grade 2 or less) were present and reoperation helped in only 36%. On the other hand, if only mild or moderate neuropathy (grade 3 or better) was present along with severe pain, the response to reoperation was favorable in 87%. Even though the chance of recovery with severe loss is low, reoperation is often the only treatment alternative available besides tendon transfer for clawing.[26]

These results compare favorably to those reported by some contemporaries.[14,25,38] Despite this, it was surprising that so much objective improvement occurred. This was not only in the patients without previous operation that were spontaneous cases, but also in those with a history of trauma to the elbow and in those patients who had had a previous operation.

Regarding follow-up on two of these patients from this earlier series which was analyzed and published several years ago, one patient was returned to the operating room 24 hours postoperatively for a hematoma, with subsequent improvement postoperatively. We also know of one patient who underwent reoperation elsewhere for "scar" 6 months following our neurolysis.

REFERENCES

1. Adelaar RS, Foster WC, and McDowell C: The treatment of the cubital tunnel syndrome. J Hand Surg 9A:90–95, 1984.
2. Bauwens P: Electrodiagnostic definition of the site and nature of peripheral nerve lesions. Ann Phys Med 5:149–152, 1960.
3. Branch C, Kelly D, and Lynch G: Surgical exposure of peripheral nerves. In: Wilkins R and Rengachary S, Eds: Neurosurgery, vol. 2. New York, McGraw-Hill, 1985.
4. Brand P: Tendon transfer in the forearm. In: Flynn J, Ed: Hand Surgery. Baltimore, Williams & Wilkins, 1966.
5. Brooks DM: Nerve compression by simple ganglia. J Bone Joint Surg [Br] 34:391–400, 1952.
6. Broudy AS, Leffert RD, and Smith RJ: Technical problems with ulnar nerve transposition at the elbow: Findings and results of reoperation. J Hand Surg 3A:85–89, 1978.
7. Brown WF, Ferguson GG, Jones MW, et al.: The location of conduction abnormalities in human entrapment neuropathies. Can J Neurol Sci 3:111–122, 1976.
8. Buck-Gramcho D: Evaluation of perineurial repair with nerve injuries. In: Jupiter J, Ed: Flynn's Hand Surgery. Baltimore, Williams and Wilkins, 1991.

9. Bunnell S: Surgery of the Hand. Philadelphia: JB Lippincott, 1964.

10. Chang KS, Low WD, Chan ST, et al.: Enlargement of the ulnar nerve behind the medial epicondyle. Anat Rec 145:149–155, 1963.

11. Childress H: Recurrent ulnar nerve dislocation at the elbow. J Bone Joint Surg [Am] 38:978–984, 1956.

12. Craven PR Jr. and Green DP: Cubital tunnel syndrome. Treatment by medial epicondylectomy. J Bone Joint Surg [Am] 62:986–989, 1980.

13. Dellon AL: Operative techniques for successful management of ulnar nerve entrapment at the elbow. Contemp Orthop 16:17–24, 1988.

14. Dellon AL: Review of treatment results for ulnar nerve entrapment at the elbow. J Hand Surg 14A:688–700, 1989.

15. Dellon AL: Pitfalls in interpretation of electrophysiological testing. In: Gelberman R, Ed: Operative Nerve Repair and Reconstruction. Philadelphia: JB Lippincott, 1991.

16. Dellon AL: Techniques for successful management of ulnar nerve entrapment at the elbow. Neurosurg Clin N Am 2:57–73, 1991.

17. Dellon AL and Mackinnon SE: Injury to the medial antebrachial cutaneous nerve during cubital tunnel surgery. J Hand Surg [Br] 10:33–36, 1985.

18. Dellon AL, Mackinnon SE, Hudson AR, et al.: Effect of submuscular versus intramuscular placement of ulnar nerve: Experimental model in the primate. J Hand Surg [Br] 11:117–119, 1986.

19. DiVincenti FC, Moncrief JA, and Pruitt BA Jr.: Electrical injuries: A review of 65 cases. J Trauma 9:497–507, 1969.

20. Ebeling P, Gilliatt RW, and Thomas PK: A clinical and electrical study of ulnar nerve lesions in the hand. J Neurol Neurosurg Psychiatry 23:1–9, 1960.

21. Eckman PB, Perlstein G, and Altrocchi PH: Ulnar neuropathy in bicycle riders. Arch Neurol 32:130–132, 1975.

22. Fannin TF: Local decompression in the treatment of ulnar nerve entrapment at the elbow. J R Coll Surg Edinb 23:362–366, 1978.

23. Feindel W and Stratford J: The role of the cubital tunnel in tardy ulnar palsy. Can J Surg 1:287–300, 1958.

24. Forshell KP and Hagstrom P: Distal ulnar nerve compression caused by ganglion formation in the Loge de Guyon. Case report. Scand J Plast Reconstr Surg 9:77–79, 1975.

25. Foster RJ and Edshage S: Factors related to the outcome of surgically managed compressive ulnar neuropathy at the elbow level. J Hand Surg [Am] 6:181–192, 1981.

26. Friedman RJ and Cochran TP: Anterior transposition for advanced ulnar neuropathy at the elbow. Surg Neurol 25:446–448, 1986.

27. Froimson AI and Zahrawi F: Treatment of compression neuropathy of the ulnar nerve at the elbow by epicondylectomy and neurolysis. J Hand Surg [Am] 5:391–395, 1980.

28. Gay JR and Love JG: Diagnosis and treatment of tardy paralysis of the ulnar nerve. J Bone Joint Surg [Am] 29:1087–1097, 1947.

29. Gelberman R: Ulnar tunnel syndrome. In: Gelberman R, Ed: Operative Nerve Repair and Reconstruction. Philadelphia, JB Lippincott, 1991.

30. Gilliatt RW and Sears TA: Sensory nerve action potentials in patients with peripheral nerve lesions. J Neurochem 21:109–118, 1958.

31. Gilliatt RW and Thomas PK: Changes in nerve conduction with ulnar lesions at the elbow. J Neurol Neurosurg Psychiatry 23:312–320, 1960.

32. Goldner J: Function of the Hand Following Peripheral Nerve Injuries. Am Acad Orthop Surg Instruct Course Lectures 10. Ann Arbor, MI: JW Edmonds, 1953.

33. Grabb WC: Management of nerve injuries in the forearm and hand. Orthop Clin N Am 1:419–431, 1970.

34. Gross MS and Gelberman RH: The anatomy of the distal ulnar tunnel. Clin Orthop 238–247, 1985.

35. Grube BJ, Heimbach DM, Engrav LH, et al.: Neurologic consequences of electrical burns. J Trauma 30:254–258, 1990.

36. Grundfest H, Oester Y, and Beebe G: Electrical evidence of regeneration. In: Woodhall B, Beebe G, Eds: Peripheral Nerve Regeneration. Veterans Administration Monograph. Washington, DC, US Government Printing Office, 1957.

37. Haase J, Bjerre P, and Simesen K: Median and ulnar nerve transections treated with microsurgical interfascicular cable grafting with autogenous sural nerve. J Neurosurg 53:73–84, 1980.

38. Hagstrom P: Ulnar nerve compression at the elbow. Results of surgery in 85 cases. Scand J Plast Reconstr Surg 11:59–62, 1977.

39. Hubbard J: The quality of nerve regeneration. Factors independent of the most skillful repair. Surg Clin N Am 52:1099–1108, 1972.

40. Hudson AR, Berry H, and Mayfield FH: Chronic injuries of peripheral nerves by entrapment. In: Youmans J, Ed: Neurological Surgery, 2nd edn., vol. 14. Philadelphia, WB Saunders, 1982.

41. Hunt J: Occupational neuritis of the deep palmar branch of the ulnar nerve. J Nerv Ment Dis 35:673, 1908.

42. Kempe L, Ed: Operative Neurosurgery, vol. 2, New York, Springer-Verlag, 1970.

43. Kim DH, Han K, Tiel RL, et al.: Surgical outcomes of 654 ulnar nerve lesions. J Neurosurg 98:993–1004, 2003.

44. Kleinert HE and Hayes JE: The ulnar tunnel syndrome. Plast Reconstr Surg 47:21–24, 1971.

45. Kline DG and Hackett ER: Reappraisal of timing for exploration of civilian peripheral nerve injuries. Surgery 78:54–65, 1975.

46. Kline DG and Hudson AR: Complications of nerve repair. In: Greenberg L, Ed: Complications In Surgery. Philadelphia, JB Lippincott, 1985.

47. Kline D and Nulsen F: Management of peripheral nerve injuries producing hand dysfunction. In: Jupiter J, Ed: Flynn's Hand Surgery. Baltimore: Willliams & Wilkins, 1991.

48. Kline DG, Hackett ER and LeBanc HJ: The value of primary repair for bluntly transected nerve injuries: Physiological documentation. Surg Forum 25:436–438, 1974.

49. Kline D, Kim D, Hun K, et al.: Guyon canal: response to letter to the editor in Neurosurgical Forum. J Neurosurg 100:168–169, 2004.

50. Kumura J: Electrodiagnosis in Diseases of Nerve and Muscles: Principles and Practices. Philadelphia, FA Davis, 1983.

51. Learmonth J: A technique for transplanting the ulnar nerve. Surg Gynecol Obstet 75:792–801, 1942.

52. Leffert RD: Anterior submuscular transposition of the ulnar nerves by the Learmonth technique. J Hand Surg 7A:147–155, 1982.

53. Lewis GK: Trauma resulting from electricity. J Int Coll Surg 28:724–738, 1957.

54. Litter J: Tendon transfers and arthrodesis in combined median and ulnar nerve paralysis. J Bone Joint Surg [Am] 31:225–234, 1949.

55. Livingston W: Evidence of active invasion of denervated areas by sensory fibers from neighboring nerves in man. J Neurosurg 4:140–145, 1947.

56. Mackinnon SE and Dellon A: Surgery of the Peripheral Nerve. New York: Thieme Medical Publishers, 1988.

57. Mackinnon SE and Dellon A: Ulnar nerve entrapment at the elbow. In: Mackinnon SE and Dellon AL, Eds: Surgery of the Peripheral Nerve, New York: Thieme Medical Publishers, 1988.

58. Mallett BL and Zilkha KJ: Compression of the ulnar nerve at the wrist by a ganglion. Lancet 268:890–891, 1955.

59. McGowan AJ: The results of transposition of the ulnar nerve for traumatic ulnar neuritis. J Bone Joint Surg [Br] 32:293–301, 1950.

60. Michon J, Amend P, and Merle M: Microsurgical repair of peripheral nerve lesions: A study of 150 injuries of the median and ulnar nerves. In: Samii M, Ed: Peripheral Nerve Lesions. New York, Springer-Verlag, 1990.

61. Millesi H, Meissl G, and Berger A: The interfascicular nerve-grafting of the median and ulnar nerves. J Bone Joint Surg [Am] 54:727–750, 1972.

62. Moberg E: Objective methods for determining the functional value of sensibility in the hand. J Bone Joint Surg [Br] 40:454–476, 1958.

63. Murphey F, Kirklin J, and Finlaysan A: Anomalous innervation of the intrinsic muscles of hand. Surg Gynecol Obstet 83:15–23, 1946.

64. Neblett C and Ehni G: Medial epicondylectomy for ulnar palsy. J Neurosurg 32:55–62, 1970.
65. Nicholson OR and Seddon HJ: Nerve repair in civil practice; results of treatment of median and ulnar nerve lesions. Br Med J 33:1065–1071, 1957.
66. Omer G: Tendon transfers for the reconstruction of the forearm and hand following peripheral nerve injuries. In: Omer G and Spinner M, Eds: Management of Peripheral Nerve Problems, Philadelphia: WB Saunders, 1980.
67. Parks BJ: Postoperative peripheral neuropathies. Surgery 74:348–357, 1973.
68. Pollock LJ and Davis L: Peripheral Nerve Injuries. New York, Paul B Hoeber, 1933.
69. Riordan DC: Tendon transplantations in median-nerve and ulnar-nerve paralysis. J Bone Joint Surg [Am] 35:312–320, 1953.
70. Sakellarides H: A follow-up study of 172 peripheral nerve injuries in the upper extremity in civilians. Am J Orthop 44A:140–148, 1962.
71. Samii M: Use of microtechniques in peripheral neurosurgery: experience in over 300 cases. Tokyo: Igoku-Shoin, 1975.
72. Seddon H: Surgical Disorders of the Peripheral Nerves. Baltimore, Williams and Wilkins, 1972.
73. Shea JD and McClain EJ: Ulnar-nerve compression syndromes at and below the wrist. J Bone Joint Surg [Am] 51:1095–1103, 1969.
74. Siegel DB and Gelberman RH: Ulnar nerve: Applied anatomy and operative exposure. In: Operative Nerve Repair and Reconstruction, New York, JB Lippincott, 1991.
75. Speed JS and Knight RA: Peripheral nerve injuries. In: Campbell's Operative Orthopaedics, vol 1. St. Louis, CV Mosby, 1956.
76. Spinner M and Kaplan EB: The relationship of the ulnar nerve to the medial intermuscular septum in the arm and its clinical significance. Hand 8:239–242, 1976.
77. Strickland JW, Idler RS, and Deisignore JL: Ulnar nerve repair. In: Operative Nerve Repair and Reconstruction. New York, JB Lippincott, 1991.
78. Stromberg WB, McFarlane RM, Bell JL, et al.: Injury of the median and ulnar nerves: 150 cases with an evaluation of Moberg's ninhydrin test. J Bone Joint Surg [Am] 43:717–730, 1961.
79. Struthers J: On some points in the abnormal anatomy of the arm. Br For Med Chir Rev 14:170–179, 1854.
80. Sunderland S: Funicular suture and funicular exclusion in the repair of severed nerve. Br J Surg 40:580–587, 1953.
81. Sunderland S: Nerve and Nerve Injuries. Baltimore, Williams and Wilkins, 1968.
82. Terzis J, Daniel R, and Williams H: Intraoperative assessment of nerve lesions with fascicular dissection and electrophysiological recordings. In: Omer G and Spinner M, Eds: Management of Peripheral Nerve Problems. Philadelphia, WB Saunders, 1980.
83. Tindall S: Chronic injuries of peripheral nerves by entrapment. In: Youmans J, Ed: Neurological Surgery, 3rd edn. Philadelphia, WB Saunders, 1990.
84. Wilson DH and Krout R: Surgery of ulnar neuropathy at the elbow: 16 cases treated by decompression without transposition. J Neurosurg 38:780–785, 1974.
85. Woodhall B, Nulsen F, White J, et al.: Neurosurgical implications. In: Woodhall B and Beebe G, Eds: Peripheral Nerve Regeneration, Veterans Administration Monograph, Washington, DC: US Government Printing Office, 1957.
86. Zachary R: Results of nerve suture. In: Seddon HJ, Ed: Peripheral Nerve Injuries. London, Her Majesty's Stationary Office, 1954.

Ulnar nerve

10

Combined upper extremity nerve injuries

Robert J. Spinner and David G. Kline

OVERVIEW

- Not surprisingly, management of these injuries can be more complex then solitary nerve injury.
- Injuries resulting in lesions in continuity sometimes have one or more nerves that are regenerating and others that are not. Properly sorting out these lesions for neurolysis versus repair is extremely important.
- Reconstructive procedures are especially important in this subset of injuries.
- Complete injuries involving both median and ulnar nerves are difficult to reverse, especially when the lesions are at a proximal level.

Combined nerve lesions result in greater deficit than solitary ones. Such loss is very difficult to reverse. Return to work may be challenging. Nerve surgery may improve function to varying degrees but, even in the best situations, typically not to pre-injury status. Rehabilitation is demanding and lengthy, not only for the patient but also for those caring for the patient, and remains a critical part of the equation. Evaluation and sequential follow-up with physical and occupational therapists are necessary to maximize functional recovery and prevent soft tissue contractures. Rehabilitative programs should focus on range of motion, strengthening, and sensory re-education. Consultation with reconstructive surgeons should be considered; tendon transfers and other soft tissue or bony procedures may be available to augment function, especially in situations when neural recovery has been incomplete.

Because these combined nerve lesions are so complex, they have been tabulated as individual cases in Tables 10-1 through 10-5 so that individual management and outcomes can be studied.

COMBINED MEDIAN/ULNAR INJURIES AT ARM LEVEL

Combined median/ulnar injuries formed a relatively large category. This injury pattern is due to the nerves' relative juxtaposition to each other throughout their anatomic course in the upper extrem-

ity. This was especially evident in the upper arm, where muscle wounds, lacerations, fractures, contusions, and even iatrogenic causes involved both median and ulnar nerves (Table 10-1). Of the 22 patients with upper arm median/ulnar nerve palsies studied and operated on, 12 (>50%) had undergone a prior operation. In six cases, this was a vascular repair, while in four the wounds had prior extensive debridement. Preoperative loss was also complete in the distribution of both the median and ulnar nerves in 13 cases. Initial loss included all hand intrinsic muscles. This produced severe clawing of all fingers, or "main en griffe" (Fig. 10-1). Unless rehabilitative exercises, nighttime splinting, or aggressive management was initiated early, the end result was a poor one.

In the missile wound group of eight cases, half were caused by shotgun injury and half by single bullet and any fragments of metal or bone created by the impact. The interval between injury and operation was relatively brief and averaged 3–4 months. Although those neural elements having complete preoperative loss usually had repair, there was one exception because of a nerve action potential (NAP) across the lesion. This median nerve had a neurolysis despite complete loss preoperatively. Recovery was excellent, as it was for the ulnar nerve despite a proximal suture repair. Average grade for the median nerve in this subset of combined injuries was 4.0, and for the ulnar nerve, it was 3.3.

Lacerations involving median and ulnar nerves at the upper arm level were usually blunt and sent late for repair. Average interval between injury and repair was almost 5 months. Most (80%) of these combined lesions were complete preoperatively. Despite laceration as a mechanism, one ulnar and two median neuromas were in continuity, had NAPs, and required only neurolysis. Results, as with the combined missile wounds, were best for median nerve distribution muscles and less for ulnar ones (Fig. 10-2).

Contusion associated with fracture, blunt blows, or more sustained compression usually did not require operation. However, in five cases selected for operation involving both median and ulnar nerves, half of the injured elements required either suture or graft repair.

Two patients had iatrogenic injury resulting from an arteriovenous fistula constructed at an arm level for renal dialysis. Both had incomplete loss but also very painful paresthesias. This was caused

Table 10-1 Combined median/ulnar nerve injuries – upper arm

| Age | Sex | Mechanism | Prior operation | Loss | | Injury–op interval | Operation | | Results | | F (yr) |
				Median	Ulnar		Median	Ulnar	Median	Ulnar	
50	M	Shotgun	Vas rep	C	C	3 mon	G	G	3	2	2
32	M	Shotgun	Vas rep	C	C	4 mon	S	S	4	3	5
30	M	Shotgun	Debride	I	C	3 mon	N	S	3–4	2–3	1.5
32	M	Shotgun	None	C	C	5 mon	G	S	3–4	3	5.5
23	M	GSW	Debride	I	I	6 mon	N	N	5	3–4	3
44	M	GSW	None	C	C	3 mon	N	S	5	4	9
6	M	GSW	None	C	I	4 mon	S	N	4–5	5	17
6	F	GSW	None	C	C	1.5 mon	S	S	4	3	9
42	M	Laceration	Debride	C	I	3 mon	G	N	4	4–5	2.5
24	M	Laceration propeller	Vas rep	C	C	5.5 mon	S	S	3	2	8
28	M	Laceration	Vas rep	C	C	1 mon	G	S	3–4	2–3	2
45	F	Laceration	Vas rep	C	C	3 mon	N	S	4	3	II
23	M	Laceration/dune buggy	Vas rep	I	C	5 mon	N	G	4–5	2	2
22	M	Laceration	Debride	C	C	4 mon	G	S	4	3–4	6.5
22	M	Compound fracture	Neurolysis	C	C	1 mon	G	G	3	2	5
48	M	Fracture	None	C	C	4 mon	N	N	4	4	5.5
25	M	Fracture	None	C	C	II mon	G	G	2–3	2	5
27	M	Contusion	None	C	I	5 mon	S	N	4	4	3
65	F	Compression	None	I	I	2 wk	N	N	2–3	2–3	I0
36	M	A-V fistula for dialysis	CT Release	I	I	8 mon	N	N	4–5	4–5	4
60	F	A-V Fistula for dialysis	None	I	I	1 mon	N	N	4	3	3
38	M	Venipuncture swelling	Pain	C	C	11 mon	G	G	2–3	2	2

GSW, gunshot wound; Cmpd, Compound; Vas rep, vascular repair; CT, carpal tunnel; F(x), fracture; N, neurolysis and in case of ulnar elbow forearm, transposition as well; G, graft; S, suture; Split, partial suture or graft repair nerve, remainder had neurolysis; 1°, primary repair or immediate repair; 2°, secondary repair; C, complete loss of motor and sensory function; I, incomplete loss of motor and sensory function distal to level of injury; N/A, not applicable; F, follow-up.

by compression and scar enveloping proximal median and ulnar nerves. Fortunately, both patients improved with removal of the fistula and neurolysis of the nerves. In neither case was there clinical or electrical evidence of a superimposed or confusing peripheral neuropathy owing to renal disease or the dialysis process itself, or a "steal" phenomenon. The combination of injury or compression by an arteriovenous fistula at the forearm level involving median and radial nerves was seen in several other cases. This more periph-

eral compressive neuropathy is discussed further under median/radial lesions in this chapter.

CASE SUMMARY – COMBINED MEDIAN/ULNAR ARM LEVEL INJURY

This 44-year-old male sustained a .38-caliber handgun wound to the medial midarm area. At admission to the hospital, he had loss of radial pulse and a

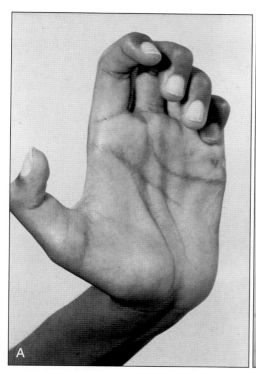

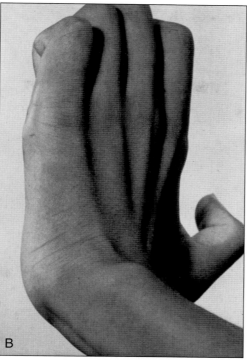

FIGURE 10-1 **(A)** "Main en griffe" hand caused by combined median and ulnar nerve injuries. Fingers and thumb are clawed, and thenar as well as hypothenar atrophy is evident. **(B)** Interosseous atrophy is evident on the dorsum of the same hand.

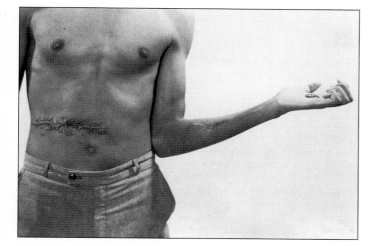

FIGURE 10-2 Combined median and ulnar nerve injury caused by a gunshot wound that crossed the patient's abdomen and penetrated the forearm. In his hand, the patient is holding the bullet that injured both the median and ulnar nerves.

complete median and ulnar nerve palsy. Using a saphenous vein graft, a repair of the brachial artery was done by the vascular service. Median and ulnar nerves were noted to be bruised and stretched but in continuity.

There was no clinical or electromyographic evidence of reversal of loss, so the area was re-explored about 3 months later. An NAP could be recorded across a median neuroma in continuity. One portion of the median nerve appeared to be more severely involved than the rest. As a result, the nerve was split into four bundles of fascicles. One bundle did not transmit and was replaced with two medial antebrachial cutaneous grafts 3.8 cm in length. Neurolysis alone was done for the remaining bundles which transmitted an NAP. The ulnar lesion did not transmit an NAP, so it was resected. Length was made up by mobilization

and transposition of the ulnar nerve. The ulnar nerve was mobilized to the junction of the upper and middle thirds of the forearm and then the distal stump was tunneled beneath the flexor carpi ulnaris and pronator teres. An end-to-end suture of the ulnar nerve was thus accomplished.

Follow-up at 1 year and 3 months gave an overall grade of 3 for the median nerve and 1 to 2 for the ulnar nerve. By 4 years, median nerve function graded 4 to 5 and ulnar, surprisingly, graded 3 to 4.

COMMENT

Initially and at the time of vascular repair, median and ulnar nerves were noted to be in continuity despite bruising, and therefore were not resected, and this was appropriate. Equally important is the need to explore even known lesions in continuity if there is no evidence of clinical or electromyographic improvement by 3 months or so.

COMBINED MEDIAN/ULNAR INJURIES AT THE ELBOW/FOREARM LEVEL

This was the second largest category of combined nerve injuries of the upper extremity (Table 10-2). Most of the nerves involved by laceration had complete loss and required repair. Although the average interval between injury and operative repair was relatively long, one sharp laceration by glass involving both nerves at the elbow level could be repaired acutely. Follow-up has extended to only 1.5 years on this case, but recovery grades by that time already averaged level 3. Whether the ulnar nerve had neurolysis or repair, it was transposed and placed deep to forearm muscles.

There were six combined lesions associated with fractures of the humerus or radius-ulna (Fig. 10-3). One distal humeral fracture was associated with a Volkmann ischemic contracture. A late neurolysis (at 11 months) done in conjunction with a flexor recession (slide) gave an incomplete result after 25 months of follow-up. In the other five fracture-associated cases, neurolysis of both nerves

Table 10-2 Combined median/ulnar nerve injuries – elbow/forearm

Age	Sex	Mechanism	Prior operation	Loss		Injury–op interval	Operation		Results		F (yr)
				Median	Ulnar		Median	Ulnar	Median	Ulnar	
26	M	Laceration/glass	Vas rep	C	I	5 mon	G	Split	4	3–4	11
21	M	Laceration/glass	None	C	C	None	S	S	3	3	I.5
24	M	Laceration/MVA	1° repair	C	C	7 mon	G	S	3–4	2	2.5
28	M	Laceration/glass	1° repair	C	I	14 mon	G	N	3–4	3	2.5
23	M	F(x) humerus	F(x) repair	C	I	4.5 mon	G	N	2	4–5	3
5	F	F(x) humerus	None	I	I	3M	N	N	4	4	6Y
29	F	F(x) humerus	Neurolysis	C	I	4 mon	Split	N	2–3	3–4	I
25	M	Volkmann	F(x) repair	C	C	11 mon	N	N	2–3	2–3	3
35	M	F(x) radius/ulna	1° ulnar repair	I	C	8 mon	N	S	5	3	9
10	F	F(x) radius/ulna	None	C	I	6 mon	N	N	4	3–4	3
46	M	Operative compression	Neurolysis ulnar	I (Severe loss)	I (Severe loss)	I yr	N	S	4	3	2.5
59	M	Operative compression	N/A	I	I	I3 yr	N	Split	5	3–4	2
56	M	Cardiac	N/A	I	I	2 mon	N	N	5	4–5	2
34	M	Electrical	Debride	C	I	10 mon	G	N	3–4	5	2.5

GSW, gunshot wound; Cmpd, Compound; Vas rep, vascular repair; CT, carpal tunnel; F(x), fracture; N, neurolysis and in case of ulnar elbow forearm, transposition as well; G, graft; S, suture; Split, partial suture or graft repair nerve, remainder had neurolysis; 1°, primary repair or immediate repair; 2°, secondary repair; C, complete loss of motor and sensory function; I, incomplete loss of motor and sensory function distal to level of injury; N/A, not applicable; F, follow-up.

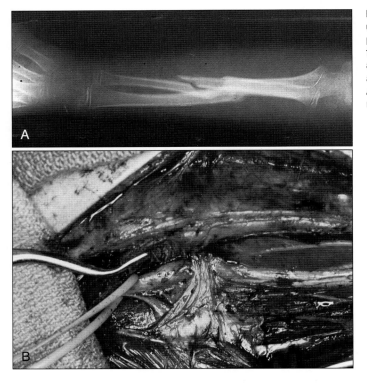

FIGURE 10-3 (A) Severe midforearm-level fractures of radius and ulna, associated with midforearm-level median and ulnar nerve palsies. **(B)** At operation 5 months after injury, median nerve was found entrapped by callus and scar. Ulnar nerve had a similar appearance. After external neurolysis, both nerves transmitted a nerve action potential beyond the injury site, so repair was not necessary. Almost full recovery occurred over the next 4.0 years. Proximal median is to the left and distal median to the right.

based on positive NAPs could be done. Recovery in the distribution of these nerves was, as expected, good. One other element could have a split repair, but only two of ten nerves required suture. Results in this group of combined median and ulnar nerve lesions associated with fractures were good. The case with a 1-year follow-up is progressing well, but further follow-up is needed. Both the laceration and fracture groups involving median and ulnar nerves at this level did surprisingly well (Fig. 10-4).

Iatrogenic cases were caused by compression or were secondary to prior operation or injection injury from cardiac catheterization. Loss was incomplete, but because of pain, an operation was done. Four of six involved elements had neurolysis, one a split repair, and one a suture. Results were good. The electrical injury was an unusual case caused by contact of an elbow with an extremely high-voltage source. Debridement of extensive soft tissue damage of volar and dorsal forearm areas had been done relatively acutely. Despite a late graft repair of the median nerve at 10 months after injury, overall median grade was 3 to 4 by 2.5 years of follow-up. Ulnar nerve function returned completely, but loss was incomplete in the early months after injury, grading 3, and only neurolysis and transposition of this nerve were done.

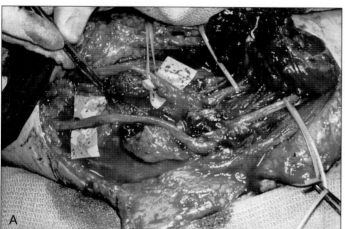
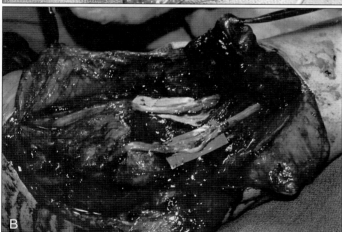

FIGURE 10-4 **(A)** Transecting injuries to median and ulnar nerves at elbow. **(B)** Ulnar nerve *(below)* required graft repair, whereas median nerve *(top)* required split repair. This case is not included in Table 10-2 but outcome for median nerve was excellent (grade 4), whereas that for ulnar nerve was grade 3 by 3 years postoperatively.

CASE SUMMARY – ELBOW-LEVEL LACERATION TO MEDIAN AND ULNAR NERVES

A 22-year-old male fell, and his arm went through a plate glass window. He required immediate repair of the brachial artery and biceps tendon. The nerve ends were tagged with tantalum clips, and the limb was casted. The patient had complete loss of both median and ulnar nerve function. The only muscle partially spared was pronator teres, which graded 3. Two weeks later, we explored the wound. Median and ulnar nerve stumps had retracted. After trimming these, four medial antebrachial cutaneous nerve grafts, measuring 6.5 cm in length, were used to bridge the gap in the median nerve. The gap in the ulnar nerve was made up by mobilization and anterior transposition and, as a result, an end-to-end suture repair of this nerve could be done. The immediate postoperative period was uncomplicated.

When seen for a 6-year follow-up, the patient could make a fist and could enclose his flexed fingers with his thumb. If he extended the fingers, the little finger tended to abduct. In the median nerve distribution, he had excellent pronation, flexor digitorum superficialis, flexor digitorum profundus (index and middle fingers), and flexor pollicis longus. Abductor pollicis brevis and opponens pollicis graded 3 to 4, and median sensation was 3. Overall median nerve grade was 4. In the ulnar nerve distribution, he recovered excellent flexor carpi ulnaris and flexor digitorum profundus (ring and little fingers), and even hypothenar muscles graded 4. Interossei and lumbricals were 3, and adductor pollicis was 3 to 4. Sensation graded 3, and overall ulnar nerve grade was 3 to 4. He could localize stimuli, but two-point discrimination remained poor. He would look at his hand when he used it for fine tasks, and he still had trouble picking up fine objects and buttoning clothes. He could use the hand to turn door knobs and could also turn the lid on a jar. As an owner of a grocery store, he stocks shelves and cuts meat. He says he can use the hand if necessary to write with a pen or pencil, but his grip is somewhat different because he uses more fingers to balance the grip of the pen on the thumb than before.

COMMENT

Even though the eventual result in this case was good, the patient was a candidate for immediate, primary repair since the injury was both transecting and sharp. The 2-week delay prevented an end-to end repair from being accomplished. Results from end-to-end repair (without tension) are superior to those achieved when an interpositional graft is used.

COMBINED MEDIAN/ULNAR INJURIES AT WRIST LEVEL

Most acute lacerations to the median and ulnar nerves at the wrist level by attempted suicides were cared for at a primary hospital, and thus our experience with this fairly frequent injury is relatively limited. However, five combined lesions that were cared for by us were caused by laceration (Fig. 10-5). Three cases had primary repair and have fared well, although ulnar nerve grades are 3 in two of these patients, and 2 to 3 in the other. Two cases had primary repair of both nerves and some flexor tendons done elsewhere within 24 hours of injury. Because of poor recovery, secondary exploration was done, and two of the four nerves required repeat suture (Table 10-3). Hypothenars recovered function, but interossei and lumbricals could contract only against gravity.

Two cases had pain problems associated with Colles' fractures and combined median/ulnar nerve palsies at the wrist level. Pain as well as function improved postoperatively in both of these patients. One was killed in another unrelated vehicular accident 2.5 years later.

There were two electrical injuries involving both of these nerves at the wrist level (Fig. 10-6). One had complete loss and required graft repair; the other had incomplete loss but severe pain, had a neurolysis, and noted improvement in the pain, either because of operation or simply with the passage of time.

No patient with complete loss in the ulnar nerve distribution gained more than a 3 as a postoperative grade. It seemed difficult to restore *strong* interosseous and lumbrical function, not only at this level, which was disappointing, but also at higher levels, which was not as surprising.

COMBINED MEDIAN/ULNAR/RADIAL INJURIES AT ARM LEVEL

Simultaneous injury of all three of these outflows without brachial plexus involvement was unusual, but did occur in four instances

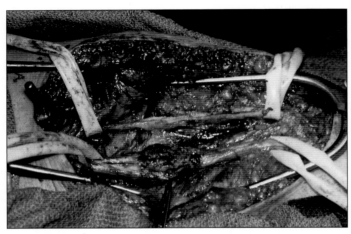

FIGURE 10-5 Combined injury involving both median and ulnar nerves at the level of the wrist.

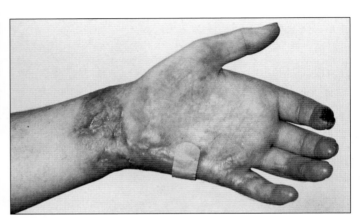

FIGURE 10-6 Severe electrical injury involving median and ulnar nerves at the wrist.

Table 10-3 Combined median/ulnar injuries – wrist level

| Age | Sex | Mechanism | Prior operation | Loss | | Injury–op interval | Operation | | Results | | F (yr) |
				Median	Ulnar		Median	Ulnar	Median	Ulnar	
14	F	Laceration/glass	None	C	C	None	S	S	3–4	3	5.5
12	M	Laceration/knife	None	C	C	None	S	S	4	3	7
28	M	Laceration/knife	None	C	C	None	S	S	4	2–3	2.5
35	F	Laceration/glass	1° repair	I	I	6 mon	S	N	4	3	6
47	M	Laceration/glass	1° repair	I	C	8 mon	N	S	4–5	3	5
75	M	Colles' (Fx)	N	I	I	19 mon	N	N	3 (pain better)	3–4	Died at 2.5
10	M	Colles' (Fx)	None	I	C	4 mon	N	S	4–5 (pain better)	3	7
55	F	Crush	N	I	I	3 yr	N	N	4–5	4–5	8
46	M	Electrical	Debride	C	C	8.5 mon	G	G	3–4	2–3	5
34	M	Electrical	Debride	I	I	5 mon	N	N	3–4 (pain better)	3	2

GSW, gunshot wound; Cmpd, Compound; Vas rep, vascular repair; CT, carpal tunnel; F(x), fracture; N, neurolysis and in case of ulnar elbow forearm, transposition as well; G, graft; S, suture; Split, partial suture or graft repair nerve, remainder had neurolysis; 1°, primary repair or immediate repair; 2°, secondary repair; C, complete loss of motor and sensory function; I, incomplete loss of motor and sensory function distal to level of injury; N/A, not applicable; F, follow-up.

(Table 10-4). Mechanisms were diverse, but three of the four patients had required earlier vascular repair. Two patients required repair of each injured element; the third had graft repair of two elements but only neurolysis of the involved ulnar nerve; and the fourth was able to have neurolysis of all three elements (Fig. 10-7). The individual case data are summarized in Table 10-4. Median and radial nerve distribution recovery was, as might be expected, superior to that for the ulnar nerve.

COMBINED MEDIAN/RADIAL INJURIES AT ELBOW/FOREARM LEVEL

Although at least eight examples of this combination of injuries were seen by us, it was surprising that this did not occur more frequently because the two nerves are in close proximity at this level. A variety of mechanisms were responsible for the injury in the cases studied, including fractures with a Volkmann contracture, shotgun wounds, laceration, venipuncture, and iatrogenic injury related to construction of an arteriovenous fistula (Table 10-5). Five prior operations had been done. Interval between injury and operation averaged 6.2 months. Eleven elements had neurolysis based on NAP recordings, four despite complete loss in their distribution preoperatively. There were five graft repairs. Average follow-up in this group at this level was 4.2 years.

Fortunately, radial nerve grades were excellent, because median and ulnar nerve recovery is significantly less useful without the presence of radial nerve function (or a satisfactory substitution with a splint). Median nerve recovery had an average grade of 3.2.

CASE SUMMARY – LACERATION WITH ARTERIOVENOUS MALFORMATION OF BRACHIAL ARTERY

A 19-year-old sustained a glass shard injury to the right antecubital fossa. He initially had a vein graft repair of his brachial artery. Median and radial nerve repair had been done elsewhere 9 months previously, and he had had a secondary procedure 8 weeks later for an arteriovenous fistula at the brachial artery repair site. For some reason, a bypass procedure was done, but the fistula was not excised. This bypass was a venous graft from upper arm brachial artery to radial artery. He presented to us with the following functional grades: in the radial

nerve distribution, brachioradialis 2, wrist extension 2, no finger or thumb extension; in the median nerve distribution, pronator 5 but flexor digitorum superficialis 3 to 4, no flexor profundus to the index finger, no flexor pollicis longus, no thenar intrinsics, no median-innervated lumbricals, and absent median sensation and sweating; in the ulnar distribution, hypothenar and hand intrinsics all graded 3.

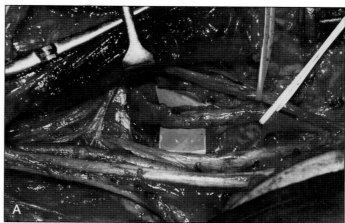

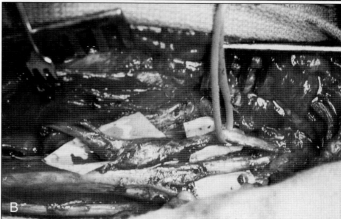

FIGURE 10-7 **(A)** Sorting out contusive injuries involving radial as well as median and ulnar nerves along the proximal and medial aspect of the arm requires careful dissection and a lot of patience. **(B)** Contused nerves at arm level secondary to gunshot wound.

Table 10-4 Combined median/ulnar/radial nerve injuries – upper arm

Age	Sex	Mechanism	Prior op	Loss			Operation				Results		
				Median	Ulnar	Radial	Interval	Median	Ulnar	Radial	Median	Ulnar	Radial
24	M	GSW	Vas rep	C	C	C	3 mon	S	S	G	3	2	3
26	M	Stab Wd.	Vas rep	C	C	C	4 mon	G	G	G	3–4	2	3
26	M	Crush	Vas rep	C	C	C	3 mon	G	N	G	3	3	3
25	M	Contusion/ swelling	None	C	C	C	1 yr	N	N	N	3	2–3	3

GSW, gunshot wound; Cmpd, Compound; Vas rep, Vascular repair; CT, carpal tunnel; F(x), fracture; N, neurolysis and in case of ulnar elbow forearm, transposition as well; G, graft; S, suture; Split, partial suture or graft repair nerve, remainder had neurolysis; 1°, primary repair or immediate repair; 2°, secondary repair; C, complete loss of motor and sensory function; I, incomplete loss of motor and sensory function distal to level of injury; N/A, not applicable; F, follow-up.

Table 10-5 Combined median/radial injuries – elbow/forearm

Age	Sex	Mechanism	Prior op	Loss Median	Loss Radial	Injury–op interval	Operation Median	Operation Radial	Results Median	Results Radial	FIY
27	M	Shotgun	Vas rep	C	C	3 mon	G	G	3	3–4	3
19	1.1	Laceration A-V fistula	1° repair artery, median nerve, & radial nerve	C	I	8 mon	G	N	5	5	10
23	M	F(x) radius ulna	F(x) repair	C	I	4.5 mon	G	N	2	4–5	1
20	F	Volkmann	None	C	C	6 mon	N	N	2–3	3–4	7
28	M	Volkmann	Fasciotomy	C	I	8 mon	G	N	3	4	5
58	F	A-V fistula for dialysis	None	C	I	6 mon	N	N	3	4	2.5
49	M	A-V fistula for dialysis	CT release	I (Severe loss)	C (Severe loss)	8 mon	N	N	2–3	3	3
46	M	Venipuncture	None	I	I	6 mon	N	N	4–5	5	2.5

GSW, gunshot wound; Cmpd, Compound; Vas rep, vascular repair; CT, carpal tunnel; F(x), fracture; N, neurolysis and in case of ulnar elbow forearm, transposition as well; G, graft; S, suture; Split, partial suture or graft repair nerve, remainder had neurolysis; 1°, primary repair or immediate repair; 2°, secondary repair; C, complete loss of motor and sensory function; I, incomplete loss of motor and sensory function distal to level of injury; N/A, not applicable; F, follow-up.

Table 10-6 Results of solitary radial, median, and ulnar nerve injuries by procedure done and level of lesion* (collected over a 15-year period ending in 1985)

Level	Partial or complete transection Primary suture	Secondary suture	Secondary graft	Split repair	Resection	In continuity + NAP Neurolysis	Split repair	−NAP Neurolysis	Suture	
Upper arm										
Radial	5/4	8/6	5/3	0/0	0/0	19/19	0/0	0/0	10/8	11/7
Median	3/2	1/1	8/4	0/0	0/0	21/19	1/1	0/0	5/5	6/4
Ulnar	4/2	2/1	1/0	2/2	0/0	10/9	1/1	3/1	3/2	5/2
Elbow level										
Radial	3/3	2/1	3/2	0/0	0/0	10/9	0/0	0/0	2/2	615
Median	2/2	2/1	3/3	0/0	0/0	30/28	0/0	0/0	4/3	9/6
Ulnar	6/4	10/7	311	0/0	1/0	36/24	1/1	0/0	9/7	4/2
Forearm or wrist										
PIN radial	3/3	2/2	715	0/0	0/0	19/18	0/0	0/0	2/1	5/4
Wrist median	13/11	2/1	2/2	0/0	0/0	15/14	0/0	0/0	11/9	615
Wrist ulnar	6/3	2/2	1/1	1/1	1/0	8/8	1/1	0/0	3/2	3/1
TOTALS	45/34	31/22	33/21	3/3	2/0	168/148	3/3	3/1	49/39	55/36

Intraoperative angiography showed continued fill from a varix arising from the brachial artery repair which still had flow through it despite the prior attempt to bypass this. A single varix arising from the artery was coagulated, then ligated and excised, and the vascular problem subsided. The original injury site was encased in a heavy vascular scar. The median nerve, on exposure, had a large neuroma in continuity. NAP recording showed a good NAP proximal to the neuroma, a smaller one to the midpoint of the neuroma, but no NAP beyond. Despite some proximal and distal mobilization, a gap of 2.8 cm remained after the resection of the neuroma. This was closed with eight pieces of sural nerve 3.2 cm in length. Histology confirmed an arteriovenous malformation and a neurotmetic Sunderland grade IV lesion in continuity to the median nerve. Scar was removed from around the radial nerve at the elbow level and from the ulnar nerve proximal to the olecranon notch.

Postoperative angiography showed resolution of the malformation and flow through both the original repair and the bypass. At clinical and electromyographic follow-up 4 years postoperatively, he presented with recovery of full wrist and finger function in the radial distribution; full hand intrinsic function in the ulnar nerve distribution; and full flexor digitorum superficialis, flexor digitorum profundus, and flexor pollicis longus function, plus partial recovery (2 to 3) of abductor pollicis longus, opponens pollicis, and lumbrical function in the median nerve distribution. Median nerve sensation graded 4.

COMMENT

Arteriovenous fistulae or pseudoaneurysms involving nerve usually require resection and occlusion so that adequate decompression is obtained.

SUMMARY

This surprisingly large category of nerve lesions is difficult to summarize because of the many combinations as well as the differing levels, injury mechanisms, and operations done. As a result, we have reported data from individual cases seen prior to 1994 in the tables and have grouped these as median/ulnar (46 cases), median/ulnar/radial (4 cases), and median/radial (8 cases) injuries at various levels. Operative experience with another 19 combined upper extremity lesions since 1994 has had similar outcomes. Axillary and musculocutaneous nerve lesions seen in combination with proximal median, radial, or ulnar lesions are addressed in the chapters on the brachial plexus. Despite some impressive results, at least as judged by the LSUMC whole nerve grading system, it was difficult for patients to regain a pre-injury level of function. Exceptions were injuries in which the radial nerve was severely injured but could be repaired, damage was more partial to median or ulnar nerves, and such partial loss reversed spontaneously. The combined median/ulnar injuries were especially devastating if loss in both distributions was complete. This resulted in "main en griffe" or clawing of all the fingers. Despite this deformity, repair of one or both nerves was worthwhile, even at proximal levels. In any combined case, it was especially important to ascertain whether any lesions in continuity could be spared complete or even partial resection by performing intraoperative nerve action potential studies. Overall recovery was, as expected, better if one or more nerves involved in a combined injury could have a neurolysis based on operative electrical evidence of either partial injury or significant regeneration. Intensive physical and occupational therapy is especially important in limbs with combined nerve injuries to prevent soft tissue contractures and promote strengthening. Tendon transfer and other reconstructive procedures which can augment function, should be considered relatively early, but may be performed later as long as the affected joints are sufficiently supple.

The results recorded in this chapter for combined or multiple lesions involving median, ulnar, and radial nerves should be compared with results collected over a similar 15-year period but affecting solitary nerves in the arm (Table 10-6).

11

Lower extremity nerve injuries

Daniel H. Kim and Judith A. Murovic

OVERVIEW

- Four hundred and twelve lesions involving the sciatic nerve at the buttock and thigh levels were managed at Louisiana State University Health Sciences Center (LSUHSC). Many injuries occurred at a proximal level, including the area of the sciatic notch, buttock, and thigh. Most patients with fracture and contusion-associated lesions and gunshot wounds (GSWs) involving the sciatic nerve were evaluated periodically for 2 to 5 months before exploration with intraoperative nerve action potential (NAP) recording and repair. The nerve was usually split into peroneal and tibial divisions to allow for separate evaluation and repair of each division, as indicated. This was important for most sciatic lesions in continuity, whether at a buttock or thigh level. In contrast, an attempt was made to repair sharp transections of the sciatic nerve as acutely as possible and when this could be achieved, the outcomes were excellent.
- The results of management of tibial division injuries were excellent, even if graft repair was necessary, and were universally good for neurolysis based on a positive intraoperative NAP recording across the lesion. Exceptions were lesions that had their origin at a pelvic level and extended through the sciatic notch to the buttock level, and a few lengthy lesions in continuity at buttock or thigh levels.
- Peroneal division laceration, GSW, and local iatrogenic injuries did much better than stretch injuries, even if end-to-end suture anastomosis or graft repair was necessary. Neurolysis based on a positive intraoperative NAP also resulted in good functional results. Repair led to enough recovery in approximately 30% of cases such that use of a kick-up foot brace was no longer necessary.

APPLIED ANATOMY

The sciatic nerve is formed from the anterior and posterior divisions of the L4, L5, S1, and S2 spinal nerves and the anterior division of S3 (Fig. 11-1). The anterior divisions form the tibial nerve and the posterior divisions, the peroneal nerve, and these two divisions join to form the sciatic nerve. At a buttock level, the two divisions of the sciatic nerve either envelop the piriformis muscle, i.e. one division is on top and the other below the muscle, or the divisions first combine to form the sciatic nerve, which then lies beneath or anterior to the piriformis muscle.

The posterior elements give rise to the superior and inferior gluteal nerves in the pelvis, which exit the pelvis via the sciatic notch to innervate the gluteus maximus and medius (Fig. 11-2). Next, the major branch to most of the hamstring muscles arises proximal to or in the sciatic notch region from the tibial division, the exception being the lateral hamstring, or short head of the biceps, which arises from the peroneal division of the sciatic nerve further distally in the proximal thigh. Branches to the gluteal muscles and gluteal vessels and the piriformis and hamstring musculature leave the sciatic notch in conjunction with the sciatic nerve. Dissection at this level of the sciatic notch is difficult due to the contiguous nature of these muscles and the gluteal vessels and vasculature to the nerves, which require careful dissection.

The thigh-level posterior femoral cutaneous nerve (Fig. 11-2) has a separate, but similar course to the sciatic nerve, lying posterior to the sciatic nerve and deep to the gluteus maximus muscle and becoming more superficial at the gluteal crease. The posterior femoral cutaneous nerve innervates the skin of the posterior thigh and leg for a variable distance toward the knee.

After arising proximal to or in the sciatic notch region as described, the major branch to most of the hamstring muscles travels through the buttocks, close to the tibial or medial division of the sciatic nerve. On reaching the upper thigh level this hamstring branch is medial to the sciatic nerve. Here the nerve to the short head of the biceps, also called lateral hamstring muscle, is found lateral to the sciatic nerve. At the upper thigh the major branch to most of the hamstrings divides to supply these hamstring muscles: the long head of the biceps, the semitendinosus, semimembranosus, and the ischial portion of the adductor magnus muscles (Figs 11-3, 11-4).

As described, while one or more branches to the hamstring muscles arise(s) from the sciatic nerve's tibial division, the fourth hamstring muscle, the lateral hamstring (Figs 11-3, 11-4), also called the short head of the biceps, is supplied by the peroneal division of the sciatic nerve. Thus, a lateral hamstring weakness, or

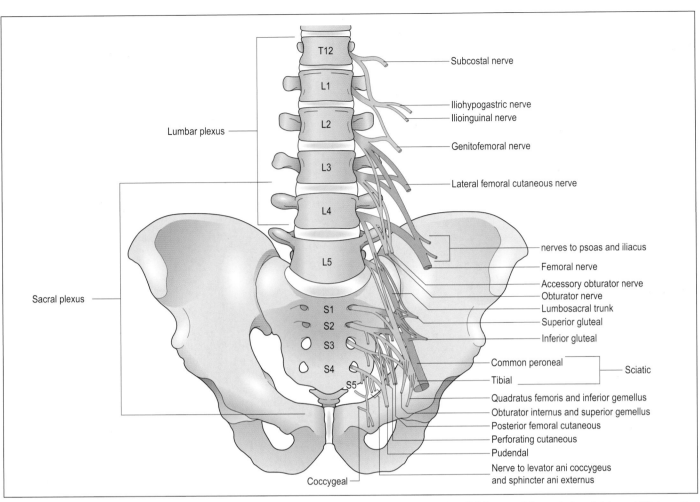

FIGURE 11-1 The lumbosacral plexus of which the L4, L5, S1, and S2 anterior and posterior divisions and the anterior division of S3 form the sciatic nerve.

The Sciatic Nerve with Gluteus Maximus Dissected and Reflected.

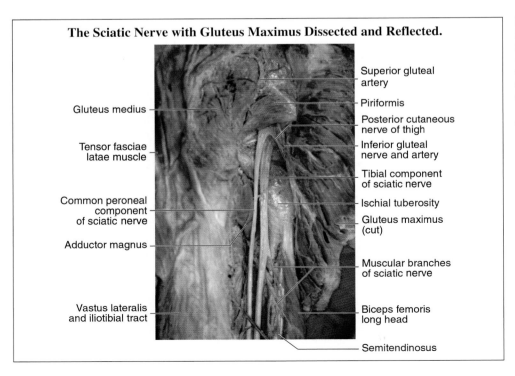

FIGURE 11-2 The gluteus maximus has been resected, and the sciatic nerve is shown entering the gluteal region through the greater sciatic foramen below the piriformis muscle. It then lies on the ischium. The nerve to the quadratus femoris is deep to it, and the posterior cutaneous nerve of the thigh is superficial. (From Kline DG, Hudson AR, and Kim DH: Atlas of Peripheral Nerve Surgery. Philadelphia, WB Saunders, 2001.)

The Sciatic Nerve at the Thigh Level.

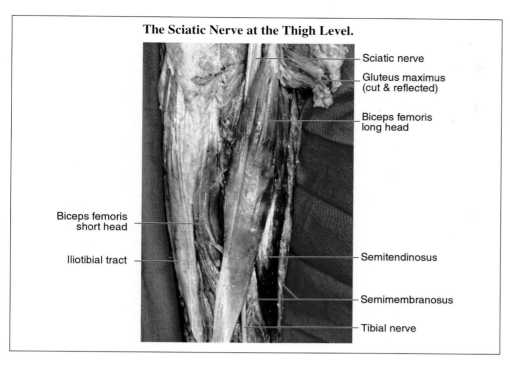

- Sciatic nerve
- Gluteus maximus (cut & reflected)
- Biceps femoris long head
- Semitendinosus
- Semimembranosus
- Tibial nerve

Biceps femoris short head

Iliotibial tract

FIGURE 11-3 A cadaver specimen showing a posterior view of the left leg and the site of the sciatic nerve at the thigh level, which here is covered superficially by the adductor magnus (not seen) which is lateral to the semimembranosus and semitendinosus and the long head of the biceps femoris muscles. (From Kline DG, Hudson AR, and Kim DH: Atlas of Peripheral Nerve Surgery. Philadelphia, WB Saunders, 2001.)

Divisions of the Sciatic Nerve Seen with Biceps Femoris Retracted.

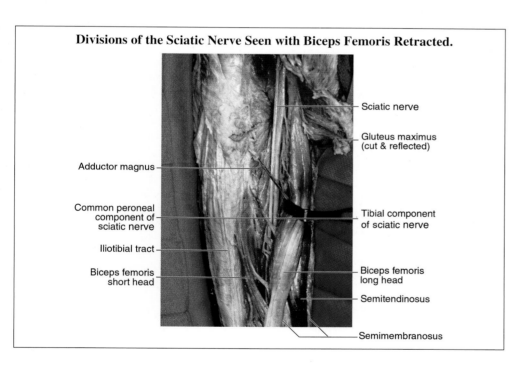

Adductor magnus

Common peroneal component of sciatic nerve

Iliotibial tract

Biceps femoris short head

- Sciatic nerve
- Gluteus maximus (cut & reflected)
- Tibial component of sciatic nerve
- Biceps femoris long head
- Semitendinosus
- Semimembranosus

FIGURE 11-4 A view similar to Figure 11-3, though now the biceps femoris long head is retracted and the adductor magnus partially removed. The sciatic nerve divisions can then be visualized, as shown. (From Kline DG, Hudson AR, and Kim DH: Atlas of Peripheral Nerve Surgery. Philadelphia, WB Saunders, 2001.)

paralysis accompanied by a foot drop, likely represents a proximal peroneal division injury.

The sciatic divisions lie on top of, or dorsal to, the obturator internus, gemelli, and quadratus femoris in the midportion of the buttocks and enter the thigh deep between the medial and lateral hamstring muscles. As the sciatic nerve proceeds distally, it bifurcates into tibial and peroneal nerves (Fig. 11-5), deep to the hamstrings at the junction of the middle and lower thirds of the thigh. Injury at or close to these levels can involve the tibial and/or peroneal nerve(s).

CLINICAL PRESENTATION AND EXAMINATION

The sciatic nerve and additionally the femoral nerve, discussed in another chapter, each with their separate anatomical course, are the two major motor and sensory innervations of the lower extremity. Except at a pelvic level, both nerves are unlikely to be injured concomitantly. If either nerve complex is injured alone, however, the ability to weight-bear with the involved extremity continues in spite of some paresis. For example, if the sciatic nerve is injured

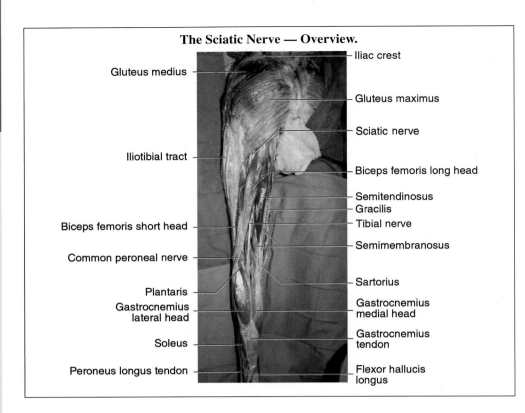

The Sciatic Nerve — Overview.

Gluteus medius

Iliotibial tract

Biceps femoris short head

Common peroneal nerve

Plantaris

Gastrocnemius lateral head

Soleus

Peroneus longus tendon

Iliac crest

Gluteus maximus

Sciatic nerve

Biceps femoris long head

Semitendinosus
Gracilis
Tibial nerve
Semimembranosus

Sartorius

Gastrocnemius medial head

Gastrocnemius tendon

Flexor hallucis longus

FIGURE 11-5 A cadaver specimen showing the posterior left buttock and thigh and the sciatic nerve as it enters the posterior thigh at the inferior border of the gluteus maximus. At the junction of the upper two-thirds and lower one-third of the thigh, the tibial and peroneal divisions separate to form their respective tibial and common peroneal nerves. (From Kline DG, Hudson AR, and Kim DH: Atlas of Peripheral Nerve Surgery. Philadelphia, WB Saunders, 2001.)

below the hamstring branches, but the femoral nerve is functional, the patient can flex the leg at the knee using the hamstring muscles supplied by the hamstring branches of the sciatic nerve and extend the leg and lock the knee using the femoral-supplied quadriceps muscles. With a kick-up foot brace to substitute for loss of foot dorsiflexion by the tibialis anterior muscle, in turn innervated by the sciatic nerve's deep peroneal branch, the patient can bear weight and walk with a surprisingly normal gait.

Conversely, most patients with an intact sciatic outflow are able to compensate for a complete femoral palsy. The patient learns to throw out the thigh or lower leg, although the knee cannot be locked. The hamstrings provide knee flexion, and the foot with its intact gastrocnemius-soleus muscles' plantar flexion and dorsiflexion gives good stability. Thus, this compensatory role of the femoral nerve in sciatic dysfunction is a favorable factor in sciatic and other lower extremity nerve injuries. Another positive factor is that two of three major motor territories are served by the tibial and femoral nerves, which can regenerate very well with proper management.

Despite these favorable considerations, distances required for regeneration from the injury site to significant motor inputs are some of the greatest in the body. As a result, the time required for regrowth is lengthy and when fibers reach innervational input sites, irreversible atrophy or replacement by fibrosis or fat may have occurred. In addition, although the peroneal nerve is similar to the radial nerve, i.e. the peroneal nerve supplies extensor muscles and its sensory inputs are relatively unimportant. Unlike the radial nerve, though, results gained by spontaneous regeneration after injury or from repair can be relatively poor. Another factor limiting recovery is the high association of sciatic nerve injury with serious bony or vascular damage in the leg.[11,33]

Buttock-level sciatic nerve injury with or without loss of the hamstring branches can give variable patterns of weakness in a tibial and/or peroneal division distribution. It is rare for lesions at this level to involve branches to the gluteus maximus and medius muscles, with the exception of the occasional penetrating injury near the sciatic notch. It is also unusual for a buttock-level sciatic injury to totally paralyze the hamstring muscles. Thus, since the glutei are not usually paretic, the proximal level of the lesion may be evidenced by paresis of the lateral hamstring, i.e. short head of the biceps femoris. Interestingly, it is known that the peroneal division already carries fibers at a buttock level, which are destined for the more distal hamstring complex.[14] A complete sciatic injury at buttock level gives the more certain loss of plantar flexion, foot inversion, toe flexion, and toe spread. There is also lack of foot eversion and dorsiflexion and toe extension.

The peroneal division rather than the tibial division is often preferentially injured at a high proximal level. Reasons for this are unclear; however, it may be related to the peroneal division's more lateral position relative to the tibial division and thus its greater exposure to stretch/contusion during blunt trauma such as fractures or hip dislocations.[34] It seems to be preferentially involved, however, if the sciatic nerve is injured by injection at the buttock level, as well. Of interest, loss with peroneal division injury at a buttock level can include weakness in inversion, since a fascicle destined for the posterior tibialis muscle via the tibial division may travel a short proximal distance in the peroneal division.

Sunderland has listed other possible reasons for the peroneal division's more frequent involvement and difficulty in attaining recovery.[40] These factors include a relatively poor blood supply, its relative lateral position close to the hip joint with increased exposure to injuring forces, a decreased amount of connective tissue between fascicles as compared with the tibial division, and its relative tethering, especially at the fibular head. Recovery also requires coordinated reinnervation along the course of the peroneal nerve-supplied long extensor muscles of the lower leg's anterior compartment.

The examination to detect a sciatic palsy is relatively straightforward. In a sitting position, the patient is asked to flex the knee, at which time the examiner can palpate and visualize contractions of the lateral and medial hamstrings. With the leg extended and with gentle pressure against the sole of the foot, the examiner can evaluate plantar flexion and can use the other hand to palpate the gastrocnemius-soleus muscles in the calf. Inversion of the foot and flexion and spread of the toes should be tested, and dorsiflexion or extension of the foot can be seen and the anterior tibial muscle palpated. The ability to evert the foot by the peronei muscles is determined, as is extension of the great toe by the extensor hallucis longus muscle and the second to fifth toes by the extensor digitorum longus muscle. Response to touch and pinprick on the sole of the foot are examined. The saphenous branch of the femoral nerve may supply skin distal to the medial malleolus and loss in this distribution should not be misinterpreted as due to a sciatic nerve deficit.

ELECTROPHYSIOLOGICAL STUDIES

ELECTROMYOGRAPHY

A pelvic-level lesion is suggested by denervational changes in the glutei, quadratus femoris, or obturator muscles. To differentiate pelvic plexus injury from proximal sciatic nerve injury, a careful electromyogram (EMG) study of a proximal sciatic lesion will show denervational changes in distal lower extremity muscles. A penetrating buttock wound can affect gluteal nerves or muscles and the sciatic nerve; thus, a clinical history and examination are also important accompaniments to the EMG. Two additional caveats are as follows: first, percutaneous needle sampling of muscles such as the piriformis, the quadratus femoris, and sometimes the glutei is not always practical; second, branches to the quadratus femoris and glutei muscles can originate at a pelvic level and leave with the sciatic nerve through the notch. These latter nerves can thus be injured by a more distal lesion.

A related electrodiagnostic challenge centers on the hamstring muscles. The proximal tibial division is the source of a large branch to all the hamstring muscles with the exception of a branch to the short head of the biceps, which is supplied by the peroneal division. The former hamstring branch travels parallel to the sciatic nerve at a buttock-to-proximal thigh level, but is often spared despite serious injury to the sciatic nerve at that level. As a result, only a few of the LSUHSC series' patients with buttock-level sciatic lesions had semimembranosus, semitendinosus, or large head of the biceps loss, either by clinical or electrical examination. On the other hand, if loss was in a peroneal distribution, a search for and finding of denervational changes in the lateral hamstring muscle, i.e. short head of the biceps, suggested a more proximal sciatic lesion, rather than a more distal peroneal nerve lesion.

The gastrocnemius muscle was the most valuable to study electrically for early recovery of sciatic function, since electrical and clinical recovery is much quicker in this tibial-innervated muscle compared with the superficial peroneal-innervated peronei muscles. Unfortunately, recovery in the tibial distribution's gastrocnemius-soleus muscle does not promise recovery in the peroneal-innervated evertor or dorsiflexor muscles. Nascent or reinnervational changes in tibial-innervated muscles are also more likely to presage useful recovery than such changes in peroneal-innervated muscles. In some cases, enough fibers may return to the peroneal-innervated muscles in the anterior compartment, however, to compensate for the delayed reversal of denervation. There may be too few fibers or fibers of insufficient size, myelination, and perhaps most importantly, reinnervational complexity, to restore peroneal function, however.

In addition to the gastrocnemius-soleus muscles, the usual muscles sampled for tibial division or tibial nerve injuries include the tibialis posterior muscle, which provides foot inversion, and the flexor hallucis longus, the great toe flexor muscle. Muscles sampled for the peroneal division or peroneal nerve are usually the peroneus longus and brevis muscles, which together provide foot eversion, the anterior tibialis muscle, which is the foot dorsiflexor muscle, and the extensor hallucis longus and extensor digitorum longus muscles, which extend the great toe and the second to fifth toes, respectively. Reinnervation and its accompanying electrical changes do not always proceed in an orderly fashion down these two cascades of muscles, especially with injury to the peroneal nerve. For example, the superficial peroneal-innervated peronei and deep peroneal-innervated extensor digitorum longus muscles may recover; however, the deep peroneal-innervated anterior tibialis and extensor hallucis muscles may not. Even the tibial division can display electrical and clinical peculiarities as far as reinnervation is concerned: tibialis posterior muscle recovery may not approach that seen with the gastrocnemius-soleus muscles, and flexor digitorum longus muscle recovery may, if it occurs at all, be superior to that of the flexor hallucis longus muscle.

The occasional painless foot drop associated with a lateral disc herniation with L5 nerve root compression can sometimes be differentiated from peroneal division injury not only by magnetic resonance imaging (MRI) or computed tomography (CT) scan findings in the spine, but also by documenting denervation of the paraspinal and posterior tibialis muscles, as well as anterior tibialis muscle denervation on EMG testing.[36] By comparison, an inappropriate lumbar laminectomy can be all too easily performed if the peroneal nerve is not appreciated as the true site of pathology.

Partial lesions to the sciatic complex, whether caused by compression or more direct injury, tend to maximally affect more distal muscles, just as with similar radial, median, and ulnar nerve lesions.[13] As a result, the electromyographer may have to sample toe flexor and extensor muscles or, on occasion, foot intrinsic muscles to document milder sciatic lesions, particularly those caused by compression.

SURGICAL EXPOSURE

BUTTOCK-LEVEL SCIATIC NERVE

For the surgical approach to the buttock-level sciatic nerve the patient is placed in the prone position, which also maximizes positioning for harvesting one or both sural nerves.[26] The knee is padded, the leg is mildly flexed on the thigh, and a folded sheet is placed under the anterior iliac crest on the side of the dissection, which tends to rotate the buttock up and somewhat medially.

The skin incision for the buttock-level exposure is curvilinear and begins at the posterior inferior iliac spine and continues around the lateral buttock. The incision must begin sufficiently superiorly, so that after the gluteal muscle is retracted medially, the notch is displayed without difficulty (Fig. 11-6).[35] If exposure of the sciatic nerve beneath the buttock and in the proximal thigh is necessary, the incision is extended into the buttock crease and then down the

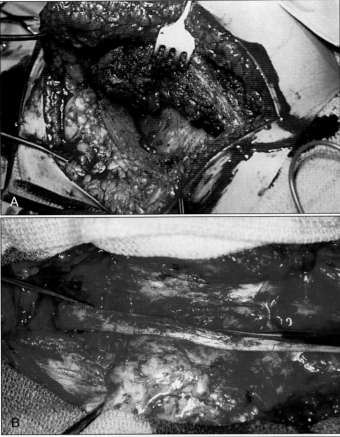

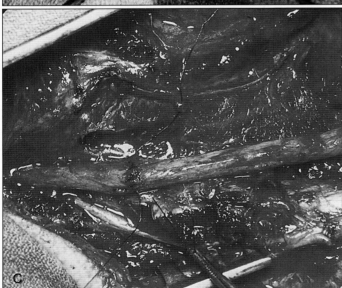

FIGURE 11-6 **(A)** The exposure of sciatic nerve at the level of the buttock includes transection of the lateral gluteus maximus and medius muscles, leaving a cuff of muscle laterally to which to sew back. Here, a rake is being used to retract the left buttock musculature medially. The patient is prone and the back is to the left with the thigh to the right. **(B)** A contusion of the sciatic nerve is shown close to the sciatic notch area, which is to the left. The thigh is to the right. **(C)** Suture of the sciatic nerve at a buttock level after resection of neuroma in continuity is seen. The injury to this nerve was caused by contusion associated with hip fracture.

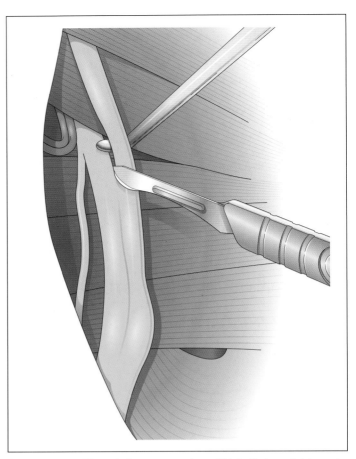

FIGURE 11-7 The sciatic nerve can be split into its two divisions at the buttock level using a scalpel as shown. (From Kline DG, Hudson AR, and Kim DH: Atlas of Peripheral Nerve Surgery. Philadelphia, WB Saunders, 2001.)

posterior midline of the thigh. The sciatic nerve can always be identified at this point, and followed up to the sciatic notch area. If necessary the nerve can be split into its two divisions (Fig. 11-7).

For exposure of the sciatic nerve at the sciatic notch, the gluteus maximus muscle and a portion of the medius muscle are separated close to the lateral pelvic brim and mobilized and retracted medially with rakes or Richardson retractors to expose the nerve up to the sciatic notch. A rim of gluteal muscle should be left laterally and tagged by heavy sutures attached to their needles to facilitate later closure. There is a somewhat avascular plane beneath the gluteal musculature and posterior to the neural structures, which can be followed medially to the sciatic nerve. Care must be taken with the dissection to preserve the hamstring branch, which lies somewhat medial and superior to the main sciatic nerve. As one approaches the area of the sciatic notch, gluteal nerves and gluteal vessels also need to be preserved, since the innervation of the gluteus medius muscle is critical to the stability of the hip joint (Fig. 11-8). The gluteus medius is the "deltoid muscle" of the hip and maintains the pelvis whenever the patient weight-bears solely on that limb.

Gluteal vessels high in the region of the notch must be ligated or coagulated prior to their division, since open vessels can retract

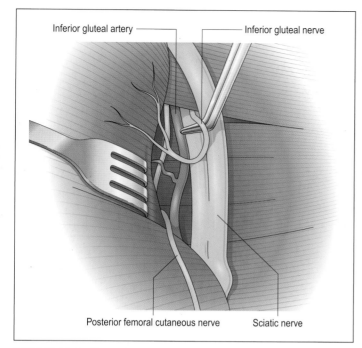

Inferior gluteal artery — Inferior gluteal nerve

Posterior femoral cutaneous nerve — Sciatic nerve

FIGURE 11-8   The sciatic nerve's inferior gluteal branch is shown as are the deeper hamstring and posterior femoral cutaneous nerves of the thigh. (From Kline DG, Hudson AR, Kim DH: Atlas of Peripheral Nerve Surgery, Philadelphia, 2001, WB Saunders Company.)

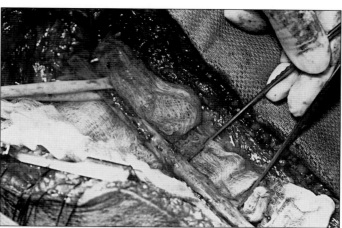

FIGURE 11-9   The long head of the biceps muscle has been displaced to expose a severe compressive lesion of the sciatic nerve at a midthigh level. This unusual circumstance occurred in a female accountant who habitually sat forward on an unpadded wooden chair without using the back rest. As a result, much of her weight compressed the posterior right thigh, and she developed a severe and progressive sciatic palsy involving both divisions. There was local tenderness and a Tinel sign at the midthigh level. The nerve action potential (NAP) amplitude and velocity, although somewhat reduced and slowed, were easily measured down to the tip of the forceps. There was a marked drop in NAP amplitude and slowing of the velocity to 20 m/sec beyond this point, with these reductions being most prominent between the two forceps tips. An external neurolysis was performed.

into the pelvis and bleed unchecked. This would then require an emergent transabdominal approach and a difficult pelvic dissection to correct.

THIGH-LEVEL SCIATIC NERVE

The approach to the sciatic nerve located in the thigh is relatively straightforward. A mildly curvilinear posterior thigh skin incision is preferred. This incision may be taken in a lateral and curved direction around the edge of the buttock for more proximal exposure or extended into the popliteal fossa for more distal exposure of the sciatic complex. At the thigh level, the hamstring muscles are readily split in the midline and retracted with Weitlaner self-retaining, Army-Navy or Richardson retractors. The long head of the biceps lies between the operator and the sciatic nerve and this muscle is easily mobilized, displaying the sciatic nerve in the posterior thigh (Fig. 11-9).

Sharp dissection with a No. 15 scalpel blade mounted on a long-handled knife is supplemented by the use of Metzenbaum scissors. Such dissection is used to expose the nerve in a circumferential fashion proximal and distal to the injury site after which dissection is performed from either end of the exposure toward the injury site. More distal hamstring branches and major collateral vessels to the sciatic nerve are spared, although the latter can be sacrificed if necessary. After intraoperative stimulation and recording on lesions in continuity is undertaken, the sciatic nerve can be split into its two divisions, each being evaluated independently (Fig. 11-10). The natural plane between the two divisions can be visualized with the aid of loupes or a low-power setting of the microscope. Devel-

oping this plane is carried out by placing Penrose drains around the two nerves and gently spreading the divisions apart from a caudal to a cephalad direction so that the more proximal whole sciatic nerve is split into its two divisions. If there is difficulty in developing this plane, the tibial and peroneal nerves can be isolated in the popliteal fossa and traced proximally. If the sciatic nerve is found to bifurcate at a mid-thigh or higher level, this portion of the dissection becomes easier.

RESULTS

BUTTOCK-LEVEL SCIATIC NERVE

The grading criteria for the LSUHSC series in this chapter are listed in Tables 11-1 and 11-2. Results are reported by injury or lesion category, by operations at a buttock or thigh level, and by surgical techniques performed (Tables 11-3 and 11-4). There are only a few series of sciatic injuries of any size previously reported,[8,9,19,22] and a number of articles attempt to summarize management.[2,4,21,25,28,46] Most series concentrate on GSWs involving the sciatic nerve.[6,23,29–31] Tumors are not included in the LSUHSC results cited in the tables, but are sometimes referred to in the text.

Injection injury

Forty-two percent of the sciatic lesions were at a buttock level, with injection injury the largest category of sciatic lesions here (Table 11-3). Injection injury patients are often thin or chronically ill and thus debilitated[7] and have a poor gluteal soft tissue covering

215

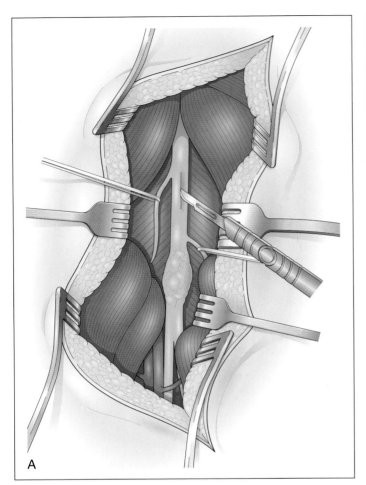
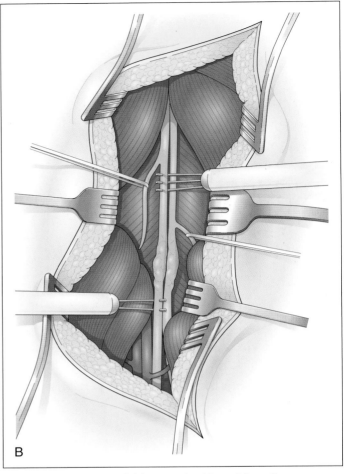

FIGURE 11-10 **(A)** The thigh-level sciatic nerve is shown in this drawing, being split into its two divisions proximal to an injury site. **(B)** Stimulating and recording electrodes are shown being placed across the tibial portion of an injury in continuity. This is done after splitting the entire sciatic nerve into its two divisions as the result of a conducted intraoperative NAP. (From Kline DG, Hudson AR, and Kim DH: Atlas of Peripheral Nerve Surgery. Philadelphia, WB Saunders, 2001.)

Table 11-1 LSUHSC motor grading system for the buttock and thigh-level peroneal divisions

Grade	Evaluation	Description
0	Absent	No or little function in the short head of biceps; no peroneal function; no AT, no EHL or ED function
1	Poor	Short head of the biceps contracts; no distal peroneal-innervated muscle function
2	Fair	Short head of the biceps contracts; peroneus muscles contract against gravity or better; no trace of AT; no other distal motor function
3	Moderate	Short head of biceps contracts; peroneus muscles are grade 3 or better; AT contracts against gravity, but the function of EHL & ED for toes usually absent
4	Good	Short head of biceps and peroneus muscles contract, as does AT, which is grade 3 or better; EHL & ED may have trace function
5	Excellent	Short head of biceps & peroneus muscles contract; AT grade 4 or better; EHL & ED contract at least against gravity

LSUHSC, Louisiana State University Health Sciences Center; AT, anterior tibialis; EHL, extensor hallucis longus; ED, extensor digitorum.

Table 11-2 LSUHSC motorsensory grading system for the buttock and thigh-level tibial divisions

Grade	Evaluation	Description
0	Absent	No gastrocnemius-soleus function; no inversion, no toe flexion; little or no sensation on the plantar surface of the foot
1	Poor	Trace gastrocnemius, but no other tibial muscle function; trace to poor plantar sensation
2	Fair	Gastrocnemius contracts against gravity only; plantar surface sensation usually grade 2 or better
3	Moderate	Gastrocnemius-soleus contracts against gravity and some force; trace or better inversion; plantar sensation is grade 3 or better
4	Good	Gastrocnemius contracts against moderate resistance; inversion grade 3 or better; either a trace or no toe flexion; sensation grade 4 or better
5	Excellent	Gastrocnemius has full function; inversion grade 4 or better; toe flexion present; plantar sensation grade 4 or better

LSUHSC, Louisiana State University Health Sciences Center.

Table 11-3 Operative results for buttock-level sciatic nerve injuries in 175 patients*

Type of injury	No. of patients	Neurolysis**		Suture		Graft	
		Tibial***	Peroneal	Tibial	Peroneal	Tibial	Peroneal
Injection	64	50/42	50/34	4/3	3/1	7/4	8/2
Fracture/dislocation	26	14/12	9/6	0/0	0/0	9/6	11/3
Contusion	22	22/20	22/18	0/0	0/0	0/0	0/0
Compression	19	19/18	19/15	0/0	0/0	0/0	0/0
GSW	17	8/7	8/6	4/3	4/1	5/3	5/1
Hip arthroplasty	15	8/6	8/2	0/0	0/0	7/4	7/1
Laceration/stab wound	12	3/3	3/3	3/2	3/1	6/4	6/2
Totals	175	124/108	119/84	11/8	10/3	34/21	37/9

*Values are expressed as the number of cases managed surgically/number of cases with recovery to ≥ grade 3. This table does not include tumors. For a given case, both divisions were not necessarily tabulated, unless there was a deficit or severe pain at the start in that distribution.

**Neurolysis was based on presence of an NAP across the lesion.

***Tibial and peroneal refer to tibial division and peroneal division.

No., number; GSW, gunshot wound.

predisposing to injection injury, especially if a long needle is used outside the upper outer quadrant of the buttocks (Fig. 11-11). There are two patterns of onset of pain and disability after such an injury to the sciatic nerve. Most frequent is the almost immediate onset of radicular pain and paresthesias with some degree of distal deficit. The less frequent pattern, occurring in 10% of patients, is a delayed onset of radicular pain, paresthesias, and deficit appearing minutes to several hours after the injection, which may or may not have produced severe local pain shortly after administration.[15] These two patterns suggest the possibility that occasionally a noxious drug does not need to be injected directly into the nerve to damage it, but rather may be deposited within epineurium or perhaps even adjacent to the nerve, and with time it diffuses into the intrafascicular structure.

To date, only 39% of patients with sciatic injection injuries seen at LSUHSC have warranted operation. Partial injuries sparing some tibial and peroneal division function can usually be treated with vigorous physical therapy, pain medications, and time. Because of

persistent symptoms, similar injuries may occasionally require exploration and external or internal neurolysis, which may or may not relieve pain. More complete lesions to the sciatic nerve as a whole or to one division alone may benefit from relatively early exploration. Intraoperative stimulation and recording of NAPs is performed and, if present, differential neurolysis of each division is carried out and, if then absent on one division, that division is resected and sutured. If NAPs are absent across the whole nerve, then the lesion is resected and repaired. The best time for such exploration is 3–5 months after the injection injury. If resection and suture are indicated for the peroneal division, the results are poor, but better with tibial division repair (Fig. 11-12). If a division is thought to be nonreparable, even resection may not help the pain associated with some injection injuries. One of the patients in the LSUHSC series who had resection of a segment of a buttock-level peroneal division eventually had a sympathectomy with some relief, even though the pain was not of a classic, sympathetically mediated nature.

Table 11-4   Operative results for thigh-level sciatic nerve injuries in 178 patients*

Type of injury	No. of patients	Neurolysis**		Suture		Grafts	
		Tibial***	Peroneal	Tibial	Peroneal	Tibial	Peroneal
GSW	62	27/27	27/24	14/14	14/10	21/18	18/9
Femur fracture	34	17/15	17/11	1/1	1/0	16/12	16/4
Laceration/stab wound	32	6/6	6/5	14/12	14/10	12/10	12/8
Contusion	28	23/21	23/16	0/0	0/0	5/3	3/1
Compression	12	12/12	12/10	0/0	0/0	0/0	0/0
Iatrogenic	10	10/10	10/9	0/0	0/0	0/0	0/0
TOTALS	178	95/91	95/75	29/27	29/20	54/43	49/22

*Values are expressed as number of cases managed surgically/number of cases with recovery to ≥ grade 3. This chart does not include tumors. For a given case, both divisions were not necessarily tabulated unless there was a deficit or severe pain at the start in that distribution.

**Neurolysis was based on presence of an NAP across the lesion.

***Tibial and peroneal refer to tibial division and peroneal division.

No., number; GSW, gunshot wound.

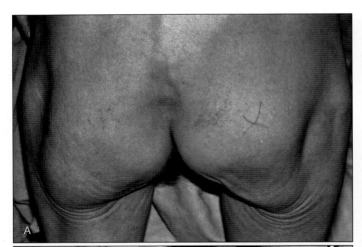

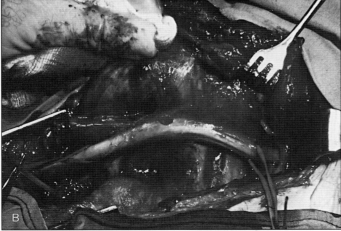

FIGURE 11-11   (A) The presumed injection site which resulted in a sciatic palsy is shown in the right buttock of a thin and cachectic individual. **(B)** In this intraoperative photograph, the sciatic nerve is adherent to the underside of the gluteus musculature at the injection site.

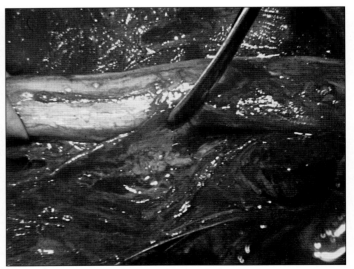

FIGURE 11-12   This individual required resection and repair of one division of the nerve at the buttock level because of an injection injury by morphine. Note the appearance of the tissue adjacent to the injected segment of the nerve.

In this LSUHSC series of injection injuries, the majority of patients treated conservatively improved. These cases usually had incomplete or partial loss in the distribution of one or both divisions. Pain was a problem in most cases, but usually responded to conservative management. Sixty-four patients had surgical intervention. The results of neurolysis if indicated based on NAP recordings were that 76 of 100 divisions improved. Four (57%) of seven divisions requiring end-to-end suture anastomosis repair and six (40%) of 15 divisions requiring graft repair had substantial recoveries. Eighteen patients (11%) had complete loss clinically and by EMG, but because they had NAPs across their lesions, neurolysis was performed and they eventually improved.

CASE SUMMARY – INJECTION INJURY

A 52-year-old woman received an injection of a morphine-related drug in the right buttock. She had pain radiating down the posterior thigh to the calf and foot and the onset of an immediate sciatic palsy. Within a few days, some degree of foot dorsiflexion returned, but there was no plantar flexion. An EMG at 4 weeks after the injection injury showed partial denervational change in the peroneal distribution muscles and severe denervational change in the tibial-innervated muscles. At neurological examination 4 months later, peroneal-innervated muscles were grade 3, tibial-innervated motor and sensory function was absent, and hamstring muscle function was normal. An EMG was similar to that done at 1 month after injury and showed no nascent activity.

Exploration of the sciatic nerve at the buttock level revealed a swollen nerve, especially along its medial aspect, i.e. tibial division. An intraoperative NAP was recorded across the sciatic lesion, so it was split into its tibial and peroneal divisions, and both divisions appeared to transmit an NAP. The main hamstring branch, however, was adherent to the side of the tibial division, and after this was dissected free, there was no NAP conducted through the tibial division. As a result, the tibial division was resected, and three 5.8 cm grafts were placed. The resected segment showed degenerated axons with marked epineurial and interfascicular fibrosis and the endoneurium was thickened. Only fine axons were present, and they were mixed with a moderately heavy proliferation of scar tissue. An external neurolysis alone of the peroneal division was done.

Follow-up at 26 months showed considerable restoration of calf girth with circumferential measurements equal bilaterally at 12 cm below the patella. Plantar flexion and inversion were both grade 3. There was no toe flexion present. Sensation on the sole was protective only. She had maintained excellent peroneal-innervated function.

COMMENT

Some injection injuries, even to the sciatic nerve at a buttock level, may be operative candidates. In this case, tibial loss predominated, and repair of this division was helpful. Pain may also sometimes be helped, especially if the tibial division is involved. Lesions due to injection are not always focal, and if resection is indicated by operative electrical studies, it must be lengthy enough to encompass the entire involved segment.

Fracture-dislocation of the hip

Injury to the buttock-level sciatic nerve was frequently caused by a fracture-dislocation of the hip (Table 11-3; Fig. 11-13), or by attempts to repair it. Buttock-level sciatic nerve injury has been found to occur most commonly when the femoral head is dislocated posteriorly.[10]

In the literature, the frequency of injury of the sciatic nerve associated with a fracture-dislocation of the hip or an acetabular fracture has been reported to be 10–19%.[10,16,17,37,38] This mechanism of proximal injury to the sciatic complex has been reported fairly frequently.[1,18,24,43] Real-time nerve monitoring has been advocated during acetabular fracture and complex total hip repairs to prevent iatrogenic sciatic nerve injury.[5,32,39] The patient presenting with a complete sciatic palsy caused by a fracture or dislocation of the hip sometimes has resolution of the tibial division loss, but seldom of the peroneal division deficit. Thus, peroneal division loss usually predominated in this series and, if complete at the start, seldom was reversed either in the nonoperative or operative cases. Three (27%) of 11 patients with graft repair of the buttock-level peroneal division had enough recovery to obviate the need for a kick-up foot brace. Six (67%) of nine patients undergoing neurolysis of the peroneal divisions at that level improved because NAPs were present across their lesions intraoperatively, and thus the

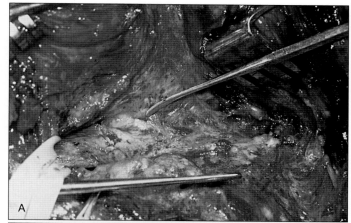

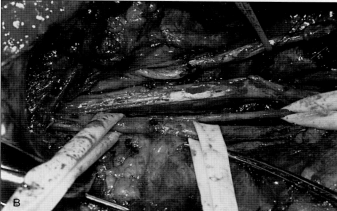

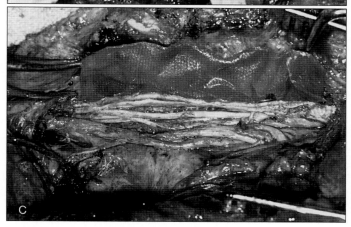

FIGURE 11-13 **(A)** This is an intraoperative photograph of the usual scar involving sciatic nerve in the notch area and associated with hip dislocation with proximal fracture of the femoral head. **(B)** After neurolysis on another buttock-level lesion associated with a fracture, the intraoperative NAP stimulation and recording was positive, so the nerve was split into its two divisions. Penrose drains are seen on the peroneal division, which had a high or proximal bifurcation. A plastic loop is on the hamstring branch; the tibial division is between it and the peroneal division. **(C)** The tibial division had transmitted an NAP, and an internal neurolysis was done. The peroneal division was repaired by sural grafts.

divisions were shown to be regenerating adequately. Significant peroneal return including some eversion and dorsiflexion resulted in these cases attaining a grade 3 or greater functional outcome. Toe extension was seldom regained, except in a few cases in which early spontaneous regeneration was evident.

Either conservative management or operation, if correctly chosen, led to a significant degree of tibial division recovery in the majority of patients. Nine (45%) of 20 graft repairs succeeded and 14 tibial divisions undergoing neurolysis based on the presence of intraoperative NAPs across their lesions had some useful degree of recovery, i.e. plantar flexion of grade 3 or better, inversion, and protective sensation on the sole of the foot. It was unusual for any patient to regain toe flexion or foot intrinsic function.

CASE SUMMARY – FRACTURE-DISLOCATION OF THE HIP

A 23-year-old male was injured in an oil rig accident when his left leg was caught by a drill and wrapped around it, and the right leg was drawn in and twisted as well. The patient sustained both a dislocation of the left hip, which was relocated a few hours later, and a right midshaft femoral fracture, which was pinned after several weeks of balanced skeletal traction. The accident resulted in an initially complete left lower extremity sciatic palsy and, after a few weeks, a small degree of plantar flexion returned. When seen at LSUHSC 4 months later, the medial hamstrings were grade 3 to 4, but the lateral hamstrings were only a trace. Plantar flexion was grade 3, but there was no foot inversion or toe flexion. Sensation was absent on the sole of the foot. Peroneal-innervated muscles were completely paralyzed. EMG showed a complete denervational pattern in the sciatic distribution, except for the partially denervated gastrocnemius-soleus muscles. There were no nascent units, even in tibial-innervated muscles.

The sciatic nerve at the buttock level was surgically exposed 4.5 months after injury. A lesion in continuity measuring 3.6 cm began close to the sciatic notch portion of the nerve and extended inferiorly and an NAP could be recorded both across this lesion and several centimeters distal to it. The nerve was split into its two divisions and re-recording showed an NAP across the tibial half of the nerve, even though it was firm and swollen, but not across the peroneal half. An internal neurolysis was done on the tibial division, and the peroneal division lesion was resected. A 3.2 cm gap was replaced by four sural grafts 3.8 cm (1.5 inches) in length (see Fig. 11-18). Buttock gluteal muscles were reattached laterally, other soft tissues were closed, and the limb was neither casted nor placed in a splint. Ambulation was begun 24 hours postoperatively with the help of a kick-up orthosis.

Follow-up at 4 years showed excellent tibial division return. Plantar flexion was grade 5 and inversion grade 4, but toe flexion remained absent. Sensation on the sole of the foot was grade 3 to 4. Both lateral and medial hamstrings were grade 5. In the peroneal distribution, eversion was grade 2 to 3, but there was no dorsiflexion of the foot or toe extension. The patient still uses a kick-up foot brace, but only when he is most active. Follow-up at 6 years showed improved eversion, but anterior tibialis was only grade 2, and there was no toe extension.

COMMENT

This case shows the usual clinical course and results of a severe proximal sciatic injury complication after hip injury. Toe flexion is seldom regained, and practical dorsiflexion of the foot is extremely difficult to obtain.

Contusive injury and gunshot wound

The contusive injuries undergoing operations were caused by falls on the buttocks and vehicular accidents and were characterized by incomplete loss on neurological examination and pain unresponsive to medications, physical therapy, or time (Table 11-3). Occasional painful sciatica was caused by an embedded gunshot shell fragment or a piece of bone from a fracture secondary to a GSW (Fig. 11-14). Operative manipulation sometimes helped the pain. Whether pain was helped or not, eventual function was excellent in 38 (86%) of 44 elements managed by neurolysis.

By comparison, most of the GSWs involving the sciatic nerve at a proximal level caused severe loss of function that usually did not improve over a 2–5-month period. Neurolysis based on positive intraoperative NAPs led to the expected good results in 13 (81%) of 16 divisions managed in this fashion in patients who had sustained GSWs. End-to-end suture anastomosis or graft repairs were necessary for 18 divisions (Fig. 11-15). Significant recovery occurred in six (67%) of nine tibial divisions using end-to-end suture anastomosis and graft repairs, but in only two (22%) of nine peroneal divisions using the same techniques (Fig. 11-16).

CASE SUMMARY – GUNSHOT WOUND

This 10-year-old male sustained a shotgun blast to the right buttock with severe soft tissue loss and extensive lengthy injury to the sciatic nerve. Several months after his injury he required shortening of the femur to remove necrotic non-healing bone and at the same time had a secondary end-to-end suture anastomosis repair of both the tibial and peroneal divisions of the sciatic nerve. The patient was placed in a hip spica cast postoperatively. Follow-up 8 years later showed recovery of tibial function with an overall grade for that nerve of 3 to 4. As expected, there was very little peroneal recovery. The patient is now in college and wears a kick-up foot brace.

COMMENT

If possible, bony fixation should be achieved prior to nerve repair even though both are done at the same operation.

Laceration/stab wound

This was a favorable category of injury even at a proximal level (Table 11-3). Because of the nature of the injury, a relatively early operation for a buttock-level sciatic nerve injury due to a laceration or stab wound was always indicated. One patient refused operation and did not recover function. Results with end-to-end suture anastomosis or graft repairs were usually favorable. Unlike contusion or stretch involving the sciatic nerve at this level, which required longer grafts, grafts, when necessary, were relatively short and seldom exceeded 3.8–5.0 cm in length. Two (67%) of three tibial division end-to-end suture anastomosis repairs and four (67%) of six graft repairs recovered to grade 3 or better, whereas only one

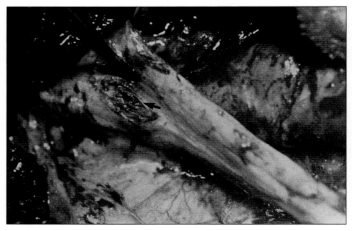

FIGURE 11-14 A shell fragment (*arrow*) is shown embedded in the tibial division of the sciatic nerve close to the region of the notch. This patient had excellent peroneal function and partial tibial function which was grade 3 to 4, but had severe neuritic pain with some degree of an autonomic component. The latter was helped by removal of the fragment, but the patient subsequently required a sympathectomy for more complete relief of pain.

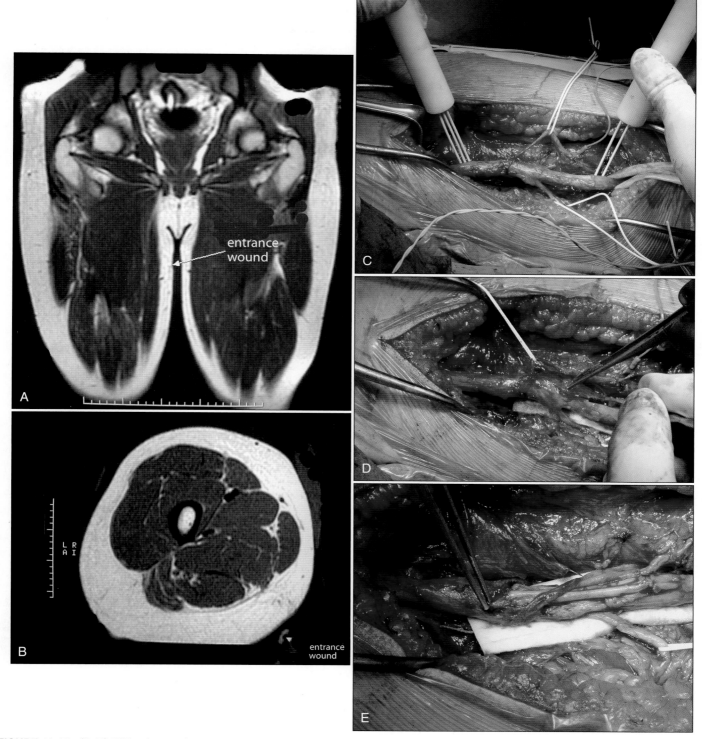

FIGURE 11-15 **(A, B)** MRIs of a gunshot wound involving the sciatic nerve are seen with the entrance wound as shown. **(C–E)** Intraoperative NAP testing showed no transmission of NAPs, thus the neuroma was resected and 5 grafts were placed using a grouped fascicular repair.

(33%) of three and two (33%) of six peroneal division repairs at this level recovered to grade 3 or better grade using the same end-to-end suture anastomosis and graft repair surgical techniques, respectively.

Retraction of nerve ends occurred despite a relatively sharp mechanism for transection in most of these cases, and grafts were sometimes necessary because of a delay in repair. In addition, even though there was a preoperative complete loss in the distribution of the sciatic nerve, contusion and thus a lesion in continuity was found in one patient with sciatic nerve laceration. Intraoperative NAPs were recorded across both divisions of this lesion, and this led to neurolysis with eventual satisfactory recovery.

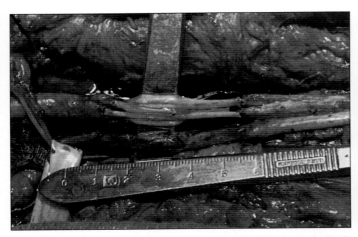

FIGURE 11-16 A split repair of the sciatic nerve close to the buttock crease in the nerve injured by a gunshot wound is seen. In this case, the peroneal division (*bottom*) transmitted an NAP but the tibial division (*top*) did not. Five grafts 4.5 cm in length were sewn into place using a grouped interfascicular repair.

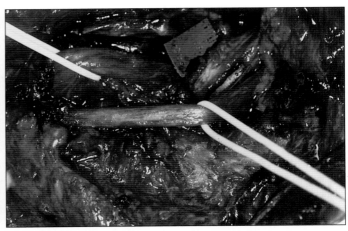

FIGURE 11-17 Exposure of the left sciatic nerve in the region of the notch, as seen intraoperatively. The origin of the tibial (*upper loop*) and peroneal (*lower loop*) divisions has been split by the piriformis muscle under the short ruler at the top right of the photograph. This child had presented with a progressive peroneal palsy associated with gluteal wasting and was thought to have a piriformis syndrome.

CASE SUMMARY – LACERATION/STAB WOUND

This 4-year-old female had learned to climb her family's refrigerator shelves to get to the top shelf. One day, shortly after a glass jar had fallen and shattered, she fell backward, landing on her buttocks. A shard of glass was driven into her left buttock, and she sustained an immediate complete sciatic palsy. She was referred several weeks later for surgical exploration at which time the nerve was found transected 2.5 cm distal to the sciatic notch. The nerve stumps had retracted and a 3.8 cm gap resulted after trimming of the proximal and distal neuromas. Both stumps were split into tibial and peroneal divisions, and each of these into several groups of fascicles. The gaps were bridged with grouped interfascicular grafts using sural nerve. Seven 4 cm grafts were placed. Follow-up at age 8 found an overall grade of 4 for the tibial nerve and a grade of 2 for peroneal nerve.

COMMENT

Although performed secondarily, buttock-level repair was especially rewarding in this young girl with a sharp injury. Had facilities and experienced personnel been available locally, this would have also been a good case for primary, i.e. early, repair.

Entrapment and iatrogenic injury

Though entrapment resulting from the piriformis syndrome has been reported,[3,12,42] this was rare in the LSUHSC experience with only two examples over a 25-year period (Fig. 11-17). One patient was helped by operation and removal of the piriformis muscle, and the other was not.

Iatrogenic injuries of the buttock-level sciatic nerve, other than those cases associated with hip repair, are unusual. Compression can occur as a result of proximal placement of nerve stimulators for the treatment of pain, and scarring associated with such a device may require a secondary operation.[27] One patient in this series had neurolysis for such scarring after removal of a stimulator at buttock level.

Although alluded to under the prior section entitled Fracture-dislocation of the hip, sciatic palsy related to hip fracture repair does occur. Unless transection or suture ligation of the nerve is

suspected, the patient is usually followed for several months. If there is no sign of recovery, the nerve is explored and intraoperative NAP recordings done unless transection is found.

THIGH-LEVEL SCIATIC NERVE

The cases of buttock- and thigh-level sciatic nerve lesions evaluated were divided approximately equally at these levels. While there were 175 buttock-level divisions, there were 178 divisions of the thigh-level sciatic nerve that had surgical intervention. Those thigh-level operative lesions included 62 patients with GSWs, 34 with fractures, usually of the femur, 32 with laceration or stab wounds, and 28 with contusive lesions. There were 12 compressive lesions and 10 iatrogenic injuries.

At a thigh level, injuries to the sciatic nerve can produce one of several outcomes: a lesion that causes injury resulting in either total or incomplete injury to both divisions, or an injury that is complete to one division with either incomplete or no involvement of the other division, or an incomplete injury of one division with no involvement of the other. This observation made it important to split the nerve into its two divisions whenever there was a lesion in continuity. Each division could then be evaluated individually by stimulation as well as by NAP stimulation and recording techniques.[20] If relative sparing or regeneration was proven by NAP recording, then external neurolysis sufficed: 91 (87%) of 105 tibial divisions at the thigh level undergoing neurolysis based on intraoperative recordings recovered to grade 3 or better (Table 11-2). This was also the case with the peroneal divisions, 75 (79%) of 95 having physiological evidence of early regeneration or relative sparing recovered.

If the injury was lengthy or if transection with retraction of stumps was present, graft placement to avoid distraction was the predominant method of repair (Fig. 11-18).[44] A number of more focal lesions could be resected and repaired by end-to-end suture anastomosis with relative immobilization of the limb for 3–4 weeks postoperatively. Twenty-seven (93%) of 29 end-to-end suture anastomosis repairs to the tibial division at this level had at least a functional level of plantar flexion and return of protective sensation

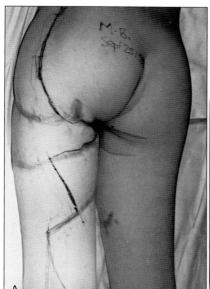

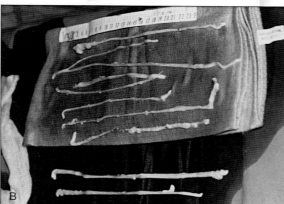

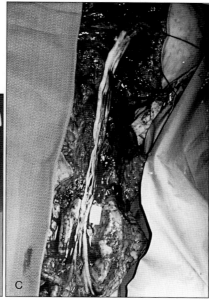

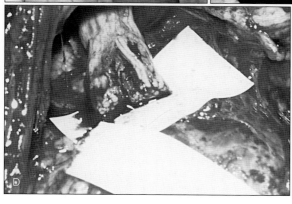

FIGURE 11-18 **(A)** A multiple-level propeller injury involving the left sciatic nerve at the thigh level is shown. The proposed incision for exposure has been drawn through and around some of the healed lacerations. **(B)** Allografts harvested from a cadaver donor are shown laid out on a drape. **(C)** Grafts 20 cm in length were sewn into place. **(D)** The proximal stump neuroma had been resected back to an excellent fascicular pattern. The patient was kept on immunosuppression therapy for 2 years and has regained some sensory return to the sole of the foot at 3 years after the injury. (From Mackinnon S and Hudson A: Clinical application of peripheral nerve transplantation, Plast Reconst Surg 90:4:695–699,1992.)

on the sole of the foot. Even graft repairs of this division at this level fared exceptionally well, with grade 3 or better recoveries in 43 (80%) of 54 repairs. As might be expected, peroneal division repairs did not have as satisfactory outcomes as tibial division repairs, but 20 (69%) of 29 patients with suture repairs recovered enough function to eliminate the need for a kick-up foot brace. The success rate for the peroneal division was less with graft repairs: only 22 (45%) of 49 patients remained free of a brace. These figures make it important to protect the peroneal division while operating on incomplete lesions involving the sciatic nerve, especially if there is partial injury or relative sparing of this division.

Gunshot wound

Gunshot wounds, which were frequent injuries to the thigh-level sciatic nerve, had surprisingly good outcomes and the literature supports this finding, as well.[41] A relatively aggressive approach included the exploration of those patients without significant spontaneous recovery within the first 3–5 months post injury (Fig. 11-19).[45] As can be seen in Table 11-2, all tibial divisions and all but three peroneal divisions selected for neurolysis based on NAP recordings recovered to grade 3 or better levels. Fourteen (100%) of 14 tibial and 10 (71%) of 14 peroneal divisions having end-to-end suture anastomosis repairs recovered. Results with graft repairs were less favorable: 18 (86%) of 21 tibial and nine (50%) of 18 peroneal divisions recovered adequately.

Fracture

Results in this category were comparable to those seen with GSWs to this level (Table 11-4). Fifteen (88%) of 17 tibial and 11 (65%) of 17 peroneal divisions undergoing neurolysis based on the presence of an intraoperative NAP recovered acceptably. End-to-end suture anastomosis and graft repairs succeeded frequently, except for the peroneal division, in which 12 (75%) of 16 grafts and one end-to-end suture anastomosis repair failed to produce a good result. Those patients not having surgery recovered tibial function better than peroneal function.

Laceration/stab wound

As at a buttock level, sharp injuries at the thigh level responded well, especially if repaired acutely. The incidence of such lesions was surprisingly high and occurred because of patients being pushed or falling through plate glass windows. Each of four limbs in three patients had a guillotine-like injury in which the limb was sectioned posteriorly through all soft tissue, hamstring muscles, and sciatic nerve to the femur. Whenever it was possible, primary repair within 72 hours was favored, for these as well as for other sharp injuries in which transection was suspected. Because of referral patterns, such acute repair was not always possible, but if it could be done, end-to-end suture anastomosis rather than graft repair was performed, and results were some of the best seen for completely injured sciatic nerves. Repair of blunt transections was delayed for several weeks or undertaken later if the referral had been late (Fig. 11-20).

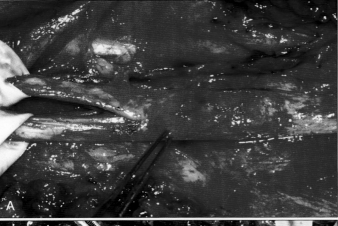

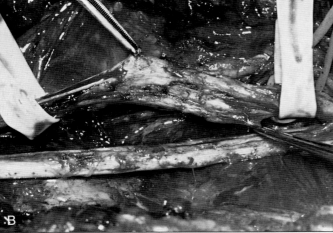

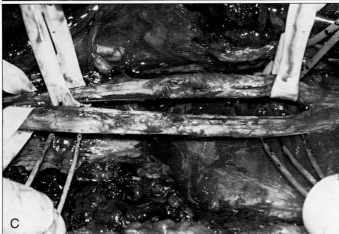

FIGURE 11-19 **(A)** A typical lesion in continuity is seen at a midthigh level caused by a gunshot wound. **(B)** Because the lesion transmitted an NAP, it was split into its two divisions. **(C)** Each division was then evaluated by NAP recordings. Stimulating electrodes are to the right and recording ones to the left.

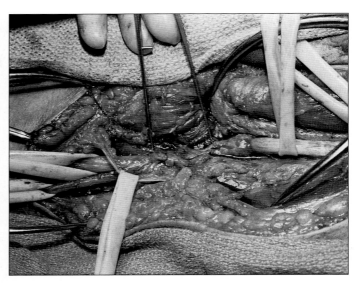

FIGURE 11-20 A blunt transection of the sciatic nerve at the level of the thigh was explored several months after injury. The stumps were not only neuromatous, but had retracted several centimeters, as shown by the spread tips of the forceps. A sural graft repair was necessary.

REFERENCES

1. Adams JC: Vulnerability of the sciatic nerve in closed ischiofemoral arthrodesis by nail and graft. J Bone Joint Surg [Br] 46:748–753, 1964.
2. Aldea PA and Shaw WA: Lower extremity nerve injuries. Clin Plast Surg 13:691–699, 1986.
3. Banerjee T and Hall CD: Sciatic entrapment neuropathy. J Neurosurg 45:216–217, 1976.
4. Bateman JE: Trauma to Nerves and Limbs. Philadelphia, WB Saunders, 1962.
5. Black DL, et al.: Somatosensory-evoked potential monitored during total hip arthroplasty. Clin Orthop 262:170, 1991.
6. Bristow WR: Injuries of peripheral nerves in two World Wars. Br J Surg 34:333, 1947.
7. Clark K, Williams P, Willis W, et al.: Injection injury of the sciatic nerve. In: Ojemann RG, Ed: Clin Neurosurg 17:111, 1970.
8. Clawson DK and Seddon HJ: The late consequences of sciatic nerve injury. J Bone Joint Surg [Br] 42:213–225, 1960.
9. Clawson DK and Seddon HJ: The results of repair of the sciatic nerve. J Bone Joint Surg [Br] 42:205–213, 1960.
10. Fassler PR, Swiontkowski MF, Kilroy AW, et al.: Injury of the sciatic nerve associated with acetabular fracture. J Bone Joint Surg [Am] 75:1157, 1993.
11. Fried G, Salerno T, Brown HC, et al.: Management of the extremity with combined neurovascular and musculoskeletal trauma. J Trauma 18:481–486, 1978.
12. Gelmers H: Entrapment of the sciatic nerve. Acta Neurochir (Wien) 33:103–106, 1976.
13. Gentilli F and Hudson AR: Peripheral nerve injuries: Types, causes, grading. In: William RH and Rengachary SS, Eds: Neurosurgery, vol 2. New York, McGraw Hill, 1985.
14. Haymaker W and Woodhall B: Peripheral Nerve Injuries. Principles of Diagnosis, 2nd edn. Philadelphia, WB Saunders, 1953.
15. Hudson AR, Kline DG, and Gentilli F: Peripheral nerve injection injury. In: Management of Peripheral Nerve Problems. Philadelphia, WB Saunders, 1980.
16. Hunter GA: Posterior dislocation and fracture-dislocation of the hip. A review of fifty-seven patients. J Bone Joint Surg [Br] 51:38–44, 1969.
17. Jacob JR, Rao JP, and Ciccarelli C: Traumatic dislocation and fracture dislocation of the hip. A long-term follow-up study. Clin Orthop 249:263, 1987.
18. Johnson EW Jr and Vittands IJ: Nerve injuries in fractures of the lower extremity. Minn Med 52:627–633, 1969.
19. Kline D: Operative management of major nerve lesions of the lower extremity. Surg Clin N Am 52:1247–1262, 1972.

20. Kline DG, Kim D, Midha R, et al.: Management and results of sciatic nerve injuries: a 24-year experience. J Neurosurg 89:13–23, 1998.

21. Kline DG, Tiel R, Kim D, et al.: Lower extremity nerve injuries. In: Omer G Jr, Spinner M, and Van Beek AL, Eds: Management of Peripheral Nerve Problems. Philadelphia, WB Saunders, 1980.

22. MacCarty CS: Two-stage autograft for repair of extensive damage to the sciatic nerve. J Neurosurg 8:319–322, 1951.

23. Marcus NA, Blair WF, Shuck JM, et al.: Low-velocity gunshot wounds to extremities. J Trauma 20:1061–1064, 1980.

24. McLean M: Total hip replacement and sciatic nerve trauma. Orthopedics 9:1121–1127, 1986.

25. Millesi H: Lower extremity nerve lesions. In: Terzis J, Ed: Microreconstruction of Nerve Injuries. Philadelphia, WB Saunders, 1987.

26. Millesi H: Nerve grafts: Indications, techniques and prognosis. In: Omer G, Spinner M, and Van Beek AL, Eds: Management of Peripheral Nerve Problems. Philadelphia, WB Saunders, 1998.

27. Nielson KD, Watts C, and Clark WK: Peripheral nerve injury from implantation of chronic stimulating electrodes for pain control. Surg Neurol 5:51–53, 1976.

28. Omer GE Jr: Results of untreated peripheral nerve injuries. Clin Orthop163:15–19, 1982.

29. Omer G Jr: Nerve injuries associated with gunshot wounds of the extremities. In: Gelberman R, Ed: Operative Repair and Reconstruction. Philadelphia, JB Lippincott, 1991.

30. Paradies LH and Gregory CF: The early treatment of close-range shotgun wounds to the extremities. J Bone Joint Surg [Am] 48:425–429, 1966.

31. Pollack LJ and Davis L: Peripheral nerve injuries, the sciatic nerve, the tibial nerve, the peroneal nerve. Am J Surg 18:176–193, 1932.

32. Pring ME, Trousdale RT, Cabanela ME, et al.: Intraoperative electromyographic monitoring during periacetabular osteotomy. Clin Orthop 158:164, 2002.

33. Rich NM and Spencer FC: Vascular Trauma. Philadelphia, WB Saunders, 1978.

34. Rizzoli H: Treatment of peripheral nerve injuries. In: Coates JB and Meirowsky AM, Eds: Neurological Surgery of Trauma. Washington DC, Office of the Surgeon General, Department of the Army, 1965.

35. Seletz E: Surgery of Peripheral Nerves. Springfield, Illinois, Charles C Thomas, 1951.

36. Singh N, Behse F, and Buchthal F: Electrophysiological study of peroneal palsy. J Neurol Neurosurg Psychiatry 37:1202–1213, 1974.

37. Stewart MJ, McCarroll HR Jr, and Mulhollan JS: Fracture-dislocation of the hip. Acta Orthop Scand 46:507–525, 1975.

38. Stewart MJ and Milford LW: Fracture-dislocation of the hip; an end-result study. J Bone Joint Surg [Am] 36:315–342, 1954.

39. Stone RG, Weeks LE, Hajdu M, et al.: Evaluation of sciatic nerve compromise during total hip arthroplasty. Clin Orthop 26:31–35, 1985.

40. Sunderland S: Nerves and Nerve Lesions. Edinburgh, Churchill Livingstone, 1978.

41. Taha A and Taha J: Results of suture of the sciatic nerve after missile injury. J Trauma 45:340–344, 1998.

42. Wagner FC: Compression of the lumbosacral plexus and the sciatic nerve. In: Szabo R, Ed: Nerve Compression Syndromes: Diagnosis and Treatment. Thorofare, NJ, Slack, 1989.

43. Weber ER, Daube JR, and Coventry MB: Peripheral neuropathies associated with total hip arthroplasty. J Bone Joint Surg [Am] 58:66–69, 1976.

44. Whitcomb B: Separation at the suture site as a cause of failure in regeneration of peripheral nerves. J Neurosurg 3:399–406, 1946.

45. White JC: Timing of nerve suture after a gunshot wound. Surgery 48:946–951, 1960.

46. Wood MB: Peripheral nerve injuries to the lower extremity. In: Operative Nerve Repair and Reconstruction. Philadelphia, JB Lippincott, 1991.

TIBIAL NERVE

OVERVIEW

- There were 135 tibial nerve lesions in the Louisiana State University Health Sciences Center (LSUHSC) series presented in this chapter. The traumatic injury category, which excluded patients with tarsal tunnel syndrome and tumors, had 71 lesions. There were 46 cases of tarsal tunnel syndrome, and 18 patients underwent surgery for nerve sheath tumors. The patients were managed operatively between 1967 and 1999.
- Of 22 tibial nerve lesions not in continuity, a functional recovery of grade 3 or better was achieved in 4 (67%) of 6 patients who required end-to-end suture repairs and 11 (69%) of 16 patients who required graft repairs.
- One hundred and thirteen tibial nerve lesions in continuity underwent external or internal neurolysis or resection of their lesions. A few had end-to-end suture anastomosis or graft repairs. Direct intraoperative recording of nerve action potentials (NAPs) guided the management of these lesions.
- Among 113 patients with lesions in continuity, 76 (81%) of 94 patients underwent neurolysis, 5 (83%) of 6 had suture anastomosis repair and 11 (85%) of 13 patients who had graft repair all recovered function to grade 3 or better.
- Repair results were best in patients with recordable NAPs treated by external neurolysis and were poor in a few patients with very lengthy lesions in continuity and in patients with tarsal tunnel syndrome having reoperations.

Surgical exploration and repair of tibial nerve lesions including nerve sheath tumors and tarsal tunnel syndrome achieved excellent outcomes in the LSUHSC series.

APPLIED ANATOMY

The tibial nerve arises from the medial half of the sciatic nerve, usually at the middle to distal one-third of the thigh. The nerve is deep to the hamstring muscles, which are on either side of the posterior compartment of the thigh and in the popliteal fossa the nerve lies posterior to the popliteal artery and vein. A medial hamstring branch occasionally leaves the tibial nerve at this level. More commonly, sensory branches to the proximal calf may arise before the nerve reaches its first major innervational site, particularly as it courses through the popliteal fossa.

The tibial nerve runs beneath the gastrocnemius-soleus muscle group, giving a profusion of branches to it and the plantaris, popliteus, and tibialis muscles (Fig. 11-21). Such branches begin to define themselves as separate tibial branches proximal to the superior edge of the gastrocnemius-soleus complex.

A deep or posterior tibial branch accompanies the tibial artery and vein and runs through the leg medial and posterior to the tibia and posterior to the intermuscular septum separating the anterior from the posterior compartments. The posterior tibial nerve carries fibers destined for the foot, but gives off branches in the more proximal leg to supply the flexor digitorum longus and flexor hallucis longus muscles. As the posterior tibial nerve approaches the ankle, it courses inferior to the medial malleolus. At this level, it passes beneath the flexor retinaculum (Fig. 11-22) and branches into the medial and lateral plantar nerves (Fig. 11-23), though these nerves can also arise and be well-defined before the posterior tibial nerve reaches the malleolus. The lateral plantar nerve runs deep in the instep and supplies some foot intrinsic muscles and sensation

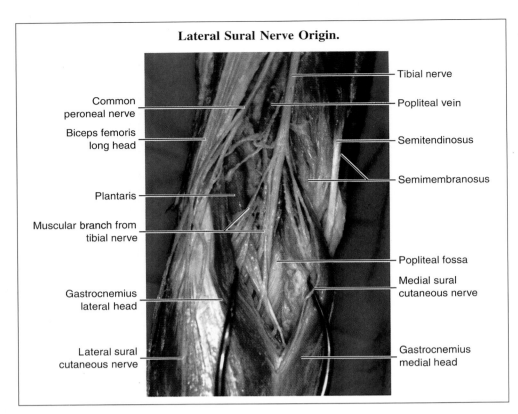

Lateral Sural Nerve Origin.

Common peroneal nerve

Biceps femoris long head

Plantaris

Muscular branch from tibial nerve

Gastrocnemius lateral head

Lateral sural cutaneous nerve

Tibial nerve

Popliteal vein

Semitendinosus

Semimembranosus

Popliteal fossa

Medial sural cutaneous nerve

Gastrocnemius medial head

FIGURE 11-21 A close-up view of the left leg at the inferior apex of the popliteal fossa. As the tibial nerve leaves the popliteal fossa, it descends deep to the lateral and medial heads of the gastrocnemius muscles. The tibial nerve gives branches to the heads of the gastrocnemius muscle and plantaris muscle seen above and also to the soleus, popliteus, and tibialis muscles. (From Kline DG, Hudson AR, and Kim DH: Atlas of Peripheral Nerve Surgery. Philadelphia, WB Saunders, 2001.)

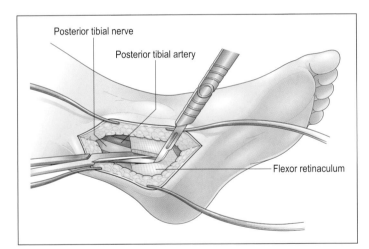

Posterior tibial nerve

Posterior tibial artery

Flexor retinaculum

FIGURE 11-22 The flexor retinaculum is shown being sectioned to expose the posterior tibial nerve as it passes beneath the medial malleolus. (From Kline DG, Hudson AR, and Kim DH: Atlas of Peripheral Nerve Surgery. Philadelphia, WB Saunders, 2001.)

for the lateral portion of the sole of the foot. The medial plantar branch provides sensation to the medial plantar surface of the foot and input to the abductor hallucis and flexor digitorum brevis muscles. A third branch, the calcaneal nerve, can usually be found to arise either proximal to these latter nerves or to branch from the medial plantar nerve. The calcaneal nerve can have numerous anatomic variations.[5,9] Injury to the medial and lateral plantar nerves may spare sensation on the heel of the foot.

TARSAL TUNNEL

The tarsal tunnel is a fibro-osseous space located posterior to the medial malleolus. It has a bony floor formed by the medial talar surface, the sustentaculum tali, and the medial calcaneal wall. The roof of the tarsal tunnel is formed by the flexor retinaculum, a thin, fibrous tissue that has its origin from the medial and inferior aspect of the medial malleolus and inserts into the periosteum of the medial tuberosity of the calcaneus. The base of the flexor retinaculum corresponds to the superior border of the abductor hallucis muscle.[19]

The posterior tibial, flexor digitorum longus, and flexor hallucis longus tendons are located within the tarsal tunnel, each with its own synovial sheath. The tendons are contained within a separate fibro-osseous compartment formed by fibrous projections from the undersurface of the flexor retinaculum.[7,8,10] The tibial nerve enters the tarsal tunnel between the overlying flexor retinaculum and the underlying tendon sheaths of the posterior tibial, flexor digitorum longus, and flexor hallucis longus muscles. The tibial nerve and artery are often attached to these sheaths through surrounding areolar tissue. The tarsal tunnel is narrowest at its distal portion where it is conjoined with the fascia of the abductor hallucis longus muscle. The nerve at this level can be entrapped, causing a tarsal tunnel syndrome which is the most common entrapment neuropathy of the tibial nerve.[14] Magnetic resonance imaging may be helpful in identifying soft tissue pathological conditions within the tarsal tunnel.[21]

CLINICAL PRESENTATION AND EXAMINATION

The sural nerve, which can arise from the tibial and/or peroneal nerves, supplies the lateral foot. The saphenous nerve, a branch of

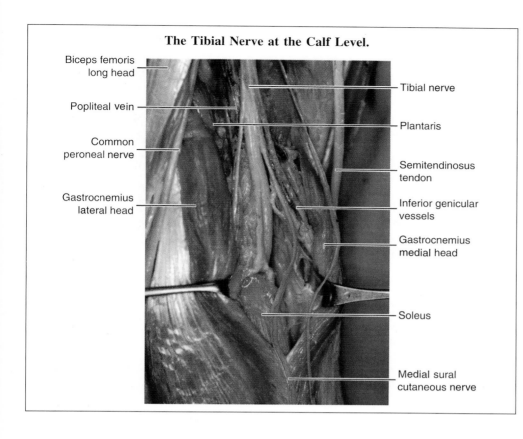

The Tibial Nerve at the Calf Level.

Biceps femoris long head

Popliteal vein

Common peroneal nerve

Gastrocnemius lateral head

Tibial nerve

Plantaris

Semitendinosus tendon

Inferior genicular vessels

Gastrocnemius medial head

Soleus

Medial sural cutaneous nerve

FIGURE 11-23 A left medial ankle dissection showing the tibial nerve as it branches into the medial and lateral plantar nerves. The flexor retinaculum shown in Figure 11-22 has been removed. (From Kline DG, Hudson AR, and Kim DH: Atlas of Peripheral Nerve Surgery. Philadelphia, WB Saunders, 2001.)

the femoral nerve, supplies an area below the medial malleolus. The posterior tibial nerve gives rise to the calcaneal and lateral and medial plantar nerves, which provide important sensory supply to the heel and plantar aspects of the feet, respectively. Sensory loss on the bottom of the foot can therefore be part of the clinical findings of severe tibial palsy. Thus, with complete tibial division injury, sensory loss on the sole and heel of the foot is marked and an insensitive foot is a problem until enough sensation returns to be protective (Fig. 11-24).[3]

Blisters, ulcers, and ultimately osteomyelitis can occur unless the patient is instructed to inspect the involved foot daily and to wear footwear that prevents excessive pressure on the ball and heel of the foot. Partial injury to the tibial complex is often very painful. Causalgia can be a major complication of tibial nerve injury, but even if this does not occur, the mixture of hyper- and hypoesthesia and neuritic pain that results can be disabling.[15,16]

Although foot intrinsic muscle loss is not a serious sequela of tibial dysfunction, it can result in clawing of the toes, similar to that which occurs in the hand with some distal ulnar, and especially combined ulnar and median, nerve injuries. Some patients can abduct the great toe on the healthy side. If this is the case, the intact side can be compared with the injured side. Inversion of the foot, also a tibial function, can sometimes be partially mimicked by co-contraction of the peroneal-innervated anterior tibialis and the usually stronger gastrocnemius-soleus muscles.

Unlike the peroneal-innervated muscles, the gastrocnemius-soleus muscles contract effectively after a relatively small number of fibers regenerate to them and connections are re-formed between the axons and motor end plates. Input sites for effective contraction are relatively proximal in this muscle complex. As a result, with effective regeneration of a knee-level tibial nerve injury, gastrocnemius-soleus contraction may begin recovery by 4–5 months

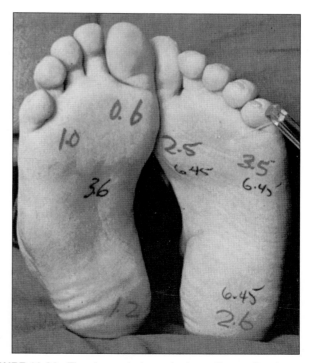

FIGURE 11-24 The above photograph shows the results of comparative sensory tests on the soles of the feet. The left foot, seen to the viewer's right, is in a limb that had lengthy 23 cm allografts for multiple-level propeller-blade injuries to the sciatic nerve from the buttock to the knee and required a higher vibration threshold to obtain a response. (From Mackinnon S and Hudson A: Clinical application of peripheral nerve transplantation. Plast Reconstr Surg 90:695–699, 1992.)

and with a mid-thigh-level lesion, by 6–9 months. The examiner must ask the patient to extend the leg before he or she presses down with the foot to ensure that the foot is not being passively pushed down by hip and knee muscles. Early contraction of the gastrocnemius-soleus muscle group can be palpated in the proximal posterior compartment of the leg.

Initial recovery of plantar flexion with buttock-level sciatic lesions, covered in the chapter on the sciatic nerve, may require a year or more. The speed of recovery depends on the severity of the injury, the capacity for spontaneous recovery, and the need for end-to-end graft repair. Inversion is more difficult to obtain, especially with proximal division injury and toe flexion, and other intrinsic foot function may not occur at all, even with a thigh-level tibial lesion. Tibial repair at any level, however, is always worthwhile provided there is a proven poor potential for spontaneous regeneration. This is not only because there is great opportunity for recovery of plantar function, so important for push-off in walking, but also because at least protective sensation to the sole of the foot can be regained.

Ankle-level injuries may involve the distal tibial nerve. As described, as the tibial nerve approaches the ankle it gives off a calcaneal branch supplying the heel of the foot. Just distal to the medial malleolus, the nerve divides into the medial and lateral plantar branches, which supply sensation to the sole of the foot and intrinsic motor function to the toes and foot.

ELECTROPHYSIOLOGICAL STUDIES

Both clinical and electromyogram (EMG) evidence of recovery of the gastrocnemius-soleus muscles and sometimes posterior tibialis is much more common than reversal of denervation in the foot muscles.

Conduction velocity studies are of value for a suspected posterior tibial entrapment in the foot, i.e. tarsal tunnel syndrome.[6] Mixed motor and sensory conduction velocity studies are accurate in 90–100% of patients.[9] As with the peroneal nerve entrapments, it is important to compare values from the involved foot with those in the contralateral limb.[2] The extreme values and the normal limits are far less precisely defined than they are for carpal tunnel studies.[17]

An accurate clinical examination should be performed and electrical studies should be used to supplement these findings.[8] This is important because true tarsal tunnel syndrome is an infrequent diagnosis,[12] and other causes for foot pain must be eliminated.[13]

Sensory nerve action potentials (SNAPs) can be evoked by toe stimulation and recorded from the posterior tibial nerve proximal to the ankle. Though well-performed sensory studies reflect more severe conductive changes earlier than do motor studies in the tarsal tunnel syndrome,[18] after more proximal stimulation of the nerve, muscle action potentials can also be recorded from foot intrinsic muscles. Needle sampling of foot intrinsic muscles can be painful, but are a necessity if loss is severe or sensory potentials are not recordable.

SURGICAL EXPOSURE

The surgical exposure of the proximal portion of the tibial nerve is straightforward. An incision is made in the popliteal fossa in the midline between the hamstring muscles and is extended distally to run laterally behind the knee in the popliteal crease. Dissection must be carefully done in order to isolate the tibial nerve from the

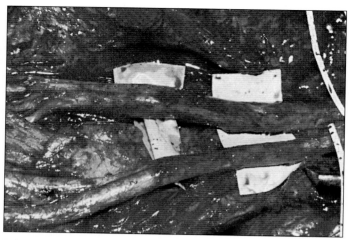

FIGURE 11-25 An intraoperative photograph of a contusive injury to the tibial and peroneal nerves behind the knee is seen here. This injury was caused by a blown-out hydraulic door. Acutely, the patient required a vascular repair and both nerves subsequently required graft repair. The tibial nerve is at the top and the peroneal nerve is at the bottom.

popliteal artery and vein without injury to these important vascular structures (Fig. 11-25). The surgeon can usually dissect out the nerve without the necessity of skeletonizing the artery, unless there has been or there is a need for a concomitant vascular repair. Branches running to the gastrocnemius-soleus muscles and the deeper posterior tibial nerve destined for the ankle and foot can be readily isolated with Penrose drains or plastic loops.

Dissection of the nerve in the lower leg is more difficult, but if only a short proximal distance is needed, some of the gastrocnemius-soleus mass can be partially elevated at its superior and medial borders to expose the deeper and more distal few centimeters of posterior tibial nerve. Most leg-level lesions requiring surgery, however, need to be approached by a medial leg incision posterior to the tibia and anterior to the bulk of the gastrocnemius-soleus muscles. This requires an up-and-down incision paralleling the palpable posterior edge of the tibia (Fig. 11-26). This is a deep dissection (Fig. 11-27), and if injury has involved the deep popliteal artery or vein as well as the nerve, the operation is not an easy one. Proximal and distal vascular control by plastic loops or small vascular clamps may be necessary before neuromatous nerve or transected nerve stumps can be dissected free.

Exposure of the posterior tibial nerve at the ankle is more straightforward than at the leg level. It can be found medial to the Achilles tendon and proximal to the medial malleolus where it can be traced beneath the medial malleolus by dividing the overlying flexor retinaculum. Exposure of the posterior tibial nerve at this level, though often compared with that of the median nerve in the carpal tunnel, is much more complex, and thus the dissection is more tedious (Fig. 11-28). The tibial artery has a serpiginous course, and arterial and venous branches intertwine with the nerve as it forms the medial and lateral plantar and calcaneal nerves. Magnification and use of the bipolar forceps and many Penrose drains or vascular loops for retraction help, as does patience in dissection. For entrapments at this level, the nerve and its branches must be entirely cleaned circumferentially to provide a bed for the nerves and branches free of scar or compressive tissues. This includes sectioning the overlying muscle and its fascial edge in the instep portion of the foot.

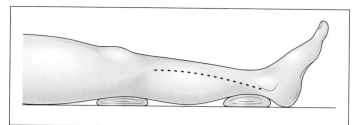

FIGURE 11-26 This incision is used to expose the tibial nerve and accompanying vessels in the calf or leg. (From Kline DG, Hudson AR, and Kim DH: Atlas of Peripheral Nerve Surgery. Philadelphia, WB Saunders, 2001.)

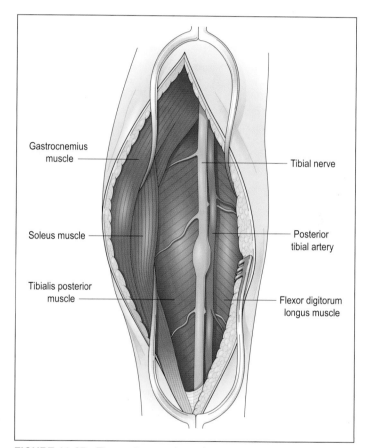

Gastrocnemius muscle

Tibial nerve

Soleus muscle

Posterior tibial artery

Tibialis posterior muscle

Flexor digitorum longus muscle

FIGURE 11-27 The gastrocnemius-soleus muscles have been incised as shown along the lower edge of the tibia and then mobilized and deflected downward. The tibial nerve, artery and vein are then dissected at a midleg level. This is a deep dissection and a difficult one, even with good retraction. (From Kline DG, Hudson AR, and Kim DH: Atlas of Peripheral Nerve Surgery. Philadelphia, WB Saunders, 2001.)

RESULTS

KNEE AND LEG LEVELS

The grading scale to gauge functional postoperative outcomes was based on the LSUHSC system and is shown in Tables 11-5 and 11-6.

The tibial nerve injury is a favorable one to manage. Similar experiences have been reported by others, even for war wounds. Results in the LSUHSC series were also good, providing a proper

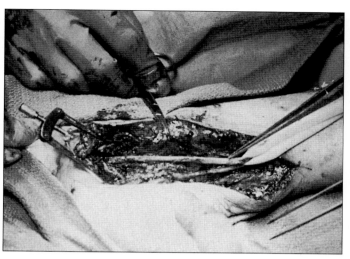

FIGURE 11-28 The posterior tibial nerve has been exposed, as seen in this intraoperative photograph, at the level of the ankle. The dissection was extended to the level of the instep.

Table 11-5 The LSUHSC grading system for motor function of the tibial nerve

Grade	Evaluation	Description
0	Absent	No gastrocnemius-soleus function; no toe flexion
1	Poor	Trace of gastrocnemius-soleus function; no other tibial muscle function
2	Fair	Gastrocnemius contracts against gravity only
3	Moderate	Gastrocnemius contracts against moderate resistance; trace or better inversion
4	Good	Gastrocnemius contracts against moderate resistance; inversion is grade 3 or better
5	Excellent	Gastrocnemius has full function; inversion is grade 4 or better; toe flexion is present

LSUHSC, Louisiana State University Health Sciences Center.

decision was made regarding the need for either surgery or conservative management.[11] If the lesion was partial or was shown to be regenerating by intraoperative electrical studies, results with neurolysis were excellent, with 19 (95%) of 20 patients achieving grade 3 or better recovery (Table 11-7). Results with repair, whether by suture or graft, were equally good. Seventeen (94%) of 18 patients with end-to-end suture anastomosis and graft repairs achieved grade 3 or better functional level.

Lacerations or penetrating injuries not related to gunshot wounds (GSWs) were usually caused by knives or glass. In one case, a lawn mower struck a wire and a piece of the wire was driven into the popliteal space, partially lacerating and contusing the tibial nerve. Motor loss was also partial, but pain was the main feature in this case. Fortunately, internal neurolysis and a split repair ameliorated the pain, and 2 years later both motor and sensory functions were grade 4.

The other relatively large categories of posterior tibial injuries were contusion or crush without fracture and fracture-associated contusion and stretch. Slightly less than half of these lesions required operation, because either the tibial lesion was partial or there was substantial recovery in the early months following injury. Nine (53%) of 17 patients with contusion injuries, although having lesions of some length, transmitted NAPs and underwent only neurolysis. There was good recovery in 8 cases. The one contusion that did not recover with neurolysis was associated with a compartment syndrome.

Iatrogenic causes of injury were associated with vascular repairs and both open and closed operations on the knee joint. Unless transection was observed by the original surgeon or suspected at LSUHSC, such lesions were managed for 3–4 months with physical therapy, outpatient follow-up visits, and periodic EMG testing.

If there was no improvement, as was the case with six lesions, then exploration and intraoperative electrical recordings were performed. Recovery occurred in all six operative cases.

If denervation is severe in the tibial distribution, great care must be taken of the sole of the foot. Well-designed shoes with a good fit are mandatory, and sometimes special shoes and support are necessary to prevent ulceration.[3]

CASE SUMMARY – LEG-LEVEL TIBIAL NERVE

A 17-year old male sustained a chain saw injury to his medial leg at its midpoint. The leg wound was debrided acutely, and pieces of wood, dirt, and some tibial bone chips were removed. The tibial nerve was found to be transected and the ends were marked with suture. The tibial artery was repaired by a vein graft. When seen by our service 5 days later, his wound was healing well. Plantar flexion was grade 5 and inversion was grade 3, but there were no toe flexion or foot intrinsic functions. Sensation on the sole of the foot was absent. At exploration, care had to be taken to protect the repaired artery. Neuromas were trimmed and the gap bridged with four grafts, 7.6 cm in length. No cast or splint was used.

The patient was begun on ambulation several days later. Follow-up at 5 years showed improved, but still diminished sensation on the sole of the foot, fully restored inversion, and some but still poor, i.e. grade 2 to 3, toe flexion.

COMMENT

Repair of this nerve at this level is worthwhile provided that enough sensation returns to the sole of the foot so that it is not hyperesthetic to touch and/or weight bearing.

ANKLE LEVEL

Ankle-level injuries involving the posterior tibial and/or plantar nerves were often associated with fracture (Figs 11-29, 11-30), but occasionally were caused by blunt contusion or by GSW without fracture. Thirty-three such injuries had operations because of severe pain with or without sensory disturbances on the soles of the feet. Three patients sustained blunt transections and required delayed repair by grafts.

Fifteen ankle-level injuries underwent only external neurolysis and 11 (73%) of these had improvement in pain. Three patients with especially severe neuritic pain had internal neurolysis. Two

Table 11-6 The LSUHSC grading system for sensory function of the tibial nerve

Grade	Evaluation	Description
0	Absent	Little or no sensation on the plantar surface of the foot
1	Poor	Plantar hyperesthesia or paresthesia
2	Fair	Plantar surface sensation is "sufficient for grip and slow protection" or less
3	Moderate	Response to touch and pin in autonomous zones localized, but not normal with some overresponse
4	Good	Response to touch and pin in autonomous zones localized, but not normal with no overresponse
5	Excellent	Near-normal response to touch and pin

LSUHSC, Louisiana State University Health Sciences Center.

Table 11-7 Knee- and leg-level operative tibial nerve injuries – incidence/results*

	Patient no.	Neurolysis	Suture	Graft
Laceration	12	3/3	2/2	7/6
Contusion with fracture	10	6/6	0/0	4/4
Contusion without fracture	7	3/2	0/0	4/4
Iatrogenic	6	5/5	0/0	1/1
Gunshot wound	3	3/3	0/0	0/0
Totals	38	20/19	2/2	16/15

*Total cases/number of operative cases recovering to a grade 3 or better result.

No., number.

were helped and the third patient had to have resection of the posterior tibial nerve, gaining partial improvement in pain, despite an insensate sole of the foot.

Including the blunt transection and contusive GSW and iatrogenic injuries involving the ankle-level tibial nerve, 11 patients had graft repairs varying from 4 to 9.2 cm in length. Seven patients regained a sensory grade of 3 or better on the sole of the foot, but only three had return of any degree of foot intrinsic muscle function. Table 11-8 summarizes the results of operations on injured posterior tibial nerves at the ankle level. If neurolysis was done based on a positive NAP across the lesion, pain was not always

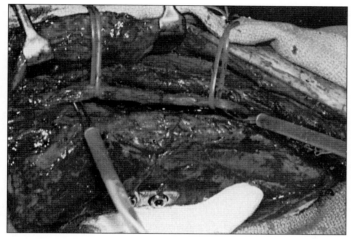

FIGURE 11-29 This posterior tibial nerve near the ankle was contused in association with a tibial fracture. The screw associated with the instrumentation of the fracture can be seen at the bottom of the photograph. Electrodes were placed on either side of the lesion, as shown above, and the nerve conducted an NAP. After neurolysis, the patient eventually experienced a nearly full recovery.

helped; however, in most cases further improvement in sensory and sometimes foot intrinsic muscle function occurred.

TARSAL TUNNEL LEVEL

Forty-six feet in 43 patients with the diagnosis of tarsal tunnel syndrome underwent operations. Those patients selected for an initial operation to release the tarsal tunnel had a history of painful paresthesias on the sole and sometimes the heel of the foot. A Tinel sign producing paresthesias on the bottom of the foot was usually elicited inferior to the medial malleolus and sometimes proximally or distally in the region of the instep. Sometimes there was either a mild hypoesthesia, or mixed hyper- and hypoesthesias on the sole or heel of the foot. Toe flexion and foot intrinsic function were spared in the majority of cases unless there had been a prior operation or ankle or foot injury as a precipitating factor, or if symptoms had been long-standing. Sensory conduction studies from the toes or instep to the tibial nerve proximal to the malleolus were abnormal. Most foot disorders are not due to tarsal tunnel syndrome, so care must be taken in making this diagnosis.

The operation included exposure of the nerve and its branches well above and below the ankle (Figs 11-31 to 11-33). A complete external neurolysis was always done, along with sectioning of the flexor retinaculum and origin of the abductor hallucis muscle and splitting of the muscles of the instep. In 28 patients without prior operation, the outcome following external neurolysis was excellent-to-good in 22 (79%) and fair-to-poor in 6 (21%). Eighteen cases of tarsal tunnel syndrome had undergone prior neurolysis and attempted decompression of the posterior tibial nerve elsewhere, yet experienced recurrent or worsening symptoms. Repeat neurolysis at LSUHSC sometimes helped the pain, paresthesias, and dysfunction. Four (40%) of ten patients who had reoperations in which external neurolysis was performed showed improvement. Five patients underwent internal neurolysis to relieve severe neuritic pain following prior surgery. Surgical results were satisfactory

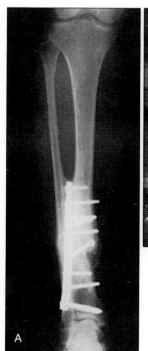

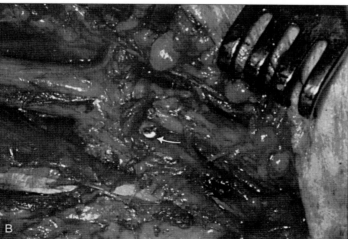

FIGURE 11-30 **(A)** This radiograph shows a severe fixated distal tibial fracture in a patient with complete posterior tibial palsy. **(B)** In addition to a severe stretch and contusive injury to the nerve, one of the screw tips was found in the nerve (*arrow*) when it was explored. A graft repair was necessary. Compare this lesion with that in Figure 11-29.

Table 11-8   Ankle-level operative tibial nerve injuries – incidence/results*

	Pt. no.	Neurolysis	Suture	Graft	Resection result
Contusion with fracture	19	9/7	2/1	5/3	3/3
Contusion without fracture	8	5/3	2/2	1/1	0/0
Blunt transection	3	0/0	0/0	3/2	0/0
Gunshot wound	2	1/1	0/0	1/1	0/0
Iatrogenic	1	0/0	0/0	1/0	0/0
Tarsal tunnel syndrome	46	34/26	5/2	0/0	7/4
Totals	79	49/37	9/5	11/7	10/7

*Results given as total cases/number with significant sensory recovery and relief of pain (if significant preoperatively); if resected, those with improved pain.

Pt., patient; No., number.

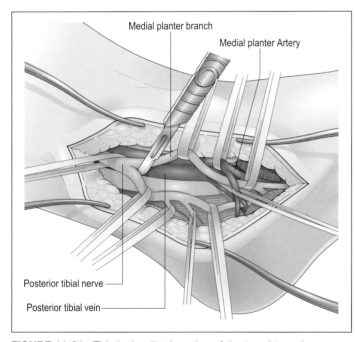

FIGURE 11-31   This is the distal portion of the tarsal tunnel exposure. Here, lateral and medial plantar branches are split apart by the scalpel as shown. Vessels are dissected and retracted separately. (From Kline DG, Hudson AR, and Kim DH: Atlas of Peripheral Nerve Surgery. Philadelphia, WB Saunders, 2001.)

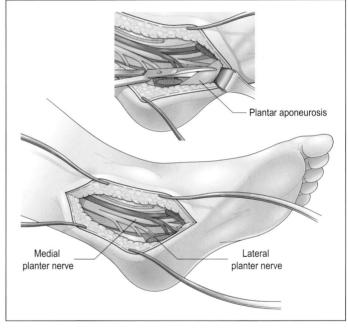

FIGURE 11-32   The completed tarsal tunnel dissection is shown. The inset shows the sectioning of soft tissues and muscle in the instep using a Metzenbaum scissors. (From Kline DG, Hudson AR, and Kim DH: Atlas of Peripheral Nerve Surgery. Philadelphia, WB Saunders, 2001.)

in only two (40%) of these patients. Seven patients had resection of the posterior tibial nerve due to severe intra- and extraneural scarring following multiple previous operations to relieve severe neuritic pain and paresthesias associated with a hypersensitive foot. Pain was helped dramatically in four (57%) cases and moderately in three (43%). Hypoesthesia was substituted for hyperesthesia on the sole of the foot and, surprisingly, each patient not only maintained plantar flexion and inversion of the foot as expected, but often some amount of toe flexion and occasionally even foot intrinsic muscle function. Ulceration of the sole has not occurred over an average of 3.2 years of follow-up.

CASE SUMMARY – TARSAL TUNNEL SYNDROME

This 79-year-old woman developed a tingling and burning sensation on the soles of both feet. This progressed and it became difficult for her to bear weight, causing her to become wheelchair-bound. There was no background of diabetes or alcohol misuse. Posterior tibial nerve conduction across the tarsal tunnel was 31 m/sec on the left and 36 m/sec on the right. At operation, both nerves were flattened and grayish in color from just distal to the medial calcaneus into the insteps of both feet. A complete external neurolysis of both nerves was done. Operative NAP conduction across these segments was in the mid-twenties and

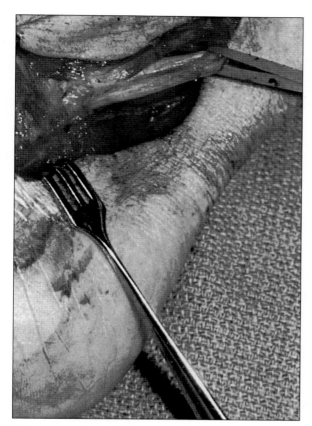

FIGURE 11-33 A posterior tibial nerve proximal to the malleolus exhibits an unusually high division into the medial and lateral plantar nerves. The tarsal tunnel has not yet been exposed.

Table 11-9 Operative tumors of the tibial nerve

	Patient no.	Resection and neurolysis*	Resection and grafts*
Schwannomas	12	11/10	1/0
Neurofibromas	6	5/5	1/0
Total	18	16/15	2/0

*Results are given as total patients/number of patients recovering to grade 3 or better.

was slower than in the preoperative studies, probably because it was done over a shorter segment of pathologic nerve.

Fortunately, she did well with this procedure. Although the toe intrinsic muscles remained weak, toe flexion was improved and she had good sensation on the soles of the feet. By 3 weeks postoperatively, she was able to bear weight and to walk without difficulty. Follow-up was over a 2-year period, and she continued to do well.

COMMENT

The diagnosis of carpal tunnel syndrome is easier to make and to treat than tarsal tunnel syndrome. If both the clinical and electrical findings agree with a tarsal tunnel syndrome, then a thorough neurolysis of the nerve and its plantar branches will help. It is important to exclude diabetic and alcoholic neuropathies and to be certain that the foot has an adequate blood supply before operating on this condition.

TUMORS

Eighteen patients with nerve sheath tumors arising from the tibial nerve underwent gross total surgical resections with preservation of preoperative function (Table 11-9). The tumors included 12 schwannomas and six solitary neurofibromas. Solid and sometimes cystic masses of different sizes were verified by computed tomography (CT) or magnetic resonance imaging (MRI) scans near the popliteal fossa. Eleven (92%) of 12 schwannomas were successfully resected, with preservation of preoperative function. One patient required graft repair after a wide resection for a recurrent tumor with extensive fascicular involvement. Of 12 patients with

schwannomas, seven (58%) had intact preoperative strength. Of these seven, six (86%) maintained full strength and one (14%) decreased to a 4–5 motor strength. Of five patients (42%) with preoperative weakness usually due to prior unsuccessful attempt at excision, three (60%) had improved strength, one (20%) was unchanged, and one (20%) became weaker. In six (50%) of the 12 patients with schwannomas, a radicular component of spontaneous pain was localized to the site of the tumor. Of these patients, five (83%) had complete resolution of their pain on follow-up evaluations, but one (17%) had only partial resolution. Of the six patients who were without preoperative pain, one (17%) had an onset of some postoperative pain, but it was not severe. Six patients with solitary neurofibromas without von Recklinghausen's disease underwent surgery for tumor resection. Five (83%) of six neurofibromas were resected completely without difficulty; however, one patient required graft repair after resection. Of the six patients, four (67%) had intact function before surgery. Of these, three (75%) maintained normal function, whereas one (25%) had some degree of postoperative weakness. Of two patients who presented with weakness, one (50%) experienced improvement and a patient who needed graft placement (50%) became worse. Of the five patients who presented with pain, all reported either no change or improvement after surgery.

SUMMARY

In summary, there were 135 tibial nerve lesions in the LSUHSC series presented in this chapter. The traumatic injury category, excluding the patients with tarsal tunnel syndrome and tumors, had 71 lesions and accounted for the most injuries. There were 46 cases of tarsal tunnel syndrome, and 18 patients underwent surgery for nerve sheath tumors. Of 22 tibial nerve lesions not in continuity (Table 11-10), a functional recovery of grade 3 or better was achieved in 4 (67%) of 6 patients who required end-to-end suture repairs, and 11 (69%) of 16 patients who required graft repairs. One hundred and thirteen tibial nerve lesions in continuity underwent primarily external or internal neurolysis or resection of their lesions. A few had end-to-end suture anastomosis or graft repairs. Direct intraoperative recording of NAPs guided management of the lesions. Among the 113 patients with lesions in continuity, 76 (81%) of 94 patients underwent neurolysis, five (83%) of six had suture repair and 11 (85%) of 13 patients who had graft repair recovered function to grade 3 or better. Repair results were best in patients with recordable NAPs treated by external neurolysis and were poor in a few patients with very lengthy lesions in continuity and in patients with tarsal tunnel syndrome having reoperations.

Table 11-10 Tibial nerve lesion categories and types of surgery performed in 135 cases

Lesion category/type of surgery	No. treated surgically	No. with grade ≥3 outcome (%)
Not in continuity		
Suture repair	6	4 (67)
Graft repair	16	11 (69)
In continuity		
NAP present		
External neurolysis	85	71 (84)
Internal neurolysis	9	5 (56)
NAP absent		
Suture repair	6	5 (83)
Graft repair	13	11 (85)

Surgical exploration and repair of tibial nerve lesions including tarsal tunnel syndrome and nerve sheath tumors achieved excellent outcomes, which agrees with the findings of others in the literature.[1,4,20]

REFERENCES

1. Aldea PA and Shaw WA: Lower extremity nerve injuries. Clin Plast Surg 13:691–699, 1986.
2. Borges LF, Hallett M, Selkoe DJ, et al.: The anterior tarsal tunnel syndrome. Report of two cases. J Neurosurg 54:89–92, 1981.
3. Brand PW and Ebner JD: Pressure sensitive devices for denervated hands and feet. A preliminary communication. J Bone Joint Surg [Am] 51:109–116, 1969.
4. Cimino WR: Tarsal tunnel syndrome: review of the literature. Foot Ankle 11:47–52, 1990.
5. Dellon AL and Mackinnon SE: Tibial nerve branching in the tarsal tunnel. Arch Neurol 41:645–646, 1984.
6. de Seze S, Dreyfus P, Denis A, et al.: Electromyography in the tarsal tunnel syndrome. Rev Rhum Mal Osteoartic 37:189–195, 1970.
7. DiStefano V, Sack JT, Whittaker R, et al.: Tarsal-tunnel syndrome. Review of the literature and two case reports. Clin Orthop 88:76–79, 1972.
8. Edwards WG, Lincoln CR, Bassett FH 3rd, et al.: The tarsal tunnel syndrome. Diagnosis and treatment. JAMA 207:716–720, 1969.
9. Havel PE, Ebraheim NA, Clark SE, et al.: Tibial nerve branching in the tarsal tunnel. Foot Ankle 9:117–119, 1988.
10. Janecki CJ and Dovberg JL: Tarsal-tunnel syndrome caused by neurilemmoma of the medial plantar nerve. A case report. J Bone Joint Surg [Am] 59:127–128, 1977.
11. Kim DH, Cho YJ, Ryu S, et al.: Surgical management and results of 135 tibial nerve lesions at Louisiana State University Health Sciences Center. Neurosurgery 53(5) 1114–1125, 2003.
12. Lam SJ: Tarsal tunnel syndrome. J Bone Joint Surg [Br] 49:87–92, 1967.
13. Lassmann G, Lassmann H, and Stockinger L: Morton's metatarsalgia. Light and electron microscopic observations and their relation to entrapment neuropathies. Virchows Arch A Pathol Anat Histol 370:307–321, 1976.
14. Lau JT and Daniels TR: Tarsal tunnel syndrome: a review of the literature. Foot Ankle Int 20:201–209, 1999.
15. Long DL: Electrical stimulation for relief of pain from chronic nerve injury. J Neurosurg 39:718–722, 1973.
16. Mitchell SW, Morehouse GR, and Keen WW: Gunshot Wounds and Other Injuries of Nerves. Philadelphia, JB Lippincott, 1964.
17. Nobel W: Peroneal palsy due to hematoma in the common peroneal nerve sheath after distal torsional fractures and inversion ankle sprains. J Bone Joint Surg [Am] 48:1484–1495, 1966.
18. Oh SJ, Kim HS, and Ahmad BK: The near-nerve sensory nerve conduction in tarsal tunnel syndrome. J Neurol Neurosurg Psychiatry 48:999–1003, 1985.
19. Sarrafian SK: Anatomy of the foot and ankle: Descriptive, topographical, functional. In: Sarrafian SK, Ed: Nerves. Philadelphia, JB Lippincott, 1993:365–383.
20. Trumble T and Vanderhooft E: Nerve grafting for lower-extremity injuries. J Pediatr Orthop 14:161–165, 1994.
21. Zeiss J, Fenton P, Ebraheim N, et al.: Magnetic resonance imaging for ineffectual tarsal tunnel surgical treatment. Clin Orthop 264:264–266, 1991.

COMMON PERONEAL NERVE

OVERVIEW

- During 141 operations for peroneal nerve stretch injury at Louisiana State University Health Sciences Center (LSUHSC), 121 nerves underwent external neurolysis based on a positive nerve action potential (NAP). One hundred and seven (88%) of 121 peroneal nerve injuries at the knee level undergoing external neurolysis based on a positive NAP recovered to grade 3 or better. Return of function began earlier than in the group of patients with end-to-end suture anastomosis or graft repairs; contraction of the peronei muscles was usually evident by 6 months and the anterior tibialis muscle by 12–14 months.

- If the injury had transected or pulled apart the nerve, end-to-end suture anastomosis repair was often not possible. However, if such a repair could be performed, recovery was good. Sixteen (84%) of a total of 19 knee-level peroneal nerves having end-to-end suture anastomosis repair had a grade 3 or better outcome.

- One hundred and thirty-eight patients with a variety of peroneal nerve injuries required graft repair. Fifty-seven (41%) of these 138 had a grade 3 or better outcome. Many patients continued to require a kick-up brace to provide optimal ambulation. This was also true of patients reaching a grade 3 level for those patients who were more comfortable in a brace, often despite eversion and dorsiflexion against some resistance.

- In the LSUHSC series, functional recovery after graft repair was dependent on the length of grafts necessary to close a gap. Seventy-five percent of those with grafts 6 cm or less in length reached a grade 3 recovery, while only 38% of those with grafts 6–12 cm in length reached the same level of recovery. Patients with grafts longer than 13 cm in length reached grade 3 only 16% of the time. These results can be compared with an earlier series reported by Seddon in which repair by suture or grafts had been done. Recovery of dorsiflexion averaged only 34.7%, but included peroneal lesions at all levels.

- The peroneal nerve innervates slender antigravity muscles such as the anterior tibialis, extensor communis, and extensor hallucis longus muscles. These muscles require multiple-site input for effective antigravity function, i.e. coordinated firing must be regained. It is difficult for regeneration to reconstruct this pattern of innervation.

Tendon transfer or partial fusion of the ankle can sometimes ameliorate the foot drop seen with peroneal palsy and this approach has been combined with graft repair of the nerve by Millesi with good results. Those patients having such an operation and managed at LSUHSC did best if they were young, slender individuals in whom there was less weight-bearing on the foot. If peroneal nerve injury is lengthy, such a substitutive approach can be more efficacious than a lengthy graft repair.

THE COMMON PERONEAL NERVE

In a recent review of 5777 trauma patients, 162 sustained a total of 200 peripheral nerve injuries. Of the 200 peripheral nerve injuries, 79 were in the lower extremity and the common peroneal nerve (CPN) was the most frequently injured nerve.[10] The CPN is superficial as it passes lateral to the surgical neck of the fibula, and it is at this point that the nerve is most susceptible to injury. Since the peroneal division is fixed proximally at the sciatic notch and at the fibular neck, the nerve is less able to accommodate stretch, which also results in a propensity to injury.[14]

Sunderland and Bradley studied 10 cadaveric specimens and found that in the popliteal region the CPN fascicle number was 7.5 and at the proximal fibular level this number increased to 18.2. The amount of connective tissue was 49% in the popliteal fossa and decreased to 31.5% at the fibular level.[13] Thus, the number of fascicles more than doubles and the percentage of connective tissue decreases distally and, therefore, the maximal load that the CPN may sustain before reaching its elastic limit is less than the tibial nerve in this same region. This suggests that when the CPN is subjected to the same force it is more susceptible to injury than the posterior tibial nerve in the same location, i.e. the internal arrangement of the nerve make it less able to absorb axially directed forces at the knee level.

APPLIED ANATOMY

The sciatic nerve bifurcates into the CPN and the tibial nerve at the middle to distal third of the thigh; thus, the level of the sciatic bifurcation, i.e. the take-off of the CPN from the sciatic nerve, varies. The CPN includes the nerve above, at, and below the head of the fibula and the nerve's superficial and deep branches in the lower leg. Close to its origin or sometimes somewhat proximal to it, one or more branches leave to form the sural nerve, either complemented or not by a branch from the tibial nerve. The CPN runs obliquely across the plantaris muscle from the popliteal fossa apex to the lateral popliteal fossa to lie over the head and neck of the fibula. As the nerve approaches the fibular head, it sometimes lies beneath the medial edge of the tendon of the long head of the biceps (Fig. 11-34). It then curves around the proximal peroneus longus muscle then over the posterior rim of the fibular head traveling to the anterior leg, at which point it divides into deep and superficial branches (Figs 11-35, 11-36).

The deep branch of the CPN quickly divides after passing over and around the head and neck of the fibula beneath the fibrous lateral edge of the peroneus longus muscle (Fig. 11-37). The initial branch supplies the anterior tibialis muscle and later branches innervate the extensor digitorum longus and extensor hallucis longus muscles. Some individuals have a peroneus tertius muscle and the deep branch may supply this muscle as well. The deep branch again divides into medial and lateral branches at the foot. The medial branch continues as a sensory branch supplying a small area of skin over the first dorsal web space of the foot, while the lateral branch innervates the extensor digitorum brevis and extensor hallucis brevis muscles.[6]

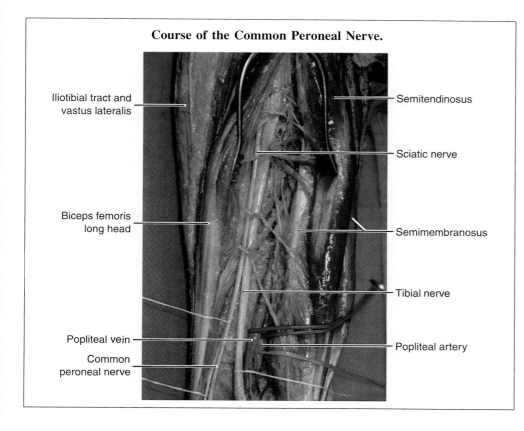

Course of the Common Peroneal Nerve.

Iliotibial tract and vastus lateralis

Biceps femoris long head

Popliteal vein

Common peroneal nerve

Semitendinosus

Sciatic nerve

Semimembranosus

Tibial nerve

Popliteal artery

FIGURE 11-34 A posterior view of the left leg popliteal fossa shows the common peroneal nerve passing from its apex, where it is medial to the biceps tendon, to the back of the head of the fibula. (From Kline DG, Hudson AR, and Kim DH: Atlas of Peripheral Nerve Surgery. Philadelphia, WB Saunders, 2001.)

Superficial Peroneal Nerve.

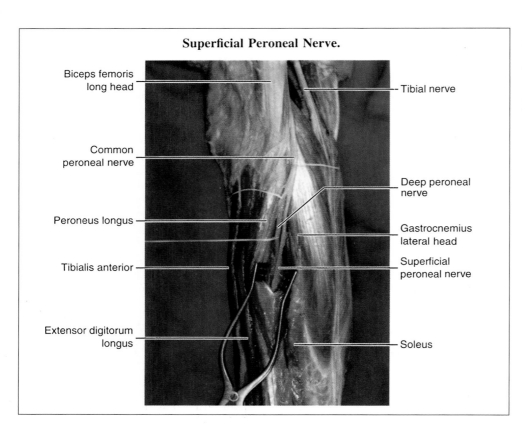

Biceps femoris long head — Tibial nerve

Common peroneal nerve

Deep peroneal nerve

Peroneus longus

Gastrocnemius lateral head

Tibialis anterior

Superficial peroneal nerve

Extensor digitorum longus

Soleus

FIGURE 11-35 A posterolateral view of the left leg depicts the common peroneal nerve in the distal popliteal fossa where it pierces the peroneus longus and divides into its superficial and deep peroneal nerve branches. (From Kline DG, Hudson AR, and Kim DH: Atlas of Peripheral Nerve Surgery. Philadelphia, WB Saunders, 2001.)

Terminal Branches of Common Peroneal Nerve at the Popliteal Fossa.

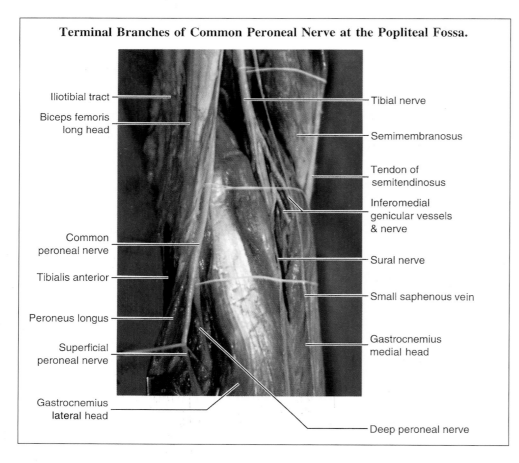

Iliotibial tract — Tibial nerve

Biceps femoris long head

Semimembranosus

Tendon of semitendinosus

Inferomedial genicular vessels & nerve

Common peroneal nerve

Sural nerve

Tibialis anterior

Small saphenous vein

Peroneus longus

Superficial peroneal nerve

Gastrocnemius medial head

Gastrocnemius lateral head

Deep peroneal nerve

FIGURE 11-36 A close-up view of the superior portion of Figure 11-35. (From Kline DG, Hudson AR, and Kim DH: Atlas of Peripheral Nerve Surgery. Philadelphia, WB Saunders, 2001.)

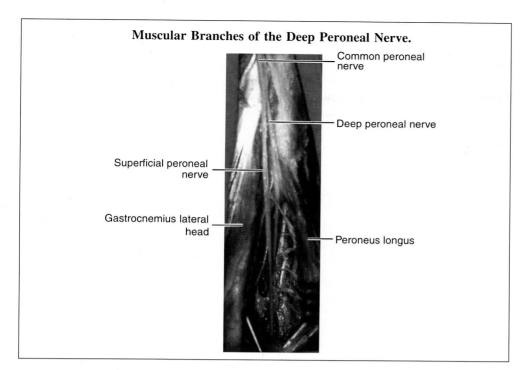

Muscular Branches of the Deep Peroneal Nerve.

Common peroneal nerve

Deep peroneal nerve

Superficial peroneal nerve

Gastrocnemius lateral head

Peroneus longus

FIGURE 11-37 A lateral view of the left leg shows the muscular branches of the deep peroneal nerve. (From Kline DG, Hudson AR, and Kim DH: Atlas of Peripheral Nerve Surgery. Philadelphia, WB Saunders, 2001.)

The superficial peroneal branch takes a relatively straight course, lying beneath the fascia and a portion of the peronei muscles. This superficial branch supplies the peroneus longus then brevis muscles and descends between the two heads of these peronei muscles. The superficial peroneal branch, as its name implies, gradually attains a more superficial position in the distal one-third of the lower leg at the midpoint where the peronei muscles blend into their tendons. This branch lies between these tendons and the lateral edge of the gastrocnemius-soleus muscle. The superficial peroneal nerve then bifurcates into the medial and lateral branches in front of the ankle joint.[3] As the nerve approaches the ankle, it is located anterolaterally and branches to supply cutaneous sensation to the anterolateral lower leg and ankle and the dorsum of the foot.

CLINICAL PRESENTATION AND EXAMINATION

Other than loss of the lateral hamstring, i.e. short head of the biceps femoris, with high peroneal-division injuries, important muscles innervated by this nerve are located below the knee, as with the tibial nerve.

Injury to the CPN or to both its superficial and deep branches causes weakness of the deep branch-innervated ankle and toe dorsiflexors. The ankle dorsiflexors include the anterior tibialis and peroneus tertius muscles, and the toe extensors include the extensor hallucis brevis and longus muscles which extend the great toe, and the extensor communis muscles which extend the second through fifth toes. Loss of toe extension is of less consequence since the shoe mitigates the importance of this function. Fortunately, the use of a shoe dorsiflexion splint insert or, for heavier and more active individuals, a spring-loaded kick-up foot brace built into a shoe, can substitute for foot extensor loss. These devices are so effective that many patients, after adapting to them, are unwilling to accept the uncertainties of results from repair of the CPN, especially if the lesion is severe.

With complete CPN injury, paresis of the superficial branch-innervated ankle evertors also occurs. These muscles include the peroneus longus and brevis muscles. The superficial branch of the CPN arises immediately distal to the fibular head.

The injury to the deep branch also results in decreased sensation in the region between the great and second toes. Involvement of the superficial branch results in decreased sensation in the antero-lateral calf and dorsum of the foot. The variable sensory loss on the dorsum of the foot associated with complete peroneal injury is of less functional consequence than is loss with tibial nerve injury where there is continuous contact of the tibial-innervated sole of the foot upon ambulation.

With knee-level injury and subsequent successful regeneration, contraction of the peronei muscles can begin by 3–5 months. The contraction of the peronei muscles can be palpated and observed. Muscles lateral to the proximal fibula can be seen to contract slightly on attempted eversion, and tightening of the tendon behind and above the lateral malleolus can be seen. Recovery of the anterior tibialis muscle does not usually occur until 9–12 months after injury, and return of the extensor hallucis longus muscle takes even longer. With early recovery of the anterior tibialis muscle, its tendon may be seen to tighten as it passes over the dorsum of the foot. The remainder of the toes may not recover extension after severe peroneal nerve injuries, even at the level of the knee.

A review of buttock- and thigh-level injuries follows. As described in a prior chapter, repair of the peroneal division at a buttock level seldom results in significant peroneal motor recovery. On the other hand, if the lesion at this level is one that permits spontaneous regeneration, even though complete, then recovery of both foot eversion and dorsiflexion can occur.

Injury at the thigh level can appear as an incomplete injury to the whole sciatic nerve, but instead it may be a complete injury to the peroneal or tibial division with sparing of function of the other. The level of bifurcation of the sciatic nerve in the thigh is variable. As stated in the chapter on the sciatic nerve, branching usually occurs at the junction of the middle and distal thirds of the thigh, but in the LSUHSC experience, the bifurcation occurred at a higher level in one-third of the cases. Recovery of the peroneal-innervated muscle function is also difficult to obtain with a thigh-level repair. When recovery does occur, return of some peronei muscle function may not take place for 6 months or more, and early contraction of the anterior tibialis muscle may not occur until after a year or more.

Injury at the level of the knee usually results in either a tibial or peroneal nerve palsy. If loss is complete, the clinical presentation is straightforward. Tibial nerve involvement causes a complete loss of inversion and plantar flexion and hypoesthesia on the sole of the foot and peroneal nerve involvement results in a lack of eversion and extension of the foot and toes.

Injury, especially penetrating injury near the head of the fibula, can damage the superficial branch of the peroneal nerve and spare the deep branch or vice versa. To reiterate, the superficial branch innervates the peronei muscles that evert the foot, and the deep branch innervates the extensors of the foot and toes.

The origin of the sural nerve can be predominantly from either the peroneal and/or tibial nerve. Proximal involvement of the sciatic nerve's peroneal and/or tibial divisions may also affect the sural sensory distribution. As stated above, a complete midthigh-level sciatic injury can involve total loss of distal muscles innervated by the tibial and peroneal divisions, and thus sural sensory function is often lost as well. With regard to sciatic nerve involvement at this midthigh level, hamstring muscle function is totally spared unless this function is compromised by direct muscle injury. Examples of the latter in the LSUHSC series are cases in which there was direct hamstring muscle injury, including several patients who sustained guillotine injuries not only to nerves but to the hamstring muscle groups as well.

Because of overlap for the saphenous and sural nerves, there is no autonomous sensory zone in which loss is reliable, even with a complete CPN injury. If sensory loss occurs, it is usually over the dorsum of the foot, particularly just proximal to the web space between the great and second toes.

Anterior compartment injury can involve a variable portion of the deep peroneal branches, depending on the level of injury. By comparison, posterior compartment injury of the tibial nerve in the leg can affect sensation on the sole of the foot and toe flexion and spread, but sometimes spares gastrocnemius-soleus muscle function, because branches to this large muscle complex enter at the proximal calf level.

ELECTROPHYSIOLOGICAL STUDIES

ELECTROMYOGRAPHY

Denervational changes in the peronei and anterior tibialis muscles and toe extensors indicate an axonotmetic or neurotmetic lesion of the peroneal nerve or its more proximal sciatic division. Nascent potentials and even a reduced number of fibrillations and denervational potentials especially in the peronei muscles promise, but unfortunately do not guarantee, return of dorsiflexion, although they favor it.

NERVE CONDUCTION STUDIES

These tests are of greatest value for entrapment or compression of the peroneal nerve over the head or neck of the fibula. It is impor-

Table 11-11 The LSUHSC muscle grading system for knee-level CPN injuries

Grade	Evaluation	Description
0	Absent	No palpable muscle contraction
1	Poor	Palpable contraction of peronei or anterior tibial muscles
2	Fair	Peronei or anterior tibial muscles contract against gravity
3	Moderate	Peronei and anterior tibial muscles contract against gravity and some resistance
4	Good	Peronei and anterior tibial muscles contract against moderate resistance
5	Excellent	Peronei and anterior tibial muscles contract against great resistance

LSUHSC, Louisiana State University Health Sciences Center; CPN, common peroneal nerve.

tant, when possible, to compare conduction in the symptomatic limb with the contralateral non-involved extremity.

The effective study of peroneal nerve entrapment usually includes stimulation of the nerve well proximal to the head of the fibula.[1] Latencies are then determined for conduction to the peronei muscles and to a more distal muscle such as the extensor hallucis longus. With entrapment, conduction velocities are slowed to both, but usually more so to the peronei than to more distal muscles. Latencies remain prolonged, often for years, even after successful neurolysis and relief of compressive bands or tissues and as a result, clinical evaluation, including careful grading of anterior compartment muscles (Table 11-11), is of greater value as an index of recovery than postoperative conductive studies. The latter, however, should not be neglected if there is failure of improvement or a plateau in clinical recovery.

SURGICAL EXPOSURE

For surgical exposure of the peroneal nerve, the patient is placed prone with cushions beneath the knee and ankle. For the more common lesions at the level of the fibula, a curvilinear incision is made extending from a point medial to the lateral hamstring in the lateral lower thigh, to the posterior head of the fibula and on towards the anterior compartment of the leg (Fig. 11-38). An alternative is a midline posterior distal thigh incision combined with a transverse incision in the popliteal space that runs laterally and then over the head of the fibula onto the leg. Occasionally, the lateral tendon of the biceps inserting onto the head of the fibula may resemble the peroneal nerve as it courses down to cross the neck of the fibula.

As the proximal portion of the incision is deepened, the lateral hamstring (the short head of the biceps) is moved laterally away from the underlying peroneal nerve (Fig. 11-39). A key portion of the deep dissection occurs just below the surgical neck of the fibula where the superficial and deep branches are exposed. The posterior edges of the peronei fasciae and muscles are cleared by sharp

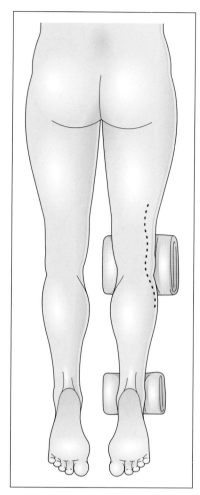

FIGURE 11-38 A drawing of the curvilinear incision is seen for a peroneal nerve lesion at the level of the right fibula, as described in the text. (From Kline DG, Hudson AR, and Kim DH: Atlas of Peripheral Nerve Surgery. Philadelphia, WB Saunders, 2001.)

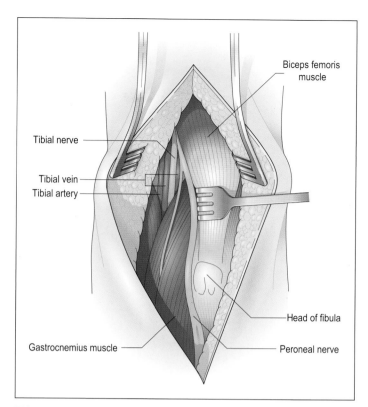

FIGURE 11-39 Exposure of the proximal peroneal nerve is carried out by moving the medial edge of the lateral hamstring muscle laterally away from the underlying peroneal nerve. (From Kline DG, Hudson AR, and Kim DH: Atlas of Peripheral Nerve Surgery. Philadelphia, WB Saunders, 2001.)

dissection, retracted, and partially split inferiorly to expose the superficial branch. With the help of a narrow Penrose drain placed around the peroneal nerve at the level of the neck of the fibula, the deep branch is traced around the fibula. Magnification and dissection onto the underside or anterior side of this branch helps, as does the use of plastic loops around the branches. Small vessels are coagulated by a bipolar forceps and fine neural branches going to the knee joint can be sacrificed if necessary to gain length along the course of the deep branch. Mobilization of the deep branches is necessary to enable "leveling-off" of the surgical neck of the fibula. This is done by dissecting away soft tissue from the posterior aspect of the surgical neck of the fibula to a depth of approximately 0.5 inches around the neck using a periosteal elevator (Fig. 11-40A). Resection of the head of the fibula is performed with a Leksell rongeur (Fig. 11-40B).

There is no reason for a small or focal exposure of the peroneal nerve and its branches, since short incisions and exposures are generally to be avoided in nerve surgery. Even with adequate exposure, it may be difficult to define a viable distal stump or branch to the tibialis anterior muscle. Nerve action potential recording is paramount to avoid needless resection, because functional regeneration after repair is limited. On the other hand, if, despite gross

continuity, the lesion has a severe injury and does not conduct, the possibility of significant spontaneous recovery is nonexistent and, as a result, a correct decision about resection is paramount.

RESULTS

At LSUHSC there were 278 knee-level operative peroneal nerve lesions that were analyzed for mechanism of injury, surgical technique used for repair, and functional outcome. The LSUHSC muscle grading system (Table 11-11) was used to document pre- and postoperative functional outcomes.

STRETCH CONTUSION

The largest injury category for the peroneal nerve at the knee level was caused by stretch/contusion (Table 11-12), and these traction injuries involving the peroneal nerve remain very difficult to manage successfully.[5,9] Stretch injury not only damages the nerve over a length, but can rupture the vasa nervorum, causing bleeding into the nerve sheath and a compressive hematoma resulting in ischemia.[7,9] Also, considerable connective tissue damage may occur with severe stretch injuries, which can lead to both intra- and extraneural scar formation.

Most stretch/contusion injuries in this LSUHSC series were caused by vehicular accidents or sports such as football, and usually occurred in relatively young individuals. Many peroneal palsies were associated with serious injury to the knee joint or surrounding structures (Fig. 11-41).

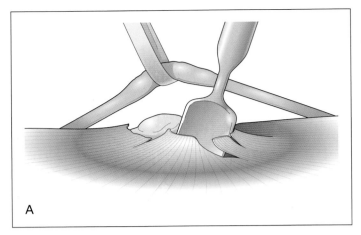

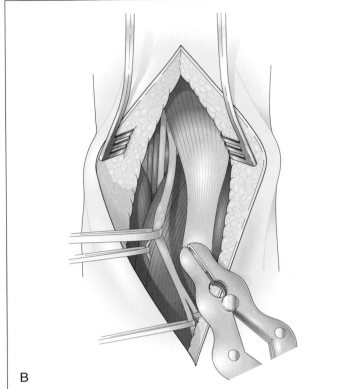

FIGURE 11-40 **(A)** The periosteal elevator dissection of the soft tissues from the posterior aspect of the surgical neck of the fibula. **(B)** A Leksell rongeur is used to resect the head of the fibula. The injured peroneal nerve and its distal superficial and deep branches have been displaced. (From Kline DG, Hudson AR, and Kim DH: Atlas of Peripheral Nerve Surgery. Philadelphia, WB Saunders, 2001.)

Table 11-12 Results of CPN traumatic injury**

Type of injury	Pt. no.	Neurolysis	Suture	Graft		
Stretch/contusion (– fx/dislocation)	141	56	0	85		
Laceration	39	3	14	22		
Entrapment	30	26	0	4		
Stretch/contusion (+ fx/dislocation)	22	10	2	10		
Compression	21	16	0	5		
Iatrogenic	13	6	0	7		
GSW	12	4	3	5		
Functional outcomes				**Graft size**		
				<6 cm	6–12 cm	13–24 cm
Total	278	121/107 (88%)*	19/16 (84%)	36/27 (75%)	64/24 (38%)	38/6 (16%)

*Number of patients having surgery/number of patients with postoperative grade 3 or better results.

CPN, common peroneal nerve; fx/dislocation, fracture or dislocation; +, with; – without.

**Abstracted from Kim D, Murovic J, Tiel R, Kline D: Management and outcomes in 318 operative common peroneal lesions at LSUHSC, Neruosurgery 54(6): 1421–1429, 2004

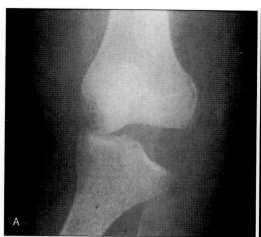

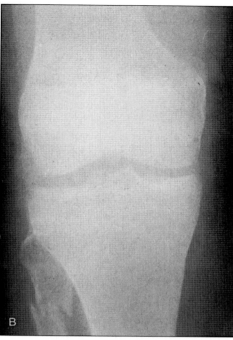

FIGURE 11-41 These are common bony injuries associated with stretch injuries involving the peroneal nerve: a severe dislocation of the knee joint **(A)** and a fracture of the neck of the fibula **(B)**. These patients both had devastating, lengthy stretch injuries of the peroneal nerve.

Some of these traction injuries did not have operative intervention because of late referral, i.e. at 1 year after injury, or because of spontaneous and relatively early recovery. Of those having operations, the interval between injury and operation was 4–9 months.

Fifty-six (40%) of the 141 operative stretch/contusion injuries without fracture/dislocations underwent neurolysis because of partial but significant injuries on presentation or because, despite more complete clinical and EMG loss, there was early evidence of significant regeneration by intraoperative NAP stimulation and recording. In 85 (60%) of 141 patients having operations for stretch/contusion injuries without fracture/dislocations, interfascicular graft repair was necessary because of total nerve distraction (Fig. 11-42) or, more frequently, lengthy severe lesions in continuity that did not transmit NAPs (Fig. 11-43). Graft lengths varied but were placed into one of three categories: <6 cm, 6–12 cm, and 13–24 cm. Graft lengths for successful cases were usually <6 cm in length and were shorter than in those cases without sufficient recovery. This was similar to the findings by Durandeau et al. that in 14 knee-level peroneal nerve lesions repaired using grafts, only patients repaired with grafts less than 5–8 cm in length had good results.[2]

Those 22 (16%) of 141 operative nerves injured by stretch, but in association with fracture or dislocation and requiring operation, had a similar fate, although two had lesions which were shorter in length and could be sutured. Both of these patients recovered significant dorsiflexion of the foot.

Fractures associated with stretch injuries usually involved the head of the fibula and tibial plateau. Such lesions tended to be more focal than those associated with knee dislocation with or without ligamentous tears. As a result, even if grafts were necessary, recovery was better with fracture-related injuries than in those patients with stretch injuries associated with dislocation of the knee or severe ligamentous injury.

LACERATION/STAB WOUND

Six (15%) of 39 lacerations to soft tissues involving the knee-level peroneal nerve were found to have left the nerve in continuity. In 3 (8%) cases undergoing operations, an NAP was recorded across the lesion and significant recovery resulted from neurolysis (Fig. 11-44). End-to-end suture anastomosis or epineurial suture repair was possible in 14 (36%) transections, and recovery to grade 3 or better was achieved (Fig. 11-44). Most of these patients had primary repair within 72 hours of sustaining a sharp injury. Grafts were necessary in 22 (56%) patients, with five recovering to grade 3 function. Most of these patients had blunt transecting injuries caused by propellers, fan blades, or shards of metal (Fig. 11-45).

GUNSHOT WOUND

The category of gunshot wound (GSW) was a relatively favorable one compared with that of stretch injury, because some of the lesions were more focal. Twelve (4%) of 278 patients with knee-level peroneal nerve lesions had surgery for injuries due to GSWs and the indication was lack of functional recovery by clinical or EMG evaluations. Nine (75%) of 12 patients with GSW injuries had contusive lesions in continuity and the other three (25%) of 12 had experienced complete peroneal nerve transections. Four (33%) of 12 GSW injuries had recordable intraoperative NAPs and underwent neurolysis. These four had excellent recoveries to grades 4 and 5 by 20 months, despite complete preoperative functional loss. Three patients had end-to-end suture anastomosis repairs after focal resection of their lesions. Five (42%) of 12 patients with peroneal nerve GSW injuries underwent repair with nerve grafts.

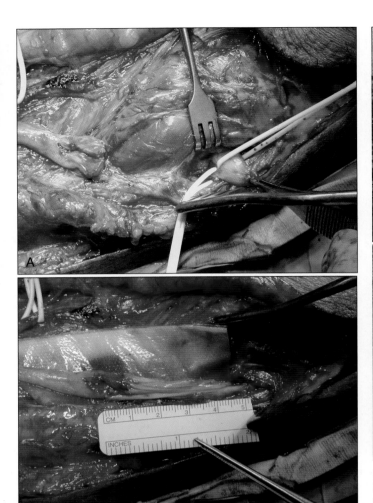

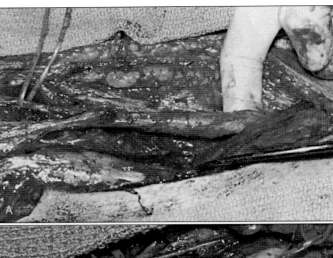

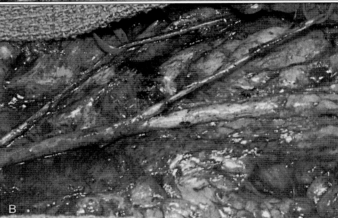

FIGURE 11-42 **(A)** An intraoperative photograph shows a common peroneal nerve lesion not in continuity, which was transected due to a stretch and avulsion injury. The proximal stump is to the left. The distal stump consisting of the deep and superficial peroneal nerves, each encircled with a Vasoloop, is to the right. **(B)** An interfascicular nerve graft repair is shown, which was performed after resection of a neuroma. Five sural nerve grafts, 5 cm in length were used for the graft repair.

FIGURE 11-43 **(A)** A segment of a stretch/contusion injury caused by a motorcycle accident involved the peroneal nerve. The lesion extended from the surgeon's gloved finger to the superficial and deep branches exposed to the left. In this case, the nerve was both swollen and firm. **(B)** A peroneal nerve which sustained a stretch injury from a ski accident. The nerve was thinned out and narrowed over an 11 cm segment. Neither lesion transmitted an NAP 5 months after injury, and both were resected and repaired using lengthy sural grafts.

ENTRAPMENT

The differential diagnosis of spontaneous peroneal nerve entrapment at the neck of the fibula includes L5 spinal radiculopathy. This distinction must be made carefully because mistakes in diagnosis of these widely separated sites of pathology are not infrequent.

A past history of trauma involving the knee (Fig. 11-46) or occasionally a postural habit such as frequently sitting with legs crossed can serve as contributing factors, but most of the LSUHSC patients undergoing operations for peroneal nerve entrapment did not have this antecedent history.[8,16]

Twenty-six (87%) of 30 patients undergoing surgical exploration for peroneal nerve entrapment injuries had neurolysis performed with sectioning of overlying soft tissue, including fascial edges or ligamentous structures.[15] Partial fibulectomy was routinely performed by leveling off the surgical neck of the fibula with a rongeur.

After neurolysis above and below the fibular head, NAP recordings were made from the deep and superficial peroneal nerve branches.

Four (13%) patients required graft repairs, with sural grafts 5–10 cm in length. These graft repairs were necessary after one to three operations performed elsewhere had failed to halt progression of neurological deficit. Two recovered function to grade 3 at 26 and 30 months, respectively. One patient who presented with a complete foot drop recovered full motor function after neurolysis; however 2.5 years later, the foot drop recurred. At reexploration, a nontransmitting segment of neuroma was resected and sural grafts 9 cm in length were used to replace a segment of nerve near the fibular neck. After 2 years, the patient again recovered to a grade 3 function.

Loss resulting from entrapment was not always readily reversed by operation. In fact, if loss was severe on presentation, operative intervention often did not improve function. Functional status was usually stabilized by operation, but in a few cases this was not so and some of these patients even progressed despite our operative neurolysis.

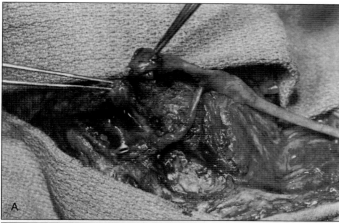

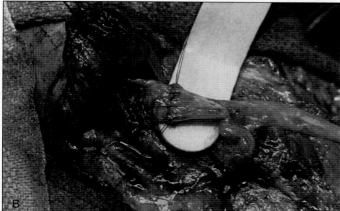

FIGURE 11-44 **(A)** A laceration of the peroneal nerve caused by a knife wound just distal to the head of the fibula is seen in this intraoperative photograph. **(B)** The end-to-end suture anastomosis repair with a 6–0 prolene suture was performed within 72 hours of injury. The head of the fibula was then leveled off and waxed before closing the soft tissues.

COMPRESSION AND TUMOR

Twenty-one (8%) of the total of 278 peroneal nerve injury patients undergoing operative intervention had surgery for compression. Most compressions of knee-level peroneal nerve were caused by poor positioning during the administration of an anesthetic or malposition of an extremity associated with alcohol or drug-induced stupor. In addition, fibular exostosis sometimes involved this nerve (Fig. 11-47). Loss of function was often progressive, usually painless, and surgery was not always successful in reversing the loss resulting from compression.

Other causes of compression included arteriovenous malformations and compartment syndromes involving the leg caused by soft tissue swelling and/or a tight cast.

Sixteen (76%) of 21 patients with compression of the peroneal nerve underwent neurolysis after intraoperative NAPs indicated regeneration across the lesion. Five (24%) patients had graft repairs.

Forty patients with tumors intrinsic to the peroneal nerve were evaluated and had surgery. Many patients, i.e. 16 (40%) of 40, in the tumor category had ganglion cysts involving the peroneal nerve. Recent observations by Spinner et al. on a large number of peroneal nerve ganglion cysts from several institutions suggest a connection between the synovial-lined tibiofibular joint and the deep branches

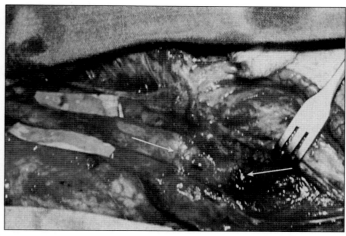

FIGURE 11-45 An accident involving a propeller caused this injury to the peroneal nerve at the point where it passes over the head of the fibula. The injury site, bracketed by white arrows, was repaired with sural nerve grafts 5 weeks after injury.

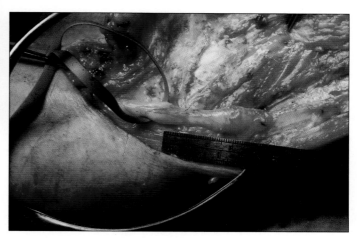

FIGURE 11-46 A left peroneal nerve with an area of narrowing and swelling on either side of the constriction. This patient had received a contusive blow behind the knee in the past and over a period of several years developed a progressive peroneal palsy. The palsy was considered to be the result of a trauma-induced entrapment. The lesion conducted an NAP, and thus a neurolysis was performed. (Courtesy of Dr. Jack Hurst, Lafayette, LA.)

of the peroneal nerve as the origin for these lesions.[12] Peroneal nerve ganglion cysts occur most frequently near the top of the fibula.[4,11]

There were 10 schwannomas, one of which was malignant, and six neurofibromas, one of which was associated with von Recklinghausen's disease. MRI or CT near the knee joint was used to show lesions that were solid, sometimes cystic, and of various sizes. These 16 patients with benign neural sheath tumors had their tumors removed in most cases without the need for repair. The malignant schwannoma was treated with a wide local resection followed by irradiation. There were two osteochondromas, two neurogenic sarcomas, two localized hypertrophic neuropathies (LHN), also called "onion bulb" disease, and one desmoid and one glomus tumor. Of the two patients with LHN involving the peroneal nerve at the knee level, one recovered some function after resection of the lesion and graft repair and one did not.

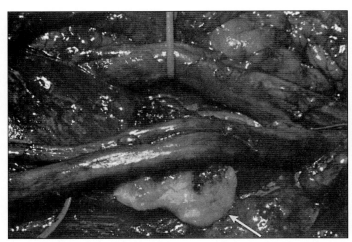

FIGURE 11-47 A peroneal nerve is seen to be entrapped by a bony exostosis near the head of the fibula (*arrow*). The posterior tibial nerve is at the top of the figure and the peroneal nerve is at the bottom.

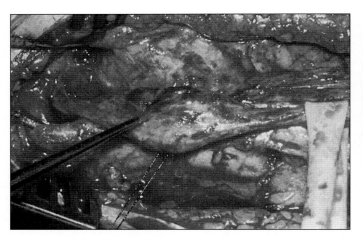

FIGURE 11-48 A large neuroma in continuity of the peroneal nerve as shown occurred after resection of a hemangioma involving the nerve. This lesion was located behind the knee of a 17-year-old girl. The neuroma transmitted an NAP, but required a split graft repair: the inferior portion of the nerve also transmitted an NAP, but the superior portion did not and was replaced by sural grafts. Over a 3.5-year period, the patient gained peroneal function to a grade 4 level.

A hemangioma involving the peroneal nerve was resected; however, secondarily, a large neuroma that transmitted an NAP formed in continuity and required a split graft repair (Fig. 11-48).

IATROGENIC (INCLUDING INJECTION INJURY)

Two patients sustained injection injuries to the peroneal nerve at the level of the knee. Both lesions were relatively mild and did not require operation. Open or arthroscopic knee procedures were the most common causes of iatrogenic knee-level peroneal nerve injuries. After waiting for 4 months, 13 patients with iatrogenic injuries without signs of regeneration underwent exploratory operations and were found to have lesions in continuity (Fig. 11-49). Six (46%) of the 13 patients with iatrogenic injuries underwent external neurolysis due to transmittable NAPs across the lesions and 7 (54%) of 13 patients had graft repairs.

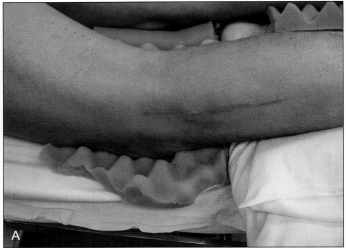

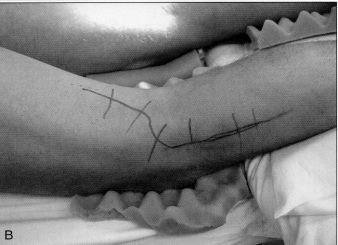

FIGURE 11-49 **(A)** The scar from an open operation on the proximal fibula during which the common peroneal nerve was lacerated. **(B)** The iatrogenic injury in **(A)** was repaired by using a modification shown of the usual incision, which incorporates the prior incision.

REFERENCES

1. Berry H and Richardson PM: Common peroneal nerve palsy: A clinical and electrophysiological review. J Neurol Neurosurg Psychiatry 39:1162–1171, 1976.
2. Durandeau A, Piton C, Fabre T, et al.: Results of 14 nerve grafts of the common peroneal nerve after a severe valgus strain of the knee. J Bone Joint Surg [Br] 79(Suppl I):54, 1997.
3. Farhan M: Nerve entrapment of the branches of the superficial peroneal nerve. J Bone Joint Surg [Br] 83(Suppl III):340, 2001.
4. Harbaugh KS, Tiel RL, and Kline DG: Ganglion cyst involvement of peripheral nerves. J Neurosurg 87:403–408, 1997.
5. Highet WB and Holmes W: Traction injuries to the lateral popliteal and traction injuries to peripheral nerves after suture. Br J Surg 30:212, 1943.
6. Mackinnon SE and Dellon A: Other lower extremity nerve entrapments. In: Surgery of the Peripheral Nerve. New York, Thieme Medical Publishers, 1988.
7. Meals RA: Peroneal-nerve palsy complicating ankle sprain. Report of two cases and review of the literature. J Bone Joint Surg [Am] 59:966–968, 1977.
8. Nagler S and Rangell L: Peroneal palsy caused by crossing the legs. JAMA 133:755–761, 1947.

9. Nobel W: Peroneal palsy due to hematoma in the common peroneal nerve sheath after distal torsional fractures and inversion ankle sprains. J Bone Joint Surg [Am] 48:1484–1495, 1966.

10. Noble J, Munro CA, Prasad V, et al.: Analysis of upper and lower extremity peripheral nerve injuries in a population of patients with multiple injuries. J Trauma 45:116–122, 1998.

11. Nucci F, Artico M, Santoro A, et al.: Intraneural synovial cyst of the peroneal nerve: report of two cases and review of the literature. Neurosurgery 26:339–344, 1990.

12. Spinner RJ, Atkinson JL, Harper M, et al.: Recurrent intraneural ganglion cyst of the tibial nerve. Case report. J Neurosurg 92:334–337, 2000.

13. Sunderland S and Bradley KC: Stress–strain phenomena in human peripheral nerve trunks. Brain 84:102–119, 1961.

14. Thoma A, Fawcett S, Ginty M, et al.: Decompression of the common peroneal nerve: experience with 20 consecutive cases. Plast Reconstr Surg 107:1183–1189, 2001.

15. Vastamaki M: Decompression for peroneal nerve entrapment. Acta Orthop Scand 57:551–554, 1986.

16. Woltman HL: Crossing the legs as a factor in the production of peroneal palsy. JAMA 93:670–672, 1929.

SURAL NERVE

OVERVIEW

- Eighteen operative sural nerve lesions from Louisiana State University Health Sciences Center (LSUHSC) are presented.
- The most common sural nerve injury was that of laceration. There were seven such injuries, five of which were due to accidents involving glass and two resulted from knife wounds. This was followed in number by gunshot wounds, which involved the sural nerve in three instances and necessitated surgery. Two sural nerve injuries were due to venous stripping and ligation and two resulted from orthopedic procedures. There were two neuromas of the sural nerve from injuries due to blunt trauma, one sural nerve biopsy-related neuroma and one contusion/crush injury.
- When the sural nerve sustained an injury resulting in the formation of a neuroma, the treatment was lengthy excision of the sural nerve above and below the neuroma. Repair was not performed since sensory loss from excision in the distribution of the sural nerve was of little functional consequence and repair could lead to a painful neuroma in continuity.
- The most common reason for exposure of the sural nerve was to harvest it for grafts, and the technique for this is delineated in this chapter.

APPLIED ANATOMY

The sural nerve is a major lower extremity sensory nerve, which supplies the skin of the posterolateral distal one-third of the leg and dorsolateral side of the foot including the last toe. Various mechanisms cause injuries to the sural nerve. It is also commonly harvested for use in graft repairs.

The sural nerve originates in the popliteal fossa from varying portions of the peroneal and tibial nerves in the popliteal fossa. Sometimes its entire origin is from one nerve (Fig. 11-50), and that usually is the peroneal nerve. It also can originate from the junction of a branch of the tibial nerve, the medial sural cutaneous nerve and the anastomotic, also called communicating, branch of the peroneal nerve.[2,4,5,7,8] It runs between the two heads of the gastrocnemius muscle beneath the gastrocnemius fascia to the juncture of the upper-third and middle-third of the leg where it pierces the fascia to become subcutaneous (Fig. 11-51). It joins the lateral sural nerve and then angles obliquely towards the lateral calf at the distal one-third of the leg. As the sural nerve approaches the ankle it lies

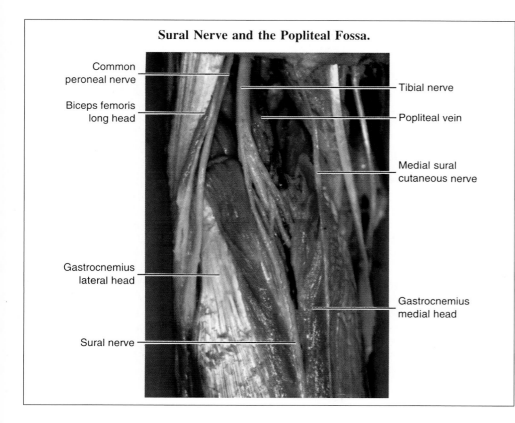

Sural Nerve and the Popliteal Fossa.

Common peroneal nerve — Biceps femoris long head — Gastrocnemius lateral head — Sural nerve — Tibial nerve — Popliteal vein — Medial sural cutaneous nerve — Gastrocnemius medial head

FIGURE 11-50 The sural nerve takes its origin from variable portions of the peroneal and tibial nerves in the popliteal fossa. Sometimes, its entire origin is from one nerve, usually the peroneal nerve. In this cadaveric specimen of the left popliteal fossa the nerve of origin, however, is the tibial nerve. The sural nerve is shown descending between the two heads of the gastrocnemius.

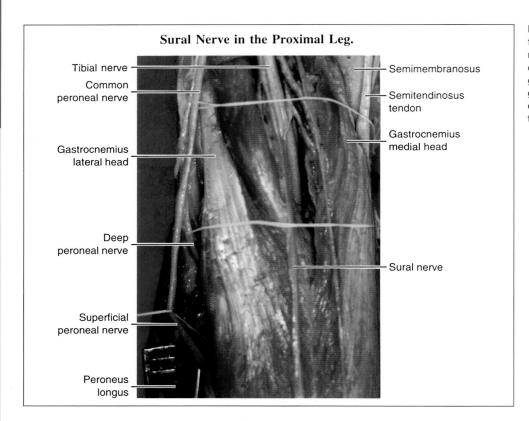

Sural Nerve in the Proximal Leg.

Tibial nerve

Common peroneal nerve

Gastrocnemius lateral head

Deep peroneal nerve

Superficial peroneal nerve

Peroneus longus

Semimembranosus

Semitendinosus tendon

Gastrocnemius medial head

Sural nerve

FIGURE 11-51 Leaving the popliteal fossa at the inferior angle, the sural nerve shown here in a left leg cadaveric specimen descends in the groove between the two heads of the gastrocnemius muscle and pierces the deep fascia proximally in the leg to join the lateral sural nerve.

lateral to the gastrocnemius tendon, i.e. the Achilles tendon. Its location at this point was found to be 7 cm above the tip of the lateral malleolus in a study of 17 cadavers by Lawrence and Botte.[5] The nerve then runs forward below the lateral malleolus and continues as the lateral dorsal cutaneous nerve along the lateral foot and last toe (Fig. 11-52). It communicates on the dorsum of the foot with the intermediate dorsal cutaneous nerve of the superficial peroneal nerve; in the leg, its branches communicate with those of the posterior femoral cutaneous nerve from the sacral plexus.

CLINICAL PRESENTATION AND EXAMINATION

Patients with sural nerve injuries usually present with lateral ankle "pins-and-needles" sensations and a concomitant hypersensitivity to light touch or loss of sensation in a sural nerve distribution.[8] Patients with sural nerve injuries in the LSUHSC series also presented with painful neuromas involving the sural nerve, which were sometimes palpable. Neuromas were found to occur at multiple sites along the course of the sural nerve in the case of surgical scars related to saphenous vein stripping.[9] A Tinel sign is usually elicitable by tapping the site(s) of the neuroma(s), and result(s) in paresthesias in the distal sural distribution in the foot.

Examination reveals an antalgic gait with a hesitancy to bear weight on the affected heel. A decreased sensation to touch and pinprick along the lateral ankle and foot is usually found on sensory examination. A hypersensitivity to touch in the sural nerve distribution may also be found.

Compression of the sural nerve in the posterior aspect of the leg resulting in calf pain is another possible presentation and has been reported in 13 athletes by Fabre et al.[3] This site, at the level of the superficial sural aponeurosis at the junction of the middle and lower

thirds of the leg, is not a common location for sural nerve compression injury.

ELECTROPHYSIOLOGICAL STUDIES

Bilateral sural nerve conduction is orthodromically studied from the ankle to the calf. When necessary it is sometimes also studied in the proximal calf to knee area and from the fifth metatarsal to the ankle region.

The electrophysiological study in a patient with sural nerve injury at the ankle reveals an absence or decrease of the 14 cm antidromic sural sensory response recording at the involved ankle. The percentage of nerve compromise is determined by comparison of the sensory nerve action potential (SNAP) amplitude of the involved side with the healthy side. An absence of the sural nerve response implies a conduction block or possible axonotmesis or neurotemesis affecting the sural sensory fibers.[9]

SURGICAL APPROACH

Most sural nerve injuries do not require operative intervention, but persistent pain and sensory symptoms may prompt surgery, especially if there is tenderness and a Tinel sign over the course of the nerve.

To harvest this nerve for graft repair, a prone approach when the patient is already in this position for a sciatic nerve exposure or posterior approach to the radial or axillary nerves. A stockinette is used to cover the foot, leg, and thigh.

When the patient is supine, a position used for many nerve dissections, exposure of the sural nerve is more difficult. A stockinette is again used to cover the foot, leg, and thigh; however, the leg is flexed at the knee and towels and towel clips are used to hold the

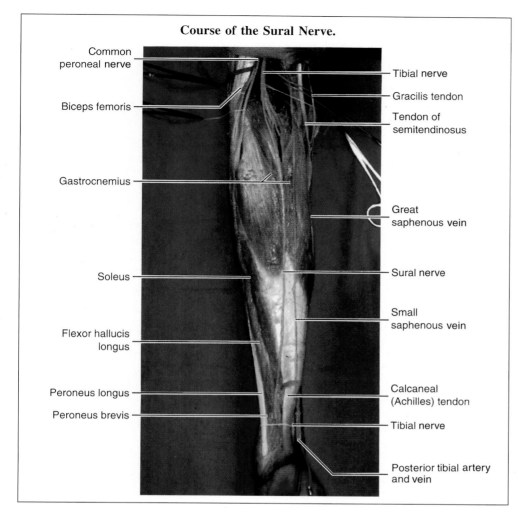

Course of the Sural Nerve.

Common peroneal nerve

Biceps femoris

Gastrocnemius

Soleus

Flexor hallucis longus

Peroneus longus

Peroneus brevis

Tibial nerve

Gracilis tendon

Tendon of semitendinosus

Great saphenous vein

Sural nerve

Small saphenous vein

Calcaneal (Achilles) tendon

Tibial nerve

Posterior tibial artery and vein

FIGURE 11-52 The sural nerve descends lateral to the calcaneus tendon to the region between the lateral malleolus and the calcaneus, accompanied by the short saphenous vein. Distal to the lateral malleolus, the sural nerve runs along the lateral border of the foot and ends at the lateral side of the last toe of the foot. It supplies the posterior and lateral skin of the distal third of the leg and the lateral border of the foot including the entire last toe. The sensory supply to the last toe is shared with the tibial nerve's lateral plantar nerve.

foot flat on the operating table. Knee and leg are then partially adducted by a sheet or towel placed around the knee and held by a towel clip to the contralateral leg's drapes. A folded sheet is placed under the ipsilateral buttock to aid in the necessary internal rotation of the leg in order to expose the calf.

In either the prone or supine position, a curvilinear incision is made on the posterior calf and is extended to the lateral ankle (Fig. 11-53). Alternatively, the sural nerve can be exposed by using multiple incisions on the posterolateral leg (Fig. 11-54). At the ankle level the nerve is located between the lateral malleolus and the Achilles tendon. The nerve can be traced proximally by sharp dissection with a scalpel or Metzenbaum scissors, with care taken to preserve its branches. The sural nerve can be easily confused with the lesser saphenous vein at this level, since the nerve travels along with this vein here[6] and is often crossed by venous or arterial branches. The overlying gastrocnemius and soleus fasciae may need to be opened as the nerve approaches the upper one-third of the leg and then the popliteal area. Too much traction on the sural nerve may cause damage to the peroneal or tibial nerves.

SURAL NERVE HARVESTING FOR USE IN GRAFT REPAIRS

The sural nerve commonly has one or more branches emanating outward at its distal aspect which supply sensory input to the lateral foot. Proximally, many branches are seen; however, the branches originate from the tibial, peroneal or, less commonly, the main sciatic nerve. The latter branches may or may not combine to form the sural nerve.

The width of the sural nerve may not always be of a good caliber, and thus, fine branches may of necessity be used. Alternatively, the opposite limb may be a source of a better caliber of sural nerve.

Using fine forceps and scissors, the fascia and fat are removed from the graft after its harvest, while it is kept moist on a towel. The sural nerve and its branches are then placed in sterile normal saline. The defect to be bridged by the graft is measured and the required length of graft is cut from the sural nerve. Each graft must be approximately 10% longer than the gap length to allow for retraction. Removal of the sural nerve for graft harvest results in a small zone of sensory loss in a non-weight-bearing portion of the lateral edge of the foot, which is usually not bothersome.[1]

SURAL NERVE INJURY

If the sural nerve sustains an injury, the treatment is a lengthy excision of the sural nerve above and below the neuroma, the latter of which has usually formed in such an injury. Repair should not be performed, since sensory loss from excision in the distribution of the sural nerve is of little functional consequence and repair could lead to another painful neuroma in continuity. The nerve is

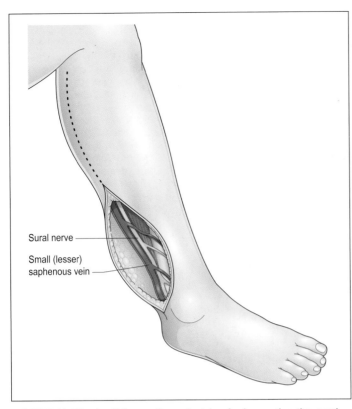

FIGURE 11-53 A mildly curvilinear incision for harvesting the sural nerve for graft repairs is made at the posterior calf and extends to the lateral ankle. At the ankle level the nerve is located between the lateral malleolus and the Achilles tendon. It is easily confused with a vein at this level, since they travel together and the sural nerve is often crossed by venous or arterial branches. Once identified, the nerve is surgically traced proximally.

Sural nerve

Small (lesser) saphenous vein

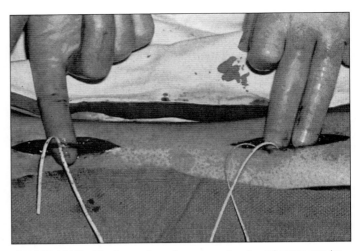

FIGURE 11-54 The harvesting of a segments of sural nerve can be accomplished by using multiple incisions rather than a single long incision on the posterolateral leg, as shown in the intraoperative photograph above.

Table 11-13 Operative sural nerve injuries

Mechanisms of injury	Number of operative cases
Glass laceration	5
Gunshot wound	3
Knife wound	2
Blunt laceration	2
Venous stripping/ligation	2
Orthopedic operations	2
Contusion/crush injury	1
Sural nerve biopsy	1
Totals	18

sharply sectioned well above the injury site, and the neuroma and some of the distal nerve removed, as well. Next, the proximal stump is visualized under loupes. The individual fascicles of the proximal stump are grasped with a fine bipolar forceps and coagulated in order to seal them. The proximal stump is left to retract under fascia and/or muscle. To date, although neuromas have recurred in a few cases, they are not painful and may be managed conservatively without reoperation.

RESULTS

The most frequent operative injury involving the sural nerve in the LSUHSC series was laceration injury due to glass in five cases and knife wounds in two patients (Table 11-13; Fig. 11-55). Gunshot wounds to the lower leg resulted in painful neuromas of the sural nerve in three patients, which required surgical excision. Venous stripping and ligation necessitated operative repair of two sural nerves and orthopedic operations also resulted in two sural nerve injuries. Wire from a lawn mower and another blunt trauma injury caused neuromas in two sural nerves, one of which was at the popliteal region close to the sural nerve take-off from the peroneal nerve. There was one contusion/crush injury, and one sural nerve biopsy resulted in a neuroma which required repair.

CASE SUMMARY – SURAL INJURY

A 30-year-old physician had congenital venous varicosities with venous insufficiency of the leg. He had had three venous strippings and ligations in the past. Several months after the last venous operation, he had the onset of pain radiating down the lateral lower leg to the ankle. Resection of a sural neuroma and repair of the nerve had been carried out elsewhere; however, within a year he had recurrence of pain and discrete tenderness. There were also complaints of painful tingling and "electric shock" sensations in the same distribution as the pain, whenever the repair site was bumped, or "pins-and-needles" sensations if clothing or a breeze touched these areas.

On examination, there was hyperesthesia and hyperpathia distal and also proximal to the repair site. Tapping at the repair site produced a Tinel sign, but so did tapping or deep palpation just below the knee and just inferior to the popliteal fossa. There were a number of transverse healed incision sites up and down the leg.

At surgical exploration, we found a sural suture neuroma in continuity in the distal leg. We could record no nerve action potential (NAP) across this, nor could we record an NAP proximal to the lesion. As a result, we followed the sural nerve

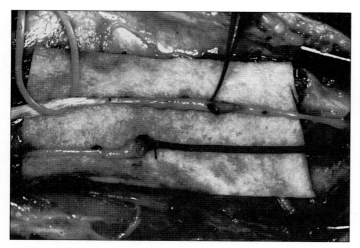

FIGURE 11-55 An intraoperative photograph of two portions of a sural nerve removed from the posterior calf: (top) this section of sural nerve was erroneously sewn at an outside hospital to a tendinous slip (to the left and encircled by a vasoloop) during a sural nerve laceration repair. A distal sural neuroma resulted (pointed out by a plastic dark loop) to the right of the anastomosis (bottom) a second distal sural neuroma (to the left of the illustrative plastic loop) was also found in another section of the nerve.

proximally to where the nerve lay beneath the gastrocnemius and soleus fasciae. A second neuroma was found on the sural nerve just below the knee. There was no NAP recordable across this lesion either. Both neuromas and intervening sural nerve were resected and a long segment of nerve was removed.

The patient has had excellent relief of his symptoms despite hypoesthesia along the lateral foot. The hyperesthesia is not bothersome to him. Histological examination of resected tissues showed a distal suture neuroma, a smaller but still quite disorganized proximal neuroma, and intervening nerve with axons that were less than 5 μm in diameter.

COMMENT

Many transections of the sural nerve do not lead to neuromas that are exquisitely tender and painful. For example, harvest of the sural nerve for use as a graft seldom results in a painful neuroma. The etiology of a resulting painful neuroma is not well understood. Nonetheless, in well-selected cases in which pain is an issue, resection of the neuroma as well as a length of nerve can be effective.

REFERENCES

1. de V. Theron F, Peach SA, and Ackerman C: Donor site morbidity of sural nerve grafts. J Bone Joint Sur [Br] 83(Suppl):2, 2001.
2. Eastwood DM, Irgau I, and Atkins RM: The distal course of the sural nerve and its significance for incisions around the lateral hindfoot. Foot Ankle 13:199–202, 1992.
3. Fabre T, Courjaud X, Benquet B, et al.: An unusual cause of chronic pain of the posterior aspect of the leg: Compression of the sural nerve in 22 operated cases. J Bone Joint Surg [Br] 83(Suppl I):40, 2001.
4. Huene DB and Bunnell WP: Operative anatomy of nerves encountered in the lateral approach to the distal part of the fibula. J Bone Joint Surg [Am] 77:1021–1024, 1995.
5. Lawrence SJ and Botte MJ: The sural nerve in the foot and ankle: an anatomic study with clinical and surgical implications. Foot Ankle Int 15:490–494, 1994.
6. Nakajima H, Imanishi N, Fukuzumi S, et al.: Accompanying arteries of the lesser saphenous vein and sural nerve: anatomic study and its clinical applications. Plast Reconstr Surg 103:104–120, 1999.
7. Ortiguela ME, Wood MB, and Cahill DR: Anatomy of the sural nerve complex. J Hand Surg [Am] 12:1119–1123, 1987.
8. Refaeian M, King JC, and Dumitru D: Isolated sural neuropathy presenting as lateral ankle pain. Am J Phys Med Rehabil 80:543–546, 2001.
9. Seror P: Sural nerve lesions: a report of 20 cases. Am J Phys Med Rehabil 81:876–880, 2002.

PELVIC PLEXUS

OVERVIEW

- Surgery for injury to the lumbar plexus, which provides femoral outflow, gave better results than that for the sacral plexus, which provides sciatic (including peroneal and posterior tibial division) outflow. Nonetheless, several lacerations involving the sacral plexus were managed with some recovery. Most of these operations were done with the help of a general, vascular or gynecological surgeon.
- The pelvic plexus group of 43 operative cases of femoral nerve injuries from Louisiana State University Health Sciences Center (LSUHSC) was a challenge to manage. The functional loss of the iliacus and quadriceps muscles in these cases is especially disabling, because of the lack of substitutes for their functions. Fortunately, proper management can lead to functional, although incomplete, recovery in most cases, even though the femoral nerve is a mixed sensory-motor nerve. This may be because the muscles innervated by the femoral nerve are large and close to both the injury and potential repair site. In the LSUHSC series, failures occurred: (1) in cases in which it was necessary for grafts to be long and to extend from the pelvic to thigh level, and (2) in the elderly whose nerves required repair rather than neurolysis. Loss from iatrogenic causes was the largest category of injury: herniorrhaphy, appendectomy, a gynecological procedure, hip repair, and femoral popliteal bypass can lead to a femoral palsy.
- The resection, rather than decompression, of the lateral femoral cutaneous nerve was favored at LSUHSC. This bias is, in part, the result of a number of such nerves requiring resection after prior unsuccessful decompression not only elsewhere, but also by ourselves.

PELVIC PLEXUS ANATOMY AND CLINICAL CORRELATIONS

The pelvic plexus, also called lumbosacral plexus, consists of the lumbar and sacral plexi. The anatomy for each plexus will be detailed along with specific anatomy and clinical correlations for the major nerves comprising each plexus. The results of the LSUHSC experience will also be presented for each plexus and its components at the end of this section of the chapter.

LUMBAR PLEXUS

The lumbar plexus originates from the anterior primary rami (APR) of the L1, L2, L3, and L4 nerves, with L1 receiving a branch from the subcostal nerve originating from T12.

Each APR of L1, L2, and L4, but not L3, splits into an upper and lower branch. The L1 APR does not form an anterior and posterior division; however, the lower branch of L2, the upper branch of L4, and the entire L3 split into anterior and posterior divisions.

The L1 APR upper branch divides into the iliohypogastric and ilioinguinal nerves. The L1 APR lower branch is joined by the L2 APR upper branch to form the genitofemoral nerve.

The anterior divisions of the L2 lower branch and each L3 and L4 upper branch contribute to the obturator nerve. Each posterior division of L2 and L3 divides into a small and large branch: the small branch from each join to form the lateral femoral cutaneous nerve; the large branch from each are joined by the L4 posterior division to form the femoral nerve.

Thus, lumbar plexus injuries can result in variable patterns of loss related to the sensory dermatomes and muscle mytomes corresponding to the above roots.

Since the spinal cord ends at the L1 level of the spine, both the anterior and posterior divisions of the various roots, i.e. the motor and sensory divisions, respectively, have a variable length within the spinal canal. The sensory divisions or roots are the central extensions of the dorsal root ganglia and do not regenerate after injury. The motor division or roots have the potential for regeneration, even though they are in the spinal canal. The two divisions combine within the intervertebral portion of the nerve root canal and exit the foramen as a single motor sensory spinal nerve, just as the brachial plexus roots do in the neck.

Knowledge of both the radicular and more peripheral anatomy is required, so that the site of injury or disease can be accurately localized. If both the femoral and obturator nerve distributions are dysfunctional the lesion is most likely in the pelvic plexus. If one or the other distribution is dysfunctional then the lesion is more peripheral.

ILIOHYPOGASTRIC NERVE

The iliohypogastric nerve passes through the psoas muscle and anterior to the quadratus lumborum muscle to reach the area superior to the iliac crest. There it lies between the transversus abdominis and internal oblique muscles, which it partially supplies. The nerve penetrates the internal and external oblique muscles as it extends anteriorly. Its sensory distribution is through a lateral cutaneous branch to the skin of the superior gluteal region and through an anterior branch to the lower abdominal skin above the pubis.

Injury to the iliohypogastric nerve is usually iatrogenic and specifically due to abdominal procedures. A lesion involving this nerve causes a sensory deficit or painful paresthesias in the distributions of the lateral cutaneous branch and the anterior branch, as described above.

ILIOINGUINAL NERVE

The ilioinguinal nerve travels around the trunk below the iliohypogastric nerve and laterally is located between the transverse and internal oblique muscles. Part of its medial course is along, but superior to, the inguinal ligament. It then courses through the superficial inguinal ring and external spermatic fascia. This nerve supplies the internal oblique and transversalis muscles in addition to the iliohypogastric nerve supply to these muscles. The ilioinguinal nerve supplies the cutaneous sensation to the skin of the upper thigh medial to the femoral triangle and also the skin over the symphysis pubis and, in the male, the dorsal penis and the upper scrotum, and, in the female, the mons and labia majora.

The ilioinguinal nerve can be inadvertently injured during pelvic or lower abdominal procedures, especially herniorrhaphies. It may also be entrapped by scar formed in the region of this nerve after these procedures. The presentation after injury is a sensory deficit or painful paresthesias in the distribution of the sensory supply as described.

GENITOFEMORAL NERVE

The genitofemoral nerve, unlike the iliohypogastric and ilioinguinal nerves, takes a straight inferior and somewhat caudal course along with the iliac vessels. The nerve then forms two branches. A genital branch innervates the cremaster muscle and a portion of scrotal skin in the male and the round ligament in the female. The femoral branch penetrates the fascia of the thigh to supply sensation to the skin in the region of the femoral triangle.

Mechanisms of injury to the genitofemoral nerve include iatrogenic injury, specifically hysterectomy and herniorrhaphy, and blunt trauma.

Since the genitofemoral nerve's genital branch innervates the ipsilateral cremaster muscle, which retracts the testis on that side and the femoral branch supplies the ipsilateral femoral triangle skin sensation, if there is injury involving these branches, a decreased cremasteric reflex involving these components is found.

Operation(s) on these three nerves, i.e. the ilioinguinal, iliohypogastric, and/or genitofemoral, is reserved for patients with severe disabling pain not responding to pharmacologic agents and time. Injury is usually associated with a prior operation such as a herniorrhaphy and/or gynecologic procedure (see specific chapters on these nerves).

INTRAPELVIC FEMORAL NERVE

The femoral nerve is one of the major outflows of the lumbar plexus. After its formation by the posterior divisions of the L2, L3, and L4 APRs, it courses for 8–10 cm within the pelvis in a retroperitoneal position, lying superolateral to the psoas and medial to the iliacus muscles.

The iliacus muscle, supplied by short branches from the posterior femoral nerve, and the psoas muscle, innervated by L1 and L2, converge to form the iliopsoas muscle. The iliopsoas is the major flexor of the thigh.

The femoral nerve also generates branches to the sartorius muscle. The origin of the sartorius branch is variable, though it usually arises from the distal intrapelvic portion of the femoral nerve. The function of the sartorius muscle can be inferred from the fact that it arises from the anterior superior iliac spine and inserts on the upper medial tibia. This muscle provides an upward and rotational elevation of the thigh as the heel is raised to the opposite knee.[12] Testing this muscle helps to localize the level of the femoral nerve injury.

As the femoral nerve leaves the pelvis, it passes beneath the inguinal ligament lateral to the femoral artery and vein. At this point, the nerve is in a separate fascial compartment and is more easily identified by proximal dissection to the thigh. Several centimeters distal to the ligament, the femoral nerve divides into a number of finger-like branches supplying the quadriceps muscle, which is composed of the rectus femoris and the vastus lateralis, medius, and intermedius muscles. Sensory contributions from the femoral nerve go to the anteromedial thigh, and also form the saphenous nerve, which courses obliquely along the medial thigh and knee and then branches to supply the medial surface of the lower leg and the medial aspect or instep region of the foot.

A pelvic-level femoral nerve palsy can be due to a penetrating lower abdominal injury caused by a gunshot wound, motorcycle handlebars, or a stab wound. Iatrogenic causes include injury to the femoral nerve during packing of the pelvis and manipulation of the pelvic contents in association with bleeding during a lower abdominal operation. A pelvic hematoma related to anticoagulation can injure the femoral nerve as can femoral artery manipulation during angiography.

Another common cause of intrapelvic femoral nerve injury is surgical section of a portion of the plexus for tumor removal. These tumors are often benign schwannomas or neurofibromas.

The femoral nerve can be mistaken for the lateral femoral cutaneous nerve and inadvertently resected during the treatment of meralgia paresthetica, or can be injured by investment with methyl methacrylate during hip repair.

The result of injury to the intrapelvic femoral nerve manifests itself by weakness of the iliacus, quadriceps, and sartorius muscles. Weakness of the iliacus muscle results in loss of hip flexion. To test the strength of the iliacus muscle, the patient is placed in a supine position. The examiner holds the leg beneath the knee with the knee flexed and asks the patient to pull the thigh up towards the abdomen or flex the hip against resistance.

The quadriceps muscle extends the knee and enables walking up stairs and having a normal gait. If there is injury to the femoral nerve, the gait is abnormal, since the knee is hyperextended by the functioning tensor fascia lata and gracilis muscles. With femoral nerve injury, loss of the knee jerk, which involves the quadriceps muscle is found on reflex testing.

Sensory loss from injury to the anterior cutaneous nerve occurs in the anteromedial thigh and is variable. Sensory loss from a saphenous nerve lesion results in sensory change on the medial lower leg and the medial aspect or instep region of the foot.

LATERAL FEMORAL CUTANEOUS NERVE

The lateral femoral cutaneous nerve emerges from the lateral border of the psoas, crosses the iliacus muscle, and at the level of the anterior superior iliac spine courses downward between the attachments of the inguinal ligament (Fig. 11-56). The relationship of the lateral femoral cutaneous nerve to the inguinal ligament is variable. The nerve can pass above, below, or through the ligament and its position relative to the anterior superior spine of the ilium is not always the same. The lateral femoral cutaneous nerve supplies sensation to the lateral thigh (Fig. 11-57).

The lateral femoral cutaneous nerve is usually injured by a stretch injury, entrapment, or during removal of a bone graft from the ilium.

If the lateral femoral cutaneous nerve is injured it can give rise to the characteristic syndrome of meralgia paresthetica. This syndrome presents with a tingling, burning pain in the lateral thigh and a frequent hyperesthesia so severe that the lateral thigh is easily irritated by clothing or touch. Patients often report normal sensibility to pinprick, but an increased and painful sensibility to testing by touch.[18]

If the pain is temporarily relieved by a local anesthetic block of the nerve and the patient tolerates the lateral thigh numbness, then the nerve can be resected, leaving the proximal end to retract retroperitoneally into the pelvis.

OBTURATOR NERVE

The obturator nerve originates from the anterior divisions of the L2, L3, and L4 roots. It reaches the medial border of the psoas muscle, travels below or deep to the iliac vessels, and takes a vertical course toward the obturator foramen (Fig. 11-58). There the obturator nerve divides into an anterior or superficial branch which supplies the adductor longus and brevis muscles, and a posterior or deep branch which supplies the obturator externus and adductor magnus muscles.

Damage to the obturator nerve can occur as part of a lumbosacral plexus injury or, less commonly, as an isolated palsy associated with

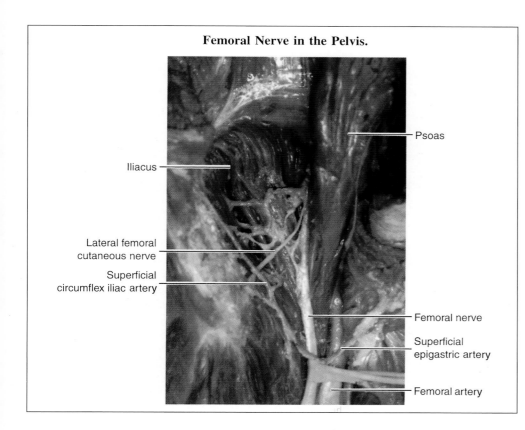

Femoral Nerve in the Pelvis.

Iliacus

Lateral femoral cutaneous nerve

Superficial circumflex iliac artery

Psoas

Femoral nerve

Superficial epigastric artery

Femoral artery

FIGURE 11-56 A cadaveric specimen depicts the intrapelvic femoral nerve as it descends in the groove between the psoas and iliacus muscles, covered by the iliacus fascia. The femoral nerve gives branches to the iliacus muscle, as shown.

Lateral Femoral Cutaneous Nerve Origin.

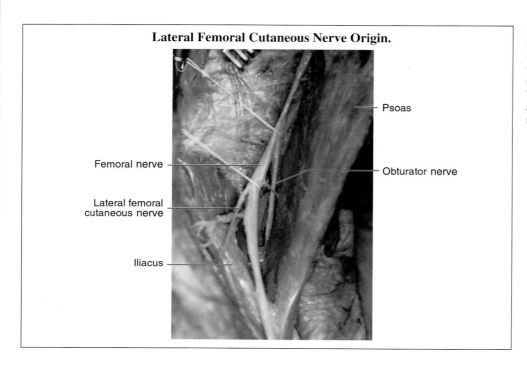

- Psoas
- Femoral nerve
- Obturator nerve
- Lateral femoral cutaneous nerve
- Iliacus

FIGURE 11-57 The lateral femoral cutaneous nerve is shown, in this cadaveric dissection, as it emerges from the lateral border of the psoas major below the iliolumbar ligament. The nerve crosses the iliacus muscle as it travels toward the anterior superior iliac spine.

Course of the Obturator Nerve in the Pelvis.

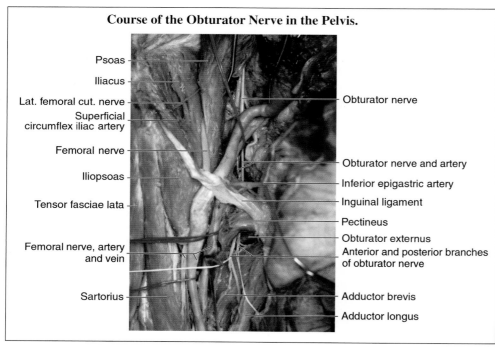

- Psoas
- Iliacus
- Lat. femoral cut. nerve
- Superficial circumflex iliac artery
- Femoral nerve
- Iliopsoas
- Tensor fasciae lata
- Femoral nerve, artery and vein
- Sartorius
- Obturator nerve
- Obturator nerve and artery
- Inferior epigastric artery
- Inguinal ligament
- Pectineus
- Obturator externus
- Anterior and posterior branches of obturator nerve
- Adductor brevis
- Adductor longus

FIGURE 11-58 The obturator nerve is seen, in this cadaveric specimen, to reach the medial border of the psoas muscle after it diverges laterally from the lumbosacral trunk and passes behind the common iliac artery and lateral to the internal iliac vessels.

a pelvic fracture. Even less frequently, a lesion can occur secondary to surgical injury. Sometimes the surgeon will section the nerve purposely as a treatment for the scissors gait seen with spasticity.

Since the adductor magnus is also innervated by the sciatic nerve and the adductor longus is innervated at times by the femoral nerve, complete loss of thigh adduction with complete atrophy of these two muscles is seldom seen with obturator nerve injury. Gait, however, is mildly disturbed, since the leg is externally rotated or tends to swing outward when the patient walks.

Sensory loss is quite variable and unreliable as an index of involvement of this nerve. Loss is sometimes present in a patchy distribution in the lower medial thigh, but at other times normal sensation is found on examination.

SACRAL PLEXUS

The sacral plexus has contributions from: (1) the lumbosacral trunk, formed by a lower branch from the L4 APR and the L5 anterior division; (2) the anterior division of the S1 APR; and (3) portions of the anterior divisions of the S2, S3, and S4 APR (Fig. 11-59).

There are 12 named branches of the sacral plexus. Seven branches contribute to the supply of the buttock and lower limb, namely: (1) the sciatic nerve, consisting at this level of the peroneal and tibial divisions; (2) the superior gluteal and (3) inferior gluteal; (4) the posterior femoral cutaneous; (5) the perforating cutaneous nerves and nerves to the (6) quadratus femoris and inferior

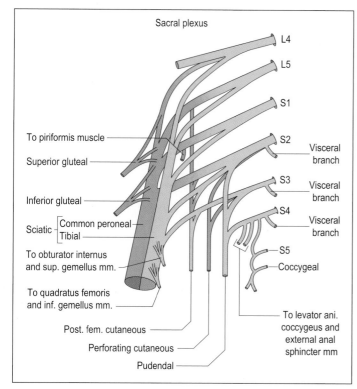

Sacral plexus

To piriformis muscle

Superior gluteal

Inferior gluteal

Sciatic — Common peroneal / Tibial

To obturator internus and sup. gemellus mm.

To quadratus femoris and inf. gemellus mm.

Post. fem. cutaneous

Perforating cutaneous

Pudendal

L4
L5
S1
S2 — Visceral branch
S3 — Visceral branch
S4 — Visceral branch
S5
Coccygeal

To levator ani. coccygeus and external anal sphincter mm

FIGURE 11-59 A schematic drawing depicts the sacral portion of the pelvic (lumbosacral) plexus.

gemellus; and (7) the obturator internus and superior gemellus muscles. The other five named branches supply pelvic structures: (1) the nerve to the piriformis; (2) the nerve to the levator ani and coccygeus; (3) the nerve to the sphincter ani muscles; (4) the pelvic splanchnic nerves; and (5) the pudendal nerve.

The peroneal division of the sciatic nerve is formed by (1) an L4 posterior division, which is formed from a lower branch off the L4 APR, and (2) the posterior divisions of the L5, S1, and S2 APRs. The superior and inferior gluteal nerves are formed from branches of each of the above posterior divisions.

The tibial division of the sciatic nerve is formed from the L4, L5, S1, and S2 anterior divisions of their APRs.

The posterior femoral cutaneous nerve is formed from one branch each of the S1 posterior and S2 anterior divisions of the S1 and S2 APRs.

The perforating cutaneous nerve is formed by an additional posterior ramus, each branching off the anterior divisions of the S2 and S3 APRs, the S3 branching after the origination of the visceral and pudendal posterior branches.

The muscles anterior to the sciatic nerve and just distal to the sciatic notch help provide hip stability. Nerve branches to these muscles are as follows: the quadratus femoris and inferior gemellus nerves are rami emanating from the beginning of the tibial division of the sciatic nerve; the obturator internus and superior gemellus nerves are branches off the area of the merging of the L5, S1, and S2 anterior divisions just proximal to the formed tibial division of the sciatic nerve.

The sacral plexus lies deep and medial in the pelvis, overlying the sacroiliac and sacrococcygeal junctions. The following plexus nerves exit the pelvis for the most part through the greater sciatic foramen: the sciatic, "hamstring," gluteal, and posterior cutaneous nerves, whereas the pudendal nerve reaches the perineum through the lesser sciatic foramen.

As with the lumbar portion of the pelvic plexus, loss with sacral plexus injuries is variable. One can identify the contributions involved in a sacral plexus injury if the sensory dermatomes and myotomes innervated by the various lumbar and sacral roots are kept in mind, especially in the lower extremity.

GLUTEAL NERVES

As the gluteal nerves leave the sciatic notch, the superior gluteal nerve travels lateral to the sciatic nerve and upward to supply the gluteus medius and minimus muscles. The inferior gluteal nerve exits the sciatic foramen medial to the sciatic nerve and supplies the gluteus maximus.

The superior gluteal nerve supplies the gluteus medius and minimus muscles, which aid in the abduction and medial rotation of the thigh at the hip joint. With injury to this nerve, the leg tends to rest in an outwardly rotated position in the recumbent patient, and during walking, the trunk is bent toward the side of the palsy. On standing on the affected leg, the contralateral pelvis drops down, causing a discrepancy in the height of the two anterior superior iliac spines.

An injury specifically to the inferior gluteal nerve, which supplies the gluteus maximus muscle, results in weak extension of the hip. The patient has difficulty arising from a sitting position or climbing steps. With sagging of the muscle belly, the infragluteal fold is decreased or lost, and atrophy of the buttock is obvious with time.

Operative work in the area of the sciatic notch requires experience since injury to vessels such as the superior gluteal artery can result in their retraction into the pelvis where a life-threatening clot can form.

In addition, it is important to spare as many of the gluteal nerves as possible. The anatomy of the piriformis muscle relative to the sciatic nerve can be quite variable at this level. Lateral section of this muscle seldom suffices and a segment of it usually has to be removed beginning within the sciatic notch area and extending laterally.

PUDENDAL (PUBIC) NERVE

The pudendal nerve, also called the pubic nerve, exits the pelvis through the sciatic foramen between the piriformis and the coccygeus muscles and lies on the sacrospinous ligament. Branches include the inferior rectal and perineal nerves and the dorsal nerve of the penis in the male or the clitoris in the female. It supplies sensation to the perineum and portions of the scrotum and penis in the male and in the female, the labia including the mucous membranes of the urethra, and the perianal region. Motor fibers supply the external sphincter of the anus, and both the bulb and the corpus spongiosus of the penis.

The pudendal nerve is seldom injured in an isolated fashion, but loss can occur in its distribution if the sacral plexus is injured, sometimes secondary to a gynecological operation.

Because of its input to the external sphincter of the bladder and the anus, the pudendal nerve is concerned with the voluntary control of urination and defecation and the maintenance of urinary and fecal continence.

SURGICAL APPROACHES

LUMBAR PLEXUS

Operations on the pelvic plexus are difficult, especially if nerve injury or tumor is involved. The lumbar plexus is usually approached by a flank, muscle-splitting, retroperitoneal approach. This can be carried out through an anterior flank or abdominal wall incision and is combined with femoral nerve exposure in the femoral triangle.

Figure 11-60A illustrates the piriformis muscle site of origin on the anterior sacrum. The originating muscle fibers interdigitate at the anterior sacral foramina. The muscle runs laterally through the greater sciatic notch to attach to the proximal end of the femur. The L4–L5 trunk traverses the sacroiliac joint to join the remaining spinal nerves of origin of the sciatic nerve. The sciatic nerve is formed on the anterior surface of the piriformis muscle and then leaves the sciatic notch below this muscle. This is the point at which the sciatic nerve is visible to the surgeon operating on it from a conventional posterior approach. By incising the piriformis and trimming away part of the bone of the notch area, the surgeon is able to reach the point in the pelvis shown by the arrow from the posterior route. If a more medial approach to the sciatic nerve and spinal nerves is needed, the approach is through the pelvis and its concomitant limited operating space. The peritoneal reflection for the rectum is medial and, for a pelvic approach, large branches of the internal iliac veins must be controlled as the spinal nerves of S1, S2, and S3 are exposed.

The femoral nerve is also seen in Figure 11-60A to be lateral to the psoas muscle as the psoas muscle and femoral nerve run forward to pass under the inguinal ligament. The psoas muscle must be retracted medially so that the femoral nerve's spinal nerves of origin can be dissected out. These spinal nerves are accompanied by branches of the lumbar arteries, which have risen from the posterior aspect of the aorta. The surgeon must take care not to misidentify the psoas minor tendon as the femoral nerve.

SACRAL PLEXUS

The sacral plexus exposure is usually difficult and is carried out with the help of a general or vascular surgeon or gynecological surgeon via a transperitoneal approach. Mobilization of the descending colon and sometimes the peritoneal reflection of the rectum must be undertaken. The ureter as well as the iliac vessels must be identified and protected. Figure 11-60B shows the sciatic nerve as it exits the greater sciatic notch under the piriformis muscle as viewed from this posterolateral position. The inferior gluteal nerve and artery can be seen to be closely applied to the sciatic nerve. As stated earlier in this section of the chapter, this inferior gluteal nerve supplies the gluteus maximus muscle. The inferior gluteal artery is a branch of the internal iliac artery and divides into branches soon after it comes into view as seen from the posterior approach. This artery should be carefully managed and if injured, controlled with care, as it may retract into the pelvis and continue hemorrhaging there. The superior gluteal nerve can be seen in Figure 11-60B to exit posteriorly above the piriformis muscle. Its accompanying artery, the superior gluteal, as with the inferior gluteal, must be handled with great attention. The superior gluteal nerve supplies both the gluteus medius (the "deltoid" of the hip joint) and the gluteus minimus and also the tensor fascia lata. In assessing patients with femoral nerve injury, contraction of the tensor fascia lata, which results in traction applied to the iliotibial tract can be mistaken for quadriceps contraction, which is supplied by the femoral nerve.

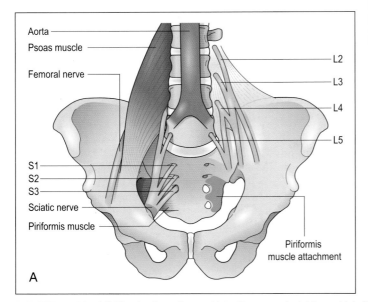

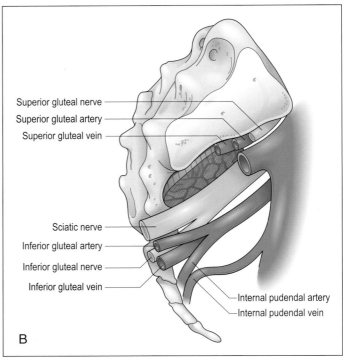

FIGURE 11-60 **(A)** The lumbar plexus. Note the cross-hatching which illustrates the piriformis muscle attachment. The arrow points to the pelvic site which is approachable from posteriorly by incising the piriformis muscle and trimming away part of the bone of the notch area. **(B)** Posterolateral view of the sacral plexus. The inferior and superior gluteal arteries, nerves, and veins are illustrated here and described in the text.

RESULTS

PELVIC PLEXUS INJURY

Pelvic plexus injuries are unusual[3] and appear in the literature as series of case reports or solitary cases.[21] There are a few small series.

Alsever[1] published a case report of a patient with a lumbosacral plexopathy sustained during gynecologic surgery. Luzzio et al.[14] published the first case in the literature of a lumbosacral plexopathy from an internal iliac artery pseudoaneurysm, which occurred after renal transplantation. The patient presented with back and limb pain and a foot-drop, and the plexopathy was confirmed electrodiagnostically.

Tung et al.[21] recently published a case report of a 16-year-old who sustained pelvic and sacral fractures in a motor vehicle accident. After orthopedic injury stabilization, his right gluteal and hamstring muscles were found to be paretic and he had no motor-sensory function below the knee. Two months later he underwent lumbosacral plexus reconstruction using a nerve graft from his L5 and S1 nerve roots proximal to the inferior gluteal nerve and distal to a branch to the hamstring muscles. After 2 more months, his recovering saphenous nerve was transferred to the sensory component of the posterior tibial nerve by using cabled sural nerve grafts to restore sole of the foot sensation. After 2.5 years, he experienced reinnervation of his gluteal and hamstring muscles and could perceive vibration in the sole of his foot. With a foot-drop splint, the patient ambulates well and is able to ski.

Cardosi et al.[4] reported a series of 1210 patients undergoing major pelvic surgery, of which 23 (1.9%) sustained a postoperative neuropathy. Injuries involved nine obturator, five ilioinguinal/iliohypogastric, four genitofemoral, and three pelvic-level femoral nerves; however, there were only two lumbosacral plexus injuries.

Siegmeth et al.[17] studied 126 patients with severe pelvic trauma and found 10 (8%) patients who had long-term neurological dysfunction of the lumbosacral plexus after nerve injuries sustained at the time of trauma. Casanas Sintes and Serra Catafau[5] presented 17 (15%) injuries of the lumbosacral plexus in 115 patients presenting with pelvic ring fractures.

Chiou-Tan et al.[6] evaluated the electrophysiological presentations of 29 patients with lumbosacral plexopathies associated with gunshot wounds (GSWs) and motor vehicle accidents. They noted that in contradistinction to GSWs of the brachial plexus in which many areas of the brachial plexus are typically involved, the injury pattern in their patients with GSWs involving the lumbosacral plexus were more discrete.

Ismael et al.[11] also presented 19 patients with lower plexus injury involving S2–S4 occurring postpartum. All patients in their series presented with urinary, anorectal, or sexual dysfunction after vaginal delivery. There were no associated lower limb sensorimotor deficits, in contradistinction with what is to be expected from the published literature for other pelvic plexus cases. All patients had electrophysiological abnormalities. These findings included signs of denervation in the perineal muscles, prolonged or absent bulbocavernosus reflex latencies in 17 (89%) and two (11%) patients, respectively, and one (5%) patient, who had abnormal somatosensory-evoked potentials of the pudendal nerve. All patients had normal pudendal nerve terminal motor latencies. Urodynamic studies disclosed low urethral closure pressure in half of the patients. Using the electrophysiological data, the authors were able to more precisely identify the site of the proximal plexus lesions.

Lang et al.[13] published a series of 10 patients with mostly traction injuries to the lumbosacral plexus, which had occurred due to severe trauma resulting in pelvic fractures. In most of the cases the roots of the cauda equina of the lumbosacral plexus had ruptured, and repair with nerve grafts in these were performed. In cases in which proximal stumps of the plexus could not be retrieved, palliative nerve transfers using lower intercostal nerves or fascicles from the femoral nerve were carried out. The patients in this series recovered basic lower extremity function such as unsupported standing and walking.

A review of the oncological literature pertinent to the lumbosacral plexus revealed one case of perineural lumbosacral plexus infiltration by systemic lymphoma presented by Moore et al.[15] Lumbar MR and abdominopelvic CT imaging did not show the lesion, while high-resolution MR neurography showed a diffusely infiltrating lumbar plexus lesion suggesting neurolymphomatosis.

With regard to neuroimaging of tumors involving the lumbosacral plexus, of 31 MRIs of 31 patients with these tumors, Taylor et al.[19] presented evidence of direct involvement of the lumbosacral plexus by tumor in 23 MRIs, and six additional MRIs showed widespread metastatic disease in the region of the plexus. Of 22 CT scans performed in these patients, however, direct involvement of the lumbosacral plexus by tumor was seen in only 13 patients. The authors stated that MRI was thus more sensitive than CT in diagnosing cancer-induced lumbosacral plexopathy. Electromyography can be of great value in these cases, especially if irradiation has been used and there is a question of irradiation plexitis.

The pelvic plexus has been reported to be involved by hematomas caused by heparinization for thrombosis, phlebitis, or pulmonary embolus, and in patients with disseminated intravascular coagulation (Fig. 11-61).[7,22]

The experience at LSUHSC has included 66 cases of pelvic plexus injuries (Table 11-14). There were 34 such injuries due to iatrogenic causes, 15 associated with pelvic fractures, some of which had accompanying lumbar or hip fractures, and 11 were caused by GSW injuries to the pelvic plexus.

Patients with fractures and incomplete pelvic plexus loss have been treated expectantly and have had acceptable results. We have followed these patients who had pelvic, usually sacral, plexus involvement secondary to pelvic fractures and most of these have improved at least partially without operation.

There have been exceptions, since some GSWs and pelvic fracture-associated lesions have required surgery. Results have been variable, but if a repair was necessary, results were generally acceptable for lesions involving the lumbar plexus outflow and poor for those of the sacral plexus.

Pelvic plexus palsies associated with pelvic fractures, as well as lumbar or sacral fractures should be evaluated by MRI, which may depict the presence of a meningocele. Figure 11-62 shows the meningocele, as well as a myelogram. A meningocele usually impedes successful repair, especially at that level, just as in brachial plexus injury (Fig. 11-63).[2,8,16]

The hallmark of panpelvic plexus involvement is a combined sacral nerve and femoral or obturator nerve involvement. Branches leading to the ilioinguinal, genitofemoral, saphenous, and lateral femoral cutaneous nerves can be involved, but usually are not. Injury and entrapment of these latter nerves are more likely to occur with distortion of the lower abdominal inguinal or upper thigh anatomy.

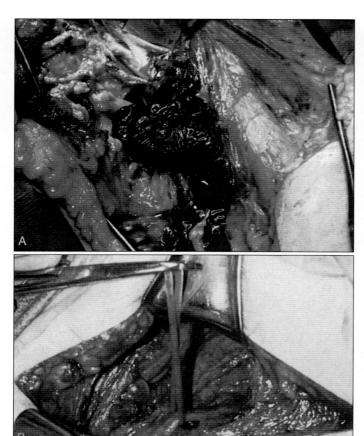

FIGURE 11-61 **(A)** An intraoperative photograph shows a clot due to anticoagulation that resulted in a femoral palsy. **(B)** A retroperitoneal exposure of the pelvic portion of a femoral nerve that had been severely compressed by a retroperitoneal clot.

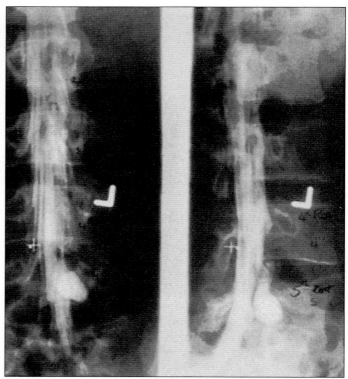

FIGURE 11-62 **(A)** A radiographic view showing a large meningocele involving the L5 root and a smaller abnormality involving the L4 root. This patient had a severe pelvic plexus stretch injury associated with multiple fractures of the pelvis. **(B)** An axial T_2-weighted image is seen of a meningocele to the left of the thecal sac, which is being compressed to the right. This lesion began at the site of the nerve root injury, indicated nerve root sleeve disruption and has extended intraspinally.

Table 11-14   Pelvic plexus injuries

Mechanisms of injury	No. of operative cases
Iatrogenic injury	34
Pelvic +/− lumbar fracture or hip fracture	15
Gunshot wound	11
Stab/laceration	5
Stretch avulsion	1
Totals	66

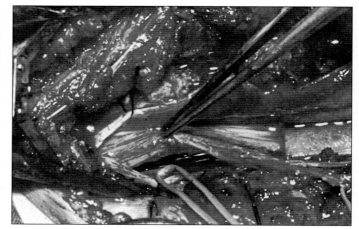

FIGURE 11-63   This is an intraoperative photograph of an exposure of the cauda equina in a child with a pelvic plexus stretch injury. Several nerve roots were extended by grafts placed through the intervertebral foramina to the iliofemoral outflow. This required a two-staged procedure. The first stage was a laminectomy, which exposed the cauda equina. Grafts were attached to the proximal cauda equina. Sutures at the distal ends of the grafts were then placed through the intervertebral foramina at several levels using Keith needles. The iliofemoral outflow at a pelvic level was then exposed by a flank and retroperitoneal approach. The Keith needles, sutures, and grafts were pulled into the pelvis and the grafts were then sewn to the pelvic portion of the femoral nerve.

One of the LSUHSC patients had a large recurrent intraspinal neurofibroma at the L3–L4 level with tumor in the pelvis, as well as in a greatly dilated intervertebral foramen at that level. The origin was thought to be from a spinal nerve in the pelvis with extension into the spinal canal. Because of extensive intraspinal recurrence, an attempt at total excision was elected. After subtotal removal of the intraspinal portion of the tumor to the level of the intervertebral foramen, the pelvic portion was resected using a transabdominal approach in conjunction with the general surgery

Table 11-15 Pelvic-level femoral nerve injuries and nerve grade results*

Mechanisms of injury	No. of cases	Neurolysis/ result**	Suture/ result**	Graft/ result**
Iatrogenic causes				
Abdominal surgery	13	9/9	0/0	4/2
Hip surgery	6***	2/2	0/0	4/1
Arterial bypass	4	2/2	0/0	2/1
Angiography	1	1/1	0/0	0/0
Laparoscopy	1	1/1	0/0	0/0
Hip or pelvic fracture	10****	4/4	0/0	6/3
GSW	5	2/2	0/0	3/1
Laceration	2	0/0	0/0	2/2
Lumbar sympathectomy	1	0/0	0/0	1/1
Total	43	21/21	0/0	22/11

*Patients undergoing neurolysis were grade 0–2 preoperatively and those having suture or graft were grade 0 preoperatively.

**Number of operations/those reaching grade 3 or better.

***Functional loss was complete preoperatively in all cases.

****Functional loss was sometimes incomplete preoperatively and was accompanied by severe pain; after intraoperative neurolysis function and pain improved.

Does not include intrapelvic femoral nerve tumors and cystic lesions.

service. The psoas muscle was split to locate the tumor, which was enucleated, sparing most, but not all of the spinal nerve input to the femoral nerve.

A number of patients with sacral plexus neurofibromas and schwannomas have undergone operations at LSUHSC in which these tumors were successfully removed. One female patient presented with dyspareunia. A mass was not palpable by vaginal or rectal examination; however, digital percussion of the lateral vaginal wall gave paresthesias into the vagina and medial thigh. This latter finding, combined with the patient's history of a mediastinal neurofibroma removed in the past, led to exploration of the sacral portion of the plexus where a solitary neurofibroma was found and successfully excised. Several other unsuspected neurofibromas were found attached to the intestinal mesentery and omentum, presumably arising from autonomic fibers.

Some other tumors of nerve sheath origin in the pelvis have been exceptionally large and have required extensive exposure of the pelvic contents, including mobilization of the bowel, identification of the ureter and protection of aortoiliac vessels and plexus nerves. For these cases a general or gynecological surgeon can provide the initial exposure and mobilize the abdominal contents.

If the sacral plexus or deep pelvis is to be explored, a transabdominal approach is favored. A lateral muscle-splitting extraperitoneal approach similar to that used for lumbar sympathectomy is also available if the lesion involves the lumbar rather than sacral plexus.

During secondary attempts at repair of plexus element injury at LSUHSC after resection elsewhere of intrapelvic tumors, which are often unsuspected subrenal neurofibromas, there has sometimes been an inability to find a proximal end of the plexus element for graft repair.[9]

PELVIC-LEVEL FEMORAL NERVE INJURY

In the LSUHSC series of 43 pelvic-level femoral nerve injuries (Table 11-15), iatrogenic causes were the most common etiology and included 25 (58%) cases. Of these 25 there were 15 (60%) femoral nerve injuries that underwent neurolysis and all 15 had functional outcomes of greater than or equal to grade 3. There were no suture repairs in this subgroup and only four (40%) of 10 graft repairs had a good outcome. The majority of iatrogenic injuries occurred as the result of bleeding during lower abdominal operations necessitating packing of the pelvis or manipulation of pelvic contents.

Vascular repairs secondarily involved the femoral nerve in four cases and these repairs were usually aortofemoral bypasses. Exposure of the injured femoral nerve at the time of repair was difficult because the bypass had to be protected. In most cases, more normal femoral nerve had to be located proximal to the inguinal ligament at a pelvic level and then traced by sharp dissection through the scar associated with the vascular repair. In some of the vascular cases neural damage began at a pelvic level because nerve there had been directly injured by a needle or catheter or a hematoma had dissected beneath the inguinal ligament to involve the pelvic portion of the nerve.

The intrapelvic femoral nerve was also injured from a pelvic hematoma related to either anticoagulation or femoral artery manipulation during angiography. Laparoscopy resulted in one injury, as well.

Hip fractures were a cause of intrapelvic femoral nerve injury in 10 patients. Of 10, four (40%) had neurolysis and all had good functional outcomes. Graft repair results in only 50% of these injuries having the same good outcomes.

At LSUHSC, another cause of pelvic-level femoral nerve palsies was related to penetrating lower abdominal injuries resulting from GSWs, of which there were five. Two patients had neurolysis and did well. There were no suture repairs and only one of three GSW injuries repaired by graft had a good functional outcome.

Other mechanisms of injury seen at LSUHSC included penetrating lower abdominal injuries, of which there were two, and these were secondary to injuries from motorcycle handlebars and stab wounds.

Another frequent cause of pelvic-level femoral nerve injury is surgical section of a portion of the plexus during the removal of a benign neurofibroma or schwannoma.

The femoral nerve can also be mistaken for the lateral femoral cutaneous nerve and can be inadvertently resected in the treatment of meralgia paresthetica, or it can be injured by being incorporated with methyl methacrylate during hip repairs, as evidence by two LSUHSC cases. In each case, a lengthy segment of nerve had to be replaced by sural grafts, and the functional results were poor.

Radiation plexopathy is less frequent than that involving the brachial plexus but it does occur.[10,20] The three patients seen by us have been managed conservatively, but have required intensive pain management and have had progressive loss of leg function. Identification of the femoral and other nerves within the pelvis may be difficult, especially if there has been pelvic injury or prior surgery. For the femoral nerve, dissecting it out at the inguinal ligament level and then tracking it proximally may help.

AUTONOMIC SUPPLY IN THE PELVIC REGION

The peripheral autonomic nervous system in the lumbosacral region consists of the lumbar portion of the thoracolumbar sympathetic nervous system and the sacral portion of the craniosacral parasympathetic nervous system.

The small-caliber, myelinated preganglionic fibers of the lumbar portion of the thoracolumbar sympathetic nervous system originate in the intermediolateral column and form the white communicating rami. These fibers synapse with the postganglionic neurons collected into two paravertebral ganglionic chains and with several single prevertebral ganglia on each side of the vertebral column. The postganglionic fibers pass via gray communicating rami to the T5 to L2 nerves and supply blood vessels, hair follicles, and sweat glands of the limbs and form plexi that supply the bladder and sex organs. The postganglionic fibers of the prevertebral ganglia form plexi which innervate the pelvic viscera. There are four to six lumbar sympathetic ganglia which supply the pelvic organs and the legs.

The sacral parasympathetic efferent fibers originate in the S2, S3, and S4 sacral segments' lateral horn cells. The preganglionic fibers which emanate from these cells are long and travel with the sacral nerves. The fibers synapse in ganglia that lie within the walls of the bladder, and other pelvic organs.

REFERENCES

1. Alsever JD: Lumbosacral plexopathy after gynecologic surgery: case report and review of the literature. Am J Obstet Gynecol 174:1769–1777; discussion 1777–1768, 1996.
2. Barnett HG and Connolly ES: Lumbosacral nerve root avulsion: report of a case and review of the literature. J Trauma 15:532–535, 1975.
3. Birch R, Bonney G, and Wynn Parry: Surgical Disorders of the Peripheral Nerves, 2nd edn. London: Churchill Livingstone, 1998.
4. Cardosi RJ, Cox CS, and Hoffman MS: Postoperative neuropathies after major pelvic surgery. Obstet Gynecol 100:240–244, 2002.
5. Casanas Sintes J and Serra Catafau J: Injuries of the lumbosacral plexus in the fracture of the pelvic ring. J Bone Joint Surg [Br] 79(Suppl 2):251, 1997.
6. Chiou-Tan FY, Kemp K Jr, Elfenbaum M, et al.: Lumbosacral plexopathy in gunshot wounds and motor vehicle accidents: comparison of electrophysiologic findings. Am J Phys Med Rehabil 80:280–285; quiz 286–288, 2001.
7. Gilden DH and Eisner J: Lumbar plexopathy caused by disseminated intravascular coagulation. JAMA 237:2846–2847, 1977.
8. Harris WR, Rathbun JB, Wortzman G, et al.: Avulsion of lumbar roots complicating fracture of the pelvis. J Bone Joint Surg [Am] 55:1436–1442, 1973.
9. Hudson AR, Hunter GA, and Waddell JP: Iatrogenic femoral nerve injuries. Can J Surg 22:62–66, 1979.
10. Iglicki F, Coffin B, Ille O, et al.: Fecal incontinence after pelvic radiotherapy: evidences for a lumbosacral plexopathy. Report of a case. Dis Colon Rectum 39:465–467, 1996.
11. Ismael SS, Amarenco G, Bayle B, et al.: Postpartum lumbosacral plexopathy limited to autonomic and perineal manifestations: clinical and electrophysiological study of 19 patients. J Neurol Neurosurg Psychiatry 68:771–773, 2000.
12. Kline D: Diagnostic approach to individual nerve injuries. New York: McGraw Hill, 1985.
13. Lang EM, Borges J, and Carlstedt T: Surgical treatment of lumbosacral plexus injuries. J Neurosurg Spine 1:64–71, 2004.
14. Luzzio CC, Waclawik AJ, Gallagher CL, et al.: Iliac artery pseudoaneurysm following renal transplantation presenting as lumbosacral plexopathy. Transplantation 67:1077–1078, 1999.
15. Moore KR, Blumenthal DT, Smith AG, et al.: Neurolymphomatosis of the lumbar plexus: high-resolution MR neurography findings. Neurology 57:740–742, 2001.
16. Moossy JJ, Nashold BS Jr, Osborne D, et al.: Conus medullaris nerve root avulsions. J Neurosurg 66:835–841, 1987.
17. Siegmeth A, Mullner T, Kukla C, et al.: Associated injuries in severe pelvic trauma. Unfallchirurg 103:572–581, 2000.
18. Stevens H: Meralgia paresthetica. Arch Neurol Psychiatry 77:557–574, 1957.
19. Taylor BV, Kimmel DW, Krecke KN, et al.: Magnetic resonance imaging in cancer-related lumbosacral plexopathy. Mayo Clin Proc 72:823–829, 1997.
20. Thomas JE, Cascino TL, and Earle JD: Differential diagnosis between radiation and tumor plexopathy of the pelvis. Neurology 35:1–7, 1985.
21. Tung TH, Martin DZ, Novak CB, et al.: Nerve reconstruction in lumbosacral plexopathy. Case report and review of the literature. J Neurosurg (Pediatric 1) 102:86–91, 2005.
22. Young MR and Norris JW: Femoral neuropathy during anticoagulant therapy. Neurology 26:1173–1175, 1976.

FEMORAL NERVE

OVERVIEW

- One hundred operative femoral nerve lesions at intrapelvic and thigh levels from Louisiana State University Health Sciences Center (LSUHSC) are presented as a guide to the management of femoral nerve lesions.
- The most common injury mechanism for this nerve was iatrogenic, which mainly occurred after hernia and hip operations, followed by arterial bypass and gynecological procedures and angiography. Other categories of nerve injury mechanisms were

hip or pelvic fractures in 19, gunshot wounds in 10 and lacerations in eight.

- The femoral nerve tumors were neurofibromas in 16 patients, schwannomas in nine, ganglion cysts in two, neurogenic sarcomas in two, and a leiomyosarcoma.
- Forty-four patients had neurolysis. Some of these patients had recordable nerve action potentials (NAPs) across their lesions in continuity, despite severe distal loss. Others with recordable NAPs had mild loss, but also had a pain problem, which was helped in some cases by neurolysis.
- Thirty-six patients had lengthy sural nerve graft repairs for mostly proximal pelvic-level injuries and some recovery of useful function occurred.
- Eight of nine thigh-level end-to-end suture anastomosis repairs improved to good functional levels. Most of the tumors were resected with preservation of preoperative function.

INTRODUCTION

The femoral nerve (Fig. 11-64) is one of the major outflows of the lumbar plexus and has its origin from the anterior divisions of the L2, L3, and L4 spinal nerves. The nerve has an 8–10 cm retroperitoneal course in the pelvis, lying initially in the groove formed between the anterolateral aspect of the psoas major muscle and the medial border of the iliacus muscle (Fig. 11-65). At this intrapelvic level, the proximal femoral nerve supplies the iliacus muscle, the major flexor of the hip via short branches arising from the posterior surface of the nerve (Fig. 11-65). The anterior motor segment of the femoral nerve also innervates the pectineus and the so-called "tailor" muscle, or sartorius muscle. The sartorius muscle (Figs 11-64, 11-66) is innervated by the more distal intrapelvic femoral nerve, though this is variable, and this muscle provides a portion of the upward and rotary lift of the thigh as the heel is raised to the opposite knee.[5]

The femoral nerve emerges from beneath the lower one-third of the lateral border of the psoas major muscle approximately 4 cm above the inguinal ligament[9] and descends beneath the iliacus fascia between the psoas and iliacus muscles. It passes under the inguinal ligament (Fig. 11-66) and into the femoral triangle. The nerve

remains beneath the fascial extension of the iliacus fascia in a separate fascial compartment during its relatively short course in the thigh and is easily identified here (Fig. 11-67). The nerve continues in the femoral trigone lateral to the femoral vein. The femoral triangle is bounded superiorly by the inguinal ligament, laterally by the sartorius muscle, and medially by the adductor longus muscle. Lymph nodes also lie close to the nerve at this level.

Dissection 3–4 cm distal to the inguinal ligament may be more difficult because the larger main nerve divides at this point into numerous smaller motor, sensory, and mixed motor-sensory branches (Fig. 11-68). The motor branches are destined for the quadriceps muscle, which includes the rectus femoris, vastus lateralis, vastus medius, and vastus intermedius, all of which extend the knee, while the sensory branches transmit anterior thigh sensation inclusive of much of the skin on the medial knee.

The saphenous nerve, a large sensory branch, arises from the anteromedial femoral nerve close to the inguinal ligament. This nerve descends in the thigh at a subcutaneous level and supplies sensory fibers to the skin around the medial knee. As the saphenous nerve descends in the leg it supplies sensation to the medial leg and to the instep region of the foot via several branches. The saphenous nerve is usually accompanied by one of the saphenous veins and occasionally by small arterioles.

Other nerves in the inguinal area include the lateral femoral cutaneous nerve, which arises from the L1 and L2 spinal nerves and courses obliquely through the pelvis lateral to the femoral nerve, but medial to the ilioinguinal and genitofemoral nerves.

CLINICAL PRESENTATION AND EXAMINATION

The neurological examination for femoral nerve injury or neuropathy is straightforward. The grading characteristics used for the pelvic- and thigh-level femoral nerve are found in Table 11-16.

The iliopsoas tendon can be readily seen and palpated in the groin as the patient attempts to flex the hip. As with the iliopsoas muscle, accurate grading of the quadriceps can be achieved;

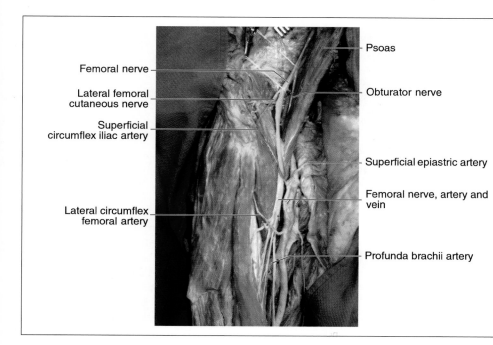

Femoral nerve

Lateral femoral cutaneous nerve

Superficial circumflex iliac artery

Lateral circumflex femoral artery

Psoas

Obturator nerve

Superficial epiastric artery

Femoral nerve, artery and vein

Profunda brachii artery

FIGURE 11-64 An overview of the right femoral nerve as it passes from the intrapelvic region to the anterior compartment of the thigh. (From Kline DG, Hudson AR, and Kim DH: Atlas of Peripheral Nerve Surgery. Philadelphia, WB Saunders, 2001.)

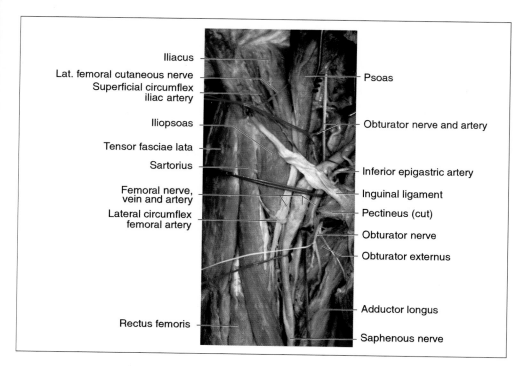

Iliacus
Lat. femoral cutaneous nerve
Superficial circumflex iliac artery
Iliopsoas
Tensor fasciae lata
Sartorius
Femoral nerve, vein and artery
Lateral circumflex femoral artery
Rectus femoris

Psoas
Obturator nerve and artery
Inferior epigastric artery
Inguinal ligament
Pectineus (cut)
Obturator nerve
Obturator externus
Adductor longus
Saphenous nerve

FIGURE 11-65 An intrapelvic view of the femoral nerve is shown as it descends between the psoas and iliacus muscles. Short branches of this nerve supply the iliacus muscle at this level. (From Kline DG, Hudson AR, and Kim DH: Atlas of Peripheral Nerve Surgery. Philadelphia, WB Saunders, 2001.)

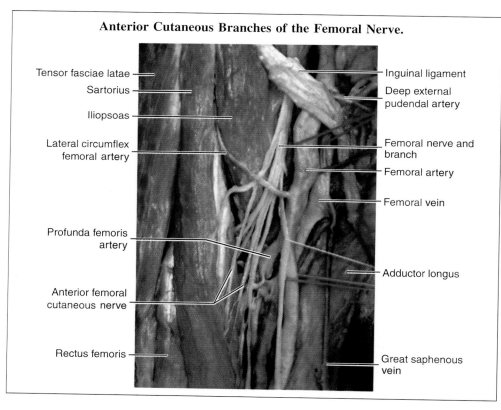

Anterior Cutaneous Branches of the Femoral Nerve.

Tensor fasciae latae
Sartorius
Iliopsoas
Lateral circumflex femoral artery
Profunda femoris artery
Anterior femoral cutaneous nerve
Rectus femoris

Inguinal ligament
Deep external pudendal artery
Femoral nerve and branch
Femoral artery
Femoral vein
Adductor longus
Great saphenous vein

FIGURE 11-66 The femoral nerve is shown as it passes beneath the inguinal ligament and remains beneath the iliacus fascia. The femoral triangle is apparent. (From Kline DG, Hudson AR, and Kim DH: Atlas of Peripheral Nerve Surgery. Philadelphia, WB Saunders, 2001.)

however, the examiner must be aware that the tensor fascia lata, supplied by the superior gluteal nerve, may provide some extension of the leg when the quadriceps is absent or very weak. If this is occurring, the examiner can usually see the patient tensing the lateral thigh skin and underlying soft tissues, rather than the anterior thigh mass.

Large muscles such as the iliopsoas and the quadriceps can be readily graded for strength of contraction, while the sartorius muscle is more difficult to assess. The sartorius muscle allows the attainment of a cross-legged position while sitting. By placing the heel of the limb to be tested on top of the contralateral knee and having the patient rotate the thigh up and medially, one can sometimes see and palpate this muscle's tendon.

The quadriceps muscle is best tested with the patient seated. The anterior thigh can be easily palpated as the patient extends the knee.

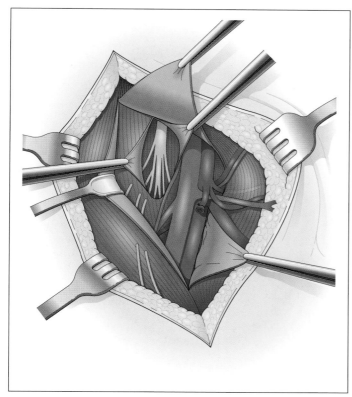

FIGURE 11-67 This is a drawing of the left femoral nerve, demonstrating the need to open the iliacus fascia for exposure of the nerve in its position lateral to the femoral artery and vein at the level of the inguinal ligament.

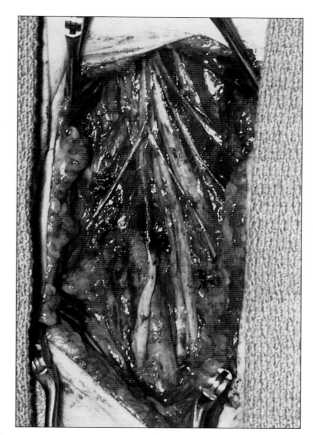

FIGURE 11-68 This operative photograph shows the exposure of the extrapelvic portion of the femoral nerve below the inguinal ligament. This nerve had been contused and the patient had a painful partial femoral neuropathy. Note the profusion of branches at the thigh level. (From Kim DH and Kline DG: Surgical outcomes for intra- and extrapelvic femoral nerve lesions. J Neurosurg 83:783, 1995.)

Thigh adduction is provided by the three adductor muscles, the adductor longus, brevis, and magnus, which are innervated by the obturator nerve, rather than by the femoral-innervated quadriceps. Abduction and some extension are provided by the more posteriorly located gluteus maximus and medius muscles, which are innervated by the gluteal nerves.

ELECTROPHYSIOLOGIC STUDIES

Electrophysiologic studies of the femoral nerve may include attempts to sample iliacus function and that of three portions of the quadriceps, i.e. the lateral, intermediate, and medial muscle groups.[2] If the nerve is partially injured or regrowing, it can be stimulated at the level of the inguinal ligament, and an attempt can be made to measure the latencies of any evoked muscle action potentials recorded from the quadriceps.

The saphenous nerve, since it is a sensory nerve, can be assessed by evoking sensory nerve action potentials (SNAPs) at a skin level by stimulating over the instep of the foot and recording over the medial knee or sometimes more proximally over the anteromedial thigh.

SURGICAL EXPOSURE

Femoral nerve exposure is helped by flexing the knee to 30–45 degrees and supporting the posterior knee by a pillow or rolled sheets. If pelvic exposure of the nerve is anticipated, a few folded sheets are placed beneath the ipsilateral buttock as well.

The initial incision is placed in the femoral triangle in a vertical direction extending from the inguinal ligament to the junction of the upper and middle thirds of the thigh (Fig. 11-69). The more medial femoral artery requires isolation, as does a portion of the femoral vein and its branches. Some of these branches may require ligation or bipolarization in the process of exposing the femoral nerve branches along the thigh. The main femoral nerve is encircled by a Penrose drain, and its branches with plastic loops.

If the injury involves the intrapelvic femoral nerve, a pelvic exposure is made by a retroperitoneal approach combined with dissection of the nerve in the femoral triangle (Fig. 11-70). After exposure in the triangle, the nerve is traced retroperitoneally by sectioning the inguinal ligament and then curving the soft tissue incision laterally. The lower abdominal and flank musculature is split as much as possible in the direction of its fibers to expose the peritoneum, which is then dissected away from the lateral and posterior false pelvis in an extraperitoneal fashion. The retroperitoneal space can usually be swept medially with the gloved hand and then the intraperitoneal abdominal contents and the abdominal wall can be retracted superiorly and somewhat medially by a Deaver or large Richardson retractor. During this portion of the dissection, the lateral femoral cutaneous nerve must be carefully spared as it runs medial to the anterior superior spine of the ilium and beneath the lateral portion of the inguinal ligament. Care should also be taken with ilioinguinal and genitofemoral nerves.

Table 11-16 Nerve grading system for the pelvic-level femoral nerve*

Grade	Evaluation	Description
0	Absent	No iliopsoas or quadriceps contraction
1	Poor	Trace iliopsoas; usually no quadriceps contraction
2	Fair	Iliopsoas contraction against gravity; trace quadriceps
3	Moderate	Iliopsoas contraction against gravity; some pressure and quadriceps contraction against gravity
4	Good	Contraction of both iliopsoas and quadriceps against moderate pressure
5	Excellent	Contraction of both iliopsoas and quadriceps against considerable pressure

*Grading system developed at Louisiana State University Health Sciences Center (LSUHSC).

Nerve grading system for the thigh-level femoral nerve*

Grade	Evaluation	Description
0	Absent	No quadriceps contraction
1	Poor	Trace quadriceps contraction, but not against gravity
2	Fair	Contraction of quadriceps against gravity
3	Moderate	Iliopsoas contraction against gravity and some pressure
4	Good	Quadriceps contraction against moderate pressure
5	Excellent	Quadriceps contraction at full strength

*Grading system developed at Louisiana State University Health Sciences Center (LSUHSC).

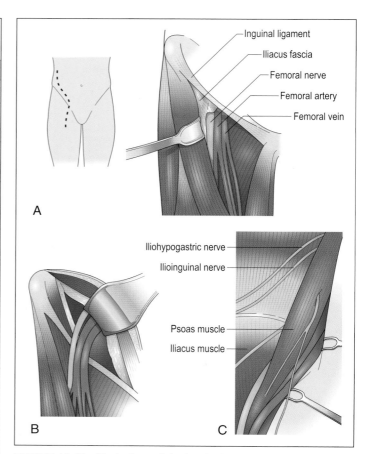

FIGURE 11-69 Illustrations of the inguinal and pelvic level femoral nerve surgical exposures. Inset: The skin incision is shown beginning in the femoral triangle. It crosses the inguinal ligament, continues into the abdominal right lower quadrant (RLQ) and runs towards the flank. **a.** The exposure of the femoral nerve (n), artery (a) and vein in the femoral triangle are seen. The iliacus fascia must be opened to expose the femoral nerve at this level (m = muscle). **b.** Transection of the inguinal ligament has been carried out as well as division of the RLQ abdominal musculature. A large abdominal retractor is shown sweeping the peritoneum, some of the retroperitoneal fat, and the abdominal contents medially. The femoral nerve and iliac vessels are depicted at an intrapelvic level. **c.** The intrapelvic portion of the femoral nerve and its relationship to the psoas and iliacus muscles are shown. The ilioinguinal and iliohypogastric nerve origins are seen superiorly and the genitofemoral nerve and some of its branches are seen to the right. (From Kim DH and Kline DG: Surgical outcomes for intra- and extrapelvic femoral nerve lesions. J Neurosurg 83:783, 1995.)

Since the incision is initially kept close to the inguinal ligament and then curved laterally and the dissection is kept retroperitoneally, these nerves should not be encountered until high in the flank.

In the pelvis, the formation of the femoral nerve by the anterior divisions of the spinal nerves has already been discussed. The nerve must be carefully dissected along the course of the iliopsoas muscle. The iliac vessels and the ureter lie more medially and must be excluded from the dissection. Smaller vessels coursing with the pelvic portion of the femoral outflow can usually be isolated from the femoral nerve and spared.

If exposure of the spinal nerves and the proximal divisions from which the femoral nerve is formed is necessary, a more direct approach through a lateral flank using a muscle-splitting incision is advisable. This approach is identical to that used for a lumbar sympathectomy. The patient is placed in a partial lateral decubitus position with a roll or support under the region of the flank to be exposed. Skin and subcutaneous tissues are opened in the lateral flank with a somewhat oblique incision beginning beneath the lateral rib cage and extending inferiorly towards the anterior iliac crest or midportion of the inguinal ligament. External and internal oblique and transversalis muscles are split in the direction of their fibers and retracted by Gelpi, mastoid, or other self-retaining retractors. The peritoneum is then dissected away from the retroperitoneal fat, and the retroperitoneal space is dissected by gloved fingers or a sponge stick until the iliopsoas muscle is located. The anterior surface of the vertebral column lies at the midline, medial to the iliopsoas muscle. The iliopsoas originates from the transverse processes. Spinal nerves usually penetrate through some of the psoas to form the upper pelvic plexus and, further distally, the femoral nerve. The sympathetic chain lies over the anterolateral vertebral column between the medial edge of the psoas muscle and the midline of the anterior surface of the lumbosacral vertebral bodies.

RESULTS

The results provided in previously published series have been limited in their size and/or number and their lack of detail.[1] It is apparent, however, from such reviews that this is a relatively favor-

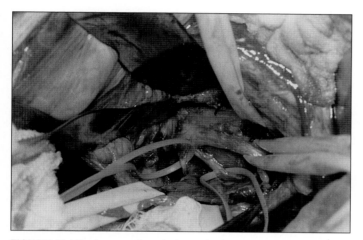

FIGURE 11-70 An operative photograph shows the dissection of the intrapelvic femoral nerve. Major branches to the iliacus and psoas muscles are encircled by small plastic loops. A Penrose drain to the right is around the femoral nerve, which is elevated away from the psoas muscle. (From Kim DH and Kline DG: Surgical outcomes for intra- and extrapelvic femoral nerve lesions, J Neurosurg 83:783, 1995.)

able nerve for management.[8,10-12,14] Table 11-17 summarizes the injury mechanisms and results in 89 operative femoral injuries in the series of patients from LSUHSC.

LACERATION

Eight femoral nerve lacerations required operative intervention. Two of these lacerations were at the pelvic level and six were at the thigh level. One injury at the pelvic level was the result of an accidental lower abdominal stab wound inflicted by a pair of scissors. Other pelvic- or thigh-level injuries were caused by falls on broken glass or, in one instance, a stab wound from a kitchen knife. In retrospect, some of these femoral nerve injuries might have been repaired acutely or primarily because it had seemed at the time of delayed exploration that the transections were sharp and relatively neat. Because of the delay in referral, most were repaired secondarily. In one of these cases, repair had been attempted acutely, but the distal stump had been sewn into the side of the femoral artery at the level of the inguinal ligament. At the time of a secondary repair seven months later, it was found that the proximal stump had retracted into the pelvis, was displaced medially, and had formed a large neuroma. After taking down the distal stump from the artery and trimming the neuroma on the proximal stump, a gap of 10 cm remained, and this was closed with interfascicular grafts. Acceptable recovery of the quadriceps to grade 4 occurred, but this degree of recovery required 4 years to attain.

GUNSHOT WOUND

The ten gunshot wounds (GSWs) involving the femoral nerve were of low caliber, and this permitted survival because there were no major vascular injuries (Figs 11-71, 11-72). Two patients with pelvic-level lesions had neurolysis with subsequent good recovery.

Table 11-17 Femoral nerve injury mechanisms and nerve grade results*

Mechanisms of injury	Pt. no.	Neurolysis/result**		Suture/result**		Graft/result**	
		Thigh	Pelvis	Thigh	Pelvis	Thigh	Pelvis
Iatrogenic etiology							
Herniorrhaphy	10	7/7	0/0	2/2	0/0	1/1	0/0
Hip surgery	10	1/1	2/2	1/1	0/0	2/1	4/1
Gynecological surgery	8	0/0	6/6	0/0	0/0	0/0	2/1
Arterial bypass	8	1/1	2/2	0/0	0/0	3/3	2/1
Angiography	7	6/6	1/1	0/0	0/0	0/0	0/0
Abdominal surgery	5	0/0	3/3	0/0	0/0	0/0	2/1
Appendectomy	2	0/0	1/1	0/0	0/0	0/0	1/1
Laparoscopy	1	0/0	1/1	0/0	0/0	0/0	0/0
Lumbar sympathectomy	1	0/0	0/0	0/0	0/0	0/0	1/1
Hip or pelvic fracture	19	5/5	4/4	2/1	0/0	2/1	6/3
GSW	10	0/0	2/2	1/1	0/0	4/3	3/1
Laceration	8	2/2	0/0	3/3	0/0	1/1	2/2
Totals	89	22/22	22/22	9/8	0/0	13/10	23/12

*Does not include 30 femoral nerve tumors.

**Number of operations/those achieving ≥ grade 3 function.

Pt. no., patient number.

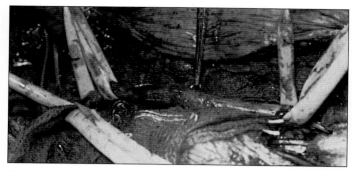

FIGURE 11-71 A gunshot wound involving a segment of a femoral nerve at the level of the inguinal ligament is seen in this intraoperative photograph. The pelvic segment is to the left and the thigh segment is to the right. When operated on 6 months after injury, a graft repair was necessary.

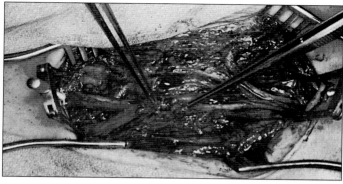

FIGURE 11-73 The photograph illustrates a femoral nerve injury secondary to an iliofemoral arterial bypass. Resection and graft repair were necessary.

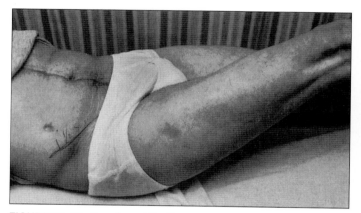

FIGURE 11-72 Function of the iliopsoas and some quadriceps function were recovered after an intraperitoneal graft repair of a gunshot wound injury to the femoral nerve which had been performed 1.5 years earlier.

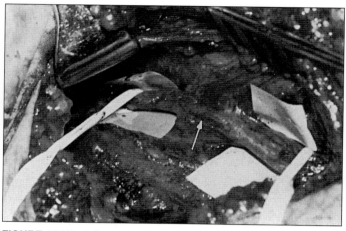

FIGURE 11-74 A femoral nerve at the pelvic level is depicted here after an injury by a retractor during the course of an abdominal operation.

In one case with complete clinical and EMG loss, an NAP was transmitted across the lesion in continuity at 7 months after injury. Only neurolysis was performed and recovery was satisfactory. There were three patients with pelvic-level GSWs who had graft repairs with only one recovery to grade 3. The patient with the good recovery had suffered an extensive shotgun wound to the abdomen involving bladder and bowel, which led to an acute exploration and repair of these injuries. Secondary graft repair of the femoral nerve after resection of the lengthy intrapelvic lesion in continuity resulted in grade 3 quadriceps recovery.

There were five patients with thigh-level GSW injuries to the femoral nerve. One patient had an end-to-end suture anastomosis repair and had a good outcome and three of four patients having graft repairs achieved grade 3 functional outcomes, as well.

IATROGENIC

The most frequent etiology of injury to the femoral nerve was iatrogenic and was related mainly to herniorrhaphy, hip surgery, arterial bypass (Fig. 11-73), gynecological surgery, events related to angiography, or abdominal surgery (Fig. 11-74). There was one injury associated with a lumbar sympathectomy.

Involvement of the femoral nerve by direct injury, scar, or suture as the result of hernia repair usually occurred at the level of the inguinal ligament and there were 10 patients with this procedure

as the etiology of their femoral nerve injury. Neurolysis helped pain in two cases with incomplete loss and there was, as expected, a recordable NAP across these lesions. Three other patients with more severe loss before operation had neurolysis because of the presence of an NAP, and as a result recovered. In one case, suture was found not only around, but in nerve. Grafts 5 cm in length were required for repair, and the quadriceps was grade 3 at follow-up 3 years later.

Femoral palsy has been previously reported as a complication of total hip replacement.[13,15] A number of cases of contusion and stretch associated with hip operations required operation at LSUHSC. Three patients with positive NAPs had neurolysis; however, most had negative NAP recordings and required a repair (Fig. 11-75). There were a few cases of femoral palsy associated with hip repair that were caused by neural encasement with methyl methacrylate. In these cases, a lengthy segment of nerve had to be replaced by sural nerve grafts and results were poor.

During resections of endometriosis-associated cysts and during salpingo-oophorectomies and hysterectomies, eight patients developed femoral nerve palsies at a pelvic level, probably due to retraction-caused stretch and compression. Six patients had external neurolysis because of positive NAPs across their lesion found at the time of operation and the other two with absent NAPs underwent graft repair. All six patients undergoing neurolysis did well, while one of two patients having graft repair had a good outcome.

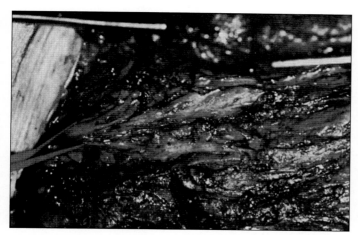

FIGURE 11-75 This intraoperative photograph shows a severely contused femoral nerve just distal to the inguinal ligament. This patient had a hip replacement operation. A graft repair was necessary.

Table 11-18 Pelvic- and thigh-level femoral nerve tumors

Tumor type	No. of tumors
Benign	
Neurofibroma	26
Schwannoma	9
Ganglion cyst	2
Malignant	
Neurogenic sarcoma	2
Leiomyosarcoma	1

Aortofemoral bypasses were vascular repairs in which the femoral nerve was secondarily and adversely involved. Exposure of the injured femoral nerve at the time of nerve repair was difficult because the bypass had to be protected. In most of these cases, more normal femoral nerve had to be located proximal to the inguinal ligament at a pelvic level and then traced by sharp dissection through scar associated with the vascular repair. In some of the vascular cases, neural damage began at a pelvic level because nerve there had sustained direct injury by a needle or catheter or a hematoma had dissected beneath the inguinal ligament to involve the pelvic portion of the nerve. Identification of the distal femoral branches, particularly if repair by grafts was necessary, was especially difficult. This was usually accomplished by carefully splitting the atrophied muscle fibers of the midportion of the quadriceps in a segmental, longitudinal fashion.

An elderly lady was found to have a large femoral artery pseudoaneurysm that was discovered 7 months after angiography despite a persistent early-onset complete femoral palsy. The pseudoaneurysm was resected, a lengthy neural graft repair was required, and only grade 1 to 2 quadriceps function was obtained at 1.5 years, postoperatively. The extent of her vascular injury had been so great that an arterial bypass had to be routed from the opposite femoral artery across the lower abdomen to the distal femoral artery on the injured side.

A pediatric patient had a large pseudoaneurysm of the femoral artery as the result of a cardiac catheterization. After resection of the pseudoaneurysm, she required a graft repair extending from the pelvic portion of the nerve to that in the thigh. Neurological function was regained in this patient.

In other cases associated with angiography, loss was incomplete, but pain and paresthesias were a problem despite vigorous physical therapy and pharmacologic management. Neurolysis seemed to ameliorate the pain syndrome in most of these cases.

STRETCH/CONTUSION IN HIP OR PELVIC FRACTURE

Stretch/contusion associated with hip or pelvic fracture was a large category of injury and included 19 patients. By comparison, however, brachial plexus stretch injuries are more frequent than pelvic plexus stretch injuries; a stretch injury involving the femoral nerve alone and unassociated with a more widespread pelvic plexus lesion was relatively infrequent. Nine patients had neurolysis based on a positive NAP and all recovered. One of two patients having end-to-end suture anastomosis repairs recovered substantial function. The other patient had a reversal of pain after resection of a lesion in continuity, but recovery of the quadriceps was only to grade 1 to 2. Eight patients had graft repairs with two at the thigh level and five at the pelvic level. Four of the eight patients recovered femoral function to grade 3 or higher. One of the graft repair patients required 9 cm sural nerve grafts and although recovery was gained to grade 3, individual muscle grades were better for the iliopsoas than for the quadriceps muscles.

TUMOR

There were 26 neurofibromas and nine schwannomas, which involved the femoral nerve (Table 11-18). Two additional tumors were neurogenic sarcomas, one of which was a malignant schwannoma involving a femoral sensory branch at the mid-thigh level, which was treated by wide local resection and local irradiation. The patient has remained free of recurrence. There were two ganglion cysts with a presumed origin in the hip joint. One patient had a large leiomyosarcoma involving the femoral nerve, which was resected with graft repair of the pelvic-level nerve; this patient has had extensive intra-abdominal recurrence 1.5 years after a gross total resection of tumor and the involved nerve. Most of the tumors were resected with preservation of preoperative function.

OTHER MECHANISMS OF INJURY

Spontaneous pelvic hematomas associated with anticoagulation or hemophilia can cause femoral neuropathy.[4] Fortunately, most of these neuropathies are usually reversible without surgery. There were exceptions, though, and a severe, complete palsy may suggest the need for early evacuation of the clot and/or blood.

The saphenous nerve was sometimes inadvertently injured during the course of venous stripping and ligation or occasionally during operative procedures around the knee (Fig. 11-76). This type of iatrogenic involvement has been previously reported.[3] The saphenous nerve, which is entirely sensory, originates from the femoral nerve in the proximal anterolateral thigh and descends in the medial thigh and leg as one or more branches. Injury at any point along its course can lead to a painful neuroma. At LSUHSC a wide

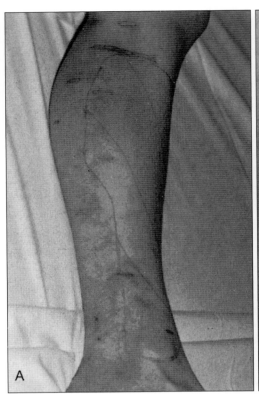
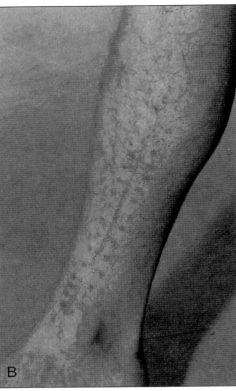

FIGURE 11-76 **(A)** Saphenous nerve injuries are seen at several levels associated with venous stripping and ligation. The sensory loss is outlined. The nerve was resected from the knee to the ankle because of painful paresthesias. **(B)** Another mechanism of saphenous injury shown here is harvesting of a saphenous vein for arterial repair.

excision of the neuroma and attached scar and removal of the nerve well proximal and distal to the injury site has been carried out in these cases, rather than repair. This nerve serves a functionally less important sensory territory than the tibial or even peroneal nerves, and attempts to resect the neuroma and repair the nerve can lead to another painful neuroma as the suture or graft site matures. Occasionally, a mass such as a lipoma, cyst, or, in one patient, a venous aneurysm, involved this nerve, but there has not been a case of a spontaneous entrapment unassociated with injury seen at LSUHSC.[6,7]

REFERENCES

1. Birch R and Wynn Parry CB: Results. London, Churchill Livingstone, 1998.
2. Calvery JR and Mulder DW: Femoral neuropathy. Neurology 10:963–967, 1960.
3. Cox SJ, Wellwood JM, and Martin A: Saphenous nerve injury caused by stripping of the long saphenous vein. Br Med J 1:415–417, 1974.
4. Fernandez-Palazzi F, Hernandez SR, De Bosch NB, et al.: Hematomas within the iliopsoas muscles in hemophilic patients: the Latin American experience. Clin Orthop 19:24, 1996.
5. Kline D: Diagnostic Approach to Individual Nerve Injuries, vol 2. New York, McGraw Hill, 1985.
6. Luerssen TG, Campbell RL, Defalque RJ, et al.: Spontaneous saphenous neuralgia. Neurosurgery 13:238–241, 1983.
7. Mozes M, Ouaknine G, and Nathan H: Saphenous nerve entrapment simulating vascular disorder. Surgery 77:299–303, 1975.
8. Osgaard O and Husby J: Femoral nerve repair with nerve autografts. Report of two cases. J Neurosurg 47:751–754, 1977.
9. Pham LH, Bulich LA, and Datta S: Bilateral postpartum femoral neuropathy. Anesth Analg 80:1036–1037, 1995.
10. Rakolta GG and Omer GE Jr: Combat-sustained femoral nerve injuries. Surg Gynecol Obstet 128:813–817, 1969.
11. Rizzoli H: Treatment of peripheral nerve injuries. Washington DC, Office of the Surgeon General, Department of the Army, 1965.
12. Seddon H: Surgical Disorders of the Peripheral Nerves. Baltimore, Williams and Wilkins, 1972.
13. Solheim LF and Hagen R: Femoral and sciatic neuropathies after total hip arthroplasty. Acta Orthop Scand 51:531–534, 1980.
14. Sunderland S: Nerves and Nerve Lesions. Edinburgh, Churchill Livingstone, 1978.
15. Weber ER, Daube JR, and Coventry MB: Peripheral neuropathies associated with total hip arthroplasty. J Bone Joint Surg Am 58:66–69, 1976.

SAPHENOUS NERVE

OVERVIEW

■ Twenty-two patients with operative saphenous neuralgias underwent surgery at the Louisiana State University Health Sciences Center (LSUHSC) and Stanford Medical Center.

■ The most common injury to the saphenous nerve (SN) was venous stripping and ligation procedures, of which there were 14 such cases. This was followed in number by three cases of entrapment/contusion injury involving the SN. The SN was lacerated during operative procedures around the knee in two instances. Occasionally, a mass such as a lipoma, cyst, and a venous aneurysm can involve this nerve; however in the present series, two saphenous nerve schwannomas and a solitary neurofibroma were removed.

■ Spontaneous entrapment is usually associated with injury, which at any point along the course of the SN can lead to a painful neuroma.[11,19] In these cases, a wide excision of the neuroma and attached scar and removal of the nerve well proximal and distal to the injury site, rather than SN repair, is carried out. The SN serves a functionally less important sensory territory than the tibial or

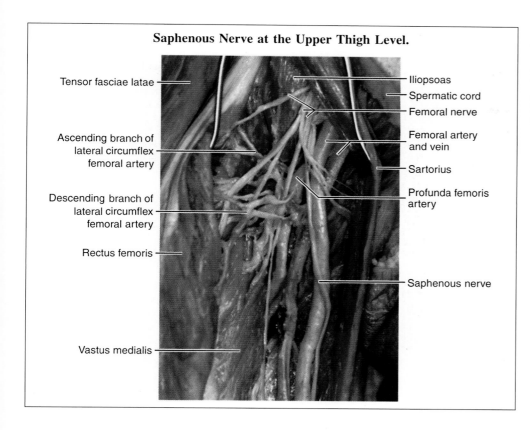

Saphenous Nerve at the Upper Thigh Level.

Tensor fasciae latae

Ascending branch of lateral circumflex femoral artery

Descending branch of lateral circumflex femoral artery

Rectus femoris

Vastus medialis

Iliopsoas

Spermatic cord

Femoral nerve

Femoral artery and vein

Sartorius

Profunda femoris artery

Saphenous nerve

FIGURE 11-77 A cadaveric dissection illustrates the saphenous nerve arising from the femoral nerve, crossing anteriorly to the femoral artery from a lateral to medial direction and exiting the femoral triangle at its inferior apex to enter the adductor canal.

peroneal nerves, and attempts to resect the neuroma and repair the nerve can lead to another painful neuroma as the suture or graft site matures.

APPLIED ANATOMY

The saphenous nerve has L3 and L4 as its spinal components and is the longest sensory branch of the femoral nerve. The SN arises near, but distal to, the inguinal ligament and accompanies the femoral artery, first anterolaterally then anteromedially through the femoral triangle (Fig. 11-76).[3,16,22]

The SN and femoral artery exit the femoral triangle at its inferior apex to enter the adductor canal, also called the subsartorial canal of Hunter, or Hunter's canal (Fig. 11-77). The canal is located approximately 10 cm proximal to the medial femoral condyle.[21,31] The anterolateral wall of Hunter's canal is formed by the vastus medialis and the posterior aspect is formed by the adductor longus and magnus muscles. The roof of the canal is bridged anteromedially by the vastoadductor membrane, a fibrous tissue under the sartorius muscle, the latter of which covers the proximal aspect of the canal.[15] This canal is the most common site of entrapment of the SN. The SN crosses the femoral artery from lateral to medial in Hunter's canal. At the distal end of the canal, the SN leaves the femoral artery.

After leaving Hunter's canal, the SN descends vertically in an S-shaped fashion along the medial side of the knee (Fig. 11-78).[27] The SN then gives off an infrapatellar branch, which courses most commonly posterior to the sartorius muscle and then emerges from its posterior border.[7] The infrapatellar branch then pierces the fascia lata between the tendons of the sartorius and gracilis muscles (Fig. 11-79). The SN and its infrapatellar branch are subcutaneous from this point. The infrapatellar branch supplies the prepatellar

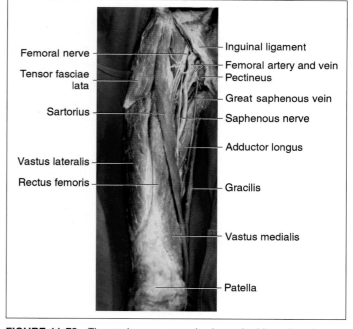

Femoral nerve

Tensor fasciae lata

Sartorius

Vastus lateralis

Rectus femoris

Inguinal ligament

Femoral artery and vein

Pectineus

Great saphenous vein

Saphenous nerve

Adductor longus

Gracilis

Vastus medialis

Patella

FIGURE 11-78 The saphenous nerve is shown in this cadaveric specimen at a midthigh level. The saphenous nerve and femoral artery enter the adductor canal approximately 10 cm proximal to the medial femoral condyle. At the distal end of the canal it leaves the femoral artery, piercing the fibrous roof, and joins the saphenous vein.

medial and anterior skin of the knee. The branch also establishes connections around the knee proximally with the medial and intermediate femoral cutaneous nerves, distally with other branches of the saphenous nerve and laterally with the lateral cutaneous femoral nerve to form a patellar plexus.

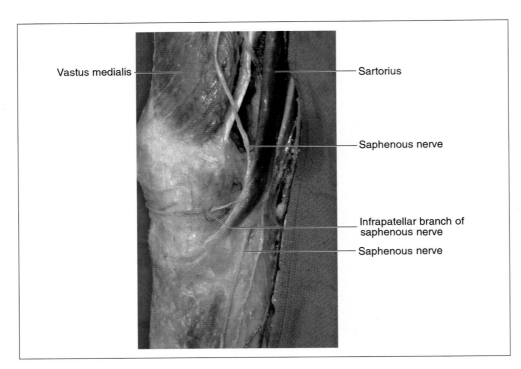

FIGURE 11-79 A cadaveric dissection showing the saphenous nerve at the knee level. Here, the nerve has left the adductor canal and is descending vertically in an S-shaped manner along the medial knee beneath the posterior border of the sartorius muscle. The nerve pierces the fascia lata between the tendons of the sartorius and gracilis muscles to become subcutaneous.

Vastus medialis

Sartorius

Saphenous nerve

Infrapatellar branch of saphenous nerve

Saphenous nerve

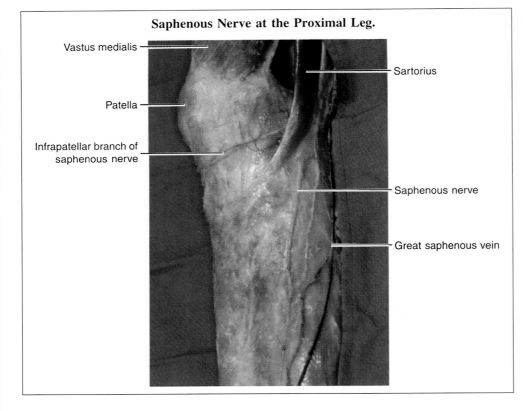

Saphenous Nerve at the Proximal Leg.

Vastus medialis

Patella

Infrapatellar branch of saphenous nerve

Sartorius

Saphenous nerve

Great saphenous vein

FIGURE 11-80 At the proximal leg, this cadaveric specimen illustrates the infrapatellar branch of the saphenous nerve. This branch pierces the sartorius and fascia lata to supply the prepatellar skin. The saphenous nerve's infrapatellar branch establishes connections around the knee as outlined in the chapter.

The SN may end at the knee and be replaced in the leg by a branch of the tibial nerve. Usually, however, it descends with the long saphenous vein along the medial side of the leg (Fig. 11-80) and in the leg's lower third it divides into two branches (Fig. 11-81). One branch continues along the tibia to end at the ankle and the other branch passes anterior to the ankle and is distributed to the medial aspect of the foot, sometimes reaching the metatarso-phalangeal joint of the great toe.

The saphenous nerve and its branches thus supply the sensation of the medial leg, ankle, and arch of foot.[8,10,15,30]

CLINICAL PRESENTATION AND EXAMINATION

Patients with SN injury at the level of Hunter's canal complain of lower medial knee pain radiating to the medial calf and into the

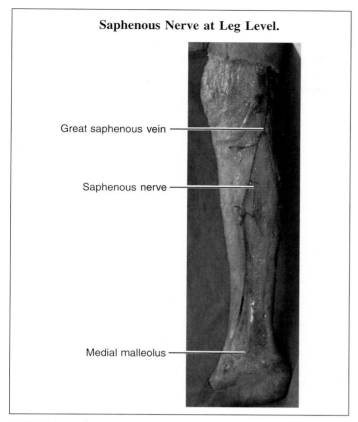

Saphenous Nerve at Leg Level.

Great saphenous vein —

Saphenous nerve —

Medial malleolus —

FIGURE 11-81 The saphenous nerve descends with the saphenous vein along the medial side of the leg towards the medial malleolus as seen in this cadaveric dissection of the right leg showing the saphenous nerve at the leg level.

Table 11-19 Saphenous nerve injuries (n=22)

Mechanism of injury	Pt. no.	Neurectomy	Neurolysis
Saphenous vein graft harvesting	14	12	2
Entrapment/contusion	3	2	1
Laceration	2	2	
Tumor*	3		
Totals	22	16	3

Pt. no., patient number.

*Tumor included two schwannomas and one solitary neurofibroma.

Table 11-20 The LSUHSC grading system for saphenous nerve sensory function

Grade	Evaluation	Description
0	Absent	No response to touch, pinprick, or pressure in the ipsilateral lateral knee, lateral calf and instep of the foot
1	Bad	Testing produces hypoesthesia or paresthesia; deep pain recovery in autonomous zones
2	Poor	Sensory response sufficient for slow protection; sensory stimuli mislocalized with overresponse
3	Moderate	Response to touch and pinprick in autonomous zones; sensation mislocalized and not normal with some overresponse
4	Good	Response to touch and pinprick in autonomous zones; response localized, but sensation not normal; no overresponse
5	Excellent	Near normal response to touch and pinprick in the entire field including autonomous zones

ankle, then the arch of the foot. Patients may alternately complain of a deep aching sensation in the distal thigh.[29]

Dysfunction of the SN from injury at this level does not cause motor dysfunction, since the SN has no motor fibers. Pre- and postoperative evaluations can be performed using the LSUHSC sensory grading system (Table 11-19). There is a loss of sensation from below the knee to the medial shin and on to the arch of the foot.

The nerve can also be compressed at it travels between the sartorius and gracilis muscles near their insertions.

SURGICAL APPROACH

Some patients with a saphenous distribution of pain and paresthesias improve with non-surgical management; however, some do not. The patients more likely to be helped by an operation are those with a Tinel sign which is maximal at a specific site on the nerve and which usually correlates with a history of injury at that level.

The surgical treatment of SN entrapment involves exposure of the SN in Hunter's canal by an incision approximately 10 cm proximal to the patella and anterior to the sartorius muscle. The interval between the quadriceps and sartorius muscles is developed. The next layer encountered is the fascia between the vastus medialis and the adductor magnus, which is incised to expose the SN.

SURGICAL TECHNIQUES

There is still a discrepancy in the literature as to whether neurolysis of the nerve or neurectomy gives the best result in saphenous neuralgia.[4,6,9,14,24] One of the more detailed reports on surgical management of this condition concluded that neurectomy gave a more predictable result than neurolysis in a series of 13 SN operations.[31] The main problem with division of the SN is the distal anesthesia, which some patients find quite annoying. Both techniques were used in the 22 LSUHSC and Stanford Medical Center patients (Table 11-20).

If neurolysis is carried out, all fascial bands around the SN must be divided in the more distal regions of the subsartorial canal. If neurectomy is performed, the nerve is divided proximal to the fascia in the canal between the vastus medialis and adductor magnus muscles. The best management for the cut proximal nerve is to place it under an adjacent muscle belly, so that any neuroma will be less likely to cause future problems. Then, a lengthy segment of distal nerve is resected to diminish distal attraction for axonal autografts.

If the nerve is compressed at it travels between the sartorius and gracilis muscles near their insertions, it can either be released or divided.

A frequent problem in sports-related injuries is the formation of a neuroma of the SN's infrapatellar branch. This branch can be irritated by repetitive movement of the knee or by direct pressure, and a neuroma is formed which causes symptoms. The surgical approach is via a straight incision over the neuroma, which is then excised, and the infrapatellar branch is dissected fairly proximally and then divided.

SAPHENOUS NERVE INJURY

A review of the recent literature reveals that the most common mechanism of injury to the SN is the greater saphenous vein stripping procedure (Fig. 11-82). External phleboextractors (EPs) have been used to replace total and short stripping of the great saphenous vein and have improved the results with reference to SN injury.

The saphenous nerve can be injured at the site of a venectomy scar. Fifteen cases of saphenous neuralgia in the distribution of the descending branch of the SN in the foreleg after coronary artery bypass graft (CABG) at the venectomy scar site have also been described.[2,11,23]

Defalque and McDanal[5] described nine cases of proximal saphenous neuralgia due to harvesting of saphenous vein grafts for venous CABG (Fig. 11.77).

Saphenous nerve injury can also occur during arthroscopic procedures at the knee.[25,28] The largest known series of the results of arthroscopy to date was a retrospective study of procedures performed by members of the Arthroscopy Association of North America (AANA). In this study Small documented 97 SN injuries in association with 375 069 knee arthroscopies.[26]

In another large retrospective study of arthroscopic knee procedures also carried out by the members of the AANA, Small[26] reported that of 121 nerves injured during knee arthroscopies, 97 (80%) involved the SN.

In a survey of surgeons at one institution,[20] two nerve injuries were reported after knee arthroscopy and both involved the SN. Sherman et al.[25] reviewed the results of 2640 knee arthroscopies and reported that eight (53%) of 15 neurological complications were directly associated with an anteromedial or posteromedial portal and involved the SN.

The SN can also be injured during meniscal repairs.[13] In a prospective study of 8791 knee arthroscopies performed by 21 surgeons experienced in the use of arthroscopy, there was only one neurological complication and this was an SN injury that was noted subsequent to a medial meniscal repair.[27] Barber[1] reported five saphenous neuropraxias after 23 meniscal repairs, or a 22% prevalence. The low prevalence of serious injury (0.01%) was attributed to the high level of expertise of the surgeons and to a refinement of the operative technique that allowed better protection of neurovascular structures. A new procedure, called the two-pin-based ROBODOC® procedure, requires a pin implantation into a patient's medial femoral condyle to register the femur.[18] Over 50% of the

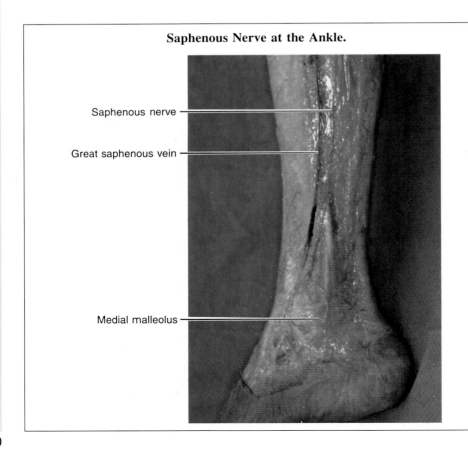

Saphenous Nerve at the Ankle.

Saphenous nerve

Great saphenous vein

Medial malleolus

FIGURE 11-82 A cadaveric dissection of the saphenous nerve at the ankle shows the nerve dividing into two branches. One branch continues along the tibia to the ankle and the other passes anterior to the ankle to the skin on the medial side towards the metatarsophalangeal joint.

patients in whom this procedure was performed reported severe knee pain. Twenty cadaver specimens were then used by the same authors to further study this procedure.[18] A 12 mm titanium screw with a 5 mm diameter was implanted into the medial femoral condyle of the cadaveric specimens. In 55% of cases there was injury to three different nerves, the SN, its infrapatellar branch, and anterior cutaneous branches of the femoral nerve. The injuries were caused by cutting of the nerve or by the screw itself. It was concluded that an anatomic region with fewer nerves should be chosen for the distal pin in the ROBODOC® procedure.

Direct trauma to the SN in contact sports from a force sufficient to disrupt the medial support structures of the knee can cause a saphenous neuralgia. A spontaneous nontraumatic saphenous neuralgia has also been described in the literature in six patients due to entrapment of the nerve in the subsartorial canal.[12] This syndrome can occur in the pediatric age group as well: Nir-Paz reported four cases in two 10-year-olds, an 11-year-old and a 15.5-year-old girl.[17]

RESULTS

In the LSUHSC and Stanford Medical Center series, there were 19 patients with operative saphenous neuralgias who underwent surgery between 1967 and 2002.

In this series, the SN was injured inadvertently during the course of venous stripping and ligation in 14 instances. Neurectomy was carried out in 12 of these cases. In one of these cases the nerve was resected from the knee to ankle level because of painful paresthesias. Neurolysis was performed in the other two patients.

There were three cases of entrapment/contusion injury involving the SN, which resulted in saphenous neuralgias. Neurectomy was performed in two of the three cases and neurolysis in one. Spontaneous entrapment is usually associated with injury, which at any point along the course of the SN can lead to a painful neuroma. In these cases we have favored wide excision of the neuroma and attached scar and removal of the nerve well proximal and distal to the injury site, rather than SN repair. The SN serves a functionally less important sensory territory than the tibial or peroneal nerves, and attempts to resect the neuroma and repair the nerve can lead to another painful neuroma as the suture or graft site matures.

The SN was lacerated during operative procedures around the knee in two instances. Neurectomy was the surgical technique used in both cases.

Occasionally, a mass such as a lipoma, cyst, or venous aneurysm can involve this nerve. In this present series, however, two schwannomas and one solitary neurofibroma were removed.

Most patients in this series had satisfactory relief of pain and paresthesias, but it should be stressed that careful selection of patients for operative intervention is very important.

REFERENCES

1. Barber FA: Meniscus repair: results of an arthroscopic technique. Arthroscopy 3:25–30, 1987.
2. Chauhan BM, Kim DJ, and Wainapel SF: Saphenous neuropathy: following coronary artery bypass surgery. NY State J Med 81:222–223, 1981.
3. Conrad P and Gassner P: Invagination stripping of the long and short saphenous vein using the PIN stripper. Aust NZ J Surg 66:394–396, 1996.
4. Deese J and Baxter D: Compressive neuropathies of the lower extremity. J Musculoskel Med 5:678–695, 1988.
5. Defalque RJ and McDanal JT: Proximal saphenous neuralgia after coronary artery bypass graft. Anesth Analg 80:620–621, 1995.
6. Dumitru D and Windsor R: Subsartorial entrapment of the saphenous nerve of a competitive female bodybuilder. Physician Sportsmed 17:116–125, 1989.
7. Ebraheim NA and Mekhail AO: The infrapatellar branch of the saphenous nerve: an anatomic study. J Orthop Trauma 11:195–199, 1997.
8. Kline DG and Hudson AR: Nerve Injury, 1st edn. Philadelphia, WB Saunders, 1995.
9. Kopell H and Thompson W: Peripheral entrapment neuropathies. Baltimore, MD, Williams and Wilkins, 1963.
10. Lancet T: Cutaneous nerve distribution to the leg. Lancet 346:830, 1995.
11. Lederman RJ, Breuer AC, Hanson MR, et al.: Peripheral nervous system complications of coronary artery bypass graft surgery. Ann Neurol 12:297–301, 1982.
12. Luerssen TG, Campbell RL, Defalque RJ, et al.: Spontaneous saphenous neuralgia. Neurosurgery 13:238–241, 1983.
13. Macnicol M: The Problem Knee. Oxford, Butterworth-Heinemann, 1995.
14. McCrory P and Bell S: Nerve entrapment syndromes as a cause of pain in the hip, groin and buttock. Sports Med 27:261–274, 1999.
15. McCrory P, Bell S, and Bradshaw C: Nerve entrapments of the lower leg, ankle and foot in sport. Sports Med 32:371–391, 2002.
16. Morrison C and Dalsing MC: Signs and symptoms of saphenous nerve injury after greater saphenous vein stripping: prevalence, severity, and relevance for modern practice. J Vasc Surg 38:886–890, 2003.
17. Nir-Paz R, Luder AS, Cozacov JC, et al.: Saphenous nerve entrapment in adolescence. Pediatrics 103:161–163, 1999.
18. Nogler M, Maurer H, Wimmer C, et al.: The risk of nerve injury through ROBODOC's distal pin in the medial femoral condyle. J Bone Joint Surg [Br] 83(Suppl I):80, 2001.
19. Pyne D, Jawad AS, and Padhiar N: Saphenous nerve injury after fasciotomy for compartment syndrome. Br J Sports Med 37:541–542, 2003.
20. Rodeo SA, Forster RA, and Weiland AJ: Neurological complications due to arthroscopy. J Bone Joint Surg [Am] 75:917–926, 1993.
21. Romanoff ME, Cory PC Jr, Kalenak A, et al.: Saphenous nerve entrapment at the adductor canal. Am J Sports Med 17:478–481, 1989.
22. Rutgers PH and Kitslaar PJ: Randomized trial of stripping versus high ligation combined with sclerotherapy in the treatment of the incompetent greater saphenous vein. Am J Surg 168:311–315, 1994.
23. Schnall B and San Luis F: Saphenous neuropathy following coronary artery bypass surgery. Orthopedic Rev 8:121–122, 1979.
24. Senegor M: Iatrogenic saphenous neuralgia: successful therapy with neuroma resection. Neurosurgery 28:295–298, 1991.
25. Sherman OH, Fox JM, Snyder SJ, et al.: Arthroscop – "no-problem surgery." An analysis of complications in two thousand six hundred and forty cases. J Bone and Joint Surg [Am] 68:256–265, 1986.
26. Small N: Complications in arthroscopy: the knee and other joints. Committee on Complications of the Arthroscopy Association of North America. Arthroscopy 2:253–258, 1986.
27. Small NC: Complications in arthroscopic surgery performed by experienced arthroscopists. Arthroscopy 4:215–221, 1988.
28. Spicer DDM, Blagg SE, Unwin AJ, et al.: An anatomical study of the saphenous nerve and its infragenicular branch in relation to arthroscopically assisted hamstring anterior cruciate ligament reconstruction. J Bone Joint Surg [Br] 82(Suppl III):247, 2000.
29. Taber KH, Duncan G, Chiou-Tan F, et al.: Sectional neuroanatomy of the lower limb II: leg and foot. J Comput Assist Tomogr 25:823–826, 2001.
30. Wartenberg R: Digitalgia paresthetica and gonyalgia paresthetica. Neurology 4:106–115, 1954.

31. Worth RM, Kettelkamp DB, Defalque RJ, et al.: Saphenous nerve entrapment. A cause of medial knee pain. Am J Sports Med 12:80–81, 1984.

GENITOFEMORAL NEURALGIA

OVERVIEW

- There were 10 genitofemoral neuralgias managed at LSUHSC which were analyzed (Table 11-21). The side of the lesion, sex and age were found to be equal. L1 and L2 nerve blocks had resulted in complete or substantial decrease in pain before neurectomy was recommended.
- Six of 10 patients had neuralgias due to iatrogenic injuries. Vasectomy and hysterectomy procedures each resulted in two of the six iatrogenic neuralgias. One neuralgia each was sustained after herniorrhaphy and gynecological surgery. Four of the 10 patients had injury to the genitofemoral nerve after blunt abdominal trauma.
- Retroperitoneal genitofemoral neurectomy was performed in all genitofemoral neuralgia patients after conservative therapy failed. This procedure resulted in considerable pain relief in all patients, whether their injury was iatrogenic or due to trauma.

DIAGNOSIS AND MANAGEMENT

Genitofemoral neuralgia is a syndrome presenting with chronic pain and paresthesias in the distribution of the genitofemoral nerve. Magee first described the syndrome of genitofemoral causalgia in 1942,[5] while Lyon in 1945 suggested the term genitofemoral neuralgia.[4] Only 25 cases of genitofemoral neuralgias were reported in the world's literature as of 1987; thus, it is not a common syndrome.[8]

Genitofemoral neuralgia can occur after inguinal herniorrhaphy, appendectomy, caesarean section, or trauma to the lower quadrant of the abdomen or inguinal regions. Nerve injury arising during inguinal herniorrhaphy may have different causal mechanisms leading to residual neuralgia. These include section or stretch of a nerve, electrocoagulation, stricture due to ligation, entrapment of the nerve in scar tissue, or irritation by proximity to a zone of inflammation. Neural stretching of the genital branches of the genitofemoral nerve can occur when the spermatic cord is handled while searching for a herniated peritoneal sac, or during placation of the fascia transversalis. The systematic ligation of the cremasteric artery, advocated by some authors, also carries a risk of injury to the genital branch of the genitofemoral nerve unless the latter has been clearly identified prior to artery ligation.

It is thought that fibrous adhesions may entrap small branches and twigs of the nerve in the region of previous surgery or blunt trauma. This has been documented in the literature as adhesions of the cecum or terminal ileum to the genitofemoral nerve, as well as adherence of the lumboinguinal branch of the genitofemoral nerve to fibrotic tissue in the femoral canal.[4,5]

The symptoms are an intermittent or constant burning sensation and pain in the inguinal region, which usually spread to the skin of the genital region and upper medial thigh. The symptoms are exacerbated by walking, running, stooping, climbing stairs, and by hip hyperextension while lying down. Hip flexion may decrease the burning dysesthesias and pain. Sometimes tenderness along the inguinal canal ring may occur and hyperesthesia can be present in the distribution of the nerve in the lower abdominal quadrant and upper medial thigh, lateral to the pubic tubercle.

The patient with genitofemoral neuralgia does not usually have an elicitable Tinel sign, while ilioinguinal entrapment, which may present in a similar manner, may have one. Local nerve blocks, in the case of the ilioinguinal neuralgia, or specific blocks, in the case of genitofemoral nerve, can also be done to determine the precise nerve that is involved. Thus, if an ilioinguinal nerve entrapment or, in some cases, injury or neuroma in the abdominal wall is responsible for the pain, a local block of that nerve through the lower anterior abdominal wall should alleviate the symptoms. If the pain is not relieved, then proximal genitofemoral injury could be responsible for the pain. L1 and L2 spinal nerves can be blocked through a paravertebral route with 0.5% bupivacaine and 7.5% lidocaine with epinephrine at a concentration of 1 : 200 000. By performing separate control and peripheral blocks and observing for pain relief, the distinction between genitofemoral and ilioinguinal neuralgias can be made.

Many patients have had their pain managed by repeated local injections, nerve stimulators, and pain medications. If these conservative measures have failed, surgical intervention to alleviate the pain may be indicated. Neurectomy of the genitofemoral nerve is the treatment of choice and, if performed via an extraperitoneal approach, may allow for an easier exploration of the nerve proximal to the site of adhesions.

DIFFERENTIAL DIAGNOSIS

The differential diagnosis of groin pain after inguinal area surgical procedures in addition to the described postoperative ilioinguinal and/or iliohypogastric nerve and genitofemoral entrapment syndromes includes abdominal cutaneous nerve entrapment syndrome, hernias of the incisional, inguinal, and femoral types, lymphadenopathy, broad ligament neuritis, pelvic sympathetic syndrome, abdominal muscle strain, periostitis of the pubic tubercle, and strain of the pectineal muscle.[1] Other possibilities which may mascarade as iliohypogastric or ilioinguinal neuralgias include hip or genitourinary disease and camptocormia or psychogenic etiologies.[5]

SURGICAL ANATOMY

The genitofemoral nerve is a mixed nerve with a preponderance of sensory fibers. Its main root originates from L2 and is constantly present, while the slender, inconsistently present accessory root

Table 11-21 Mechanism of genitofemoral nerve injuries

Mechanism of injury	Genitofemoral nerve
Iatrogenic	
Hysterectomy	2
Vasectomy	2
Herniorrhaphy	1
Gynecological	1
Surgery	
Blunt trauma	4
Total	10

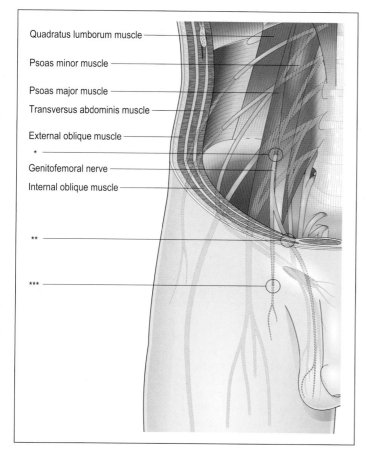

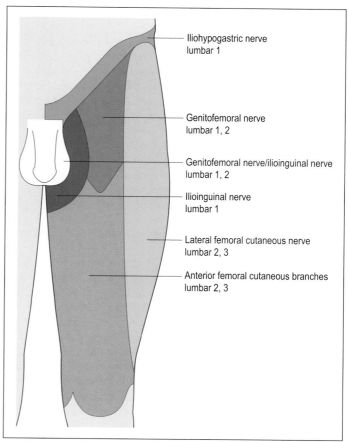

FIGURE 11-83 This is an illustration of the genitofemoral nerve which is shown to pierce the psoas major at *, which is at the level of the L3–L4 intervertebral disc space. The nerve then descends along the anterior surface of the psoas muscle. Before passing through the transverses abdominus and internal oblique muscles, shown at **, it divides into its two terminal branches, the genital and femoral branches. The femoral branch passes through the fascia lata at *** lateral to the femoral artery. The genital branch enters the inguinal canal, runs along the posteromedial spermatic cord and leaves the inguinal canal as shown through the superficial orifice to terminate in the scrotum or mons pubis and labia majora. It also supplies the cremaster muscle.

FIGURE 11-84 The sensory distribution of the genitofemoral nerve as well as that of the iliohypogastric, ilioinguinal, lateral femoral cutaneous nerve, and femoral nerve are shown. (From Murovic J, Kim D, Tiel R, and Kline D. Surgical management of 10 genitofemoral neuralgias at LSUHSC. Neurosurgery 56:2, 300, 2005.)

originates from the anterior branch of the L1 nerve. The genitofemoral nerve travels obliquely between the two muscle bellies of the psoas muscle and perforates the psoas major at the level of the intervertebral disc lying between the third and fourth lumbar vertebrae (Fig. 11-83). It descends along the anterior surface of the psoas muscle. As the nerve passes through the lumbar region it crosses behind the ureter. It takes a straight inferior and somewhat caudal course along with the iliac vessels into the region of the internal iliac fossa. Slightly posterior to and at a variable distance above the inguinal ligament, it divides into its two terminal branches, the genital and femoral branches.

The femoral branch is a cutaneous nerve and branches of it descend and follow the external iliac artery, remaining lateral to it. The femoral branch continues behind the inguinal ligament, and through the fascia lata into the femoral sheath, lateral to the femoral artery. This branch supplies the skin over the femoral triangle (Fig. 11-84), which is bounded superiorly by the inguinal ligament, laterally by the sartorius muscle, and medially by the

adductor longus muscle. The femoral branch communicates with the intermediate cutaneous nerve of the thigh.

The genital branch crosses the lower end of the external iliac artery and enters the inguinal canal through the internal inguinal ring. Within the canal, it runs along the posterior medial surface of the spermatic cord, and along with the cremasteric artery lies in apposition to the superficial sheath surrounding the cord. It leaves the inguinal canal through the superficial sheath surrounding the cord. It leaves the inguinal canal through the superficial orifice to terminate in the skin of the scrotum in men and the mons pubis and labia majora in women (Fig. 11-84).[2,3,8] It also supplies the cremaster muscle in men, as well.

There is great variability in the anatomy of the genitofemoral nerve. Occasionally, the main nerve may divide within the substance of the psoas muscle and the two terminal branches may emerge separately from the anterior surface of the muscle. Additional variations were found by Bergman et al., who studied 200 cadavers and found that the genitofemoral nerve was a single trunk in 80% and two separate branches, genital and femoral, in 20%.[1] The single trunk may arise from L1 or L2 and L3 and if there are two trunks, these may arise from L1 and L2 or L1, L2, and L3. The second lumbar nerve was represented in every case in the Bergman et al. publication and the third lumbar was represented in 0.75% of cases. The level of division into terminal branches was also highly variable.

Other authors have documented anatomical variations as well. Salama and Chevrel found a genital branch of the genitofemoral nerve in 18 of 25 cadaveric dissections and in the seven other cases it was absent and could not be demonstrated, nor even the spermatic cord.[7] In cases where this genital branch was absent, an accessory ramus from the iliohypogastric or ilioinguinal nerve was found. In three cases, the accessory ramus arose from the genital branch of the ilioinguinal nerve with the iliohypogastric nerve providing the innervations to the pubic region. In the four other cases, the accessory ramus arose from a common trunk between the genital branches of the iliohypogastric and ilioinguinal nerves. It was noted that the accessory ramus displayed the same course and distribution as the genital branch it replaced. In all dissections, the genital branch of the genitofemoral nerve entered the inguinal canal through the deep orifice.

Great variation of the genitofemoral sensory nerves to the inguinal region is also common, with free communication between branches of the genitofemoral, ilioinguinal, or iliohypogastric nerve.[6] Other scenarios may occur, such as the genitofemoral nerve or either of its genital branch and the lateral cutaneous or the anterior femoral nerve may replace the femoral branch. The branches of the genitofemoral may replace or join the ilioinguinal nerve. The genital branch may bypass the deep inguinal ring running superficial to it in the aponeurosis of the external abdominal oblique muscle. The femoral branch may replace or join the lateral or middle cutaneous nerve. On occasion, the femoral branch has an extensive distribution to the skin of the upper two-thirds of the thigh. The genital branch may supply the lower fibers of the internal abdominal oblique and transverse muscles.

SURGICAL MANAGEMENT

A lateral extraperitoneal approach to the genitofemoral nerve is the preferred surgical approach. For a right-sided neuralgia, the patient was placed in a supine position with elevation of the right thorax and hip on folded sheets. A transverse flank incision, similar to that utilized for a lumbar sympathectomy, was used to approach the genitofemoral nerve.

The incision was begun slightly above and lateral to the umbilicus and extended several centimeters to the anterior axillary line. The external and internal oblique muscles were split using cutting cautery and the transversus abdominis muscle divided in line with its fibers. The extraperitoneal fat and peritoneum were retracted medially and the retroperitoneum exposed, while a plane anterior to the quadratus lumborum and psoas major muscles was defined and developed. The ureter was identified and protected. The genitofemoral nerve was identified as it exited the psoas muscle along its medial edge. The nerve was stimulated with a nerve stimulator and contractions of the cremaster muscle were observed prior to resection. Nerve was sectioned proximal to the assumed site of entrapment of injury and a 23 cm segment of nerve which usually included its bifurcation was resected. The wound was then closed.

Because of frequent abnormal variations in the point of nerve bifurcation, identification of both branches was made to ensure transection of the proximal genitofemoral nerve trunk. Once the branches of the genitofemoral nerve pass into the region of the internal inguinal ring or femoral canal, their respective distal branches are too small to allow precise identification.

RESULTS

There were 10 patients who had surgery at LSUHSC for genitofemoral neuralgia. The mechanisms of injury to the genitofemoral nerve included six iatrogenic injuries. Vasectomy procedures antedated two of the six genitofemoral neuralgias due to iatrogenic injuries, and hysterectomy resulted also in two patients with similar nerve injuries. There was one genitofemoral neuralgia each after herniorrhaphy and gynecological surgery. Four patients sustained injury to the genitofemoral nerve after blunt abdominal wall trauma.

Genitofemoral neurectomy was performed in all cases after conservative measures had failed to alleviate the patients' discomfort. Neurectomy was predicated by a good result with L1 and L2 nerve blocks in each case. Neurectomy resulted in considerable pain relief in all 10 patients, whether their injury was iatrogenic or due to trauma.

DISCUSSION

A thorough history and physical examination must be done in patients with inguinal pain following surgery. In patients being evaluated for genitofemoral neuralgia, a local block of the ilioinguinal nerve should be performed. If complete or substantial relief of pain is achieved with an ilioinguinal nerve block, surgical re-exploration of the original inguinal incision associated with the neuralgia and ilioinguinal nerve identification are indicated. If no relief of pain occurs with the ilioinguinal nerve block, then a genitofemoral block, which is more difficult, is done. As described earlier, the genitofemoral nerve arises from the L2 and to a lesser extent L1 nerves and with a specific block of the L1 and L2 spinal nerves the genitofemoral and a variable portion of the ilioinguinal nerves are blocked. By performing separate blocks and observing pain relief, the distinction between genitofemoral or ilioinguinal neuropathy can be made. If an L1 and L2 block results in pain relief, genitofemoral nerve exploration should be considered. If partial relief is achieved with both blocks, consideration should be made for surgical exploration of both nerves.

Side effects of neurectomy include hypoesthesia of the scrotum or labium majorus, and/or skin over the femoral triangle, and loss of the cremasteric reflex. The hypalgesia may resolve, though the absence of the cremasteric reflex may remain.[3] By performing the nerve excision through an extraperitoneal rather than intraperitoneal approach, operative complications can be minimized.

CONCLUSION

Genitofemoral neuralgia is an uncommon lesion; however, its dysesthesias can prove recalcitrant to conservative measures. Genitofemoral neuralgia must be carefully differentiated from ilioinguinal neuralgia, which presents in a similar manner, by using local ilioinguinal nerve blocks versus L1 and L2 nerve blocks if the former block proves not to ameliorate the symptoms and findings. Neurectomy in 10 cases of genitofemoral neuralgia patients at LSUHSC resulted in considerable pain relief in all patients.

REFERENCES

1. Bergman RA, Afifi, AK, and Miyauchi R: Genitofemoral Nerve. Virtual Hospital, University of Iowa Health Care, 2002.

2. Harms BA, DeHawas DR Jr, and Starling JR: Diagnosis and management of genitofemoral neuralgia. Arch Surg 110:339–341, 1984.

3. Laha RK, Rao S, Pidgeon CN, et al.: Genitofemoral neuralgia. Surg Neurol 8:280–282, 1977.

4. Lyon E: Genitofemoral causalgia. Can Med Assoc J 53:213–216, 1945.

5. Magee K: Genitofemoral causalgia (A new syndrome). Can Med Assoc J 46:326–329, 1942.

6. Mandelkow H and Loweeneck H; The iliohypogastric and ilioinguinal nerves. Distribution in the abdominal wall, danger areas in surgical incisions in the inguinal and pubic regions and reflected visceral pain in their dermatomes. Surg Radiol Anat 10:145–149, 1988.

7. Salama J, Chevrel JP: The Anatomical Basis of Nerve Lesions Arising During the Reduction of Inguinal-Hernia. New York, Spring-Verlag, 1983.

8. Starling JR, Harms BA, Schroeder ME, et al.: Diagnosis and treatment of genitofemoral and ilioinguinal entrapment neuralgia. Surgery 102:581–586, 1987.

ILIOINGUINAL AND ILIOHYPOGASTRIC NERVE INJURY AND ENTRAPMENT

OVERVIEW

- The major etiology for these painful palsies is prior surgery, usually for hernia, although appendectomy, iliac crest bone harvest, and gynecologic and urologic procedures can also be responsible.
- In addition to sensory disturbances in the inguinal, groin, scrotal, and inner thigh areas, denervational change can be present in the pyramidalis if ilioinguinal nerve is seriously injured.
- Anesthetic blocks of one or more of these nerves can be helpful in selecting patients for surgery.
- Patients in this series of cases had neurectomy done at the level of the abdominal wall. This was combined with removal of scar tissue, heavy sutures or clips to secure mesh, and sometimes removal of a portion of mesh used to reconstruct the abdominal wall.
- Preoperative study of the anatomic courses of these two nerves as well as their anatomic variations is important.
- A more proximal retroperitoneal approach to these nerves can be done but was not utilized in this series of cases.

The primary operation which results in these two neuralgias is inguinal hernia repair, which, at an annual rate of 2800 herniorrhaphies per 1 million people, is one of the most common operations performed in the United States. The incidence of persistent symptoms of neuralgia is quite low, however, and is estimated to be 0–8% after open and 0–10% after laparoscopic hernia repairs.[3,4] In one report of 939 inguinal hernia repairs, 2.8% still had significant pain and 1.4% remained disabled at 3 years.[5]

In addition to herniorrhaphy, other abdominal procedures which may result in injury to these nerves include appendectomy, iliac crest bone graft harvesting, gynecological surgery, including transverse or paramedian incisions for hysterectomy, and urological operations.

Mechanisms of injury to a sensory branch(es) of the iliohypogastric and/or ilioinguinal nerves resulting from the above procedures can include partial or complete section, crush, stretch/contusion, or electrocoagulation.[9] Secondary damage to a sensory nerve may also result from cicatricial compression and neuroma formation and from irritation by an adjacent inflammatory process such as a suture granuloma.[12]

Mechanisms of nerve injury specific to certain procedures include entrapment of nerves by suture or metallic staples used to affix prosthetic material during laparoscopic hernia repairs. Stretch of the genital branches of the iliohypogastric and ilioinguinal nerves can occur when the spermatic cord is handled during hernia repairs and during the search for a herniated peritoneal sac, and stricture of these nerves may occur when the conjoined tendon is mobilized or the aponeurosis of the external oblique is sutured.[10]

Patients with ilioinguinal or iliohypogastric neuralgias present with chronic groin pain and paresthesias. The discomfort may extend to the medial thigh and, additionally, in men to the scrotum or testicle, and in women to the labia majora. Thus, the diagnostic triad of nerve entrapment or neuromas of the ilioinguinal or iliohypogastric nerves consists of: (1) burning or lancinating pain near the precipating operation's incision that radiates to the area supplied by the nerve, (2) clear evidence of impaired sensory perception in the involved nerve territory, and (3) pain that is relieved by infiltration with anesthetic in the area of the nerve.

CHARACTERISTICS OF INGUINAL PAIN

Acute pain after herniorrhaphy or after any other abdominal procedure is related to the patient's age, is in proportion to the extent of the procedure, and can be associated with anxiety and activation of the sympathetic nerve system. This type of pain is usually readily managed with analgesics and subsides as the surgical wound heals. Some patients, however, develop chronic disabling pain which lasts longer than 4 weeks after surgery and is out of proportion to the apparent pathology. In most, the condition resolves spontaneously within 4–6 months, but in some it may progress to a chronic, disabling pain, which is the type of pain addressed in this chapter. In addition to occurring immediately after surgery, the neuralgia can occur after months or years. In 23 patients with a painful ilioinguinal and/or iliohypogastric nerve entrapment syndrome managed by Stulz and Pfeiffer, 10 patients had manifestation of the pain immediately after the operation, in four cases it occurred after more than 6 months, and in nine it occurred after 4 pain-free years.[11]

The pain of ilioinguinal or iliohypogastric neuralgia is usually described as burning and sharp in nature, but without spontaneous paroxysms, and is more or less persistent. Hyperesthesia and hyperpathia occur in areas innervated by the nerve(s). If a neuroma is present, percussion can cause severe lancinating pain. Body movements often aggravate the pain, while some body positions may actually alleviate the discomfort. Thus, the pain is intensified by forcible stretching of the hip joint, coughing, sneezing, Valsalva's maneuver, or movements that increase the tension in the abdominal muscles. The patient frequently adopts a posture that eases discomfort, with slight flexure of the hip and a slight forward inclination of the trunk.

There may be impairment of groin sensory perception i.e. dys-, hyper-, or hypoesthesia and these dysesthesias sometimes occur in a band extending from the iliac crest into the root to the penis, the proximal zone of the scrotum or labia majora and on the inside and anterior surfaces of the thighs.[11]

In women with chronic pelvic pain, careful abdominal wall examination should be performed to look for trigger points, which manifest as areas of discrete hyperalgesia and when palpated with fingertip pressure elicit sharp pain that can refer to distant dermatomes. Tenderness on bimanual examination does not always equal visceral pathology. Somatic pain generators can be misdiagnosed as ovarian, uterine, or bladder pathology. The entire peripheral nerve could be etiological or there may be isolated neuromas causing discomfort.

CLINICAL EXAMINATION

In the evaluation of groin neuralgia one must focus on a history of prior infection, trauma, back or other chronic pain, psychiatric disorders, or previous scrotal or inguinal surgery, since these events give insight into possible etiologies of the neuralgia and lend support to the diagnosis. The social history regarding the ability to work and financial compensation due to pain are important, at times, as well. Most of the patients included in this present study were referred to LSUHSC after other mechanical etiologies of groin pain were eliminated. However, on physical examination, the following entities may exist and be the cause of the neuralgias, including: tumor, intermittent testicular torsion, varicocele, hydrocele, spermatocele, or inguinal hernia. Thus, if there are complaints or findings in the history and physical examination referable to a mass lesion and it has not already been obtained, scrotal ultrasound should be performed to rule out structural abnormalities.

SURGICAL ANATOMY

THE ILIOINGUINAL NERVE

This is a mixed nerve with both motor and skin sensory functions which arises from L1 with contributing filaments from the T12 spinal nerve, the nerve then runs beneath the peritoneum (Fig. 11-85). Muscle branches innervate the lowest portions of the transversus abdominis and internal oblique muscles and their fasciae. A distal branch also innervates the pyramidalis muscle, which a well-trained electromyographer can sometimes sample and find denervation when there has been serious injury to the nerve. A narrow strip of skin over the iliac crest is innervated by a recurrent branch. It follows the path of the iliohypogastric nerve, then moves away and continues slightly caudally and parallel to it. Unlike the iliohypogastric, it does not give off a collateral branch, whereas its two terminals, the abdominal and genital branches, follow the same course and distribution as those of the iliohypogastric nerve. It crosses the two internal abdominal muscles leaving the internal oblique at a point slightly medial and caudal to it. It continues below the aponeurosis of the external oblique abdominal muscle, and travels towards the symphysis and pubic region (Fig. 11-86). When it travels within the inguinal canal, the nerve lies below the spermatic cord or round ligament of the uterus, and accompanies either one through the superficial abdominal ring where it leaves these structures. At this level, the fibers may be too small to be seen. Branches occasionally fan out over the spermatic cord. The ilioinguinal sensory distribution is a ribbon-shaped area over the inguinal region up to the iliac crest, and the region over the symphysis, the root of the penis, the proximal parts of the scrotum or the labia majora and a small adjacent zone of the anterior part and the medial upper thigh and the skin of the groin.

THE ILIOHYPOGASTRIC NERVE

The iliohypogastric nerve is a mixed nerve which arises from the anterior branch(es) of the L1 nerve and frequently the T12 nerve.

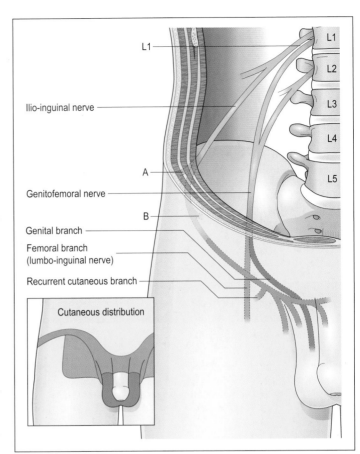

FIGURE 11-85 The course and distribution of the ilioinguinal and genitofemoral nerves. As the ilioinguinal nerve courses along the crest of the ilium it gives off branches (A, B) to abdominal muscles. The cutaneous distribution of each of the nerves is indicated in the inset. From Kopell HP, Thompson WA, Peripheral Entrapment Neuropathia, Williams & Wilkins, Baltimore 1963.

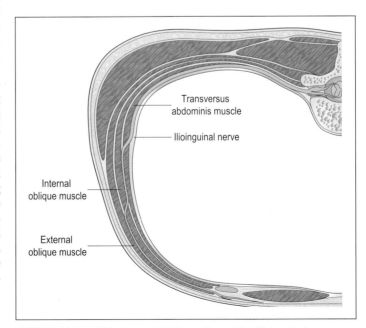

FIGURE 11-86 This is an axial illustration of the ilioinguinal nerve showing the nerve crossing the transversus abdominus muscle (1st step of a two-stepped line) then internal oblique muscle (2nd step) as shown.

It emerges along the lateral margin of the psoas muscle to pass anterior to the quadratus lumborum. The nerve perforates the transversus abdominis muscle above the iliac crest and divides into two terminal branches, an abdominal and a genital branch.

The abdominal branch of the iliohypogastric nerve is found up to 3 cm medial to the anterior superior iliac spine between the transversus abdominis and internal oblique muscles. In the region slightly above the deep orifice of the inguinal canal, it pierces the internal oblique muscle. It next runs between the internal oblique and external oblique muscles to reach the lateral margin of the rectus abdominis at a point 4 cm lateral to midline where it penetrate the aponeurosis of the external oblique muscle. Posterior to the rectus abdominis muscle, the abdominal branch gives off a lateral and a medial cutaneous ramus to supply the skin of the anteroinferior part of the abdomen. In its course through the abdominal wall, the abdominal branch of the iliohypogastric anastomoses with its homolog arising from the ilioinguinal and with the T12 intercostal nerve to give off numerous rami distributed to the muscles of the anterolateral part of the abdominal wall. The lateral cutaneous branch of the iliohypogastric nerve leaves the nerve at the lateral summit of the iliac crest between the internal oblique and the transversus abdominis muscles and supplies the skin above the tensor fasciae latae.[6]

The genital branch of the iliohypogastric follows the same course as the abdominal branch between the transversus abdominis and internal oblique muscles. At the level of the anterosuperior iliac spine, it perforates the internal oblique muscle and runs inferiorly and medially within the anterior wall of the inguinal canal at a level slightly above the inguinal ligament. In the inguinal region, the genital branch runs along the deep surface of the external oblique fascia anterior to the internal oblique muscle and lies between the spermatic cord and the conjoined tendon. At the level of the superficial orifice of the inguinal canal, this nerve branch enters the subcutaneous tissue and distributes to the skin of the pubic region, the medial part of the groin, and the upper medial part of the thigh.

ANATOMICAL VARIATIONS

In a study by Rab et al., who analyzed 64 halves of 32 cadavers, there were four types of distributions of the cutaneous branches of the ilioinguinal nerve in the inguinal and ventromedial thigh regions.[7] Type A, the most common distribution, occurred in 44% of the cadavers. In this type, the ilioinguinal nerve gave no sensory distribution to the scrotal/labial and ventromedial thigh areas, but rather there were was dominance of the genitofemoral nerve in these regions. In type B, which occurred in 28% of 64 cadaver halves, there was a dominance of the ilioinguinal nerve, and the genitofemoral nerve shared a branch with the ilioinguinal nerve, giving motor fibers to the cremaster muscle in the inguinal canal. There was, however, no sensory branch to the groin. In type C, found in 20% of cadavers, the ilioinguinal nerve had sensory branches to the mons pubis and inguinal crease together with an anteroproximal part to the root of the penis or labia majora. There was, however, a dominance of the genitofemoral nerve. The ilioinguinal nerve was found to share a branch with the iliohypogastric nerve. In type D, which occurred in 8% of cadavers, cutaneous branches emerged from both the ilioinguinal and the genitofemoral nerves. Additionally, the ilioinguinal nerve innervated the mons pubis and inguinal crease together with a very anteroproximal part of the root of the penis or labia majora.[7]

TREATMENT

An initial trial of conservative therapy for iliohypogastric and/or ilioinguinal neuralgias should be undertaken using analgesics, antidepressants, anticonvulsants, and anxiolytics. Other modalities may be tried including transcutaneous electrical nerve stimulation (TENS), antiinflammatory agents such as systemic prednisolone acetate or repeated local injections with or without betamethasone diproprionate, along with regional nerve blocks or physical therapy.

Surgical therapy in the form of neurectomy was the surgical technique that was used with some success in the 33 neuralgia patients presented in this chapter. In these patients, the involved nerve was identified by local anesthetic nerve blocks, since the iliohypogastric and ilioinguinal nerves can be easily blocked in the groin. If ilioinguinal and/or iliohypogastric nerve block(s) relieve the pain, these nerves should be explored in the groin, and removed along with any offending lesion. When the nerve is completely encased in scar tissue, neurolysis rarely results in lasting relief from pain because with time there is renewed scar formation. In the paper by Stulz and Pfeiffer, neurolysis of the iliohypogastric nerve was attempted, but did not help.[11]

Other surgical techniques described in the literature for management of these syndromes include cicatricotomies, and Rauck et al. described an open cryoanalgesic technique used in 11 male patients with chronic inguinal neuralgia uncontrolled by conventional management techniques. Prior to cryoanalgesia, all patients demonstrated pain relief with ilioinguinal local anesthetic nerve blocks. The mechanism of pain relief in cryoanalgesia is thought to be that it causes Wallerian degeneration and subsequent regeneration of the axon. In the Rauch et al. study, four patients had postherniorrhaphy pain and the etiology of pain was idiopathic in seven.[8] Duration of pain relief was from 1 week to 11 months and the duration of sensory change was 1 week to 5 months with a mean of 33 days.

Orchiectomy has been found to be successful in 75% of 45 patients with orchialgia in a study by Davis et al.,[2] although there are other reports that 80% of 48 patients continued to have significant scrotal pain after orchiectomy.[1] Denervation of the spermatic cord, consisting of division of the ilioinguinal nerve along with spermatic branches of the genitofemoral nerve and autonomic fibers of the cord, was reported in 27 men with testicular pain, with 76% complete pain relief, 9.1% partial relief, and no relief in 15%.

The abdominal incision from the original procedure resulting in the neuralgia is extended toward and just short of the anterior superior iliac spine, exposing the iliohypogastric and/or ilioinguinal nerve's(es') site(s) of muscle emergence. The external oblique muscle's aponeurosis is exposed and split in the direction of the muscle fibers and the nerve(s) can be found by raising the fascia from the internal oblique muscle. The course of the nerve(s) is traced medially and the site at which it (they) pass into scar or are trapped by suture can be seen. Neuromas are usually not visualized since the axons are not usually sectioned at the time of the original operation. After identification, the nerve is sectioned as closely as possible to the site where it leaves the retroperitoneum and is excised peripherally along with the scar tissue. At times, there may be minimal or no postoperative sensory defects, presumably since the area is supplied by adjacent nerves.[11]

An alternative is to approach the nerves by a flank incision where muscles are split. A retroperitoneal approach is then used similar

Table 11-22 Ilioinguinal and ilioinguinal/hypogastric nerve injuries (n=33)

Mechanism of injury	Ilioinguinal nerve	Ilioinguinal/ iliohypogastric nerves
Herniorrhaphy	13	3
Appendectomy	4	2
Hysterectomy	3	0
Abdominoplasty	0	3
Gynecological	0	1
Blunt trauma	3	1
Total	23	10

Table 11-23 Operative outcomes in ilioinguinal and ilioinguinal/iliohypogastric lesions (n=33)

	No cases evaluated	No. of patients with pain relief
Ilioinguinal	23	21
Ilioinguinal and iliohypogastric	10	9
Totals	33	30

to that done for a lumbar sympathectomy or for genitofemoral neurectomy. However, all the patients reported in this series were done at the level of the abdominal wall.

RESULTS

There was no predilection for the right or left side, and sex and age delineations were equal. The nerve injury involved only the ilioinguinal nerve in 23 patients while there were combined ilioinguinal/iliohypogastric nerve injuries in 10 individuals (Table 11-22). The majority, or 29 (88%) of the total of 33 patients with ilioinguinal or combined ilioinguinal/iliohypogastric neuralgias, had injuries due to iatrogenic causes and the remainder, or 4 (12%) of 33 injuries, were the result of blunt trauma to the abdominal wall.

In the isolated ilioinguinal nerve injury category, the operative procedure associated with the majority of neuralgias was herniorrhaphy after which there were 13 (57%) of 23 patients who developed ilioinguinal neuralgia. This was followed in number by four patients (17%) who were status-postappendectomy, which had resulted in ilioinguinal neuralgias. There were three (13%) hysterectomy-induced lesions. Three patients (13%) had neuralgias resulting from blunt trauma.

In the 10 combined ilioinguinal/iliohypogastric lesions, the majority, or nine (90%) of these 10 lesions, were due to iatrogenic causes and there was one patient (10%) with injury due to blunt trauma.

The diagnosis was made using physical examination, history, preoperative electromyography, and nerve blocks. Nerve blocks must have resulted in a complete or substantial decrease in pain before a recommendation for neurectomy was made. Neurectomies resulted in complete or considerable pain relief in 21 (91%) of 23 patients with ilioinguinal lesions and nine (90%) of 10 patients with combined ilioinguinal/iliohypogastric lesions (Table 11-23). The pathological reports on the resected nerve tissues showed fibrous adhesions in the majority of cases, while an occasional specimen showed nerve or scar involving a neuroma and/or foreign body, such as suture material.

The postoperative side effects were usually persistent numbness distal to the level of the nerve section and loss of the cremasteric reflex. Minor postoperative complications consisted of two superficial skin infections.

CONCLUSION

Ilioinguinal and ilioinguinal/iliohypogastric neuralgia is an infrequent condition; however, 33 patients from LSUHSC were accrued and analyzed in this study. Most were due to iatrogenic causes, with herniorrhaphy as the most common etiology of these neuralgias. After a trial of conservative measures, neurectomy was found to result in pain relief in 91% of the patients in this series.

REFERENCES

1. Costabile RA, Hahn M, and McLeod DG: Chronic orchialgia in the pain-prone patient: the clinical perspective. J Urol 146:1571–1574, 1991.
2. Davis BE, Noble MJ, Weigel JW, et a.l: Analysis and management of chronic testicular pain. J Urol 143:936–939, 1990.
3. Katkhouda N, Mavor E, Friedlander MH, et al.: Use of fibrin sealant for prosthetic mesh fixation in laparoscopic extraperitoneal inguinal hernia repair. Ann Surg 233:18–25, 2001.
4. Kennedy EM, Harms BA, and Starling JR: Absence of maladaptive neuronal plasticity after genitofemoral or ilioinguinal neurectomy. Surgery 116:665–670; discussion 670–671, 1994.
5. Kopell HP, Thompson WA, and Postel AH: Entrapment neuropathy of the ilioinguinal nerve. N Engl J Med 266:16–19, 1962.
6. Mandelkow H and Loeweneck H: The iliohypogastric and ilioinguinal nerves. Distribution in the abdominal wall, danger areas in surgical incisions in the inguinal and pubic regions and reflected visceral pain in their dermatomes. Surg Radiol Anat 10:145–149, 1988.
7. Rab M, Ebmer, and Dellon AL: Anatomic variability of the ilioinguinal and genitofemoral nerves: implications for the treatment of groin pain. Plast Reconstr Surg 108:1618–1623, 2001.
8. Rauk RL, Lafavore P, Naveira FA, et al.: Evaluation of the efficacy of open cryoanalgesia technique in the management of ilioinguinal/ hypogastric neuralgia. Anesthesiology 89(Suppl 3A):1108A, 1998.
9. Ravichandran D, Kalambe BG, and Pain JA: Pilot randomized controlled study of preservation or division of ilioinguinal nerve in open mesh repair of inguinal hernia. Br J Surg 87:1166–1167, 2000.
10. Salama J and Chevrel CP: The Anatomical Basis of Nerve Lesions Arising During the Reduction of Inguinal Hernia, vol 5. New York, Springer-Verlag, 1983.
11. Stulz P and Pfeiffer KM: Peripheral nerve injuries resulting from common surgical procedures in the lower portion of the abdomen. Arch Surg 117:324–327, 1982.
12. Wantz G: Testicular atrophy and chronic residual neuralgia as risks of inguinal hernioplasty: Surg Clin N Am 73:571, 1993.

12

Brachial plexus anatomy and preoperative physiology

Rajiv Midha

OVERVIEW

- The elements or portions of the nervous system that usually comprise the brachial plexus arise from the C5, C6, C7, C8, and TI segmental nerves.
- These elements begin as roots until they penetrate dura and then become spinal nerves as they lie in their intervertebral foramina.
- Fixation of the spinal nerves in their bony canals and their relative intraforaminal length and obliquity become important as the mechanisms involved in stretch and avulsive injuries are studied and operations are designed to attempt correction of proximal injury.
- The clinical deficits with truncal, cord, and cord-to-nerve-level injuries are relatively constant.
- An exception is the wrist and finger function remaining after combined middle and lower truncal damage. In addition, lower trunk loss sometimes involves more than hand intrinsic muscle and ulnar-distribution sensory loss.
- The pattern of loss for a single spinal nerve can also vary, especially for C6, C7, and C8. Loss from C7 injury can be surprisingly little, often only triceps weakness, as other spinal nerves carry input to muscles supplied by this element.
- Divisional-level injury can also give variable patterns of loss, depending on which truncal outflows are involved and the proportion of anterior and posterior division loss.
- The differentiation of trapezius, serratus anterior, and rhomboid loss by a thorough clinical examination of the upper back and shoulders is very important, as is testing for supraspinatus, infraspinatus, and latissimus dorsi loss.
- The clinician's understanding of plexus anatomy, its variations and response to injury, is tested by the necessity of ordering the appropriate diagnostic tests and placing them in context with the clinical examination.
- Electromyographic sampling of proximal muscles such as paraspinals, rhomboids, serratus anterior, and spinati is of help, as are carefully done sensory conduction studies if preganglionic injury is suspected.
- Denervational changes may persist for months after clinical contraction of a muscle is evident in recovery.
- In contrast, a muscle such as the deltoid or biceps may show some nascent or early reinnervational activity in the early months after injury and yet never gain enough new input to restore useful contraction.

- Plain film radiographic studies may show humeral, clavicular, scapular, rib, or spine fractures, providing some indication of the severity and level of the injury.
- Of even greater potential importance is the use of myelography for evaluation of plexus stretch injuries (including anterior–posterior, lateral, and oblique views), in spite of possible false-positive or false-negative studies.
- Thin section computerized tomography (CT) scans post-myelography and magnetic resonance imaging (MRI) studies are playing a more important role as these may display root and spinal nerve abnormalities with increasing accuracy.

SURGICAL ANATOMY

The brachial plexus originates at the level of the spine and usually includes the C5, C6, C7, C8, and T1 spinal nerves, the three trunks of the plexus, and their anterior and posterior divisions. Spinal nerves and trunks are supraclavicular, whereas divisions tend to lie beneath the clavicle. Lateral, posterior, and medial cords are infra-clavicular, as are their origins for the major nerves of the upper extremity (Fig. 12-1).

SPINAL NERVES

Several texts have thoroughly summarized the anatomy of the roots or spinal nerves as well as their variations.[7,27,31,32,38,48,59] A thorough exposition of anatomy, physiology, and the literature available on some of the nonsurgical conditions responsible for brachial plexo-pathy, such as neuralgic amyotrophy, athletic "burners or stingers" affecting the plexus, and rucksack paralysis was provided by Wilbourn.[58] We have selected the most useful surgical information from such sources as well as from our own experience.

Each individual spinal nerve or root of the plexus originates as multiple sensory rootlets from the dorsal root entry zone of the posterolateral sector of the spinal cord and usually as one ventral or motor rootlet from the ventrolateral portion of the cord. The dorsal rootlets combine, usually at the entrance of the interverte-bral foramen, to form one dorsal root per spinal segment, and the anterior or motor root enters the foramen. The foraminal course of the roots varies between 10 and 16 mm (Fig. 12-2). The dorsal

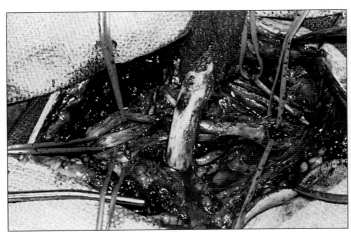

FIGURE 12-1   View of left plexus from the side of the neck and shoulder. Supraclavicular plexus is to the right of the clavicle and infraclavicular plexus is to the left. Right lower two loops are on C5 and C6 spinal nerves, and upper right loop is on the phrenic nerve. Left loops are on, from top to bottom, lateral, medial, and posterior cords. Sponges are around the clavicle so it can be moved up or down during the dissection.

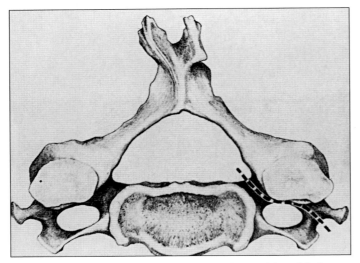

FIGURE 12-2   Intraforaminal course of spinal nerve (*dotted line*). Nerve lies posterior to foramen transversarium, which contains vertebral artery. Note that intraforaminal course of the spinal nerve is considerable. (Adapted from Sunderland S: Nerve and Nerve Injuries, 2nd edn. Edinburgh, E. Livingstone, 1984.)

root ganglion is located at an intraforaminal level and usually at its midpoint. Shortly distal to this, the anterior and posterior roots blend together to form the spinal nerve. Then, posterior primary branches (rami) go to the paraspinal muscles and a larger anterior ramus contributes to the brachial plexus.

Spinal nerve is not usually tethered within the intraforaminal canal but is bound by attachments to the cervical transverse processes.[53] Exceptions to this are the lower (C8 and T1) elements, where such attachments make the spinal nerve more likely to avulse from the spinal cord than at the higher levels. Dura changes to epineurium and is continuous with it within the foramen, and the arachnoid usually ends close to or on the posterior root ganglia.

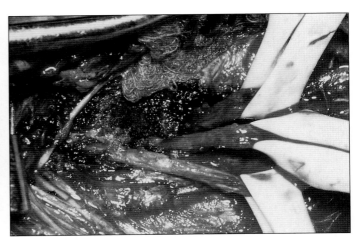

FIGURE 12-3   Dissection of spinal nerves (Penrose drains are shown around three of these) into foramina, which are to the left. The bipolar coagulator and Oxycel or Fibrillar cotton is used to control bleeding as foraminal dissection proceeds. The descending cervical plexus is seen at lower left-hand corner.

Vertebral artery originates from subclavian artery and travels superiorly to enter the foramen transversarium of C6 and to run through those of C5, C4, C3, and C2. The artery lies anterior to the spinal nerves at these levels. Small branches from this vessel supply the spinal nerves and anastomose with spinal cord vasculature. Vertebral branches also anastomose with branches from ascending cervical, deep cervical, and superior intercostal arteries.[3,28]

Within the foramen, the C5 spinal nerve gives rise to a dorsal scapular nerve branch, which supplies the rhomboids. In addition, a branch that contributes to the long thoracic nerve exits the foramen posterior to the spinal nerve. The caliber of C5 is usually smaller than that of the other spinal nerves. Exposure requires soft tissue dissection high in the neck. Descending cervical plexus must be mobilized and moved away, as must phrenic nerve. Small arteries and veins cross the root or travel with it as it exits the foramen and they must be coagulated. Dissection into the foramen requires resection of origins of the anterior scalene and resection of some of the transverse process of the fifth cervical vertebra (Fig. 12-3). The extraforaminal course of C5 is along the lateral edge of the anterior scalene, and sometimes the nerve may be partially embedded in it. C4 may make a small contribution to the plexus. Rarely, this may be substantial and thus represents a prefixed plexus (Fig. 12-4).

C6 has a slightly longer intraforaminal course than C5 but a shorter extraforaminal course before blending with C5 to form the upper trunk (Fig. 12-4).[38] The extraforaminal course of C6 is somewhat oblique and posterior to the anterior scalene. It joins C5 at the lateral edge of the anterior scalene to form the upper trunk of the plexus. Most frequently, long thoracic nerve arises from the dorsal surface of the distal portion of C6, just before it melds into the upper trunk. While C6 is the major contributor to long thoracic nerve, branches to this nerve also arise from C5 and C7, and less frequently from C8 as well as C4. The long thoracic nerve is usually posterior to the junction of C6 to upper trunk and dives inferiorly to penetrate and course through the middle scalene.

The intraforaminal portion of the C7 spinal nerve is 12–15 mm in length. Extraforaminal C7 spinal nerve has the straightest course of any of the spinal nerves of the plexus, and it blends imperceptibly into the middle trunk with little to differentiate the two

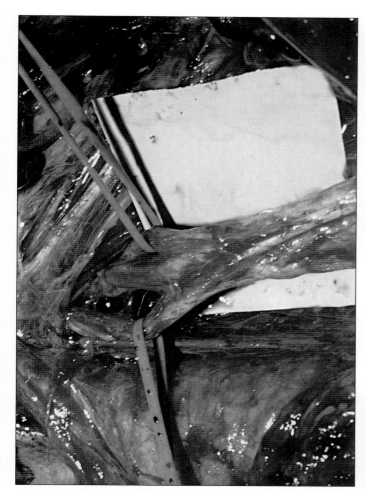

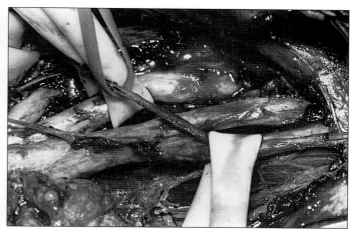

FIGURE 12-5 Exposure of proximal left supraclavicular plexus viewed from the side. Anterior scalene has been resected. Lower Penrose drain is around the C5 spinal nerve and the proximal portion of the phrenic nerve. C6 is superior to this, and its junction with C5 to form the upper trunk is readily seen. The phrenic nerve is also encircled by a plastic loop at the top left. The upper Penrose drain is around the junction of C7 to middle trunk. Nerve to subclavius muscle can be seen arising from the superior surface of the upper trunk (*left*) and taking its usual oblique course to the subclavius muscle.

FIGURE 12-4 C5 and C6 spinal nerves characteristically combine to form the upper trunk. This is a useful landmark in supraclavicular and proximal plexus surgery. This patient had an additional major contribution to upper trunk from C4 (encircled by lower plastic loop), forming a prefixed brachial plexus.

(Fig. 12-5). C7 lies posterior to the medial edge of the anterior scalene and may be adherent to it.

C8 has an intraforaminal course of 10–15 mm; after exiting its foramen, C8 combines with T1 to form the lower trunk. The course of C8 is slightly oblique, and this spinal nerve is usually larger in caliber than either T1 or C7. Its extraforaminal extent is relatively short, for it blends with T1 to form the lower trunk. It lies anterior to the middle and posterior scalene muscles, and in some cases is covered by Sibson's fascia, which extends from the transverse processes of the seventh cervical and sometimes the sixth cervical vertebra to the apical pleura. C8 root is closely covered by or accompanied by arterioles and venules or small veins, and the vertebral artery is anterior to it.

After a relatively short intraforaminal course, T1 exits its foramen and takes a transverse and somewhat curvilinear course laterally to meet C8. Both of these spinal nerves form the lower trunk (Fig. 12-6). It is at this level that rami communicantes are most likely seen coming and going from spinal nerve. These rami and their ganglia form the cervical sympathetic chain, whose largest ganglion is usually found posterior to the vertebral artery close to the latter's division from the subclavian artery. Occasionally, T2 or a contribution from it may combine with T1 or its junction with the lower trunk to help form the latter.

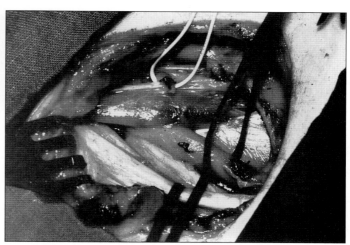

FIGURE 12-6 The right phrenic nerve is easily seen anterior to the scalenus anticus (white plastic loop). Dark loop (*top right*) is around subclavian artery, whereas to bottom right, loop is around lower trunk. The right subclavian artery and plexus, however, are inclined at a much steeper angle than normal, associated with a large cervical rib that displaced these structures laterally.

TRUNKS

The upper and middle trunks are the most readily identified portions of the supraclavicular plexus.

The upper trunk is usually adherent to and sometimes partially covered by the anterior scalene muscle. With injury, sharp dissection is necessary along the medial edge of the trunk to dissect it away from the anterior scalene (Fig. 12-7). Lateral dissection of the trunk, away from medial scalene, is usually easier. As one proceeds distally along the lateral edge of the trunk, suprascapular nerve is encountered arising from the dorsolateral surface of the distal upper trunk, just as it forms anterior and posterior divisions

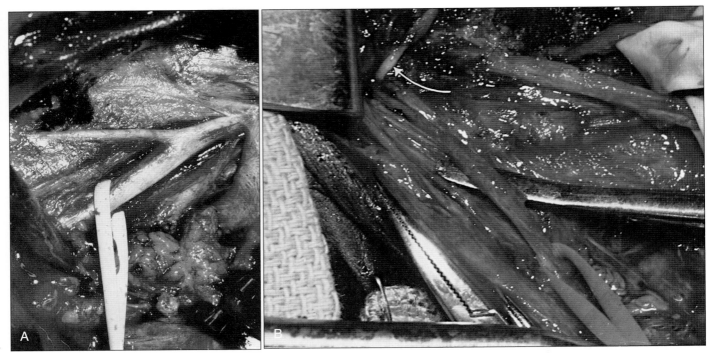

FIGURE 12-7 **(A)** Tracing this left phrenic nerve superiorly, as it lies posterior to the prevertebral fascia on the front of scalenus anticus leads the surgeon to the C5 spinal nerve and upper trunk (surrounded by white plastic loop). This may be a useful maneuver in a heavily scarred plexus, because the locus of the C5 spinal nerve then defines the plane between scalenus anticus and medius. Dissecting deeper in that plane defines the remaining spinal nerves of origin of the brachial plexus. The surgeon often has to dissect the C5 spinal nerve proximal to its contribution to the phrenic, and this is accomplished by dividing the muscle fibers of the scalenus anticus to reveal the anterior tubercles of the transverse processes of the C4 and C5 vertebrae. **(B)** Cervical plexus (beneath metal instrument) is seen coursing inferiorly in an oblique fashion from the region of the right C5 nerve root, whereas phrenic nerve (*curved arrow*) courses obliquely in a superior direction. If the surgeon tracks the phrenic nerve proximally, the origin from C3 and C4 spinal nerves can be found.

more anteriorly. This trident-like structure, with suprascapular nerve, and posterior and anterior divisions (from lateral to medial), is an excellent landmark for the termination of the upper trunk. In some cases, an anteriorly located branch to subclavius arises from the middle part of the upper trunk to run medially and somewhat obliquely to the subclavius muscle. This nerve is not infrequently mistaken for the phrenic nerve by the novice operator.

Truncal divisions vary somewhat in their relation to the clavicle, depending on the positioning of the shoulder, neck, and head on the operating table. Some exposure of these structures is helped by placing folded sheets beneath the shoulder. The head is turned somewhat toward the opposite side and elevated slightly above the chest level.[29] The dorsal scapular artery and vein, originating from or draining to subclavian vessels, cross the lower and middle trunks and branch amongst the upper trunk divisions, and may be adherent to one or more of these elements (Fig. 12-8). These constantly encountered vessels need to be either ligated or coagulated and divided for a complete dissection at these levels.

The middle trunk is found beneath the anterior scalene and is often covered by some muscular connections between the anterior and medial scalene or with scar tissue resulting from injury (Fig. 12-9). The middle trunk is usually smaller in caliber than either the upper or lower trunk. The distal middle trunk may on occasion blend into or be quite adherent to either the distal upper or the lower trunk, or occasionally to both. The posterior division of the middle trunk is usually relatively short and combines with posterior divisions from upper and lower trunks to form posterior cord distal to the clavicle. The middle trunk anterior division combines with

that from the upper trunk to form lateral cord, which, as a cord element, is usually formed proximal to the posterior cord but not as proximally as the medial cord.

The lower trunk is usually relatively short and lies somewhat behind the subclavian artery (Fig. 12-10). Exposure is helped by skeletonizing enough of the inferior surface of the subclavian artery so that it can be gently elevated by a vein retractor. Metzenbaum scissors are then used to clear the medial edge of the lower trunk and proximal medial cord away from the vessel. This trunk is usually crossed by the same sizable artery and vein (dorsal scapular) that involve the more laterally positioned middle and upper trunk divisions. Medially, vertebral artery ascends anterior to the level of the trunk and usually anterior to the T1 spinal nerve. The posterior division of the lower trunk blends with those divisions from the other trunks to help form the posterior cord.[59] The bulk of the lower trunk proceeds directly through its anterior division to form the medial cord.

DIVISIONS

Although each trunk has an anterior and a posterior division as outlined above, they can blend with other divisions before forming cords (Fig. 12-11). Sometimes one or more divisions trade bundles of nerve fibers back and forth several times.[55] In addition, the site at which cords begin distal to the clavicle can vary from patient to patient.

Separating divisions in cases in which there has been a stretch injury, gunshot wound, or prior vascular dissection can be quite

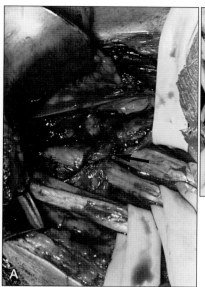

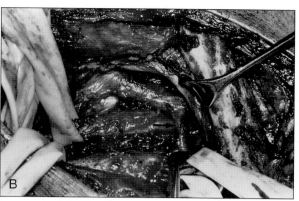

FIGURE 12-8 **(A)** Deep supraclavicular arterial and venous complex (*arrow*) originating from or terminating in subclavian vessels. These vessels cross lower and middle trunk (*below arrow*) to course posterior to divisions of upper trunk (*bottom*). Such vessels can bleed vigorously unless they are coagulated or ligated. **(B)** Subclavicular view of deep arterial origin of supraclavicular vessel (*arrow*) from subclavian artery. Clavicle is retracted superiorly by vein retractor. **(C)** The right clavicle has been displaced inferiorly to show a ligature around the external jugular junction with the subclavian vein. A Moynihan is beneath the suprascapular vessels, which usually run parallel to but beneath the clavicle. An arterial branch (dorsal scapular) from the subclavian lies superior to the lower and middle trunks at a divisional level and in this drawing goes between the divisions of the upper trunk.

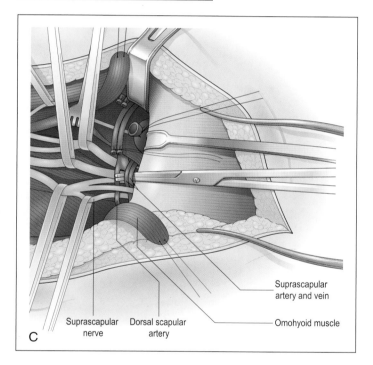

Suprascapular artery and vein

Suprascapular nerve

Dorsal scapular artery

Omohyoid muscle

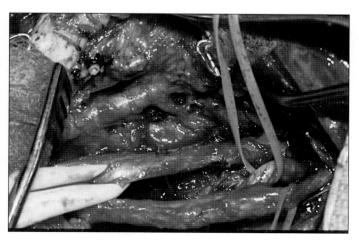

FIGURE 12-9 This dissection shows C7 to middle trunk exposed after resection of the anterior scalene muscle. Penrose drain is around the posterior division of this trunk just before it blends in with that of the upper trunk. Subclavian artery and origin of vertebral artery are seen in the top. C5 and C6 (plastic loops) and upper trunk are seen at bottom.

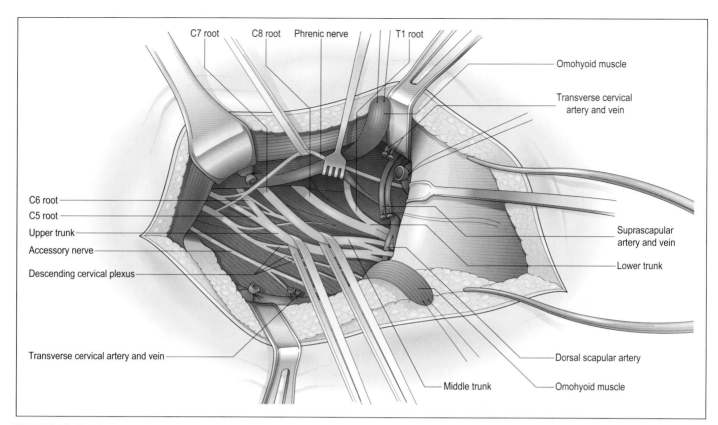

FIGURE 12-10 Further exposure of the supraclavicular plexus reveals spinal nerves, trunks, and divisions of the plexus. The take-off of the phrenic nerve from descending cervical plexus and C4 is seen, as is a contribution from C5. Deep to C6 and between that and C7 runs the long thoracic nerve, with contributions in this case from C4, C5, and C6, before the nerve penetrates the scalenus medius.

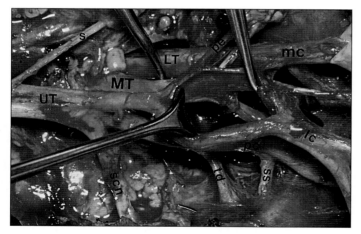

FIGURE 12-11 In this case, clavicle has been sectioned to expose divisions of trunks (lc, lateral cord; LT, lower trunk; mc, medial cord; MT, middle trunk; pc, posterior cord; pe, pectoral branches; s, nerve to subclavius; scn, suprascapular nerve; ss, subscapular (upper) nerve; td, thoracodorsal; UT, upper trunk).

difficult. The surgeon must work from trunks in a distal direction and cords in a proximal one to expose the divisions. By passing two moist and strung out 2 × 4 sponges beneath the clavicle with the help of a Moynihan or curved hemostat, the clavicle can be pulled alternatively up or down to aid dissection. With this maneuver, division of the clavicle is rarely needed, in our experience. Before passing sponges deep to clavicle, the subclavius muscle is sectioned or, more commonly, has a segment resected. If retroclavicular

vessels (suprascapular artery and vein) have not been ligated during the supraclavicular dissection, they are now isolated and ligated to prevent severe bleeding that may occur by blind passage of instrument or sponges deep to clavicle.

CORDS

These are named in relation to the axillary artery at the level of pectoralis minor (Fig. 12-12). Lateral cord is usually superficial to the artery and is the first major neural element encountered after section of the pectoralis minor muscle as one begins dissection in the infraclavicular region. It tends to run somewhat obliquely over the artery from a medial to a lateral direction but sometimes is entirely lateral to the artery. It terminates in a contribution to the median nerve and an oblique take-off running laterally to form the musculocutaneous nerve. The latter dives quickly into biceps/brachialis but usually gives off one or more coracobrachialis branches first. Variations are frequently found in the formation of musculocutaneous nerve and lateral cord branches to median and also in their relationship to medial cord branches to median.[31,32,56]

The posterior cord is deep or posterior to axillary artery (Fig. 12-13), and is best approached lateral to the axillary artery. Mobilization of the latter structures medially greatly facilitates dissection of the posterior cord and its branches. Several subscapular branches (upper and lower) usually arise from the posterior cord and run inferiorly and obliquely. A relatively sizable branch, the thoracodorsal, runs from its posterior aspect almost directly posteriorly to supply the latissimus dorsi. The thoracodorsal frequently will arise from the proximal axillary nerve or at least the portion

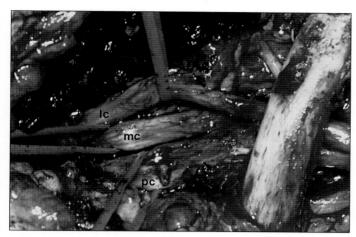

FIGURE 12-12 The three cords of the plexus. Lateral cord (lc) has been retracted superiorly, medial cord (mc) somewhat laterally to bring it superficial to the axillary artery, and posterior cord (pc) inferiorly and laterally. Clavicle is to the right.

of posterior cord destined to be the axillary nerve. The cord then divides into its two major branches, the axillary and the radial nerves. After coursing inferiorly and slightly laterally, the axillary nerve dives down to reach the quadrilateral space and eventually the deltoid muscle.

The major posterior cord outflow is the radial nerve, which runs inferiorly towards the humeral groove to wind around the humerus. It passes over and sometimes through the leaves of the subscapularis muscle.[47] A very important anatomic landmark is the medial relation between the radial nerve and the profundus branch of the axillary artery. This can be used to locate the proximal radial and differentiate it from the more lateral axillary nerve.[35] It is especially important to maintain the profundus branch with either more proximal axillary or more distal brachial arterial occlusion.

Dissection in this area is difficult and requires patience. Care must be taken not to place severe retraction against biceps/brachialis because musculocutaneous nerve runs a parallel but hidden course beneath the biceps muscle. If self-retaining retractors are to be used in this area, it is best to clear musculocutaneous nerve through upper biceps. Nerve can then be retracted anteriorly and laterally so that self-retaining retractors can be safely placed. Sometimes sacrifice of a small and insignificant coracobrachialis contributor from the musculocutaneous nerve greatly facilitates its mobilization. Dissection also needs to extend around axillary and upper brachial artery and around the profundus branch. This permits their retraction so that the relation between the cords and nerves in this area can be adequately worked out. Lateral to axillary vein and somewhat inferior to it is the medial cord, and, with injury, this nerve element can be quite adherent to vein. This requires careful dissection because holes in the vein are usually harder to repair than those in artery.

The surgeon also needs to exercise care when dissecting medial to the axillary artery as the medial and lateral pectoral nerves, arising from the medial and lateral cords, respectively, are quite small and their origin may be obscured by scar tissue. As these nerves run towards the pectoralis minor and major muscles, they exhibit considerable branching. Not infrequently, a plexus will form where branches from the medial and lateral pectoral nerves, destined for the pectoralis major, will merge together and then final branches will run towards the muscle.[4,8] Appreciation of the

detailed pectoral nerve anatomy is crucial for their safe dissection and in operations where medial pectoral nerve branches are transferred to the musculocutaneous nerve.[5]

Medial cord sends a major contribution to median nerve which wraps around the medial and superior side of the axillary artery. On occasion, this contribution to median passes beneath the artery.[44] As this contribution is given off, so are the ulnar nerve and the medial brachial and antebrachial branches. These neural structures remain medial to brachial artery as they begin their descent down the arm. Stretch injury can change the positions of trunks, cords, and nerves and their proximal to distal positions in relation to the usual anatomic landmarks of the arm.

CLINICAL EXAMINATION

A comprehensive clinical evaluation begins with an assessment of the shoulders, neck, and high back from behind with the patient erect. One can readily spot asymmetry of the shoulder girdles, dropped shoulder, or laterally rotated scapula.[1,25,49] In addition, the parascapular area is inspected for rhomboid atrophy, winging of the scapula, or atrophy of supraspinatus, infraspinatus, or deltoid. The muscular atrophy can be a true neurogenic type, from muscle denervation, or at times from disuse. The mechanics of shoulder abduction and internal and external rotation of the upper arm can be viewed from behind, as can the response of latissimus dorsi to a deep cough.[51] If there is a question of diaphragmatic paralysis, the chest can be percussed from behind, matching inspiratory tympany with that on expiration. Then, standing at the patient's side, one can recheck internal and external rotation of the arm as well as adduction of the arm by the pectoralis and other muscles. Biceps/brachialis and brachioradialis can then be tested as elbow flexors and triceps as an elbow extensor. With the elbow fully extended, pronation and supination are tested, and then wrist extension and flexion.

Hand muscle function is best tested with both the subject and the examiner seated and facing one another. The patient's hands can be placed palm up on the knees for finger flexion testing and palm down on the knees or on a flat surface to test for extension. Each hand can then be held and manipulated to test for fine muscle hand intrinsic function, presence or absence of sweating, and sensory testing.

After inspecting and testing these muscles, the examiner's attention is directed to the front of the patient's body. The neck is also inspected and palpated. Associated findings such as Horner syndrome (including ptosis, enophthalmos, miosis) or, less frequently, facial palsy should be looked for.[62] Scars in supraclavicular, infraclavicular, and axillary spaces should be inspected and palpated. Deep tendon reflexes are ascertained and compared to the contralateral extremity.

DORSAL SCAPULAR NERVE PALSY

The function of the dorsal scapular nerve is to innervate the rhomboid muscles, which pull the medial edge of the scapula upward and toward the midline (Fig. 12-14). Injury to this nerve results in atrophy and weakness of the rhomboideus major and minor and can be observed as absence of bulk medial to the scapula and between that structure and the thoracic spinal column. It is most noticeable when the subject braces his or her shoulders as if at military attention. Another method of testing rhomboids is to have the patient place hands on hips and push back against pressure on

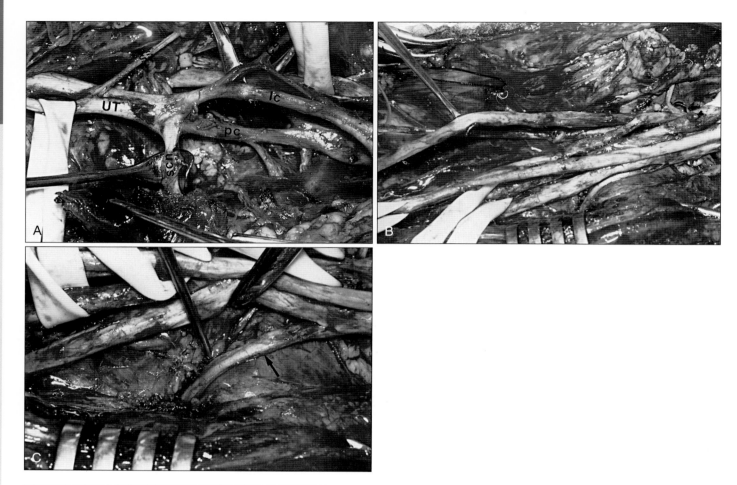

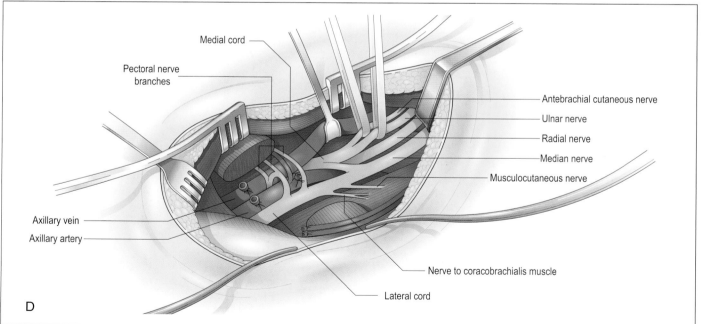

FIGURE 12-13 **(A)** Right supra- and infraclavicular plexus viewed from the side. Upper Penrose drain is around medial cord. Note rather lengthy lateral cord contribution to median. In this case, musculocutaneous nerve had a distal origin from the median complex (lc, lateral cord; pc, posterior cord; pe, medial pectoral branches; scn, suprascapular nerve; ss, subclavius branch; UT, upper trunk). **(B)** Infraclavicular plexus at a subclavicular level. Penrose to the far left is around distal median nerve. Penrose to the left of center is around axillary artery. Beneath or inferior to this Penrose is the radial nerve. Vein retractor is elevating ulnar nerve. **(C)** Closer view of course of axillary nerve (*arrow*) into proximal quadrilateral space. Radial nerve is held slightly superiorly by the tips of the Metzenbaum scissors. **(D)** The infraclavicular plexus and vessels are further exposed with the aid of Weitlaner retractors placed and opened in the pectoralis muscles. A vein retractor is displacing the inferior portion of the axillary vein. This aids dissection of the distal medial cord branches, such as its contribution to the median nerve and the antebrachial cutaneous and ulnar nerve.

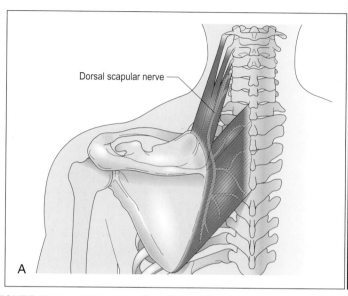

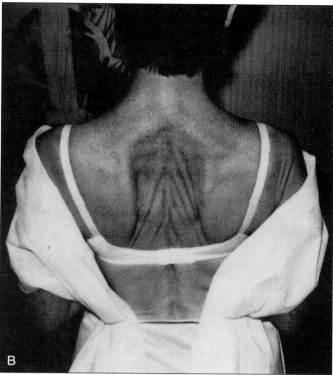

FIGURE 12-14 **(A)** Drawing of position of rhomboid muscles and usual course of dorsal scapular nerve, which arises from proximal C5 and C6 spinal nerves. Proximal course of dorsal scapular nerve is parallel to that of levator scapulae, which runs from cervical spine to superior and medial scapula. **(B)** Patient with bilateral rhomboid paralysis. (**B**, courtesy of Dr. Michael Lusk, Naples, FL.)

one or both elbows. Loss produces some winging, lateral and slight downward displacement of the scapula, and a slightly awkward abduction of the shoulder. This abduction difficulty is, however, not as profound as that seen with serratus anterior or trapezius paralysis. Because the nerve arises from the proximal intraforaminal portion of C5 and sometimes C6, loss of function from injury implies damage to the spinal nerve or root close to the spinal cord (Fig. 12-15).

LONG THORACIC NERVE PALSY

The long thoracic nerve arises from the proximal portions of the C5–7 spinal nerves and innervates serratus anterior, which pulls scapula away from the midline and forward on the posterior chest area (Fig. 12-16). Paralysis of serratus anterior gives severe winging of the scapula, both at rest and with the shoulder flexed and the elbow fully extended.[25] This differentiates it from the winging associated with spinal trapezius paralysis, in which winging is minimal when the elbow is fully extended and hand and arm push forward against resistance. With serratus anterior palsy, abduction of the shoulder is not smooth, particularly above the horizontal. If damaged in association with root or spinal nerve injury, long thoracic nerve palsy implies a very proximal loss (Fig. 12-17).[41] This is particularly so for lesions involving C5, C6, and even C7, as well as C4 if it provides input to the long thoracic nerve.

PALSY OF ACCESSORY (ELEVENTH CRANIAL) NERVE

Trapezius forms the major posterior bulk of the shoulder region, and its spinal or lower portion provides the most important dorsal

and medial support for the scapula. Muscle fibers used for shrugging the shoulder or pulling up the scapula can be roughly divided into medial, intermediate, and lateral divisions. Some accessory nerve lesions distal to the sternocleidomastoid branch may spare medial nerve or fibers, at times even some intermediate fibers, but always paralyze the lateral ones. As a result, the shoulder tends to drop or be carried lower than the contralateral normal shoulder. At times, the patient overcompensates and carries the injured shoulder higher than the normal one. Distance between the tip of the shoulder and the midline of the body usually appears shorter on the paralyzed side. With spinal segment loss of accessory nerve, the scapula wings and usually moves laterally with attempted abduction. The latter motion is unwieldy for the patient. Without the help of the spinal segment of trapezius, abduction of the arm above the horizontal is difficult and can be very painful.

Unlike the winging seen with serratus palsy, that seen with loss of the spinal segment of trapezius is brought out best by having the patient push forward or across the chest with the elbow bent or partially flexed, as opposed to pushing forward with the elbow fully extended.[49] The mechanics of shoulder abduction are severely affected by accessory paralysis. Some patients learn to substitute by rolling the forearm into a pronated position as abduction reaches the horizontal level.

Levator scapulae runs between the transverse processes of the cervical vertebrae superiorly and the superior and medial angle of the scapula inferiorly (see Fig. 12-15). This muscle receives neural input from C3, C4, and C5 and is usually spared with most plexus injuries and, of course, with accessory palsy. Thus, some ability to elevate (shrug) the shoulder is usually present even with severe plexus or accessory palsy.

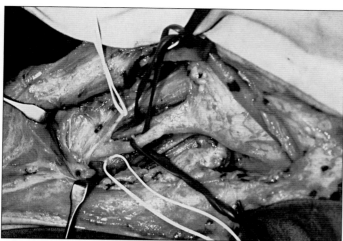

FIGURE 12-15 The right phrenic nerve has been dissected and mobilized (upper white plastic loop). This leads the surgeon to C5 and thence to C6 (dark plastic loops). This latter spinal nerve is attenuated as it flows over the edge of the transverse process. A proximal branch of C5 is the nerve to rhomboid (lower white plastic loop). Clinically, the patient had normal rhomboid function but complete loss of deltoid, biceps, and spinati function. Intraoperative stimulation of the phrenic nerve resulted in diaphragmatic contraction. As expected, stimulation of proximal C5 caused rhomboid and levator scapulae contraction, thus proving the integrity of the more proximal C5 spinal nerve. Somatosensory evoked potentials could not be recorded by stimulating C6. Nerve action potentials could not be evoked by stimulating proximal upper trunk and recording from lateral and posterior cords. The massive neuroma (*on right*) of the distal upper trunk was therefore resected, and grafts were led from C5 to musculocutaneous and axillary nerves. A distal branch of accessory nerve was attached to the suprascapular nerve by a short graft. Two years later, the patient had 50% recovery of shoulder abduction and elbow flexion.

It is rare to see paralysis of the sternocleidomastoid muscle as part of an accessory palsy. This is because branches to this large neck muscle come off proximally from the accessory nerve and run beneath that muscle to innervate it. These branches are deep and medial and are protected from most penetrating iatrogenic or spontaneous injuries. In addition, sternocleidomastoid muscle is also supplied by branches from C2, C3, and C4 spinal nerves. Further information about this important nerve is provided in the chapter devoted to it (Chapter 19).

SUPRASCAPULAR NERVE PALSY

The suprascapular nerve supplies both supraspinatus and infraspinatus and originates from the upper trunk of the plexus (Fig. 12-18). The supraspinatus is readily observable along the superior border of the spine of the scapula. This muscle provides the first 20–30 degrees of abduction of the shoulder, working in concert with deltoid and other parascapular muscles to provide shoulder abduction. If the deltoid is paralyzed, supraspinatus can be tested with gravity eliminated by placing the patient supine and asking the patient to attempt to abduct the outstretched arm away from the side. The infraspinatus is a large muscle located below the spine of the scapula. It is the principal external rotator of the shoulder and thus the upper arm. External rotation is tested by flexing the patient's forearm at the elbow and holding the tip of the elbow against the patient's side, and asking him or her to externally rotate the forearm and thus the humerus and shoulder joint laterally ("tennis backhand" motion).

AXILLARY NERVE PALSY

The axillary nerve arises from the posterior cord as it gives rise to the radial nerve (Fig. 12-19; also see Fig. 12-13). The major input of this nerve is to the deltoid. Atrophy of this large shoulder muscle is readily apparent on inspection, as is the dropped position of the head of the humerus. Loss affects abduction of the arm, especially beyond 30 degrees from the horizontal. Motor loss may or may not be accompanied by sensory change over the cap of the shoulder. Sensory change is usually present in the relatively acute injury. Within a few weeks to months, descending cervical plexus fibers sprout or branch to supply sensation in this area, so that over time, loss, if present, is relative rather than absolute. With incomplete axillary nerve involvement or partial regeneration of the nerve to muscle, some deltoid contraction may be evident by inspection or palpation. Even a little function requires a substantial degree of reinnervation, however, before the deltoid can overcome gravity, let alone pressure applied to the upper arm as abduction beyond 30 degrees is attempted.[42] Sometimes, the muscle mass of anterior deltoid contracts and yet the intermediate or posterior muscle mass is poor. Some patients can substitute for lack of this muscle by initiating abduction by a well-developed supraspinatus and then using shoulder rotators as well as the long head of the biceps to gain a good deal of forward abduction of the arm.[55] Under these circumstances, the contracting biceps tendon is discernable, and palpation of the deltoid itself shows it to be flaccid or to have minimal contraction.

With partial recovery, it is important to test the three major segments of the muscle: anterior, middle, and posterior. For example, it is difficult to gain coordinated recovery of the posterior deltoid muscle mass, and this must be tested by having the patient abduct the arm somewhat behind the plane of the body. Muscle must be not only inspected but palpated as the patient attempts to contract it, and this is best done with the patient standing or sitting erect in a chair.

THORACODORSAL NERVE PALSY

The latissimus dorsi is one of the major adductors of the shoulder. The latissimus also extends the shoulder and medially rotates the arm. This large muscle innervated by the thoracodorsal nerve can also be palpated from behind (Fig. 12-20). A deep cough should make it contract, and it is useful to place both hands on these muscles bilaterally and compare contraction. Another method of testing this muscle is to place the patient's extended and abducted arm on the examiner's shoulder and asks the patient to push down on it. Muscle can be seen contracting in the posterior axillary fold, particularly the lower portion of the fold. Teres major resides in the high axillary fold and also serves as an adductor; it is innervated by proximal subscapular branches of the posterior cord. In addition to the latissimus dorsi and teres major, pectoralis is also a powerful adductor of the arm.

PALSY INVOLVING PECTORALIS MAJOR MUSCLE

The anatomy of the pectoral nerves have already been discussed and are further illustrated in Figure 12-21. This major large muscle has several segments or heads. The bulk of the muscle adducts the arm to the side of the chest and can be observed and palpated as the elbow is brought down forcibly or against pressure to the side.

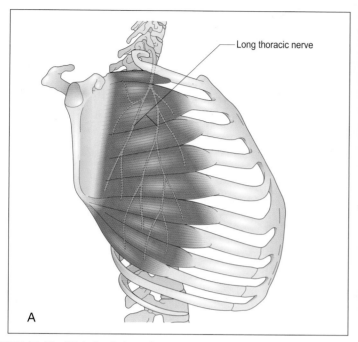

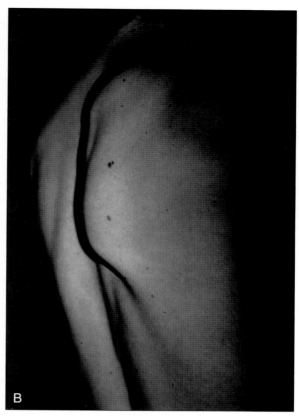

FIGURE 12-16 **(A)** Lateral view of course of long thoracic nerve beneath clavicle (not shown in this drawing) and then over the lateral rib cage, where it branches at many levels to supply the serratus anterior. **(B)** Patient with long thoracic palsy and protrusion or winging of the right scapula.

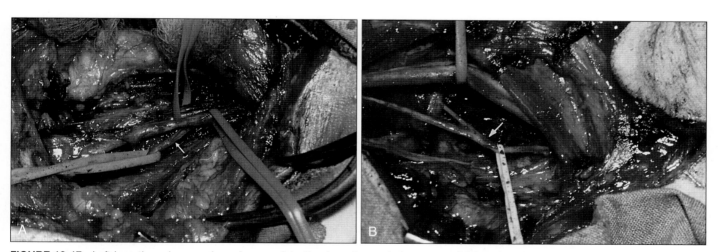

FIGURE 12-17 Left long thoracic nerve (*arrow*) seen originating from the posterior aspect of C6 and running obliquely and posteriorly beneath upper trunk. Nerve then courses through the middle scalene muscle. **(B)** Bifid origin of a right long thoracic nerve (*arrow and white plastic loop*). Upper trunk is retracted superiorly by the dark plastic loop.

The clavicular head is best tested by having the patient push down from a horizontal and anterior position of the arm with the elbow flexed.

C5 SPINAL NERVE OR ROOT

Very proximal involvement of this element paralyzes rhomboids and weakens serratus anterior, so these functions should be tested as previously outlined. The C5 spinal nerve supplies most of the suprascapular nerve's input to supraspinatus and infraspinatus. The latter muscle may also receive a little input from C6, so it may not be totally paralyzed with a C5 root lesion. Certainly, the deltoid muscle is paralyzed, because it almost always receives exclusive input from this spinal nerve. Sensory loss may be present over the cap or tip of the shoulder. Again, input or sprouting from the cervical plexus usually lessens this sensory deficit. Biceps/brachialis may also be weak, although this is a partial loss because C6 supplies this function as well.

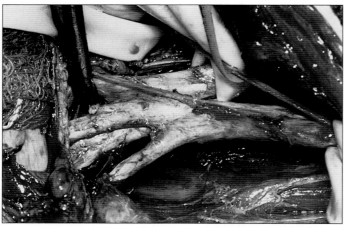

FIGURE 12-18 More distal left supraclavicular plexus showing origin of supraclavicular nerve and the posterior and anterior divisions (lateral to medial, respectively) of the upper trunk just to the right of the clavicle. Dissector is beneath the more distal middle trunk. Small-caliber nerve at top is the phrenic, whereas inferior to this, arising from upper trunk, just before divisions, is nerve to subclavius muscle.

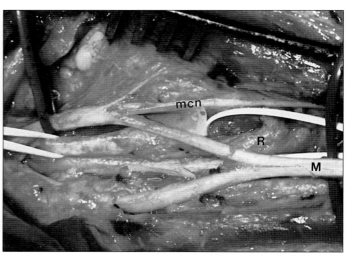

FIGURE 12-19 The medial (motor) and lateral (sensory) heads of the left median nerve (M) embrace the axillary artery. Tracing the lateral head proximally brings the operator to the origin of the musculocutaneous nerve (mcn) and a small twig destined for coracobrachialis. This patient suffered a posterior cord injury with loss of axillary and radial function. Plastic loops are passed above and below the neuroma in continuity involving posterior cord. Proximal portion of radial nerve (R) is still covered by scar.

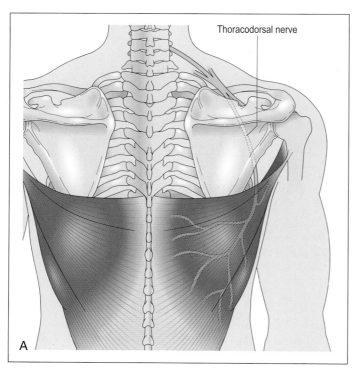

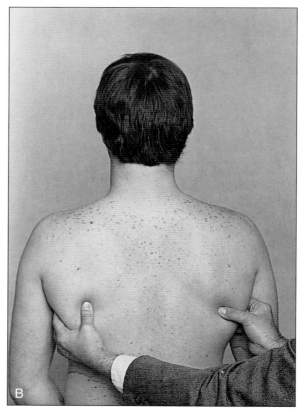

FIGURE 12-20 **(A)** Course of the thoracodorsal nerve which originates from posterior cord of plexus and then travels inferiorly to innervate latissimus dorsi. **(B)** Testing patient for latissimus dorsi palsy. Because this is a branch of the posterior cord, a patient with wrist drop but intact latissimus has a lesion in radial nerve rather than posterior cord.

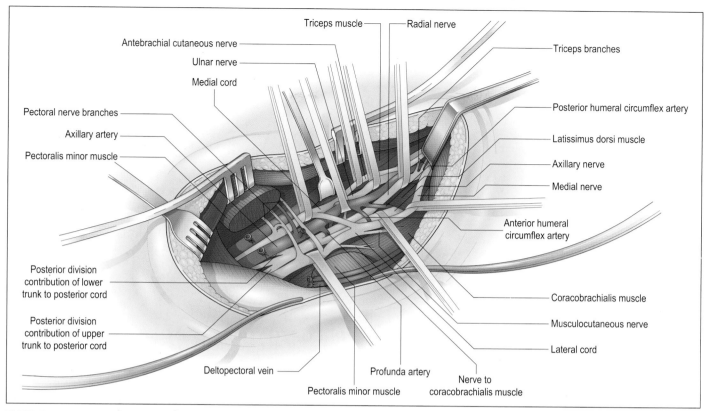

FIGURE 12-21 The entire right infraclavicular plexus is exposed. Cords of the plexus are positioned around the axillary artery and its branches, making for a challenging dissection. Note the position of the profundus arterial branch between the radial and axillary nerves. Note particularly the medial pectoral branches arising from the medial cord and their interplay with lateral pectoral branches before common branches run into the pectoralis muscles.

C6 SPINAL NERVE OR ROOT

This root provides input to biceps/brachialis, a function it shares with the C5 root. This muscle is best tested with the hand fully supinated so as to reduce elbow flexion by the brachioradialis. Biceps tendon is seen to tighten over the flexor surface of the elbow, and the contracting muscle belly is most prominent at the midhumeral level. The C6 root also supplies brachioradialis, which is a strong flexor of the elbow, especially when the hand is halfway between pronation and supination. The brachioradialis can be readily observed and palpated on the lateral aspect of the proximal forearm and elbow. C6 supplies the supinator, a muscle deeply located in the proximal third of the forearm. Because biceps can also provide supination, true supinator function should be tested by first extending or straightening out the elbow completely. The patient's hand is then placed in a pronated position and held by the examiner as the patient attempts to supinate it or turn it palm up. C6 can also supply some of the triceps, although the major input to this muscle is from C7. Outflow from C6, as from most of the roots, also contributes to the pectoralis major, which is the major adductor of the arm. Latissimus dorsi, another adductor, is also weak or totally paralyzed with a C6 lesion.

UPPER TRUNK

Because upper trunk is formed by C5 and C6, loss with a complete lesion of this element includes paralysis of supraspinatus, infraspi-natus, deltoid, latissimus dorsi, biceps/brachialis, brachioradialis, and supinator. The posture of the upper extremity and hand is that of an Erb's palsy. Partial lesions often produce loss of deltoid, whereas biceps/brachialis may be weak but not totally paralyzed. Anatomical variations at this level affecting function of muscles such as biceps or deltoid are much less common than at an infra-clavicular level.

C7 SPINAL NERVE AND MIDDLE TRUNK

The C7 root or spinal nerve forms the entire middle trunk, most of whose fibers go to the radial portion of the posterior cord through the posterior division. These fibers supply most of the triceps. This large muscle extends the forearm at the elbow joint. The examiner can gently grasp the muscle belly on the posterior upper arm and resist extension of the forearm with the opposite hand. To eliminate gravity for testing of this muscle as well as biceps, the patient can be placed supine and flexion and extension of the forearm gently resisted. Fibers from the posterior division of the middle trunk may also provide input to extensor carpi radia-lis, and sometimes to extensor carpi ulnaris as well. These muscles dorsiflex the wrist. The extensor carpi radialis does this in a radial direction and extensor carpi ulnaris in an ulnar direction. C7 may also provide some fibers to extensor communis or extensor pollicis longus, or both. Because of this, one or more digits may be weak but not paralyzed in extension, as input to these muscles from C8 is considerable.

Nerve fibers going to the anterior division of the middle trunk are carried to the lateral cord and (via the median nerve) can supply the pronator teres as well as wrist and finger flexors. The pronator teres is tested with the elbow extended, holding the hand in a supinated position and rotating it against resistance into a palm-down position. Wrist flexion and finger flexion can readily be tested and should be separated as to flexor superficialis and flexor profundus function.

Loss in this distribution varies with C7 or middle trunk injury. C7 contributes primarily to muscles supplied by one or more other roots, so isolated injury to C7 often leads only to paresis rather than paralysis and may produce no discernable loss (other than partial triceps weakness).[22]

C8 SPINAL NERVE

Finger and thumb extensors as well as flexors to wrist and fingers primarily receive input from this important root. It also supplies a variable amount of input to hand intrinsic muscles, sharing this function with the T1 root. Loss therefore usually includes weakness or paralysis of extensors to thumb, forefinger, and long finger. Flexor profundi to the latter two digits are weak or paralyzed. Intrinsics are weak or paralyzed, especially thenar intrinsics such as abductor pollicis brevis and opponens pollicis. Testing procedures for these muscles are found in the chapters entitled "Ulnar Nerve" and "Median Nerve" (Chapters 9 and 8, respectively). Sensory loss or decrease is in the ulnar distribution and may involve the ring finger and even the little finger.

T1 SPINAL NERVE

This root supplies hand intrinsics, especially those of the hypothenar eminence, including the abductor digiti minimi and opponens digiti minimi. Interossei, lumbricals, and adductor pollicis are weak or absent. Flexor profundi to the little and ring fingers may also be weak unless there is a predominant C8 input to these muscles. C8 is, however, more likely to supply flexor profundus input to the forefinger and long finger. The sensory field is again that of the little finger and sometimes the ring finger but may

include skin over the hypothenar eminence and on the ulnar side of the forearm.

LOWER TRUNK

The anterior division of the lower trunk goes to the medial cord, which provides input to all of the ulnar nerve and partial input to the median nerve, especially to the thenar intrinsics and lumbricals to the forefinger and long ringer. The most reproducible deficit with complete injury to this element is loss of all hand intrinsics, including those in the ulnar and median distribution. With time, there is obvious atrophy of interossei and muscles of hypothenar and thenar eminence. There is a variable degree of finger and wrist flexor loss, especially to flexor digitorum profundi. In addition, there may be some extensor loss because the posterior division of this trunk goes to the posterior cord, which supplies radial nerve. The portion of radial outflow most likely to be weak is that to extensor communis and pollicis longus.[29] In some patients, there may also be loss of extensor carpi ulnaris.[35] Some or all of the flexor profundi can be involved but less frequently than the finger extensors.

PREOPERATIVE ELECTRICAL STUDIES OF BRACHIAL PLEXUS LESIONS

Although a thorough physical examination of the involved limb as well as the clinical examination of the patient as a whole are paramount, well-selected electrical and imaging studies play an important role in the assessment of brachial plexus lesions.

SPECIAL ELECTROMYOGRAPHIC STUDIES

For supraclavicular palsies, the major question to be answered is how far proximal or medial the injury extends on the spinal nerves and roots (Fig. 12-22). Special electromyographic (EMG) studies are of some help in this regard.[60] Nonetheless, the following electrical studies must always be interpreted in the context of the clinical findings and can never substitute, even in part, for a thorough clinical examination.

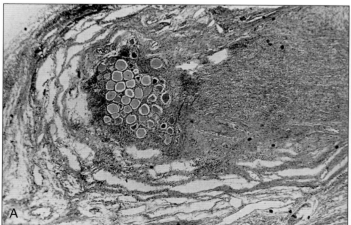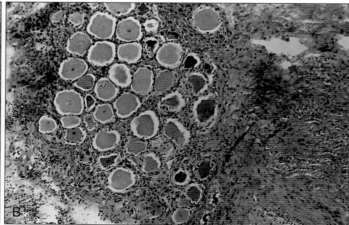

FIGURE 12-22 Histologic findings associated with proximal damage to spinal nerve(s). **(A)** Low-power view of Masson stain of section of a proximal spinal nerve. There is very little axonal structure; heavy scar is seen to the right and ganglion cells to the left. **(B)** Higher-power view. Presence of ganglion cells indicated that spinal nerve had been pulled down into the foramen, and, thus, this element had preganglionic as well as postganglionic injury.

PARASPINAL MUSCLE SAMPLING

These large posterior muscles are supplied by posterior spinal branches that originate at a foraminal level, so denervation in their distribution implies proximal spinal nerve or root injury.[9] Because there is overlap in their input to muscle, even severe denervation does not necessarily mean that one or more plexus roots are not damaged more laterally and at a reparable level.[61] Not infrequently, C5, and sometimes also C6, has extraforaminal injury, and yet more proximal injury to C7, C8, and T1 can give extensive paraspinal denervational change. Nonetheless, widespread denervation of these muscles remains a relatively important finding, suggesting very proximal spinal nerve or root injury. On the other hand, C3, C4, and at times also C2 may contribute to superior paraspinal muscles, so denervation may not be as widespread as one might think, even in the less common situation in which C5 or C6 or both are damaged quite proximally. Sampling must be done at a number of levels and by an experienced electromyographer.

SERRATUS ANTERIOR AND RHOMBOIDS

Although loss in these muscles is usually quite evident on clinical examination, sampling of their activity may be necessary. This is not an easy task because serratus is deep to the scapula and requires a very experienced electromyographer for its assessment. It is all too easy to place the tip of the EMG needle into an intercostal muscle, which lies just deep to serratus. In the reverse sense, because the spinal or lower segment of the trapezius overlies some of the rhomboids, the diagnostician has to be sure the needle is deep to trapezius before sampling of rhomboids is begun.

SENSORY NERVE ACTION POTENTIAL RECORDING

Presence of a sensory nerve action potential (SNAP) recorded at skin level along the dipole of a peripheral nerve such as ulnar, median, or radial, providing loss is complete in the distribution of the nerve stimulated, suggests preganglionic injury of one or more dorsal roots.[6,20,39] If sensory loss is complete in either the ulnar or median distribution and yet a SNAP is recorded, this means one or more dorsal posterior roots feeding the nerve have been injured between the dorsal root ganglion and the spinal cord. Injury at this site does not lead to degeneration of the ganglion's more distal afferent fibers, so the nerve is still capable of conducting electrical impulses even though there is no central connection. Lack of a central connection can be inferred at the operating table by stimulation of more distal spinal nerve and inability to record a somatosensory evoked potential or evoked cortical response from the spine or scalp (Fig. 12-23).[13,30,37,52]

Some clinicians have also suggested that the presence of a Tinel sign on percussion or deep palpation of the supraclavicular space when there is complete loss distal to this level indicates a central connection of at least some spinal nerve fibers.[36,44] Estimates for this number vary, but it may be as few as 100 fibers or so; this is a relatively small number of axons, and effective and functional regeneration requires a much larger number of nerve fibers. Unfortunately, this is also the case when somatosensory and cortical response recordings are evoked, even by operative stimulation of spinal nerves after stretch injury. Such responses can be present even though only a few hundred fibers have a central connection.

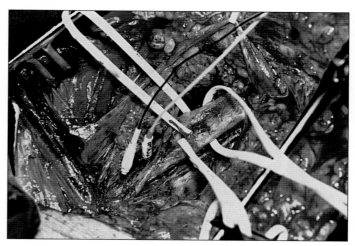

FIGURE 12-23 The integrity of spinal nerves can be checked by stimulation through electroencephalographic needles placed directly in proximal nerve. The recording of somatosensory evoked potentials through posterior superior cervical skin electrodes or contralateral scalp electrodes indicates that at least the posterior rootlets of the spinal nerves are attached to the spinal cord and hence can be used, after transection, as proximal stumps for attachment to grafts in appropriate cases.

Because each of the peripheral nerves usable for this type of study has three or more dorsal root contributions, the presence of a SNAP does not necessarily mean that all of the contributing roots are damaged at a preganglionic level.[35,54]

An attempt to make the SNAP more specific is by stimulating distal fingers at sensory sites considered to be more precise for given roots. Little and ring finger digital nerves can be stimulated by ring electrodes to correspond with T1 and C8 dorsal roots, middle finger to correspond with C7, and index finger or thumb to correspond with C6. The difficulty is that there is overlap peripherally in terms of input, especially to long finger, index finger, and thumb. A SNAP recorded by stimulating the long finger and recording from the median nerve could be caused by a dorsal root lesion of C8 or even C6 rather than C7. A SNAP recorded by stimulating the index finger and recording from median nerve could be caused by a dorsal root lesion of C7 in addition to or rather than C6. Stimulating little and ring fingers and recording from ulnar nerve are more certain for assessment of the C8 and T1 roots. Although controversial, there is in our experience neither a precise enough nor exclusive enough site to stimulate or record for a C6 distribution SNAP. In addition, neither axillary nerve nor suprascapular nerve can be stimulated precisely enough, let alone recorded from, to be certain of evaluation of the C5 root.[35]

In summary, the presence of a SNAP in the distribution of a nerve with complete clinical loss strongly implies a preganglionic injury. However, the absence of a SNAP in the distribution of a nerve with plexus dorsal root input does not exclude preganglionic injury. If an injury is extensive enough, as frequently happens, it damages both the pre- and postganglionic segments of the root. In these cases, the sensory fibers do degenerate, and no SNAP is recorded even though root-level damage extends close to the spinal cord.[10] Moreover, electrical evidence of preganglionic injury to the dorsal root does not guarantee that the ventral root is damaged as severely and as closely to the spinal cord, although it does strongly suggest it.[58]

OTHER ELECTROMYOGRAPHY CONSIDERATIONS

Sampling of other muscles may help the clinician ascertain the location and extent of a plexus lesion or, in other cases, suggest the possibility of recovery even though there is no clinical evidence of this. For example, loss of deltoid and biceps/brachialis function may suggest an upper trunk lesion, but the latter is more certain if supraspinatus and infraspinatus are also denervated. These same muscles along with biceps/brachialis should be sampled when looking for early recovery after an upper trunk lesion. Even under favorable circumstances, the deltoid is slow in regaining input. The larger, more bulky biceps shows earlier electrical and clinical recovery.[20] With a complete upper trunk lesion, brachioradialis and supinator also lose input, and the electromyographer may decide to sample those muscles as well.

C7 and middle trunk lesions may display a variety of electrical findings. The triceps usually has denervational changes, although it may also receive input from C6 and, surprisingly often, even from C8. A similar problem exists with specificity if extensor muscles such as extensor carpi radialis and ulnaris, extensor communis, and extensor pollicis longus are sampled. These muscles usually receive C7 outflow, but often also have considerable input from C8,[57] especially the extensor communis and extensor pollicis longus. A similar problem exists with sampling the flexor profundi; because of variable input from both C7 and C8, denervational changes within these muscles can suggest C8 or C7 injury or both. By comparison, lower trunk lesions cause loss in all hand intrinsics, including those of the thenar eminence. Clinical loss and electrical changes may also involve extensor communis and some of the flexor profundus system.[35,55] Unfortunately, the same is usually the case with medial cord lesions, so it may be difficult for either the clinician or electromyographer to differentiate these two close but different levels.

After serious plexus injury, it may take many months for certain electrical signs of recovery to occur. Undue delay while awaiting reversal of denervational change may make the timing for surgical repair inopportune. Nonetheless, with some injuries, recovery in the distribution of one or more elements may become evident in the early months. This makes repeated electrical as well as clinical study worthwhile.

IMAGING STUDIES OF BRACHIAL PLEXUS INJURIES

PLAIN RADIOGRAPHS

The beginner in this field rapidly gains an appreciation of the value of these studies. Special attention should be given to the clavicle, scapula, and shoulder joint including humeral bone, ribs, and the cervical spine. With blunt injury in which the plexus has been stretched, there is a high association with fracture and dislocation.[17,43] Alternatively, there can be severe plexus injury without any history of shoulder dislocation or radiographic presence of a fracture.[11] One cannot conclude that the fracture site localizes the level of the lesion.[16] Instead, the force fracturing the bone is often maximal at a site distant from the plexus; moreover, plexus damage is often proximal to the fracture site. Exceptions may be provided by complex depressed clavicular fractures, which on occasions involve plexus maximally at that level.

Fracture-dislocations of the cervical spine are often associated with myelopathy but can also be associated with severe plexus stretch on one side or the other. If seen with either blunt or penetrating injuries, transverse process fractures augur poorly for the root or spinal nerve involved at that level. Damage usually extends proximally close to spinal cord on that element or adjacent ones and may not be reparable. With penetrating wounds and transverse process fracture, there may also be vertebral arterial injury. Associated vascular injury of this nature may not be evident without arteriography (or magnetic resonance angiography), and even a negative study does not completely rule out vascular injury. Fractures of the lamina of the vertebral column are more likely to be associated with myelopathy than those of the spinous processes, and vertebral body fractures bode poorly for reparability of roots at that level if loss is in their distribution and is caused by stretch/contusion.

Rib fractures can result from severe contusive blows to the chest as well as the plexus. These can be associated with pneumothorax or hemothorax as well as a usually severe and lengthy lesion to the plexus.

On occasion, a fracture can mimic palsy because it prevents motion of a portion of the affected extremity. A good example was provided by a middle-aged woman who was referred for persistent "axillary palsy" some 7 months after she experienced a crushing injury to the shoulder. A humeral neck fracture had been treated for 7 weeks by a Valpeau type of sling. It was presumed healed, and, in addition, an electromyographer thought the deltoid showed denervational changes. When she was examined in New Orleans, she could not abduct her right shoulder beyond 10 degrees, and the deltoid muscle did seem somewhat shrunken but not completely so. EMG needle sampling of the deltoid, however, showed no denervation. As a result, the right shoulder and arm were X-rayed with the arm at the side and then with it held abducted to 90 degrees by the technician. As can be seen in Figure 12-24, there was nonunion of this proximal humeral fracture and, as a result, the arm could not be effectively abducted. The shoulder was readily stabilized operatively by an orthopedist, and, after a period of immobilization, almost full shoulder abduction was regained.

ANGIOGRAPHY AND VENOGRAPHY

These studies are probably done more often than is needed in the management of plexus palsies.[58] Even so, we cannot be too critical of their use, particularly if penetrating injuries involving upper arm, shoulder, or neck are present. Angiography is certainly indicated if there is absence of a radial or carotid pulse, an expanding mass in the area of the wound, or presence of a bruit or a thrill in the area of the wound. Occlusion or vascular avulsion is usually localized as to level by an arteriogram because there is no filling beyond the injury site. Under these circumstances, collateral filling of more distal vessels is seen surprisingly early, especially with lesions at the axillary level. In other cases, distal axillary and brachial vessels may be filled in a retrograde fashion through the profundus vessel.

Pseudoaneurysms are usually caused by a hole or laceration in the wall of the vessel which leads to a dissection by blood into tissues that invest the artery. These lesions are more commonly seen with gunshot wounds that involve the infraclavicular plexus and occasionally with a stab or glass wound to that area. Angiography cannot always be relied on to fill the aneurysm, because it is a false one and the site of leakage tends to seal off. More commonly,

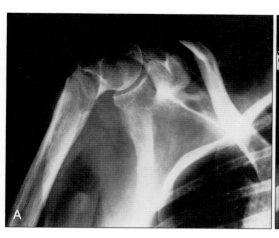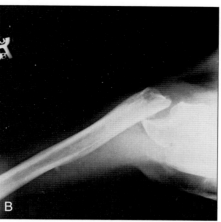

FIGURE 12-24 Radiographs of shoulder of patient referred because of "axillary palsy" and presumed paralysis of the deltoid following a humeral fracture thought to be healed. Inability to abduct the arm was due to malunion of a humeral fracture which was not very evident **(A)** until the arm was passively abducted and a radiograph **(B)** was taken in that position. (From Kline D and Hudson A: Acute injuries of peripheral nerves. In: Youmans J, Ed: Neurological Surgery. Philadelphia, WB Saunders, 1990).

the intimal surface is irregular at the original site of the injury to the vascular wall.[35] As a result, the contrast column has partial interruption or appears irregular at this level. Nonetheless, in about half of the pseudoaneurysm cases seen in our clinic, the preoperative angiogram was thought to be normal. In some cases, the diagnosis was suspected because of the presence of a pulsatile mass in the axilla or shoulder region with or without the presence of a bruit. In other cases, the lesion was discovered at the time of exploration for neural repair.

Less often, arteriography is indicated for vascular injury associated with stretch/contusion.[35,41] Associated vascular injury, especially if it involves the subclavian artery, denotes a particularly severe stretch to the plexus.[43] This is because a blunt or stretch injury involving vessels as well as plexus has usually severely distracted the shoulder and arm, resulting in a lengthy and proximal neural injury. This makes the probability of direct repair of a significant portion of the plexus lesion less likely than in one without vascular injury, but it does not completely exclude repair as a possibility. Sometimes, those repairing the vascular injury report their observations concerning the status of the plexus elements with regard to continuity or noncontinuity or obvious contusion or hemorrhage. More often, referral sources report one or more nerves being torn apart with one end seen but not the other, or nerves without a specific anatomic designation "running along and appearing bruised or hemorrhagic." Such reports should be weighed carefully but should not prevent neural exploration nor force it when it is too early to evaluate the regenerative ability of nerve lesions in continuity.

Although frequently negative, arterial and venous angiograms are still widely used in patients with suspected thoracic outlet syndrome.[46] Venous and sometimes arterial injections are done with the arm at the side and then with the arm abducted 90 degrees. Occlusion or constriction of flow suggests a vascular thoracic outlet problem but seldom proves it outright. Such associated vascular abnormalities are more likely to be present if there are vascular as well as neural symptoms, presence of a bruit or thrill, especially with abduction, and, sometimes, a positive Adson test (see Chapter 18, "Thoracic Outlet Syndrome").

A rare disorder is entrapment of axillary nerve near the quadrilateral space. This can be associated with posterior circumflex humeral artery or axillary arterial branch occlusion when the arm is hyperabducted and the axillary artery injected.[42] This is known as the quadrilateral space syndrome of Cahill. Patients have shoulder pain and paresthesias and sometimes a milder degree of shoul-der abduction weakness than is seen with more severe axillary nerve injury. Palpation of the quadrilateral space by compression behind the posterior deltoid usually produces severe pain and tenderness. The symptoms are caused by neural compression of the axillary nerve with shoulder abduction rather than by vascular compression. Occlusion or narrowing of the circumflex humeral vessels is, nonetheless, a useful marker for the entity.

MYELOGRAPHY

This is a diagnostic study primarily of use for stretch/contusion injuries in which there is a question of nerve root avulsion.[11] Several early papers were seminal in the application of this technique to this injury.[45,48] Despite the more recent development of computerized tomography (CT) and magnetic resonance imaging (MRI) scans, such studies, even with subarachnoid placement of contrast, can easily miss small meningoceles unless the transverse slices are very thin. Presence of meningoceles on a root sleeve suggests but does not prove either avulsion of that root from the spinal cord or damage in continuity of the root very close to cord.[26,50] Presence of this finding on a root suggests but again does not prove that damage can also be quite proximal on other roots, particularly those adjacent to the level of the meningocele.[14] Proximal damage may be present even if there are no myelographic abnormalities at levels adjacent to one with a meningocele. On occasion, however, the root at the level of a meningocele is either quite intact or, less commonly, injured lateral to the intervertebral foramen.[33] Conversely, a root can be damaged close to cord or even avulsed from cord without a meningocele being present.[62]

In summary, myelography for stretch injuries to the plexus has both a false-positive and a false-negative incidence.[12] Despite this, the myelogram does provide some indication of how proximal the injury is. This in turn suggests the probability that in cases where meningoceles are present, especially on the lower roots, they will not be reparable. However, meningoceles at the lower levels do not mean that spinal nerves at a higher level, especially C5 and C6, cannot be repaired. We therefore use the presence of meningoceles on myelography as an indication that the injury is likely proximal but do not consider them a contraindication to plexus exploration.

Other myelographic findings associated with root avulsion or very proximal stretch include widening of the cord from contusion or edema. For this reason, if a myelogram is done in the week or two after injury, a narrowing of the contrast column on one or both sides of the cervical gutter can be present with or without menin-gocele. The contrast column in the gutter may be thicker than normal after several weeks because of spinal cord shrinkage. In still other cases, enough contrast may exit a damaged root sleeve to form a linear collection of contrast material at an epidural or sub-dural level. Thus, even if there is no myelopathy, presence of one or more findings such as these augurs poorly for repair of the roots, at least at the levels at which these abnormalities are seen.

CT AND MRI SCANS

These studies have their greatest application for tumors either arising in plexus or secondarily compressing it.[19] Especially useful is the MRI with contrast by gadolinium.[18,34] Unfortunately, those unfamiliar with the field of stretch injury to the plexus often try to substitute CT or MRI scans for myelography. Poorly done scans, with thick slice acquisition and using techniques not sensitive for the appreciation of the nerve root junction with the spinal cord and spinal nerve within the foramen, are all too frequently seen. Improving quality of CT and MRI studies is hopefully reversing this trend.

CT scans following subarachnoid contrast injection when positive at nerve root levels can be quite dramatic with stretch injuries.[40] Earlier studies, using thin section CT scans, following myelography, demonstrated superior nerve root resolution and ability to detect avulsion compared to MRI.[12] Newer MRI tech-niques, incorporating coronal and oblique slices of the neck and shoulder and phase array surface coils are improving the ability of these techniques to image the brachial plexus.[2,15,23,24,34] More recent studies from centers with dedicated protocols for brachial plexus imaging demonstrate greatly improved sensitivity of MRI for evalu-ating nerve root avulsions.[15,21] Over time, as these techniques become widely applied and accepted, MRI will likely replace myelography and postmyelography CT for the imaging of brachial plexus avulsion.

In cases of presumed thoracic outlet syndrome, myelography, CT scans (postmyelography), or MRI scans, may be useful in excluding more proximal lesions such as cervical disc, tumor, or spondylytic disease. As the sensitivity of MRI continues to improve, it is hoped that it will allow more precise imaging of the plexus and the offending soft tissue and bony compressive element in thoracic outlet syndrome.[2,24]

REFERENCES

1. Aids to the examination of the peripheral nervous system. London, Baillière Tindall, 1986.
2. Aagaard BD, Maravilla KR, and Kliot M: Magnetic resonance neurography: magnetic resonance imaging of peripheral nerves. Neuroimaging Clin N Am 11:viii, 131-viii, 146, 2001.
3. Abdullah S and Bowden RE: The blood supply of the brachial plexus. Proc R Soc Med 53:203–205, 1960.
4. Aszmann OC, Rab M, Kamolz L, et al.: The anatomy of the pectoral nerves and their significance in brachial plexus reconstruction. J Hand Surg [Am] 25:942–947, 2000.
5. Blaauw G and Slooff AC: Transfer of pectoral nerves to the musculocutaneous nerve in obstetric upper brachial plexus palsy. Neurosurgery 53:338–341, 2003.
6. Bonney G and Gilliatt RW: Sensory nerve conduction after traction lesion of the brachial plexus. Proc R Soc Med 51:365–367, 1958.
7. Bowden REM, Abdullah S, and Gooding MR: Anatomy of the cervical spine, membranes, spinal cord, nerve roots, and brachial plexus. In: Wilkinson MF, Ed: Cervical Spondylosis and other Disorders of the Cervical Spine. Philadelphia, WB Saunders, 1967.
8. Brandt KE and Mackinnon SE: A technique for maximizing biceps recovery in brachial plexus reconstruction. J Hand Surg [Am] 18:726–733, 1993.
9. Bufalini C and Pescatori G: Posterior cervical electromyography in the diagnosis and prognosis of brachial plexus injuries. J Bone Joint Surg [Br] 51:627–631, 1969.
10. Burkholder LM, Houlden DA, Midha R, et al.: Neurogenic motor evoked potentials: role in brachial plexus surgery. Case report. J Neurosurg 98:607–610, 2003.
11. Campbell JB: Peripheral nerve repair. Clin Neurosurg 17:77–98, 1970.
12. Carvalho GA, Nikkhah G, Matthies C, et al.: Diagnosis of root avulsions in traumatic brachial plexus injuries: value of computerized tomography, myelography, and magnetic resonance imaging. J Neurosurg 86:69–76, 1997.
13. Celli L and Rovesta C: Electrophysiologic intraoperative evaluations of the damaged root in tractions of the brachial plexus. In: Terzis J, Ed: Microreconstruction of Nerve Injuries. Philadelphia, WB Saunders, 1987.
14. Davies ER, Sutton D, and Bligh AS: Myelography in brachial plexus injury. Br J Radiol 39:362, 1966.
15. Doi K, Otsuka K, Okamoto Y, et al.: Cervical nerve root avulsion in brachial plexus injuries: magnetic resonance imaging classification and comparison with myelography and computerized tomography myelography. J Neurosurg 96:277–284, 2002.
16. Dolene W: Intercostal neutralization of the peripheral nerves in avulsion plexus injuries. Clin Plast Surg 11:143–147, 1984.
17. Drake CG: Diagnosis and treatment of lesions of the brachial plexus and adjacent structures. Clin Neurosurg 11:110–127, 1964.
18. Ganju A, Roosen N, Kline DG, et al.: Outcomes in a consecutive series of 111 surgically treated plexal tumors: a review of the experience at the Louisiana State University Health Sciences Center. J Neurosurg 95:51–60, 2001.
19. Gebarski KS, Glazer GM, and Gebarski SS: Brachial plexus: anatomic, radiologic, and pathologic correlation using computed tomography. J Comput Assist Tomogr 6:1058–1063, 1982.
20. Gilliatt R: Physical injury to peripheral nerves, physiological and electrodiagnostic aspects. Mayo Clin Proc 56:361–370, 1981.
21. Grant GA, Britz GW, Goodkin R, et al.: The utility of magnetic resonance imaging in evaluating peripheral nerve disorders. Muscle Nerve 25:314–331, 2002.
22. Gu Y, Xu J, Chen L, et al.: Long term outcome of contralateral C7 transfer: a report of 32 cases. Chin Med J (Engl) 115:866–868, 2002.
23. Gupta RK, Mehta VS, Banerji AK, et al.: MR evaluation of brachial plexus injuries. Neuroradiology 31:377–381, 1989.
24. Hayes CE, Tsuruda JS, Mathis CM, et al.: Brachial plexus: MR imaging with a dedicated phased array of surface coils. Radiology 203:286–289, 1997.
25. Haymaker W and Woodhall B: Peripheral nerve injuries, 2nd edn. Philadelphia, WB Saunders, 1956.
26. Heon M: Myelogram: A questionable aid in diagnosis and prognosis of brachial plexus components in traction injuries. Conn Med 29:260–262, 1965.
27. Hollingshead WH: Anatomy for surgeons, vol. 3: The Back and Limbs, 2nd edn. New York, Harper & Row, 1969.
28. Hovelacque A: Anatomic des nerfs craniens et rach, diens et du systeme grand sympathique. Paris, Doin, 1927.
29. Hudson AR and Tranmer BI: Brachial plexus injuries. In: Wilkins RH and Rengachary SS, Eds: Neurosurgery. New York, McGraw Hill, 1985.

30. Jones SJ: Diagnostic value of peripheral and spinal somatosensory evoked potentials in traction lesions of the brachial plexus. Clin Plast Surg 11:167–172, 1984.

31. Kaplan EB and Spinner M: Normal and anomalous innervation patterns in the upper extremity. In: Omer GE and Spinner M, Eds: Management of Peripheral Nerve Problems. Philadelphia, WB Saunders, 1980.

32. Kerr AT: The brachial plexus nerves of man, the variation in its formation and its branches. Am J Anat 23:285, 1918.

33. Kewalramani LS and Taylor RG: Brachial plexus root avulsion: role of myelography – review of diagnostic procedures. J Trauma 15:603–608, 1975.

34. Kichari JR, Hussain SM, Den Hollander JC, et al.: MR imaging of the brachial plexus: current imaging sequences, normal findings, and findings in a spectrum of focal lesions with MR-pathologic correlation. Curr Probl Diagn Radiol 32:88–101, 2003.

35. Kline DG, Hackett ER, and Happel LH: Surgery for lesions of the brachial plexus. Arch Neurol 43:170–181, 1986.

36. Landi A and Copeland S: Value of the Tinel sign in brachial plexus lesions. Ann R Coll Surg Engl 61:470–471, 1979.

37. Landi A, Copeland SA, Parry CB, et al.: The role of somatosensory evoked potentials and nerve conduction studies in the surgical management of brachial plexus injuries. J Bone Joint Surg [Br] 62:492–496, 1980.

38. Leffert RD: Brachial plexus injuries. London, Churchill Livingstone, 1985.

39. Licht S: Electrodiagnosis and electromyography. New Haven, CN, E Licht, 1971.

40. Marshall RW and De Silva RD: Computerised axial tomography in traction injuries of the brachial plexus. J Bone Joint Surg [Br] 68:734–738, 1986.

41. McGillicuddy JE: Clinical decision making in brachial plexus injuries. Neurosurg Clin N Am 2:137–150, 1991.

42. McKowen HC and Voorhies RM: Axillary nerve entrapment in the quadrilateral space. Case report. J Neurosurg 66:932–934, 1987.

43. Midha R. Epidemiology of brachial plexus injuries in a multitrauma population. Neurosurgery 40:1182–1189, 1997.

44. Millesi H: Surgical management of brachial plexus injuries. J Hand Surg [Am] 2:367–378, 1977.

45. Murphey F, Hartung W, and Kirklin J: Myelographic demonstration of avulsing injuries of the brachial plexus. Am J Epidemiol 58:102–105, 1947.

46. Pang D and Wessel HB: Thoracic outlet syndrome. Neurosurgery 22:105–121, 1988.

47. Pernkopf E: Atlas of topographical and applied human anatomy, vol. 1, head and neck. Philadelphia, WB Saunders, 1980.

48. Robles J: Brachial plexus avulsion. A review of diagnostic procedures and report of six cases. J Neurosurg 28:434–438, 1968.

49. Seddon HJ: Surgical Disorders of the Peripheral Nerves. Baltimore, Williams & Wilkins, 1972.

50. Simond J and Sypert G: Closed traction avulsion injuries of the brachial plexus. Contemp Neurosurg 50:1–6, 1983.

51. Stevens J: Brachial plexus paralysis. In: Codman EA, Ed: The Shoulder. Boston, T. Todd, 1934:332–381.

52. Sugioka H, Tsuyama N, Hara T, et al.: Investigation of brachial plexus injuries by intraoperative cortical somatosensory evoked potentials. Arch Orthop Trauma Surg 99:143–151, 1982.

53. Sunderland S: Meningeal-neural relations in the intervertebral foramen. J Neurosurg 40:756–763, 1974.

54. Synek VM and Cowan JC: Somatosensory evoked potentials in patients with supraclavicular brachial plexus injuries. Neurology 32:1347–1352, 1982.

55. Terzis J, Liberson WT, and Maragh H: Motorcycle brachial plexopathy. In: Terzis J, Ed: Microreconstruction of Nerve Injuries. Philadelphia, WB Saunders, 1987.

56. Uysal II, Seker M, Karabulut AK, et al.: Brachial plexus variations in human fetuses. Neurosurgery 53:676–684, 2003.

57. Warren J, Gutmann L, Figueroa AF Jr, et al.: Electromyographic changes of brachial plexus root avulsions. J Neurosurg 31:137–140, 1969.

58. Wilbourn AJ: Brachial plexus disorders. In: Dyck PJ and Thomas PK, Eds: Peripheral Neuropathy, 3rd edn. Philadelphia, WB Saunders, 1993.

59. Wolock B and Millesi H: Brachial plexus – applied anatomy and operative exposure. In: Gelberman RH, Ed: Operative Nerve Repair and Reconstruction. Philadelphia, JB Lippincott, 1991.

60. Yiannikas C, Shahani BT, and Young RR: The investigation of traumatic lesions of the brachial plexus by electromyography and short latency somatosensory potentials evoked by stimulation of multiple peripheral nerves. J Neurol Neurosurg Psychiatry 46:1014–1022, 1983.

61. Zalis AW, Oester YT, and Rodriquez AA: Electrophysiologic diagnosis of cervical nerve root avulsion. Arch Phys Med Rehabil 51:708–710, 1970.

62. Zorub DS, Nashold BS Jr, and Cook WA Jr: Avulsion of the brachial plexus. I. A review with implications on the therapy of intractable pain. Surg Neurol 2:347–353, 1974.

13

Suprascapular nerve injury and entrapment

David G. Kline and Daniel H. Kim

OVERVIEW

- The suprascapular nerve (SSN) enters the scapular area beneath the suprascapular ligament, and a deep and lateral surgical exposure located superior to the scapular spine is required for section of the ligament.
- The nerve can less frequently be entrapped in the region of the spinoglenoid notch.
- Forty-two patients with SSN injuries and entrapments at the supraclavicular notch underwent surgery between 1970 and 2002.
- The SSN injuries and entrapments were associated with occupational overuse in 19 patients, sports-related injury in 16 and direct trauma in four. Three cases had removal of ganglion cysts at the supraclavicular notch which had caused nerve compression.
- Function of the supraspinatus muscle usually recovered to a better level than that of the infraspinatus after surgery, but the latter usually reached a grade of 3.

INTRODUCTION

The suprascapular nerve (SSN) is a branch of the brachial plexus upper trunk and contains fibers from C5 and C6.[12,19] The SSN courses laterally in the shoulder deep to the trapezius and omohyoid muscles and passes through a narrow foramen, the suprascapular notch and its roof, the suprascapular ligament, also called the superior transverse scapular ligament (STSL) (Figs 13-1, 13-2). In the region of the suprascapular notch, the suprascapular artery passes over the superior aspect of the STSL. Branches of the SSN normally supply the supraspinatus muscle in the supraspinatus fossa, as well as the shoulder joint and the acromioclavicular joint.[43] As described by Spinner et al., however, the SSN branch to the supraspinatus can pass at times superior to the suprascapular ligament.[38]

The SSN continues through a second notch, the spinoglenoid notch which has as its roof the inferior transverse scapular ligament (ITSL), also known as the spinoglenoid ligament (Fig. 13-1). The nerve then winds around the lateral border of the scapular spine to enter the infraspinous fossa where it terminates in two branches to the infraspinatus muscle and smaller branches to the shoulder joint and the scapula.[28,43]

A cutaneous branch was described in the anatomical literature more than 20 years ago[18,21,29] and begins either under or just distal to the STSL or from the superior branch of the nerve to the supraspinatus muscle. This branch courses superolaterally along the supraspinatus muscle, passing anterior to the coracoacromial ligament toward the acromion tip, and pierces the deltoid muscle to become subcutaneous. The SSN cutaneous branches are present in the proximal one-third of the arm and are thought by some to be contained within the axillary nerve at a subcutaneous site.[2,21,29]

INJURY MECHANISMS

The SSN can be impinged against the sharp inferior border of the STSL ligament at its site of angulation at the suprascapular notch. Though there is no translational motion, this indentation mechanism of injury occurs during scapular excursions and has been termed the "sling effect" by Rengachary et al.[33] The angulation is exaggerated even further during movements of the scapula involving cross-body abduction or adduction which happens during a variety of activities involving upper extremity movement.[3] The ensuing inflammation further reduces the free area in this notch already constrained by the overlying STSL.[31]

Patients with SSN entrapment frequently complain of severe scapular and parascapular pain for a period of time. These patients can be baseball pitchers,[15,35] football,[37] handball,[36] or volleyball players,[7,13,20,25,44] weight lifters,[1,47] and dancers,[26] all of whom experience repetitive SSN trauma from shoulder depression and abduction. Workers required to carry heavy objects, such as meat-packers[41] or newsreel cameraman,[24] are at risk for SSN injury, as well.

Other injury mechanisms include stretch injury, direct trauma via scapular, humeral or midshaft clavicular fractures[46] and anterior shoulder dislocations,[42] entrapment by tight ligaments[5] or a bone spur or bridge over the suprascapular or spinoglenoid notches.[11] Ganglion cysts can entrap the SSN nerve, as well.[4,16,17,23,27,28,30,32,39,40,45]

Rare causes of SSN entrapment at the suprascapular notch included in the literature are a hematoma associated with a fracture, synovial and Ewing's sarcomas, chondrosarcoma, metastatic renal cell carcinoma,[14] and a lipoma of the suprascapular notch.[19]

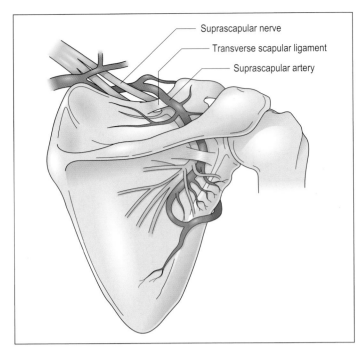

FIGURE 13-1 A drawing of the course of the suprascapular nerve and artery viewed from a posterior vantage point. The usual entrapment site is beneath the transverse scapular ligament, also called the suprascapular ligament. Occasionally, the nerve can be entrapped at or distal to the level of the scapular notch, which is also called the glenoid notch. The usual loss in the later instance involves the infraspinatus muscle with sparing of the supraspinatus muscle function.

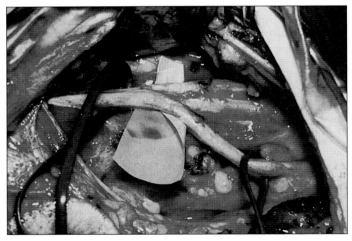

FIGURE 13-2 The right suprascapular nerve (SSN) (encircled by the Vasoloop to the right) is shown intraoperatively. It leaves the upper trunk (depicted by the Vasoloop encircling the upper trunk to the left) as the trunk begins to divide into its anterior and posterior divisions. As the SSN travels laterally, it runs beneath or deep to the inferior belly of the omohyoid muscle and beneath the trapezius muscle. The nerve then traverses the suprascapular notch, where it lies beneath the transverse scapular ligament (TSL), also called the suprascapular ligament. Dissection to that level becomes difficult with an anterior approach because the clavicle in the front and the upper border of the scapula behind impinge upon the operative space. Though the TSL can be sectioned by an anterior procedure, the lesion is more easily approached from behind.

The distal SSN branches supplying the infraspinatus muscle can also undergo impingement as they wind around the lateral scapular spine and travel through the spinoglenoid notch and its roof which is formed by the ITSL.[43] The incidence of SSN entrapment here, however, remains controversial, though it has recently been increasingly cited in the literature as an etiology in some cases of SSN entrapment.[22] This entrapment would result in isolated infraspinatus muscle atrophy, usually without pain, since the distal portion of the SSN is purely a motor nerve while the more proximal SSN contains motor and sensory fibers.[21]

Ide et al.[22] investigated 115 shoulders of cadavers and measured the width of the ITSL and the maximal distance to bone and nerve. The ligament width varied from 1.8 to 9 mm (mean, 5.4 mm). It was membranous in 69 (60%), a true ligament in 25 (21.7%) and was absent in 21 (18.3%) cadaver shoulders. The maximal distance from ligament to bone varied from 3.0 to 11.1 mm (mean, 5.7 mm) and the distance from ligament to nerve also varied from 0.1 to 7 mm (mean, 3.1 mm). There was thus a considerable variation in distances from ligament to bone and from ligament to nerve. The instances of the minimal distances of ligament to bone and ligament to nerve in some cadavers may be evidence that in some patients there is a congenital predisposition to developing SSN injury or entrapment. The converse is also true: in 18.3% of cadavers the ligament was absent; thus, the distal SSN is not at risk for entrapment in these individuals.

In another study by Demirhan,[9,10] 14 (61%) of 23 cadaveric shoulders had a non-membranous spinoglenoid ligament and during cross-body adduction and internal rotation of the glenohumeral joint, the SSN was found to be stretched underneath this ligament. Fibrils of the spinoglenoid ligament were seen to interact with the posterior aspect of the capsule.

Bektas et al.[6] studied 32 cadaveric shoulders and presented their work in 2003 in the paper "Spinoglenoid septum: a new anatomic finding." A thin, loose, and weak spinoglenoid ligament was seen in only five shoulders; however, a septum they termed the spinoglenoid septum, formed by the thickening of the fascial cover of the distal third of the supraspinatus and infraspinatus muscles, was seen in the remaining shoulders. This septum originated from the spinoglenoid notch and extended into the posterior capsule. The SSN was observed to pass between the bony margin of the spinoglenoid notch and the medial concave margin of the spinoglenoid septum. Thus, this septum may be another cause of dynamic compression of the SSN.

CLINICAL PRESENTATION AND EXAMINATION

Entrapment of the SSN results in a diffuse, deep, aching pain in the posterior and lateral aspects of the shoulder and the arm which, especially in the early weeks, can be quite severe. The pain may be due to compression of SSN fibers destined for the glenohumeral and acromioclavicular joints or to atrophy of the supraspinatus and infraspinatus muscles. As quickly as the pain originates and as severe as it is, it usually suddenly disappears after denervation has occurred. The patient then notes difficulty with the supraspinatus muscle's initial 30 degrees of abduction of the upper arm and/or the infraspinatus' external rotation of the shoulder. Inspection of the posterior shoulder at this point usually reveals atrophy of the spinati, which is pathognomonic when observed.

Compression of the SSN in the spinoglenoid tunnel in the cases presented in the literature causes functional impairment of the infraspinatus muscle alone, which is often minimal and pain is absent, since the distal SSN is a pure motor nerve.[21] In the variant described by Spinner et al.,[38] in which the supraspinatus branch of the SSN passes superior to the suprascapular ligament at the suprascapular notch, a similar isolated infraspinatus weakness occurs, but with pain, since the proximal SSN is a mixed motor/sensory nerve. Thus, a differentiating feature between these two sites of entrapment is the absence or presence of pain. Concurrent SSN entrapment at both the suprascapular notch and spinoglenoid notch is infrequent.

NEUROIMAGING

In cases of suspected SSN injury or entrapment, anteroposterior and lateral cervical spine plain X-rays should be performed to document other possible non-SSN-related etiologies of the patient's symptoms and findings, such as spinal cord or root lesions. The plain film X-ray beam can be directed 15–30 degrees caudally toward the suprascapular notch to determine its size. This angulation removes the superimposition of the clavicle, the scapular spine, and the ribs.[34] Plain films of the shoulder are indicated in appropriate cases of trauma to this area to rule out a scapular fracture as the cause of the SSN injury or entrapment.

Cervical spine magnetic resonance imaging (MRI) is carried out to eliminate a C4–C5 herniated disc as the source of presenting symptoms and findings. A shoulder MRI defines a focal mass causing SSN entrapment such as a ganglion cyst or tumor.

ELECTROPHYSIOLOGICAL STUDIES

Electromyography enables a positive diagnosis of suprascapular notch-related SSN injury and demonstrates denervation potentials in the supra- and infraspinatus muscles, with changes in the latter usually being more severe and widespread than in the former. Stimulation at Erb's point and recording from supra- or infraspinatus muscles, though controversial as an electrodiagnostic study, may show delayed conduction. Normal latencies from Erb's point to supraspinatus have a relatively large range, from 1.7 to 3.7 msec, so it is best to compare the affected side with the contralateral asymptomatic side.

If the SSN is involved by brachial plexitis, there is usually other loss in the distribution of the brachial plexus, or the long thoracic or accessory nerves. The suprascapular involvement in such cases is not helped by surgery.

SURGICAL EXPOSURE

Conservative therapy consisting of the avoidance of muscular activity is recommended for patients with pain alone, while surgery is reserved for patients with intractable pain, weakness, and atrophy. Surgical intervention for this entity is difficult since the point of entrapment is deep, and as a result, illumination and magnification are useful. Palpation of the scapula on a skeletal model before the operation to appreciate the location of the suprascapular and glenoid notches is helpful. Also to be kept in mind is that the bony anatomy may vary.

The position for the patient with a suprascapular neuropathy can be either supine or prone. The preferred position in our cases was to place the patient in a supine position with the head supported by a donut and the head and thorax elevated 30–45 degrees by raising the head of the operating table (Fig. 13-3A). The shoulder area was then slightly elevated further by placing folded sheets beneath the patient's interscapular region. In this position the spine of the scapula and the supra- and infraspinatus muscles are accessible to the surgeon standing at the head of the operating table.

A transverse incision is made parallel and slightly anterior to the scapular spine and carried toward the tip of the shoulder. After dissection through the subcutaneous layers, the trapezius fibers are divided. The supraspinatus muscle is either split in the direction of its fibers or separated from the superior aspect of the scapular spine and retracted forward. Sometimes, it is advantageous to dissect around the supraspinatus and circumscribe it with a Penrose drain. The muscle can then be alternately displaced anteriorly and posteriorly.

Dissection deep to the supraspinatus muscle with a curved hemostat exposes the transverse and oblique course of the suprascapular ligament, which angles from a medial location anteriorly to a lateral one posteriorly (Fig. 13-3B, C). Sometimes, identification of the suprascapular notch is helped by identifying the SSN just proximal to its entry to the scapular notch and then tracing it along with its vessels anteriorly to the suprascapular notch region. At a depth of 8–10 cm, the nerve was found beneath this ligament, sometimes with the supraspinatus branch and often with a suprascapular artery branch superficial to it. The SSN takes an oblique course, running on top of the dorsal superior scapular bone and angling from a medial location anteriorly to a lateral one posteriorly. The usual area of entrapment where the nerve passes beneath the ligament is opened by placing a fine-tipped Moynihan placed beneath the ligament above the nerve and dividing the ligament with a No. 15 scalpel blade on a long-handled plastic knife. Vasa-loops can be placed around the nerve and if necessary the nerve can be dissected proximally and outward through the scapular notch. After neurolysis of the nerve, the muscular and fascial layers are sutured closed with 2–0 and 3–0 resorbable sutures. A drain is seldom necessary.

If the site of injury or entrapment is inferior to the spine, the nerve is cleared in its path around the lateral edge of the scapular spine and through the spinoglenoid notch. Here, a portion of infraspinatus muscle whose fibers run parallel to the superior surface of the scapular spine is detached transversely from the spine, leaving a cuff to which to sew back. Some of the superior and lateral infraspinatus muscle is swept away from the inferior surface of the scapular spine to expose the lateral spine of the scapula from below. The muscle-splitting approach for both the supra- and infraspinatus muscles has been used in each of three cases of ganglion cysts. In these instances, a ganglion cyst had compressed the nerve in the suprascapular notch region and was located both above and below this structure, as well as within it.

The notch apertures may be increased with osteotomies if there is an inadequate notch size found during direct intraoperative observation.[8]

RESULTS

The mean follow-up period for the 42 surgically treated injuries was 18 months (range 12–48 months). There were 39 SSN injuries and entrapments and three additional cases of compression due to ganglion cysts (Table 13-1). All 42 injuries and entrapments

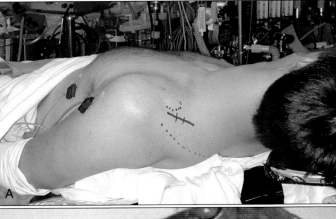

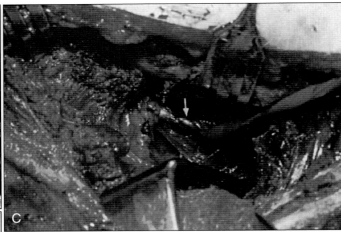

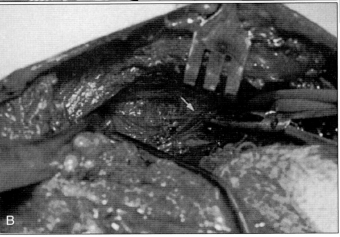

FIGURE 13-3 **(A)** The intraoperative photograph shows the positioning of the patient and planned incision for exposure of the left suprascapular nerve (SSN) by a posterior approach. The outlined incision line runs parallel to and slightly superior to the scapular spine and should extend laterally to the acromion–scapular junction. The coracoid process is outlined superior to the incision with a dotted line, as is the scapular spine below the incision. **(B)** A curved hemostat is shown placed under the ligament (*white arrow*) and superior to the SSN on the right side. The supraspinatus muscle has been split in the direction of its fibers to gain this exposure. **(C)** A Vasoloop has been placed around the SSN (*white arrow*) after the release of the ligament on the right side.

Table 13-1 Etiologies of SSN injury/entrapment (n=42)

Etiology	No. of patients (%)
Occupation	19 (45%)
Sports related	16 (38%)
Direct trauma	4 (10%)
Ganglion cysts	3 (7%)
Total	42 (100%)

SSN, suprascapular nerve; No., number.

including those due to ganglion cysts were at the site of the suprascapular notch.

Thirty-one patients (78%) of the 39 with SSN injuries and entrapments at the suprascapular notch excluding the patients with ganglion cysts presented with weakness of both the supraspinatus and infraspinatus muscles (Table 13-2) and mild to moderate pain. Eight patients (21%) of 39 patients with SSN injuries and entrapments presented with grade 3 motor strength of the spinati muscles accompanied by persistent severe pain preoperatively.

The results of preoperative motor testing for the 31 patients with spinati weakness included supraspinatus muscle strength ranging from grade 0 to less than grade 2 of 5; infraspinatus muscle weakness in these patients on motor examination was grade 0 to 2.

The motor function of the supraspinatus muscle in these 31 patients improved postoperatively to grade 4 or better in 28 patients (90%) of the 31 cases and three patients (10%) improved to grade 2 to 3. Postoperatively, motor function of the infraspinatus muscle improve in 10 (32%) to better than grade 3, in 14 (45%) to grade 2 to 3, and seven (23%) had an improvement to only grade 1.[21]

In eight patients with persistent severe pain which was present preoperatively the pain improved postoperatively in seven of eight patients (99%). The motor strength remained the same or improved to grade 4.

The three patients with ganglion cysts removed from the scapular notch region retained good motor strength postoperatively (Fig. 13-4).

Results in 42 cases, then, have been quite satisfactory. Decreased pain and increased shoulder mobility have been almost uniformly obtained. The function of the supraspinatus muscle usually recovered to a better level than that of the infraspinatus muscle. Exceptions were provided by three patients who had the onset of their palsy associated with scapular fracture. Here, recovery of function was not as good, although pain seemed to be helped in two of the three cases having surgery with neurolysis of the SSN, as well as section of the suprascapular notch ligament.

Table 13-2 LSUHSC criteria for grading suprascapular nerve injury

Grade	Evaluation	Description
0	Absent	No muscle contraction of the supraspinatus or infraspinatus
1	Poor	Some supraspinatus contraction* and infraspinatus usually without contraction
2	Fair	Supraspinatus contraction against gravity and infraspinatus contracts, but not against gravity**
3	Moderate	Supraspinatus contraction against gravity and some force and infraspinatus contracts against gravity
4	Good	Supraspinatus and infraspinatus contraction is against moderate force
5	Excellent	Good recovery of supraspinatus and infraspinatus function

LSHUSC, Louisiana State University Health Sciences Center.

*The contraction of the supraspinatus muscle can be felt and sometimes seen.

**The contraction of the infraspinatus muscle can be seen and felt.

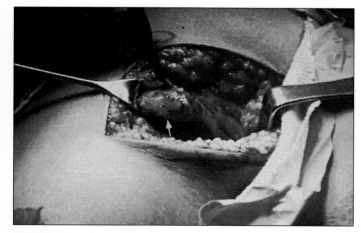

FIGURE 13-4 A ganglion cyst (*white arrow*) involving the right suprascapular nerve is shown being removed intraoperatively.

REFERENCES

1. Agre JC, Ash N, Cameron MC, et al.: Suprascapular neuropathy after intensive progressive resistive exercise: case report. Arch Phys Med Rehabil 68:236–238, 1987.
2. Ajmani ML: The cutaneous branch of the human suprascapular nerve. J Anat 185 (Pt 2):439–442, 1994.
3. Antoniadis G, Richter HP, Rath S, et al.: Suprascapular nerve entrapment: experience with 28 cases. J Neurosurg 85:1020–1025, 1996.
4. Antoniou J, Tae SK, Williams GR, et al.: Suprascapular neuropathy. Variability in the diagnosis, treatment, and outcome. Clin Orthop 386:131–138, 2001.
5. Asami A, Sonohata M, and Morisawa K: Bilateral suprascapular nerve entrapment syndrome associated with rotator cuff tear. J Shoulder Elbow Surg 9:70–72, 2000.
6. Bektas U, Ay S, Yilmaz C, et al.: Spinoglenoid septum: a new anatomic finding. J Shoulder Elbow Surg 12:491–492, 2003.
7. Carlson CT and Frankovich R: Arm weakness – volleyball. Med Sci Sports Exerc 30:132, 1998.
8. Cummins CA, Messer TM, and Nuber GW: Suprascapular nerve entrapment. J Bone Joint Surg [Am] 82:415–424, 2000.
9. Demirhan M: Spinoglenoid ligament (letter). J Bone Joint Surg [Am] 82:599–600, 2000.
10. Demirhan M, Imhoff AB, Debski RE, et al.: The spinoglenoid ligament and its relationship to the suprascapular nerve. J Shoulder Elbow Surg 7:238–243, 1998.
11. Edelson JG: Bony bridges and other variations of the suprascapular notch. J Bone Joint Surg [Br] 77:505–506, 1995.
12. Ferranti F: Medical Management of Chronic Shoulder Pain. Philadelphia, Lippincott Williams & Wilkins, 1999.
13. Ferretti A, Cerullo G, and Russo G: Suprascapular neuropathy in volleyball players. J Bone Joint Surg [Am] 69:260–263, 1987.
14. Fritz RC, Helms CA, Steinbach LS, et al.: Suprascapular nerve entrapment: evaluation with MR imaging. Radiology 182:437–444, 1992.
15. Gambrell R: Shoulder pain – baseball. Med Sci Sports Exerc 30:95, 1998.
16. Ganzhorn RW, Hocker JT, Horowitz M, et al.: Suprascapular-nerve entrapment. J Bone Joint Surg [Am] 63:492–494, 1981.
17. Green JR, Freehill MQ, and Buss DD: Diagnosis and treatment of ganglion cysts about the shoulder. Techniques Shoulder Elbow Surg 2:100–105, 2001.
18. Harbaugh KS, Swenson R, and Saunders RL: Shoulder numbness in a patient with suprascapular nerve entrapment syndrome: cutaneous branch of the suprascapular nerve: case report. Neurosurgery 47:1452–1455; discussion 1455–1456, 2000.
19. Hazrati Y, Miller S, Moore S, et al.: Suprascapular nerve entrapment secondary to a lipoma. Clin Orthop 411:124–128, 2003.
20. Holzgraefe M, Kukowski B, and Eggert S: Prevalence of latent and manifest suprascapular neuropathy in high-performance volleyball players. Br J Sports Med 28:177–179, 1994.
21. Horiguchi M: The cutaneous branch of some human suprascapular nerves. J Anat 130:191–195, 1980.
22. Ide J, Maeda S, and Takagi K: Does the inferior transverse scapular ligament cause distal suprascapular nerve entrapment? An anatomic and morphologic study. J Shoulder Elbow Surg 12:253–255, 2003.
23. Inokuchi W, Ogawa K, and Horiuchi Y: Magnetic resonance imaging of suprascapular nerve palsy. J Shoulder Elbow Surg 7:223–227, 1998.
24. Karatas GK and Gogus F: Suprascapular nerve entrapment in newsreel cameramen. Am J Phys Med Rehabil 82:192–196, 2003.
25. Khan AM, Guillet MA, and Fanton GS: Volleyball: rehabilitation and training tips. Sports Med Arthroscop Rev 9:137–146, 2001.
26. Kukowski B: Suprascapular nerve lesion as an occupational neuropathy in a semiprofessional dancer. Arch Phys Med Rehabil 74:768–769, 1993.
27. Levy P, Roger B, Tardieu M, et al.: Cystic compression of the suprascapular nerve. Value of imaging. Apropos of 6 cases and review of the literature. J Radiol 78:123–130, 1997.
28. Moore TP, Fritts HM, Quick DC, et al.: Suprascapular nerve entrapment caused by supraglenoid cyst compression. J Shoulder Elbow Surg 6:455–462, 1997.
29. Murakami T, Ohtani O, and Outi H: Suprascapular nerve with cutaneous branch to the upper arm. Acta Anat Nippon 52:96, 1977.

30. Piatt BE, Hawkins RJ, Fritz RC, et al.: Clinical evaluation and treatment of spinoglenoid notch ganglion cysts. J Shoulder Elbow Surg 11:600–604, 2002.

31. Post M: Diagnosis and treatment of suprascapular nerve entrapment. Clin Orthop 368:92–100, 1999.

32. Rachbauer F, Sterzinger W, and Frischhut B: Suprascapular nerve entrapment at the spinoglenoid notch caused by a ganglion cyst. J Shoulder Elbow Surg 5:150–152, 1996.

33. Rengachary SS, Burr D, Lucas S, et al.: Suprascapular entrapment neuropathy: a clinical, anatomical, and comparative study. Part 3: comparative study. Neurosurgery 5:452–455, 1979.

34. Rengachary SS, Neff JP, Singer PA, et al.: Suprascapular entrapment neuropathy: a clinical, anatomical, and comparative study. Part 1: clinical study. Neurosurgery 5:441–446, 1979.

35. Ringel SP, Treihaft M, Carry M, et al.: Suprascapular neuropathy in pitchers. Am J Sports Med 18:80–86, 1990.

36. Rochwerger A, Franceschi J, and Groulier P: Cyst of the coracoid notch causing compression of the suprascapular nerve in a sportsman. J Bone Joint Surg [Br] 79(Suppl I):44, 1997.

37. Rollenhagen BL and Reeder MT: Musculoskeletal-football 617. Med Sci Sports Exerc 29:108, 1997.

38. Spinner RJ, Tiel RL, and Kline DG: Predominant infraspinatus muscle weakness in suprascapular nerve compression. J Neurosurg 93:516, 2000.

39. Takagishi K, Maeda K, Ikeda T, et al.: Ganglion causing paralysis of the suprascapular nerve. Diagnosis by MRI and ultrasonography. Acta Orthop Scand 62:391–393, 1991.

40. Van Zandijcke M and Casselman J: Suprascapular nerve entrapment at the spinoglenoid notch due to a ganglion cyst. J Neurol Neurosurg Psychiatry 66:245, 1999.

41. Victor M and Ropper AH: Adams and Victor's Diseases of the Peripheral Nerves. New York, McGraw Hill, 1997:1432.

42. Visser CP, Coene LN, Brand R, et al.: The incidence of nerve injury in anterior dislocation of the shoulder and its influence on functional recovery. A prospective clinical and EMG study. J Bone Joint Surg [Br] 81:679–685, 1999.

43. Weinfeld AB, Cheng J, Nath RK, et al.: Topographic mapping of the superior transverse scapular ligament: a cadaver study to facilitate suprascapular nerve decompression. Plast Reconstr Surg 110:774–779, 2002.

44. Witvrouw E, Cools A, Lysens R, et al.: Suprascapular neuropathy in volleyball players. Br J Sports Med 34:174–180, 2000.

45. Wong P, Bertouch JV, Murrell GA, et al.: An unusual cause of shoulder pain. Ann Rheum Dis 58:264–265, 1999.

46. Yu JS and Fischer RA: Denervation atrophy caused by suprascapular nerve injury: MR findings. J Comput Assist Tomogr 21:302–303, 1997.

47. Zeiss J, Woldenberg LS, Saddemi SR, et al.: MRI of suprascapular neuropathy in a weight lifter. J Comput Assist Tomogr 17:303–308, 1993.

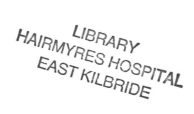

14

Lacerations of the brachial plexus

Daniel H. Kim and Judith A. Murovic

OVERVIEW

- If the mechanism of injury is penetrating or cutting and functional loss is complete in the distribution of one or more elements of the brachial plexus, continuity may still be maintained in one or more of the elements exhibiting distal loss. In some cases, this is because of partial transection of the element(s); in others, it results from contusion without partial division. If possible, these lesions are best treated in a delayed fashion so that intraoperative nerve action potential (NAP) studies can be used to document the presence or absence of regeneration or recovery.

- If the mechanism of injury is sharp, circumstances mandate early repair within 72 hours after injury. Sorting out brachial plexus injuries at the time of soft tissue or vascular repair is more straightforward than after delay and the onset of scarring. Length is not lost to retraction and an end-to-end suture anastomosis repair can almost always be achieved after minimal trimming of each stump. As a result, outcome in this category for the Louisiana State University Health Sciences Center (LSUHSC) series of brachial plexus lacerations is one of the best of all plexus injuries, even for elements generally viewed as unfavorable for repair. Delay in referral led to secondary suture or was more likely to make grafts necessary in this category. Such repairs did not fare as well as the primary end-to-end suture anastomosis repairs.

- Injury in which transection of one or more brachial plexus elements is thought to be caused by a blunt mechanism is best managed surgically after a delay of several weeks. This gives time for delineation of the extent of injury to the proximal and distal stumps of the plexus so that both can be trimmed back to healthy tissue. With time, transected plexus stumps retract; therefore, if acute exploration for vascular or soft tissue repair presents the opportunity, stumps should be "tacked down" to maintain length. At the time of secondary repair, end-to-end suture anastomosis repair is thus likely to be achieved. Grafts were often necessary in this subset, and results were not as good as those for end-to-end suture anastomosis repair either in this blunt mechanism category or with sharp transection if repair was delayed.

- If early operation for suspected vascular injury is carried out, it is very important to isolate and to protect the neural structures which are not only injured themselves, but are often adherent to the involved vessels.

INTRODUCTION

A laceration of the tissues surrounding the brachial plexus has the potential to transect a portion of the plexus, which happens more frequently, or at times the entire brachial plexus. Transecting injuries tend to be either sharp, which prompts an acute neural repair, or blunt, which can be repaired in a delayed manner.[1,5,10,23,25]

Mechanisms responsible for lacerations of the brachial plexus in the series from Louisiana State University Health Sciences Center (LSUHSC) included injuries from knives and glass, which were classified as sharp and accounted for injuries to 83 plexal elements. Most knife wounds (Fig. 14-1) resulted from criminal acts perpetrated by others and were inflicted with kitchen or hunting knives. Glass injuries (Fig. 14-2) were caused by falls through glass windows and by exploding glass in factory or automobile accidents.

Injuries from auto metal fragments, fan or motor blades, and chain saws were classified as blunt and occurred in 61 plexus elements (Fig. 14-3). More focal penetrations of the neck or shoulder leading to brachial plexus injury from mechanisms such as animal bites have been included under the blunt laceration category.

A variety of vascular lesions associated with penetrating injuries of the brachial plexus have been described in the literature.[7,20,21,25] In the LSUHSC series included in this chapter, one-third of the laceration category injuries were explored acutely because of clinically suspected or angiographically proven vascular injuries. These vascular injuries included partial or complete transections of major vessels with hematomas. Pseudoaneurysms or arteriovenous fistulae were not seen acutely, but were found in several patients explored in a delayed fashion.

PRINCIPLES OF MANAGEMENT

The fundamental goal of managing lacerating injuries of the brachial plexus is to establish an accurate diagnosis as soon as possible and attempt to improve the prognosis. This requires the urgent restoration of circulation, stabilization of associated fractures, adequate exposure of lesions due to lacerations with operative physiological monitoring and relatively early nerve repair. Surgeons should also

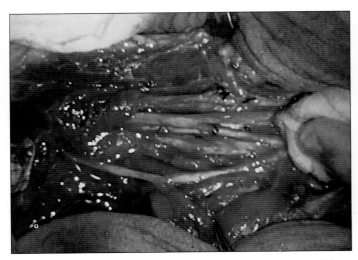

FIGURE 14-1 This supraclavicular plexus was totally transected by a knife. It was repaired with end-to-end suture anastomosis relatively acutely. Stumps required minimal trimming, and there was no tension while performing the repair.

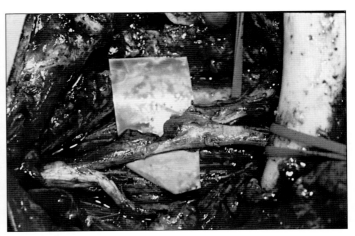

FIGURE 14-2 A partial transection of a brachial plexus upper trunk by a shard of glass is seen here. Due to a delayed referral, surgery was performed some weeks post-injury. A split repair was carried out using sural nerve grafts.

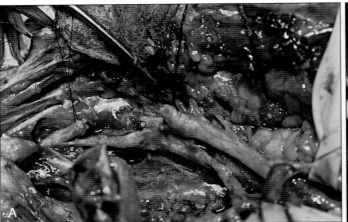

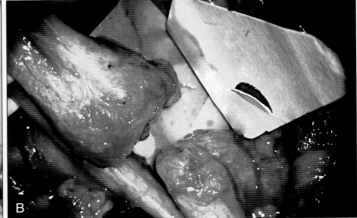

FIGURE 14-3 **(A)** The plexus had been transected bluntly near the clavicle, which was divided to provide this exposure. **(B)** A more sharply transected plexus element is seen in another patient.

be aware of laceration-associated vascular injuries because their incidence is higher in open wounds.

Thorough and repeated physical examinations are necessary to detect progressive injuries to the head, chest, and abdomen associated with lacerating injuries of the brachial plexus. When there is clinical suspicion of damage to the aortic arch, arteriography is essential, since it must be remembered that a knife does not respect tissue planes. Angiography is not always necessary before urgent surgery, however. An arterial injury associated with a lacerating injury to the brachial plexus is indicated by frank bleeding from an open wound; an expanding swelling with or without a bruit suggests an arteriovenous fistula. The clinical diagnosis of rupture of the axillary artery in a high-energy closed infraclavicular lacerating lesion is usually straightforward. The posterior triangle of the neck is not swollen, but there is an enlarging swelling below the clavicle and the subclavian pulse can be felt, though there is no brachial pulse. In such a case, angiography might cause an unnecessary delay before exploration and vascular repair.

The presence of a Tinel sign elicited by tapping the supraclavicular area can be quite useful in differentiating between spinal nerve transection or rupture and root avulsion.[15] A positive Tinel sign, which is perceived by the patient as tingling in an anesthetic arm or hand, usually indicates transection or rupture rather than avulsion.

A less contaminated wound allows primary repair of all structures; thus, a sharp nerve transection in a stable, clean soft-tissue environment can be treated successfully by primary end-to-end suture anastomosis repair or, less frequently, by graft repair. Standard techniques are used, i.e. epineurial or grouped fascicular repair with fascicular coaptation. Minimal suture material is utilized to reduce the chance of fibrosis at the juncture. The principles of nerve repair dictate that the coaptation of severed ends be free of interposed fibrous or other soft tissue and be without tension at the repair site. The early and competent repair of clean stab wounds involving C5 to C7 (Fig. 14-4) can confidently be expected to yield a return of function to close to normal levels. Under these circum-

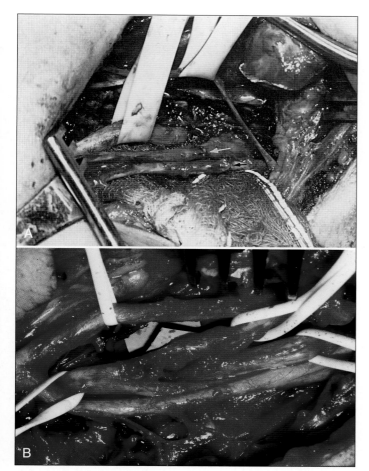

FIGURE 14-4 (A) These C5 (*black arrow*) and C6 (*white arrow*) spinal nerves were transected by a knife wound at the point where they unite to form the upper trunk. They were repaired 4 hours after injury by end-to-end suture anastomosis repair with 6–0 prolene. **(B)** A stab wound that involved the middle trunk of the plexus (*arrow*) is seen in this intraoperative photograph and was explored at 1 month. This lesion was resected, and an end-to-end suture anastomosis repair was performed. This lesion could have been repaired acutely had there been the opportunity to do so.

stances, however, even an accurate repair of C8 and T1 results in some, but far from normal, recovery of hand function.

The treatment of the severely contaminated wound on the other hand, requires an entirely different approach. The principles of treatment, as defined by Robert Jones, were implemented by surgeons in the First World War and included debridement, wound excision, and delayed primary closure. The wound was never closed primarily.

The course of action followed at the present time includes stabilization of the skeleton, which is achieved for the humerus by an external fixator, restoration of the circulation by a reversed vein graft tunneled away from the wound, and adequate wound debridement. At 48 hours, a second examination of the wound should lead to further debridement. Necrotic bone must be removed and the wound may then be ready for closure, preferably by a myocutaneous flap. In such cases, nerves should be repaired only after all dead tissue has been debrided and the risk of sepsis has been overcome.

The methods and techniques employed to treat the nerve lesion include neurolysis, primary or delayed end-to-end suture anastomosis repair, nerve grafting, and nerve transfer. If restoration of function to the injured nerve is deemed impossible, tendon transfers and joint stabilization procedures may be considered and, in certain severe cases, amputation and a prosthetic fitting may be necessary.

Neurolysis is usually performed when operative inspection and nerve action potential (NAP) recording indicate function or the potential for it. Releasing the nerve from a scarred bed and providing a favorable soft tissue environment may help to support axonal regrowth.

With transections, thorough debridement of the ends back to healthy nerve tissue is also a prerequisite for success. Following debridement, mobilization of the proximal and distal stumps can overcome 2–3 cm gaps, permitting repair without tension. Some alignment of the fascicles is also important. This is best accomplished by the gross inspection and matching of proximal and distal topographies using longitudinally oriented blood vessels at an epineurial level. Special staining techniques are available for the identification of sensory and motor fascicles within the nerve to enable more precise alignment.[26]

Direct repair may not be feasible because of loss of nerve tissue. This may be the result of the traumatic injury itself, the resection of a large neuroma in continuity, or the debridement of fibrotic stumps, all of which can create a gap greater than 3 cm.[17] Under these conditions, attempted repair will create undue tension at the repair site and result in a subsequent suboptimal outcome. Nerve grafting provides the solution to this situation because the results of a properly performed nerve graft far exceed those of an improperly performed direct repair. Factors that affect the success of nerve grafting include the length of the graft segment, adequacy of the soft tissue bed for vascular invasion, graft survival, and the time from injury to grafting.[18]

Dunkerton and Boome summarized their experience with 64 stab wounds of the brachial plexus and recommended grafting even in early injury cases.[5] They concluded that primary nerve grafting produced better results than end-to-end anastomotic suture repair, even in fresh cases. They also deduced that lesions of the C5 and C6 roots recovered better than those of more distal roots or spinal nerves. At LSUHSC, however, end-to-end anastomotic suture repair is favored when it can be performed with minimal tension.

Common sources of nerve grafts include sural, lateral antebrachial cutaneous, and the anterior division of the medial antebrachial cutaneous nerves. Other donor sources include the sensory branch of the radial nerve and the posterior cutaneous nerve of the arm.

Vascularized nerve grafting has been performed in an attempt to limit failure related to ischemic change of a long graft, particularly when the bed is poorly vascularized and scarred. A vascularized nerve graft diminishes endoneurial scarring by maintaining the Schwann cell population and decreasing fibroblast infiltration, both of which lead to an increased rate of axonal regeneration.[4] A variety of donor sites have been described for the vascularized nerve graft. Doi et al. used a vascularized sural nerve graft based on either the cutaneous branch of the peroneal artery or the muscular perforating branch of the posterior tibial artery, and recommended a vascularized nerve graft for a nerve gap of more than 6 cm.[4] Gailliot and Core[6] described the vascularized serratus anterior intercostal nerve graft, and Koshima et al.[14] reported the use of a free vascularized deep peroneal nerve graft with anterior tibial vessels. Because of the time required for these procedures and the limited clinical series, vascularized nerve grafts should be considered as a salvage procedure only.

GRADING NEURAL FUNCTION

In the LSUHSC series of lacerations of the brachial plexus, preoperative neural function was graded for each individual plexus element and then the grades for the involved elements were combined and averaged (Table 14-1).[13] The LSUHSC grading system was used to give more extensive functional recovery classifications than the British Medical Research Council (MRC) system, as well as being a precise method for evaluating both proximal and distal recovery of motor function.

Postoperative recovery grades ranging from 0 to 5 for the various patterns of brachial plexus laceration injuries were also calculated for each element and were aggregated and averaged to obtain the overall grade. Successful outcomes were defined as grade 3 or higher and good and excellent recoveries were represented by grades 4 and 5, respectively.

ELECTROPHYSIOLOGICAL STUDIES

After transection of a nerve, the distal stump can transmit stimuli to muscle and involve muscle contraction for up to 72 hours. Axonal discontinuity results not only in predictable pathological features, but also in time-related electrical changes that parallel the pathophysiology of denervation. Wallerian degeneration results in the emergence of spontaneous electrical discharges or fibrillations

that appear at least 3 weeks after the injury; therefore, a needle electromyogram should be postponed for several weeks. In addition to fibrillations, larger potentials, that are denervation potentials, can be seen. With time and successful regeneration, the number of fibrillations and denervation potentials decrease, and nascent potentials may be present.

A needle electromyogram of the paraspinal muscles, which are innervated by the dorsal rami of the spinal roots, should also be routinely performed, since denervation of these muscles provides strong evidence of avulsion of the corresponding roots.

Some surgeons find the use of intraoperative somatosensory evoked potentials (SSEPs) useful to verify a suspected avulsion of a root or to determine whether resection of a neuroma and interposition nerve grafting should be performed.[8,12,19] The advocates of this intraoperative electrophysiological technique believe that root avulsion is definitely excluded only if direct stimulation of the individual surgically exposed nerve root elicits reproducible cortical somatosensory evoked potentials.[16]

Others believe that intraoperative transcranial electrical motor evoked potentials can be of use in assessing the connectivity of the roots to the spinal cord.[27] Intraoperative stimulation proximal to a lesion in continuity may produce muscle contraction distally, which implies there are some fibers in continuity. Lack of response implies either discontinuity or insufficient time for regenerating axons to have reached their designated organs. Therefore, the use of intraoperative bipolar stimulating and recording electrodes to identify

Table 14-1 The LSUHSC* grading system by element of brachial plexus

Overall grading		
Grade	Evaluation	Description
0	Absent	No muscle contraction
1	Poor	Proximal muscles contract but not against gravity
2	Fair	Proximal muscles contract against gravity and distal muscles do not contract; sensory grade, if applicable, is usually <2
3	Moderate	Proximal muscles contract against gravity and some resistance; some distal muscles contact against gravity; sensory grade, if applicable is usually 3
4	Good	All muscles contract against gravity and some resistance; sensory grade, if applicable, is 3 or 4
5	Excellent	All muscles contract against moderate resistance; sensory grade, if applicable, 4
Sensory grading		
Grade	Evaluation	Description
0	Absent	No response to touch, pin, or pressure
1	Poor	Testing produces hyperesthesias or paresthesias; deep pain recovery in autonomous zones
2	Fair	Sensory response sufficient for grip and slow protection, sensory stimuli mislocalized with some overresponse
3	Moderate	Response to touch and pin in autonomous zones, sensation mislocalized and not normal, with overresponse
4	Good	Response to touch and pin in autonomous zones, response localized but not normal; however, there is no overresponse
5	Excellent	Near-normal response to touch and pin in entire field of plexus element including autonomous zones; stimuli were accurately localized

*LSUHSC, Louisiana State University Health Sciences Center.

propagation of an action potential along the course of a nerve is very helpful. The electrodes are held 3–6 cm apart and the point distally where the action potential is lost represents the most proximal extent of the lesion. Resection of the neuroma and nerve graft are required to restore continuity and the potential for return (Fig. 14-5).

As the result of experience with both SSEP and NAP recordings at LSUHSC, currently the latter is used almost exclusively for lacerations in continuity (Fig. 14-6), gunshot wounds (GSWs), and supra- (Fig. 14-7) and infraclavicular stretch injuries.

RESULTS

There were 71 patients with lacerations involving the brachial plexus examined at LSUHSC and 201 plexus elements were judged to be seriously injured. Brachial plexus lacerations were either sharp and caused by knives or glass, or blunt and caused by automobile metal, fan and motor blades, chain saws, or animal bites. One-third of patients with lacerating injuries to the brachial plexus underwent acute surgical exploration because of suspected or angiographically proven vascular injuries. Sharp transections accounted for injuries of 83 plexus elements and blunt transections, 61 (Table 14-2). There were 57 plexus elements in 20 patients in whom the lesions were in some degree of continuity, despite a lacerating or penetrating mechanism.

Twenty-six elements were associated with a positive NAP across the lesion and were treated with neurolysis. Of these 26 elements, 24 (92%) recovered to a grade 3 or better level of function. Nine elements in which the NAP recording showed no transmission beyond a lesion in continuity were treated with delayed suture anastomosis repair. Of these nine elements, seven (78%) recovered to a grade 3 or better level of function. Graft repair was performed on 22 other elements, 17 (77%) of which recovered to a similar functional grade. This level of function was achieved in 48 (84%) of the 57 involved elements.

When referrals were expedited and surgery occurred within 72 hours, the outcome was favorable for 83 sharp transections. Twenty-five (81%) of 31 primary suture anastomotic repairs recovered to a grade 3 or better level of function. Due to delays in referral or transport, the repair of 40 sharply transected elements was delayed (Fig. 14-8). In this group, in which graft rather than suture was necessary because of stump retraction, the overall recovery rate was 53%. Of 12 elements in which end-to-end-anastomotic suture repair was delayed, 8 (67%) did well. Overall, a grade 3 or better level of function was achieved in 54 (65%) of the 83 involved elements.

Repairs were delayed by choice in lesions from blunt transections because the extent of damage was initially difficult to assess accurately. Thus, 56 of 61 blunt transections required graft repair of which 25 (45%) had a grade 3 or better functional outcome. Secondary suture was possible in only five cases and three (60%) of these had this level of functional recovery. In this category, the overall recovery of grade 3 or better levels of function was 28 (46%) of 61.

RECOMMENDATIONS

Primary, i.e. acute, repair is advised for sharply transected plexus elements, whereas secondary, or delayed repair is reserved for bluntly transected injuries (Fig. 14-9) or for those suspected to be

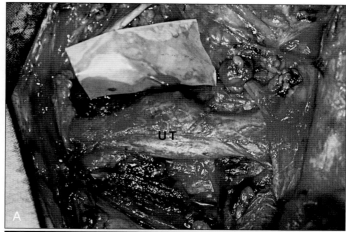
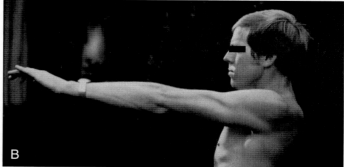
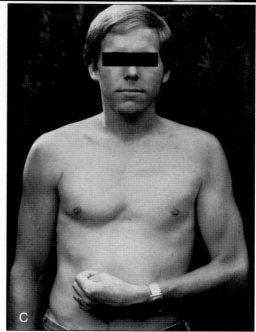

FIGURE 14-5 **(A)** A large left upper trunk neuroma is shown, which resulted from a partial laceration due to a chain saw injury. The lesion was explored and repaired secondarily at 1 month using sural nerve grafts. The patient experienced restitution of grade 4 function in the arm **(B, C)**.

in continuity.[13] Most authors agree that urgent repair is indicated for sharp lacerations of the plexus, especially if the loss of function is complete in the distribution of one or more elements.[2,22,24,26] The advantages of such primary or acute repair for sharply transected plexus injuries are numerous.[3,11] Epineurial suture is more likely to

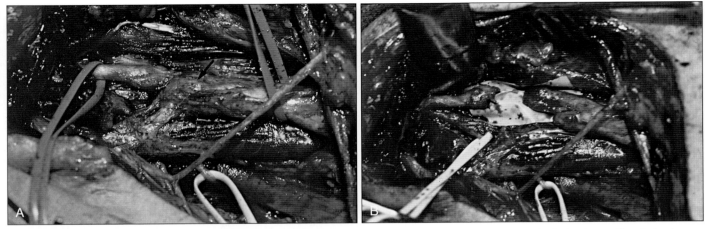

FIGURE 14-6 **(A)** A penetrating glass wound that involved the upper trunk (*arrow*) and left the plexus in continuity is shown. The darker loop to the left is around C5, and the white loop to the right is pulling a more superficial sensory nerve laterally. **(B)** Despite gross continuity, this was a complete lesion that did not transmit an NAP. As a result, it was resected, and in this intraoperative photograph, stumps are shown prior to a graft repair.

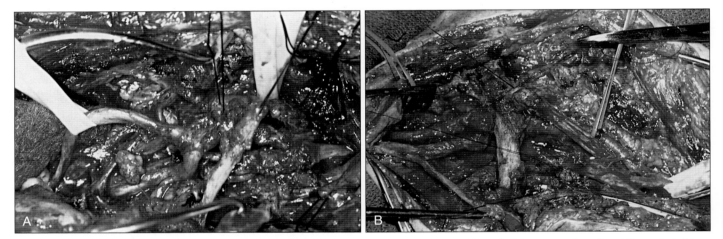

FIGURE 14-7 **(A)** A transection of the supraclavicular plexus caused by a chain saw is seen. The clavicle was sectioned and the ends held apart by a Gelpi retractor. The trunks are to the right and the cords to the left. Surgical exposure was made 1 month after injury because this was a blunt transection. An end-to-end suture anastomosis repair was achieved by trimming the proximal and distal stumps with mobilization of the cord, cord-to-nerve segments, and trunks to make up length. The sectioned clavicle was then pinned. **(B)** In another chain saw injury shown here, the plexus was also totally divided, but repair was undertaken without sectioning the clavicle. Grafts were necessary, however.

Table 14-2 Outcomes of surgery for 71 patients with brachial plexus lacerations

	In continuity	Sharp transection	Blunt transection	Totals
No. of operative plexus cases	20	28	23	71
No. of plexus elements	57	83	61	201
Neurolysis/results	26/24	0/0	0/0	26/24
Primary suture results	0/0	31/25	0/0	31/25
Secondary suture/results	9/7	12/8	5/3	26/18
Secondary graft/results	22/17	40/21	56/25	118/63
Total elements/results	57/48	83/54	61/28	201/130

Primary, repair within 72 hours of injury; secondary, delayed repair after several weeks; No., number; NAPs, nerve action potentials.

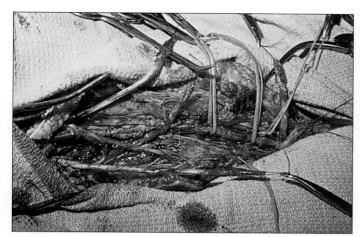

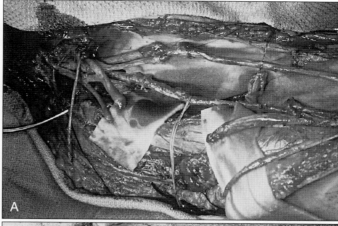

FIGURE 14-8 This intraoperative photograph shows a sharp transection of the plexus at a cord level that was repaired in a delayed fashion, but might have been more readily addressed at the time of the acute arterial repair. An end-to-end suture anastomosis repair of each element was obtained with the help of proximal and distal plexus neurolysis and mobilization.

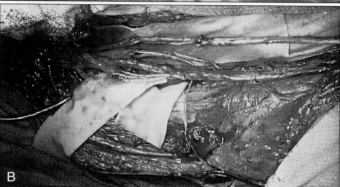

FIGURE 14-9 **(A)** A propeller injury that had transected the plexus in a blunt fashion at the cord-to-nerve level is seen in this intraoperative photograph. The clavicle is to the left, and the hand is to right. The loop surrounds the axillary-to-brachial artery segment, which had required an acute repair. **(B)** Because of retraction, as well as the need to trim the stumps of the neuromas, grafts shown here were necessary when the injury was repaired at 3.5 months.

be possible than graft repair. In this series, better outcomes were achieved in patients with sharp injuries who received only an end-to-end suture anastomosis repair compared with patients whose surgical treatment was delayed, resulting in the need for grafts. As with GSWs to the brachial plexus, early intervention is indicated for increasing neurological deficit, which can be associated with a progressive pain syndrome. This presentation may be due to a hematoma, arteriovenous fistula, or pseudoaneurysm. As pointed out by Sunderland,[9,26] follow-up beyond 5 years in this group of patients and in the GSW series gives occasional evidence of sustained late regeneration.

If repair is to be delayed because of a blunt injury, then stumps should be "tacked down" by suture to adjacent fascial or muscle planes so that retraction is lessened and secondary repair can be achieved by epineurial suture repair rather than by graft repair.[9,11] Delay of repair for blunt injuries permits the damage in each stump to delimit itself. It then becomes apparent how much resection is needed to provide healthy tissue for anastomosis. The disadvantage of delaying repair is that the nerve may retract and lose some of its elasticity if it has not been "tacked down" acutely, in which case graft repair becomes necessary.

In the LSUHSC series, the value of primary or acute repair in carefully selected sharply injured cases is quite evident. This may also be due in part to the fact that these elements had a less severe up-and-down injury than the blunt transections. Nonetheless, elements sutured end-to-end in a delayed fashion, if this could be achieved, did almost as well. Graft repairs fared less well, but this again can be also attributed to the fact that these were more serious injuries.

CASE SUMMARY – LACERATIONS OF THE BRACHIAL PLEXUS

This 18-year-old, right-handed woman was stabbed from behind in the left paracervical area with a long knife. She immediately noticed absence of movement of the shoulder girdle and loss of elbow flexion. The entrance wound was sutured at her local hospital. Cervical spine X-ray films and a computed tomography (CT) scan showed fractures of the left C5 and C6 transverse processes

and some of the facet structures, and CT myelography showed poor filling of the left C6 root sleeve.

When examined 3 months after injury, the patient had total paralysis of the left supraspinatus, infraspinatus, deltoid, biceps, brachioradialis, and supinator muscles. The remaining muscles of the left upper extremity were functioning, but were slightly weak and there was no Horner's sign. Because of the proximal and complete injury of the C5 and C6 nerve roots, it was decided to explore the plexus by a posterior subscapular approach and spinal nerves and trunks were thus exposed from behind. The elements were scarred but still in continuity, although the upper trunk was reduced to scarred threads of neurofibrous tissue. Extensive scar tissue was removed up to and into the neural foramina. During the C4–C5 and C5–C6 foraminotomies, a lacerated vertebral artery was found to be occluded by organized clot and scar. The vessel ends were cauterized. The C5 and C6 roots were injured at the site of their emergence from the dural sac. The C6 nerve root was scarred medial to its dural exit, whereas some fascicular structure remained in the C5 root. Four sural nerve grafts, each 3.8 cm long, were placed between the C5 root and the distal portion of the upper trunk.

The patient's postoperative course was uneventful. Examination at 14 months after repair revealed that the supraspinatus muscle was grade 3, the infraspinatus and deltoid muscles grade 1, and the biceps grade 2, but there was no brachioradialis muscle function. Subsequent follow-up evaluation at 3 years indicated further improvement in shoulder abduction, with the deltoid muscle grade 3 to 4, and forearm flexion (biceps and brachioradialis muscles) were grade 3. She could now use this arm to carry her school books.

REFERENCES

1. Amine AR and Sugar O: Repair of severed brachial plexus: A plea to ER physicians. JAMA 239:1039, 1976.

2. Birch R, Bonney G, and Wynn Parry CB: Surgical Disorders of the Peripheral Nerves. Edinburgh, Churchill Livingstone, 1998:157–207.

3. Brooks DM: Peripheral Nerve Injury. London, HM Stationery Office, 1954.

4. Doi K, Tamaru K, Sakai K, et al.: A comparison of vascularized and conventional sural nerve grafts. J Hand Surg Am 17:670–676, 1992.

5. Dunkerton MC and Boome RS: Stab wounds involving the brachial plexus. A review of operated cases. J Bone Joint Surg [Br] 70:566–570, 1988.

6. Gailliot RV Jr and Core GB: Serratus anterior intercostal nerve graft: A new vascularized nerve graft. Ann Plast Surg 35:26–31, 1995.

7. Galen J, Wiss D, Cantelmo N, et al.: Traumatic pseudoaneurysm of the axillary artery: Report of 3 cases and literature review. J Trauma 24:350–354, 1984.

8. Holland NR and Belzberg AJ: Intraoperative electrodiagnostic testing during cross-chest C7 nerve root transfer. Muscle Nerve 20:903–905, 1997.

9. Kline DG: Perspectives concerning brachial plexus injury and repair. Neurosurg Clin N Am 2:151–164, 1991.

10. Kline DG, Hackett ER: Reappraisal of timing for exploration of civilian peripheral nerve injuries. Surgery 78:54–65, 1975.

11. Kline DG and Hudson AR: Nerve Injuries: Operative Results for Major Nerve Injuries, Entrapments, and Tumors. Philadelphia, WB Saunders, 1995.

12. Kline DG and Hudson AR: Diagnosis of root avulsions. J Neurosurg 87:483–484, 1997.

13. Kline DG and Judice DJ: Operative management of selected brachial plexus lesions. J Neurosurg 58:631–649, 1983.

14. Koshima I, Okumoto K, Umada N, et al.: Free vascularized deep peroneal nerve grafts. J Reconstr Microsurg 12:131–141, 1996.

15. Landi A and Copeland S: Value of the Tinel sign in brachial plexus lesions. Ann R Coll Surg Engl 61:470–471, 1979.

16. Landi A, Copeland SA, Parry CB, et al.: The role of somatosensory evoked potentials and nerve conduction studies in the surgical management of brachial plexus injuries. J Bone Joint Surg [Br] 62:492–496, 1980.

17. Millesi H: Brachial plexus injuries. Management and results. Clin Plast Surg 11:115–120, 1984.

18. Millesi H: Brachial plexus injuries. Nerve grafting. Clin Orthop 237:36–42, 1988.

19. Murase T, Kawai H, Masatomi T, et al.: Evoked spinal cord potentials for diagnosis during brachial plexus surgery. J Bone Joint Surg [Br] 75:775–781, 1993.

20. Nichols IS and Lillehei KO: Nerve injury associated with acute vascular trauma. Surg Clin N Am 68:837–852, 1988.

21. Robbs J and Naidoo K: Vascular compression of brachial plexus following stab injuries to neck (letter). S Afr Med J 60:345–346, 1981.

22. Seddon HJ: Peripheral Nerve Injuries. London, HM Stationery Office, 1954.

23. Seddon H: Surgical Disorders of Peripheral Nerves. Baltimore, Williams & Wilkins, 1972.

24. Spinner RJ and Kline DG: Surgery for peripheral nerve and brachial plexus injuries or other nerve lesions. Muscle Nerve 23:680–695, 2000.

25. Sunderland S: Nerves and Nerve Injuries. New York, Churchill Livingstone, 1978.

26. Sunderland S: Nerve Injuries and Their Repair: A Critical Reappraisal. Edinburgh, Churchill Livingstone, 1991.

27. Turkof E, Millesi H, Turkof R, et al.: Intraoperative electroneurodiagnostics (transcranial electrical motor evoked potentials) to evaluate the functional status of anterior spinal roots and spinal nerves during brachial plexus surgery. Plast Reconstr Surg 99:1632–1641, 1997.

15

Gunshot wounds to the brachial plexus

Daniel H. Kim

OVERVIEW

■ Gunshot wounds (GSWs) to the brachial plexus most often cause lesions in continuity, though about 10% can transect elements.

■ The force associated with the injury varies depending on missile caliber and acceleration, and range at which the firearm was shot.

■ In this series, the criteria used for the selection of neural operation as the mode of treatment were: (1) the loss of function was complete and persistent in the distribution of one or more of the elements, (a) no improvement was detected clinically or by electromyogram in the early months following injury, (b) the loss of function was in the distribution of at least one element usually helped by operation, such as C5, C6, C7, the upper or middle trunk, or the lateral or posterior cords or their outflows, and (c) surgery was not performed on injuries with loss restricted to the lower element(s); other indications for surgery were that there was (2) incomplete loss of function attended by pain that was not alleviated pharmacologically; (3) pseudoaneurysm, clot, or fistula involving the plexus; and (4) true causalgia requiring sympathectomy.

■ Each plexus injury must be evaluated by the element(s) involved and not just according to the plexus as a whole. Incomplete loss in the distribution of an element does not guarantee recovery of others and, moreover, recovery in the distribution of an element does not guarantee recovery of others.

■ Intraoperative nerve action potential (NAP) stimulation and recording studies are important for the identification of those elements needing resection. Although the majority of lesions in continuity with complete preoperative loss of function were treated by resection in the Louisiana State University Health Sciences Center (LSUHSC) series because of the absence of NAPs, a significant number were spared because recordings showed evidence of regeneration.

■ In the LSUHSC series in this chapter, approximately 70% repaired by end-to-end suture anastomosis and more than 50% of lesions repaired by grafts had successful outcomes.

■ The best outcomes were achieved with upper trunk and lateral and posterior cord lesions, but recovery occurred with some C7 to middle trunk and medial cord to median nerve repairs. Results with lower trunk and most medial cord lesions were poor unless early regeneration was proven by intraoperative NAPs, in which case either neurolysis or split repair could be performed.

■ Often, an associated vascular injury will warrant emergency repair. In addition to a transection of a major vessel, GSWs to the

brachial plexus can produce a pseudoaneurysm or arteriovenous fistula, each of which can compress the plexus and produce progressive loss of function and severe pain. Injured elements need to be dissected and gently moved away from the area of vascular repair. It may also be necessary to perform a second operation for NAP stimulation and recording and appropriate neural repair.

■ In the LSUHSC series there was a low incidence of serious complications, but the decision for surgical intervention must always be weighed with the knowledge that complications and poor outcomes are possible. It is also essential that surgery be supplemented by intensive physical therapy, lengthy follow-up, and reconstructive or rehabilitative measures.

■ Surgery is warranted for selected GSWs to the plexus.

INTRODUCTION

Gunshot wounds (GSWs) are the second largest category of injuries involving the brachial plexus following those of stretch/contusion. There has been interest in reporting the management of these intricate lesions during wartime;[4,8,24–26,31] however, there have been fewer cases of GSWs to the brachial plexus reported in times of relative world peace, despite a sizable number of cases related to civil disturbance.[1,2,14,21,23] The management of civilian GSW injuries to the brachial plexus has changed since World War II.[6,11,19,27,28,33] Many elements left in continuity at the time of injury do not improve with time, as was the former philosophy. Successful repair, however, is now possible when indicated since the advent of intraoperative electrical techniques to evaluate lesions in continuity, and the re-emergence of the use of nerve grafts. The necessity for repair and efficacy of neurolysis are now more certain.[16]

To illustrate the current management of GSWs to the brachial plexus, a relatively large series of patients sustaining such injuries between 1968 and 1998 were evaluated at Lousiana State University Health Science Center (LSUHSC). There were one hundred and eighteen patients who sustained GSWs that resulted in 293 plexal element injuries, while 51 patients had GSWs not requiring surgery on the plexus. Patient ages ranged from 18 to 62 years, with a median age of 34 years. Each patient's sex, neurological status, type of injury, presentation, and prior treatment of the injury were recorded before surgery. Electrophysiological studies were conducted preoperatively and these, along with details of the surgical procedure used at LSUHSC, intraoperative electrophysiological and pathological findings, and postoperative functional status, were recorded. The minimum follow-up period was 18 months with a mean follow-up period of 42 months. Most of the 293 surgically treated plexal elements had some gross continuity when surgically exposed. Of the 118 patients with plexus injuries, who had surgical intervention, 12 cases (10%) had lower root and trunk injuries.

Most wounds in the LSUHSC civilian series were from bullets, but some were from shell fragments, and all were caused by handguns, shotguns, and rifles. Included were .22-, .38- and .45-caliber and even .470-magnum wounds. While low-velocity missile injuries may display a significant return of function within a few months,[35] many of the LSUHSC penetrating missiles, although of small caliber, had relatively high velocities. Thus, many cases in which high-velocity missiles were involved failed to recover spontaneously in the LSUHSC cases, although the older literature concerning GSWs to the brachial plexus emphasizes that many such lesions do so.[5,30] Because soft tissue damage relates not only to missile or fragment size, but also to the cube of its velocity, damage to nerve and other structures was extensive, just as with war-time injuries.[3,7,12] About half of the wounds were associated with crimes, and the rest were related to hunting accidents or, more frequently, to poor handling of weapons. About one-sixth of these wounds were inflicted during unsuccessful suicide attempts.

The initial management of GSWs resulting in plexus-related palsies in general, and also for patients in the LSUHSC series, consists of three main components: local wound care, tetanus toxoid administration, and the institution of antibiotics.

Many patients had angiography in an effort to rule out vascular injury and this was often performed even in the absence of any clinical signs of vascular compromise (Fig. 15-1A). In some cases, there had been a hospital or institutional policy that made angiography a requirement for any patient with a penetrating wound of the neck or shoulder; however, not every patient having relatively acute exploration for suspected vascular injury had undergone prior angiography. In some cases, persistent wound bleeding, usually of an arterial nature, an expanding soft tissue hematoma, or an absent radial pulse with or without other findings suggesting vascular injury had led to acute exploration.

ASSOCIATED INJURIES

There was a high incidence of associated injuries with the LSUHSC series of GSWs to the brachial plexus, and these associated injuries had relatively acute operations for their repair (Fig. 15-1B). Vascular injuries and their exploration for repair were the most frequent concomitant insults requiring acute procedures and were of two categories.

The first category of vascular injury was the larger and included those explorations performed acutely for suspected major vascular interruption. Indications for exploration included: (1) a penetrating wound of the neck, shoulder, or upper arm; (2) diminished or absent brachial or radial pulses; (3) a cool hand; (4) an expanding mass or sizable hematoma; (5) persistent bleeding from the wound; and (6) progressive swelling of a distal extremity due to ischemia or venous insufficiency. In most of these cases, in the LSUHSC patients, angiography performed before an operation had demonstrated vessel compromise or occlusion. Some wounds, however, with suspected vascular injury as well as injury to nerve were explored acutely without preoperative angiography, usually because of persistent bleeding from the wound or an expanding hematoma. Repairs to major arteries varied from simple suture repairs to the use of vein or synthetic graft replacements. The status of the plexal elements was not consistently noted when a wound was explored in an emergent fashion. In a few cases, acute repair of transected neural elements was attempted, but as subsequent studies or operation suggested, this seldom led to a good result. In some cases, transected elements were "tacked down" to adjacent fascial planes. This technique appeared to be effective in maintaining the length of the neural structures. Unfortunately, secondary operation for plexus repair sometimes revealed that neural elements had been incorporated by suture into the vascular repair.

The second category of vascular injury was pseudoaneurysm, which was less frequent, harder to diagnose, and not easy to treat. Diagnosis was usually suspected because of: (1) pain increasing in intensity and duration; (2) progressive neural loss; (3) the presence of a thrill and/or bruit; and (4) a palpable mass. A positive angiogram for a pseudoaneurysm showed irregularity or roughening of a portion of most commonly the axillary artery, without contrast-filling of the aneurysm. At exploration, a large mass of variably organized and often encapsulated clot was found encircling usually the axillary artery and displacing the cords and cord-to-nerve

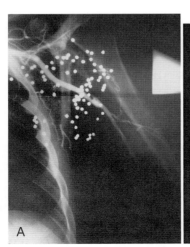
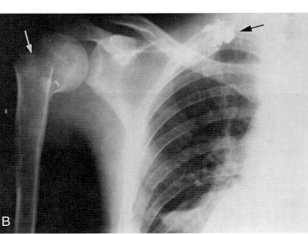

FIGURE 15-1 **(A)** An angiogram of a patient with a shotgun injury to the left brachial plexus. **(B)** A chest and shoulder plain X-ray of a patient with severe plexus palsy. Missile fragments are noted by the black arrow and a humeral fracture by the white arrow.

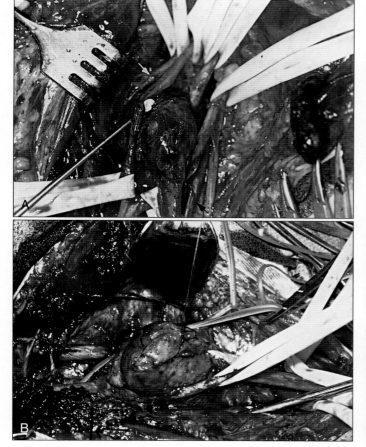

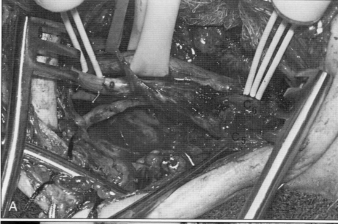

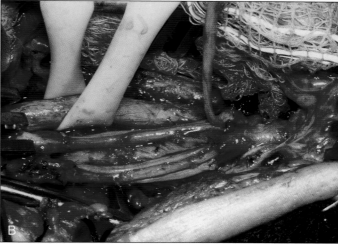

FIGURE 15-2 **(A)** A pseudoaneurysm of the axillary artery secondary to a gunshot wound can be seen. The dissector is beneath the lateral cord contribution to the median nerve. The medial cord contribution traveled beneath the more distal axillary artery in this case. The ulnar nerve is marked by a black arrow and the musculocutaneous nerve by a white arrow. This was a severe stretch injury of the lateral and medial cord contributions to the median nerve and the posterior cord. Most of the loss was reversed by removal of the pseudoaneurysm and neurolysis of the plexus. **(B)** A large organized clot associated with another pseudoaneurysm caused by a gunshot wound is seen. In this case, some of the cord and cord-to-nerve elements required repair after resection of the pseudoaneurysm.

FIGURE 15-3 **(A)** A missile wound injury to C5, C6, and the upper trunk. Function had not improved clinically or electrically by 5 months after injury. Operative stimulation and recording showed only a small nerve action potential from a portion of the C6 outflow to the upper trunk. This was split off and spared resection; the rest of the C6 and all of the C5 outflow to the upper trunk were replaced by grafts. **(B)** One graft remains to be attached distally.

connections of the plexus (Fig. 15-2). To isolate and gain control of the proximal and distal axillary artery and the profundus, i.e. deep brachial vessel, dissection of these vessels above, below, and distally was required. The covering of the organized clot could then be opened after dissecting the neural elements free from its capsule. Repair of the vessel was usually straightforward, i.e. the vascular rent was oversewn in most instances, but occasionally had to be patched by a portion of a vein. Interposition vein graft repair was sometimes needed, but only rarely.

In a study completed and reported in 1989 from LSUHSC, 141 patients with GSWs to the brachial plexus were evaluated.[16] Thirty vascular procedures had been performed in 90 cases that eventually had surgery due to severe neural loss or pain. This incidence of vascular procedures was much lower for the supra- than for the infraclavicular lesions and much higher in those requiring neural operation than in the 51 patients not having surgery. Either venous or synthetic vascular grafts were placed in 24 cases. Other associ-

ated injuries in this series required orthopedic procedures in the early days after injury. These associated operations included six for proximal humeral or glenohumeral joint fractures (Fig. 15-3) and several relatively acute repairs of comminuted clavicular fractures. Several other patients required clavicular stabilization at the time of neural repair by either pinning or wiring. The severity of injury in this group of plexus patients is further supported by the fact that eight required early thoracotomy and six others required placement of a chest tube.

Stewart and Birch[32] in their series of missile injuries to the brachial plexus also found that major vascular lesions (24%) and chest injuries (38%) predominated. Three patients underwent emergency neurovascular repair. One other patient required repair of an esophageal laceration and another of a pharyngeal wound. Five patients required stabilization of humeral or clavicular fractures. Injury to the spinal cord occurred in three patients and two others with complete plexal lesions had an associated intradural injury and the other had a Brown-Séquard syndrome due to spinal cord injury.

PAIN MANAGEMENT

Management of pain is difficult in GSWs to the brachial plexus and was also an issue in the LSUHSC series of cases. There were a few patients who had true causalgias, who were helped permanently by repeated sympathetic blocks, or temporarily by sympathetic blocks, but required eventual cervical sympathectomy for more permanent relief. These patients with causalgia had severe pain and also autonomic disturbances, usually in the hand. More importantly, they could not stand to have the hand touched or manipulated, even if their attention was distracted. Most of these patients had had a trial of phenoxybenzamine or similar sympatholytic agents and such management had failed. Others authors have had greater success with such a pharmacological approach to causalgia associated with GSWs.[12,15]

More difficult to manage than the patients with causalgia in this series were those with severe dysesthesias and often some degree of hyperpathia. These patients had severe neuritic pain, rather than pain related to the sympathetic system. Nonetheless, manipulation of the sympathetic system had often been tried elsewhere, but usually had failed. Some of these patients were helped by a combination of sympatholytic agents and further time. Nevertheless, some patients had operations a number of months after injury for pain of a noncausalgic nature in the hope that neurolysis and manipulation of the plexus would help their pain syndrome. Half of the time such an approach did just that, but the other half of the time, it did not.

The institution of range of motion exercises as early as possible was an important step in the management of all cases. If paralysis was incomplete, a more structured, regular system of physical therapy was instituted.

Three distinct patterns of severe pain have been recognized by other authors, which include neurostenalgia, post-traumatic neuralgia, and central pain.[32] Neurostenalgia is pain caused by persistent compression, distortion, tethering, or ischemia of a nerve. The rapid relief of neurostenalgia after liberating nerve trunks from an entrapment in scar tissue or callus, or after removal of a missile fragment, is characteristic. Post-traumatic neuralgia is pain which occurs after a nerve injury that is usually partial in nature. It is not sympathetic in origin and does not respond to a sympathetic block or sympatholytic agents. It usually responds to a local anesthetic block of a nerve trunk proximal to the lesion. Central pain is from injury to the roots of the brachial plexus central to the dorsal root ganglion in their intradural course, or from injury to the spinal cord itself. Interestingly, in a recent publication regarding the above pain patterns, repair of the nerve and vascular lesions abolished, or significantly relieved, severe pain in 33 of 35 patients (94%) with various types of pain patterns.[32]

Another alternative for pain control is the dorsal root entry zone (DREZ) procedure, which in a long-term study showed satisfactory results.[29] Amputation for pain control is rarely required and, if carried out, is often not successful.

GRADING OF NEURAL FUNCTION

In the LSUHSC series, preoperative neural function was graded from 0 to 5 for each individual plexal element, and the grades were combined and averaged for the elements involved to give a whole plexus grade (Table 15-1).[19] The LSUHSC grading system was used to give more extensive functional recovery classifications, and it was a more precise method for evaluating both proximal and distal recoveries of motor function than the British Medical Research Council (MRC) system. Each plexus injury had to be evaluated by the element(s) involved and not just according to the plexus as a whole. Incomplete loss or recovery in the distribution of an element does not guarantee recovery of others.[16]

Likewise, postoperative recovery grades using the same grading system for the various patterns of brachial plexus injuries or tumors were calculated for each element and were then combined and averaged to obtain the overall grade. Successful outcomes were defined as grade 3 or higher, and good and excellent recoveries as grades 4 and 5, respectively. If an element was considered irreparable and no attempt had been made to lead outflow from the proximal portion or to neurotize the element, it was excluded from the calculations. Irreparable situations usually correlated with the C8–T1 roots or lower trunk elements. Some grades, therefore, which had been applied to the supraclavicular flail arm series reflect averaged grades for muscles at C5, C6, and C7 only. Despite this, the data still reflect the difficulties encountered in restoring neural function to patients with flail arms.

Each clinical assessment was augmented by radiological and electrodiagnostic studies. Plain X-ray films of the neck and shoulder were important for evaluating associated injuries and the diaphragm level was checked by a review of chest X-ray films. Angiography was performed in some cases of suspected vascular injuries. More than 95% of the patients had undergone preoperative nerve conduction (NCV) studies and electromyographic (EMG) examinations. During surgery all lesions with some degree of physical continuity underwent direct electrical stimulation above and below the lesion, as well as NAP recordings.[17] The results of histological studies of resected neural tissue were correlated with preoperative clinical findings and the results of intraoperative electrical studies. Postoperative follow-up included outpatient visits during which the strengths of individual muscles and muscle groups were graded and EMG examinations were performed. Almost all patients returned for at least one postoperative visit. Further follow-up was accomplished by subsequent visits, telephone calls, and/or contact via mail. In cases in which follow-up beyond 18 months was not possible, the patient's postoperative status was represented by findings from the last documented clinic visit.

PATIENT SELECTION FOR OPERATION

Because most civilian GSWs to the plexus do not transect elements, but rather contuse, bruise, or stretch them, the majority of GSW plexus cases were managed conservatively for 2–5 months (Table 15-2). A thorough baseline clinical examination was essential. Electromyography was deferred for 3–4 weeks. Patients were then re-evaluated on at least one occasion in subsequent months to see if there were clinical signs of reversal of loss or electrical evidence of reinnervation. For this reason, the average injury-to-operative interval was 17 weeks. Since most patients came from states other than Louisiana for their initial evaluation and subsequent operation, these individuals could not always be scheduled at 2–4 months, which was considered to be an optimal interval between injury and operation. The reason for neural operation was usually because loss in the distribution of one or more elements of the plexus failed to improve in the early months after injury and this occurred in the majority of the operative patients (Fig. 15-4). Other indications for surgery were pseudoaneurysm, clot, or fistula compressing or involving the plexus. Remaining indications included

Table 15-1 The LSUHSC grading system by element of brachial plexus

Overall grading		
Grade	**Evaluation**	**Description**
0	Absent	No muscle contraction
1	Poor	Proximal muscles contract, but not against gravity
2	Fair	Proximal muscles contract against gravity and distal muscles do not contract; sensory grade, if applicable, is usually <2
3	Moderate	Proximal muscles contract against gravity and some resistance; some distal muscles contract against gravity; sensory grade, if applicable, is usually 3
4	Good	All muscles contract against gravity and some resistance; sensory grade, if applicable, is 3 or 4
5	Excellent	All muscles contract against moderate resistance; sensory grade, if applicable, is 4
Sensory grading*		
Grade	**Evaluation**	**Description**
0	Absent	No response to touch, pin, or pressure
1	Poor	Testing produces hyperesthesia or paresthesias; deep pain recovery in autonomous zones
2	Fair	Sensory response sufficient for grip and slow protection, sensory stimuli mislocalized with some overresponse
3	Moderate	Response to touch and pin in autonomous zones, sensation mislocalized and not normal, with overresponse
4	Good	Response to touch and pin in autonomous zones, response localized but not normal; however, there is no overresponse
5	Excellent	Near normal response to touch and pin in entire field including autonomous zones

*Where applicable, such as at C8, T1, lower trunk, lateral cord, and medial cord.

Table 15-2 Gunshot wounds – criteria for selection for a neural operation

1. Complete loss in the distribution of at least one element and:
   a. No improvement clinically or by EMG in early months after injury;
   b. Loss should be in the distribution of at least one element usually helped by operation such as C5, C6, C7, upper or middle trunk, lateral or posterior cords or their outflows;
   c. Injuries with loss in lower element(s) only did not have surgery. However, if there was also loss in other element(s) likely to be helped by operation, then they were repaired whenever possible.

2. Incomplete loss where pain could not be controlled pharmacologically. In addition, when completely injured elements underwent surgery, those elements incompletely injured were dissected out and also checked by NAP recordings.

3. Pseudoaneurysm, clot, or fistula involving plexus.

4. True causalgia requiring sympathectomy.

---

noncausalgic pain not responding to pharmacological management and true causalgia requiring sympathectomy.

INTRAOPERATIVE ELECTROPHYSIOLOGICAL STUDIES

The recording of NAPs for supraclavicular plexus lesions was performed intraoperatively by using a tripolar stimulating electrode placed directly on an extradural spinal nerve, and a bipolar recording electrode placed on a segment of a more distal plexus element

such as the trunk or its division(s).[13] Stimulating and recording electrodes were separated by 3–6 cm.[34]

If a spinal nerve was regenerating adequately and 3–4 months had elapsed since injury, an NAP with a low amplitude and slow conduction was recorded.[17] If the nerve was not regenerating, the trace was flat. If there was a preganglionic injury to the dorsal root due to a GSW involving the spine, the NAP was recordable but exhibited a relatively large amplitude and rapid conduction compared with the findings of a regenerative potential.[13,34] Such an NAP could be recorded because sensory fibers distal to the dorsal

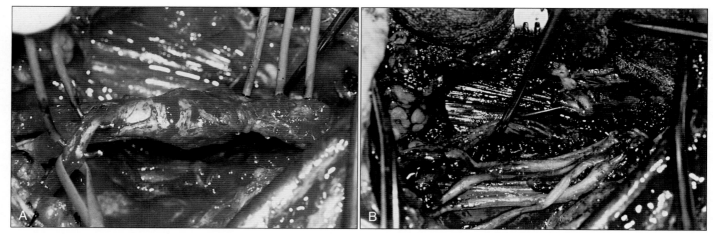

FIGURE 15-4 **(A)** A gunshot wound has caused severe injury to the upper trunk. At this point, C5 is being stimulated (*right*), and recording electrodes have been placed on the supraclavicular nerve (*left*). **(B)** There was no transmission through any portion of this lesion, so a graft repair was necessary. The middle trunk is shown retracted by an instrument superior to the graft; it had transmitted an NAP, so underwent only a neurolysis.

root ganglion had been spared, despite a more proximal disconnection from the spinal cord and complete clinical loss of function distal to the lesion. On the other hand, if there was severe postganglionic damage to the root or to the extradural spinal nerve, or if there was both pre- and postganglionic damage, no NAP was recorded.

If a regenerative NAP was found, only neurolysis was performed. If there was no NAP, resection of the spinal nerve and the more distal and involved plexus element(s) was performed. Thus, when NAP traces were flat or preganglionic, the spinal nerve, i.e. extradural root, was sectioned back toward the dura mater.[18] With the aid of magnification, the spinal nerve was exposed proximally by removing some of the bone structure around the element. If sectioning did not allow visualization of fascicles from which to lead out grafts, graft repair at that level was not attempted. In cases in which the roots were avulsed or severely damaged at an intradural level, the proximal extradural root or spinal nerve was scarred on cross-section and did not usually have discernible fascicles. If fascicles were found, however, grafts were led out from that level. In the event there was doubt about fascicular structure, a frozen section of the proximal stump of the spinal nerve was examined.[22]

If the spinal nerve was stimulated close to its foraminal exit and recording electrodes were placed over the upper posterior cervical spine or the scalp corresponding to the contralateral motor area, a somatosensory response was recorded if the posterior or dorsal root at that level was intact. Such a somatosensory evoked potential (SSEP) or evoked cortical potential indicated an intact dorsal root, although the results of animal studies have indicated that as few as 100 intact fibers can produce such a response.[36] If the SSEP or evoked cortical potential of the dorsal root was positive, there was usually, but not always, continuity to the ventral, i.e. motor, root.

Recent work has advocated percutaneous magnetic stimulation of the motor strip and recording from the spinal nerve as a test of the integrity of the ventral root. Experience at LSUHSC and that of others with this procedure, however, are too nascent for inclusion in this series. Despite experience with both SSEP and NAP recordings, the latter is currently used at LSUHSC almost exclusively, not only for lacerations and GSWs in continuity but also for supra- and infraclavicular stretch injuries. NAP recordings were also used to sort out infraclavicular plexus GSW injuries. Often, partially injured or less involved elements at this level could be tested just to ensure that electrodes and recording equipment were working.

OPERATIVE APPROACH

In the LSUHSC experience the operative approach was usually an anterior one.[9,19] A posterior subscapular procedure with resection of the first rib was used for 12 cases (10%) of GSWs to the lower roots and trunk.[10]

Exposure of injured elements was usually performed by sharp dissection using a No. 15 blade on a slender, long-handled knife or by a long pair of Metzenbaum scissors. Dissections were done under magnification, usually provided by 3.5-power eye loupes. Neural and vascular structures both proximal and distal to the injury site were exposed if possible. This permitted not only an optimal approach to the wound site, but also placement of electrodes for operative stimulation and recording of NAPs. In patients with shotgun or high-power rifle wounds or extensive prior surgery for vascular or neural repair, a lengthy up-and-down exposure was necessary.

SUPRACLAVICULAR INJURY

Injuries at a supraclavicular level were usually approached anteriorly through an oblique neck incision extending from the lateral border of the sternocleidomastoid muscle to the clavicle. Supraclavicular or transverse cervical vessels were isolated and ligated, the supraclavicular fat pad was mobilized laterally and the anterior scalene region was totally dissected or skeletonized. The phrenic nerve, if still intact, was dissected out and mobilized medially so that the upper trunk could be dissected away from the anterior scalene muscle (Fig. 15-5). The anterior scalene muscle was usually resected so that C7 to the middle trunk and the lower elements could be exposed. Exposure of the divisions required dissection beneath the clavicle, ligation of the suprascapular artery and vein, and usually resection of the subclavius muscle. By passing sponges around the clavicle, the latter could be pulled somewhat inferiorly to permit this division-level dissection.

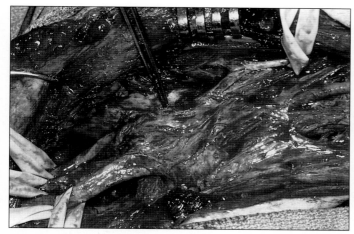

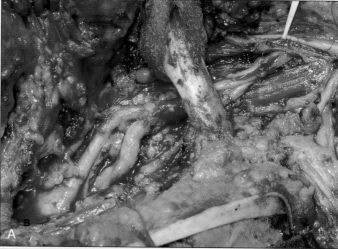

FIGURE 15-5 A severe scar is seen to involve the cords of the brachial plexus and axillary vessels at an infraclavicular gunshot site. The initial operative step was isolation of the axillary artery and then the axillary vein and major neural elements above and below the area of scar. Each element was dissected out of the scar and, if not found to be transected was electrically tested. Despite severe preoperative loss that was complete in the lateral and posterior cord distribution and incomplete in that of medial cord, each of these plexus elements transmitted nerve action potentials and thus were either regenerating well or originally only partially injured.

Generally, the supraclavicular dissections were easier to accomplish than those below the clavicle because the subclavian artery and vein lay inferior to the major portion of the dissection site and, if needed, could be readily retracted with a vein retractor. Below the clavicle, the axillary artery, which was often injured or previously repaired, was at the core of the plexus lesion and had to be cleared and protected.

INFRACLAVICULAR INJURY

Injuries centered at an infraclavicular level were approached by splitting the pectoralis major muscle close to the deltopectoral groove. The deltopectoral vein was usually ligated as it crossed to reach the axillary vein close to the clavicle. The pectoralis minor muscle was divided or, for proximal infraclavicular lesions, retracted inferiorly by a Richardson retractor. Vessels overlying the cords were coagulated or ligated and then divided. The subclavius muscle was also divided, or more commonly, a segment was removed. The clavicle could be mobilized somewhat and moved slightly superiorly by passing sponges beneath it and using them as slings to displace the clavicle superiorly. Again, as with a supraclavicular approach, if an infraclavicular lesion necessitated the same exposure of divisions requiring dissection beneath the clavicle, the suprascapular vessels were isolated, ligated, and divided.

Self-retaining retractors such as Adsons were placed in either the pectoralis minor or pectoralis major muscle on either side of the deltopectoral groove and opened to expose a large area of the infraclavicular space. The initial element seen was the lateral cord, usually lying superolateral to the axillary artery. Because of the higher incidence of vascular injury associated with GSWs at this level, the lateral cord as well as the posterior and sometimes medial cords were adherent to vessels and occasionally one or more neural elements had been inadvertently incorporated into the vascular repair.

Dissection at an infraclavicular level for many GSWs was tedious because of the need to skeletonize the axillary artery and some-

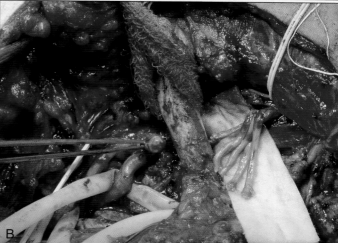

FIGURE 15-6 Gunshot wound to plexus. **(A)** An extensive stretch injury was found to involve the upper trunk to the lateral cord. **(B)** A graft repair was necessary because no NAP was transmitted through any portion of this lesion.

times the axillary vein (Fig. 15-6). Rents or tears in these vessels often had to be repaired or re-repaired in the process of dissecting the plexus elements away from the vessels. The most difficult part was the isolation of the posterior cord and its distal course as it divided into the axillary and radial nerves. The isolation of the branches coming off these elements including those to the triceps, latissimus dorsi, and subscapularis muscles was also tedious if scar tissue heavily involved the posterior wall of the infraclavicular space.

Dissection at this level was also sometimes difficult because of the intimate relationships of the lateral and especially the medial cord contributions to the median nerve as they wrapped around or were adherent to the axillary artery. If there was physical injury to the musculocutaneous outflow from the lateral cord to the biceps/brachialis muscles, dissection had to be precise, especially laterally. Small coracobrachialis branches run laterally from the lateral cord to the musculocutaneous nerve junction or very proximal musculocutaneous nerve and were spared whenever possible.

There were 12 cases in which GSWs involved roots or spinal nerves close to the spine. These patients had surgery via a posterior subscapular approach with resection of the first rib and exposure of the involved roots or spinal nerves medial to their dural exit.[10,20]

END-TO-END SUTURE ANASTOMOSIS REPAIR

Once an element was determined to have no recordable conduction and a short nerve gap was found after resection, end-to-end epineurial repair was performed. The same procedure was used for a transection in which end-to-end opposition could be gained with minimal tension. When the gap was too great for end-to-end repair, autografts, usually sural nerve, were harvested and a grouped interfascicular repair was performed (Fig. 15-7). Grafts were frequently necessary for lengthy lesions in continuity and not associated with recordable NAPs or when stumps of transected nerves were retracted and could not be approximated without tension.

A split repair was performed when a portion of the element's cross-section was more involved or damaged than the rest. If no NAP was recorded across the more damaged segment after it was split away, it was resected and a graft repair was performed. Excess scar tissue was removed from the segment to be spared, with care taken to preserve as much fascicular structure as possible.

RESULTS

In the LSUHSC series, there were 118 patients with plexus injuries due to GSWs. Most of the 293 plexus elements which were surgically treated had some gross continuity found on surgical exposure. Only 8% of elements with complete loss distal to the lesion were found to have total physical disruption during surgical exploration.

Some lesions in continuity recovered spontaneously, while others showed no signs of reversal or reinnervation after several months. In these cases, exploration and intraoperative NAP recording were performed. Of the 293 in-continuity elements that were explored and evaluated, 120 had recordable NAPs and, in response to neurolysis, function improved to grade 3 or better in 94% of these cases (Table 15-3). Elements that did not have early evidence of regeneration usually required repair (Fig. 15-8). Thus, 156 (77%) of the 202 elements suspected to be completely injured required resection and repair, as indicated by intraoperative electrical evaluation (Fig. 15-9). Pathological examination of the resected specimens confirmed neurotmesis or grade IV injuries based on the Sunderland classification.

Repairs were relatively effective for predictable elements such as the upper trunk and the C5 and C6 nerve roots, and for lateral and posterior cords and their outflows. Acceptable results were achieved in 73 (54%) of 135 lesions with complete loss repaired by grafts and in 14 (67%) of 21 cases repaired by end-to-end suture anastomosis. In this series, the functional outcomes of graft repair were as satisfactory as end-to-end suture anastomosis repair, perhaps because the grafts used were relatively short, i.e. 1–2.5 inches. Recovery occurred in severe C8, T1, lower trunk, and medial cord injuries when the nerve was in continuity and NAPs were recordable. Graft or end-to-end suture anastomosis repair of these elements did not result in useful recovery, except in a few pediatric cases.

Stewart and Birch[32] also concluded that predictable results could be achieved in the repair of C5, C6, and C7 and of the lateral and posterior cords, but the prognosis for complete lesions of the plexus associated with damage to the cervical spinal cord was particularly poor. Of the 91 elements preoperatively assessed as having incomplete loss, at LSUHSC, intraoperative stimulation and NAP studies documented that nine were not regenerating adequately.

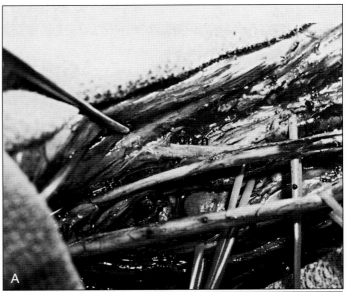

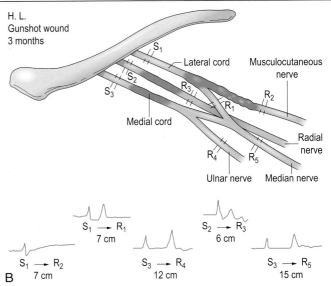

FIGURE 15-7 **(A)** This intraoperative photograph shows a gunshot wound at the level of the cords. The most serious damage was to the junction of the lateral cord (lc) and musculocutaneous nerve (mcn) (the dissector tip points to the entry of the damaged mcn into the biceps muscle). No nerve action potentials (NAPs) transmitted along this segment, although they did transmit to the median nerve. This segment of damage was resected and repaired by grafts. **(B)** A drawing of operative findings, including NAP studies is depicted here. Fortunately, the medial cord, which was determined by preoperative clinical and electrical evaluation to be severely involved, transmitted an NAP (S_3 to R_4, S_3 to R_5). The posterior cord was less involved and, as expected, transmitted an NAP (S_2 to R_3). Because the lateral cord transmitted to the median nerve (S_1 to R_1), but not to the musculocutaneous nerve (S_1 to R_2), its contribution to the median nerve was dissected proximally. Grafts were placed from the lateral cord to the musculocutaneous nerve only.

These discrepancies were usually due to a variation in anatomy at the infraclavicular level. These lesions required end-to-end suture anastomosis or graft repair.

The best outcomes were achieved with upper trunk and lateral and posterior cord lesions, but recovery occurred with some C7 to middle trunk (Fig. 15-10) and medial cord to median nerve repairs.

Table 15-3 Outcomes of surgery for 118 patients with GSW injuries to the brachial plexus (n=293 elements)

Type of lesion	Neurolysis*	Suture**	Graft**
Lesions with complete loss (202 elements)	46/42 (91%)	21/14 (67%)	135/73 (54%)
Lesions with incomplete loss (91 elements)	82/78 (95%)	6/5 (83%)	3/2 (67%)
Total	128/120 (94%)	27/19 (70%)	138/75 (54%)

Results are given as the total number of elements/the number of elements recovering to ≥ grade 3.

*Neurolysis was based on the presence of an NAP across a lesion in continuity.

**Suture or graft repair was based on the absence of an NAP across a lesion in continuity. A few graft repairs were performed in lesions conducting an NAP in which split graft repairs were carried out.

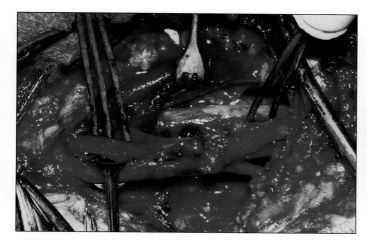

FIGURE 15-8 A gunshot wound to the upper trunk is shown. C5 (to the left) was stimulated and recording electrodes (to the right) were placed on the anterior division of the upper trunk. This truncal lesion, which was exposed 3.5 months after injury, required resection and repair. The outcome was favorable: at 3.5 years, the biceps muscle was grade 4 to 5, the pronator muscle and wrist and finger flexor muscles were grade 3 to 4, and the sensation within the median distribution was grade 4.

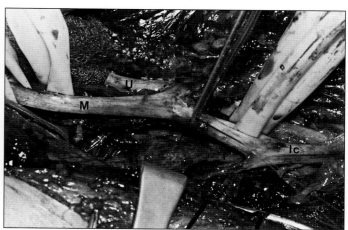

FIGURE 15-9 Shown is a severe lesion in continuity to the posterior cord, which did not transmit a nerve action potential (NAP). The nerve required resection and graft repair. The functional loss of the musculocutaneous-innervated muscle was complete preoperatively, but the element transmitted an NAP across the injury. A neurolysis was performed. The musculocutaneous nerve is displaced by the retractor in this figure (lc, lateral cord; M, median; U, ulnar). (From Kline DG: Civilian gunshot wounds to the brachial plexus. J Neurosurg 70:166–174, 1989.)

Results with lower trunk and most medial cord lesions were poor unless early regeneration was proved by intraoperative NAPs, in which case either neurolysis or split repair could be performed.

Surgery is therefore warranted for selected GSWs to the plexus.

CASE SUMMARIES – GUNSHOT WOUND TO THE BRACHIAL PLEXUS

CASE 1

A 55-year-old, right-handed warehouse manager was shot in the left shoulder by a .35-caliber pistol at close range. The bullet entered the supraclavicular space, fractured the clavicle and the first two ribs, and a shell fragment lodged in the posterior subscapular area. Initially, he had a flail arm. After angiography showed normal axillary and subclavian artery blood flow, the entrance wound was debrided at a local hospital to remove shell fragments and pieces of fractured clavicle.

When seen 6 weeks later, he had total paralysis of the supraspinatus, infraspinatus, deltoid, biceps/brachialis, triceps, brachioradialis, pronator teres, supi-

nator, and wrist and finger extensor muscles. Wrist and finger flexion, including the flexor pollicis longus muscle were graded as 2 to 3, and the interosseus muscles were grade 3. There was no function of the lumbrical muscles of the hand or of the thenar intrinsic muscles and there was sensory loss in the C5, C6, and C7 distributions, with relative sparing of C8 and T1.

Electromyography showed extensive denervational changes involving all muscles, with most severe changes in the C5, C6, and C7 distributions. Exploration was performed almost 3 months after the injury, through anterior supraclavicular, as well as infraclavicular approaches. The comminuted, callused portion of the clavicle was resected and after extensive scar tissue was removed, the spinal nerves, trunks, and cords of the plexus were exposed. All elements were in continuity, but were scarred. No NAPs could be recorded by stimulating the C5, C6, and C7 nerves and recording from the anterior and posterior divisions of the upper and middle trunks; and in addition there were no distal muscle contractions on stimulation of these elements. On the other hand, stimulation of either C8 or T1 elicited a small amount of wrist flexion and moderate-sized NAPs could be recorded from the medial cord. External neurolysis alone was performed on C8, T1, and their outflows and portions of C5, C6, and C7 nerves and all of the upper and middle trunks were resected. Eleven grafts, 5–6.4 cm in length,

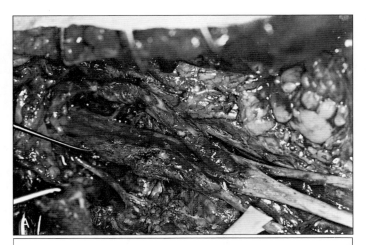

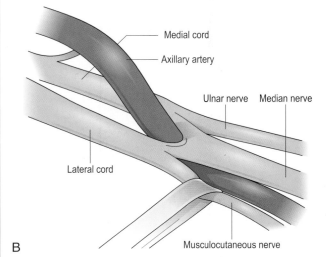

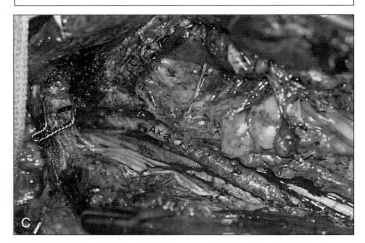

FIGURE 15-10   (A) This gunshot wound involved the lateral and posterior cords. An arterial repair had been acutely performed, and unfortunately, the posterior wall of the artery had been sewn to the lateral and some of the posterior cords. **(B)** The accompanying drawing depicts the major relationships between some of the plexus elements and the artery. **(C)** The lateral cord segment required repair. Grafts are in place in the lateral cord distribution. The clavicle had been divided because the proximal suture site for the grafts was immediately below the clavicle (Ax a, axillary artery). (Reprinted in part from Kline DG, Judice DJ: Operative management of selected brachial plexus lesions. J Neurosurgery 58:631–649, 1983.)

(labels in B: Medial cord, Axillary artery, Ulnar nerve, Median nerve, Lateral cord, Musculocutaneous nerve)

were then placed from C5 to the suprascapular nerve, C5 to the lateral and posterior cords, C6 to the lateral and posterior cords, and C7 to the posterior cord and a portion of the medial cord. The clavicle was wired together and soft tissues were closed over a Penrose drain. The drain was removed on the third postoperative day and the patient was discharged on the seventh day with instructions for physical therapy.

The patient was seen on several occasions for follow-up evaluation. At 5 years postoperatively, muscle testing gave the following results: supra- and infraspinatus muscles were grade 3 to 4, the deltoid muscle was grade 3, the biceps/brachialis muscles were grade 4, the triceps muscle was grade 3, pronation/supination was grade 3, and wrist extension was grade 4. Extension of the finger and thumb, however, was absent. Wrist and finger flexors were grade 4, interosseus and lumbrical muscles were grade 4, and thenar intrinsic muscles were grade 3. Although touch and pinprick were decreased in the thumb, fore-, and long fingers, the patient could localize stimuli in these areas well. He considered a tendon transfer to improve work-needed finger and thumb extension; however, since he was able to work and use this arm and hand quite well, he did not wish to have this done. He has recovered to grade 4 for the C5, C6, and upper trunk repairs and to grade 3 for the C7 and middle trunk repairs.

COMMENT

This was a fortunate result from a very severe GSW to the plexus. If loss, especially that in the C5, C6, and C7 distribution or their outflow, does not improve spontaneously in the early months after the injury, exploration and intraoperative recording are in order.

CASE 2

This 22-year-old, right-handed mechanic sustained a wound in the right shoulder from a shotgun blast at close range. Acutely, he required a subclavian-to-brachial artery nonanatomical saphenous vein bypass graft and immobilization of the arm for a humeral fracture. Some voluntary contraction of the hand muscles was initially noted. Subsequent EMG showed complete denervation of the deltoid and biceps muscles as well as muscles innervated by the radial and median nerves, but only partial denervation of the hand intrinsic muscles. Evaluation at LSUHSC showed findings similar to those described by the referring institution. Supraspinatus and infraspinatus muscles were grade 3 to 4. Deltoid power was absent as were biceps/brachialis and brachioradialis muscle strengths. The triceps muscle functioned, but was weak and was grade 3. There was no finger, thumb, or wrist extension and pronation and supination were absent. Wrist flexion was provided by the flexor carpi ulnaris muscle, which was grade 3. Finger flexion was quite weak, although the flexor digitorum profundi of the ring and little fingers were grades 2 to 3, as were the hand intrinsic muscles in the ulnar distribution. All median-innervated muscles had absent function, There was hypoesthesia in the median and radial nerve distributions and less hypoesthesia in an ulnar distribution. These findings did not change over the next 6 weeks.

The patient underwent exploration of the infraclavicular plexus through an anterior approach 5.5 months after the injury. The entire shoulder to upper arm area was found to have multiple, scattered "shot" and all elements were surrounded by heavy scar tissue.

The pectoralis major and minor muscles were divided to provide adequate exposure. A segment of the lateral cord to musculocutaneous nerve was missing and was replaced by two sural grafts, each 5 cm in length. A longitudinal portion of the lateral cord to median nerve transmitted a small NAP, but the remainder did not; thus, a split repair of the lateral cord was carried out such that a portion was replaced with a 5 cm graft, and the remainder of the element underwent neurolysis.

A large neuroma in continuity involving the posterior cord to radial nerve exhibited no NAP on proximal stimulation and distal recording; thus, it was resected and replaced with three 6.4 cm sural grafts. The posterior cord to the axillary nerve transmitted an NAP, so only neurolysis was performed.

Despite heavy scarring around and some firmness in the medial cord and its outflows, NAPs could be recorded for all medial cord outflows, except the medial cord to median nerve. After a thorough external neurolysis, an antebrachial sensory segment was fashioned into two 3.8 cm grafts which were placed from the medial cord to the median nerve. The medial cord to ulnar nerve had only external neurolysis. The pectoralis major, but not minor, muscle was repaired, and the large wound was closed in multiple layers without a drain. The patient was given antibiotics postoperatively and remained afebrile. He was discharged to his referring facility for physical therapy on the ninth postoperative day.

The patient was seen on several occasions during the first postoperative year and was noted to have early recovery of deltoid function. He returned to work as a service station manager, using mainly his left arm, with assistance from the right.

By 2 years postoperatively, the biceps/brachialis muscles were grade 3 to 4, and the pronator muscle was grade 4. Median and ulnar nerve functions had improved dramatically. Follow-up evaluation 6.5 years after injury documented shoulder abduction to 110 degrees with loss of axillary soft tissue restricting further abduction. Biceps/brachialis, brachioradialis, and triceps muscle functions were excellent. There was excellent pronation and partial supination and wrist extension was grade 3 to 4. Finger and thumb extension was absent. There was a slight tendency to claw the fingers, but overall motor strength for specific elements were grade 4 for the muscles innervated by the axillary nerve, lateral cord to musculocutaneous nerve, lateral cord to median nerve, medial cord to median nerve, and the posterior cord to radial nerve was grade 3 to 4.

He now uses his right arm daily in his work including writing with his right hand, even though it tires readily.

COMMENT

If previous vascular surgery has resulted in a nonanatomical placement of a vascular graft, the surgeon must avoid injury to the graft. Repair of the pectoralis minor may compromise neural suture lines and is usually not done. The pectoralis major, however, is carefully repaired. Drains must be placed meticulously so as to not displace grafts by their suction and must subsequently be removed with care for the same reason.

REFERENCES

1. Bateman JE: The Shoulder and Neck, 2nd edn. Philadelphia, WB Saunders, 1978.
2. Binns JH and Wynn Parry CB: Successful repair of a complete brachial plexus lesion. Injury 2:19, 1970.
3. Black AN, Burns BD, and Zuckerman S: An experimental study of the wounding mechanism of high velocity missiles. Br Med J 2:872–874, 1941.
4. Brooks DM: Open wounds of the brachial plexus. J Bone Joint Surg [Br] 31:17–33, 1949.
5. Brooks DM: Peripheral nerve injuries. Medical Research Council Special Report Series, HMSO, 1954:418–429.
6. Brown AK: Gunshot wounds then and now. J R Coll Surg Edinb 34:302–309, 1989.
7. Callender GR: Wound ballistics – mechanism of production of wounds by small arms, bullets and shell fragments. War Med 3:337–342, 1943.
8. Davis L, Martin J, and Perret G: The treatment of injuries of the brachial plexus. Ann Surg 125:647–657, 1947.
9. Davis DH, Onofrio BM, and MacCarty CS: Brachial plexus injuries. Mayo Clin Proc 53:799–807, 1978.
10. Dubuisson AS, Kline DG, and Weinshel SS: Posterior subscapular approach to the brachial plexus. Report of 102 patients. J Neurosurgery 79:319–330, 1993.
11. French LA: Clinical experience with peripheral nerve surgery with special reference to the results in early nerve repair. MS Thesis, University of Minnesota, 1946.
12. Ghostine SY, Comair YG, Turner DM, et al.: Phenoxybenzamine in the treatment of causalgia. J Neurosurg 60:1263–1268, 1984.
13. Happel LT and Kline DG: Nerve lesions in continuity. In: Gelberman R, Ed: Operative Nerve Repair and Reconstruction, vol 1. Philadelphia, JB Lippincott, 1991.
14. Hudson AR and Dommissee I: Brachial plexus injury: Case report of gunshot wounds. Can Med Assoc J 117:1162–1164, 1977.
15. Jebara VA and Saade B: Causalgia: A wartime experience – report of twenty treated cases. J Trauma 27:519–524, 1987.
16. Kline DG: Civilian gunshot wounds to the brachial plexus. J Neurosurg 70:166–174, 1989.
17. Kline DG and Happel LH: Penfield Lecture: A quarter century's experience with intraoperative nerve action potential recording. Can J Neurol Sci 20:3–10, 1993.
18. Kline DG and Hudson AR: Diagnosis of root avulsions. J Neurosurg 87:483–484, 1997.
19. Kline DG and Judice DJ: Operative management of selected brachial plexus lesions. J Neurosurg 58:631–649, 1983.
20. Kline DG, Kott J, Barnes G, et al.: Exploration of selected brachial plexus lesions by the posterior subscapular approach. J Neurosurg 49:872–880, 1987.
21. Leffert RD: Brachial Plexus Injuries. New York, Churchill Livingstone, 1985.
22. Malessy MJ, van Duinen SG, and Feirabend HK: Correlation between histopathological findings in C-5 and C-6 nerve stumps and motor recovery following nerve grafting for repair of brachial plexus injury. J Neurosurg 91:636–644, 1999.
23. Nakaras A: The surgical management of brachial plexus injuries. In: Daniels RK and Terzis JK, Eds: Reconstructive Microsurgery. Boston, Little, Brown, 1977.
24. Nelson KG, Jolly PC, and Thomas PA: Brachial plexus injuries associated with missile wounds of the chest. A report of 9 cases from Viet Nam. J Trauma 8:268–275, 1968.
25. Nulsen FE and Slade WW: Recovery following injury to the brachial plexus. In: Woodhall B and Beebe GW, Eds: Peripheral Nerve Regeneration: A Follow-up Study of 3,656 World War II Injuries. Washington, DC, US Government Printing Office, 1956.
26. Omer GE: Injuries to nerves of the upper extremity. J Bone Joint Surg [Am] 56:1615–1627, 1974.
27. Omer GE: The prognosis for untreated traumatic injuries. In: Omer GE, Spinner M, and Van Beek A, Eds: Management of Peripheral Nerve Problems, 2nd edn. Philadelphia, WB Saunders, 1998.
28. Ordog GJ, Balasubramanium S, Wasserberger J, et al.: Extremity gunshot wounds: Part one – Identification and treatment of patients at high risk of vascular injury. J Trauma 36:358–368, 1994.
29. Samii M and Moringlane JR: Thermocoagulation of the dorsal root entry zone for the treatment of intractable pain. Neurosurgery 15:953, 1984.
30. Seddon HJ: Peripheral Nerve Injuries. London, HM Stationery Office, 1954.
31. Seddon HJ: Surgical Disorders of the Peripheral Nerves. Baltimore, Williams & Wilkins, 1972.
32. Stewart MP and Birch R: Penetrating missile injuries of the brachial plexus. J Bone Joint Surg [Br] 83:517–524, 2001.
33. Sunderland S: Nerves and Nerve Injuries, 2nd edn. Edinburgh, Churchill Livingstone, 1978.
34. Tiel RL, Happel LH, and Kline DG: Nerve action potential recording method and equipment. Neurosurgery 39:103–109, 1996.
35. Vrettos BC, Rochkind S, and Boome RS: Low velocity gunshot wounds of the brachial plexus. J Hand Surg [Br] 20:212–214, 1995.
36. Zhao S, Kim DH, and Kline DG: Somatosensory evoked potentials induced by stimulating a variable number of nerve fibers in rat. Muscle Nerve 16:1220–1227, 1993.

16 Stretch injuries to brachial plexus

Rajiv Midha

OVERVIEW

- Management of these frequently encountered lesions is one of the most controversial areas in medicine and surgery.
- As with other plexus lesions, it is most important to evaluate them in terms of complete and incomplete loss for each and every plexus element.
- Incomplete loss, significant sparing, or early recovery can lead to a good spontaneous recovery in that element's distribution. Yet, other and more seriously stretched or avulsed elements may not recover.
- Multiple signs of severe proximal injury and evidence supporting avulsion, particularly of C5, C6, and C7, argue against a successful direct repair of the plexus.
- Limitations to the precision of some findings such as paraspinal denervation, positive sensory potentials, and even abnormal myelography point to the continuing importance of intraoperative exploration, evaluation, and electrical studies.
- In the entire experience, we followed a selective route and tried to study the value of direct repair for stretch injuries chosen for operation.
- Neurotization using the descending cervical plexus, the accessory nerve, pectoral branches, and intercostal nerve has been added with increasing frequency to any direct repair possible.
- Grading recovery of function in plexus injuries where multiple elements were involved has been difficult, but an attempt has been made to do this using the Louisiana State University Health Sciences Center (LSUHSC) system to gain some determination of the value of direct repair.
- C5, C6 distribution stretches have a relatively low incidence of avulsion, recover sometimes spontaneously, and may include severe damage to C7. These injuries are excellent candidates for direct repair, aided by neurotization, with very good results.
- C5, C6, C7 distribution stretches have more roots avulsed than do C5, C6 stretches, recover spontaneously with less frequency, and have a variable loss of wrist and finger movement. Nonetheless, some of these lesions are also good candidates for direct repair with acceptable results.
- C5 through T1 distribution stretches are difficult to help by direct repair, although almost 50% of those selected for operation regain some usable shoulder and arm function. Graft repair from a single root (often C5) is frequently augmented with neurotization in these cases.

- There is an immense spectrum of presentations regarding reparability of roots or spinal nerves in the C5 through T1 stretches, and this affects outcome in a variable fashion.
- Many infraclavicular plexus stretch injuries do not recover spontaneously and require operation.
- Results with repair of lateral and posterior cords and their outflows, such as the musculocutaneous and axillary nerve, are surprisingly good. As expected, medial cord recovery is poor if resection and repair are necessary. Repair of medial cord to median lesions is, however, useful in the majority of cases.
- It is unusual for the suprascapular nerve to sustain isolated direct injury, but loss in its distribution is a frequent concomitant of C5, C6, and upper trunk injuries.
- Stretch injuries affecting both axillary and suprascapular nerves in an isolated fashion (rather than C5, C6, and/or upper trunk) is relatively common. The suprascapular portion usually improves with time and seldom requires repair although the axillary nerve often does need exploration and repair.
- Lacerating and iatrogenic injuries, particularly involving proximal spinal nerve to trunk levels, are well managed via a posterior subscapular approach for exploration and repair.

INTRODUCTION

In spite of intense interest in and literature generated about brachial plexus injuries, and specifically those caused by stretch/contusion, in the last several decades, there is not unanimity concerning the management of these difficult problems. Some authors still believe that there is little indication for surgery, whereas others feel all cases should be operated on.[103] Some surgeons still urge relatively early amputation, at least for the flail or totally paralyzed arm.[62] Other clinicians, including ourselves, try to select those cases more likely to respond to plexus repair for operation.[44,45] There is also a diversity of operative procedures and combinations of them for such plexus palsies. Direct repair, usually with the help of grafts, is sought by a variety of approaches for roots or spinal nerves that can be repaired in this fashion.[1,4,48,55] Attempts at direct neural repair can also be combined with neurotization if other nerves, such as higher cervical roots, descending cervical plexus, accessory, phrenic, or intercostal nerves, are led to distal inputs with or without intervening grafts.[2,37,51,76,109] A few surgeons tend to prefer a neurotization procedure as the initial operation because more direct repair is either not possible or frequently fails.[14,23,108] Other surgeons utilize relatively early reconstructive procedures, such as fusion of glenohumeral joint which still permits some shoulder mobility, and, if possible, flexoroplasty or pectoralis or latissimus dorsi transfer to provide some elbow flexion.[6,16,53]

Because there is such a diversity of opinion and variety of approaches available, we will first review a selected portion of the vast literature on stretch injuries before presenting our own results. The accompanying figures for the next section depict some of the different combinations of stretch injuries we have encountered and how they have been managed.

BACKGROUND FOR STRETCH/CONTUSION INJURIES

MECHANISTIC ISSUES

The most common lesion of the plexus is that caused by stretch/contusion, usually secondary to motor vehicular accidents, particularly those involving motorcycles.[21,26] Although a high proportion of severe plexus injuries in trauma patients are caused by vehicular accidents,[66] other traumatic etiologies result in many injuries.[19] In a review of 39 patients with sports injuries involving the plexus, football was responsible for nine and bicycling for seven.[43] There were four skiing and sledding accidents, four equestrian injuries, seven water sport-related injuries, and eight injuries related to other sports such as wrestling, gymnastics, and golf. Regardless of the setting, the head and neck are usually forcefully pushed in one direction and shoulder and arm in another direction.[27,71] This results in severe stretch to soft tissues, including nerve and, less frequently, vessels (Figs 16-1 to 16-3).[33,119]

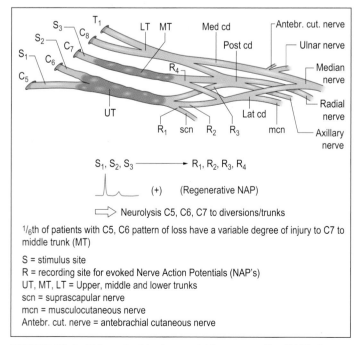

FIGURE 16-1 This patient had recordable regenerative NAP's from C5, C6 and C7 innervated structures at five months despite loss of supraspinatus infraspinatus, deltoid, biceps brachioradialis, and supination. Since 1/6th of patients with C5/C6 loss also have injury to C7, C7 to middle trunk also had NAP recordings made from it.

CONSERVATIVE MANAGEMENT AND NATURAL HISTORY

Regardless of the mechanism of injury, a conservative, nonsurgical approach predominated historically. Leffert has nicely summarized the literature of the early 1900s.[52] These early authors included Thoburn, Kennedy, Clark, Taylor, Prout, A. S. Taylor, Forester, Sever, Sharp, Jepson, and Stevens. Many of the cases reported were birth palsies, but some were adult traction injuries. Some

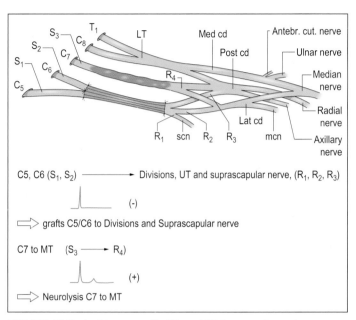

FIGURE 16-2 In this case with C5 and C6 loss, graft repair was needed. NAP traces from C5/C6 to divisions of upper trunk were flat and while C7 to middle trunk had a recordable response.

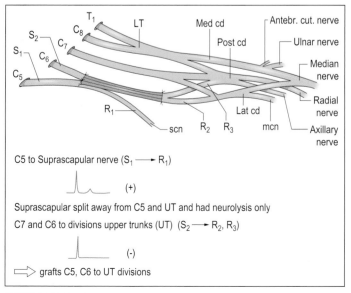

FIGURE 16-3 C5 to suprascapular nerve had a recordable NAP so was split off and spared whereas C5 and C6 to divisions had flat traces and grafts were placed. C7 was not involved in this case.

success with surgery was reported, but as a whole, the relatively poor outcomes were discouraging.[96] On the other hand, it has always been obvious that spontaneous functional regeneration is limited with severe injuries and that the possibilities for reconstructive surgery are often small. Amputation can occasionally permit the use of a prosthesis.[84] Unfortunately, the amputees seldom use such devices, especially if amputation is done at a very proximal level. This makes this type of surgery only ablative in nature (Fig. 16-4).

Some review of the prior half century of literature regarding spontaneous recovery of function without surgery is necessary. In 63 cases injured by stretch reported by Barnes in 1949, 14 had only a C5 and C6 deficit, and 11 of these recovered some biceps and a little shoulder function in a spontaneous fashion.[5] In addition, 11 of 19 with C5, C6, and C7 root damage had some return of wrist and finger extension, biceps, and some shoulder abduction. Prognosis, however, was poor for complete palsies involving all the plexus elements, and the latter observation was confirmed by Bonney in 1959.[10] In his series of 19 patients with complete lesions of the entire plexus followed for 2 years, there was very little return of function. If recovery did occur, it was delayed for 12–24 months and was to proximal muscles only. Fifteen patients underwent exploration electively to determine prognosis. Each of the stretched elements was found to be in continuity, and no repairs were done. At that time, Bonney concluded that suture or grafting could be advised only if plexus was found to be torn apart and not if continuity was present. In 1962, P. E. Taylor found 90 stretch injuries reported in the literature and thought that 50 were adequate for study: 17 incomplete and 33 complete.[104] In the complete group, 60% regained no function at all.

Leffert and Seddon reviewed 31 closed brachial plexus injuries in which there was no fracture of the clavicle, swelling, or indura-

tion in the supraclavicular space; paralysis of muscles innervated by the dorsal scapular, suprascapular, or long thoracic nerves; or Homer syndrome.[54] In comparison with other series, this was a mildly injured group of patients with a predominately infraclavicular level of injury. The investigators, as a result, concluded that conservative management was in order. On the other hand, Alnot found that a number of infraclavicular lesions required operation.[3] Most cases done in his series involved posterior cord to radial nerve or axillary nerve, but a few involved lateral cord or lateral cord to musculocutaneous nerve or medial cord outflows.

Wynn Parry reported on a number of patients who were not operated on, but who were re-examined 5 or more years after injury.[114] In 36 patients treated conservatively who had complete C5 and C6 lesions, two-thirds recovered some degree of elbow flexion and one-third recovered some shoulder abduction (Figs 16-5, 16-6). In 50 patients with complete C5, C6, and C7 lesions, one-third recovered some degree of elbow flexion and some shoulder abduction. In 84 patients with complete C5 through T1 lesions, only 20% recovered elbow flexion, 16% elbow extension, and 7% finger flexion. From our perspective, however, spontaneous positive results do not seem to be quite this frequent. Perhaps this reflects a referral bias, as we are sent only the more serious cases. Those with very early recovery are probably treated conservatively elsewhere. This certainly seems to be the case with some series reported by neurologists. Nagano et al.'s figures on patients with postganglionic lesions of variable severity, reported in 1979, indicated good or excellent spontaneous recovery in more than 40% of patients.[72] Unfortunately, in our experience, such is usually not the case if initial loss is complete in the distribution of two or more roots.

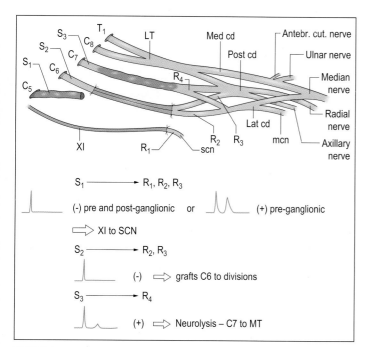

FIGURE 16-4 C5 had irreparable injury so distal accessory nerve was sewn to suprascapular nerve and grafts were used to replace C6 outflows.

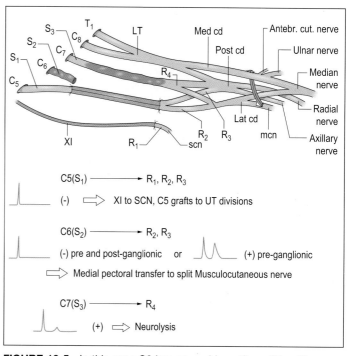

FIGURE 16-5 In this case C6 has no usable outflow. C5 outflow was led to the divisions of the upper trunk while distal accessory nerve was sewn to the suprascapular nerve. In addition, medial pectoral branches were sewn to a split musculocutaneous nerve.

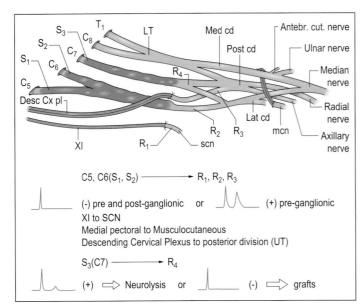

FIGURE 16-6   In this example both C5 and C6 had either preganglionic or pre- and postganglionic injury. As a result, accessory nerve was sewn to suprascapular nerve and medial pectoral branch(es) was transferred to musculocutaneous nerve. Then descending cervical branches were sewn to the posterior division of the upper trunk.

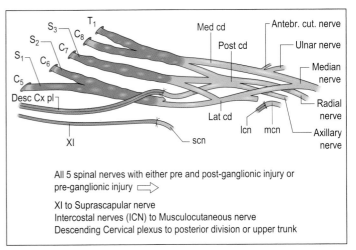

FIGURE 16-7   Flail arm cases are the most difficult to repair. Here the five plexus roots had either pre- or postganglionic injury. The accessory nerve was sewn to the suprascapular nerve, intercostals (usually three) were placed to musculocutaneous nerve, and descending cervical plexus was sewn to posterior division of the upper trunk.

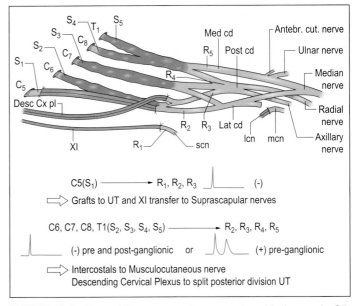

FIGURE 16-8   Four of five nerve roots were not usable for repair. C5 was however usable for outflow and grafts were placed to distal upper trunk. Then accessory was sewn to suprascapular nerve, descending cervical plexus to posterior division of upper trunk, and intercostals to musculocutaneous nerve.

MUSCULOSKELETAL RECONSTRUCTIVE APPROACHES

Yeoman and Seddon reported on patients with severe multiple-root injuries who had reconstructive orthopedic procedures.[118] Results were so poor that they recommended amputation and use of a prosthesis, even though Hendry was somewhat more optimistic about reconstructive orthopedic procedures in an earlier report.[31] On the other hand, Ransford and Hughes provided a 10-year follow-up on 20 patients with complete plexus palsies and noted that amputation did not relieve pain and that patients with prostheses seldom used them.[85] Nonetheless, a few authors still advocate early amputation for serious stretch injuries.[62]

In 1973, Zancolli and Mitre summarized their experience with latissimus dorsi transfer to substitute for biceps loss.[120] This and other muscle transfers have occasionally been useful if some function in the distribution of the plexus is spared to begin with or returns with time.[53,100,101] Experience with grafts for plexus lesions during the World War II period reported by Seddon and Brooks and by Nulsen and Slade gave limited encouragement for repair of these difficult lesions.[81]

There is little question that reconstructive and substitutive operations can be of value in some well-selected cases.[34,36] The difficulty with their use in the usual stretch injury is that there is often no muscle that works well enough to shift or move to provide substitution. Nonetheless, in cases in which loss remains complete in the C5–C6 distribution and yet C7 and lower root function are spared, a flexorplasty, in which either forearm flexors are slid proximally to originate above elbow or triceps is used to substitute for biceps, can be quite effective in restoring flexion of the elbow[15,40,63] Less frequently, recovery or sparing of enough pectoralis major or latissimus dorsi permits use of these muscles as a substitute for biceps/brachialis.[16,20] If, with upper root or spinal nerve damage, some

forearm flexion can be regained but the shoulder remains paralyzed, then glenohumeral fusion of the shoulder can be done. This places the arm at an effective partially abducted, forward flexed, and internally rotated position.[87,113] Muscle transfers, especially using extensions from the trapezius, have been attempted to provide shoulder abduction, but usually with less success than with fusion.[30]

In some cases in which repaired stretch injuries either spare or recover some forearm and hand function, tendon transfers can be done, particularly to improve wrist and finger extension (Figs 16-7 to 16-9).[85,115]

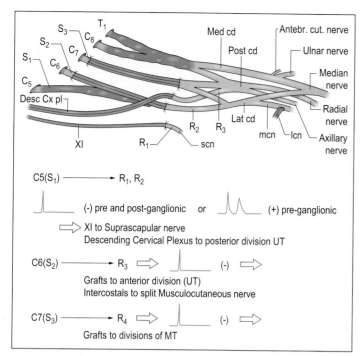

FIGURE 16-9 In this case, C6 had usable outflow whereas C5 did not; grafts could also be led out from C7 to divisions of the middle trunk. Accessory nerve was sewn to suprascapular nerve and since there was some potential regenerative input from proximal C6, intercostals were sewn to a split musculocutaneous nerve.

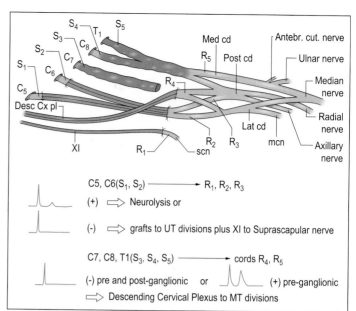

FIGURE 16-10 A relatively favourable flail arm example where C5 and C6 outflows were either regenerating or could be replaced by grafts. Accessory was still placed to suprascapular nerve while descending cervical plexus was sewn to distal middle trunk C7, C8 and T1 had pre- or postganglionic responses and were not reparable.

DIRECT BRACHIAL PLEXUS REPAIRS

Lusskin and Campbell urged a more aggressive approach for blunt injuries to the plexus than most earlier authors.[58] They indicated that neurolysis alone improved the outcome, as had Davis et al., who reported on this procedure for penetrating wounds in 1947.[22] Lusskin and Campbell also recommended use of autografts.

A relatively aggressive but still selective approach was followed by Narakas.[74,76] Of 615 patients with stretch injuries, 237 were selected for operation. Four operations were for prognosis only, 4 were done on an emergency basis, 20 resulted in external neurolysis only, 13 had fascicular neurolysis, and 127 had autogenous, usually sural nerve grafts, placed. In 26 other instances, neurotization procedures using intercostal nerves were done, and 33 patients had such procedures as well as direct grafting of the plexus. Forty patients also had tendon transfers, 7 had a second operation, 18 had vascular repairs, and amputations were done in 8. A good result, as deemed by Narakas, occurred in 41% of his operated cases. Of the 143 patients with supraclavicular lesions repaired by grafts who had 3 or more years of follow-up, only 15 had good results, and 30 had fair results. Narakas concluded that despite high magnification it was impossible to tell if scarred fascicles represented healed lesions or obstacles to regeneration, but intraoperative electrical recordings were not used. The author agreed with earlier suggestions that it was worthwhile to graft the pathways of the upper three roots, whereas grafts of pathways leading to the median nerve gave only fair or more often poor results. Repair of the lower elements, although giving flexor carpi ulnaris return, did not restore hand intrinsic function. Roughly one-half of the patients having transfer of intercostal nerves, with or without sural grafts to the more distal portions of the plexus, benefited from the

surgery. However, they had improvement only in recovery of a single function, which was usually elbow flexion. More recently, Hentz and Narakas (1988) provided further useful data about their results with stretch injuries producing flail arms (Figs 16-10, 16-11).[32]

Millesi reported on 54 stretch injuries operated on between 1964 and 1972.[69,70] He did not believe that myelography was useful, did not use intraoperative recording, and preferred operative exposure and direct microscopic inspection. Eighteen patients had a complete brachial plexus palsy caused by root-level lesions, with some of the roots avulsed and others with infraganglionic or lateral lesions suitable for graft repair. Twelve of these patients had lost physical continuity in all roots whereas six had some continuity, especially in the lower roots. Useful shoulder recovery occurred in 5 of 18, elbow flexion in 9, triceps alone in 4, and wrist and finger movement in 2. With complete lesions caused by more peripheral lesions, 6 of 13 had acceptable shoulder recovery, 7 had elbow function, and 5 had some degree of wrist and finger recovery. With partial palsy caused by variable root lesions, 3 of 10 recovered shoulder function, 7 elbow function, and 3 wrist and finger function. With partial palsies caused by more peripheral lesions, 7 of 10 patients obtained return of shoulder function, 8 of 9 recovered elbow function, 3 of 6, wrist, and 3 of 8, finger flexion. Millesi provided a partial update on his results in both 1984 and 1988, and considering the severity of these lesions his results remain excellent. He still relies on relatively early microscopic inspection of the elements to determine whether to resect those in continuity or not. Millesi also believes internal neurolysis improves function in some stretch injuries to the plexus. The latter tenet is not accepted by all and certainly has not been our experience.

In 1982, Sedel reported on 139 plexus injuries operated on between 1972 and 1980.[95] Sixty-three patients had enough follow-up for analysis, including 32 complete lesions involving all elements of the plexus and 31 incomplete ones. Repairs were done in 48

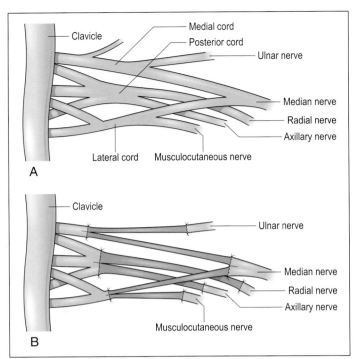

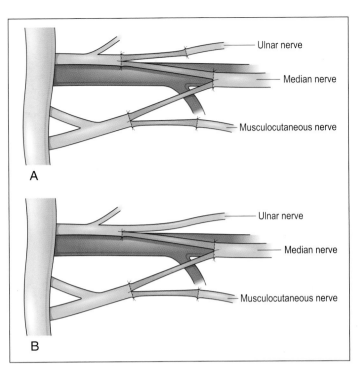

FIGURE 16-11 **(A)** Infraclavicular cord and cord-to-nerve level brachial plexus. **(B)** Entire plexus at cord and cord-to-nerve level is replaced by grafts. No attempt is made to repair input to brachial and antebrachial cutaneous nerves. Instead, they as well as sural nerves are used as donor grafts.

FIGURE 16-12 A fairly common scenario is partial infraclavicular stretch injury involving lateral and medial cords and their outflows with relative sparing of posterior cord. **(A)** Outflows to musculocutaneous, median, and ulnar nerves have received grafts from lateral and medial cords. **(B)** Both medial and lateral cord input to median required repair, but that to ulnar nerve did not.

cases and neurolysis alone in 15. An attempt was made to compare operative results with those in a group of patients treated conservatively. Those patients operated on had higher grades of recovery. All roots and elements in continuity had only a neurolysis because intraoperative recording techniques were not used. His experience with transferring other nerves into more distal plexus was disappointing. Sedel updated some of these data a few years later.[94]

In 1983, Stevens and colleagues reported on 25 patients with plexus injuries operated on over a 32-year period.[102] Five of those repaired resulted from stretch/contusion, four complete to all roots and one incomplete. Partial recoveries were obtained in a few cases by transposition of intact proximal plexus elements into degenerated but noncorresponding distal elements without the use of grafts.

In a series of 171 plexus injuries operated on between 1968 and 1980, 60 patients with stretch/contusion injury were reported by Kline and Judice in 1983.[48] The authors felt that it was important to follow each patient for 4 or 5 months before operation to look for clinical signs of recovery of function and, on electromyographic (EMG) evaluation, to search for evidence of reinnervation. As a result, cases with significant improvement in the early months were not operated upon. Selection for operation also excluded cases with high probability of multiple nerve root avulsions, based on clinical, myelographic, and electrical criteria. These criteria further evolved with a larger and more recent experience and have been subsequently reported.[41,44,45] At the time of operation for the more severe cases, intraoperative stimulation and recording techniques were used to ascertain whether injured elements required resection or were regenerating.

As a result of this selective process, 148 stretched and contused elements that were surgically evaluated were reported in 1983 (Figs 16-12, 16-13). The majority of elements operated on (114) were thought to be completely injured according to preoperative

clinical and EMG testing. These cases were done by the classic anterior approach, although in the interim some were approached posteriorly if exposure of spinal nerves, especially lower ones close to dura, was desired.[50] Intraoperative NAP studies showed 31 of the spinal nerves to be regenerating or, in two cases, partially injured to begin with. These elements had only a neurolysis, and 26 recovered to a grade 3 or better functional level. Of the 58 elements that could be surgically repaired, only four could be repaired by direct suture, and two of these had significant recovery. Three elements had a split repair, in which a portion of the element received a neurolysis and a portion was replaced by grafts, and each recovered. Success with graft repair was slightly less than 50% and, surprisingly, compared well with patients having gunshot wounds to the plexus in cases in which grafts were necessary. This may be because a higher percentage of elements viewed as favorable for repair received repair in the stretch series than in the gunshot wound series.

Even after excluding stretch injuries thought not to be reparable, 25 elements in 12 cases were still not reparable because of medial or proximal root injury or damage over an excessive length. In only five patients was this true of all plexus elements. Partial repair was possible in the other seven cases. Nevertheless, histologic sections of the proximal stump of roots of several of these patients showed a mixture of heavy scarring with only fine axons and presence of many ganglion cells. Such was also the case with several other patients in whom preoperatively it was considered that all the plexus was capable of repair by grafts from root to cord level. If heavy scarring and ganglion cells were seen, function did not result despite placement of technically satisfactory grafts.

In the five patients with total distraction of the plexus at a root level, three were not reparable either because of very proximal and severe root damage or because the gaps extended from the root

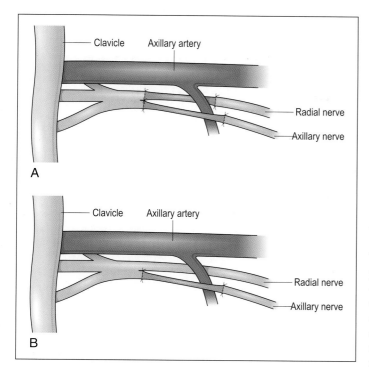

FIGURE 16-13 Posterior cord and one or two of its outflows can be damaged by stretch/contusion with relative sparing of lateral and medial cord structures. **(A)** Input to both radial and axillary nerves required replacement by grafts. **(B)** Input to axillary nerve only was replaced. Although it does occur, an isolated posterior cord to radial injury requiring repair is much less common.

level well down into the upper arm. In the other two patients, the upper roots could be used as lead-out for repair. Results were best in patients with C5, C6, and/or C7 lesions in whom myelography was normal or showed meningoceles only on one or more lower roots. Repair of upper elements by grafts resulted in biceps, brachialis, brachioradialis, and sometimes some degree of deltoid, supraspinatus/infraspinatus, and triceps function. Almost 40% of patients who preoperatively had complete loss in the distribution of all five roots gained partial recovery of upper root function after graft repair.

Bonney and associates published their experience with a small series of vascularized grafts to replace upper plexus elements.[11] The ulnar nerve was usually used because it was distal to a preganglionic injury involving the C8 and T1 roots. The authors were enthusiastic about their early results. At this time, their results seem no better than those more readily accomplished by use of nonvascularized sural interfascicular graft repairs. Support for the latter approach continues to grow, with relatively recent reports from many European countries as well as Australia and New Zealand.[8,13,37–39,87,92,98,99]

Several investigators have carefully evaluated the fascicular anatomy of the various plexus elements in an attempt to make graft repair more specific.[9,97,103] The merits of such a microscopic approach, however, remain to be proven.

NERVE TRANSFERS

Nerve transfers (also referred to as "neurotization") involve the repair of a distal denervated nerve element using a proximal foreign nerve as the donor to reinnervate the distal targets. Its use for the repair of brachial plexus injuries has recently been extensively

reviewed.[64] The concept is to sacrifice the function of a (lesser valued) donor muscle to revive function in the recipient nerve and muscle that will undergo reinnervation.[67,75] The anatomical and physiological principles that underlie nerve transfers are relatively straightforward. Since motor recovery has been the main goal, the choice of a donor nerve or plexus element that has a reasonable aliquot of motor fibers is required.[77] The loss of the muscle denervated by transferring the donor nerve must not represent loss of important or critical function.[57] Obviously, the value of the neuromuscular element to be reinnervated must greatly exceed the utility of the sacrificed one.

The first report of neurotization in an attempt to restore injured plexus function was by Tuttle in 1913.[111] A review of the historical precedent as well as the anatomical basis and rationale for nerve transfers in brachial plexus surgery were enunciated most clearly almost 30 years ago by Narakas.[75] Since then, nerve transfers have become increasingly popular and utilized for the repair of brachial plexus injuries, especially where the proximal motor source of the denervated element is absent because of avulsion from the spinal cord.[89,90,99] Increasingly advocated too is the use of transfers in situations where the proximal motor source is available but the regeneration distance is so long that the outcome would be poor;[28,29] a nerve transfer into the denervated distal nerve stump close to the motor end-organ would then restore function, which otherwise would not be possible.[79]

There are several important principles to adopt in order to maximize outcome in nerve transfers, the first of which is to reinnervate the recipient nerve as close to the target muscle as possible. A good example of this is the transfer of an ulnar nerve fascicle directly to the biceps branch of the musculocutaneous, in close proximity to its entry into the muscle.[82] The second principle is to perform a direct repair, without intervening grafts, a tactic that seems to be associated with improved outcomes, as reported convincingly with intercostal–musculocutaneous transfers.[39,60,73,88,112] The third principle is to utilize combinations of similarly behaving neuromuscular units, maximized when agonist donor and recipient are chosen, as cortical readaptation is the physiological basis for functional recovery.[59,61] This may also be the physiological underpinning that explains why intraplexal (example: medial pectoral–musculocutaneous) nerve donors may garner superior results as compared to extraplexal (example: intercostal–musculocutaneous) nerves.[12,90] The last principle, not so different from all nerve surgery (assuming that nerve is irreparably damaged and thus incapable of spontaneous functional regeneration),[67,68] where prolonging axotomy and target denervation is associated with progressively poorer outcomes,[28,29] is to perform the transfer surgery as early as possible to maximize outcomes.[80,90,93]

Much of the literature related to brachial plexus surgery is in the form of retrospective case reviews, anecdotal experiences, a few and rare prospective studies, and no randomized studies of different surgical techniques. Moreover, the field has been in considerable evolution with traditional direct plexal repairs[41,46] being gradually replaced by a much more liberal use of nerve transfers.[7,35,64,99,110] The use of nerve transfers has been a significant advance in the field of brachial plexus nerve reconstructive surgery, for stretch injuries, with many different ingenious transfers associated with improved results, reported and reviewed recently.[7,12,35,47,62,64,99,116]

A meta-analysis conducted on the nerve transfer literature noted that for restoration of shoulder abduction it is best to use an accessory nerve transfer to the suprascapular nerve, while for elbow flexion, intercostals without graft should be used.[64] In the grim scenario of complete avulsions, the addition of a contralateral C7 transfer with an interposed vascularized ulnar nerve graft directed to the entire or perhaps the lateral root of median nerve in the axilla could be considered.[106] Alternatively, some lower intercostals or cervical plexus elements could be directed to the sensory aspect of the median nerve. This set of transfers is certainly appropriate for the situation where the patient has a complete flail arm with all five spinal nerve roots avulsed. However, it is most important in the case of the completely flail arm patient to ensure that the C5 or any other upper spinal nerve is in fact avulsed and not ruptured extraforaminally.[41,46] To deny an intraplexal repair from a useable C5, C6, or C7 spinal nerve to its distal outflow would be a disservice, given the relatively poor number of extraplexal transfer possibilities available. In some cases, the repair from C5 or C6 to distal elements can be augmented by the transfers of accessory and intercostal nerves.[41]

While the above strategy is appropriate for the panplexus injury, the tactics are very different for the isolated Erb's palsy. For example, if C5 and C6 are avulsed but C7 is injured at a postganglion level, intraplexal graft repairs from the C7 may be used to help reinnervate the shoulder abductors and elbow flexors, but then accessory transferred to suprascapular and medial pectoral branches to a split musculocutaneous nerve can supplement the repair. A combination of distal accessory to suprascapular, ulnar nerve fascicle to biceps nerve (perhaps augmented by a portion of medial pectoral nerve via graft to brachialis nerve),[110] and long head of triceps nerve orthorocodorsal (if functional) to the anterior portion of the axillary nerve could be performed.[7] While such transfers appear promising, outcomes over the long term and in sufficient numbers of patients have not been reported. Hence, same workers have combined neurotization for spinal nerves not reparable with direct repair of spinal nerves where there is useful outflow. Results with such combined repairs appear better in those cases than in those with neurotization alone.[41] In summary, modern nerve reconstruction of brachial plexus stretch injuries often combine direct plexal (graft) repair with neurotization, as dictated by the individual findings for each case.[41,47,116]

The results from management of stretch injuries involving different sets and combinations of brachial plexus elements are reported in the subsequent section of this chapter.

MANAGEMENT OF PAIN ASSOCIATED WITH PLEXUS STRETCH INJURIES

Central destructive lesions to brain or spinal cord can sometimes control the severe pain associated with some plexus stretch injuries.[56,91] Dorsal root entry zone lesions as advanced and practiced by Nashold and co-workers are, in their hands, relatively effective for the severe, unremitting deafferentation pain seen with plexus stretches.[78] Most severe pain associated with plexus stretch injuries lessens or leaves altogether in the early months after injury. This pain can sometimes be helped by institution of early physical therapy and especially range of motion exercises and use of amitriptylline and/or Gabapentin.[42,65] Other cases associated with severe pain appear to be aided by operation on the plexus, especially if some movement is restored.[8,69,105] There are cases, however, in which the neuritic and at times phantom limb pain persists for several years or more, and then dorsal root entry zone lesions are indicated. There are potential complications such as paralysis and respiratory insufficiency, and their incidence varies according to the series presented and techniques used.[25,107] This and other central

procedures for pain should be done only in carefully selected patients.

CRITERIA FOR SELECTING PATIENTS FOR EXPLORATION AND REPAIR OF SUPRACLAVICULAR BRACHIAL PLEXUS STRETCH INJURIES

Not all patients with severe stretch injury involving the plexus can, at the present time, be meaningfully helped by an operation. This is especially so in complete avulsion cases, where direct repair is not feasible and nerves available for successful neurotization are very limited.

For the usual case with serious paralysis of the plexus, we evaluate the patient as early as possible. This includes grading any residual motor or sensory function in the extremity and obtaining a baseline set of electrodiagnostic studies at 3 or 4 weeks after injury. Special attention is given to assessing proximally innervated muscles such as paraspinal muscles, rhomboids, serratus anterior, and supraspinatus. In addition, it is most important to define how complete the injury and loss are to each element of the plexus involved. Significant, incomplete loss in the distribution of an element usually improves with time, but complete loss often does not. In addition to radiographs of associated bones such as spine, scapula, clavicle, ribs, and shoulder joint including humerus, a chest film is important to note the relative positions of the diaphragm and to exclude injury to the phrenic nerve. The patient is usually followed for about 3–4 months with periodic clinical and electromyographic examinations. If significant function does not begin to recover, then the patient has a myelogram and post-myelogram cervical computed tomography (CT) scan, if that has not already been done.[17,117]

The patient is then operated on if there are not too may contraindications to exploration and if there is a possibility of direct repair of at least a portion of the plexus at levels favorable for repair, which are usually C5, C6, C7, and their more distal outflows (Table 16-1). One advantage to a delay of several months in exploring stretch injuries to the plexus relates to the fact that often there is physical continuity to one or more of the plexus elements. These elements have not been avulsed from the spinal cord or distracted more laterally but require time for even adequate spontaneous regeneration to occur. Even direct intraoperative recordings cannot with certainty exclude adequate regeneration in these elements, especially those with lengthy lesions in continuity, until 3–4 months from the time of injury. Such a delay has to be balanced against the advantage provided by earlier repair done within weeks of the injury. The problem with earlier surgery is that even intraoperative electrical techniques have difficulty assessing fairly the need for resection. In addition, those cases capable of spontaneous recovery in the distribution of one or more elements may have them prematurely resected and replaced by grafts if operation is done too early. In any case, maintenance or recovery of a good range of motion in all involved joints is paramount while awaiting operation.

There are some findings which make the possibility of direct repair less likely. The presence of one such finding should seldom prevent exploration, although serious spinal cord injury at the plexus level usually does. However, such findings, especially if multiple, usually make direct repair with significantly useful outcome less likely (Table 16-1). Nonetheless, if there is doubt, it is probably better to explore these lesions. The opportunities for other reconstructive or neurotization procedures are not very good

Table 16-1 Relative contraindications for exploration and direct repair of plexus stretch injuries

Evidence of proximal spinal nerve injury at multiple levels, especially the upper levels; included is extensive paraspinal denervation by electromyogram, rhomboid, serratus anterior, or diaphragmatic paralysis.
Presence of sensory nerve action potentials elicited by stimulation of and recording from multiple peripheral nerves (median, radial and ulnar), whose sensory domain is anesthetic.
Presence of pseudomeningoceles at multiple spinal nerve levels, especially the upper levels.
Presence of extensive fractures of the cervical spine or serious cervical myelopathy.
Injury limited to the C8–T1 spinal nerves or their outflows.
Referral of the patient a year or more after injury.
Cases in which there has been severe scapular or thoracic distraction, especially if there has been subclavian artery avulsion.

in most patients, or only help one portion of the paralyzed limb. Unfortunately, direct repair may also not lead to enough return to muscles to make them usable for transfer. This is because the yield in terms of significant muscle power is relatively low, especially when an attempt is made to reinnervate a completely flail arm.

Winging of the scapula as a result of long thoracic nerve palsy and serratus anterior loss suggests a very proximal lesion of C5, C6, and C7 spinal nerves. The long thoracic nerve usually arises from the distal intraforaminal portion of C6 but can also receive proximal spinal nerve branches of C5 and sometimes C7 or even C8 or C4. For a similar reason, rhomboid paralysis suggests a proximal spinal nerve lesion of C5 and C6 because the dorsal scapular nerve has a proximal intraforaminal origin from these structures. It is unusual, however, for these losses to be present in adult stretch injuries unless there has been severe scapular or thoracic dissociation.

In 20 LSUHSC patients having C5 root injury close to the spine and confirmed at the operating table, clinical examination and EMG showed normal or near normal rhomboid, serratus anterior, and paraspinal function despite severe more distal losses. At operation seven C5 roots were avulsed and the other 13 had proximal traction injuries with heavy scar but were in continuity. It was postulated that the angled takeoff of the posterior primary roots, the long thoracic nerve, and the dorsal scapular nerve spared their axons for the large traction forces delivered more directly to the C5 fibers. Thus, preserved innervation of axial musculature in the C5 myotome does not exclude otherwise severe injury to this nerve root or spinal nerve. (Andrew Change, John England, Austin Sumner, David Kline, Robert Tiel-personal contribution "Sparing of Axial Muscles in Traumatic Cervical Root Avulsions" AANS poster-2004 Meeting)

Even though the phrenic arises usually from C3 and C4 spinal nerves, it often has input from C5 and, in any case, is adherent and often incorporated into a portion of C5 as the latter exits its foramen. Thus, if the diaphragm is paralyzed in the case of blunt and non-penetrating injury to the neck and supraclavicular plexus, relatively proximal damage to C5 is often present. Moreover, if C5

is damaged proximally, so often is C6 and even C7, and yet these are the very levels responding best to direct repair if it can be achieved.

Another clinical finding suggesting a proximal level of injury is the presence of Horner syndrome. This suggests but does not prove proximal involvement of the T1 and frequently the C8 spinal nerve also. However, there is a false-positive and false-negative incidence of correlation of Horner syndrome with the non-reparability of T1 and C8 spinal nerves. Like meningoceles on a myelogram, though, this finding usually means a proximal and thus irreparable lesion at these lower levels. Nonetheless, the presence of Horner syndrome does not necessarily mean that more proximal spinal nerves such as C5, C6, and C7 are not more laterally injured and thus reparable. Similar arguments can be marshaled for and against the value of myelography in this setting, and are summarized elsewhere in this and other chapters. Similarly, sensory NAP recordings, which can provide evidence of preganglionic injury fairly effectively in lower spinal nerves such as C8, T1, and sometimes C7, are not as reliable to evaluate either C5 or C6, and yet these are the spinal nerves of the plexus we would like to know the most about.

STRETCH INJURY RESULTS

GRADING AND OVERALL RESULTS

The majority of stretch-injured patients selected for operation were done by a classical anterior approach. Most of the proximal stretch injuries required both a supraclavicular and infraclavicular anterior approach. Most cord and cord-to-nerve injuries were, of course, approached anteriorly. A small number of stretch/contusive lesions had a posterior approach, as detailed at the end of this chapter.

Over a 30-year period (1968–1998), approximately 2500 patients with brachial plexus lesions were evaluated, and somewhat over 1000 patients with these lesions were surgically managed at LSUHSC (Table 16-2).[41] Approximately 50% of these, or 509 cases, represent stretch injuries and are discussed further in this chapter. Follow-up on this group of patients was extremely difficult to obtain. These individuals were especially mobile, often had changed addresses, and did not always maintain contact with family, friends, or referring physicians.[18] In addition, because at least 18 months of follow-up was desired, some operated patients were not far enough along to include.

A standardized (LSUHSC) grading system was used for assessing outcome of operated patients (Table 16-3). This system differs from the British Medical Research Council (MRC) system in that the LSUHSC grade 3 includes at least some muscle contraction against mild resistance as well as gravity while grade 2 is against gravity only, which would be an MRC 3. Favorable outcomes were, therefore, in our view, patients with element(s) recovering to an LSUHSC grade of 3 or better level, not an MRC grade 3 level.

Postoperative or recovery grades for the various patterns of supraclavicular stretch injuries operated on were initially calculated for each element, usually at root or spinal nerve level. These grades (ranging from 0 to 5) were then added together and averaged to obtain the overall grade. For example, if the postoperative grades in a patient with a C5 and C6 stretch injury were 3.5 in the C5 distribution and 4.0 in the C6 distribution, then the average would be 3.75, and the overall grade would be 3 to 4. If the initial lesion was a C5, C6, and C7 stretch injury and postoperative grades were

Table 16-2 Brachial plexus lesions surgically treated at LSUHSC between 1968 and 1998 (modified from Kim et al.)[41]

Type of lesion	No. of lesions (%)
Stretch/contusion	509 (50)
Supraclavicular	366
Infraclavicular	143
GSW	118 (12)
Laceration	71 (7)
TOS	160 (16)
Nerve sheath tumor	161 (16)
Total	1019 (100)

Table 16-3 Grading system by element of brachial plexus

Grade	Description
	Overall grading
0	No muscle contraction
1 (poor)	Proximal muscles contract but not against gravity
2 (fair)	Proximal muscles contract against gravity and distal muscles do not contract; sensory grade, if applicable, is usually ≤2
3 (moderate)	Proximal muscles contract against gravity and some resistance; some distal muscles contract against gravity; sensory grade, if applicable, is usually 3
4 (good)	All muscles contract against gravity and some resistance; sensory grade, if applicable, is 3 or 4
5 (excellent)	All muscles contract against moderate resistance; sensory grade, if applicable, is 4
	*Sensory grading**
0 (absent)	No response to touch, pin, or pressure
1 (bad)	Testing produces hyperesthesia or parasthesias; deep pain recovery in autonomous zones
2 (poor)	Sensory response sufficient for grip and slow protection, sensory stimuli mislocalized with some overresponse
3 (moderate)	Response to touch and pin in autonomous zones, sensation mislocalized and not normal, with overresponse
4 (good)	Response to touch and pin in autonomous zones; response localized but not normal; however, there is no overresponse
5 (excellent)	Normal response to touch and pin in entire field of plexus element including autonomous zones

*Where applicable, such as C8, T1, lower trunk, lateral cord, and medial cord.

C5 = 2, C6 = 4, and C7 = 3, then the average grade would be 3. If elements were considered irreparable and no attempts were made to lead outflow from the proximal portions of other elements to those damaged or to neurotize them, then these elements were excluded from the calculations. This situation usually applied to C8–T1 to lower trunk elements, so some of the grades in the flail arm series of operated patients reflect averaged grades for C5, C6, and C7 muscles. Despite this, we believe that the data accurately reflect the difficulties encountered in restoring neural function to the patient with a flail arm, because it was usually more difficult to repair or find outflows or substitutes for C7, C6, and sometimes C5 in the patients with C5–T1 lesions than in those with C5, C6, C7 or C5–C6 lesions.

Supraclavicular stretch injury patterns included spinal nerves C5–6 (15%), C5–7 (20%), and C5–T1 (57%), or other more unusual patterns such as nerves at C8–T1 or C7–T1 (8%). Table 16-4 provides the overall postoperative grades at 18 or more months after operation in 366 supraclavicular stretch injuries with various preoperative distributions. Notably, the most common scenario (208 cases) is the patient with a completely flail arm (C5–T1 loss). The difficulties in obtaining satisfactory results in the flail arm patient, by direct graft repair, are evident. Only 35% of such patients recovered to an average postoperative grade of 3 or better. Results from repair of patients having isolated upper plexus injuries (C5–6 or C5–7) were somewhat better. However, it is also evident that outcomes with direct repair of many stretch injuries are less than optimal. This has prompted us to add nerve transfers to direct repair whenever possible in recent years, as discussed in subsequent sections.

RESULTS OF OPERATION ON C5 AND C6 STRETCH INJURIES

There were 55 patients in this category (Table 16-5). Loss was complete in the C5–C6 distribution (no supra- or infraspinatus, and no deltoid, biceps, brachioradialis, or supinator function) and had persisted for 4 or more months in virtually all of these cases operated upon. A significant subset (8) of these patients, who had a C5–C6 pattern of loss but intact function of the rest of the arm, were found to have serious involvement of C7 spinal nerve at the time of operation (Figs 16-14, 16-15). In exceptional cases, C7 had been avulsed despite no clinical loss in the C7 distribution. In the remaining cases, the nerve was in continuity but an NAP could not be recorded. The C7 spinal nerve was resected in these cases, and a graft repair from the C7 proximal stump was done. Postoperatively, there was no increased clinical deficit. Histologic examination of the resected nerves showed them to be neurotmetic. One possible explanation was that these plexi were postfixed. Against this theory is that C5 and C6 were in each instance dissected out and at least at their dural exits had, as well as could be determined, normal volume. More likely as a theory is the occasional dominance of C8 input not only to wrist extensors but also to the triceps. These observations concerning C7 are important, for if it is not functional and yet not injured close to the spinal cord, it can be used to supplement lead-out from C5 and/or C6 by use of grafts.

Most (43 patients) of the C5–C6 lesions selected for operation required graft repair (Table 16-5). Those not having avulsion of both roots and grafts placed from both C5 and C6 (34 patients) to the anterior and posterior divisions of the upper trunk represent the largest subgroup. The results were generally very good in these 34 patients, with useful function obtained in the vast majority. For

Table 16-4 Overall postoperative functional grades in patients with 366 supraclavicular plexus stretch injuries

Initial loss of function	Postoperative grade									
	0	1	1–2	2	2–3	3	3–4	4	4–5	Totals
C5–6[a]	1	0	0	0	6	14	18	9	7	55
C5–7[a]	1	0	0	2	14	23	20	9	6	75
C5–T1[a]	21	8	15	29	62	40	20	13	0	208
C5–8[a]	0	0	0	0	0	1	1	0	0	2
C6–T1[a]	0	0	0	1	0	2	1	0	0	4
C7–T1[a]	0	0	0	0	1	1	0	0	0	2
C8–T1[a]	2	3	2	2	0	2	0	0	0	11
C8–T1[b]	0	0	0	0	0	0	2	2	3	7
C7–T1[b]	0	0	0	0	0	1	1	0	0	2
Total	25	11	17	34	83	84	63	33	16	366

[a]Complete or nearly complete loss.

[b]Incomplete loss.

Table 16-5 Outcomes of surgery for 55 stretch injuries to the C5 and C6 nerves with complete loss of function

Operation	No. of patients	Average outcome (no. of patients)
Grafts of C5 & C6 nerves	34	Grade 3 (19) Grade 3–4 (7) Grade 4 (8)
C5 nerve grafts, C6 nerve avulsed, descending cervical plexus used*	5	Grade 2–3
C5 nerve avulsed, C6 nerve grafts, descending cervical plexus used†	2	Grade 3–4
C5 and C6 neurolysis (NAPs present)	12	Grade 3–4
C5 neurolysis, C6 nerve grafts	2	Grade 3–4

*Patients who underwent these procedures might have done better had medial pectoral branch transfer to the musculocutaneous nerve been added. Four patients who were surgically treated after 1998 in this fashion had a mean outcome of grade 4.

†Patients who underwent these procedures might have done better had accessory nerve transfer to the suprascapular nerve been added. Two patients who were surgically treated after 1998 in this fashion had a mean outcome of grade 3.8.

instance, nine patients recovered to grade 3, eight patients to grade 4, and seven patients to grade 3 to 4. Five patients had an isolated C6 avulsion and underwent direct graft repairs to the C5 nerve with a supplemental nerve transfer from the descending cervical plexus. Outcomes in this group averaged only grade 2 to 3. In recent years (1999–2002), this group of patients underwent medial pectoral branch transfers to the musculocutaneous nerve with improved results to the biceps muscles. Two patients had a C5 avulsion and underwent graft repairs to the C6 nerve, supplemented with transfers from descending cervical plexus, resulting in recovery grade of 3 or 4, but predominantly for biceps function. More recently, several patients in this category have undergone a procedure in which the distal accessory nerve is transferred directly to the suprascapular nerves, with improved results for the supraspinatus muscle and thus shoulder abduction.

Finally, there were 12 cases in which both C5 and C6 spinal nerves had recordable NAPs despite being 4–8 months after injury with complete clinical and EMG loss (Fig. 16-16). These patients underwent neurolysis alone, and had grade 3 to 4 overall recovery, with very satisfactory results.

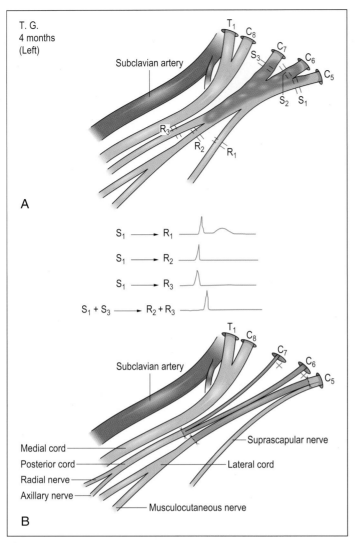

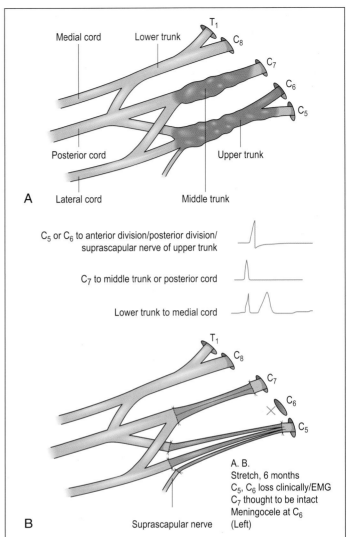

FIGURE 16-14 **(A)** This patient presented with typical C5 and C6 loss involving left arm. Function of triceps as well as wrist and finger extensors was excellent. Nonetheless, at the operating table, C7 was found to be severely injured. C5 to supraclavicular nerve was thought, based on nerve action potential studies, to be regenerating, and was spared resection. **(B)** The rest of C5 was used as a lead-out for grafts, but only a portion of C6 and C7 was usable. Postoperatively, there was no additional loss. About 1 in 6 patients with loss that appears clinically to be confined to C5 and C6 also have serious injury involving C7. Today, this repair might be supplemented by transfer of medial pectoral or a fascicle of the ulnar nerve to the musculocutaneous nerve.

Although results were generally good with C5–C6 stretch repairs, recovery was not uniform in this distribution. Forearm flexion was almost always better than shoulder abduction. The latter was seldom good enough to raise the shoulder above the horizontal. Thus, it remains important to identify patients with early spontaneous recovery and spare them from surgery. Occasionally, very lengthy grafts are necessary (Fig. 16-17). These appear to work better for biceps than deltoid recovery.

Summary of C5, C6 lesions

1. Distribution of loss is very predictable: supra- and infraspinatus, deltoid, biceps/brachialis, brachioradialis, and supinator.

FIGURE 16-15 **(A, B)** Another patient with an exact clinical pattern of C5 and C6 loss that clinically and by EMG was complete who was nonetheless found to also have complete injury to C7 at operation. If C7 to middle trunk had not been tested, the C7 outflow would not have been used to add to the graft repair. Medial pectoral could also have been transferred to a split musculocutaneous nerve to aid the repair.

2. Almost 30% regain significant function spontaneously. Signs of this are usually evident by 3–4 months after injury.
3. Despite apparent clinical and (preoperative) electrical sparing, C7 may be found to be seriously involved at operation in 15% of cases. If C7 is resected because of an absent NAP in this setting, postoperative loss is not increased and yet C7 can be used to supplement the repair.
4. This is the most favorable group of serious stretch injuries to repair with direct nerve grafts.
5. Direct repair of one or both spinal nerves is likely. Need for neurotization is less likely than with other injury patterns.
6. Neurotization using descending cervical plexus to supplement the C5 or C6 lead-out is of limited added benefit. Other forms of neurotization (medial pectoral or ulnar fascicle to musculocutaneous and accessory to suprascapular) are currently favoured.[41]

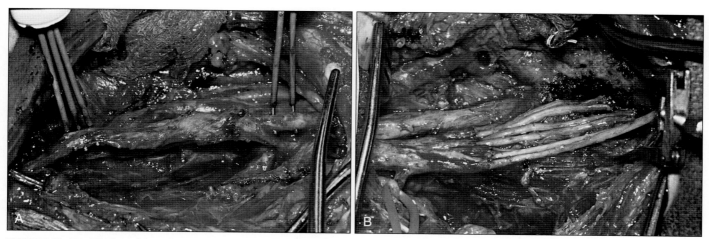

FIGURE 16-16 **(A)** Right C5 and C6 stretch injury extending into upper trunk. Clavicle is to the right. After exposing spinal nerves and more distal elements, nerve action potential recordings were done. Here, C5 is being stimulated (to the left), and recording electrodes are on one of the upper trunk divisions (to the right). **(B)** Graft repair of another but left-sided C5–C6 stretch injury. Sural grafts run from an intraforaminal level of both C5 and C6 to distal upper trunk. Less injured or involved C7 to middle trunk is seen in the background. Plexus is viewed from the side.

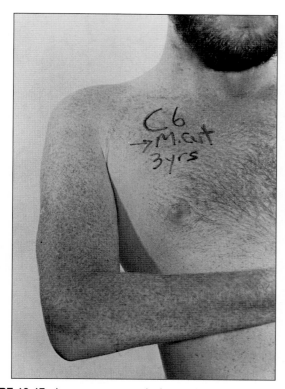

FIGURE 16-17 In severe upper spinal nerve injury over a length of plexus, a sural graft sometimes needs to be placed between C6 and the proximal cut end of the musculocutaneous nerve. The grafts are led either superficial or deep to the clavicle. This patient obtained useful elbow flexion by 3 years after such a lengthy graft.

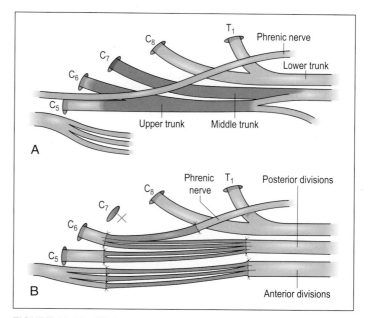

FIGURE 16-18 **(A)** Drawing depicting extent of lesion in patient with C5, C6, and C7 loss. C7 was not reparable, but C5 and C6 were **(B)**. Descending cervical plexus was also used to provide more lead-out for sural grafts which went to anterior and posterior divisions of upper and middle trunks. In this case, phrenic nerve was encased in scar, was further injured during dissection, and was repaired by a graft as well.

RESULTS OF OPERATION ON C5, C6, AND C7 STRETCH INJURIES

The 75 patients in this category had not only a C5–C6 pattern of loss but lack of triceps and some weakness of wrist and sometimes finger extension. Loss of wrist and finger extension and weakness of the flexor profundi muscle varied because of a dominant input of the C8 nerve to these muscles in some patients. This group was selected for surgical exploration and repair because they suffered complete or persistent severe clinical loss, at least in the C5–C6 distribution (Table 16-6).

Most of the C5, C6, and C7 stretch injuries selected for operation required graft repairs (Table 16-6; Fig. 16-18). There were, however, important exceptions, based on intraoperative NAP studies that supported regeneration or nerve root avulsion. If two of the three involved roots could have a neurolysis based on a positive NAP, despite complete clinical and electrical loss, results were also predictably good (Fig. 16-19). Where only one spinal nerve had a neurolysis, average recovery in that spinal nerve distribution was

Table 16-6 Outcomes of surgery for 75 stretch injuries to the C5–C7 nerves with complete loss of function

Operation	No. of patients	Average outcome
Grafts of C5, C6, & C7 nerves	31	Grade 3–4
C5 nerve grafts, C6 & C7 nerves avulsed, descending cervical plexus used*	10	Grade 2–3
C5 & C6 nerve grafts, C7 nerve avulsed, descending cervical plexus used	10	Grade 3
C5 nerve avulsed, C6 & C7 nerve grafts, descending cervical plexus used†	6	Grade 3–4
C5, C6, & C7 neurolysis (NAPs present)	18	Grade 4

*Patients who underwent these procedures might have done better had medial pectoral branch transfer to the musculocutaneous nerve been added. Three patients who were surgically treated after 1998 in this fashion had a mean outcome of grade 3.7.

†Patients who underwent these procedures might have done better had distal accessory nerve transfer to the suprascapular nerve been included as an additional step. Two patients who were surgically treated after 1998 in this fashion had a mean outcome of grade 3.5.

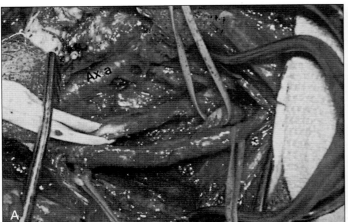

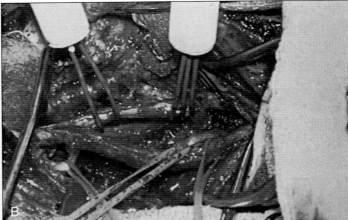

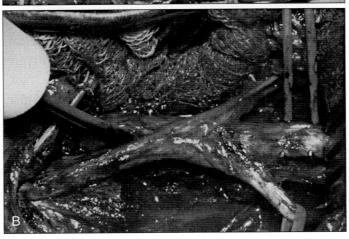

FIGURE 16-19 **(A)** Stretch injury involving left C5, C6, and C7 spinal nerves and their outflows (Ax a, subclavian artery). **(B)** Operative electrodes for nerve action potential studies are placed on C7 to middle trunk segments. **(C)** Exposure of C5, C6, upper trunk (UT), and divisions of UT in a patient with a right C5 to C7 stretch injury. Stimulating electrode is placed under the C6 spinal nerve and recording electrode (right of picture) on the anterior division of the UT. Loop displaces suprascapular nerve downward at right lower corner of photograph.

3 to 4. Overall, slightly less than 25% of the patients operated on in this category had neurolysis not only because of physical continuity of the stretched elements but because of present (regenerative) NAPs. This was despite the fact that loss clinically and electrically in their distribution was complete. These patients had very good outcomes, achieving a grade 4 overall result (Table 16-6).

The second factor playing a significant role in the outcome in these cases was the presence of avulsion injury extending to the level of the dura (Fig. 16-20). This usually affected one root (16 instances). However, in 10 cases, such injury affected two roots. As a result, in 26 cases, nerve repair was performed with grafts from only one or two proximal spinal nerves. In earlier cases (until

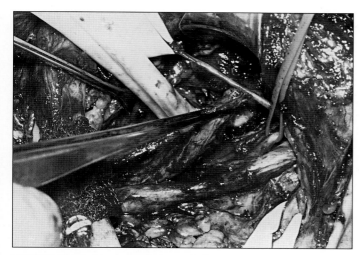

FIGURE 16-20 Meningocele beneath C7 root in a patient with a C5, C6, and C7 stretch injury. Forceps are elevating the C7 nerve root.

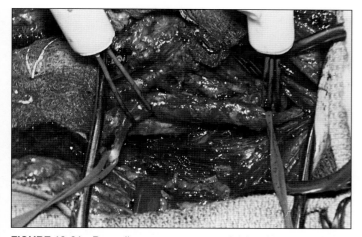

FIGURE 16-21 Recording on a severe stretch injury involving left C5, C6, and C7. Here, stimulating electrodes are on C6, and recording ones are on origin of supraclavicular nerve from upper trunk.

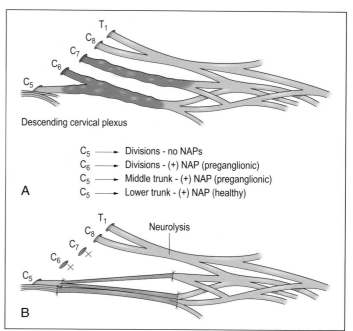

FIGURE 16-22 **(A)** Stretch injury involving proximal portions of C6 and C7 and more distal portion of C5. C8 and T1 were spared. **(B)** Despite avulsion at C6 and C7 levels, this was still a favorable injury for repair because lead-out was available from C5 as well as descending cervical plexus. A more current operation might have included transfer of medial pectoral or a fascicle of the ulnar nerve to the musculocutaneous nerve.

1988), direct repairs from the one spared nerve were supplemented by neurotization using descending cervical plexus, but outcomes from repair averaged only grade 2 to 3.

If only one root was avulsed in the C5, C6, and C7 category, neurotization was usually not felt to be necessary. Instead, grafts were led out from one or more of those roots damaged close to but not all the way to the spinal cord (Figs 16-21, 16-22). In 10 cases of isolated C7 avulsions, direct graft repairs from C5 and C6 nerves to the anterior and posterior divisions of the upper and middle trunks resulted in an average recovery of grade 3. Six patients who had C5 avulsions and received direct graft repairs to C6 and C7 nerves achieved an average recovery grade of 3.5. Grafts were not only led distally to what the root normally innervated, but also to adjacent outflows whose proximal counterparts had been avulsed. Recovery in an avulsed root's distribution by transfer of grafts from other roots ranged from grade 1 to 4, but averaged at grade 2 to 3. Thus, avulsive root injuries usually lowered the overall grades for repair of C5, C6, and C7 injuries.

In recent years (1999–2002), if usable outflow to the suprascapular nerve was poor, the accessory nerve was transferred to this nerve. If usable outflow to the biceps muscle was poor, an anastomosis was created between the medial pectoral branches and part or all of the musculocutaneous nerve (Table 16-6).

Summary of C5, C6, C7 lesions

1. Loss involves triceps, in addition to shoulder muscles, biceps/brachialis, brachioradialis, and supinator. Loss of finger extension, flexor profundi, and wrist extension is variable, since C8 input to these muscles is dominant in some patients.
2. A few cases of serious C5, C6, C7 injury (16%) improve spontaneously in the early months after injury.
3. Despite sparing of C8–T1 muscle function, opportunities for effective substitutive procedures are limited. For example, it is difficult to substitute for loss of shoulder and upper arm function. As a result, operation to attempt direct repair of the plexus with or without the addition of neurotization is usually indicated.
4. The incidence of root avulsions is much higher in this group than the C5–C6 stretch injuries.
5. In circumstances where only neurolysis is required or 2–3 spinal nerves can be directly grafted from, the outcomes are very satisfactory.
6. Direct repair of only one element frequently needs to be supplemented by neurotization.
7. Outcome is usually best for biceps/brachialis, but imperfect return there can be affected adversely by partial recovery of triceps. Supraspinatus recovery is usually better than that for deltoid.

RESULTS OF OPERATION ON C5–T1 STRETCH INJURIES

The most common stretch injury was at the C5–T1 level, which was seen in 208 patients (57%). The presenting and usually persistent symptom was total upper extremity paralysis or flail arm. This group of patients had the lowest spontaneous recovery rate (4%).

Criteria used to select these C5–T1 stretches for operation included preservation of rhomboid, serratus anterior, and diaphragmatic function. Patients with a meningocele of C4–C5, a cervical myelopathy, overwhelming medical problems, or who were evaluated by us a year or more after injury were excluded.

Not unexpectedly, approximately half of the spinal nerves or roots evaluated at the operating table had proximal irreparable damage or were avulsed at the dural level. This was despite the fact that some attempt was made to select the more favorable patients for operation and to visualize the root or spinal nerve as close to the dural level as possible in these patients (Figs 16-23, 16-24). On the other hand, despite this large number of avulsed and irreparable spinal nerves, an almost equal number were reparable or, in some instances, had a regenerative NAP. As can also be seen in Table 16-7, which shows the usual operative findings in 112

patients with flail arms, C7, C8, and T1 roots were not reparable in 31 cases, and in 34 instances C8 and T1 were not. There were also 10 cases in which C5 was the only spinal nerve reparable by direct repair. These three patterns alone accounted for about 80% of the nonreparable roots. Table 16-8 documents some of the more unusual distributions of reparable and irreparable loss. In four cases, C5, C6, C8, and T1 were reparable or had neurolysis but C7 was not reparable. In another three cases, C6 and C7 were not reparable, but C5, C8, and T1 were reparable or had a neurolysis. Still other variations can be seen in Table 16-8. This table serves to point out how diverse the patterns of both irreparable and reparable damage can be in patients with flail arms.

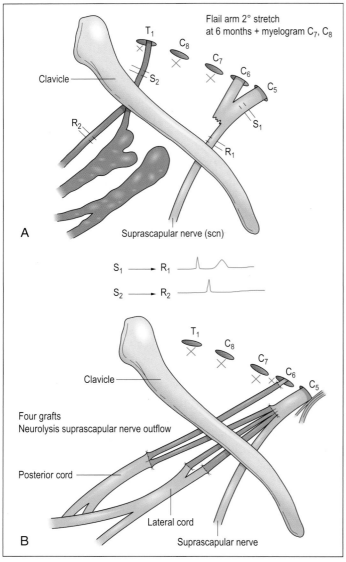

FIGURE 16-23 **(A)** Drawing of an unfortunately frequent set of findings at the operating table when the arm is flail. C5 to supraclavicular nerve was regenerating, but the rest of the supraclavicular plexus was ruptured as well as damaged back to the spinal cord. **(B)** Grafts from C5 and some of C6 were 8 cm in length. This patient might have been helped further by placing intercostal nerves to a split musculocutaneous nerve.

Table 16-7 C5 to T1 stretch injury patterns based on operative findings in 112 cases (usual distributions)

	No. cases	Description
A	34	C5, C6, C7 reparable or had neurolysis; C8, T1 not reparable
B	31	C5, C6 reparable or had neurolysis; C7, C8, T1 not reparable
C	10	C5 reparable or had neurolysis; C6, C7, C8, T1 not reparable
D	8	All roots reparable (4 cases) or had neurolysis (2 cases) or both (2 cases)
E	6	C5, C6, C7, C8 reparable or had neurolysis; T1 not reparable
F	2	C6 reparable; C5, C7, C8, T1 not reparable
G	2	No roots reparable directly nor responded to neurolysis

Table 16-8 C5 to T1 stretch injury patterns in 112 cases (unusual distributions)

	No. cases	Description
A	4	C5, C6, C8, T1 reparable or had neurolysis; C7 not reparable
B	3	C5, C8, T1 reparable or had neurolysis; C6, C7 not reparable
C	2	C5, C6, T1 reparable or had neurolysis; C7, C8 not reparable
D	2	C5, C6, C8 reparable or had neurolysis; C7, T1 not reparable
E	1	C5, C7, C8, T1 reparable or had neurolysis; C6 not reparable
F	1	C5, C7, C8 reparable or had neurolysis; C6, T1 not reparable
G	1	C5, C8 had neurolysis; C6, C7, T1 not reparable
H	1	C5, C7 reparable; C6, C8, T1 not reparable

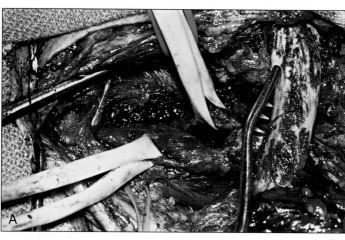

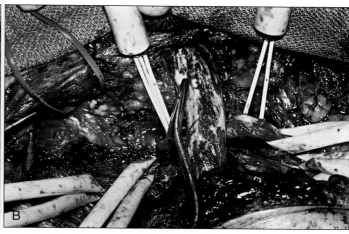

FIGURE 16-24 **(A)** Extensive stretch injury which has produced a flail arm. C5 and C6 to divisions of upper trunk did not conduct nerve action potential (NAP), nor did C7 to distal middle trunk. Lesion extended to cord levels. **(B)** Stimulation of lower trunk or C8 or T1 and recording from medial cord gave a rapidly conducting and relatively high amplitude NAP, indicating preganglionic injuries at these levels.

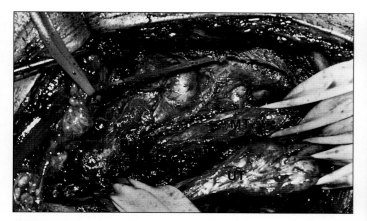

FIGURE 16-25 Stretch injury involving all elements within a heavily scarred supraclavicular space. Phrenic is retracted upward by the plastic loop; right upper Penrose is around thickened, scarred middle trunk (MT), and lower two Penroses are on the divisions of a very neurotomatous upper trunk (UT).

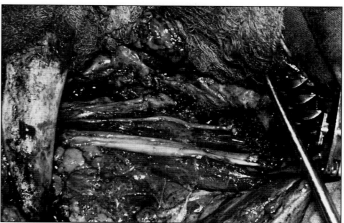

FIGURE 16-26 Grafts from C5 (3), C7 (1), C8 (3), and T1 (1) to cords in a 15-year-old with a flail arm due to a blunt stretch as well as transecting injury as a result of a motorcycle accident. Sural grafts were 12.7 cm in length and extended to the cord level. A vein graft repair of the subclavian was necessary, but the patient had no restoration of the radial pulse. Follow-up over a 3.5-year period showed recovery of biceps, brachioradialis, and some supraspinatus and deltoid.

In the most recent data analysis of cases over 30 years, 1040 spinal nerves were evaluated in 208 patients at the operating table.[41] Despite attempts to select favorable cases for repair, 470 elements had irreparable proximal damage, usually due to avulsion: 35% at the C7–C8 level, 35% at the C7–T1 level, and only 10% at the C5 level. Direct graft repairs were performed on the remaining 570 spinal nerves. Graft repair of two spinal nerves per patient was performed in 54 cases, and three or more spinal nerves per patient were repaired in 76 cases. Because regenerative NAPs were measured distal to their lesions, 35 of the patients required only neurolysis without graft repairs on one or more plexus elements. Nine patients underwent split graft repair of the C5 or C6 nerve and its outflows.

The C5–T1 lesions or flail arms were especially difficult to manage effectively. Restoration of function was often quite limited, even after an attempt was made to select patients for their operability. Although some restoration of shoulder abduction and flexion of the elbow was obtained in approximately 40% of cases and some triceps function in 30%, these operations were often salvage-like in nature (Fig. 16-25). Useful wrist or finger motion was seldom

obtained. Most of the better functional grades were due to shoulder and upper arm recovery rather than distal function. In the few exceptions, presence of not only continuity but a non-preganglionic and regenerative NAP led to neurolysis of one or more lower elements and, because of spontaneous regeneration, some subsequent degree of useful recovery of hand function occurred.

Selection for attempted direct repair of the C5 and possibly the C6 spinal nerve was carried out if possible. Cases operated on had rhomboid and serratus anterior function and did not have a meningocele at the C4–C5 level (involving C5 root or spinal nerve). In the large majority of cases, at least C5 was either regenerating or, if not regenerating, could be used to provide adequate lead-out for grafts at or after its dural exit (Fig. 16-26). If C5 was the only directly reparable root, overall grades of recovery averaged only 2. There were only a few exceptions where all roots including C5 were clearly avulsed. Recovery did not ensue in any of these patients. In a few cases, C5, C7, C8, and T1 were avulsed but C6 was not. Some recovery was gained in these cases by supplementing direct C6 repair with neurotization using descending cervical plexus and phrenic nerve as lead-outs for grafts.

A large subgroup of injuries had reparable or regenerating C5 and C6 roots despite proximal avulsions of C7, C8, and T1 roots (Figs 16-27, 16-28). These 31 cases formed the second largest subset of C5–T1 lesions selected for operation in our earlier analysis (reported in the first edition of this text). If all 31 patients are summarized regardless of length of follow-up, average recovery in the C5 distribution was 2.2. Recovery averaged 2.3 in the C6 distribution and only 1.4 in the C7 distribution. In flail arm patients with C5–C6 spinal nerve injuries that were reparable or regenerating after follow-up of 30 months and more, averaged C5 recovery was 2.7, C6 recovered to 2.9, and C7 to 1.6. Looked at another way, 11 of 19 patients in this category with follow-up of more than

30 months achieved grades of 3 or more for C5- and C6-innervated muscles (Fig. 16-29). One patient had a split repair of C5 to upper trunk with neurolysis of outflow to suprascapular nerve. Result in this patient's C5 distribution graded 4.

The largest subset of C5–T1 stretch patients operated on were those with either regenerating or reparable C5, C6, and C7 roots found at the operating table. In these 34 cases from our earlier series (first edition of this textbook), C8 and T1 were not reparable. This group was summarized for return in the distribution of various roots. C5 recovery averaged 2.4, C6 was 2.7, and C7 was 1.9. Only one patient had significant recovery in the C8 distribution, which was grade 2. In patients in this category who had 24 or more months of follow-up, C5 averaged 2.6, C6 was 2.9, and C7 remained 1.9. The data could be further analyzed in another way. In patients with 24 or more months of follow-up, 14 of 26 had recovery in both the C5 and C6 distributions averaging 3 or better. In seven of these same patients, C7 distribution recovery was 3 or better (Fig. 16-30).

As can be seen in Table 16-4, only about a third of all C5–T1 stretch injured patients gained an overall grade of 3 or better outcome. As a result, in the last few years, most patients with C5–T1 stretch injuries or flail arms have undergone neurotization (nerve transfers) in addition to any direct graft repairs. These transfers have usually involved accessory nerve to suprascapular nerve or posterior division of upper trunk and intercostal nerves to musculocutaneous nerve. As a result, grades for shoulder and biceps muscles have increased by an average of 0.85.

Similar to the C5–C6 and C5–C7 stretch injuries, intraoperative findings of regeneration (positive but not preganglionic NAPs) portended improved outcomes in the distribution of that element with a recordable response. (Figs 16-31, 16-32).

Summary of C5, C6, C7, C8, and T1 lesions

1. This most frequent pattern of loss due to stretch seen in this series of patients unfortunately produces a totally paralyzed or flail arm.
2. The incidence of spontaneous recovery of function is the lowest (only about 4%) for all patterns of severe stretch injury.
3. A combination of severe paraspinal denervation, positive sensory NAPs from several nerves, or meningoceles at three or more

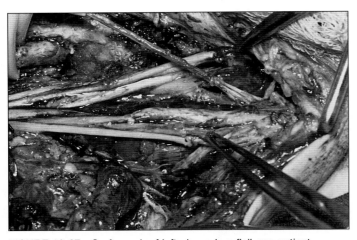

FIGURE 16-27 Graft repair of left plexus in a flail arm patient. Lengthy grafts using sural nerve were led out from descending cervical plexus and C5 and C6 spinal nerves and sutured distally to lateral and posterior cords. C7 and C8 were damaged back to the dura. Forceps point to proximal suture sites for grafts.

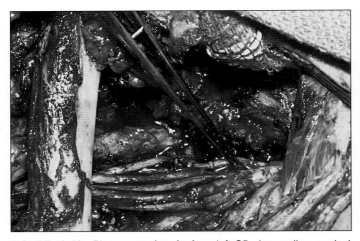

FIGURE 16-28 Placement of grafts from left C5, descending cervical plexus, and a portion of C6 to cord level just distal to the exposed clavicle. The patient had a flail arm. C7 was damaged back to the spinal dura, so one C6 graft and one of the C5 grafts were led to the middle trunk. Lower trunk is seen just above the grafts and in the middle of the photograph. It conducted typical preganglionic nerve action potentials so was not directly reparable.

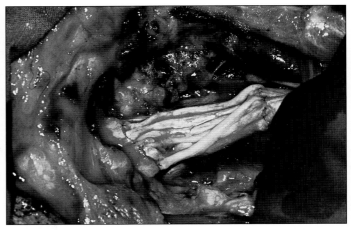

FIGURE 16-29 Graft repair in a patient with a flail arm as a result of a motor vehicle accident. Sural grafts were led from C5, C6, and descending cervical plexus to divisions of upper and middle trunk. C7 was not reparable, and C8 and T1 had preganglionic injury.

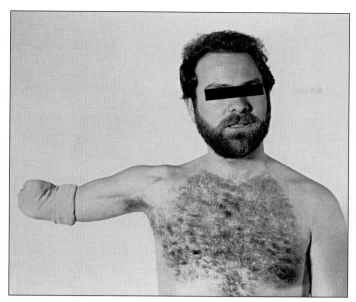

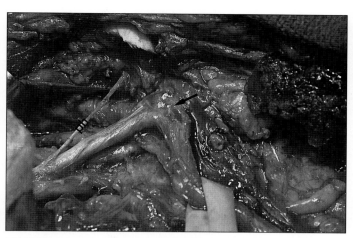

FIGURE 16-31 Stretched and distorted plexus (*arrow*) in a patient with a flail arm. Fractured and poorly healed clavicle was resected in this case. All elements conducted an operative nerve action potential, so only an external neurolysis of the plexus was done (ph, phrenic nerve).

FIGURE 16-30 This man avulsed his lower roots and damaged his upper plexus in a motorcycle accident. The upper elements were repaired and the limb was subsequently amputated through the proximal forearm. Return of strong elbow flexion, some triceps function, and shoulder abduction allowed him to use a prosthesis very successfully.

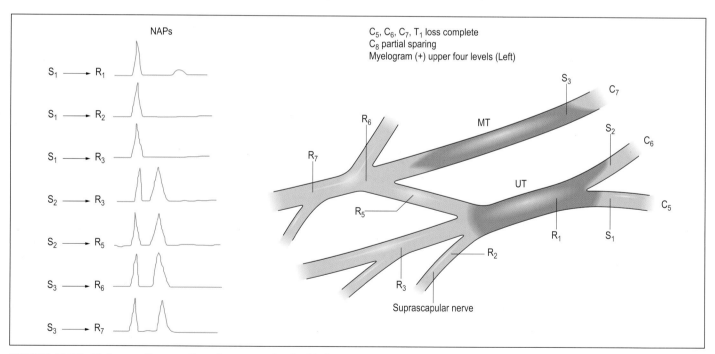

FIGURE 16-32 Flail arm with exception of some sparing in C8 distribution. As might have been predicted from the myelogram, most elements had a preganglionic injury with large, rapidly conducted nerve action potentials. Despite this, some outflow from C5 to proximal upper trunk was regenerating. Patient subsequently had a shoulder fusion but refused an attempt to neurotize biceps by use of intercostal nerves.

levels (especially if upper levels are involved), stands against success with attempted direct repair.

4. These patients are difficult to help by either direct repair and/or neurotization, and these operations are often only salvage-like in nature.

5. About a third of patients obtain useful recovery by direct repairs. Selective transfers appear to improve outcomes for shoulder and elbow function in an additional number of patients.

OTHER STRETCH PATTERNS

There were a small number of additional operative patients who had either partial loss to begin with or had only lower element,

343

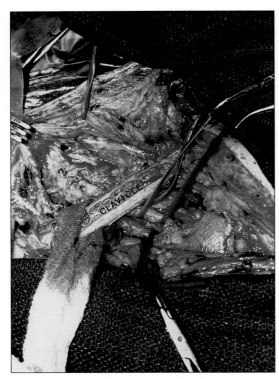

FIGURE 16-33 Lower trunk injury can be initially approached by an infraclavicular procedure. The shoulder is abducted and the artery and medial cord defined below the clavicle. Subsequently, the shoulder is adducted and the clavicle pulled down and forward by the encircling sponges, thus allowing the dissected vascular and plexus structures to be seen above the clavicle and followed medially in a safe fashion.

such as C8 and T1 loss (Fig. 16-33). They have been excluded from this analysis. The C8–T1 repairs gave uniformly poor results in four cases; another two with partial loss improved, but might have improved without surgery also. In another two cases, loss was partial in the C7, C8, and T1 distributions. Neurolysis in these cases was associated with some eventual recovery, but this again might have occurred without surgery. Graft repair of C6, C8, and T1, or C8 and T1 with neurolysis of C7 or C6 and C7 led only to significant recovery of C6 and proximal C8 innervational territories but not to recovery of fine muscle function at the level of the hand (four patients).

NEUROTIZATION FOR BRACHIAL PLEXUS STRETCH INJURIES

TORONTO EXPERIENCE

Between 1972 and 1986, 47 patients seen at the University of Toronto underwent a variety of neurotization procedures for traumatic brachial plexus palsy with root avulsion. There were 42 males and 5 females. Age at injury ranged from 14 to 34 years (mean, 22 years). Most patients were injured in traffic accidents involving a motorcycle (28), a car (6), a bicycle (3), or as a pedestrian (2). Others were injured while skiing (2), water-skiing (2), or on a snowmobile (2). One patient tripped and fell, and another was struck by a falling tree. Patients underwent surgical exploration of the brachial plexus with intraoperative nerve stimulation and recordings as well as recording of somatosensory evoked potentials to confirm root avulsion. Twenty-two patients had five roots avulsed,

and avulsion involved four roots in 2 patients, three roots in 6, two roots in 15, and one root in 2 patients.

Neurotization procedures were offered to patients with root avulsion who were young, well-motivated, presented within 9 months of injury, and whose limb was in good condition. The majority of patients had intercostal nerves extended by grafts to musculocutaneous nerve (Figs 16-34, 16-35). Some of these patients also had other neurotization procedures including the use of accessory nerve and cervical plexus.

There were no operative deaths and no significant morbidity after neurotization. Five patients developed small pneumothoraces after harvesting of the intercostal nerves, but all resolved spontaneously. There were no wound infections. None of the patients in this series was made worse by the procedure, and none developed a significant long-term pain syndrome.

The best results were achieved with neurotization of the musculocutaneous nerve with 21 (57%) of 37 patients obtaining useful elbow flexion (Fig. 16-36). Outcome was correlated with the number of intercostal nerves used as donors. If three or four intercostal nerves were connected to the musculocutaneous nerve, the outcome was much more likely to be useful elbow flexion than if only two intercostal nerves were used. There was little difference in outcome whether three or four intercostals were used. There was no significant correlation between the length of the grafts, the interval from injury to surgery, or the age of the patient and outcome. Maximum recovery took up to 24 months in some patients. There were several patients in whom the musculocutaneous nerve was torn out of the biceps and thus intercostal neurotization of this nerve was impossible (Fig. 16-37).

The restoration of active elbow flexion resulted in significant improvement in the functional abilities of these patients. Even in the presence of an anesthetic, immobile hand, active elbow flexion allowed the forearm to be used as a paperweight, as a platform on which objects could be balanced, or as a hook from which they could be hung. The hand could be used to turn simple levers.

Intercostal neurotization of the radial, median, and ulnar nerves failed to restore useful function. Neurotization of the axillary nerve fared only slightly better. Using the spinal accessory as motor donor gave modest results, but the numbers are too small to allow definitive comment. Protective sensation after neurotization by the cervical plexus was restored to part or all of the hand and fingers in 11 instances (55%). In four other cases, a degree of sensibility returned but was not sufficient to be adequately protective. We found no particular predictors of outcome for sensory recovery after neurotization.

None of the patients in this series requested amputation. A flail, anesthetic limb that is one's own seems preferable to an inanimate prosthesis. Thirty-seven patients returned to gainful employment, but only six returned to their preinjury occupations. The majority has resumed sports, and one even returned to motorcycle racing, the activity which led to her initial injury.

LSUHSC EXPERIENCE

Limited clinical outcomes with direct repair (as outlined in sections above) of plexal stretch injuries has more recently and increasingly led to the addition of nerve transfers rather than the exclusive use of direct repairs. *Emphasized is the importance of doing direct plexus repair in conjunction with nerve transfers in the same patient whenever possible.* The intent of such a "pants over vest" approach is to maximize axonal input to denervated structures. The current

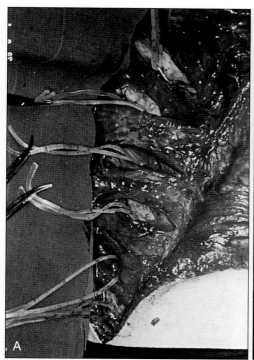
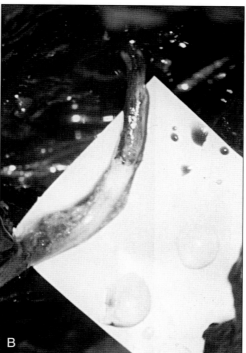

FIGURE 16-34 Intercostal neurotization to musculocutaneous and axillary nerves. **(A)** Intercostal nerves are isolated and sewn to sural nerve grafts. The graft bypasses the plexus, and the distal suture line is at the cut end of the recipient peripheral nerve **(B).**

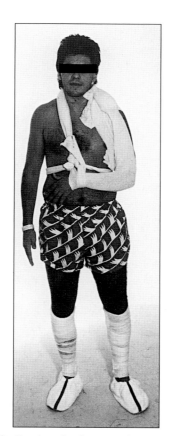

FIGURE 16-35 On the day after intercostal neurotization, the patient is out of bed. Dressings cover the wound of the initial plexus exploration, the lateral chest site of intercostal nerve surgery, and the donor sural nerve sites of both legs. Physical therapy commences 3 weeks later.

Table 16-9 Repair preference for C5–C6 stretch or C5–C6–C7 stretch injuries

Neurolysis if NAPs indicate regeneration
Direct repair if NAPs negative (flat) and proximal fascicular structure found on sectioning spinal nerve(s) plus addition of medial pectoral to split musculocutaneous nerve (for C6 avulsion) or accessory to suprascapular nerve (for C5 avulsion)
Accessory and medial pectoral transfers and less frequently descending cervical plexus transfers if NAP studies indicate preganglionic lesions or sectioning indicates pre- and postganglionic lesions of C5 and C6

algorithm (Fig. 16-38) and operative approach to these injuries and preliminary outcomes are outlined below and summarized in Tables 16-9 and 16-10.

At the time of operation for supraclavicular stretch injuries, we dissect out the elements in a 360 degree fashion and do direct recordings by stimulating proximal spinal nerve and recording from distal trunks or divisions as well as cords. If the trace is flat (absent) then injury is either postganglionic or pre- and postganglionic and we section proximal spinal nerve looking for useable fascicular structure for lead out to grafts. If NAPs are positive but small in amplitude and relatively slow in conduction, then the element is regenerating and is not sectioned. If the response has relatively high amplitude and is rapid in conduction then preganglionic injury with sensory fiber sparing is likely unless there has been preoperative clinical and/or EMG evidence of sparing in its distribution which suggests that it is an intact or partially injured element. When NAP

345

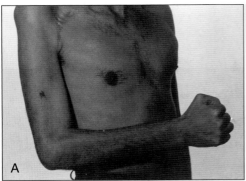
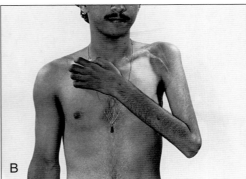
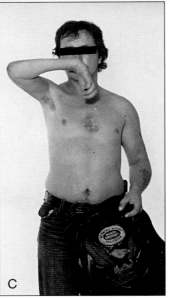

FIGURE 16-36 **(A)** Examination of a patient 2 years after intercostal neurotization for irreparable C5 and C6 injury reveals moderate elbow flexion augmenting useful hand function. **(B)** Although only a single lower root survived avulsion, another patient still felt that this degree of elbow flexion, following intercostal neurotization, was of use to him despite his severely limited hand function. **(C)** This patient avulsed all five roots on the right side. He regained sufficient elbow flexion on the right to carry his leather jacket (held in his normal left hand) over his flexed right forearm.

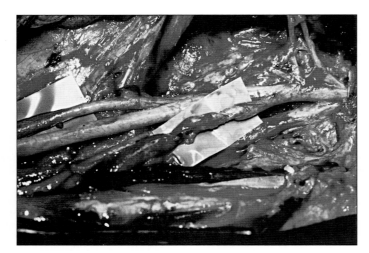

FIGURE 16-37 It is advisable to check the musculocutaneous nerve in C5–C6 avulsion cases before the intercostal nerves are dissected or sural grafts removed. This patient had sustained an associated musculocutaneous injury extending well distal into biceps from the same force that avulsed the nerve roots. The procedure was abandoned in this case. The musculocutaneous nerve is seen beneath the rubber dam.

Table 16-10 Repair preferences for C5 through T1 stretches or flail arms

Neurolysis where NAPs indicate regeneration (this is infrequent but does occur)

Direct repair, if NAPs negative and yet, on sectioning, fascicular structure is found proximally. Grafts are from proximal spinal nerves to divisions or cords. Added in are:
  Accessory to suprascapular nerve
  Descending cervical plexus to posterior division of upper trunk or middle trunk and its divisions
  Intercostals (3 or 4) to a longitudinally split portion of musculocutaneous nerve

If all 5 plexus roots are avulsed: XI to suprascapular nerve Intercostal nerves to musculocutaneous nerve Either descending cervical plexus or XI input to sternocleidomastoid placed to posterior division of upper trunk

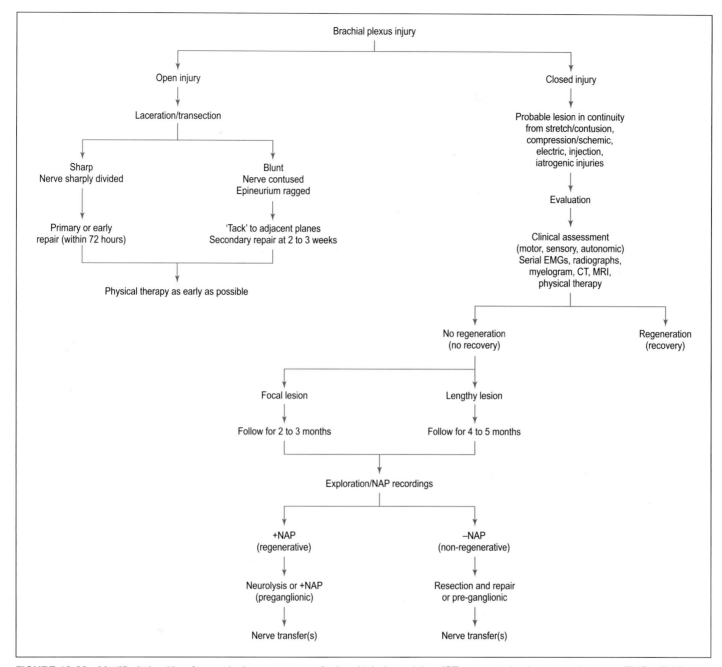

FIGURE 16-38 Modified algorithm for surgical management of a brachial plexus injury (CT, computerized tomography scan; EMGs, EMG studies). (Reproduced from Dubuisson A, and Kline DG: Indications for peripheral nerve and brachial plexus surgery. Neurol Clin 10:935–951, 1992, with permission.)

recordings are positive the element (usually spinal nerve) is not sectioned looking for fascicular structure unless visual inspection suggests the possibility of split repair, which is unusual in the stretch/contusion category. Repairs are usually done with an interfascicular technique using one or both surals as donor nerves and sometimes the antebrachial cutaneous nerves.

In the earlier experience, descending cervical plexus had been used to add to the direct repairs in 13% of the C5–C6 repairs and 27% of the C5, C6, and C7 repairs. Looking at Tables 16-5 and 16-6, which summarize outcomes for C5–C6 and C5, C6, and C7 stretches, one can see how the pattern of avulsions and whether they affected C5 or C6 or both changed outcomes. The additional value of transfer of accessory for shoulder and medial pectoral or

other transfer for biceps in a smaller cohort of patients done between 1998 and 2000 can also be seen by study of these tables. Nonetheless, it can also be appreciated that direct repairs by grafts also had much to offer.

Since the year 2000, we have added transfers to most direct plexus repairs for these severe stretch injuries. Accessory has been transferred to suprascapular nerve unless there is evidence of regeneration to it or C5 is usable as a lead-out for grafts. Nonetheless, when it has been the case, most of the C5 grafts have usually been led to the posterior division of upper trunk. We favor when possible, for C5, C6, and C7 stretch injuries, use of the medial pectoral branches to add to any direct repair we gain for elements leading to musculocutaneous nerve (see Table 16-9). In the last few years, one of the surgeons in the nerve group at LSUHSC, Dr. Robert Tiel, has used the Oberlin transfer of a fascicle of the ulnar nerve to the musculocutaneous nerve.[82] This experience, although encouraging, is too nascent to report but others have found this to be a favorable transfer. When there has been proximal direct repair with possible lead-in to musculocutaneous nerve, the latter is split in a longitudinal direction. One distal half is then used for lead-in from medial pectoral branches or ulnar nerve while the other half is left intact to receive proximal downflow. Transfers are done without an intervening graft since use of an intervening graft appears to decrease results.

In the C5–C6 stretch injury patients, medial pectoral added to musculocutaneous nerve improved grades to an averaged 4. Accessory to suprascapular transfers improved that subset of patients to 3.8. In the C5, C6, and C7 stretch injury patients, medial pectoral to musculocutaneous helped achieve an averaged grade of 3.7 while accessory to suprascapular nerve improved average grades to 3.5.

In the flail arm cases where medial pectoral or other nerves are not available for transfer, intercostal nerves have been transferred end-to-end to musculocutaneous nerve which has been sectioned proximally and then curved down distally to meet the intercostals at the level of the axilla (see Table 16-10). Accessory nerve has been mobilized so that it can be sutured directly to the suprascapular nerve which, whenever possible, is sectioned well proximally.[65] Any available direct outflow from C5, and less frequently C6 and rarely C7, has been led to posterior division of the upper trunk, posterior cord, or the portion of lateral cord going to median nerve. When direct repair of C6 outflow is judged to be feasible, the musculocutaneous nerve is split longitudinally so that intercostals are sewn into only one half of it.

COMPLICATIONS OF OPERATIONS ON STRETCH/CONTUSION INJURIES TO BRACHIAL PLEXUS

Complications included phrenic paralysis, which in most instances reversed in time but did persist beyond a year in three cases. Several patients required a chest tube postoperatively, and others had thoracocentesis. Serious wound infection was not seen in this category of injuries. All patients received perioperative and postoperative coverage by antibiotics and were sent home on an antibiotic for 7 days. Several seromas were aspirated in the early postoperative period and fortunately did not recur. Two patients required aspiration of a collection of lymph, and the wound subsequently healed with the help of a compressive dressing. Two patients collected cerebrospinal fluid at their wound sites, and these resolved by recurrent local aspiration and compressive dressing.

In the earlier years of this series, the clavicle was sometimes divided. Despite fixation, malunion occurred in several instances. In the last 20 years, the clavicle has been cleared of soft tissues, encircled by sponges, and drawn up superiorly and then down inferiorly to complete the necessary dissection of plexus beneath it. Bleeding from the vertebral artery at a foraminal level led to its surgical occlusion in five cases; in other instances the bleeding was stopped by use of the bipolar forceps and oxycel cotton. Vertebral occlusion, if necessary, was usually tolerated well. In one case, vertebral occlusion led to a delayed cerebellar and brainstem stroke in a patient who had undergone prior treatment of an ipsilateral carotid cavernous fibula by a balloon technique, and the internal carotid had subsequently occluded.

OPERATIVE RESULTS WITH INFRACLAVICULAR STRETCH AND CONTUSIVE INJURIES

These cord and cord-to-nerve lesions had a higher incidence of associated injuries than the supraclavicular stretch injuries. Axillary artery injury, shoulder dislocation or fracture, and humeral fracture were especially prevalent. Isolated axillary palsy or one associated with other cord or cord-to-nerve injuries was especially common. Table 16-11 depicts the common patterns and combinations of involvement seen with infraclavicular stretch injuries.

Unlike gunshot wounds involving plexus at an infraclavicular level, injury was less focal and thus less likely to be restricted to one level of the plexus elements alone. In other words, damage was seldom restricted to cords alone and more likely to extend from divisions to cords and to more distal nerves. As might be expected, such damage sometimes began at a divisional level and extended a variable distal distance along peripheral nerves. If repair was necessary in such instances, results were, as expected, not good because of the length and severity of the lesion in continuity.

CORD LESIONS

If injury was primarily at a divisional-to-cord or cord level alone, then lesions for purposes of analysis were categorized as those to "cords" (Figs 16-39 to 16-41). If injury extended beyond cord to peripheral nerve level, they were placed in the "cord-to-nerve" category. Stretch injuries involving cords were less common than those involving cords to nerves. Of the 143 infraclavicular brachial plexus stretch injuries, 35 cases involved 78 elements at the division or cord level (Table 16-12).

As in the gunshot wound series, elements in the lateral cord distribution, including musculocutaneous nerve to biceps, lateral cord to median outflow to proximal median-innervated forearm muscles, and median distribution sensation, did very well (Table 16-12). Despite several extensive lesions requiring lengthy grafts, overall grades in the graft category were 3.8. Neurolysis based on NAP recordings gave the expected excellent outcome, with grades

Table 16-11 Infraclavicular stretch injuries – common patterns or associated nerve lesions

No. cases	Description
33	Posterior cord to axillary alone
14	All elements including axillary
11	All elements except axillary
11	Posterior cord and axillary
7	Axillary and suprascapular
4	All elements except posterior cord
3	Lateral to musculocutaneous nerve alone
3	Lateral and medial cord to nerves
2	Lateral to musculocutaneous nerve and also posterior cord injury

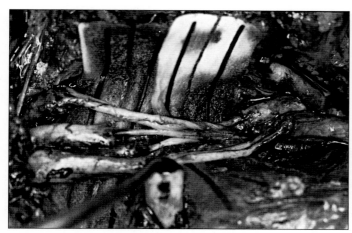

FIGURE 16-39 This plexus stretch injury was associated with a fracture of the clavicle as a result of a fall from a horse. Lesions extended from trunks to cords and were resected and replaced with grafts. Trunks are to the left and cords to the right.

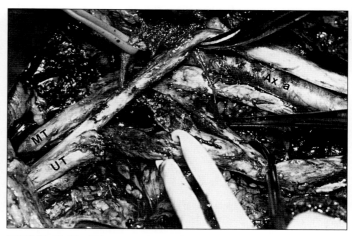

FIGURE 16-41 This unusual stretch injury involved only the posterior divisions of all three trunks. These elements did not transmit nerve action potentials, were resected, and were then replaced by grafts. Loss was to the deltoid and to all of the muscles in the radial nerve distribution (Ax a, axillary artery; MT, middle trunk; UT, upper trunk).

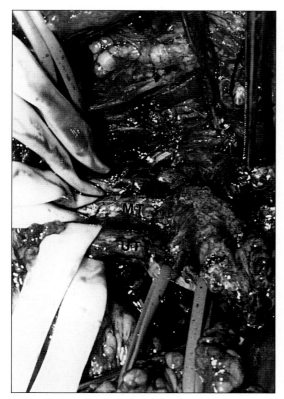

FIGURE 16-40 Stretch/contusion involving plexus at a divisional-to-cord level. Not surprisingly, this required a graft repair (LT, lower trunk; MT, middle trunk; UT, upper trunk).

medial cord, it is especially important to be certain that resection is necessary or, conversely, that it is not.

Posterior cord lesions did not do as well as lateral cord ones, but they certainly fared much better than medial cord lesions. This was despite the fact that their dissection was often complicated by adherence or incorporation of the element to a vascular repair site. In this setting, there was a need to spare or dissect out axillary and radial nerves for repair along with any retained triceps branches. Therefore, despite difficult dissections due to prior vascular repairs, 25 posterior cord lesions did much better than medial cord lesions. Graft repairs resulted in a mean grade of 3.0 and sutures a mean grade of 3.6, which was similar to split repairs. Neurolysis resulted in a mean grade of 4.1.

CORD-TO-NERVE LESIONS

Outcomes in 337 operated elements in 108 cases were studied in this category. Dissections usually extended from clavicle well down into upper arm and required preservation of major vascular structures including axillary artery, profundus artery, and axillary veins wherever possible. Despite the need for such extensive dissection, outcomes seemed to justify these procedures (see Table 16-12). Once again, it was especially important to assess each lesion in continuity by operative NAP recordings.

Lateral cord to musculocutaneous nerve
Overall average grade for outcome in this group of elements was 4.0. Not unexpectedly, neurolysis gave the better results, averaging 4.4, but several patients having neurolysis had some biceps contraction before their operation. Nonetheless, those with absent biceps preoperatively and yet a recordable NAP indicating good regeneration had an average grade of 4.0. Averaged outcome for 35 graft repairs in this category was 3.8. The occasional patient had lengthy lesions in continuity, which, after resection, required very long grafts for repair, with extremely poor recovery (Fig. 16-42).

Lateral cord to median nerve
Another favorable category for gaining recovery was injuries involving lateral cord to median nerve elements. In 49 cases, 29 had

averaging 4. Repair of lateral cord stretch injuries by suture produced a mean grade of 4.3.

By contrast, outcome was not nearly as good with the 29 medial cord stretch injuries managed (Table 16-12). Graft repairs produced a mean grade of 1.2 and suture a mean grade of 2.2. If split repair could be done, as it was in four cases, results were better and averaged 3.6. If regeneration or partial sparing could be shown by operative NAP studies, neurolysis alone gave an average recovery of 3.9. Thus, when operating on lesions in continuity involving

Table 16-12 Surgical outcome in infraclavicular plexus stretch injuries (n = 143)*

	Neurolysis**	Suture	Grafts	Split repair
Cords				
Lateral	12 / 4.5	3 / 4 .3	6 / 3.8	3 / 4
Medial	16 / 3.9	2 / 2.2	7 / 1.2	4 / 3.6
Posterior	14 / 4.1	2 / 3.6	6 / 3.0	3 / 3.5
Cords to nerves				
Lateral to musculocutaneous	20 / 4.4	0 / NA	35 / 3.8	0 / NA
Lateral to median	29 / 4.1	1 / 4	19 / 3	0 / NA
Medial to median	24 / 4.3	1 / 4	17 / 3	0 / NA
Medial to ulnar	33 / 3.6	1 / 0	13 / 1.4	1 / 2.3
Posterior to radial	29 / 4.1	1 / 0	32 / 2.7	3 / 3.5
Posterior to axillary	28 / 4.7	1 / 3	48 / 3.5	1 / 4
Totals				
Elements / results	205 / 4.2	12 / 2.3	183 / 2.8	15 / 3.6

*Number of elements /averaged grade of recovery achieved (NA, not applicable).

**Neurolysis based on a positive NAP.

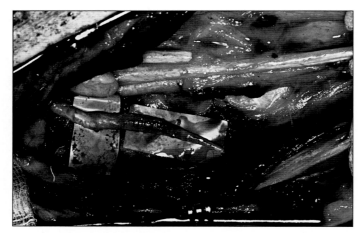

FIGURE 16-42 Most isolated musculocutaneous nerve (mcn) stretch injuries occur near the take-off form the lateral cord. On occasion, the injury also extends close to the entry point into biceps. Only a few small fascicles were found in this attenuated nerve. The clinical result was poor after graft repair.

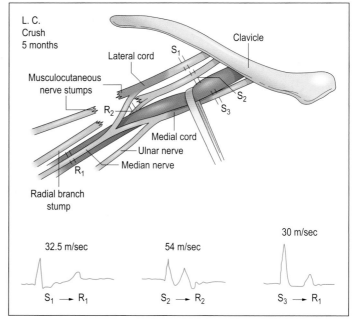

FIGURE 16-43 Drawing of contusive injury to cords and cord-to-nerve levels of the left plexus. Musculocutaneous nerve had been distracted, as had radial nerve just distal to the triceps branches. Grafts were used to repair lateral cord to musculocutaneous and posterior cord to radial nerves. NAPs were recorded from lateral cord to median (S1 to R1), posterior cord to triceps branch (S2 to R2), and medial cord to median (S3 to R1), so these elements were spared resection.

neurolysis. Hence, almost 60% of these elements demonstrated electrical evidence of regeneration at surgery. Approximately half of these had partial function in this distribution, with some pronator teres and wrist and finger flexion function before surgery. Others had an NAP across their lesion despite absence of distal function (Fig. 16-43). Recovery in this latter group averaged 3.5. These averages take into account sensory as well as motor recovery. In the former group, in which function was partial to begin with, recovery averaged 4.5. As expected, those with partial function to begin with regenerated to a level superior to those without any function at the time of surgery. Regeneration was nonetheless excellent in those patients with complete distal loss if intraoperative NAPs were present across the lesions. Graft repairs for 19 lateral cord to median nerve lesions had averaged results of 3.0 (Fig. 16-44). There were also a few cases in which lengthy (>15 cm) avulsive or stretch injury extending from lateral cord to median nerve precluded repair. As expected, no recovery occurred in these severely injured cases.

Medial cord to median nerve

Even if only some function was spared initially, or if an NAP was recordable despite complete loss, this was a surprisingly good category or subset of element injury, not only for spontaneous recovery but also for recovery after graft repair. Many patients had partial function in this distribution to begin with, and had neurolysis based on a positive NAP across the lesion, with recovery to an average grade of 4.5. When function was absent preoperatively, and yet a NAP could be recorded, a neurolysis was done and the average outcome was graded as 4.1. In the 17 cases in which function was completely absent preoperatively, and a graft repair of this element could be done, outcome averaged 3.0. There were a few cases in which the length of the injury extended from the medial cord well distal on the median nerve to elbow level, and this precluded any effective repair.

Medial cord to ulnar nerve

As might be expected, this was a difficult element to manage with success. Graft repairs did not work very well. If neurolysis could be done because of partial sparing of function or because of a positive NAP despite absence of distal function, results were acceptable. If function was partially spared in the distribution of this element, as it was in somewhat over half the neurolysis cases, outcome was good and graded an average of 4.2. If loss was complete and yet a NAP was recorded, average grade was 3.1. Results in those 13 patients in whom repair by graft or suture was attempted averaged only 1.4. A few patients had extensive injuries, precluding any attempt at repair.

Posterior cord to radial nerve

There were 65 elements in this category operated on for stretch/contusion. In about a third of cases, there was some function to begin with. As expected, NAPs across these lesions were positive and, with neurolysis and time, results had an average grade of 4.8. If function was absent but an NAP was recorded across the lesion, as it was in several instances, the average grade was 3.3. Despite evidence of regeneration at the operating table, these relatively low grades reflect the difficulty in regaining functional reinnervation of finger and thumb extensors. If graft repair was necessary because of absence of an NAP, as it was in 32 posterior cord to radial elements, average grade was 2.7. Split repairs gave slightly better results, while the rare cases in which lengthy grafts were needed gave the expected poor results.

Posterior cord to axillary nerve

These 99 operated elements included 56 that were unassociated with other serious plexus element damage (see first row of data in Table 16-13).[49] These represented isolated axillary palsies caused by stretch (Figs 16-45 to 16-47). If function was partial and neurolysis only was done, as in four cases, graded recovery was a 4.3. If function was absent but adequate regeneration was shown by intraoperative NAPs, average grade was 3.8. However, the majority of these patients had absent NAPs and required nerve repair. If suture, grafts, or split repairs were done in isolated axillary palsies (46 cases), grades averaged 3.8.

There were 11 cases of posterior cord to axillary palsies associated with suprascapular nerve palsy (Table 16-13). When associated with a closed stretch contusive injury, loss of supraspinatus, infraspinatus, and deltoid function is seldom due to C5 injury but rather to individual injuries to suprascapular and axillary nerves. In each case, suprascapular loss was either partial or had a recordable NAP across the lesion at operation. Supraspinatus and infraspinatus recovered to a satisfactory level in all cases. Despite this, 7 of these combined lesions required graft repair of the axillary nerve. Results in grafted axillary nerves in this subset averaged 3.2. The other four cases had neurolysis and recovered quite well. On rare occasion, isolated C5 stretch injury mimicked combined axillary and suprascapular stretch injuries (Fig. 16-48).

Not too unexpectedly, 14 of the axillary palsies were associated with posterior cord or posterior cord to radial palsy (Table 16-13). Axillary nerve had graft repair in nine of these cases; average result was 3.0. If neurolysis of the axillary nerve could be done, as it was in five cases, results averaged from 4.3 to 4.5.

Another 15 axillary lesions were associated with more widespread infraclavicular stretch injuries (Table 16-13). In seven cases, in which the axillary nerve component had partial function to begin with and a NAP was recordable across the lesion, the average result was 4.0. If loss was complete but at operation an NAP could be recorded, as in four cases, outcome graded 4.2. Grafts to the axillary nerve were required in seven other cases associated with other infraclavicular lesions. Average results in these cases were 3.1.

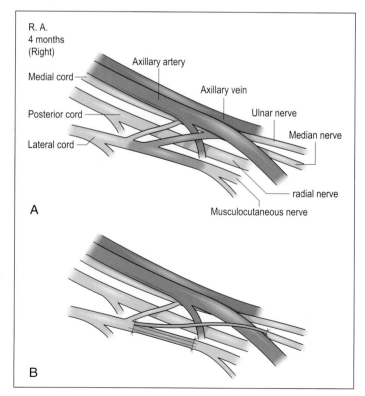

FIGURE 16-44 **(A)** Drawing of lateral cord injury involving outflow to musculocutaneous and median nerves. These lesions in continuity did not transmit nerve action potentials and were replaced by grafts. **(B)** This was a very favorable infraclavicular stretch injury for repair, and, as a result, recovery was good.

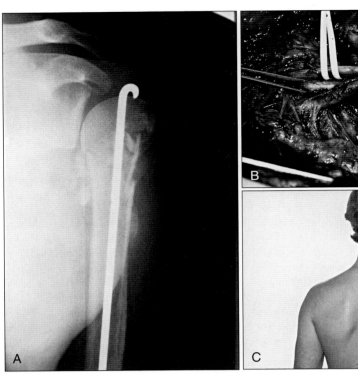

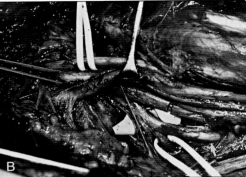

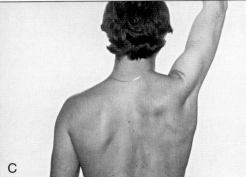

FIGURE 16-45 **(A)** Severe humeral fracture associated with a complete axillary palsy which was present before placement of rod. **(B)** Dissection of axillary nerve (white arrow) and subscapularis branch (*white loop*) below the radial nerve from an anterior approach. Radial nerve (R) is seen originating from posterior cord; vein retractor is on axillary artery (Ax a). **(C)** Recovery of function in deltoid after graft repair.

Table 16-13 Outcomes of axillary nerve repair in 99 patients[49]

Outcome	No. of nerves / mean postop LSUHSC grade			
	Partial loss & positive NAP / neurolysis*	Complete loss & positive NAP / neurolysis[†]	Resection & suture[†]	Resection & graft[‡]
Solitary axillary palsy (56 cases)	4 / 4.3	6 / 3.8	3 / 3.8	43 / 3.8[§]
Axillary palsy with suprascapular palsy (11 cases)	1 / 4.5	3 / 4.3	0 / 0	7 / 3.2
Axillary palsy with radial loss (14 cases)	3 / 4.3	2 / 4.5	0 / 0	9 / 3.0
Axillary palsy with other plexus loss (18 cases)[‖]	7 / 4.0	4 / 4.2	0 / 0	7 / 3.1
*Totals***	15 / 4.1±0.4	15 / 4.0±1.0	3 / 3.8±0.6	66 / 3.7±1.1

*The mean preoperative grade was 2.2 (range 1–4).

[†]Preoperative grade in each case was 0.

[‡]Preoperative grade in most cases was 0, except in three in which it was 1 (trace only).

[§]Includes two split repairs with a mean outcome of grade 4.

[‖]Two additional axillary nerves were exposed, but irreparable due not only to lengthy involvement, but also to distal avulsion.

**The mean values are expressed as means±SDs.

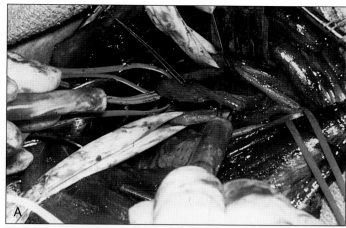

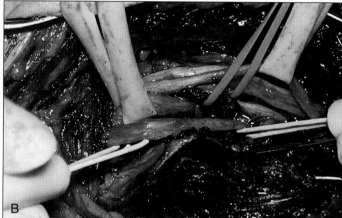

FIGURE 16-46 **(A)** Nerve action potential (NAP) testing of axillary nerve injured by stretch/contusion. This lesion had no NAP across the lesion and required resection and a graft repair. **(B)** NAP testing of another stretched axillary nerve with complete loss of deltoid for 5 months. This lesion conducted an NAP and had only neurolysis.

It is to be re-emphasized that results of repair of stretch injury to axillary nerve alone can be seen in the first row in Table 16-13 (see also Fig. 16-49).

SUMMARY OF INFRACLAVICULAR STRETCH INJURIES

1. These injuries are less frequent than supraclavicular ones, but clinical loss can be just as severe.
2. There is a high association with fractures and serious vascular injuries.
3. Some of these injuries improve spontaneously, but many do not and thus require surgery.
4. Operations can be technically more demanding than those in the supraclavicular region because there is a need to skeletonize large vessels which often have had prior repair.
5. Results of suture and graft repair are relatively favorable for lateral and posterior cord and their outflows. Repair of medial cord to median nerve often gives acceptable results.
6. Results of repair of medial cord and medial cord to ulnar nerves are poor. If resection is not needed in this distribution because of recordable NAPs across a lesion in continuity, then outcome from spontaneous regeneration can be surprisingly good.

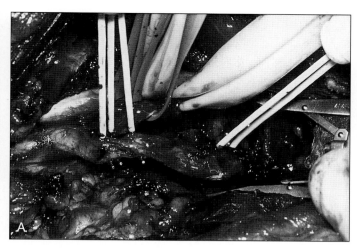

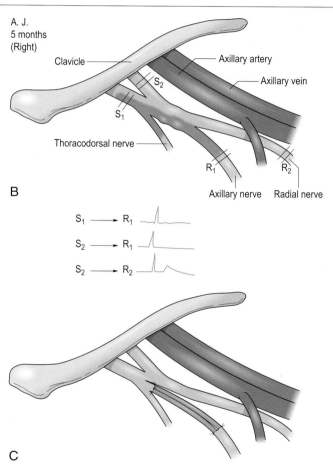

FIGURE 16-47 **(A)** Axillary stretch injury explored 5 months after a vehicular accident. No nerve action potentials were evoked and a graft repair was necessary. In **(B)**, the lesion began in posterior cord and extended into axillary nerve, so a relatively lengthy graft repair was necessary. **(C)** Medial antebrachial cutaneous nerve was used for the graft repair.

7. Axillary nerve is injured in an isolated fashion in approximately 55% of cases. Relatively common associated injuries are those to the suprascapular nerve and posterior cord to radial nerve.
8. The axillary nerve often (two-thirds of the time) requires graft repair, with associated good results in the majority of patients, but not all.

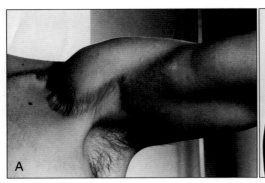

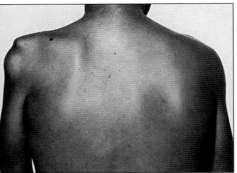

FIGURE 16-48 **(A)** Return of deltoid function and bulk 2.5 years after axillary nerve grafts 5 cm in length were placed. **(B)** The wasted left rhomboid, supraspinatus, and infraspinatus muscles in another patient indicate that the shoulder subluxation resulting from deltoid palsy is caused by a very proximal C5 spinal nerve or root injury and not an axillary stretch injury.

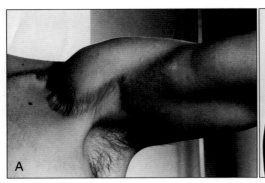

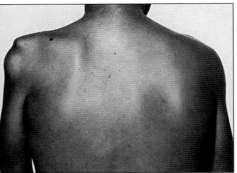

SELECTION OF INFRACLAVICULAR STRETCH INJURIES FOR OPERATION

Operation is indicated for many of these lesions because recovery is not assured without it. Patients were usually followed for 3–5 months before operation. This usually permitted recovery from the frequently associated vascular and orthopedic injuries and time for adequate soft tissue coverage if that had been disrupted by the original injury. Those selected for operation did not show early and significant clinical and/or electrical reversal of loss. Operation was more likely to be selected if loss persisted in the distribution of one or more elements which could potentially be helped by operation, particularly if repair was necessary. In practice, this usually included most of the infraclavicular elements. The major exceptions were patients in whom the major deficit was in medial cord and medial cord to ulnar loss, where loss was mild or nonexistent in other cord distributions.

COMPLICATIONS OF SURGERY FOR INFRACLAVICULAR STRETCH INJURY

Operation often had to be done despite the fact that vascular repair preexisted. Often, vascular repair had included placement of a graft from subclavian or axillary artery to brachial artery. In these cases especially, the vessels had to be carefully dissected out and preserved or re-repaired. As a result, these were difficult and prolonged dissections. Usually, re-repair could be done by the operating service, but there were several in which repeat vascular repair was necessary within 72 hours of the infraclavicular plexus surgery. These cases were done by our vascular surgery service.

Other complications included wound infection in a few cases. These infections were superficial and responded to local wound care and antibiotics. A Penrose drain was usually placed at the time of operation, but in one case, a persistent seroma required drainage. A few patients had increased deficit postoperatively, usually in the lateral cord distribution, and these improved spontaneously with time. In one patient who had increased radial distribution loss postoperatively there was, with time, improved triceps, brachioradialis, and wrist extension function, but finger and thumb extension remained poor.

POSTERIOR APPROACH TO THE BRACHIAL PLEXUS

Most of the operations done for injury in this series involved an anterior approach to the plexus. In a few selected cases in which

injury was very close to the spine or was predicted to be intraforaminal, a posterior subscapular approach was used. In these injuries operated on posteriorly, the facet joint over involved spinal nerves was usually removed by a Kerrison rongeur or a high speed drill. The spinal nerve could be more readily traced to its dural exit and thus sometimes more readily repaired by a posterior approach than if an anterior approach had been used.[29,48,50] In several cases in which injury was caused by laceration or gunshot wound, the posterior subscapular approach also permitted a repair which would have been most difficult from an anterior approach. Two of the gunshot wounds to plexus operated on posteriorly had a complete deficit at a spinal nerve level, and both patients had undergone prior anterior operations for vascular repair. The three lacerated plexus injuries operated on posteriorly were suspected to have transection of one or more spinal nerves close to their dural exit.

TRAUMATIC PLEXUS INJURIES OPERATED POSTERIORLY

Twenty-three patients were operated on posteriorly for traumatic brachial plexus palsy. There were 16 males and 7 females in this subset. Patient age ranged from 19 months to 65 years (mean age, 30 years). In 15 patients, the injuries were secondary to stretch/contusion trauma. Injury resulted from automobile or motorcycle accidents in nine cases, iatrogenic stretch/contusion trauma from a transaxillary operation in three cases, football injury in one, snowmobile accident in one, and birth-related stretch injury in one. Four injuries were caused by laceration: one from a stab wound, another by a blunt laceration of the neck with prior suture of the C6 nerve root, and yet another from transection by a scalpel during transaxillary first-rib resection, and by scissors during a neck dissection for tumor. Three patients sustained a gunshot wound to the plexus close to the spine. Each had had prior anterior explorations for presumed vascular injury and in two cases had had vascular repairs.

Preoperatively, 19 patients presented with a complete deficit in the distribution of one or more plexus elements. Six of these patients had a flail arm. An incomplete but severe and persistent deficit was present in the other 13 patients. Patients were operated on because of persistence of complete denervation in the distribution of at least one plexus element or because of severe pain, or both.

At operation, 15 patients were found to have ruptured or transected elements or absence of NAPs across a lesion in continuity. After resection of these lesions, sural grafts were placed. Neurolysis with removal of scar tissue was performed on one or more elements in seven patients because of the presence of regenerating axons proven by NAP recordings. The patient with birth injury was explored posteriorly at 19 months after injury because of complete C5–C6 loss. NAPs were recorded from the upper trunk divisions after stimulation of both C5 and C6, so only a neurolysis was performed. Recovery in this distribution began 1 year later, and follow-up evaluation at 11 years of age shows acceptable shoulder and arm function. Neurotization using the descending cervical plexus was performed in one patient with a gunshot wound to the plexus in whom the proximal plexus elements were found impossible to repair but this led to only a small amount of recovery. In another patient, an iatrogenic laceration of the C8 nerve root was treated 2 weeks after injury by end-to-end anastomoses with a little recovery of hand intrinsic function and some sensory recovery to little and ring finger.

Ten of 15 patients with graft repair had a follow-up period of at least 5 years: one patient underwent amputation of a painful flail arm, two recovered strength to only grade 1, another to grade 2, and six to a level of 3 or better. Six of seven patients treated by neurolysis had a follow-up period of at least 4 years or more: one patient made a poor recovery, three had a good recovery, and one an excellent recovery. The patient with a repeat repair of the C6 root after blunt transection and prior suture did regain biceps, grading 3 to 4 by 3 years postoperatively. One patient with a stab wound involving the dural level of C5 and C6 roots which was partially repaired by grafts via a posterior subscapular approach has made a good recovery.

OPERATIVE TECHNIQUE

Positioning of the patient

The patient is turned to a lateral decubitus position and rolled to a prone position, which brings the operative side close to the edge of the operating table. Rolls are placed laterally under the anterolateral chest wall and transversely beneath shoulders and the manubrium of the chest. Upper extremity on the operative side is partially abducted and flexed forward at the shoulder. The arm is then flexed at the elbow and placed in a padded Mayo stand at a level below that of the operating table (Fig. 16-49). Elbow, wrist, and hand are wrapped with protective pads. The operating table is then tilted up 20 degrees or so or in a reverse Trendelenburg position to allow further abduction of the shoulder and the scapula. Head is turned toward the operative side and placed on a well-padded donut or on several folded sheets, taking care to keep pressure off the orbits and to maintain the airway. The contralateral arm is padded at the elbow and placed to the side.

Surgical exposure

A curvilinear skin incision is made, centered between the thoracic spinous processes and the medial edge of the scapula (Fig. 16-50, upper center). This incision tends to protect the spinal branch of the accessory nerve and the ascending branch of the transverse cervical artery, which course close to the medial vertebral border of the scapula. The inferior portion of the trapezius muscle is divided along the entire length of the skin incision, and the edges are marked at intervals with suture for later approximation. Beneath the trapezius lie the levator scapulae muscle superiorly, the rhomboideus minor muscle intermediate in location, and the rhomboideus major muscle inferiorly (Fig. 16-51). All three of these muscles insert on the medial border of the scapula. A Kelly clamp

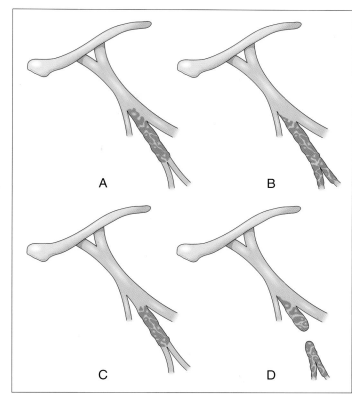

FIGURE 16-49 This drawing shows the various levels and extent of injury seen in over a 100 operative cases of axillary palsy, some of which were associated with other infraclavicular palsies and some of which were not. **(A)** Lesion usually found beginning in posterior cord and extending to but not into nerve branches. **(B)** Lesion involves axillary nerve and its branches. **(C)** Lesion restricted to axillary nerve. **(D)** Distracture stretch injury with distal branch injury requiring posterior as well as anterior approach. (From Reference 49 with permission J Neurosurgery.)

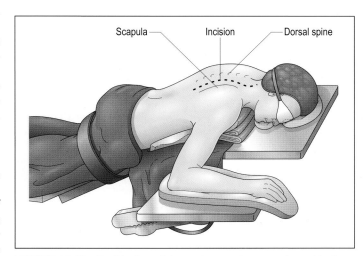

FIGURE 16-50 Positioning of the patient on the operating table for subscapular approach to the plexus. Chest rolls are placed under the chest and transversely beneath the shoulders. The arm is abducted at the shoulder, flexed at the elbow, padded, and placed on a Mayo stand. The head is turned toward the operative side and placed on a donut. The operating table is placed in a reverse Trendelenburg position 15–20 degrees above the horizontal axis.

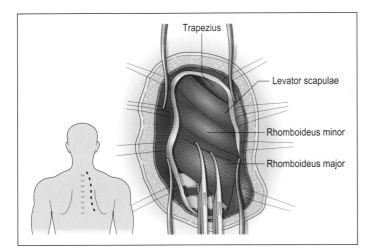

FIGURE 16-51 Diagram on left shows line of parascapular incision. On the right, the trapezius muscle has been sectioned and a portion of the rhomboid muscles are about to be sectioned between two long Kelly clamps. Divided muscle edges are marked on both sides by suture for subsequent closure. Note position of levator scapulae, which sometimes needs to be divided as well.

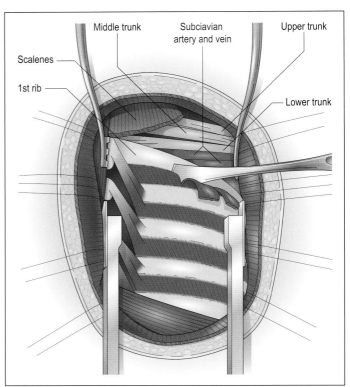

FIGURE 16-52 A self-retaining chest retractor is placed beneath the scapula laterally and embedded in the paraspinous muscles medially, then gradually opened as the arm is further abducted by lowering the Mayo stand or raising the operating table. The scalene muscles have been detached from the superior surface of the first rib, and a periosteal dissector is used to remove intercostal muscles from the inferior rib surface. Early exposure of the subclavian vessels and the trunks of the plexus are seen.

is used to dissect beneath them midway between the scapula and the spine. By dividing muscle away from the edge of the scapula, the deeper dorsal scapular nerve and ascending branch of the transverse cervical artery are protected. Segments of muscle are clamped (usually by Serrats) and sectioned between two clamps, beginning inferiorly and proceeding superiorly. If the rhomboid muscles are thick, they are split longitudinally and the two layers clamped and divided individually. Each of the edges is marked with heavy suture. Paired sutures of heavy Vicryl are placed behind each clamp and tied. The needles are left attached and the ends fastened to adjacent drapes so that subsequent approximation of divided muscle is as accurate as possible. As dissection approaches the neck, the thicker portion of the trapezius muscle can be split somewhat in a medial direction and, if necessary, the levator scapulae muscles can be clamped, divided, and marked by sutures as well. Occasionally, some of the serratus posterior muscle is also sectioned.

After division of muscles, the posterior chest wall is exposed. The surgeon then sees a relatively avascular plane beneath the scapula and with gloved fingers can create a plane between the shoulder blade and chest wall. One blade of a medium self-retaining chest retractor is placed beneath the scapula and the other is inserted into the paraspinous muscle mass. A length of the paraspinal mass can be split down to the posterior chest wall to permit firm placement of the medial blade of the thoracic retractor. The retractor is opened as the limb on the Mayo stand is lowered or the operating table is elevated to provide further abduction and external rotation of the scapula.

Ribs are then palpated. Running the fingers superiorly and over the second rib permits palpation of the first rib. Sharp dissection of intercostal muscles on the caudal side of the rib and the scalene muscles on the cephalad side, as well as use of an Alexander periosteal elevator and Doyen rib dissectors, helps to clear the rib of soft tissues (Fig. 16-52). The first rib is removed from the costotransverse articulation posteriorly to the costoclavicular ligament anteriorly.

Leksell rongeurs or sometimes a rib cutter is used to resect the rib and periosteum. Resection of the posterior portion of the second rib is sometimes useful in exposing the first rib in very large patients or for large tumors extending into the mediastinum. Bone edges should be carefully manicured and waxed to minimize injury to pleura or surrounding tissues. The posterior and middle scalene muscles are released from their insertions and are resected to their origin from the transverse spinous processes. The spinal nerves and the trunks of the brachial plexus are exposed after removal of these muscles superiorly (Fig. 16-53). The spinal nerves and divisions are further exposed by following the trunks medially and then laterally. The extraspinal course of the nerve roots is dissected back to the spine. Some elevation and retraction of the paraspinous muscle mass exposes lateral posterior spine overlying the intraforaminal course of the spinal nerve roots.

A Weitlander retractor can be placed on the second rib and in the superior soft tissues of the neck to open up the supraclavicular space posterior to the plexus. A malleable chest retractor can be placed over the apical pleura to protect it as the posterior portion of the first rib is removed between the T1 and C8 nerve roots. The lower trunk is then isolated from the underlying subclavian artery and exposed circumferentially. Dissection of the plexus can then proceed medially along its spinal nerves and laterally along its truncal divisions. The middle trunk is isolated next and, if necessary, the upper trunk. The long thoracic nerve is visible as it originates from the posterior aspect of the C6, or sometimes C5 and C7 spinal nerves as well as C6, and can be protected.

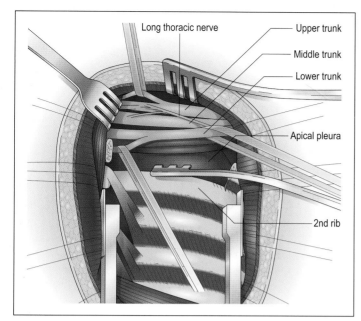

FIGURE 16-53 After resection of the first rib and scalene muscles, one blade of a Weitlander or similar retractor is placed against the superior surface of the second rib and the other blade in the superior soft tissues of the neck. Paraspinal muscles are retracted by a large rake so as to expose the spinal nerves or roots. If necessary, either Kerrison rongeurs or a high-speed drill can be used to remove overlying facets to provide exposure of roots close to their dural exits.

With this exposure, the phrenic nerve is anterior to both the upper trunk of the brachial plexus and the anterior scalene muscle, which is usually not divided during this procedure. Nerve roots or spinal nerves are dissected free in a circumferential fashion. The use of Penrose drains around the various elements, including the spinal nerves, to gently retract them helps in the dissection. If indicated, intraoperative NAP recordings can then be obtained. Lateral dissection can extend to divisions, but it is difficult to gain much exposure of the cord level of the plexus with this posterior approach.

If necessary, the facet joint can be removed using a high-speed drill or Kerrison rongeurs to expose the intraforaminal course of the spinal nerve. In most cases, the nerve can be traced to its dural exit by careful bites with a Kerrison rongeur, keeping the rongeur footplate superficial to the nerve but not compressing it. The vertebral artery lies anteriorly, so the spinal nerve roots can be readily unroofed without fear of serious bleeding. More laterally, the subclavian artery is anterior and inferior to the lower trunk of the brachial plexus, and the subclavian vein is anterior to both. Both vessels are identified early in the dissection and can be readily dissected away from the lower trunk and its divisions and easily protected. If more than two facet joints are removed, the area of bone removal is subsequently filled in with methyl methacrylate.

After such a plexus procedure, it is important to achieve meticulous closure of the wound by approximation of the divided but previously marked muscles. Anatomic re-approximation of the different muscle planes of the greater and lesser rhomboid muscles, as well as most of the lower portions of the trapezius and levator scapulae muscles, is necessary. Good hemostasis must be obtained. A Penrose drain is sometimes placed with one end deep to the muscle closure and superior to the apical pleura. The other end of the drain is then brought out posteriorly through a separate stab

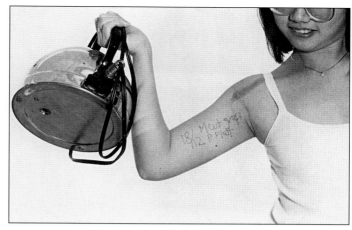

FIGURE 16-54 This gymnast suffered an iatrogenic injury to the musculocutaneous nerve during an anterior shoulder repair. Eighteen months after graft repair of the musculocutaneous nerve, she had regained useful elbow flexion.

wound. Any pleural rents must be repaired. The integrity of the pleural repair is tested by filling the wound with saline and having the anesthetist perform a Valsalva test. A chest tube is seldom needed. The reader is referred to the published report of Dubuisson, Kline, and Weinshel[24] for further technical information.

IATROGENIC PLEXUS INJURIES

Operations or other medical procedures resulting in brachial plexus injury are not uncommon (Fig. 16-54). The consequences may be severe, particularly if the injury is either ignored or not corrected in a timely fashion. The list of operations or medical maneuvers done on or around the neck and shoulder is a large one. We have evaluated and attempted to correct a variety of different injuries to the plexus caused by iatrogenic mechanisms. This has included division of plexus or a plexus element by scalpel, scissors, or rongeur; crush injury caused by a hemostat or a retractor; traction injury by retractors or other surgical instruments or from hyperabduction of the shoulder; compressive injury from the surgeon or assistant leaning on the patient; suture or bone hardware in or around the plexus; clot or pseudoaneurysm resulting from angiography; and even injection and laser injuries. Besides injuries associated with direct operations on the neck and shoulder, injuries have also been seen with thorascopic approaches for sympathectomy and transaxillary approach for first rib resection.

Whenever possible, we used the same criteria to select patients for surgery and to time operations as used for other plexus lesions caused by noniatrogenic transection and stretch, contusion, or compression. Because of the nature of these injuries and the referral logistics involved, acute repair of surgically sharp plexus transections was seldom possible (Fig. 16-55). Exceptions were provided by an occasional local case in which transection of one or more plexus elements was recognized and help was sought by the operating surgeon while the patient was still anesthetized. Outcomes were best in these cases, but it must be kept in mind that these were sharply divided plexus elements that were ideal candidates for primary end-to-end repair. If one or more bluntly transected or torn elements were found in such a case, the contused stumps were tacked down to adjacent fascial levels; a secondary delayed repair was then done several weeks later when stumps could be more accurately trimmed back to healthy tissue. Some of these lesions

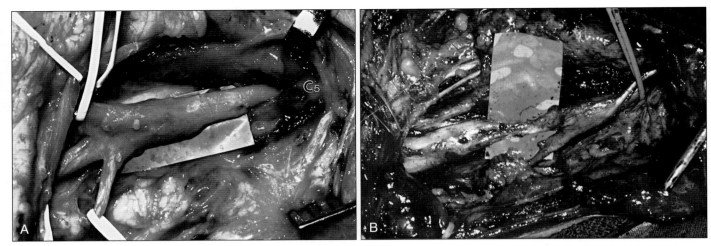

FIGURE 16-55 **(A)** Relatively sharp section of C5 spinal nerve with a scalpel during the course of a scalenotomy for thoracic outlet syndrome. Proximal stump of C5 is seen to the right, and suprascapular nerve and divisions of the plexus are seen to the left at the time of a delayed repair. **(B)** Inadvertent supraclavicular plexus injury during the course of a neck dissection, and when explored, these bluntly shredded elements were found.

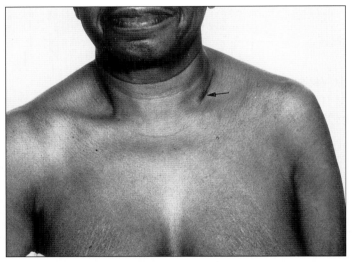

FIGURE 16-56 A left "scalenotomy" was performed on this patient who suffered from carpal tunnel syndrome. Postoperatively, the patient could neither abduct the left shoulder nor flex the left elbow. The upper trunk had been accidentally divided and subsequently required repair by sural grafts.

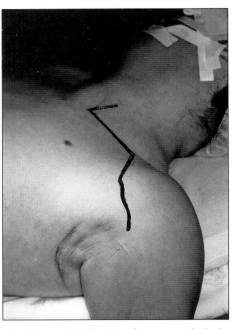

FIGURE 16-57 Planned skin incision for a supraclavicular and infraclavicular plexus exploration marked out before draping the patient. In this case, the patient had sustained a plexus injury as a result of transaxillary resection of the first rib. The surgical scar for that operation can be seen in the patient's axilla.

required graft repair, as did some sharp as well as blunt injuries referred for repair after some delay of time (Fig. 16-56).

Most of the iatrogenic injuries to plexus were blunt and led to lesions in continuity. If clinical or electrical improvement did not occur in the early months postoperatively, then the plexus was explored and intraoperative NAP studies were used to make a decision for or against resection and repair (Fig. 16-57). Unfortunately, some categories of operative complications of the plexus involved C8, T1, and lower elements and their outflows such as medial cord, proximal ulnar, and, less frequently, proximal median nerves. As might be expected, gaining useful results in these categories was very difficult. Functional results even with careful repair were poor if associated with thoracic outlet operations, such as transaxillary first rib resection, in which the iatrogenically injured elements were usually lower trunk or medial cord. Despite these functionally poor results, repair, if indicated by exploration and intraoperative electrical studies, was still worthwhile if the lesion

was accompanied by severe neuritic pain. Cleaning up the operative site and resection of the iatrogenic lesion often reduced the pain.

If suture was found to be encircling or in a plexus element, removal without resection and repair of the involved nerve sometimes helped but often did not unless an NAP could be transmitted beyond the lesion (Fig. 16-58). If orthopedic hardware or manipulation directly involved an element in a patient selected for operation because of persisting severe loss, repair of that element rather than neurolysis was usually necessary although not always possible (Fig. 16-59).

One subset of 13 patients thought to have thoracic outlet syndrome had undergone 15 prior operations done elsewhere, including 12 transaxillary and three supraclavicular plexus dissections.

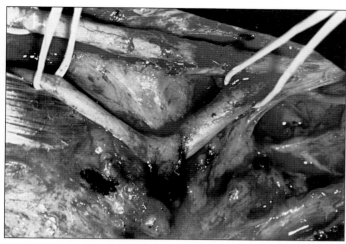

FIGURE 16-58 Kinking and distortion of left axillary nerve by a suture. Radial nerve lies above the axillary nerve. (Proximal is to the right and distal to the left.) Note swelling of the nerve proximal to the point of distortion. The segment of nerve involved by suture did not transmit an NAP and required resection. Nerve was then repaired.

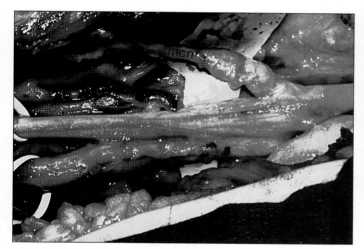

FIGURE 16-59 In this case, a good bit of the right musculocutaneous nerve (mcn) had been avulsed from the biceps during a Putti-Platt operation. This made a useful repair of this element difficult. Less involved plexus elements are seen below musculocutaneous nerve (mcn).

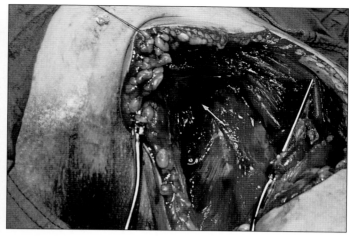

FIGURE 16-60 Blood clot at the level of the axilla (*white arrow*) as a result of an angiographic study. A compressive neuropathy of the plexus was reversed by relatively early evacuation of the clot.

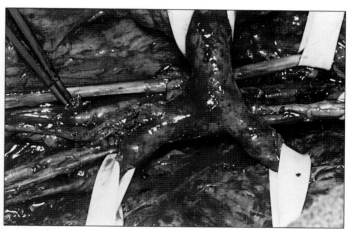

FIGURE 16-61 Compressive lesion to cords of the plexus secondary to construction of an axillary arteriovenous fistula for renal dialysis. Scar beneath the fistula and involving lateral and medial cords was severe. Fortunately, these elements conducted NAPs and were helped by neurolysis. The fistula had to be preserved because other extremity sites for dialysis had been exhausted.

These patients had mild to moderate deficits postoperatively. These are discussed in more detail in Chapter 18. The pertinent features of these cases are nonetheless summarized for this chapter.

Symptomatology included recurrence of pain in all patients. Pain was associated with mild to moderate neurologic deficit in ten patients; the EMG tracings were normal in eight, and two showed partial denervation of the C8- and T1-innervated muscles. In one patient, a cervical rib was shown on radiographic films. In each of these patients, a posterior operation was performed to further decompress the brachial plexus. Spinal nerves and plexus trunks were treated with neurolysis. Residual first ribs and, in one case, cervical rib were resected. Scar tissue was usually found involving the lower elements of the plexus. In three cases, residual bands or fascial edges of middle or minimus scalene muscle also appeared to compress the lower plexus elements. Most patients had abnormal NAP studies across the lower elements and more normal conductions and amplitudes on the upper elements. Follow-up

evaluations were available for 10 patients (mean follow-up period, 3.3 years). Nine had improvement in pain, and the one whose pain was unchanged underwent repeat neurolysis through an anterior approach with only partial improvement. Most of those patients with a preoperative mild deficit had some improvement in function on follow-up evaluation, as did those with a moderate deficit. The other patients did not show progression of their deficits on follow-up examination.

Another four patients who had undergone transaxillary first-rib removal for thoracic outlet syndrome sustained severe injury to the plexus requiring repair. These cases are considered earlier in the chapter under traumatic brachial plexus injuries operated upon by a posterior subscapular approach.

Blood clots, pseudoaneurysms, and arteriovenous fistulae involving other nerves as well as plexus have been discussed in other chapters. These complications usually involved infraclavicular plexus. Results were best if they were identified early and if plexus could be decompressed without the need for resection and repair (Figs 16-60, 16-61). See Iatrogenic injuries (Chapter 24).

Information concerning irradiation plexitis and those patients selected for plexus operation can be found in Chapter 23.

REFERENCES

1. Allieu Y, Privat JM, and Bonnel F: L'exploration chirurgicale et le traitement des paralysies du plexus brachial. Paris, Reunion Annuelle de la Societe Francaise de Neurochirurgie, 1980.
2. Allieu Y, Privat JM, and Bonnel F: [Neurotization with the spinal nerve (nervus accessorius) in avulsions of roots of the brachial plexus]. Neurochirurgie 28:115–120, 1982.
3. Alnot JY: Infraclavicular lesions. Clin Plast Surg 11:127–131, 1984.
4. Alnot JY, Jolly A, and Frot B: Traitement direct des lesions nerveuses dans les paralysies traumatiques du plexus brachial chez l'adult. Int Orthop 63:82–90, 1981.
5. Barnes R: Traction injuries of the brachial plexus in adults. J Bone Joint Surg 31:10–16, 1949.
6. Barr JS, Freiberg JA, Colonna PC, et al.: A survey of end results on stabilization of the paralytic shoulder. J Bone Joint Surg 24:699–710, 1942.
7. Bertelli JA and Ghizoni MF: Reconstruction of C5 and C6 brachial plexus avulsion injury by multiple nerve transfers: spinal accessory to suprascapular, ulnar fascicles to biceps branch, and triceps long or lateral head branch to axillary nerve (1). J Hand Surg [Am] 29:131–139, 2004.
8. Birch R: Traction lesions of the brachial plexus. Br J Hosp Med 32:140–143, 1984 (See also Birch R, Bonney G, Wynn Parry C. Surgical Disorders of Peripheral Nerves. New York, Churchill Livingstone, 1998).
9. Bonnel F: Microscopic anatomy of the adult human brachial plexus: an anatomical and histological basis for microsurgery. Microsurgery 5:107–118, 1984.
10. Bonney G: Prognosis in traction lesions of the brachial plexus. J Bone Joint Surg [Br] 41:4–35, 1959.
11. Bonney G, Birch R, Jamieson AM, et al.: Experience with vascularized nerve grafts. Clin Plast Surg 11:137–142, 1984.
12. Brandt KE and Mackinnon SE: A technique for maximizing biceps recovery in brachial plexus reconstruction. J Hand Surg [Am] 18:726–733, 1993.
13. Brophy BP: Supraclavicular traction injuries of the brachial plexus. Aust NZ J Surg 48:528–532, 1978.
14. Brunelli G and Monini L: Neurotization of avulsed roots of brachial plexus by means of anterior nerves of cervical plexus. Clin Plast Surg 11:149–152, 1984.
15. Carroll RE and Hill NA: Triceps transfer to restore elbow flexion. A study of fifteen patients with paralytic lesions and arthrogryposis. J Bone Joint Surg [Am] 52:239–244, 1970.
16. Carroll RE and Kleinman WB: Pectoralis major transplantation to restore elbow flexion to the paralytic limb. J Hand Surg [Am] 4:501–507, 1979.
17. Carvalho GA, Nikkah G, Matthies C, et al.: Diagnosis of root avulsions in traumatic brachial plexus injuries. Value of computerized tomography, myelography and magnectic resonance imaging. J Neurosurg 86:69–76, 1997.
18. Choi PD, Nova KCB, Mackinnon SE, et al.: Quality of life and functional outcome following brachial plexus injury. J Hand Surg [Am] 22:605–612, 1997.
19. Clancy WG, Brand RL, and Bergfield JA: Upper trunk brachial plexus injuries in contact sports. Am J Sports Med 5:209–216, 1977.
20. Clark JP: Reconstruction of biceps brachialis by pectoralis muscle transplantation. Br J Surg 34:180, 1946.
21. Davis DH, Onofrio BM, and MacCarty CS: Brachial plexus injuries. Mayo Clin Proc 53:799–807, 1978.
22. Davis L, Martin J, and Perret G: The treatment of injuries of the brachial plexus. Ann Surg 125:647–657, 1946.
23. Dolenc VV: Intercostal neurotization of the peripheral nerves in avulsion plexus injuries. Clin Plast Surg 11:143–147, 1984.
24. Dubuisson AS, Kline DG, and Weinshel SS: Posterior subscapular approach to the brachial plexus. J Neurosurg 79:319–330, 1993.
25. Fazl M, Houlden DA, and Kiss Z: Spinal cord mapping with evoked responses for accurate localization of the dorsal root entry zone. J Neurosurg 82:587–591, 1995.
26. Fletcher I: Traction lesions of the brachial plexus. Hand 1:129–136, 1969.
27. Frykholm R: The mechanism of cervical radicular lesions resulting from friction or forceful traction. Acta Chir Scand 102:93–98, 1957.
28. Fu SY, Gordon T: Contributing factors to poor functional recovery after delayed nerve repair: prolonged denervation. J Neurosci 15:3886–3895, 1995.
29. Fu SY, Gordon T: Contributing factors to poor functional recovery after delayed nerve repair: prolonged axotomy. J Neurosci 15:3876–3885, 1995.
30. Harmon PH: Surgical reconstruction of shoulder by multiple muscle transplantations. J Bone Joint Surg [Am] 32:583–586, 1950.
31. Hendry AM: The treatment of residual paralysis after brachial plexus injury. J Bone Joint Surg 318:42–49, 1949.
32. Hentz VR and Narakas A: The results of microneurosurgical reconstruction in complete brachial plexus palsy. Assessing outcome and predicting results. Orthop Clin N Am 19:107–114, 1988.
33. Highet J: Effects of stretch on peripheral nerve. Br J Surg 30:355–369, 1942.
34. Hoffer MM, Braun R, Hsu J, et al.: Functional recovery and orthopedic management of brachial plexus palsies. JAMA 246:2467–2470, 1981.
35. Hou Z and Xu Z: Nerve transfer for treatment of brachial plexus injury: comparison study between the transfer of partial median and ulnar nerves and that of phrenic and spinal accessory nerves. Chin J Traumatol 5:263–266, 2002.
36. Hovnanian AP: The treatment of residual paralysis after brachial plexus injury. J Bone Joint Surg [Br] 31:42–49, 1949.
37. Hudson AR and Tranmer BI: Brachial plexus injuries. In: Wilkins RH and Rengachary SS, Eds: Neurosurgery. New York, McGraw Hill, 1985.
38. Jamieson A and Hughes S: The role of surgery in the management of closed injuries to the brachial plexus. Clin Orthop 147:210–215, 1980.
39. Kawai H, Kawabata H, Masada K, et al.: Nerve repairs for traumatic brachial plexus palsy with root avulsion. Clin Orthop 237:75–86, 1988.
40. Kettlecamp DB, larson CB: Evaluation of the Steindler flexorplasty. Am J Orthop 45-A:513–518, 1963.
41. Kim DH, Cho YJ, Tiel RL, et al.: Outcomes of surgery in 1019 brachial plexus lesions treated at Louisiana State University Health Sciences Center. J Neurosurg 98:1005–1016, 2003.
42. Kingery WS: A critical review of controlled clinical trials for peripheral neuropathic pain and complex regional pain syndromes. Pain 73:123–139, 1997.
43. Kline DG and Lusk M: Management of athletic brachial plexus injuries. In: Schneider R, Kennedy J, and Plant M, Eds: Sports Injuries – Mechanisms, Prevention and Treatment. Philadelphia, Williams & Wilkins, 1985 (See also Spinner R and Kline D: Peripheral nerve injuries in athletes. In: Bailes J and Dana, Eds: Neurological Sports Medicine. Rolling Meadows, IL, AANS Publications, 2001).
44. Kline DG: Selection of brachial plexus cases for operation – based on results. In: Samii M, Ed: Peripheral Nerve Lesions. Berlin Heidelberg, Springer-Verlag, 1990:396–410.

45. Kline DG: Perspective concerning brachial plexus injury and repair. Neurosurg Clin N Am 2:151–164, 1991.

46. Kline DG and Hudson AR: Nerve Injuries: Operative Results from Major Nerve Injuries, Entrapments, and Tumors. Philadelphia, WB Saunders, 1995.

47. Kline DG and Hudson AR: Coaptation of anterior rami of C-3 and C-4. J Neurosurg 75:667–668, 1991.

48. Kline DG and Judice DJ: Operative management of selected brachial plexus lesions. J Neurosurg 58:631–649, 1983.

49. Kline DG and Kim DH: Axillary nerve repair in 99 patients with 101 stretch injuries. J Neurosurg 99:630–636, 2003.

50. Kline DG, Kott J, Barnes G, et al.: Exploration of selected brachial plexus lesions by the posterior subscapular approach. J Neurosurg 49:872–880, 1978.

51. Kotani T, Toshima Y, Matsuda H, et al.: [Postoperative results of nerve transposition in brachial plexus injury]. Seikei Geka 22:963–966, 1971.

52. Leffert RD: Brachial plexus injuries. London, Churchill Livingstone, 1985.

53. Leffert RD: Reconstruction of the shoulder and elbow following brachial plexus injury. In: Omer GE and Spinner M, Eds: Management of Peripheral Nerve Problems. Philadelphia, WB Saunders, 1980.

54. Leffert RD and Seddon H: Infraclavicular brachial plexus injuries. J Bone Joint Surg [Br] 47:9–22, 1965.

55. LeJune G, Leclercq D, Carlier A, et al.: [Direct microsurgical treatment of brachial plexus lesions (author's transl)]. Acta Chir Belg 82:251–260, 1982.

56. Levy WJ, Nutkiewicz A, Ditmore QM, et al.: Laser-induced dorsal root entry zone lesions for pain control. Report of three cases. J Neurosurg 59:884–886, 1983.

57. Luedemann W, Hamm M, Blomer U, et al.: Brachial plexus neurotization with donor phrenic nerves and its effect on pulmonary function. J Neurosurg 96:523–526, 2002.

58. Lusskin R, Campbell JB, and Thompson WAL: Post-traumatic lesions of the brachial plexus. J Bone Joint Surg [Am] 55:1159–1176, 1973.

59. Malessy MJ, Bakker D, Dekker AJ, et al.: Functional magnetic resonance imaging and control over the biceps muscle after intercostal-musculocutaneous nerve transfer. J Neurosurg 98:261–268, 2003.

60. Malessy MJ and Thomeer RT: Evaluation of intercostal to musculocutaneous nerve transfer in reconstructive brachial plexus surgery. J Neurosurg 88:266–271, 1998.

61. Malessy MJ, Thomeer RT, and van Dijk JG: Changing central nervous system control following intercostal nerve transfer. J Neurosurg 89:568–574, 1998.

62. Malone JM, Leal JM, Underwood J, et al.: Brachial plexus injury management through upper extremity amputation with immediate postoperative prostheses. Arch Phys Med Rehabil 63:89–91, 1982.

63. Mayer VL and Green W: Experiences with the Steindler flexorplasty at the elbow. J Bone Joint Surg [Am] 36:775, 1954.

64. Merrell GA, Barrie KA, Katz DL, et al.: Results of nerve transfer techniques for restoration of shoulder and elbow function in the context of a meta-analysis of the English literature. J Hand Surg [Am] 26:303–314, 2001 (See also Gabriel, E, Villavicencio A, and Friedman A: Evaluation and Surgical repair of brachial plexus injuries. Sem Neurosurg 12:29–48, 2001).

65. Merren MD: Gabapentin for treatment of pain and tremor: a large case series. South Med J 91:739–744, 1998.

66. Midha R: Epidemiology of brachial plexus injuries in a multitrauma population. Neurosurgery 40:1182–1189, 1997.

67. Midha R: Nerve transfers for severe brachial plexus injuries: a review. Neurosurg Focus 6:E5, 2004.

68. Midha R and Kline DG: Evaluation of the neuroma in continuity. In: Omer GE, Spinner M, and Van Beek AL, Eds: Management of Peripheral Nerve Problems. Philadelphia, PA, WB Saunders, 1998:319–327.

69. Millesi H: Brachial plexus injuries. Management and results. Clin Plast Surg 11:115–120, 1984.

70. Millesi H: Brachial plexus injuries: nerve grafting. Clin Orthop Rel Res 237:36–42, 1988.

71. Milton GW: The mechanism of circumflex and other nerve injuries in dislocation of the shoulder, and the possible mechanism of nerve injury during reduction of dislocation. Aust NZ J Surg 23:25–30, 1953.

72. Nagano A, Tsuyama N, Hara T, et al.: Brachial plexus injuries. Prognosis of postganglionic lesions. Arch Orthop Trauma Surg 102:172–178, 1984.

73. Nagano A, Yamamoto S, and Mikami Y: Intercostal nerve transfer to restore upper extremity functions after brachial plexus injury. Ann Acad Med Singapore 24:42–45, 1995.

74. Narakas A: Brachial plexus surgery. Orthop Clin N Am 12:303–323, 1981.

75. Narakas AO: Thoughts on neurotization or nerve transfers in irreparable nerve lesions. Clin Plast Surg 11:153–159, 1984.

76. Narakas AO: The surgical treatment of traumatic brachial plexus lesions. Internat Surg 65:521–527, 1980.

77. Narakas AO and Hentz VR: Neurotization in brachial plexus injuries. Indication and results. Clin Orthop 237:43–56, 1988.

78. Nashold BS Jr and Ostdahl RH: Dorsal root entry zone lesions for pain relief. J Neurosurg 51:59–69, 1979.

79. Nath RK, Mackinnon SE, and Shenaq SM: New nerve transfers following peripheral nerve injuries. Oper Techn Plastic Reconstr Surg 4:2–11, 1997.

80. Nikkhah G, Carvalho GA, El Azm M, et al.: Functional outcome after peripheral nerve grafting or neurotization in brachial plexus injuries (abstract). Zentralbl Neurochir (suppl):55, 1995.

81. Nulsen F and Slade WW: Recovery following injury to the brachial plexus, peripheral nerve regeneration: a follow-up study of 3,656 WW II injuries. Washington DC: US Government Printing Office, 1956.

82. Oberlin C, Beal D, Leechavengvongs S, et al.: Nerve transfer to biceps muscle using a part of ulnar nerve for C5-C6 avulsion of the brachial plexus: anatomical study and report of four cases. J Hand Surg [Am] 19:232–237, 1994.

83. Omer GE: Tendon transfer for reconstruction of the forearm and hand following peripheral nerve injuries. In: Omer GE and Spinner M, Eds: Management of Peripheral Nerve Problems. Philadelphia, WB Saunders, 1980.

84. Perry J, Hsu J, Barber L, et al.: Orthoses in patients with brachial plexus injuries. Arch Phys Med Rehabil 55:134–137, 1974.

85. Ransford AO and Hughes PF: Complete brachial plexus lesions. J Bone Joint Surg [Br] 59:417–420, 1977.

86. Richards RR: Operative treatment for irreparable lesions of the brachial plexus. In: Gelberman RH, Ed: Operative Nerve Repair and Reconstruction. Philadelphia, JB Lippincott, 1991.

87. Rorabeck CH and Harris WR: Factors affecting the prognosis of brachial plexus injuries. J Bone Joint Surg [Br] 63:404–407, 1981.

88. Ruch DS, Friedman A, and Nunley JA: The restoration of elbow flexion with intercostal nerve transfers. Clin Orthop 314:95–103, 1995.

89. Samardzic M, Rasulic L, Grujicic D, et al.: Results of nerve transfers to the musculocutaneous and axillary nerves. Neurosurgery 46:93–101, 2000.

90. Samii A, Carvalho GA, and Samii M: Brachial plexus injury: factors affecting functional outcome in spinal accessory nerve transfer for the restoration of elbow flexion. J Neurosurg 98:307–312, 2003.

91. Samii M: Dorsal root entry zone coagulation for control of intractable pain due to brachial plexus injury. In: Samii M, Ed: Peripheral Nerve Lesions. Berlin, Springer-Verlag, 1990.

92. Samii M: Use of microtechniques in peripheral nerve surgery: Experience with over 300 cases. In: Handa H, Ed: Microneurosurgery. Tokyo, Igaku-Shoin, 1975.

93. Samii M, Carvalho GA, Nikkhah G, et al.: Surgical reconstruction of the musculocutaneous nerve in traumatic brachial plexus injuries. J Neurosurg 87:881–886, 1997.

94. Sedel L: The management of supraclavicular lesions: Clinical examination, surgical procedures, results. In: Terzis J, Ed: Microreconstruction of Nerve Injuries. Philadelphia, WB Saunders, 1987.

95. Sedel L: The results of surgical repair of brachial plexus injuries. J Bone Joint Surg [Br] 64:54–66, 1982.

96. Sharpe W: The operative treatment of brachial plexus paralysis. JAMA 66:876–884, 1916.

97. Slingluff CL, Terzis J, and Edgerton M: The quantitative microanatomy of the brachial plexus in man. In: Terzis J, Ed: Microreconstruction of Nerve Injuries. Philadelphia, WB Saunders, 1987.

98. Solonen KA, Vastamaki M, and Strom B: Surgery of the brachial plexus. Acta Orthop Scand 55:436–440, 1984.

99. Songcharoen P: Brachial plexus injury in Thailand: a report of 520 cases. Microsurgery 16:35–39, 1995.

100. Steindler DA: Kinesiology of the human body. Springfield, IL, Charles C Thomas, 1955.

101. Steubdaker A: Muscle and tendon transplantation of the elbow. In: Thomson JE, Ed: Instruction Course Lecture on Reconstructive Surgery. Chicago, American Academy of Orthopedic Surgeons, 1944.

102. Stevens C, Davis D, and MacCarty CS: A 32-year experience with the surgical treatment of selected brachial plexus lesions with emphasis on reconstruction. Surg Neurol 19:334–345, 1983.

103. Sunderland S: Nerve and Nerve Injuries. Edinburgh, Churchill Livingstone, 1978.

104. Taylor PE: Traumatic intradural avulsion of the nerve roots of the brachial plexus. Brain 85:579–602, 1962.

105. Terzis J: Microreconstruction of Nerve Injuries. Philadelphia, WB Saunders, 1987.

106. Terzis JK, Vekris MD, and Soucacos PN: Outcomes of brachial plexus reconstruction in 204 patients with devastating paralysis. Plast Reconstr Surg 104:1221–1240, 1999.

107. Thomas DG and Jones SJ: Dorsal root entry zone lesions (Nashold's procedure) in brachial plexus avulsion. Neurosurgery 15:966–968, 1984.

108. Tsuyama J, Kara T, and Nagano A: Intercostal nerve crossing as a treatment of irreparable brachial plexus. In: Noble J and Galusko C, Eds: Recent development in orthopedic surgery. Manchester, England, Manchester University Press, 1987.

109. Tung TH and Mackinnon SE: Brachial plexus injuries. Clin Plast Surg 30:269–287, 2003.

110. Tung TH, Novak CB, and Mackinnon SE: Nerve transfers to the biceps and brachialis branches to improve elbow flexion strength after brachial plexus injuries. J Neurosurg 98:313–318, 2003.

111. Tuttle HK: Exposure of the brachial plexus with nerve transplantation. JAMA 61:15–17, 1913.

112. Waikakul S, Wongtragul S, and Vanadurongwan V: Restoration of elbow flexion in brachial plexus avulsion injury: comparing spinal accessory nerve transfer with intercostal nerve transfer. J Hand Surg [Am] 24:571–577, 1999.

113. Wilde AH, Brems JJ, and Boumphrey FR: Arthrodesis of the shoulder. Current indications and operative technique. Orthop Clin N Am 18:463–472, 1987.

114. Wynn Parry C: The management of traction lesions of the brachial plexus and peripheral nerve injuries to the upper limb: A study in teamwork. Injury 11:265–285, 1980.

115. Wynn Parry C: Rehabilitation of the hand. London, Butterworths, 1981.

116. Yamada S, Peterson GW, Soloniuk DS, et al.: Coaptation of the anterior rami of C3 and C4 to the upper trunk of the brachial plexus for cervical nerve root avulsion. J Neurosurg 74:171–177, 1991.

117. Yeoman PM: Cervical myelography in traction injuries of the brachial plexus. J Bone Joint Surg [Br] 50:253–260, 1968.

118. Yeoman PM and Seddon HJ: Brachial plexus injuries: treatment of the flail arm. J Bone Joint Surg [Br] 43:493–500, 1961.

119. Yoshimura M, Amaya S, and Tyujo M: Experimental studies on the traction injury of peripheral nerves. Neuro Orthop 7:1–7, 1989.

120. Zancolli E and Mitre H: Latissimus dorsi transfer to restore elbow flexion. An appraisal of eight cases. J Bone Joint Surg [Am] 55:1265–1275, 1973.

17

Plexus birth palsies

David G. Kline

OVERVIEW

- The basis of this chapter is a group of 171 newborn birth palsies in 169 patients evaluated at Louisiana State University Health Sciences Center (LSUHSC) from 1975 until 2003. Although patients were referred for consideration for plexus surgery, most palsies improved or residual loss was judged not severe enough to warrant plexus surgery. Seventy-six of these palsies were presented in some detail in the first edition of this book while another 95 palsies have been seen and followed or operated on since 1991. In both series, a long labor, use of forceps or suction, and pelvic disproportion and shoulder dystocia were common etiologic factors.

- In the more recent LSUHSC series the average birth weight in 93 babies was 9.1 lbs while their mother's averaged weight gain was 46.8 lb. Sixteen palsies (9.4%) were operated upon, usually because of failure to improve shoulder and/or biceps function by 8 months or more of age. Ninety-two of the patients not operated upon and having fairly acceptable recovery did not recover biceps until after 3 months of age. In addition, in the recent series, onset of shoulder abduction was analyzed and late onset of this function was also not unusual even though eventual shoulder function was often useful. One hundred and eleven patients had one or more years of follow-up while 67 had 3 or more years of follow-up.

- We continue to favor a fairly selective approach for operation, including following the palsied newborn for 6–9 months before operating. In general, an operation on the plexus is then done only if there is not satisfactory biceps and/or shoulder function.

INTRODUCTION

Management of birth palsies remains one of the most controversial topics in pediatrics and in pediatric nerve surgery.[11,20,24,28,77] Further studies to document the disorder's natural history, long-term outcomes from surgery, and especially better clinical criteria for proper selection for operation are still needed.[5,7,16,40]

METHOD AND RESULTS

Table 17-1 provides some of the demographic information about the more recent series of birth palsy patients. At the onset it should be recognized that the LSUHSC series is a referral-based group of patients, not hospital based. Thus, in the 1991–2003 series only 11 of 93 patients were initially seen before 3 months of age and only 23 before 6 months of age. In addition, 16 were seen at or after 2 years of age. As a result, age at initial visit to our clinic for operative cases between 1991 and 2003 averaged 8.5 months and operation, when done, was done at an average of 14 months of age. Follow-up averaged 23.5 months. As in the initial series, the majority (54%) of the birth palsies we have seen were Erb-Klumpke (C5–T1) or flail at birth and sometimes for some weeks postnatal. Other palsies were Erb's (C5–C6) or Erb's plus (C5, C6, C7) but had not improved satisfactorily from the viewpoint of the referring sources and so were referred for potential surgery. Thirty-two patients were from out of state and three were from another country.

An impairment rating scale as developed by Eng et al.[27] (Table 17-2) was used to evaluate outcomes at follow-up of 151 birth palsies seen between 1975 and 2001. As a group, their improvement rating improved substantially on follow-up. Review of Table 17-3 also illustrates a major problem with birth-palsied children and that is that it is difficult to restore normal or near-normal function either spontaneously or even with appropriate surgery. Thus, 30% of patients still had at follow-up an INR rating of either 4 or 5 in the nonoperative group and 22% in the operative group. Looked at another way, 47% in the nonoperative group reached a good (level 2) impairment rating while only 17% in the operative group did so. In part, this is due to the fact that the more severely involved patients were selected for surgery, 67% with an initial INR of 4 or 5 versus the nonoperative group where only 52% were grade 4 or 5 at the initial visit. This is one point that might favor earlier surgery rather than later selection for surgery. Later selection leaves the surgeon with the more seriously injured cases where results with plexus repair are less successful. The downside to earlier surgery on more infants, however, as pointed out by this analysis, is that selection for surgery earlier, at least based on currently available criteria, could lead to operations on infants with subsequent respectable, spontaneous recovery of function.

Thus, the efforts of Mallet, Gilbert and Tassin, Morelli, Birch and, more recently, Clarke and Waters and their associates to

Table 17-1 Birth palsies LSUHSC (1991–2003)

93 patients with 95 palsies
32 out of state
3 outside of country
Birth weight, 9.1 lb (average)
Mother's weight gain, 46.7 lb (average)
54% born with flail arm
Long labor, forceps, suction
Pelvic disproportion, gestational diabetes
Shoulder dystocia, occasional breach

develop criteria to properly select cases for operation, especially in the early months after birth and injury, are to be applauded and their systems for evaluations should be studied carefully.[7,10,16,34,49,51,67]

RECOVERY OF BICEPS AND SHOULDER FUNCTION

Table 17-4 shows that a large number of patients in the nonoperative group did not initiate biceps recovery until after 3 months of age and yet went on to have acceptable recovery of biceps function. There were even 24 who began to have recovery at 6–12 months who eventually had acceptable biceps grades. Similar conclusions could be drawn regarding onset of shoulder abduction. Such quite frequently did not initiate until 3–12 months and yet outcomes were acceptable in the nonoperative group. Table 17-5 shows initial

Table 17-2 Impairment rating scales[27]

Table impairment rating for BPP on initial physical exam.	Moderate
1 = Almost no abnormal findings + DTRs	Obvious scapula winging
	Shoulder abduction less that 90° with substitution of trapezius
2 = Slightly weak shoulder depressors	and serratus anterior in shoulder elevation.
Elbow flexion – antigravity	Uses short head of biceps with deltoid to lift arm
Good hand	Flexion contracture of elbow
Trace DTRs	Antigravity biceps
	Good wrist and finger extensors and flexors
3 = Shoulder abduction <90°	Good hand
Elbow flexion – not antigravity	Moderate to severe
"Waiter's tip" posture	Marked scapular winging
Good hand	Shoulder abduction <45°
0 DTRs	Elbow contracture, no supination
	Biceps movement negligible
4 = Shoulder – no movement	Loss of hand function
Elbow flexion – not antigravity	Severe loss of sweat and sensation
Some hand involvement	Withered arm or agnosia of the arm
0 DTRs	Severe
Some loss of sweat and sensation	Marked scapula winging
5 = Limp arm	Shoulder abduction <45°
Limp hand	Elbow contracture, no supination
Sweat and sensation	Biceps movement negligible
0 DTRs	Loss of hand function
± Horner's etc.	Severe loss of sweat and sensation
	Withered arm or agnosia of the arm
Impairment rating for brachial plexus palsy on follow-up	
Complete recovery	
Mild	
Minimal winging of scapula	
Abducts to 90° or more	
Some external rotation	
Good biceps (antigravity +)	
Minimal loss of supination	
Normal sweat and sensation	
Good hand use	

Table 17-3 Impairment rating (IR) for 151 birth palsies (1975–2001)

IR* number	Nonoperative palsies		Operated palsies	
	At initial visit (%)	At follow-up (%)	At initial visit (%)	At follow-up (%)
1	0	5	0	0
2	3	47	0	17
3	45	18	33	61
4	35	28	22	22
5	17	2	45	0

*Impairment rating based on Eng G, Binder H, Geston P, O'Donnel R.: Obstetrical brachial plexus palsy (OBPP): Outcome with conservative management. Muscle Nerve 19:884–891, 1996.

Table 17-4 Onset of biceps contraction and shoulder abduction matched to grade of contraction and degrees of abduction 1991–2003 series (84 cases)* (nonoperative)

Onset of contraction	Biceps		Shoulder abduction		
	Number of palsies	Average grade on follow-up[†]	Number of palsies	Average grade on follow-up[†]	Average degree of abduction on follow-up
<3 mon	23	3.7	27	3	85°
3–6 mon	34	3.7	33	3	75°
6–9 mon	21	3.7	17	3	70°
9–12 mon	3	4.5	5	3	86°
>12 mon	3*	3.7	2*	2	60°

*Additional child seen at 19 months with biceps=0 and shoulder abduction only 15°. Operation refused.
[†]Grades are based on the LSUHSC system, not the MRC system.

visit date in months, operative date, and follow-up in months, and eventual biceps and shoulder abduction and degrees of abduction. When looking at the average grade at follow-up for both biceps and shoulder function in our series, it should be kept in mind that 17 patients had less than 1 year of follow-up (Table 17-5). These were the more recent patients seen and sometimes operated upon between 2001 and 2004. This limitation in follow-up impacts most unfavorably the three relatively recent operative cases where follow-up time averaged only 9 months, whereas those six operated upon between 1991 and 2001 had an averaged follow-up time of 34 months. Of importance though, eight out the nine operated cases had not had onset of biceps contraction until after 6 months of age. In the nonoperative group for biceps, eventual grade was acceptable but not perfect irrespective of when contraction of biceps was first noted. However, the family of one child who had no biceps, when first seen at 19 months of age, refused operation and we do not know what outcome there would have been.

For shoulder function, eventual degrees of abduction were acceptable in the LSUHSC series and averaged 70–86% when onset of abduction was before 1 year. Six of the nine in the operative group between 1991 and 2003 did not have abduction of the shoulder begin before 9 months, the other three had it begin after 12 months.

Despite 54% of the recent series of patients presenting with a flail arm, 46 of 84 eventually had 5/5 intrinsic function using the LSUHSC grading system (Table 17-6). Twelve had 4/5 and 11 had 3/5 function, while only 15 patients had grade 2 or less function. On follow-up, this would suggest that even in the Erb-Klumpke patient, the lower elements, C8 and T1, sustain a lesser injury in most although not all cases than other elements. Follow-up in the 1991–2003 series averaged 23.5 months since some patient's were only relatively recently operated on and added to the cohort.

These figures can be compared to the LSUHSC earlier series from 1975–1991 where averaged date of operation was 19 months of age but averaged follow-up was much greater at 66 months. The grades in 16 Erb-Klumpke patients seen with lengthy follow-up in the 1975–1991 study are depicted in Table 17-7 while those for the Erb plus palsies are seen in Table 17-8.

DISCUSSION

The history of obstetrical birth palsies is fascinating and has been reviewed by many. Especially detailed is Birch, Bonney, and Wynn-Parry's chapter in the second edition of Seddon's Surgery of Peripheral Nerve[10] but others have also contributed well in this fashion.[12,28,62,64,72,74,75] Since the original early descriptions, by Smellie in 1765,[63] Danyou in 1851, Duchenne in 1872,[25] Erb in 1874,[29] and Klumpke in 1885 there have been a large number of papers published about birth palsies.[1,10] The early operative papers by Kennedy, Clark and Taylor, antedated by many years

Table 17-5 Operative newborn palsies (n=16)

1975–1991 (4 Erb-Klumpke, 3 Erb's)

Case	Initial visit (mon)	Operation (mon)	Follow-up (mon)	Averaged biceps (grade)	Averaged shoulder abduction (grade)	Averaged shoulder abduction (degrees)
1	3	9	123	3.5	3	70
2	9	18	42	3.0	4	90
3	10	12	48	3.0	3	65
4	28	36	24	2.5	2	60
5	22	24	24	3.0	4	100
6	9	14	22	2.5	2	40
7	9	12	20	4.0	3	70

1991–2003 (6 Erb-Klumpke, 3 Erb's)

Case	Initial visit (mon)	Operation (mon)	Follow-up (mon)	Averaged biceps (grade)	Averaged shoulder abduction (grade)	Averaged shoulder abduction (degrees)
1	11	12	31	2.0	2	40
2	10	1	24	2.5	2	40
3	8	8	60	4.0	3	65
4	10	12	39	3.0	3	65
5	4	12	16	2.0	2	30
6	6	22	16	4.0	3	65
7	9	15	2	1.0	0	10
8	11	14	12	3.5	3	90
9	7	20	12	2.0	0	10

Key: Biceps grades are by the LSUHSC System

Shoulder abduction

0 = 15° or less

1 = 15–30°

2 = 30–60°

3 = 60–90°

4 = 90–120°

5 = 120–180°

Table 17-6 Hand intrinsic grades at follow-up 1991–2003 (n=93 palsies)

Grade	No operation	Operation
5	46	1
4	12	1
3	11	0
2	6	3
1	5	2
0	4	2
Totals	84	9

publications about operations for the much more frequently injured adult plexus.[15,45,68] These early surgical attempts were not very successful and Gilbert and Tassin have been largely credited with restimulating interest in surgical repair by using grafts and promulgating the suggestion that if biceps did not recover by 3 months of age operation was indicated.[33,34,67] Surgeons though such as Narakus, Morelli, Raimondi, and Terzis and others had begun to study and operate on some of these unfortunate children in the 1970s and early 1980s. The Zancolli's,[80,81] Wickstrom,[78,79] and others even earlier had been doing reconstructive work for residual deficits in these unfortunate children.

There have been a number of studies of the mechanics and factors responsible for paralysis as well as the natural history of the disorder.[31,32,53,58,61,65-67,72,77] Although less frequently observed, plexus palsy can result from in utero position and/or forces and has certainly been reported after caesarean section.[6,26,52,57] Interesting

Table 17-7 Older patients 1975–1991 (76 patients)

Erb-Klumpke (follow-up muscle grades*)

Age last seen (yr)	Number	S	D	Bic	Tri	Wr	Ha
11–15	5	3.3	2.5	3.9	3.3	3.4	3.0
5–6	2	3.5	3.5	4.5	3.5	2.5	1.5
*5–6	2	3.0	3.0	3.5	3.0	2.0	1.5
4	3	2.6	1.6	2.8	2.0	1.0	0.0
3	4	3.0	2.4	3.5	3.0	2.5	1.5

*Operative cases + grades based on the LSUHSC grading system.

S, supraspinatus; D, deltoid; Bic, biceps; Tri, triceps; Wr, wrist flexion and extension; Ha, hand intrinsics.

From: Kline D and Hudson A: Nerve Injuries. Philadelphia, WB Saunders, 1995.

Table 17-8 Older patients 1975–1991 (76 patients)

Erb's (follow-up muscle grades†)

Age last seen (yr)	Number	S	D	Bic	Tri	Wr	Ha
*11	1	3.0	3.5	3.5	4.0	4.0	4.0
5	3	3.0	2.8	3.5	3.2	4.0	4.5
*5	1	2.5	2.0	3.0	5.0	5.0	5.0
4	2	3.0	2.8	4.0	3.7	4.5	5.0
3	2	4.0	3.5	4.0	4.5	4.5	5.0
*3	1	3.0	2.0	3.0	3.0	4.5	4.5

*Operative cases.

†Grades based on the LSUHSC grading system.

S, supraspinatus; D, deltoid; Bic, biceps; Tri, triceps; Wr, wrist flexion and extension; Ha, hand intrinsics.

From: Kline D and Hudson A: Nerve Injuries. Philadelphia, WB Saunders, 1995.

reflections on the value of magnetic resonance imaging (MRI), computed tomography (CT), myelography, and electromyogram (EMG) have also been published[22,30,41,71,76] In Gjorup's series with lengthy follow-up published in 1965, 21% of 103 patients had persistent serious loss.[37] This incidence was somewhat higher in Rossi's and Wickstrom's experience as it was in Eng's earlier publication.[28,56,79] Although 70% of infants had on follow-up a mild residual impairment, 22% had moderate impairment and 8% had severe deficits. In a more recent publication of Eng's group, almost all (88%) of the patients presented with upper plexus palsies while only 12% had complete plexus palsy (flail arm) at birth.[27] Of the 149 patients with follow-up using a functional classification (see Table 17-2), 72% had concordant scores over time while most with discrepant scores improved. Michelow et al. studied a group of infants who had a higher incidence of Erb-Klumpke palsies (60%) than Eng's series but found that over 80% recovered a good deal of function spontaneously.[50]

There is no question, though, that some children do not have satisfactory spontaneous recovery, and then operation may help. Thus, Birch, who has a major interest in this topic, has operated on the plexus in 147 (22%) of the 680 birth palsies he has seen.[9] Waters, Laurent Sloof, Sedel, Thomeer, Al-Quatton, Hentz and

Meyer, Piatt and Hudson and others have also operated on the plexus in the early months post birth using a variety of methods to select patients felt to need such.[2–4,18,23,42,43,46–48,54,55,60,62,64,69,77] As in adult stretch injury patients, a variety of nerve transfers have been advocated with a variable degree of success.[3,44] The problem remains who and when to select for surgery. Gilbert, Birch, and Clarke have all devised criteria but none is totally satisfactory and Clarke and others continue to work on this issue.[7,10,16,77]

There have been other attempts to simplify the selection process. For example, Waters feels that infants with antigravity biceps by 1–2 months of life recover completely by 1–2 years. On the other hand, those without antigravity biceps by 5–6 months of life have permanent, marked limitations.[7,77]

In earlier work, Clarke's group selected patients for surgery by grading five joint movements: elbow flexion and extension and wrist, finger, and thumb movement (Table 17-9).[16] Numerical scores were added to give a score between 0 and 10. If at 3 months of age the score was less than 3.5, infants were operated upon. If above 3.5, they were followed until the age of 9 months, and if biceps using a 0 to 7 scale was less than 6 they were operated upon. Of 110 patients evaluated, 26 (23%) were operated upon and 16 of these had neurolysis only.[17] Nine of these patients had Erb's

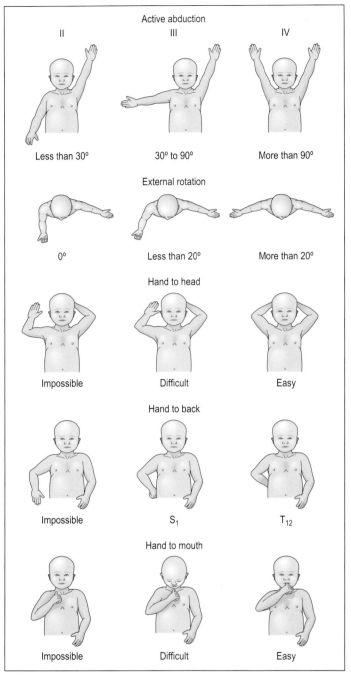

Table 17-9 Clarke's active movement grading scale

Score	Motion	Gravity
0	None	
1	Contraction, no motion	
2	Motion <$\frac{1}{2}$ range	Gravity
3	Motion >$\frac{1}{2}$ range	Eliminated
4	Full motion	
5	Motion <$\frac{1}{2}$ range	Against
6	Motion >$\frac{1}{2}$ range	Gravity
7	Full motion	

palsy and seven had total plexus palsy (Erb-Klumpke). If after exposure of a plexus element there was no conduction to muscle, the element was resected and a graft repair was done (nine cases). The nine patients with Erb's palsies who had neurolysis benefited, or seemed to, from operation, whereas the seven who had total palsy had less benefit. No attempt was made to record nerve action potentials (NAPs). More recently, even neuromas in continuity that conduct, but presumably not well, have been resected and repaired with some good outcomes.[13]

Gilbert, Tassin, and more recently Birch, classified birth palsies in a relatively straightforward fashion.[10,34,35] As pointed out by Birch et al., these categories provide a useful way to view birth palsies:

- Group 1 – The fifth and sixth cervical nerves are damaged with paralysis of deltoid and biceps. About 90% of these babies proceed to full spontaneous recovery with usually clinical evidence of recovery beginning at no later than 2 months.
- Group 2 – The fifth, sixth, and seventh cervical nerves are damaged. The long flexor muscles of the hand are working from the time of birth, but there is paralysis of extension of elbow, wrist, and digits. Perhaps 65% of these children make full spontaneous recovery; the remainder persist with serious defects in control of the shoulder. Recovery is slower, activity in the deltoid and biceps becoming clinically evident between 3 and 6 months.
- Group 3 – Paralysis is virtually complete, although there is some flexion of the fingers at or shortly after birth. Full spontaneous recovery occurs in less than one-half of these children, and most are left with substantial impairment of function at the shoulder and elbow joints, with deficient rotation of the forearm. Wrist and finger extension does not recover in about one-quarter.
- Group 4 – The whole plexus is involved. Paralysis is complete. The limb is atonic, and there is a Bernard-Horner syndrome. No child makes a full recovery; the spinal nerves have been either ruptured or avulsed from the spinal cord, and there is permanent and serious defect within the limb.

Either the Mallet[49] (Fig. 17-1) or the Gilbert system[34,35] can be used to measure shoulder function, while Morelli has devised a good grading system for the hand.[51]

Gilbert, as reported in 1995, had operated on 178 children.[33] The 65 with Erb's had good or satisfactory shoulder function in

FIGURE 17-1 Grading system proposed by Mallet. The Mallet system grades the amount of usable abduction and external and internal shoulder rotation, as well as the child's ability to reach the mouth with the hand. Affected limb is the child's right arm on the reader's left. (Adapted from Gilbert A and Tassin JL: Obstetrical palsy: A clinical, pathologic and surgical review. In: Terzis J, Ed: Microreconstruction of Nerve Injuries. Philadelphia, WB Saunders, 1987.)

80% of cases and all but one regained elbow flexion. When C5, C6, and C7 were involved 65% regained shoulder function and 70% wrist extension. However, it should be mentioned that it is not clear in how many children in this category wrist extension was totally paralyzed to begin with. Remarkable was the report that in the 54 children with total (C5–T1) paralysis, useful finger flexion was gained in 75% and intrinsic function in an amazing 50%. Again, how many children born with paralysis of the hand had relatively early spontaneous and possibly partial recovery of hand muscles before surgery was not clear.

RECONSTRUCTIVE EFFORTS

Delayed or later surgery to correct muscle imbalance makes sense. The surgeons at Texas Children's Hospital have had experience with such in over 350 children with Erb's palsy. The operation is termed the "quad procedure" because it encompasses four steps:

1. Latissimus dorsi, providing it is working, is transferred to improve external rotation and abduction;
2. Teres major is transferred to provide scapular stabilization;
3. The subscapularis muscle is released;
4. The axillary nerve has a neurolysis done.

Shenaq et al. from the Texas Medical Center have developed protocols for reconstruction, placing children into one of six categories, I through VI, depending on the extent of paralysis and the residual dysfunction.[59] Included are *late operations with neurolysis on infraclavicular nerves such as the radial, musculocutaneous, and axillary nerves.* These latter steps remain controversial, at least as to the late operative dates, and are not generally accepted. On the other hand, the reconstructive steps recommended by them for releases and transfers of muscles are more generally accepted and are also in use in various combinations by others.[8,14,19,36,39,64] The intent has been to improve abduction of the shoulder as well as external rotation, and this group reports very favorable outcomes in that regard.

The Mayo clinic workers use a great deal of physical therapy and, if need be, casting for deformities for the first year of life. In the second year, if external rotation of the shoulder is less that 45 degrees, the subscapularis is lengthened. Pectoralis major, if working, can also be lengthened by a Z-palsy. For abduction less than 90 degrees, the latissimus dorsi and teres major tendons, providing these muscles are working, can be transferred to the supraspinatus portion of the rotator cuff. Use of latissimus dorsi transfer to shoulder capsule to provide external rotation depends on some function of the deltoid and subscapulars as well as pectoralis major to provide some medial rotation.[8,70]

After the age of 2, a proximal humeral osteotomy can be done if the above steps fail.[38] Zyaoussis and Birch et al. also use osteotomy of the radius, providing wrist extension is present, so the hand can be placed in a more supinated position.[10,82] A variety of reconstructive procedures can be done for poor elbow flexion, including a Steindler recession of the flexor mass.[73] Comtet and colleagues use transfer of pectoralis minor to substitute for biceps and poor external rotation.[18] Doi and others have pioneered work on whole-muscle transfer from the leg to substitute for elbow and wrist flexion when neurotization is not possible.[21]

It is far more difficult to substitute for loss of hand function, although use of a portion of flexor carpi ulnaris if there is strong wrist flexion can provide some wrist and finger motion, especially in extension.[10] Loss of hand intrinsics, however, poses larger reconstructive problems.

SUMMARY

Waters correctly points out that the literature is confusing.[77] For example, the range of infants needing surgery varies between 10%

Table 17-10   Conclusions – LSUHSC series
Most birth palsies have acceptable spontaneous recovery
Some palsies require surgical intervention
Operative rate in this series=9%
Spontaneous biceps or shoulder recovery may not occur until 6–12 months after delivery

to 35%, timing for such plexus surgery also varies greatly, secondary and even tertiary procedures for reconstruction are done at different times by different surgeons, and their use furthermore makes it difficult to analyze outcomes of the plexus surgery done. Follow-up on operated patients, at least that published, could be longer. What is needed "are prospective multi-center studies."[77] We would, at this point in time, full heartedly agree to this stance. Our other conclusions based on our experience to date is summarized in Table 17-10.

REFERENCES

1. Adler B and Patterson RL: Erb's palsy: Long-term results of treatment in eight-eighty cases. J Bone Joint Surg [AM] 49:1052–1056, 1967.
2. Alanen M, Ryoppy S, and Varho T: Twenty-six early operations in brachial palsy. Z Kinderchir 45(3):136–139, 1990.
3. Allieu Y, Privat JM, and Bonnel F: Paralysis in root avulsion of the brachial plexus. Neurotization by the spinal accessory nerve. Clin Plast Surg 11:33–36, 1984.
4. Al-Qattan MM: The outcome of Erb's palsy when the decision to operate is made at 4 months of age. Plast Reconstr Surg 106(7):1461–1465, 2000.
5. Al-Qattan MM, Clarke HM, and Curtis CG: The prognostic value of concurrent phrenic nerve palsy in newborn children with Erb's palsy. J Hand Surg [Br] 23(2):255, 1998.
6. Al-Qattan MM, El-Sayed AA, Al-Kharfy TM, et al.: Obstetrical brachial plexus injury in newborn babies delivered by caesarean section. J Hand Surg [Br] 21:263–265, 1996.
7. Bae D, Waters PM, and Zurakowski D: Reliability of three classification systems measuring active motion in brachial plexus birth palsy. J Bone Joint Surg 85:1733–1738, 2003.
8. Bennett JB and Allan H: Tendon transfers about the shoulder and elbow in obstetrical brachial plexus palsy. J Bone Joint Surg 81:1612–1627, 1999.
9. Birch R: Surgery for brachial plexus injuries. J Bone Joint Surg [Br] 75(3):346–348, 1993.
10. Birch R, Bonney G, and Wynn-Parry CB: Birth lesions of the brachial plexus In: Surgery of Peripheral Nerve. London, Churchill Livingstone, 1998.
11. Bodensteiner JB, Rich KM, and Landau WM: Early infantile surgery for birth-related brachial plexus injuries: justification requires a prospective controlled study. J Child Neurol 9(2):109–110, 1994.
12. Boome RS and Kaye JC: Obstetric traction injuries of the brachial plexus. Natural history, indications for surgical repair and results. J Bone Joint Surg [Br] 70:571–576, 1988.
13. Capek L, Clarke HM, and Curtis CG: Neuroma-in-continuity resection: early outcome in obstetrical brachial plexus palsy. Plast Reconstr Surg 102:1555–1562, 1998.
14. Chuang DC, Ma HS, and Wei FC: A new strategy of muscle transposition for treatment of shoulder deformity caused by obstetric brachial plexus palsy. Plast Reconstr Surg 101:686–694, 1998.

15. Clark LP, Taylor AS, and Prout TP: A study on brachial birth palsy. Am J Med Sci 130:670–707, 1905.

16. Clarke HM and Curtis CG: An approach to obstetrical brachial plexus injuries. Hand Clin 11(4):563–580; discussion 580–581, 1995.

17. Clarke HM, Al-Qattan MM, Curtis CG, et al.: Obstetrical brachial plexus palsy: results following neurolysis of conducting neuromas-in-continuity. Plast Reconstr Surg 97(5):974–982; discussion 983–984, 1996.

18. Comtet JJ, Sedel L, Fredenucci JF, et al.: Duchenne-Erb palsy: experience with direct surgery. Clin Orthopaed 237:17–23, 1988.

19. Covey DC, Riodan DC, Milstead ME, et al.: Modification of the L 'Episcopo Procedure for brachial plexus birth palsies. J Bone Joint Surg [Br] 74:897–901, 1992.

20. Dodds SD and Wolfe SW: Perinatal brachial plexus palsy. Curr Opin Pediatrics 12(1):40–47, 2000.

21. Doi K: Obstetric and traumatic paediatric palsy. In: Peimer CA, Ed: Surgery of Hand and Upper Extremity, 2nd edn. New York, McGraw Hill, 1996:1443–1463.

22. Doi K, Otsuka K, Okamoto Y, et al.: Cervical nerve root avulsion in brachial plexus injuries: magnetic resonance imaging classification and comparison with myelography and computerized tomography myelography. J Neurosurg 96(3 Suppl):277–284, 2002.

23. Dol'nitzkii OV: Microsurgical operation on the brachial plexus in children. Klin Khir 6:22, 1988.

24. Donnelly V, Foran A, Murphy J, et al.: Neonatal brachial plexus palsy: An unpredictable injury. Am J Obstetr Gynecol 187(5):1209–1212, 2002.

25. Duchenne GB: Del'Electrisation Localisee et de son Application a la Pathologie et a la Therapeutique. 3rd edn. Paris, Ballière, 1872.

26. Dunn DW and Engle WA: Brachial plexus palsy: intrauterine onset. Pediatr Neurol 1:367–369, 1985.

27. Eng G, Binder H, Geston P, et al.: Obstetrical brachial plexus palsy (OBPP). Outcome with conservative management. Muscle Nerve 19:884–891, 1996.

28. Eng GD, Kock B, and Smokvina MD: Brachial plexus palsy in neonates and children. Arch Phys Med Rehabil 59:458, 1978.

29. Erb WH: Ueber eine eigenthumlishe localization von lahmungen im plexus brachialis. Verh Naturhist Med Vereins Heidelberg 1:130–139, 1874.

30. Francel PC, Koby M, Park TS, et al.: Fast spin-echo magnetic resonance imaging for radiological assessment of neonatal brachial plexus injury. J Neurosurg 83(3):461–466, 1995.

31. Geutjens G, Gilbert A, and Helsen K: Obstetric brachial plexus palsy associated with breech delivery. A different pattern of injury. J Bone Joint Surg [Br] 78(2):303–306, 1996.

32. Gherman RB, Ouzounian JG, Miller DA, et al.: Spontaneous vaginal delivery: a risk factor for Erb's palsy? (comment). Am J Obstetr Gynecol 178(3):423–427, 1998.

33. Gilbert A: Long-term evaluation of brachial plexus surgery in obstetrical palsy. Hand Clin 11(4)583–594; discussion 594–595, 1995.

34. Gilbert A and Tassin JL: Obstetrical palsy: a clinical, pathologic and surgical review. In: Terzis JK, Ed: Microreconstruction of Nerve Injuries. Philadelphia, WB Saunders, 1987:529–553.

35. Gilbert A, Razaboni R, and Amar-khodja S: Indications and results of brachial plexus surgery in obstetrical palsy. Orthop Clin N Am 190:91–105, 1988.

36. Gilbert A: Tendon transfers for shoulder paralysis in children. Hand Clin. 4:633–638, 1988.

37. Gjorup L: Obstetrical lesion of the brachial plexus. Acta Neurol Scand 42(Suppl 18):1, 1966.

38. Goddard NJ and Fixsen JA: Rotation osteotomy of the humerus for birth injuries of the brachial plexus. J Bone Joint Surg [Br] 66:257–259, 1984.

39. Green WT and Tachdijian MD: Correction of the residual deformities of the shoulder in obstetrical palsy. J Bone Joint Surg [Am] 45:1544, 1963.

40. Gu YD and Chen L: Classification of impairment of shoulder abduction in obstetric brachial plexus palsy and its clinical significance. J Bone Joint Surg [Br] 25:46–48, 2000.

41. Hasimoto T, Mitomo M, and Hirabuki N: Nerve root avulsion of birth palsy: comparison of myelography with CT myelography and somatosensory evoked potential. Radiology 178:841–845, 1991.

42. Hentz VR: Operative repair of the brachial plexus in infants and children. In: Gelberman RH, Ed: Operative Nerve Repair and Reconstruction. Philadelphia, Lippincott, 1991.

43. Hentz VR and Meyer RD: Brachial plexus microsurgery in children. Microsurgery 12(3):175–185, 1991.

44. Kawabata H, Shibata T, Matsui Y, et al.: Use of intercostal nerves for neurotization of the musculocutaneous nerve in infants with birth-related brachial plexus palsy. J Neurosurg 94(3)386–391, 2001.

45. Kennedy R: Suture of the brachial plexus in birth paralysis of the upper extremity. Br Med J 11:298–301, 1903.

46. Kline D and Hudson A: Brachial plexus birth palsies In: Nerve Injuries: Operative Results for Major Nerve Injuries, Entrapments, and Tumors. Philadelphia, WB Saunders, 1995.

47. Laurent JP, Lee R, Shenaq S, et al: Neurosurgical correction of upper brachial plexus birth injures. J Neurosurg 79(2):197–203, 1993.

48. Malessy MJ and Thomeer RT: Evaluation of intercostals to musculocutaneous nerve transfer in reconstructive brachial plexus surgery. J Neurosurg 88:266–271, 1998.

49. Mallet J: Paralysie obstetricale du plexus brachial. Traitement des sequelles. Primaute du traitement de l'epaule – Methode d'expression des resultants. Rev Chir Orthop Reparatrice Appar Mot 58(suppl 1):166–168, 1972.

50. Michelow B, Clarke H, Curtis C, et al.: The natural history of obstetrical brachial palsy. Plast Reconstr Surg 93(4):675–680, 1994.

51. Morelli E, Raimondi P, Saporiti E: Loro truttamento precoce In: Pipino F, Ed: Le Paralisi Ostetriche. Bologna, Auto Gaggi, 1984.

52. Narakus A: Obstetrical brachial plexus injuries. In: The Paralyzed Hand. Lamb D, Ed: Edinburgh, Churchill Livingstone, 1987.

53. Paradiso G, Granana N, and Maza E: Prenatal brachial plexus paralysis. Neurology 49(1):261–262, 1997.

54. Parks DG and Ziel HK: A proposed indication for primary caesarean section. Obstetr Gynecol 52:407–409, 1978.

55. Piatt JH, Hudson AR, and Hoffman HJ: Preliminary experiences with brachial plexus exploration in children: Birth injury and vehicular trauma. Neurosurgery 22:714–719, 1988.

56. Rossi LN, Vassella R, and Mumenthuler M: Obstetrical lesions of the brachial plexus. Eur Neurol 21:1, 1982.

57. Rouse DJ, Owen J, Goldenberg RL, et al.: The effectiveness and costs of elective cesarean delivery for fetal marosomia diagnosed by ultrasound. JAMA 276(18):1480–1486, 1996.

58. Sever JW: Obstetric paralysis: report of eleven hundred cases. JAMA 85:1862–1865, 1925.

59. Shenaq SM, Berzin E, Lee R, et al.: Brachial plexus birth injuries and current management. Clin Plast Surg 25(4):527–536, 1998.

60. Sherburn EW, Kaplan SS, Kaufman BA, et al.: Outcome of surgically treated birth-related brachial plexus injuries in twenty cases. Pediatr Neurosurg 27(1):19–27, 1997.

61. Sjoberg I, Etrichs K, and Bjerre I: Cause and effect of obstetric (neonatal) brachial plexus palsy. Acta Paediat Scand 77:357–364, 1988.

62. Slooff AC: Obstetric brachial plexus lesions and their neurosurgical treatment. Clin Neurol Neurosurg 95(Suppl):S73–77, 1993.

63. Smellie W: Collection of preternatural cases and observations in midwifery. London, Wilson and Durham, 1764.

64. Solomen KA, Telaranta T, and Ryoppy S: Early reconstruction of birth injuries of the brachial plexus. J Pediatr Orthop 1:367, 1981.

65. Spong CY, Beall M, Rodrigues D, et al.: An objective definition of shoulder dystocia: prolonged head-to delivery intervals and/or the use of ancillary obstetric maneuvers. Obstet Gynecol 179:934–937, 1995.

66. Stallings SP, Edwards RK, and Johnson JW: Correlation of head-to-body delivery intervals in shoulder dystocia and umbilical artery acidosis. Am J Obstet Gynecol 185:268–271, 2001.

67. Tassin JL: Paralysies obstetricales du plexus brachial: Evolution spontanee resultants des interventions reparatrices precoces. Thesis, Université Parish VII, 1983.

68. Taylor AS: Brachial birth palsy and injuries of similar type in adults. Surg Gynecol Obstet 30:494–502, 1920.

69. Terzis JK: Management of obstetric brachial plexus palsy. Hand Clin 15:717–736, 1999.

70. Vallejo GI, Toh S, Arai H, et al.: Results of the latissimus dorsi and teres major tendon transfer on to the rotator cuff for brachial plexus palsy at birth. Scand J Plast Reconstr Surg Hand Surg 36(4)207–211, 2002.

71. Van Dijk JG, Malessy MJ, and Stegeman DF: Why is the electromyogram in obstetric brachial plexus lesions overly optimistic? Muscle Nerve 21(2):260–261, 1998.

72. Van Dijk JG, Pondaag W, and Malessy MJ: Obstetric lesions of the brachial plexus muscle. Muscle Nerve 24(11):1451–1461, 2001.

73. Van Egmond C, Tonino AJ, and Kortleve JW: Steindler flexorplasty of the elbow in obstetric brachial plexus injuries. J Pediatr Orthoped 21(2):169–173, 2001.

74. Van Ouwerkerk WJ, Van der Sluijs JA, Nollet F, et al: Management of obstetric brachial plexus lesions: state of the art and future developments. Childs Nervous Sys 16(10–11):638–644, 2000.

75. Vredeveld JW, Blaauw G, Slooff BA, et al.: The findings in paediatric obstetric brachial palsy differ from those in older patients: a suggested explanation. Dev Med Child Neurol 42(3):158–161, 2000.

76. Walker AT, Chaloupka JC, de Lotbiniere AC, et al.: Detection of nerve rootlet avulsion on CT myelography in patients with birth palsy and brachial plexus injury after trauma. AJR Am J Roentgenol 167(5):1283–1287, 1996.

77. Waters PM: Comparison of the natural history, the outcome of microsurgical repair, and the outcome of operative reconstruction in brachial plexus birth palsy. J Bone Joint Surg 81(5):649–659, 1999.

78. Wickstrom J, Haslam ET, and Hutchinson RH: The surgical management of residual deformities of the shoulder following birth injuries of the brachial plexus. J Bone Joint Surg [Am] 37:27, 1955.

79. Wickstrom J: Birth injuries of the brachial plexus. Treatment of defects in the shoulder. Clin Orthopaed Rel Res 23:187–196, 1962.

80. Zancolli E: Classification and management of the shoulder in birth palsy. Orthop Clin N Am 12:433–457, 1981.

81. Zancolli EA and Zancolli ER: Reconstructive surgery in brachial plexus sequelae. In: Scheker L, Ed: The Growing Hand. London, Mosby, 2000:805–823.

82. Zyaoussis AL: Osteotomy of the proximal end of the radius for paralytic supination deformity in children. J Bone Joint Surg [Br] 45:523, 1963.

18

Thoracic outlet syndrome

David G. Kline

INTRODUCTION

Thoracic outlet syndrome (TOS) remains a controversial entrapment neuropathy to diagnose and treat.[2,5,16,36,51,73] TOS can be either vascular, when the subclavian artery and/or vein are compressed, or neurogenic, when spinal nerves C8, T1, and/or lower trunk of the brachial plexus are involved.[64] Vascular TOS is relatively rare and symptoms are related to limb ischemia (in the arterial type) or venous thrombosis and stasis (in the venous type).[21] Neurogenic TOS (NTOS) is further subdivided into two categories: "true" and "disputed."[12] True NTOS is universally acknowledged and is defined as a demonstrable, chronic C8, T1, and lower trunk brachial plexopathy, usually caused by congenital bony and soft tissue anomalies. Gilliatt described, in 1970, the characteristic features of true NTOS: thenar, hypothenar, and interossei weakness, and/or atrophy, plus ulnar and medial antebrachial cutaneous hypoesthesia in the affected arm[17] (Fig. 18-1). This constellation of clinical features, along with associated electrical findings, is now recognized as the Gilliat or, as we prefer, Gilliatt-Sumner hand (GSH). Disputed NTOS has poorly defined boundaries and many articles have been written debating its incidence, diagnostic features, and indications (if any) for surgery.

The major symptom of TOS is an achy pain in an arm which is usually but not always confined to the medial border of the arm and hand. This discomfort is sometimes but not always associated with elevation of the arm or activity of the extremity and occasionally associated with vasomotor symptoms or changes in the extremity. TOS remains a diagnosis of exclusion and its management remains confusing as well as difficult. Few symptoms generate as much controversy and emotion, both pro and con as to its existence and its surgical management, as does the thoracic outlet syndrome. To understand the passion that this syndrome evokes, some knowledge of the history and evolution of the entity may be helpful.

HISTORY

The existence of cervical ribs was known at the time of Galen but the relationship between the cervical rib and symptomatology was not recognized until much later by Hunald. In 1818, Sir Astley Cooper reported a woman with an ischemic limb attributed to "a projection of the lower cervical vertebrae towards the clavicle and consequent pressure on the subclavian artery."[8] The first surgical intervention was reported by Coote, in 1869, who removed an exostosis of the transverse process of the seventh cervical vertebra to treat a weak, ischemic hand followed by Paget's description of an axillary vein thrombosis in 1875.[9,50] The initial emphasis focused on cervical ribs being the culprit for symptoms presumably produced by vascular compromise of the upper limb. In 1910, Murphy reported a follow-up of 3 months after a new surgical procedure of first rib resection.[47] The first rib was felt to be the responsible structure for the TOS symptoms. Halstead postulated that turbulence was the etiology for poststenotic aneurysms and described his series of 716 cases of cervical ribs.[22] In 1927, Adson and Coffey promulgated the phrase "cervical rib syndrome."[1] Thirty-one patients underwent rib resection and five had a then novel operation, scalenotomy. These authors acknowledged the "frequent complications of rib resection." In the next few decades, others re-emphasized the important role the first rib and the cervical rib might play in neurovascular compression of the upper extremity (Fig. 18-2).[12,55,74]

Ochsner was the first to coin the phrase "scalenus anticus syndrome" as he reviewed reports of the anterior scalene abnormalities.[49] A similar term, "cervicobrachial syndrome," was used by Aynesworth in 1940 to encompass all causes of TOS.[3] Peet et al. are to be credited for using the current term of thoracic outlet syndrome in 1956 when they used this to express pain, numbness, and other symptoms in the upper extremity.[52] Of interest, in their series of 55 patients, 71% improved with conservative management alone. Bonney pointed out in 1965 the potential role of a scalenus medius band and also felt that a hypertrophic suprapleural membrane or Sibson's fascia could also trap lower elements.[4] Observations such as this favored an anterior approach and scalenotomies.

The pendulum swung back towards rib resection when Clagett advocated removal of the first rib as an optimal treatment as opposed to scalenotomy.[7] His description for a posterior approach

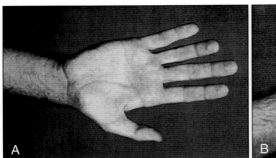

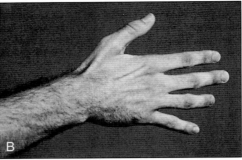

FIGURE 18-1 Gilliatt-Sumner hand. **(A)** front; **(B)** back. The thenar, hypothenar, and intrinsic hand muscles are atrophied.

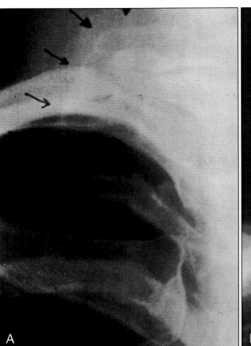

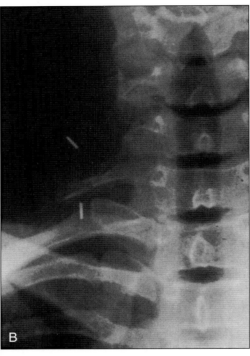

FIGURE 18-2 **(A)** Large cervical rib in a patient with symptoms of thoracic outlet syndrome (TOS). Arrows outline the extra rib. **(B)** Partially resected cervical rib in another patient whose TOS symptoms did not reverse after the initial operation. At the time of reoperation, medial scalene was still attached to the tip of the cervical rib. Note presence of metallic clips. **(C)** Radiograph of a patient who had elongated transverse processes of C7 vertebra (*arrows*) and who had bilateral first rib resection and yet recurrence of symptoms.

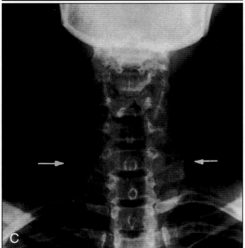

for rib resection was an adaptation from the old tuberculosis surgical literature and his impetus was predominantly dissatisfaction with a high recurrence rate in procedures of scalenotomy alone. Following this, Roos and then others described the transaxillary route for first rib resection and this has become a very popular procedure for TOS.[55] In more recent years, selection of either a supraclavicular or transaxillary approach has varied according to the personal preference of the surgeons involved with these difficult to manage patients.[5,10,36,51,61]

DEFINITION OF THE THORACIC OUTLET

Generally, the area called the "thoracic outlet" is anatomically defined as the area bound inferiorly by the lung apex, posteriorly by the spine and then the first rib which continues as its lateral border. The mediastinum forms the medial border. Superiorly, the outlet continues to the level of the fifth cervical spinal nerve and thus seems more cone-shaped.

For many anatomists, the thoracic "outlet" is felt to be the site of communication between the thorax and abdomen (inferior thoracic aperture).[54] The area between the scalene muscles and the first rib and clavicular area is as a result called "thoracic inlet." Be that as it may, the definition of inlet and outlet is, at least for vessels with blood flow, determined by the direction of that flow. Therefore, from the perspective of a subclavian vein, this region of interest is an inlet where as for the artery it is an outlet. Interestingly enough, for the nerves that suffer from compression, it is not exclusively either an inlet or an outlet to the thorax as both afferent and efferent pathways transverse this region towards the upper extremity.

Since the term thoracic outlet syndrome is so prevalent, it seems best to use it even though the etiology may be either neurogenic or vascular and the designation is not strictly correct.

SURGICAL ANATOMY

The brachial plexus elements traverse three narrow anatomical spaces from their origin at the neural foramina to the nerves in the arm. These spaces are, from proximal to distal: the interscalene triangle, the costoclavicular triangle, and the subcoracoid space.[51]

The C5 through T1 spinal nerves emerge from their respective foramina and recombine to form the upper, middle, and lower trunks of the brachial plexus. The spinal nerves and trunks are situated between the anterior and middle scalene muscles. These scalene muscles originate from the anterior and posterior tubercles of the transverse processes of the cervical vertebrae, respectively, and they both insert on the surface of the first rib. The two scalene muscles and the first rib form the interscalenic triangle, the site of entrapment for most cases of TOS.[33] The subclavian artery accompanies the lower trunk in the interscalenic triangle, in close proximity to the first rib, while the subclavian vein runs in front of the anterior scalene muscle. Congenital anatomic variations can further compromise this already narrow passage.[6,36,57] The part of the muscles inserting on the first rib may be tendinous and act as a vice for the lower elements of the plexus.[68] An acute angle or oblique take-off of the first rib, from transverse process, as occasionally seen in slender, long-necked women, may promote wedging of the artery and the lower trunk of the brachial plexus between the rib and the scalenes.[74] Other bony anomalies can be associated with TOS and include hypertrophic C7 transverse processes and cervical ribs (Fig. 18-3).[60] These bony anomalies appear to serve as a scaffold for the true culprits for neural compression, the displaced soft tissues, such as a thickened or tendinous medial border of the scalene muscle or Sibson's fascia (Fig. 18-4).[36,37] Roos, in 1976, described nine different compressive bands at various levels which might be responsible for neurovascular compression.[56] Poiterin described three separate bands felt to be potentially restrictive that cross in an anterior to posterior direction over the region where Sibson's fascia is located.[53] A very thorough assessment of these abnormalities and their potential role in TOS was provided by Luoma and Nelems in 1991.[41]

Although entrapment in the costoclavicular space is infrequent, the neurovascular bundle can become compromised by structural pathology and less frequently prolonged and strenuous physical exertion.[12,15] This area is a triangular area bordered anteriorly by the medial portion of the clavicle and underlying subclavius muscle, its tendon, and the costocoracoid ligament. It is bordered posteromedially by the first rib and the insertion of the anterior and middle scalene muscles. Posterolaterally, it is bordered by the upper scapula. Congenital abnormalities such as a straight first rib and/or a straight clavicle can compromise this space. A tight subclavius muscle, especially one with a large fascial edge, can restrict or compress the available space and directly impinge on plexus divisions. Similarly, a fractured clavicle with excessive callus formation can lead to TOS at this level.[77] Patients who have droopy shoulders habitually or secondary to an external cause may also have compromise of this space.[51,65]

During abduction of the shoulder, the coracoid process and scapula can be depressed, leading to impingement of the neurovascular bundle against the subclavius muscle and/or ligament. This maneuver, albeit rarely, can be the causative factor in irritation or compression of the nerve bundle against the lower edge of the pectoralis minor in the subpectoral minor space. Nonetheless, the subcoracoid space is rarely a site for neural compression.

Several dynamic factors can worsen the symptoms of TOS. Abduction and external rotation narrow the costoclavicular triangle and stretch the nerves across the coracoid process. Poor posture, cervicothoracic scoliosis, and malnutrition lead to acromioclavicular descent and may further compromise the brachial plexus elements.

PATHOPHYSIOLOGIC CONSIDERATIONS

Excellent reviews of the histological succession of events have been provided by Mackinnon, and Hudson et al. Nerve compression can distort the blood–nerve barrier and cause demyelination or even axonal loss, depending on the severity and duration of compression and susceptibility of the patient.[42,43] In patients with TOS, compression at the "outlet" can be an isolated phenomenon or can occur in combination with other more peripheral entrapment syndromes.[27,44] Upton and McComas introduced the "double crush theory" that suggested nerve compression proximally could lead to increased susceptibility distally due to interruption or dampening of the axoplasmic flow. The initial compression site may be asymptomatic but when combined with distal pathology, both sites may cause symptoms. This is important since those patients with "double crush," "reverse double crush," or "multiple crush" phenomenon can require additional investigation and treatment.[75] The precise pathogenesis is not always clear, but the factors leading to two levels of compromise can be biologic (diabetes or other metabolic diseases of the peripheral nervous system), structural (i.e. compression), or vascular.[24,31,62] On a cellular level, in addition to dampening axoplasmic flow, these factors could lead to impairment of distal neural microcirculation precipitated by proximal endoneurial edema, disruption of lymphatic and/or venous outflow close to the proximal region of nerve compression, and, of course, a decreased number of neurofilaments.[20,64]

In patients with TOS, release of a concomitant distal cubital or carpal tunnel may improve axonal flow and subsequently obviate the need to decompress the plexus at the outlet.[13,26,35,46] As a result, there may be significant improvement in symptoms and the potential morbidity of a procedure such as first rib resection or scalenectomy and plexus neurolysis can be obviated.

The scalene muscles can exhibit fibrosis sometimes related to cervical injury. Spasm and resultant shortening of these muscles places them at an ergonomical disadvantage.[39] This can lead to

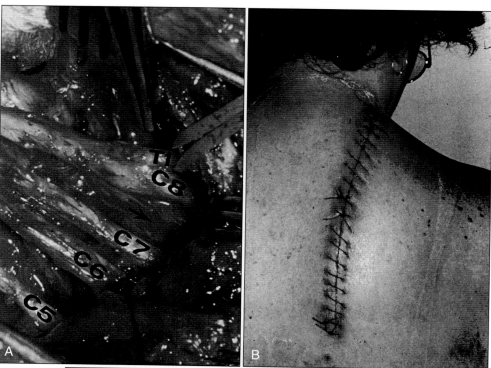

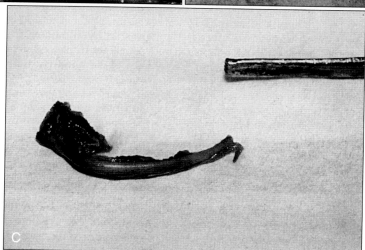

FIGURE 18-3 **(A)** Plexus exposed from a posterior subscapular approach. The cervical rib site (*arrow*) is between C8, T1, and C7 and has deformed the junction of C8 and T1. **(B)** Incision (sutured) used for a posterior subscapular approach to the plexus. **(C)** A resected cervical rib specimen from another patient.

dysfunctional and painful neck muscles and eventually to excessive stress and imbalance in other muscle groups such the trapezius.[45]

PATIENTS AND METHODS

Data were gathered on one hundred and thirty-three operations for neurogenic TOS on one hundred and twenty-five patients operated upon over the past 25 years. These patients were felt to have either true neurogenic thoracic outlet syndrome (TNTOS) or disputed neurogenic thoracic outlet syndrome (DNTOS). The patient's age, mechanism of injury if present, symptoms, physical examination, operative findings, and outcomes were recorded. Preoperatively, radiographs were reviewed and electrophysiologic studies preformed. During surgery, observations about potential areas of compression were noted and nerve action potentials were recorded by stimulating spinal nerves and recording from more distal trunks and their divisions. All patients had at least 1 year of postoperative follow-up.

TRUE NEUROGENIC THORACIC OUTLET SYNDROME

The typical patient with true neurogenic TOS is a young, slender woman with progressive weakness and atrophy of the hand muscles. Usual complaints include difficulties using the affected hand for activities requiring fine motor skills or, in later stages, inability to hold things with that hand. Pain is only occasionally present and is usually described as a dull, constant, heavy ache in the lateral neck and shoulder and radiating in the arm, but without a specific dermatomal pattern.[18,39] Paresthesias usually precede motor changes and are localized to the last two digits and the medial side of hand and forearm.

The most commonly affected muscles are the abductor pollicis brevis and the interossei followed by the opponens pollicis and the rest of the thenar muscles. While weakness is usually present in both median and ulnar distributions, the median-innervated muscles are sometimes more severely affected than the ulnar ones.[17,73]

Paresthesias and hypoesthesia involve the ulnar aspect of the hand and forearm, while the median sensory innervation is typically spared. Atrophy is commonly present in the hand intrinsic muscles (Fig. 18-5).

Electromyography (EMG) helps in the differential diagnosis by showing normal ulnar conduction across the elbow, both median and ulnar decreased compound muscle action potentials (CMAPs), and decreased ulnar sensory nerve action potentials (SNAPs), with normal median SNAPs.[11,19,28,38,73]

"DISPUTED" NEUROGENIC THORACIC OUTLET SYNDROME

The typical patient with "disputed" neurogenic TOS is a middle-aged man or woman with chronic pain in the neck, shoulder, and arm.[73] This is a much larger category of patients than those with

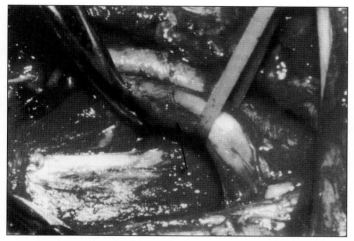

FIGURE 18-4 Fibrous edge to medial scalene which had irritated junction of C8 and T1 with lower trunk. The latter is being elevated by a loop and Metzenbaum scissors, and the arrow points to the area of irritation and some thickening of epineurium on its inferior surface.

TNTOS.[48] The pain is usually moderate to severe, and is typically exacerbated by arm abduction or elevation. Occasionally, the debut of symptoms is marked by a motor vehicle accident or work-related injury.[30] Physical examination reveals no muscle atrophy or hypoesthesia. There is usually no true motor weakness, although strength testing may be difficult secondary to pain. On occasion, there may be, on careful testing, mild weakness without atrophy in the lumbrical to the little finger or abductor digiti minimi or interossei and sometimes mild, sensory changes in the ulnar distribution. Such mild changes may be difficult to document. Usually, the EMG and conduction studies are normal and magnetic resonance imaging (MRI) studies of the plexus are also normal.[11,18,72] Somatosensory studies have been suggested by some authors as a means of showing slowed conduction across the plexus.[19,66,76] However, recordings either at a spinal or scalp level include conduction via cervical roots which may be involved by spondylosis and disc disease. Recording at "Erb's" point provides an imprecise locus and, moreover, one which may be in the area of pathology if such is present. As in patients with suspected TNTOS, X-rays to ascertain presence of a cervical rib, elongated C7 process, or abnormality of the rib or clavicle are important.

In both of these neurogenic thoracic outlet categories other conditions simulating TOS need to be excluded such as a more peripheral median or ulnar entrapment or more central cervical disc or spondylitic disease or tumor of the plexus and/or spine.

SURGICAL TECHNIQUE

In our experience, two approaches are suitable for decompression of the lower brachial plexus involved by NTOS: anterior supraclavicular and posterior subscapular. Both of them have been previously described.

ANTERIOR SUPRACLAVICULAR

The anterior supraclavicular approach is best known to most neurosurgeons.[23,26,32,35] The skin incision can be varied somewhat, depending on the size and habitus of the patient and whether there

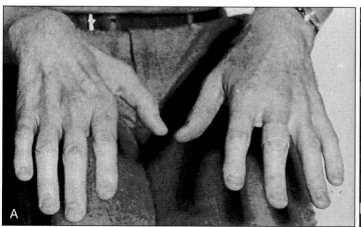
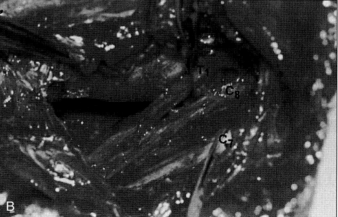

FIGURE 18-5 **(A)** Patient with bilateral Gilliatt-Sumner hands. Loss was worse on the right than left side. **(B)** Plexus in a patient with Gilliatt-Sumner hand whose spinal nerves and trunks were exposed by a posterior subscapular approach. The plexus is viewed from the head looking toward the posterior chest wall. Nerve action potentials (NAPs) recorded by stimulating T1 and C8 and recording from lower trunk were of very small amplitude and conducted at less than 30 m/sec. Stimulation of more healthy-appearing C7 and recording from the middle trunk gave a higher amplitude NAP that conducted at 60 m/sec.

has been a prior neck operation. The most commonly used is a transverse neck incision a finger's breadth superior to the clavicle and parallel to it. If some infraclavicular exposure is necessary because of patient size or habitus, a classic plexus incision is used along the lateral edge of the sternocleidomastoid muscle and then the incision is angulated inferiorly to lie in the crease of the delto-pectoral groove. An alternative is to "T" the transverse supracla-vicular incision, placing the lower limb of the "T" in the deltopectoral groove (Fig. 18-6).

The incision is then deepened to transect the platysma. The omohyoid, which is the only strap muscle running obliquely and somewhat transversely across the neck, is identified and dissected free from the underlying fat. This muscle provides the superior anatomical border of the neck's anterior triangle and separates it from the posterior triangle. The omohyoid is transected between two heavy Vicryl or silk sutures which are then used to retract the medial half up and over the sternocleidomastoid and the lower half laterally near the distal clavicle. With this exposure, the underlying fat pad needs to be dissected away from the scalene muscles and brachial plexus. The external jugular vein is mobilized, and usually ligated and transected near the clavicle. The fat pad is dissected with hemostats and Metzenbaum scissors toward an eventual lateral locus, usually by beginning beneath the lateral edge of the sternocleidomastoid.

Deep to the omohyoid muscle and fat pad, the anterior scalene muscle is identified, with the phrenic nerve running on its surface. Dissection and mobilization of the phrenic nerve with the help of a Penrose drain allows for better protection during the operation for exposure and resection of the underlying scalene muscle and neurolysis of the lower elements of the plexus. It is usually not necessary to dissect much of the C5 or C6 spinal nerves, although the more distal upper trunk and its divisions should be dissected and gently retracted laterally by Penrose drains.

Excision of the anterior scalene muscle exposes the trunks in the interscalenic triangle. Heavy silk or Vicryl sutures can be placed around the superior and inferior portion of the muscle to elevate it as the section is made superiorly and inferiorly so that a segment of the muscle can be removed. Bleeding points are coagulated and then fragments of the muscle around C7 and sometimes C6 and C5 are resected. Resection of the scalene exposes soft tissues overlying C7 and C7 to middle trunk. The subclavian artery has to be gently elevated by a vein retractor to find and dissect out the lower trunk as well as C8 and T1 spinal nerves. If the lower trunk is encased in heavy scar or is difficult to find, an infraclavicular exposure of the medial cord is helpful. The medial cord and its proximal elements of origin can then be followed and dissected away from the axillary and subclavicular vessels from beneath the clavicle to the neck level, where the lower trunk and C8 and T1 are exposed.

To reach T1, it helps to gently elevate the lower trunk with a vein retractor or Penrose drain and then to find T1 adjacent but inferior to C8. The pleural cap is in very close proximity, especially near the proximal extent of T1. If the pleura is opened, it usually can be closed without a chest tube by using 4–0 silk and a fine dural needle small enough to fit into this area.

Cervical ribs or hypertrophic C7 transverse processes are then resected, as well as fascial bands or any other soft tissue abnormali-ties compressing the C8 and T1 spinal nerves or lower trunk (Fig. 18-7). Nerve action potential recordings (NAPs) from C8 and T1 to lower trunk and from C7 to middle trunk are then performed.

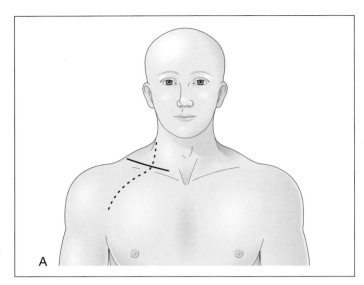

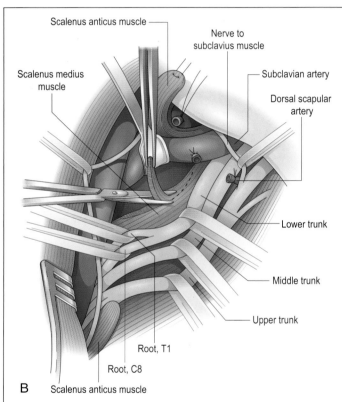

FIGURE 18-6 Illustrations depicting the anterior supraclavicular approach. **(A)** Skin incision. The commonly used incision is horizontal, parallel to the clavicle (*solid line*). Complex patients may require a supraclavicular and infraclavicular incision (*dotted line*). **(B)** Removal of band. The medial portion of the scalenus medius is resected. This exposure also permits the resection of an elongated transverse process C7 or a cervical rib. (From Kline DG, Hudson AR, and Kim DH: Thoracic outlet syndrome dissection. In: Kline DG, Hudson AR, and Kim DH, Eds: Atlas of Peripheral Nerve Surgery, 1st edn. Philadelphia, WB Saunders, 2001:51–55.)

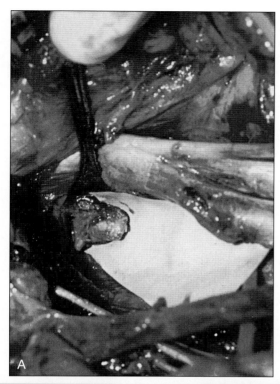

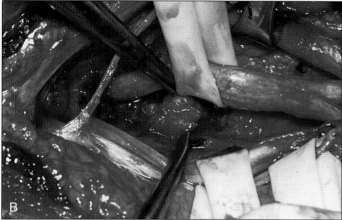

FIGURE 18-7 (A) Plexus retracted away from the tip of cervical rib beneath a rubber dam. An anterior approach was used. Medial scalene muscle and a fascial band have been removed from the tip of this bony abnormality. The bony protrusion was then removed with a rongeur. **(B)** Elongated process of C7 vertebra exposed beneath C7 spinal nerve to the middle trunk area in a patient with TOS. Lower trunk is retracted slightly by vein retractor at the top of the picture. Discoloration due to the irritative/compressive lesion can sometimes be seen on the underside of trunk.

POSTERIOR SUBSCAPULAR APPROACH

The posterior subscapular approach is reserved for complicated TOS cases: morbid obesity, large bony abnormalities (large cervical ribs or very large C7 transverse processes), or cases with previous anterior neck operations.[14,37] The patient is positioned initially in a lateral decubitus position, and then rolled into a prone position, with the operative side close to the edge of the table. Chest rolls are placed along both sides as well as transversely, beneath both

shoulders and the sternal manubrium. The arm on the operative side is then abducted, flexed at the elbow, and secured to a padded Mayo stand at a level below that of the operating table. Adequate padding of the elbow, wrist, and hand is mandatory. Further abduction of the shoulder and scapula can be obtained by tilting the operating table in a reverse Trendelenburg position. The head is partially turned towards the operative side and adequately padded, while the contralateral arm is padded at the elbow and tucked to the side.

Skin incision is slightly curved and centered between the thoracic spinous processes and the medial edge of the scapula, in order to protect the spinal branch of the accessory nerve and the ascending branch of the transverse cervical artery. The first layer to be traversed is the trapezius muscle, which is divided along the entire length of the skin incision with large Kelly or Serat clamps, in a caudal to cranial fashion. The divided muscle is then marked with heavy (0) sutures for later approximation. The sutures are placed in pairs behind each clamp and the ends are fastened to the drapes for subsequent accurate approximation. The next layer to be divided is formed by the levator scapulae, rhomboid minor, and rhomboid major muscles, all of them inserting on the medial border of the scapula. Muscle dissection should be performed away from the scapular edge, in order to protect the deeper dorsal scapular nerve and the ascending branch of the transverse cervical artery (Fig. 18-8).

The scapula is then retracted to an abducted and externally rotated position, by use of a small chest retractor. The first rib is exposed and removed by rongeurs extraperiosteally, from the costotransverse articulation to the costoclavicular ligament. Removal of the posterior and middle scalene muscles exposes the lower spinal nerves and trunks of the brachial plexus, which are freed by a complete 360 degree external neurolysis. Care must be exercised to protect the long thoracic nerve as it originates from the posterior aspect of C6 as well as branches to it from C5 and C7, and sometimes C4 spinal nerves. Potential sites of compression by soft tissue, such as a fascial edge of middle scalene, Sibson's fascia, scalenus minimus, cervical rib, or elongated C7 transverse process are removed. If necessary, the spinal nerves can be followed intraforaminally by removing part of the facet joint.[34,37] Closure of the muscle layers must be in anatomical planes, in order to minimize a winged scapula postoperatively.

It is difficult to provide complete decompression of spinal nerves close to the spine through a transaxillary approach. As a result, we did not utilize the transaxillary first rib resection for NTOS treatment. Although we do not do first rib resection for TOS, many others do.[5,29,41,57,63] In this regard, Sanders and Pearce[59] in 1989 published a comparison of transaxillary first rib resections (111 cases), anterior and middle scalenectomy (279 cases), and combined supraclavicular first rib resection with scalenectomy (278 cases).[58] At 15 years after operation, almost identical results were noted with all of these surgical procedures.

RESULTS

One hundred and twenty-five patients underwent one hundred and thirty-three operations of which 66 were through an anterior (50%) and 67 through a posterior approach. The male to female ratio was 1 : 1.6, with the most common complaint consisting of pain and paresthesias (83%). Only 36 patients (28%) had a history of trauma to the shoulder or neck. Patient demographics are listed in Table 18-1. Fifty-six patients (45%) had a previous operation for TOS

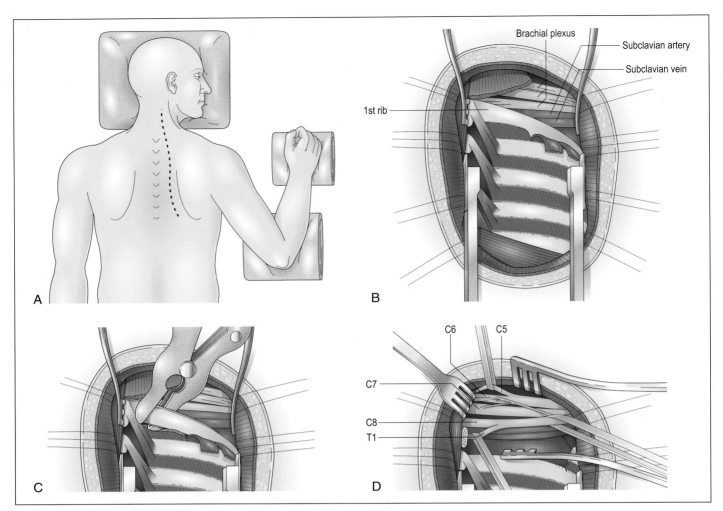

FIGURE 18-8 Illustrations depicting the posterior subscapular approach. **(A)** Skin incision. The flexed elbow and arm are placed on a Mayo stand adjacent to the operating table. This can be lowered or elevated to change the position of the scapula. The skin incision is placed halfway between the scapular edge and the thoracic spinous processes. **(B)** Scapular retraction. As the retractor is opened, the scapula is rotated laterally to expose the posterior aspect of the upper ribs. The posterior scalene muscle is detached from the superior surface of the first rib. **(C)** Exposure of inferior brachial plexus. The first rib is resected from the costotransverse articulation to the costoclavicular ligament. **(D)** Plexus after neurolysis. The C8 and T1 spinal nerves appear thin and scarred. The long thoracic nerve originates from the posterior aspect of C6 and C7 spinal nerves at this level. The subclavian vessels are located anterior to the plexus. (From Kline DG, Hudson AR, and Kim DH: Posterior subscapular approach to plexus. In: Kline DG, Hudson AR, and Kim DH, Eds: Atlas of Peripheral Nerve Surgery, 1st edn. Philadelphia, WB Saunders, 2001:41–50.)

involving the brachial plexus before their surgery at our institution (Table 18-2).

All 33 operations for TNTOS and almost all of the DNTOS operations had intraoperative nerve action potential (NAP) recordings done. The most commonly encountered findings were decreased NAP amplitude and velocity from the T1 and C8 spinal nerves to the lower trunk. In 10 patients no NAP could be elicited from the T1 root. Typically, the upper plexus elements, such as the C5 and C6 spinal nerves to upper trunk and its divisions, were not affected. In nine patients the C7 spinal nerve to the middle trunk showed slowing of conduction velocity. Upper element recordings served as controls to those recordings done on the lower elements. Most of the patients were found to have slowing of their conduction close to the spine at a spinal nerve to truncal level as opposed to more distally. Forty-two plexuses, 41 of which had DNTOS, had normal NAP recordings.

The most common findings in patients operated through an anterior approach was an elongated transverse process of C7 with or without a displaced and somewhat fibrous edge to the middle scalene (n = 23) followed by a thickened middle scalene muscle usually with a fibrous edge (n = 19) and then scar related to the prior operation (n = 16) (Fig. 18-9). The latter was found most commonly in patients operated originally anteriorly and then reoperated through the posterior approach (n = 29) (Table 18-3).

Postoperatively, after an anterior approach (Table 18-4), 37 patients had complete resolution of their pain or paresthesias and another 21 had a decrease in their symptoms. Nine patients had serious residual pain. One had new deficits with a total complication rate of 15%. Of the 67 patients operated posteriorly, 34 experienced resolution of the pain with an additional 27 experiencing some relief. Sixteen patients experienced complications (24%) (Table 18-4).

Table 18-1 Patient demographics

Unilateral TOS patients		117
Bilateral TOS patients		8
Total patients operated		125
Total operations		133
Anterior approach		66
Posterior approach		67
Gender of patients	Male	48
	Female	77
Age range at operation	11–20	13
	21–30	26
	31–40	55
	41–50	22
	51–60	14
	61–70	3
Pain and paresthesias		111
Prior cervical operation		56
History of trauma		36
Gilliat-Sumner hand		33

Table 18-2 Prior operations

Operation	Subsequent anterior approach	Subsequent posterior approach
Transaxillary first rib operation ×1	18	23
Transaxillary first rib operation ×2	2	2
Cervical rib removal	2	6
Scalenectomy	6	5
Anterior neurolysis	5	3
Thrombectomy	1	1
Sympathectomy	2	2
Cervical laminectomy	0	2
Anterior cervical fusion	3	2
Pulmonary lobectomy	0	2
Clavicle plating	1	2
Ulnar transposition	7	3
Carpal tunnel release	6	3
Needle biopsy of plexus	4	3
Clavicle resection	1	0

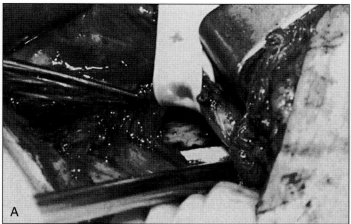

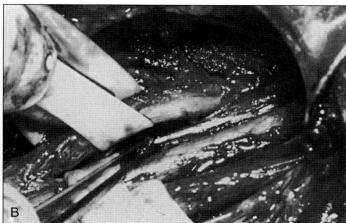

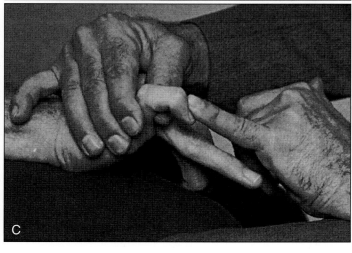

FIGURE 18-9 **(A)** View of a fibrous edge to medial scalene in a patient with left-sided thoracic outlet syndrome (TOS). This somewhat oblique band lay behind the C8 to T1 junction with lower trunk and must have been a source of irritation to it. **(B)** Fibrous edge of medial scalene beneath lower trunk of the plexus. This raphe of tissue is shown grasped by fine-toothed forceps. **(C)** Muscle most likely to be weak in a patient with true TOS. This is the lumbrical for the little or fifth finger.

Table 18-3 Gross operative findings

Finding	Anterior approach	Posterior approach
Cervical rib	2	2
Residual cervical rib	3	6
Residual first rib	2	8
C7 elongated with or without band	23	6
Medial or middle scalene bands	19	7
Other bands	8	8
Sibson's fascial band	3	3
Tight or taut plexus elements(s)	5	23
Scar involving plexus element(s)	16	29
Prior serious operative plexus injury	4	5

Table 18-4 Results and complications

Result	Anterior approach	Posterior approach
No pain/paresthesias	37	34
Partial improvement pain	21	27
Serious residual pain	8	6
Re-operation for pain	1	2
Mild motor deficit improved	9	10
Mild motor deficit unchanged	7	2
Severe motor deficit improved	7	7
Severe motor partially improved	7	10
Severe motor deficit unchanged	3	7
New deficit produced	1	1
Pleural opening (corrected at surgery)	3	4
Chest tube	0	2
Postoperative thoracentesis	2	3
Phrenic paresis	4	3
Wound infection	0	1
Scapula winging	0	4
Chylothorax	1	0
Subsequent diagnosis of syrinx	0	1

Observations made with intraoperative NAP recordings in 91 patients where abnormalities were documented are presented in Table 18-5.

OUTCOMES FOR TRUE NEUROGENIC THORACIC OUTLET SYNDROME

Between 1977 and 2001, a total of 33 plexuses underwent surgical decompression for TNTOS at LSUHSC.[67] Patients with iatrogenic or post-traumatic NTOS were not included in this retrospective analysis.[30] Results were compared to those in two other published series and are summarized in Table 18-6. An overview of the patients is presented in Table 18-7. Age ranged from 14 to 68 years (mean, 39). The minimum follow up period was 12 months, while the mean follow up period was 60 months. Neurological examination in all patients was performed and recorded. All patients had weakness and some atrophy of lumbricals, interossei, and thenar and hypothenar muscles. Three patients also had weakness of finger extension, and four had flexor profundus weakness. Sensory examination usually paralleled motor function using the LSUHSC grading system (Table 18-8), but sensory function was less reliable as an outcome parameter and therefore was not used in this study. One patient had bilateral NTOS, although the right side was more affected than the left. While most patients were in their third and fourth decade of life, nine patients were less than 30 years of age and seven patients were older than 50. Pain was absent in about one-third of the patients; when present, it was described as a dull, constant ache going down into the arm, but poorly localized.

It is notable that 14 of our patients had previous operations (Table 18-9) none of which alleviated the TOS symptoms. Patients who had undergone transaxillary first rib resection for TOS at other centers were not included in the TNTOS portion of the study, since some had had iatrogenic injury to the plexus as a result.

Table 18-10 summarizes the intraoperative findings in our 33 patients with TNTOS. In eight cases, no particular bony or soft tissue abnormality was found, but the lower elements of the plexus were felt to be "tight" or "snug" by the surgeon. Three patients had significant scarring around the inferior elements of the proximal brachial plexus, although there was no history of trauma or previous surgery in that region. Middle scalene bands were the most frequent finding. Sometimes, this correlated with thickening or what appeared to be scar on the posterior side of the lower spinal nerves' junction to lower trunk.

Cervical ribs and elongated C7 transverse processes were encountered in 14 of these patients, confirming the high incidence of bony abnormalities in patients with Gilliatt-Sumner hand (GSH). However, most commonly, these appear to serve only as a scaffold for the true culprit for compression, the soft tissue anomalies, encountered in most of the patients in our series (Table 18-10). An elongated C7 transverse process or incipient cervical rib has an associated lateral origin of the middle scalene which then courses medially to insert on the superior aspect of the first and sometimes second rib. With this configuration, the lower elements of the plexus may drape over the scalene and be irritated or entrapped, especially if the muscle has a fibrous medial edge.

All patients with TNTOS underwent intraoperative NAP recordings and the results are presented in Table 18-11. The typical patient had a markedly decreased or flat T1 to lower trunk (LT) NAP, moderately reduced C8 to LT NAP, and normal C7 to middle trunk (MT) trace (Fig. 18-10). Velocities were similarly affected, mostly in the T1 to LT traces, followed by C8 to LT traces and then C7 to MT recordings (Table 18-11). Amplitudes were recorded using a preamplifying factor that varied from one patient to another, but was maintained constant for a given patient. Therefore, in those patients who had recordings for the whole brachial plexus (mostly patients with anterior approaches), amplitudes of lower plexus elements were compared to the C5 and C6 to UT amplitudes, which were considered normal, and then expressed in percentages (Table 18-11). All patients with flat C8 to lower trunk traces also had flat T1 to lower trunk traces. Six patients also had involvement of C7 to middle trunk by NAP recordings, even though these traces were never flat. Only one TNTOS patient had normal NAP amplitudes and normal velocities for all spinal nerve to trunk levels.

Thirty-two patients had decreased velocity and/or amplitude of T1 and/or C8 to lower trunk. Six patients also had abnormality of C7 to middle trunk NAPs. Care was taken to have a distance of at least 3 cm between the stimulating and recording electrodes, in order to avoid falsely flat traces. NAP recording confirmed the involvement of C8 and T1 spinal nerves at the junction with the lower trunk, close to the spine and in the interscalenic triangle. This suggests that the injury or entrapment responsible for Gilliatt-Sumner hand occurs close to the spine, involving the spinal nerve to trunk level, rather than more laterally, between the first rib and clavicle, corresponding to trunk to divisions level.

Outcome was analyzed in terms of pain in the affected limb and motor function in the four muscle groups (thenar, hypothenar, lumbricals and interossei). Patients who experienced pain preoperatively were asked postoperatively to categorize their pain as one of the following: completely resolved, improved, unchanged, or worsened. Improvement of the motor deficit was defined as

Table 18-5	Intraoperative NAP recordings	
Patients with abnormalities		91
Decreased amplitude T1 to LT		39
Decrease CV T1 to LT		45
Flat T1 NAP trace		10
Decreased amplitude C8 to LT		31
Decreased CV C8 to LT		30
C7 to MT abnormality		9
NAP abnormal on all elements		1
NAP on patients with prior serious plexus injury		7
	(–) NAPs → grafts	4
	(+) NAPs → neurolysis	1
	(+) and (–) NAPs → split or partial graft repair	2

CV, conduction velocity; LT, lower trunk; MT, middle trunk; (+), positive, (–), negative.

Table 18-7	Gilliatt-Sumner hand patients – TNTOS	
A	Unilateral Gilliatt-Sumner hand	32
	Bilateral Gilliatt-Sumner hand	1
	Total patients operated	33
	Total operations on plexus	34
B	Anterior approach	19
	Posterior approach	15
C	Gender of patient	
	Male	19
	Female	14
D	Age of patients (years)	
	11–20	6
	21–30	3
	31–40	11
	41–50	6
	51–60	4
	61–70	3
E	Pain	
	Present	22
	Absent	11

Table 18-6	Recent studies with results from true neurogenic thoracic outlet syndrome					
Study	No. operations	Method of diagnosis	Patients with resolved pain (%)	Patients with decreased pain (%)	Complication rate (%)	Approach
Nannapaneni 2003	59	Radiographic	60	20	0	SCI
Sanders 2002	65	Radiographic	59	13	N/A	SCI, TA
Kline, Hudson 2005	133	Radiographic and EMG	53	36	18	SCI, PSc

SCI, supraclavicular neurolysis and scalenectomy; TA, transaxillary; PSC, posterior subscapular and neurolysis; N/A, not available.

Table 18-8 Louisiana State University Health Science Center grading system for C8–T1 lesions

Grade	Functional evaluation	Description
0	Absent	No function in C8–T1 distribution
1	Poor	Some but usually poor (grade 2 or less) sensation in ulnar distribution of hand; some recovery of finger extensor or finger flexor function if that had been absent previously (grade 2)
2	Fair	Finger extensors or flexors function if function was lost before (grade 3); ulnar sensation is grade 3 or better; hypothenars contract and are grade 2 or better; function of other intrinsics is trace or absent
3	Moderate	Ulnar sensation is grade 3 or better; finger extensors or flexors, if function was lost before, grade 3 or better; hypothenar muscles grade 3 or better; most other hand intrinsics contract against gravity only
4	Good	Ulnar sensation grade 3 or better; finger extensors or flexors, if function was lost before, grade 3 or better; hypothenars grade 3 or better; most other intrinsics contract against gravity and some resistance
5	Excellent	Ulnar sensation grade 4 or 5; return of any lost finger extension or flexion; all intrinsics contract against at least moderate pressure or resistance

Table 18-9 Previous operations TNTOS

Carpal tunnel release	5
Ulnar nerve transposition	3
Anterior cervical discectomy	4
Cervical laminectomy	2

Table 18-10 Intraoperative findings – TNTOS

	Anterior approach	Posterior approach
Bony abnormalities		
Cervical rib	5	1
Elongated C7 transverse process	7	1
Soft tissue abnormalities		
Middle scalene band	11	3
Sibson fascial band	1	3
Scar involving T1 and/or C8	1	2
Other bands*	3	2
"Tight" plexus	3	5

*Scalenus minimus or anterior scalene bands.

Table 18-11 Intraoperative nerve action potential recordings in TNTOS

Overview	Anterior approach	Posterior approach
Decreased amplitude/velocity T1 to LT	12	13
Decreased amplitude/velocity C8 to LT	16	13
Flat T1 to LT	5	2
Flat C8 to LT	2	1
Abnormal C7 to MT	4	2
Normal recordings	1	0
Velocity	**Range (m/s)**	**Median**
C7 to MT	25–88	47
C8 to LT	0–68	30
T1 to LT	0–50	17
Amplitude	**Range (%)***	**Median**
C7 to MT	30–100	70
C8 to LT	0–70	40
T1 to LT	0–60	30

*Compared to C5 to upper trunk nerve action potential amplitudes.

recovery of at least one grade in the LSUHSC grading system (see Table 18-8), in at least two of four muscle groups (thenar, hypothenar, lumbricals and interossei).

Table 18-12 summarizes the postoperative results at one year. Of the 21 patients who experienced pain preoperatively, six had complete resolution and 14 had partial improvement of the pain level postoperatively. Only one of the patients described his level of pain as unchanged at the 1-year follow-up visit and he did improve one grade in muscle strength.

Analysis of the pre- and postoperative motor deficit showed improvement in 12 of 14 patients who had mild deficit preoperatively and partial improvement in 14 of 20 patients with severe

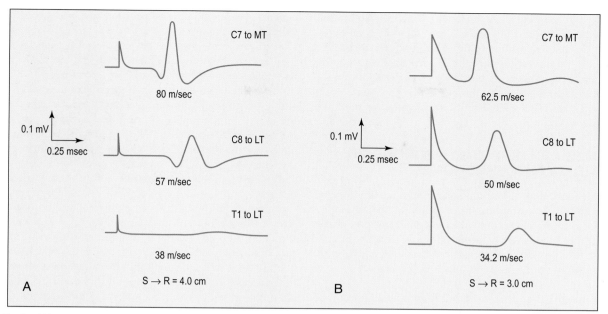

FIGURE 18-10 **(A)** Nerve action potential (NAP) tracings show a very small and slow response (*bottom tracing*) recorded from T1 to lower trunk (LT) in a patient with thoracic outlet syndrome (TOS). The response from C8 to LT was probably abnormal also, especially compared with the one recorded from C7 to middle trunk (MT). **(B)** NAP tracings in another patient with spontaneous TOS. Trace is also abnormal from T1 to LT, but less so from C8 to LT, and again that from C7 to MT is more normal.

Table 18-12 Postoperative results – TNTOS		
	Anterior approach	**Posterior approach**
Pain		
No pain/paresthesias	4	2
Partial improvement of pain	10	5
No change in pain	4	6
Serious residual pain	1	0
Required another operation for pain	0	0
Motor deficit		
Mild motor deficit improved	9	3
Mild motor deficit unchanged	1	1
Mild motor deficit worsened	0	0
Severe motor deficit improved	7	7
Severe motor deficit unchanged	2	4
Severe motor deficit worsened	0	0

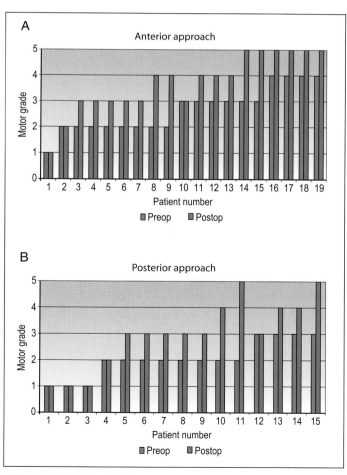

FIGURE 18-11 Graphs illustrating motor grade before surgery (Preop) and after surgery (Postop) in patients undergoing an anterior supraclavicular **(A)** or posterior subscapular **(B)** approach. Motor deficit improved in most patients.

deficit (Fig. 18-11). Disease progression was usually ameliorated by an adequate surgical decompression. None of the patients experienced new or worsening of preexisting deficits at 1-year follow-up. Patients with mild deficit were more likely to recover than the ones with severe deficit, although return to normal motor function was seldom achieved. The presence of bony abnormalities expedited the diagnosis of TNTOS but did not have significant impact on the functional outcome in this series.

One patient with an anterior approach to the brachial plexus for TNTOS experienced postoperative phrenic palsy, which had improved at the subsequent examination 6 months later. Hand motor strength improved from grade 3 to grade 4 at 1 year postoperatively. One patient with a posterior approach to the brachial plexus had an intraoperative pleural rent, which was recognized and closed primarily. Another patient with posterior approach had a moderate degree of scapular winging, which had persisted by follow-up at 1 year. This patient remained at motor grade 2 at 1 year postoperatively.

OUTCOMES FOR DISPUTED NEUROGENIC THORACIC OUTLET SYNDROME

Patients with complaints of vague medial arm pain and a plethora of other complaints are often diagnosed as having NTOS. Further investigation with physical examination and ancillary tests usually yields no hard findings indicating neural compromise at the brachial plexus level. The proper diagnosis of these patients has been the debate of many treating physicians and is called "disputed" TOS (DNTOS).

The majority of the patients operated for TOS fall in the category of disputed TOS. Surgeons who believe in this clinical entity believe that it can be caused by either compression or stretch of the brachial plexus leading to chronic irritation of the plexus with subsequent complaints. Decompression, therefore, is felt to be the solution. However, despite the fact that many clinical tests as well as electrodiagnostic findings are felt by some to have predictive value, most have failed to show any merit upon scientific scrutiny. Clinical symptoms complicating disputed TOS can be subdivided into four groups:

1. Concomitant cervical plexopathy: Posterior, lateral, and anterior neck pain; trapezial ridge pain; ear pain; temporomandibular pain; occipital pain ("migraine headache"); trapezius muscle spasm.
2. Sympathetic or central nervous system dysfunction: Facial and neck swelling; eye pain; blurred vision; eyelid droop; nonfocal syncope; hyperactive reflexes; reflex sympathetic dystrophy with livido reticularis; limb swelling; joint contractures; movement disorders (inability to initiate movement, tremor, spasms, dystonic posture); pain spread to ipsilateral lower and contralateral upper extremities.
3. Inability of plexus elements to move or glide smoothly, secondary to anomalous structures or plexus/periplexus scarring: Cervical radiculopathies; ulnar neuropathies at elbow and hand; posterior interosseous neuropathy at elbow; median neuropathies at elbow and wrist.
4. Abnormal posture (excessive descent of scapula, forward displacement of shoulder): Impingement syndrome (rotator cuff tear); trapezius spasm; biceps tendonitis; trigger points; lateral epicondylitis.[65]

Some or many of these symptoms are felt to comprise TOS; however, no evidence has been provided for such. A study performed in Washington State amongst workman compensation patients resulted in 50% of the surgical patients with presumed TOS having greater medical costs and 3 to 4 times higher likelihood of disability than those not operated upon.[73] Since that study, TOS is not recognized as a diagnosis in much of that state.

It is our belief that, considering the lack of evidence for this entity, surgical treatment should be reserved for some but not all patients. Those who develop pain and have had all of the differential diagnoses eliminated and yet have persistent symptoms despite a lengthy trial of physical and occupational therapy, or the less frequent patient with clear clinical, radiographic, or electrodiagnostic findings may be candidates for an operation.[40]

One of the major criteria for surgical decompression for DNTOS besides the typical arm pain in an abducted position is the persistence and reproducibility of symptoms on serial examinations. A follow-up of 6 months to 1 year is usually indicated before an operation is contemplated. Complex socioeconomic factors such as personality type and secondary gains from litigation should always be taken into consideration before making the decision to operate.

Some 60% of the NAP recordings done in this group of patients selected for operation had abnormalities but not as abnormal as in the TNTOS group of patients. These abnormalities involved abnormal conduction velocity from T1 to LT, C8 to LT, and less frequently C7 to MT and amplitude changes in lower plexus elements in that order of frequency. Presence of conductive abnormalities did not necessarily predict postoperative improvement in DNTOS. Patients in this category sometimes improved and sometimes did not.

ARTERIAL THORACIC OUTLET SYNDROME

Arterial lesions in the thoracic outlet occur from long-standing and intermittent vascular compression.[2] In the vast majority of cases, cervical ribs are present. Fusion of the cervical rib to the first rib or presence of a fibrous band or hypertrophic scalene muscle causes displacement of the supraclavicular course of the artery. Initially, this compression is asymptomatic but is followed by minor thromboembolic symptoms (small punctuate lesions in the fingers and thumb). In more advanced cases or with delayed diagnosis, major arterial occlusion and potential limb-threatening ischemia can occur. The more proximal the arterial insult, the better it is tolerated due to collateral supply downstream. Other symptoms in the course of the disease reported include Raynaud's phenomenon, episodic pallor, cyanosis, chronic pain, coldness, and paresthesias.[39] The initial diagnosis is made by physical examination with presence of a pulsatile mass in the supraclavicular area as a result of displacement and/or prestenotic dilatation of the artery. Auscultation as well as careful palpation can be useful, as a bruit can often be heard or a thrill felt. Hyperabduction tests such as the Adson test can reveal a decrease in arterial pressure. As developed initially for vascular compression, the Roos test can be used for exercise-induced ischemia. In the occasional patient, skin pallor, coldness of the hand and fingers, atrophy, hair loss and, in later stages, atrophy of hand intrinsics can be seen.

In the work-up, a chest and cervical spine X-ray are important to diagnose cervical ribs, an elongated transverse process of C7, and other abnormalities such as callus of the clavicle due to an old fracture. Once suspicion is raised based upon these findings, an arteriogram with the arm at the side and abducted allows the most reliable information about compromise of the subclavian artery.

Treatment relies on the obliteration of the offending structure, i.e. bands, cervical ribs, callused clavicle, etc. Occasionally, the vessel may be damaged to an extent that direct graft repair may be necessary for preservation of the vessel. This can often be accomplished through a supraclavicular approach but usually requires the input of a vascular surgeon.

VENOUS THORACIC OUTLET SYNDROME

Also known as Paget-Shroetter syndrome, the subclavian vein can be compromised upon its entry into the supraclavicular space where it empties into the innominate vein. It is located medial to the anterior scalene muscle and its thrombosis can be spontaneous (primary) or due to an anatomical constraint or after multiple iatrogenic manipulations such as subclavian catheters. Contrary to arterial TOS, venous TOS manifests itself with swelling and cyanosis of the extremity.

The diagnosis can be confirmed with duplex Doppler but dynamic venography with arm in neutral and abducted position is the gold standard. The treatment is variable depending on the age of the thrombosis and the structural abnormality of the vessel, as well as removal of any potentially constrictive structures.

COMPLICATIONS

As with any major surgical procedure, complications can and do occur. Some of the more serious ones involve loss of function in the limb or serious vascular loss (Fig. 18-12). Conservative non-operative management using exercises and posture-altering steps does work in some cases and should be tried before surgery is undertaken.

Complications can be minimized by good surgical technique. The importance of a thorough knowledge of the brachial plexus anatomy cannot be overemphasized. Adequate exposure of each element of interest, mainly C7, C8, T1 spinal nerves and middle and lower trunk, and gentle retraction with Penrose drains, avoids inadvertent damage to the neural structures and iatrogenic deficits. Special attention should be given to the phrenic nerve. The nerve should be dissected off the surface of the anterior scalene muscle over a length and gently retracted with a Penrose drain. This permits resection of a segment of the anterior scalene muscle so that exposure of the lower plexus elements is full.

The subclavian vessels also need to be exposed and protected. When retraction of the artery is necessary, a vein retractor is used. Occasionally, vascular branches, such as the dorsal scapular artery, or suprascapular nerve need to be ligated and cut; care must be exercised not to stenose the lumen of the parent vessel with a too proximal ligature on the stump of a branch.

Pleural rents can be recognized intraoperatively by filling the operative field with saline and asking anesthesia to do a Valsalva maneuver. Primary repair can usually be accomplished, but, occasionally, placement of a chest tube may be necessary for drainage of a pneumothorax.

Winged scapula is a known complication of the posterior subscapular approach. It can usually be prevented by marking the rhomboids, levator scapulae, and trapezius muscles with paired sutures as they are sectioned, thus allowing for a robust closure in anatomical planes. In addition, lateral retraction of the scapula by the thoracotomy retractor should not be overzealous so that the long thoracic nerve is not stretched.

Nine patients were seen in our clinic with serious plexus injuries due to prior operations. Procedures included transaxillary first rib resection, scalenectomy, and in one case use of a laser to attempt neurolysis and in another thorascopic neurolysis. Most of these patients required graft repair(s) (Fig. 18-13; see Table 18-5). In two cases transection of the plexus or a portion of it required suture or graft.

CONCLUSION

In our opinion, TOS is a diagnosis of exclusion. We do believe it exists and may sometimes be helped by appropriate conservative therapy and sometimes, in well-selected cases, by surgical decom-

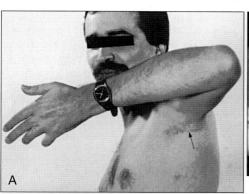
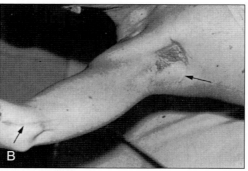
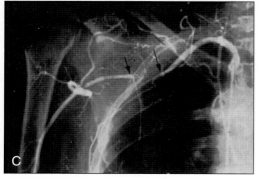

FIGURE 18-12 **(A)** Patient with thoracic outlet syndrome who has transaxillary resection (TAR) of the first rib (*arrow*) with resultant ulnar distribution palsy. **(B)** Another patient had carpal tunnel release, ulnar transposition, then TAR of the first rib. The last operation was associated with a pneumothorax, and a lower trunk injury resulted. **(C)** An axillary artery injury (*arrows*) associated with TAR.

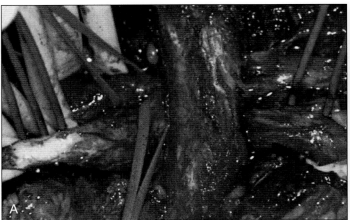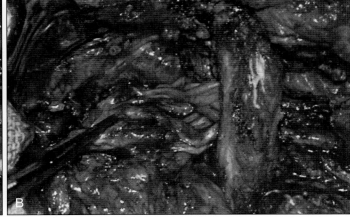

FIGURE 18-13 **(A)** An injury to the entire plexus as a result of use of a laser during a scalenectomy. Most of the plexus did not transmit an operative nerve action potential. **(B)** Most of the plexus extending from trunks to cords had to be replaced with sural grafts.

pression. Since some patients are not helped by surgery and complications can occur, a conservative and selective approach has been advocated by others and we agree with that approach.[25,69–71]

Intraoperative stimulation and recording studies on a series of 33 patients with TNTOS and in some of the 60 patients with DNTOS recorded upon showed conductive and amplitude abnormalities close to the spine and at a spinal nerve to truncal level. This suggests that when present, compression or irritation of the plexus elements, especially of C8, T1, and LT, usually occurs medially and not laterally between clavicle and first rib. Therefore, operations for TOS, whether by first rib resection, scalenectomy with or without neurolysis etc., should include dissection of elements, especially spinal nerves close to their exit from the spine. In this regard, we favor a 360 degree dissection of these lower elements, especially C8, T1, and lower trunk.

REFERENCES

1. Adson AW and Coffey JR: Cervical rib: a method of anterior approach for the relief of symptoms by division of the scalenus anticus. Ann Surg 85:839–857, 1927.
2. Axelrod DA, Proctor MC, et al.: Outcomes after surgery for thoracic outlet syndrome. J Vasc Surg 33:1220–1225, 2001.
3. Aynesworth KH: The cerviocobrachial syndrome: a discussion of the etiology with report of twenty cases. Ann Surg 111:724–742, 1940.
4. Bonney G: The scalenus medius band: A contribution in the study of thoracic outlet syndrome. J Bone Joint Surg [Br] 47:268–272, 1965.
5. Campbell JN, Naff NJ: Thoracic outlet syndrome: neurosurgical perspective. Neurosurg Clin N Am 2:227–233, 1991.
6. Cherington M and Wilbourn AJ: Neurovascular compression in the thoracic outlet syndrome. Ann Surg 230:829–830, 1999.
7. Clagett OT: Research and proresearch: Presidential Address. J Thor Cardiovasc Surg 44:153–166, 1962.
8. Cooper A: On exostosis. In: Cooper A and Travers B, Eds: Surgical Essays, part 1. London, Cox and Son, 1818:159.
9. Coote H: Exostosis of the left transverse process of the seventh cervical vertebra, surrounded by blood vessels and nerves: successful removal. Lancet 1:360–361, 1861.
10. Dale WA: Thoracic outlet compression syndrome. Critique in 1982. Arch Surg 117:1437–1445, 1982.
11. Daube JR: Nerve conduction studies in thoracic outlet syndrome (abstract). Neurology 25:347, 1975.
12. Dawson D and Hallett M: Entrapment Neuropathies, 2nd edn. Boston, Little, Brown, 1990.
13. Dellon AL and Mackinnon SE: Human ulnar neuropathy at the elbow: clinical electrical and morphometric correlations. J Reconstr Microsurg 4:179–184, 1988.
14. Dubuisson AS, Kline DG, et al.: Posterior subscapular approach to the brachial plexus. Report of 102 patients. J Neurosurgery 70:319–330, 1993.
15. Falconer M and Weddell G: Costoclavicular compression of the subclavian artery and vein: Relation to the scalenus anticus syndrome. Lancet 2:539–543, 1943.
16. Fulford PE, Baguneid MS, et al.: Outcome of transaxillary rib resection for thoracic outlet syndrome – a 10 year experience. Cardiovasc Surg 9:620–624, 2001.
17. Gilliatt RW, LeQuesne PM: Wasting of the hand associated with a cervical rib or band. J Neurol Neurosurg Psychiatry 33:615–624, 1970.
18. Gilliatt RW: Thoracic outlet compression syndrome. Br Med J 1:1274–1275, 1976.
19. Glover JL, Worth RM, et al.: Evoked responses in the diagnosis of thoracic outlet syndrome. Surgery 89:86–93, 1981.
20. Golovchinsky V: Double crush syndrome in the lower extremities. Electromyogr Clin Neurophys 38:115–120, 1998.
21. Green RM: Vascular manifestations of the thoracic outlet syndrome. Semin Vasc Surg 11:67–76, 1998.
22. Halsted WS: An experimental study of circumscribed dilation of an artery immediately distal to a partially occluding band and its bearing on the dilation of the subclavian artery observed in certain cases of cervical rib. J Exp Med 24:271–286, 1916.
23. Hardy R and Wilbourn A: Thoracic outlet syndrome. In: Wilkins R and Rengachary S, Eds: Neurosurgery. Baltimore, McGraw Hill, 1985.
24. Hebl JR, Horlocker T, and Pritchard DJ: Diffuse brachial plexopathy after interscalene blockade in a patient receiving Cisplatin chemotherapy: the pharmacologic double crush syndrome. Anesth Analg 92:249–251, 2001.
25. Horowitz SH: Brachial plexus injuries with causalgia resulting from transaxillary rib resection. Arch Surg 120:1189–1191, 1985.
26. Hudson A, Berry H, and Mayfield F: Chronic injuries of nerve by entrapment. In: Youmans J, Ed: Neurological Surgery, 2nd Ed. Philadelphia, WB Saunders, 1983.
27. Hudson A, Kline D, and Mackinnon S: Entrapment neuropathies. In: Horowitz N and Rizzoli H, Eds: Postoperative Complications of Extracranial Neurological Surgery. Philadelphia Williams & Wilkins, 1987.
28. Jerrett, SA, Cuzzone LJ, and Pasternak BM: Thoracic outlet syndrome. Electrophysiological reappraisal. Arch Neurol 41:960–963, 1984.

29. Johnson CR: Treatment of thoracic outlet syndrome by removal of first rib and related entrapments through posterolateral approach: A 25-year experience. J Thorac Cardiovasc Surg 68:536–545, 1974.

30. Kai Y, Oyama M, et al.: Neurogenic thoracic outlet syndrome in whiplash injury. J Spinal Disord 14:487–493, 2001.

31. Katz JN, Simmons BP: Carpal tunnel syndrome. N Engl J Med 346(2):1807–1812, 2002.

32. Kempe LG: Operative Neurosurgery, vol. 2. New York, Springer-Verlag, 1970.

33. Kirgis H and Reed A: Significant anatomic relations in the syndrome of the scalene muscles. Ann Surg 127:1182–1201, 1948.

34. Kline DG, Donner, TR et al.: Intraforaminal repair of plexus spinal nerves by a posterior approach: an experimental study. J Neurosurg 76:459–470, 1992.

35. Kline DG, Hackett E, et al.: Surgery for the lesions of the brachial plexus. Arch Neurol 43:170–181, 1986.

36. Kline DG and Hudson AR: Thoracic outlet syndrome In: Nerve Injuries. Philadelphia, WB Saunders, 1995:473–493.

37. Kline DG, Hudson AR, and Kim D: Thoracic outlet syndrome dissection. In: Atlas of Peripheral Nerve Surgery. Philadelphia, WB Saunders, 2001:51–55.

38. LeForestier N, Moulonguet A, et al.: True neurogenic thoracic outlet syndrome: electrophysiological diagnosis in six cases. Muscle Nerve 21:1129–1134, 1998.

39. Leffert RD and Perlmutter GS: Thoracic outlet syndrome. Results of 282 transaxillary first rib resections. Clin Orthop 368:66–79, 1999.

40. Lindgren KA: Conservative treatment of thoracic outlet syndrome: a 2 year follow-up. Arch Phy Med Rehabil 78:373–378, 1997.

41. Luoma A and Nelems B: Thoracic outlet syndrome: Thoracic surgery perspective. Neursrug Clin N Am 2(1):187–226, 1991.

42. Mackinnon SE, Dellon AL, Hudson AR, et al.: Chronic nerve compression: an experimental model in the rat. Ann Plast Surg 13:112–120, 1984.

43. Mackinnon SE, Dellon AL, Hudson AR, et al.: Chronic human nerve compression: a histological assessment. Neuropathol Appl Neurobiol 12:547–565, 1986.

44. Mackinnon SE: Double and multiple crush syndromes. Hand Clin 8:369–380, 1992.

45. Mackinnon S: Thoracic outlet syndrome. Curr Probl Surg 39:1070–1145, 2002.

46. Mayfield F and True C: Chronic injuries of peripheral nerves by entrapment. In: Youmans JR, Ed: Neurological Surgery. Philadelphia, WB Saunders, 1973:1141–1161.

47. Murphy T: Brachial neuritis caused by pressure of first rib. Aust Med J 15:582–585, 1910.

48. Novak CB, Mackinnon SE, and Patterson GA: Evaluation of patients with thoracic outlet syndrome. J Hand Surg 18A:292–299, 1993.

49. Ochsner A, Gage M, and DeBakey M: Scalenus anticus (Naffziger) syndrome. Am J Surg 28:669–695, 1935.

50. Paget J: Clinical lectures and essays. London, Longman, Greens, 1875.

51. Pang D and Wessel HB: Thoracic outlet syndrome. Neurosurgery 22:105–121, 1998.

52. Peet RM, Henderickson JD, Anderson TP, et al.: Thoracic outlet syndrome: evaluation of a therapeutic exercise program. Mayo Clin Proc 31:281–287, 1956.

53. Poitevin L: Proximal compression of the upper limb neurovascular bundle: An anatomic research study. Hand Clin 4:575–581, 1988.

54. Ranney D. Thoracic outlet: an anatomical redefinition that makes clinical sense. Clin Anat 9(1):50–52, 1996.

55. Roos DB: Transaxillary approach for first rib resection to relieve thoracic outlet syndrome. Ann Surg 163:354–358, 1966.

56. Roos DB: Congenital anomalies associated with thoracic outlet syndrome. Am J Surg 132:771–778, 1976.

57. Roos D: The thoracic outlet syndrome is underrated. Arch Neurol 47:327, 1990.

58. Sanders RJ, Monsour JW, Gerber WF, et al.: Scalenectomy versus first rib resection for treatment of the thoracic outlet syndrome. Surgery 85:109–121, 1979.

59. Sanders RJ and Pearce WH: The treatment of thoracic outlet syndrome: a comparison of different operations. J Vasc Surg 10:626–634, 1989.

60. Sanders RJ and Hammond SL: Management of cervical ribs and anomalous first ribs causing neurogenic thoracic outlet syndrome. J Vasc Surg 36:51–56, 2002.

61. Sheth RN and Belzberg AJ: Diagnosis and treatment of thoracic outlet syndrome. Neurosurg Clin N Am 12:295–309, 2001.

62. Simpson RL and Fern SA: Multiple compression neuropathies and double crush syndrome. Orthop Clin N Am 27(2):381–388, 1996.

63. Stallworth JM Quinn GJ, and Aiken AF: Is rib resection necessary for relief of thoracic outlet syndrome? Ann Surg 185:581–592, 1977.

64. Sunderland S: Nerves and Nerve Injuries, 2nd Ed. Edinburgh, Churchill Livingstone, 1978.

65. Swift TR and Nichols FT: The droopy shoulder syndrome. Neurology 34:212–215, 1984.

66. Synek VM: Diagnostic importance of somatosensory evoked potentials in the diagnosis of thoracic outlet syndrome. Clin Electroencephalogr 17:112–116, 1984.

67. Tender GC, Thomas AJ, Thomas N, et al.: Gilliat-Sumner hand revisited: a 25 year experience. Neurosurgery 55:883–890, 2004.

68. Thomas GI, Jones TW, Stavney LS, et al.: The middle scalene muscle and its contribution to the thoracic outlet syndrome. Am J Surg 145:589–592, 1983.

69. Urschel HC and Razzuk MA: The failed operation for thoracic outlet syndrome. The difficulty of diagnosis and management. Ann Thorac Surg 42:523–525, 1986.

70. Wilbourn AJ: Thoracic outlet syndrome: a plea for conservatism. Neurosurg Clin N Am 2:235–245, 1991.

71. Wilbourn A and Lederman R: Thoracic outlet syndrome surgery causing severe brachial plexopathy. Muscle Nerve 11:66–74, 1988.

72. Wilbourn A and Lederman R: Evidence for conduction delay in thoracic outlet syndrome is challenged (letter). N Engl J Med 310:1052–1053, 1984.

73. Wilbourn AJ: Thoracic outlet syndromes. Neurol Clin 17:477–497, 1999.

74. Williams AF: The role of the first rib in the scalenus anterior syndrome. J Bone Joint Surg [Br] 34:200–203, 1952.

75. Wood V, Biondi J: Double crush nerve compression in thoracic outlet syndrome. J Bone Joint Surg [Am] 72:85–87, 1990.

76. Yiannikas C and Walsh JC: Somatosensory evoked responses in the diagnosis of thoracic outlet syndrome. J Neurol Neurosurg Psychiatry 46:234–240, 1983.

77. Young MC, Richards RR, and Hudson AR: Thoracic outlet syndrome with congenital pseudoarthrosis of the clavicle: Treatment by brachial plexus decompression, plate fixation, and bone grafting. Can J Surg 31:131–133, 1988.

19

Accessory nerve

Rajiv Midha

OVERVIEW

- The vast majority of injuries involving the extracranial accessory nerve are iatrogenic in origin.
- Lymph node biopsy remains the most common operation leading to nerve injury. The other main iatrogenic cause is damage during tumor excision, with rare cases complicating carotid endarterectomy, face lift surgery, and irradiation.
- Non-iatrogenic traumatic etiologies include injuries caused by stretch/contusion, stab or glass wounds, and gunshot wounds.
- A keen appreciation of the relevant anatomy remains paramount in both avoiding nerve injury and in the surgical exploration of the non-recovering cases.
- It is extremely important to differentiate scapular winging caused by accessory palsy from that caused by long thoracic or dorsal scapular palsy. This determination can be easily made clinically by taking into account the mechanism of injury on history and a careful physical examination of the shoulder girdle, including noting where prior surgical scar is located.
- From a series of close to 200 patients evaluated with accessory nerve injury at LSUMC over a 22-year period, 122 had surgery and 111 of those operated on were available for follow-up.
- In this series of 111 operated cases, neurolysis was performed on 19 patients with lesions in continuity and positive nerve action potential (NAP) recording, with generally excellent results (Table 19-1).
- Grade 3 or better recovery was obtained in over 75% of patients having end-to-end repairs (26 cases) and interpositional graft repairs (58 cases).
- For graft repairs, it was usually possible to utilize nearby sensory nerves for this purpose, but because of extensive scarring in the neck, the sural nerve had to be harvested and utilized in somewhat less than half the grafting cases.
- Neurotization using C2 and C3 proximal input or burial of grafts from proximal accessory directly into the trapezius muscle was a less successful surgical strategy.
- Spinal accessory nerve injuries should be managed aggressively if clinical recovery does not occur, with surgical exploration and repair, allowing favorable outcomes to be achieved in most cases.

INJURY MECHANISMS

Extracranial injuries to the eleventh cranial (accessory) nerves are unusual but do occur.[5,12] The leading cause remains iatrogenic and operative (Fig. 19-1).[13,14] Most cases are associated with lymph node biopsy, but, as can be seen from Table 19-1 as well as in the literature, other associated operations include excision of neck tumors, carotid endarterectomy, plastic surgery procedures, and irradiation.[5,12,13,15,21] Distressingly, the accessory nerve remains the most frequent of the major nerves injured iatrogenically.[2,14,24]

Although more commonly spared in stretch injuries involving neck or shoulder, this nerve can be stretched either in association with plexus stretch or in isolation. Penetrating wounds from knives, glass, or gunshot can occasionally involve this nerve. Even less frequent is a more spontaneous onset which may or may not involve compression,[6] physical exertion, and a variation of Parsonage-Turner syndrome.[7] Historically, accessory palsy has also been associated with tuberculosis or scrofula of the neck and with vascular ectasias involving the nerve in the neck.[8,9] In the past, the accessory nerve was routinely sacrificed as part of a radical neck dissection, but in more recent years, many surgeons have been sparing this nerve during such dissections.[1,22]

APPLIED ANATOMY

Rootlets making up the accessory nerve arise from the lower medulla and the upper, usually four, segments of the cervical spinal cord. The cervical rootlets ascend the ventral spinal canal to join the medullary descending rootlets. They form the accessory nerve, which exits the skull through the jugular foramen. Below the base of the skull, accessory nerve lies lateral to the internal jugular vein. The nerve then courses either anterior or posterior to the internal jugular vein. Then, the nerve lies behind the stylohyoid and digastric muscles, and in front of the palpable lateral mass of the atlas. The nerve then passes through the more proximal sternocleidomastoid (SCM) muscle, which it innervates. In this area, spinal branches from C2, C3, and sometimes C4 contribute to sternomastoid innervation, so even complete injury to proximal accessory nerve does not give paralysis of the SCM.

The accessory runs from beneath the posterior or lateral border of SCM and can be identified on the posterior border of the SCM muscle, 8.2 ± 1.01 cm cranial to the clavicle in recent anatomic study of cadavers.[11] This approximates a point one-fourth to one-third of the length of the posterior border of SCM from mastoid eminence to clavicle (Fig. 19-2). It is in close juxtaposition to the great auricular nerve, which wraps around the lateral border of the SCM to course cephalad. Anatomic study of cadavers has indicated that the spinal accessory nerve almost always lies cephalad to the great auricular nerve at the level of the lateral SCM and usually within 2 cm of it, and the two nerves together form an important landmark.[19] The course of the accessory nerve can also usually be judged by palpating the C2 transverse process beneath SCM and then projecting a straight line from there to the tip of the shoulder.

The accessory nerve then courses somewhat obliquely across the posterior triangle, where it lies on the surface of the levator scapula muscle. On reaching the superior portion of the trapezius, it branches to innervate this muscle. It supplies short branches to supply the trapezius along the superior and posterior border of this muscle in the neck and longer branches to descend into the thoracic or what some authors term the spinal portion of the muscle. Occasionally, the spinal accessory nerve becomes bifid, usually where it gives off its proximal or upper trapezius muscle branches.

In some cases, branches from C2 or even C3 spinal nerves may supplement input to trapezius, especially the lower or spinal portion of that muscle.[19,20] The majority of the evidence points strongly to the fact that the main motor supply to the trapezius muscle is by the eleventh cranial nerve. Certainly, by the time the nerve is seen in the posterior triangle, it is, in our experience, the sole source of motor supply to the trapezius. Regardless of whether it has picked up contributions from the cervical plexus before entering the posterior triangle, if the accessory nerve is injured in that area, the patient will have a major trapezius motor loss.

One of the key points relating to the anatomy of the accessory nerve in the posterior triangle is the fact that it is covered only by skin and the investing fascia of the neck. It is therefore very exposed to operative injury. Cervical lymph nodes often immediately abut on the accessory nerve. Lymph nodes may lie deep to the plane of the accessory nerve, so that the nerve, in its course through the posterior triangle, runs through lymph node-bearing adipose tissue. This anatomic relation underlies the fact that the most common cause of iatrogenic accessory nerve injury seen by us is cervical lymph node biopsy (Fig. 19-3).

In diagnosing iatrogenic injuries within the posterior triangle which result in winged scapula, anatomical considerations should be taken into considerable account in distinguishing long thoracic from accessory nerve injury. The nerve to serratus anterior arises from C5, C6, and C7 spinal nerves, with the main physical contribution from the posterior surface of the C6 spinal nerve. The confluence of these three spinal nerves often occurs within the substance of scalenus medius before the named (long thoracic) nerve emerges in the lower portion of the posterior triangle. Thus, it is virtually impossible selectively to injure the nerve to serratus anterior through an incision placed directly over the course of the accessory nerve in the posterior triangle unless, of course, the plexus itself is seriously injured. Contrariwise, it is extremely easy to injure the accessory nerve through an incision placed directly over the course of that nerve.

CLINICAL PRESENTATION AND EXAMINATION

Onset of accessory nerve palsy is usually associated with pain, presumably because of atrophy of this relatively large shoulder and back muscle. The tip of the shoulder droops, and this may produce

Table 19-1 Causes of accessory nerve palsy in 111 operated cases[12]

Cause	No. of patients
Iatrogenic	
Lymph node biopsy	82
Tumor excision	19
Carotid endarterectomy	1
Plastic face lift	1
Traumatic	
Stretch	5
Laceration	3
Total	111

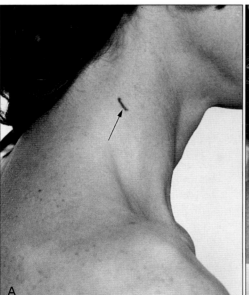
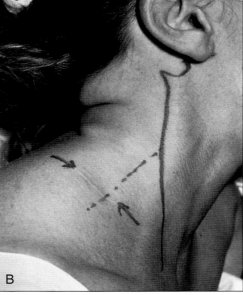

FIGURE 19-1 (A) A small lymph node biopsy incision resulted in severance of the accessory nerve. **(B)** A lower incision (*arrows pointing to scar*) in a different patient undergoing lymph node biopsy injured the nerve more distally, close to the trapezius muscle. The solid line outlines the posterior border of the sternocleidomastoid muscle, while the dotted line indicates the course of the accessory nerve.

The Accessory Nerve in the Posterior Cervical Triangle (Right).

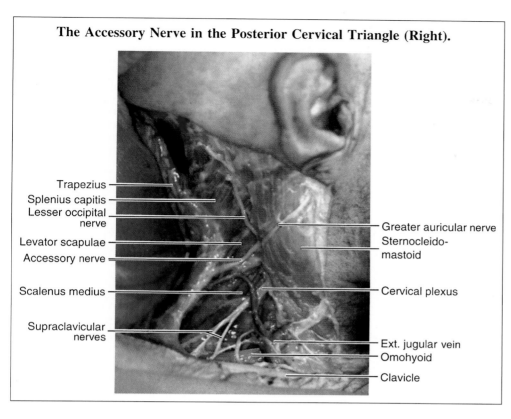

Trapezius
Splenius capitis
Lesser occipital nerve
Levator scapulae
Accessory nerve
Scalenus medius
Supraclavicular nerves

Greater auricular nerve
Sternocleido-mastoid
Cervical plexus
Ext. jugular vein
Omohyoid
Clavicle

FIGURE 19-2 Cadaveric anatomic dissection illustrating the accessory nerve and its relationship to adjacent structures. (From Kline DG, Hudson AR, and Kim DH: Eds: Atlas of Peripheral Nerve Surgery, 1st edn. Philadelphia, WB Saunders, 2001.)

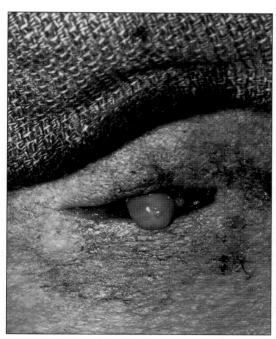

FIGURE 19-3 A small posterior triangle incision for a lymph node biopsy fortunately missed the accessory nerve. The nerve lay in the depths of the wound, just below the node and somewhat adherent to it.

traction on soft tissues of the neck, including nerves which may also be responsible for or contribute to the pain. This is variously described as a dragging or pulling sensation in the neck and can be associated with arm pain and occipital as well as posterior neck discomfort.

Patients may well ascribe their initial postoperative abnormal symptoms to the operation, such as a lymph node biopsy, itself. It is not unusual (and indeed typical) for a patient to delay recognition that something is seriously wrong for a few days or weeks. Pain may not be noticed for several weeks until the patient attempts to resume household tasks requiring normal shoulder activity. Progressively, the patient notices a decrease in strength of the affected arm and difficulty in such daily tasks as combing hair, putting on a shirt or blouse, and raising the arm above the horizontal plane.

With severe or complete palsy, the scapula wings and the patient notes, in addition to the droopy shoulder, inability to abduct the arm in a smooth fashion, especially above the horizontal (Fig. 19-4). Pushing forward with the elbow flexed or across the chest against resistance accentuates the winging associated with trapezius palsy. On the other hand, pushing forward against resistance with the shoulder joint flexed and elbow fully extended does not produce severe winging, as it would with long thoracic palsy. Some patients learn that with abduction in a lateral direction, they can turn the hand from a palm down to palm up direction and gain some further abduction above the horizontal. Others learn to throw or toss their arm out in abduction and use the force of the initiation of abduction to carry the arm past the horizontal, despite the winging and lateral deviation of the scapula.

Shrug of the shoulder is poor, although the levator scapula can substitute for this in a variable fashion, especially for more medial shoulder function. More medial trapezius may also contract because branches to this portion of the muscle may arise from a more proximal portion of the accessory beneath SCM and thus be spared with the usual more lateral nerve injury. Simple inspection shows atrophy of the superior portion of the trapezius and some, but usually not complete, winging of the scapula (Fig. 19-4B). This winging is not as severe or as complete as is seen with serratus anterior loss. Mild wasting of supra- and infraspinatus (presumably

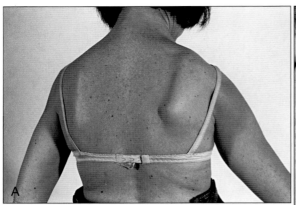
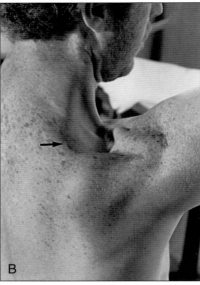

FIGURE 19-4 Clinical features of accessory nerve palsy. **(A)** Winged right scapula in a patient with iatrogenic accessory nerve injury, associated with drooping of the pectoral girdle causing the patient's brassiere strap to slide down constantly. **(B)** Severe wasting of the right trapezius muscle (*arrow*) so that the upper border of the scapula appears very prominent as seen in a different patient.

from disuse) is a common accompaniment of a wide range of disorders of the shoulder joint, including trapezius palsy. The appearance of this non-specific sort of scapular muscle wasting should not mislead the examiner to an incorrect diagnosis of brachial plexus injury, amyotrophy, or suprascapular nerve injury.

Loss of trapezius function results in lack of coordinated trapezius/serratus anterior function, which is required for rotation of the scapula during the final 90 degrees of shoulder abduction. The main complaint expressed by the patient may reflect this functional impairment. Supraspinatus and deltoid abduct the humerus to the 90-degree position, but further abduction requires rotation of the scapula. This rotation is primarily brought about by the combined action of trapezius and serratus anterior. Deltoid and supraspinatus functions are retained, but these muscles have the disadvantage of working from an unstable base and, in addition, the crucial component of scapular rotation is severely impaired by the weakness or paralysis of trapezius. A stable scapula is essential to serve as a platform for function of short muscles around the shoulder joint. The lack of scapular stability which follows trapezius palsy thus results in alteration of coordinated function of the short muscles and hence of a fluid shoulder movement. Very characteristically, patients complain of sudden "clunking" of the scapula during attempted circumduction of the shoulder. The upper border of the scapula is often prominent if the patient is viewed from behind, and there is a characteristic flattening of the tissues immediately behind the clavicle on the affected side, compared with the normal side. The wasting of trapezius should be distinguished from that affecting the rhomboid muscles (in isolated lesions of the dorsal scapular nerve). The latter results in a characteristic scalloping of the medial border of the scapula that becomes more prominent when an attempt is made to bring together the shoulder blades in a military posture. The scapular winging seen with rhomboid muscle paralysis only affects the medial border of the scapula.

ELECTROPHYSIOLOGICAL STUDIES

After a few weeks, electromyography (EMG) shows denervational changes in the trapezius. There may be some relative sparing of medial fibers, but with severe lesions there is seldom sparing of intermediate or more lateral muscle innervation. By contrast, EMG

study of SCM seldom shows denervational change.[5,17] Needle studies of the spinal portion of the trapezius muscle are difficult to do because rhomboideus major and minor are just deep to the more inferior portion of the trapezius and levator scapula to the more superior part of it.

If reinnervation occurred spontaneously in this series, its onset was usually delayed for 3–9 months. As with other muscles, early electrical signs included presence of nascent motor units and usually a simultaneous decrease in the intensity of fibrillations and denervational potentials. The muscle is usually reinnervated from above down. Only very clear-cut evidence of significant reinnervation should be allowed to delay surgical exploration. This is especially so because the results of electrodiagnostic studies do not always predict the functional outcome of patients with accessory nerve injuries.[7]

OPERATION

The re-operation follows the principles of any nerve exploration. It is usually appropriate to add vertical limbs to the previously placed skin-crease horizontal incision, which makes this secondary incision "Z-shaped." Reflection of the two somewhat triangular flaps thus created allows the posterior or more lateral border of the SCM to be cleared and the anterior border of the trapezius to be displayed. The transverse cervical and greater auricular nerves serve as guides. These auricular branches of the cervical plexus are usually easily found during the initial stages of the dissection, because they curve around the posterolateral border of SCM. The proximal stump of the accessory nerve is then usually found approximately 1–2 cm superior to these nerves. The usual pattern is that of a single nerve trunk with branches running a short distance to the anterior border of the trapezius. If the nerve injury is distal to a branch, every effort must be made to conserve that branch. On occasion, the main trunk may appear to divide, and, once again, all functioning elements must be preserved.

As a general principle, it is, as with other nerve injuries, appropriate to dissect out nerve proximal and distal to the lesion, subsequently working toward the main pathology. In accessory nerve injuries in the posterior triangle, this is a difficult maneuver. Often a mixture of scar and adipose tissue occupies the upper part of the posterior triangle between the posterolateral border of the SCM and the anterior border of the trapezius. The dissection under the operating microscope or loupes may occupy a considerable period of time as the dissector distinguishes cervical plexus and other sensory branches to the skin of the neck and auricular regions running medially from the area of the trapezius muscle, and the damaged accessory nerve (Fig. 19-5). The operation is hampered if the vertical limb placed at the medial extent of the previous horizontal incision is not extended sufficiently high. A variable-voltage nerve stimulator helps locate the proximal stump because it causes SCM contraction. The searching electrode may accidentally stimulate levator scapulae or cervical branches to it and this occurrence should not be misinterpreted as evidence of trapezius contraction.

The surgeon should be at pains to preserve the smallest of branches emanating from the proximal accessory stump, which lead to the distal nerve, because the difficulty with this operation may be that of defining an appropriate distal stump. The operator may have to search through the scar tissue on the anterior border of the trapezius to find fascicles or branches indicating motor entry points. The proximal nerve runs between sternomastoid and cleidomastoid, and the neuroma may be found enmeshed in adipose and fibrous tissue or, less frequently, as a well-defined and smoothly outlined proximal neuroma bulb.

The proximal and distal stumps are prepared in standard fashion after the appropriate electrophysiologic and microsurgical appraisal of the lesion. If a lesion in continuity is found, the standard electrical and microscopic criteria are utilized to decide for or against resection after an external neurolysis has been performed.[16] If direct stimulation of the nerve results in unequivocal trapezius contraction (i.e. in a situation in which none was seen on clinical examination), then the procedure is terminated, because this feature is consistent with an excellent prognosis. Attempts should be made to obtain nerve action potentials (NAPs) across the lesion. Sometimes this may be difficult because the distance available between proximal and distal electrode placement may be short. If the lesion in continuity transmits an NAP, the procedure should be terminated following neurolysis with the knowledge that outcomes are generally excellent (as discussed below). In the situation of a nonconducting neuroma, the lesion is resected and the nerve repaired (Fig. 19-6).

The locally available greater auricular nerve is a good donor nerve, but more frequently a more lateral branch of descending cervical sensory plexus is utilized for grafting. However, we have often harvested the sural nerve, as a considerable graft length can be obtained. The graft should be placed in a relaxed fashion to allow movement of the patient's neck postoperatively and to allow for shrinkage of graft substance (Fig. 19-7).

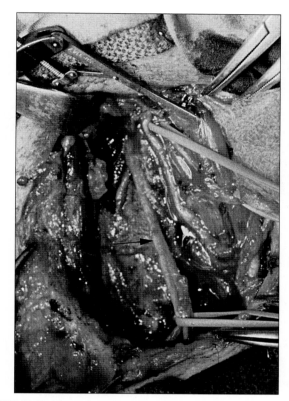

FIGURE 19-5 Dissection of an injured accessory nerve (*arrow*), with a plastic loop around adjacent cervical plexus sensory nerves to the right.

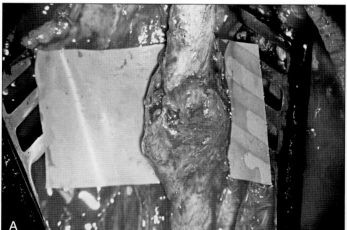
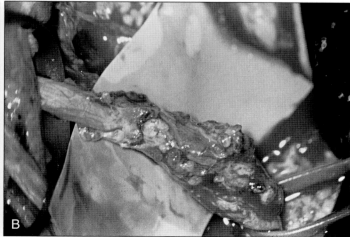

FIGURE 19-6 **(A)** Operating microscopic appearance of an accessory neuroma in continuity. This lesion failed to transmit an NAP 4 months after injury and required resection and repair. **(B)** Another severe lesion in continuity involving the accessory nerve which required resection and graft repair.

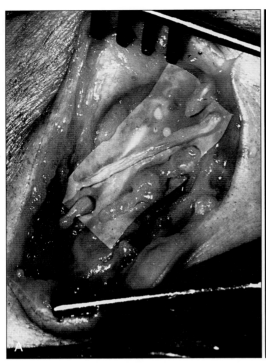
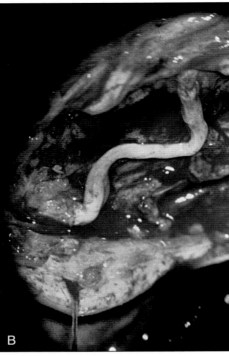

FIGURE 19-7 Operative reconstruction of accessory nerve injury. **(A)** This neuroma was resected (shown just on right side of graft), leaving a considerable gap between the proximal and distal stumps of the accessory nerve. **(B)** A sural nerve graft was used to bridge the gap, with some redundancy to allow for graft shrinkage and neck movements. This patient had recovery of the majority of trapezius function over several years.

RESULTS

Patients selected for operation usually had complete or nearly complete loss of trapezius with denervation by EMG persisting for 2 months or longer. Early experience had shown that a proportion of such lesions were in continuity *even* if the mechanism was operative injury. As a result, exploration was delayed for several months after onset of palsy in most iatrogenic injuries as well as in the stretch injuries unassociated with prior operation. Approximately one-half of such injuries were found to be in continuity. Some were regenerating and had a transmitted NAP, and thus had a neurolysis only, but the majority required resection and repair. One exception was provided by an iatrogenic case in which the surgeon involved recognized that the nerve was divided, did not repair it acutely, and sent it for secondary repair. Another exception was a case in which the pathologist reported a nerve segment of approximate caliber for accessory nerve along with the lymph node submitted. In these cases, repair was done relatively early but nonetheless secondarily. Accessory nerves injured by glass or knife wounds were also repaired relatively early or soon after they were first seen.

GRADING

For assessing results, each patient underwent a detailed clinical assessment pre- and postoperatively of motor and sensory functions of the spinal accessory nerve according to a standardized grading scheme (Table 19-2).[12] Functional assessment included measurement of active abduction of the shoulder and manual muscle testing of the trapezius. The contour, function, and strength of the trapezius muscle were assessed. The contraction of the trapezius and its ability to stabilize the scapula during a complete arc of abduction were assessed and compared with those of the normal side. Using the grading scheme illustrated in Table 19-2, a favorable functional outcome was considered for grade 3 or better recovery.

Table 19-2 Grading system to assess accessory nerve function

Grade	Clinical findings
0 (none)	Trapezius muscle contraction clinically absent
1 (trace)	Trapezius muscle contraction clinically evident but with only a flicker of movement
2 (poor)	Trapezius contracts, allowing some portion of arc of shoulder abduction movement with gravity eliminated
3 (fair)	Trapezius contracts, allowing a full arc of shoulder abduction against gravity
4 (good)	Strength of abduction against gravity and weak resistance
5 (normal)	Strength equal to the contralateral normal side

NONOPERATIVE CASES

Those patients not selected for operation usually improved significantly with time or were, as in some cases, referred very late. Other patients presented with function that was partial but was thought to be acceptable. A few patients who were treated conservatively remained unchanged over 1–2 years of further follow-up. Another patient who had injury caused by irradiation had a progressive loss of not only trapezius but also SCM function, and eventually developed a complete palsy.

Table 19-3 shows the initial grades seen in a group of 34 patients, as well as their latest grade on follow-up. Only patients with some sequential follow-up are included in this table. Average length of follow-up in this group was 16.1 months, with a range of 11 to 96 months.

OPERATIVE CASES

Table 19-4 depicts the type of operations performed in 111 patients for whom there were follow-ups of 12 months or more available. Improvement is shown by grade in Table 19-5, which includes the 103 patients who underwent neurolysis or repair. Nineteen patients had a neurolysis because the nerve was in continuity and exhibited intraoperative electrical evidence of regeneration, such as a positive NAP beyond the point of injury or trapezius contraction in response to the spinal accessory nerve stimulation. Transected nerves or those in which a nerve segment was unable to transmit an NAP required end-to-end repair or graft repair. The donor nerves for the grafts were harvested from local, cervical sensory, or greater auricular nerve, if they had suitable caliber and quality. Otherwise, the sural nerve was used.

A feature of some accessory nerve injuries is that despite meticulous dissection and exhaustive searching, either a suitable proximal or distal stump can not be isolated. These patients require either a nerve transfer or a direct nerve–muscle neurotization. These operations were performed in seven patients; five patients had the contribution of C2 and/or C3 to the sternocleidomastoid "swung down" and transferred to the distal accessory nerve when a proxi-

mal nerve trunk could not be identified;[3] two patients had the proximal nerve "blind-ended" into the muscle when a distal stump could not be identified.

Excellent results were obtained in patients who required only neurolysis, with grade 3 or better functional recovery seen in all 19 patients (100%) with an average of 23.5-months follow-up (range of 12–39 months). Eight of these patients reached grade 5. Dramatic improvements in arm abduction and normalization of shoulder posture were obtained in all these patients (Table 19-5). Nagging pain syndromes seen in thirteen of these patients also resolved. One patient had ligature material removed from the nerve followed by neurolysis and regained full bulk and function of the trapezius muscle.

Eighty-four patients with lesions not in continuity, or with lesions in continuity but across which nerve action potentials could not be recorded, underwent end-to-end suture (26 patients) or interposition graft repair (58 patients) and were seen an average of 26.9 months postoperatively (range 12–44 months; Table 19-6). Sixty-five (77%) of these patients achieved a grade 3 or better functional recovery following surgery and most of them (50 patients, 60%) reached a grade 4 or 5. With normalization of shoulder posture, these patients all reported cessation of the dragging pain noted

Table 19-3 Nonoperative case results of accessory nerve injuries (n=34*)

Grade	Initial grade	Final grade
5	0	10
4	6	11
3	14	8
2	8	2
1	4	0
0	2	3

*Initial and final grades of accessory nerve function are tabulated for a cohort of 34 patients that did not undergo surgery.

Table 19-4 Operations on 111 patients with extracranial spinal accessory nerve injury[12]

Operation	No. of patients
Graft	58
Local nerve	33
Sural nerve	25
End to end repair	26
Neurolysis	19
Neurotization (C2–C3)	5
Burial into muscle	2
Ligature removal	1
Total	111

Table 19-5 Results of surgery in 103 patients who underwent neurolysis or repair[12]

Grade	Neurolysis		Grade	Repair	
	Preoperative (n=19)	Postoperative (n=19)		Preoperative (n=84)	Postoperative (n=84)
5	0	8	5	0	11
4	0	10	4	0	39
3	0	1	3	0	15
2	0	0	2	0	9
1	2	0	1	11	7
0	17	0	0	73	3

Table 19-6 Results of surgery in 84 patients who underwent end-to-end suture or interpositional graft repair[12]

Grade	End-to-end		Graft (local)		Graft (sural)	
	Preoperative (n=26)	Postoperative (n=26)	Preoperative (n=33)	Postoperative (n=33)	Preoperative (n=25)	Postoperative (n=25)
5	0	4	0	5	0	2
4	0	16	0	12	0	11
3	0	3	0	7	0	5
2	0	2	0	4	0	3
1	5	1	4	3	2	3
0	21	0	29	2	23	1

above. Of the 26 patients who underwent end-to-end suture repair, 23 patients (88%) recovered to grade 3 or better, somewhat better recovery than patients receiving graft repairs (72%). There was no clear difference in outcome between groups receiving local (73%) and sural grafts (72%). The average graft length was 4 cm in both groups.

The five patients who underwent neurotization, in which C3 and C4 branches were swung down and sewn to grafts which were attached to distal accessory branches, had some degree of recovery after surgery. All of these patients had preoperative grades of 0 and improved to grades of 2 in three patients and 3 in two patients with an average 15-months follow-up. Two other patients who had proximal nerve buried into muscle did not improve, and their pre- and postoperative grades were both 0.

SUMMARY

If managed correctly, the outcome with accessory palsy was usually good, and this has been the case in other smaller series.[4,10,18,23,25–27] On the other hand, recovery was usually not perfect. Shoulder shrug was often recovered, but some winging of the scapula and lack of full abduction was not an infrequent outcome. Even with good recovery, the shoulder on the affected side was often carried by the patient at a lower level than on the contralateral side. Most of these patients were able to return to some type of work, but there were exceptions, particularly if the work involved heavy labor, heavy lifting, or climbing ladders.

REFERENCES

1. Becker GD and Parell GJ: Technique of preserving the spinal accessory nerve during radical neck dissection. Laryngoscope 89:827–831, 1979.
2. Birch R, Bonney G, Dowell J, et al.: Iatrogenic injuries of peripheral nerves. J Bone Joint Surg [Br] 73:280–282, 1991.
3. Braun V, Mayer M, Antoniadis G, et al.: Reconstruction of the spinal accessory nerve with an anastomosis to the dorsal C3 branch: technical note. Neurosurgery 38:208–210, 1996.
4. Chandawarkar RY, Cervino AL, and Pennington GA: Management of iatrogenic injury to the spinal accessory nerve. Plast Reconstr Surg 111:611–617, 2003.
5. Donner T and Kline D: Extracranial spinal accessory nerve injury. Neurosurgery 32:907–911, 1993.
6. Eisen A and Bertrand G: Isolated accessory nerve palsy of spontaneous origin. A clinical and electromyographic study. Arch Neurol 27:496–502, 1972.
7. Friedenberg SM, Zimprich T, and Harper CM: The natural history of long thoracic and spinal accessory neuropathies. Muscle Nerve 25:535–539, 2002.
8. Hanford JM: Surgical excision of tuberculosis lymph nodes of neck. Report of 131 patients with followup results. Surg Clin N Am 13:301–303, 1933.
9. Havelius U, Hindfelt B, Brismar J, et a.l: Carotid fibromuscular dysplasia and paresis of lower cranial nerves (Collect-Sicard syndrome). Case report. J Neurosurg 56:850–853, 1982.
10. Hudson AR: Comments on accessory nerve injury. Neurosurgery 32:911, 1993.
11. Kierner AC, Zelenka I, Heller S, et al.: Surgical anatomy of the spinal accessory nerve and the trapezius branches of the cervical plexus. Arch Surg 135:1428–1431, 2000.
12. Kim DH, Cho Y-J, Tiel RL, et al.: Surgical outcomes of 111 spinal accessory nerve injuries. Neurosurgery 53:1106–1112, 2003.
13. King RJ and Motta G: Iatrogenic spinal accessory nerve palsy. Ann R Coll Surg Engl 65:35–37, 1983.
14. Kretschmer T, Antoniadis G, Braun V, et al.: Evaluation of iatrogenic lesions in 722 surgically treated cases of peripheral nerve trauma. J Neurosurg 94:905–912, 2001.
15. Marini SG, Rook JL, Green RF, et al.: Spinal accessory nerve palsy: an unusual complication of coronary artery bypass. Arch Phys Med Rehabil 72:247–249, 1991.
16. Midha R and Kline DG: Evaluation of the neuroma in continuity. In: Omer GE, Spinner M, and Van Beek AL, Eds: Management of Peripheral Nerve Problems, 2nd edn. Philadelphia, WB Saunders, 1998:319–327.
17. Olarte M and Adams D: Accessory nerve palsy. J Neurol Neurosurg Psychiatry 40:1113–1116, 1977.
18. Osgaard O, Eskesen V, and Rosenorn J: Microsurgical repair of iatrogenic accessory nerve lesions in the posterior triangle of the neck. Acta Chir Scand 153:171–173, 1987.
19. Soo KC, Guiloff RJ, Oh A, et al.: Innervation of the trapezius muscle: a study in patients undergoing neck dissections. Head Neck 12:488–495, 1990.
20. Straus WL and Howell AB: The spinal accessory nerve and its musculature. Q Rev Biol 11:387–405, 1936.
21. Swann KW and Heros RC: Accessory nerve palsy following carotid endarterectomy. Report of two cases. J Neurosurg 63:630–632, 1985.
22. Weitz JW, Weitz SL, and McElhinney AJ: A technique for preservation of spinal accessory nerve function in radical neck dissection. Head Neck Surg 5:75–78, 1982.

23. Wiater JM and Bigliani LU: Spinal accessory nerve injury. Clin Orthop 368:5–6, 1999.

24. Wilbourn AJ: Iatrogenic nerve injuries. Neurol Clin 16:55–82, 1998.

25. Williams WW, Twyman RS, Donell ST, et al.: The posterior triangle and the painful shoulder: spinal accessory nerve injury. Ann R Coll Surg Engl 78:521–525, 1996.

26. Woodhall B: Trapezius paralysis following minor surgical procedures in the posterior cervical triangle. Ann Surg 156:375–380, 1952.

27. Wright TA: Accessory spinal nerve injury. Clin Orthop 108:15–18, 1975.

20

Reconstructive procedures

Robert J. Spinner

OVERVIEW

While the extent of reconstructive procedures is beyond the scope of this chapter, we wish to emphasize the indications, benefits, and limitations of soft tissue and bony procedures in the context of the treatment of patients with peripheral nerve and brachial plexus injuries. We have seen our patients benefit from well-indicated reconstructive procedures and well-thought-out physical therapy programs. The number of substitutive procedures developed to replace lost upper or lower limb function, and especially hand function, is a tribute to human ingenuity. While we are proponents of neural repair whenever possible, we readily recognize the difficulties in obtaining strong shoulder and elbow function in some cases, and in obtaining more distal function in many cases. Unlike nerve reconstruction, these secondary procedures have the advantage of not being time dependent.

Tendon transfer, with or without concomitant tenodesis or joint fusion, can restore useful and predictable function in patients with single nerve deficits. For example, transfer of three tendons can effectively restore wrist extension, finger extension, and thumb extension in a patient with a complete radial nerve paralysis. A surgeon may select from a variety of opponensplasties to compensate for loss of opposition in a patient with a median nerve palsy. Anti-clawing procedures combined with adductorplasties may help patients with ulnar nerve lesions. Tenodesis procedures may improve finger posture and flexion in high median or ulnar nerve palsies. Successful substitution for loss of distal thumb flexion may be achieved with a balanced tendon transfer or a thumb axis fusion. Posterior tibial transfer can be helpful to correct a footdrop deformity, if done by an experienced surgeon.

Effective substitution for brachial plexus palsies is very difficult, especially if a flail arm is present. Shoulder stability and motion may be improved with tendon transfer or fusion, if it is not regained by neural reconstruction. Elbow flexion is a major priority of reconstruction. Depending on the extent of the lesion, substitution for elbow flexion may not be possible with standard tendon transfers, including the pectoralis major, latissimus dorsi, triceps, or a Steindler flexorplasty (advancement of the flexor-pronator group to the distal humerus). Free functioning muscle transfer, which involves intricate microvascular techniques, can restore reliable elbow flexion in these cases where other options may not be available.

The importance of appropriate referral of patients to orthopedists, plastic surgeons, and hand surgeons is emphasized. These surgeons are important members of a multidisciplinary approach to patients with complex peripheral nerve and brachial plexus disorders.

INTRODUCTION

There is little question that reconstructive procedures such as tendon transfers, tenodesis, and joint arthrodesis are indicated for many severe or irreparable peripheral nerve injuries. In fact, the practical results of such reconstructive procedures are viewed by some as more successful for restoration of function than those produced by neural repair alone.[22,29,36,43] Tendon transfers may augment or provide complete function when function is insufficient or absent. In cases of a deficit limited to one peripheral nerve territory, tendon transfer(s) may provide reliable function; examples would include: opponensplasty, adductorplasty, anti-clawing procedure, flexor-to-extensor transfer, elbow flexorplasty – to name just a few. Other soft tissue or bony procedures may be applied in these single-territory peripheral nerve cases as well as combined injuries affecting peripheral nerves or the brachial plexus. Each patient's loss must be individually assessed. Peripheral nerve surgeons should be knowledgeable regarding the spectrum and the potential application of these reconstructive procedures, even if they themselves do not perform them. A skilled orthopedic, hand, or plastic surgeon should be available to offer these techniques to patients as part of a concerted team approach.

What follows is only a brief overview of this field. Further discussion on the use of reconstructive procedures and rehabilitation can be found in this book's individual chapters on various nerve injuries as well as the brachial plexus. Nuances of principles of tendon transfer, operative techniques, and rehabilitative programs will not be discussed. More detailed explanations are available and should be consulted for further information.[6,13,21,23,49,54]

BASIC PRINCIPLES OF TENDON TRANSFER

Tendon transfers have a rich history in that they have been performed with good results for over a century. Popularized for deficits from poliomyelitis, leprosy, and tetraplegia, tendon transfers are performed widely for post-traumatic neurologic conditions in which the muscle imbalance is usually static (rather than progressive as it may be in certain neuropathies, e.g. Charcot-Marie-Tooth).

Tendon transfers involve the substitution of an expendable functioning muscle or tendon for one that is nonfunctional. The goal of tendon transfer surgery is to reestablish tendon balance and replace lost function in the affected limb. In this regard, tendon transfer is analogous to nerve transfer. Tendon transfer for peripheral nerve injury is indicated when sufficient recovery has not occurred either spontaneously or after previous reconstructive attempts. In addition, it may be appropriate when local trauma to the muscle or its soft tissue bed prevents the native nerve from functioning effectively. Unlike a nerve transfer (which has an optimal period of time in which it can be performed), a tendon transfer can be done at any time (even years later), assuming that the joints involved are passively supple.

When considering a tendon transfer, several questions need to be answered:

1. What function (s) is (are) needed most?
2. What tendons are working?
3. What tendons are available for transfer?
4. How do the potential donor muscles/tendons compare to the specific muscle/tendon that is not functioning?
5. What about balance (antagonist function)?
6. What is the status of soft tissue beds?
7. When should the transfer be performed or staged?

In order to answer these questions, certain principles need to be adopted. The most critical and most achievable functions need to be prioritized: wrist control first, then grasp, pinch, and release in that order.

A careful examination will allow one to assess what muscles are functioning and which are not. Antagonist muscles are necessary to supply balance. Only expendable tendons will be included in the available list of donors. Obviously, use of a tendon transfer hinges on whether musculature with spared innervation has sufficient power so that a portion can be sacrificed or borrowed for transfer. The strength of a transferred tendon/muscle typically will lose one grade of strength after transfer. Previously denervated muscles are suboptimal for transfer, even if they have regained good function, as they may lack endurance.[36] Suitable muscles and attendant tendons must be available. For example, a patient with a brachial plexus palsy without function in forearm and wrist muscles typically may not have suitable muscles to transfer to substitute for loss of hand function, nor does the typical patient with a severe brachial plexus stretch palsy usually have suitable muscles to transfer to substitute for lack of biceps. Because of limited donors that are typically available, special care must be taken when transferring tendons. Joint fusions may increase motors that are available and can concentrate the force developed by the tendon transfer if the tendon transfer crosses multiple joints (i.e. the thumb).

Once a list of donor muscles is made, each muscle must be compared to the native muscle in terms of strength (cross-sectional muscle area), power (muscle volume), and excursion or amplitude (muscle fiber length). Ideally, the tendon transfer should be synergistic with the desired motion. Wrist extension and finger flexion are synergistic as are wrist flexion and digit extension as seen in grasp and release. For patients with a radial nerve palsy, transfer of a wrist flexor to a finger extensor would be synergistic. A single muscle should subserve a single function (one tendon – one function). The line of pull (direction of action) should be as direct as possible; occasionally, this is impossible and a pulley needs to redirect the line of pull. Use of a pulley, however, decreases strength and increases the potential for scar tissue which can diminish excursion. The point of attachment should recreate the insertion of the tendon. Optimal tension of the tendon transfer should approximate normal resting tension; tendon transfers that are too loose or too tight may function suboptimally, if at all. A technically simple procedure should be performed over a more complex one, whenever possible.

Tendon transfers should only be considered when soft tissue equilibrium exists. They should not be performed in the face of infection, edema, inflammation, unhealed bony injury, or a bad soft tissue bed. Aggressive hand therapy (or even joint releases) may be needed to improve soft tissue conditions so that tendon transfer can be performed. The limb with an injured nerve does not heal by being placed at rest for long. Early and sustained physical and occupational therapy is a must. Both the patient and the patient's family should be taught to supplement structured therapy with home exercises. In the totally paralyzed limb, range of motion activities are a necessity until recovery begins to occur. Use of direct stimulation to paralyzed muscle while awaiting recovery of peripheral nerve function has been advocated by many. To our knowledge, there is no objective or well-controlled evidence to date that the eventual result with such daily stimulation is any better than that gained from frequent passive motion of the paralyzed extremity.[31] In many cases, however, daily stimulation provides encouragement to the patient as well as his or her family, for they can see muscles contract that do not have voluntary contraction. It may also encourage an otherwise reluctant patient to attend physical therapy sessions. However, if the procedure becomes a time-consuming or painful one, it may prevent the patient from using the extremity for the functions of day-to-day living, and he or she may not even learn the substitutive and trick movements that patients learn when left to their own devices.

Timing of reconstruction is controversial. In some settings, tendon transfers may be indicated in the early weeks or months after nerve injury. On the other hand, as long as the extremity's range of motion is maintained and the limb is cared for adequately, tendon transfer or other substitutive procedures can usually be delayed until the neural regenerative process has completed itself. One must consider the level, extent, and mechanism of the injury and age of the patient. Complex reconstruction sometimes needs to be performed in a staged fashion; for example, if both flexor and extensor tendon transfers are required, a two-stage surgery is proposed.

Some prefer tendon transfers early for high injuries (e.g. radial nerve transfers) based on what may be perceived as poor outcomes with nerve reconstructions and practical limitations of effective neural regeneration from proximal injuries to distal targets. Early tendon transfers may reduce the "down time" of patients and reduce financial loss. These tendon transfers may, however, prove unnecessary if neurologic recovery occurs following neural reconstruction. Some may opt to perform transfers as "internal splints," procedures designed to provide early function, prevent deformity, and eliminate external splinting while awaiting recovery. Others prefer to perform reconstruction after recovery has maximized.

Patients must be cooperative, motivated, and well informed. In addition they must be realistic about the expectations and limitations of the proposed procedure. They must understand that tendon transfers do not improve joint contractures, edema, sensation, and neuropathic pain.

COMMON PATTERNS OF NEUROLOGIC LOSS

MEDIAN LOSS

Low median nerve palsy

Patients with a low median nerve palsy will be bothered by loss of sensation and opposition. Unfortunately, it is difficult to compensate for total loss of median-innervated sensory function. This makes an attempt at direct repair of median injury, regardless of level or extent of injury, worth a try. Further comments on sensory reinnervaton will be discussed later in the chapter.

If median nerve regeneration fails to provide satisfactory thumb opposition, several effective opponensplasty procedures are available.[16,36,40] Because thumb opposition is a complex function, various techniques have been advocated over the years using different tendons (such as the palmaris longus [Camitz], flexor digitorum superficialis [Brand], abductor digiti minimi [Huber][Fig. 20-1]; extensor indicis proprius [Burkhalter[10]], extensor carpi ulnaris [Phalen], and flexor carpi radialis [Riordan]), and various insertions into the thumb. Some of these techniques may require a tendon pulley near the pisiform, helping to reestablish a line of pull that closely mimics opposition. These procedures will fail if the line of pull is incorrectly established (Fig. 20-2) or if the first web space is contracted.

High median nerve palsy

Patients have lost flexor pollicis longus, flexor digitorum profundi to the index and/or middle digits, flexor digitorum superficialis,

and median-innervated intrinsics (especially the opponens pollicis). Less important functions are subserved by the pronator teres, palmaris longus, flexor carpi radialis, and pronator quadratus. Restoration of finger flexion and opposition are the most important functions in an effort to restore grasp and prehensile pinch. These functions can be corrected by brachioradialis transfer to the flexor pollicis longus, extensor carpi radialis longus transfer to flexor digitorum profundi to index and/or middle fingers, and extensor indicis proprius for opposition. Alternatively, side-to-side transfer of the flexor digitorum profundus of the ring and little fingers to the flexor digitorum profundus of the index and middle fingers can be performed. Proximal interphalangeal joint flexion is not essential in regaining optimal function, and a thumb interphalangeal joint fusion may also be considered in lieu of a tendon transfer.

ULNAR LOSS

Patterns of deficit vary. Some patients may not require or benefit from certain procedures, while others may depend on the resting attitude and function of the hand. Patients with low ulnar nerve lesions will experience a variable amount of clawing, loss of pinch, and weakness of grip. Profound functional loss may be attributed to diminished pinch from adductor pollicis and first dorsal interosseous muscle dysfunction.

Low ulnar nerve loss
Anti-clawing
One of the major disabilities with ulnar nerve palsy is difficulty in extending the ring finger and especially the little finger at the

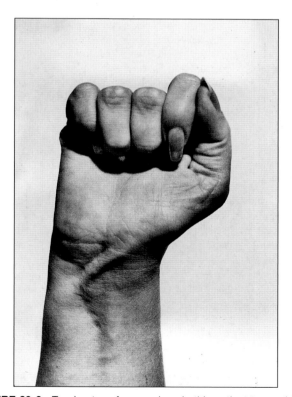

FIGURE 20-2 Tendon transfer was done in this patient to provide some abduction and opposition of the thumb for a severe median palsy. The transferred flexor digitorum superficialis tendon can be seen running subcutaneously and obliquely across the wrist. Its line of pull is suboptimal, however.

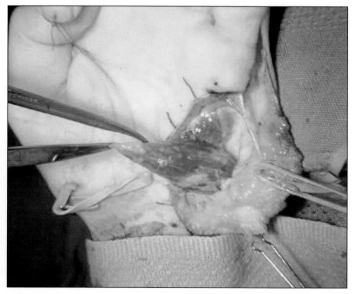

FIGURE 20-1 Huber transfer is being performed to improve opposition.

proximal interphalangeal and distal interphalangeal joints. Clawing results from the loss of intrinsic muscle function resulting in imbalance of finger extension and finger flexion. Clawing may be worse with distal ulnar nerve rather than proximal ulnar lesions because proximally innervated flexor digitorum profundi to the little and ring fingers still work and are unopposed by an effective extensor mechanism.

While clawing can be improved with splinting, patients do not use splints well. Clawing can be corrected by performing an extensor carpi radialis longus tendon extended with a four-tailed tendon graft into the lateral band of the digits (volar to the transverse metacarpal ligament) (Bunnell-Stiles technique).[40] In our experience, this technique has provided a hand with which most patients are happy regardless of whether there is significant ulnar nerve regeneration.[7,8] Such a procedure is needed for many severe ulnar lesions and should be done early enough so that fixed clawing of the fingers does not develop. Alternatively, Zancolli has described a lasso procedure using the flexor digitorum superficialis tendons to provide active flexion of the metacarpophalangeal joints.[54] A portion of the flexor digitorum superficialis is substituted for lumbrical function and is transferred through the lumbrical canals to the extensor expansions of the digits. The flexor digitorum superficialis can be extended by fascia obtained either from the plantaris or a toe flexor in the leg or the palmaris longus tendon in the forearm.

Adductorplasty

The need for performing an adductorplasty to improve key pinch is variable. A flexor digitorum superficialis tendon (middle finger preferred) can be transferred across the palm, extending and inserting into the normal adductor pollicis insertion. The extensor carpi radialis brevis or the extensor indicis proprius may also be used. A technique has been described where transfer of flexor digitorum superficialis tendons can be transferred to improve thumb adduction, improve opposition and prevent clawing.[36]

Other procedures

Other tendon transfers have been described to improve thumb–index tip pinch, restore first dorsal interosseous function or correct Wartenberg's sign. Arthrodesis of the thumb metacarpophalangeal joint may improve tip pinch.

High ulnar nerve palsy

Patient with high ulnar nerve palsy will also benefit from consideration of the procedures previously mentioned for low ulnar nerve palsy. In addition, patients with more proximal injury experience loss of little and ring finger distal interphalangeal joint flexion. This functional loss can be restored by a side-to-side transfer connecting the flexor digitorum profundus of the little and ring fingers to the index and middle fingers. Loss of flexor carpi ulnaris is not clinically important.

Sensory defects for median or ulnar nerve lesions

Nerve grafts may be successful in restoring sensation but not motor function. Some have recommended sensory nerve transfers, a procedure that has not been emphasized in the literature. As sensory recovery may occur even as long as several years after injury, this procedure should be considered. Neurocutaneous flaps, neurovascular cutaneous island pedicles, and free neurovascular cutaneous islands are other possibilities to improve sensation in the digits.

Combined palsies

Particularly difficult to treat by either reconstructive or neural operations are combined palsies, such as a combined ulnar and median palsy.[37,40] Sometimes, a combination of capsulodesis, tenodesis, tendon transfer plus arthrodesis is useful in an effort to restore grasp, pinch, and release.[30] While specific tendon transfers are similar to those performed for isolated injuries, fewer donors are available in these combined lesions, balance is harder to achieve, and more limited goals should be considered.

RADIAL LOSS

Low (posterior interosseous nerve) – finger drop

Direct neural repair is the first order of business for most serious radial injuries and is often effective. Paradoxically, tendon transfers are also much more effective for this type of neural loss than for that associated with median or ulnar nerve in cases in which nerve repairs are less successful. Loss of finger extension is easily corrected by transfer of a wrist flexor (e.g. flexor carpi radialis longus) to the digital extensors, and the palmaris longus to the extensor pollicis longus.

High radial nerve loss

High radial nerve paralysis produces severe functional deficit. Tendon transfers can be performed immediately or in a delayed fashion. Without wrist extension, grip is weakened in a palmar flexed position (Fig. 20-3). There is no extension at the metacarpophalangeal joints. In contrast, restoration of wrist extension incrementally increases grip power. Use of a dynamic splint maintaining the wrist and metacarpophalangeal joints in extension is helpful, but patients are not likely to wear them.

Transfer of median- or ulnar-innervated flexor tendons to the dorsum of the wrist and to finger and thumb extensor regions can readily provide extensor function for the limb with a radial nerve

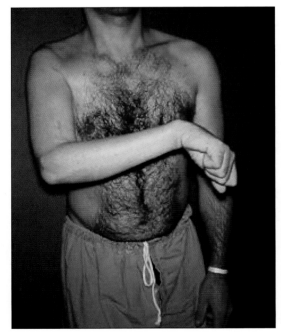

FIGURE 20-3 Wrist drop from radial nerve palsy. Grip is impaired when the wrist is held in flexion.

injury. Some workers believe that this technique can be saved until the results of nerve repair are known, especially because the radial nerve regenerates so well. Others believe just as strongly that because such a procedure is an effective substitute for radial palsy, it should be done as soon as feasible.[27,32,35] A splint or similar device is provided in the meantime to prevent contracture and to assist finger flexion. A dynamic wrist extension splint with outrigger, rubber bands, and finger slings is a particularly effective device under these circumstances (Fig. 20-4). We have usually waited and opted to have the extensor deficiencies reconstructed with tendon transfer, when recovery was incomplete or absent. However, few patients who received tendon transfers early were also pleased with their results.

Separate transfers can be accomplished to restore wrist extension, finger extension, and thumb extension. When median- and ulnar-innervated muscles are available for transfer, ample donors exist. Standard transfers include pronator teres to extensor carpi radialis brevis; flexor carpi radialis or ulnaris to extensor digitorum communis, extensor indicis proprius, and extensor digitorum minimi; and palmaris longus to extensor palmaris longus. Flexor digitorum superficialis may also be transferred to the finger extensors, or to the extensor pollicis longus when the palmaris longus is absent.

If the injury is not reparable or tendons are not available for transfer, wrist fusion in a position of slight extension is effective. Fusion places the hand in a more functional position, permitting what lumbrical function there is to extend the fingers while the median-innervated abductor pollicis brevis can pull the thumb away from the palm somewhat. Median- and ulnar-innervated flexor digitorum superficialis and profundus muscles can flex the fingers, making a fist – a function that is not very effective with wrist drop unless the wrist is provided some degree of extension.

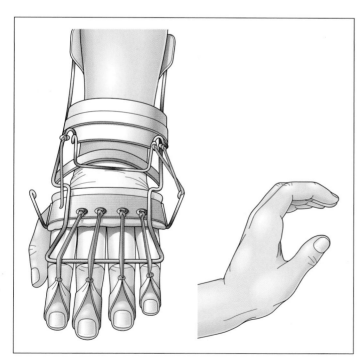

FIGURE 20-4 A brace used for radial nerve palsy, especially if median- and ulnar-innervated finger flexion is present. This is a dynamic wrist extension splint with outrigger, rubber bands, and finger pads. This brace places wrist and fingers in an optimal position (*smaller drawing*) and permits finger flexion against resistance.

Loss of brachioradialis and supinator is not usually problematic. Triceps function is not affected with midhumeral-level lesions.

Winging of the scapula
Winging of the scapula can be due to weakness of the serratus anterior, trapezius, and rhomboid muscles. The clinical presentations of these deficits appear different, are tested differently, and have been discussed elsewhere in this book. Isolated serratus anterior and trapezius dysfunction may be disabling, leading to impaired scapula stability and pain. Isolated rhomboid dysfunction is extremely rare.

Serratus anterior loss
Tendon transfer for isolated serratus anterior palsy improves scapular stability, function, and pain.[47] The sternal portion of the pectoralis major is transferred and secured to the inferior pole of the scapula. This tendon transfer decreases the winging (Fig. 20-5) and does not change the cosmetic contour of the chest wall.

Trapezius loss
Trapezius loss may be substituted for by transfer of the levator scapulae and rhomboids (Eden-Lange).[17] Results for trapezius loss and winging have not been as favorable as for serratus anterior loss.

Brachial plexus loss
Effective substitution for loss resulting from plexus injury is difficult to obtain. All too frequently, most of the muscles of the limb are severely paralyzed so that the possibilities for substitution or transfer are limited (Fig. 20-6).[34,44] To paraphrase Sterling Bunnell, a pioneer in hand surgery, "for those with nothing, even a little is a lot." Priorities for reconstruction are restoration of shoulder stability and elbow flexion.

Shoulder tendon transfer
The trapezius can be transferred to the lateral portion of the humeral head to aid abduction of the shoulder. This procedure may provide some stability and improve abduction and forward flexion of the shoulder to some degree.[41,42]

Shoulder fusion (arthrodesis)
Shoulder fusion remains a popular and frequently used reconstructive procedure, particularly for patients with severe brachial plexus palsy involving the shoulder (paralysis of deltoid and rotator cuff) when other scapular stabilizers are preserved. Some surgeons do not attempt neural reconstruction of the shoulder, opting instead to perform shoulder fusion at a later date. This approach allows axons from nerve grafts or nerve transfers to be prioritized for other functions. Many other surgeons perform shoulder fusion if neural reconstruction has been unsuccessful, and for a painful subluxated shoulder. Shoulder fusions, when properly done, do not totally fixate shoulder movement but rather permit the scapular muscles to provide improved abduction and shoulder rotation.[38] Successful shoulder fusion should retain adduction of the arm to the trunk and improve grasp. Results following this procedure are largely dependent on scapulothoracic control and are also improved with preserved pectoralis major function.[12] When performed well, shoulder fusion provides fairly predictable results, in many cases providing stability, increasing function (of abduction and forward flexion), and decreasing pain.

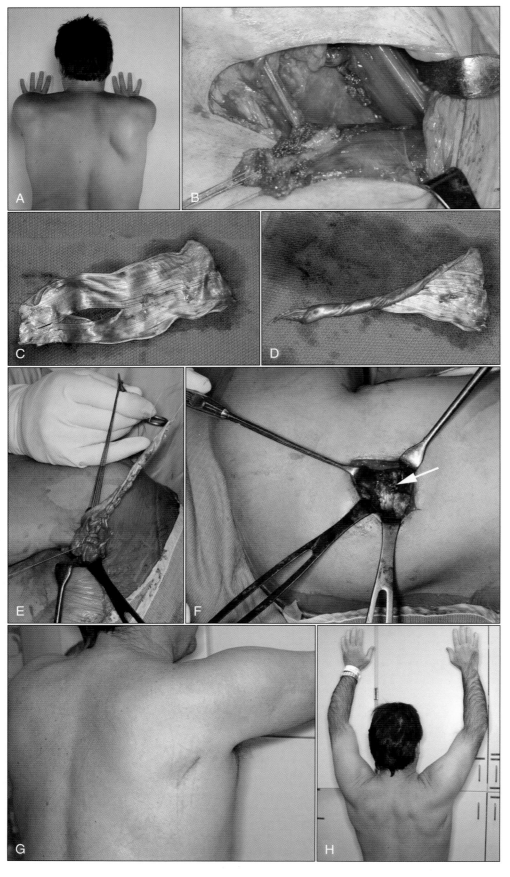

FIGURE 20-5 Winged scapula.
(A) Preoperative winging secondary to long-standing isolated serratus anterior paralysis. **(B)** The hemipectoralis major muscle is mobilized through an axillary incision. **(C)** Fascia lata is harvested and entubulated **(D)**. **(E)** The fascia lata graft is woven into the pectoralis major tendon. **(F)** The tendon graft is sutured to the inferior portion of the scapula spine which was exposed through a second incision. **(G)** The healed posterior incision is seen. The winging has been eliminated. **(H)** Postoperatively, full motion has nearly been restored.

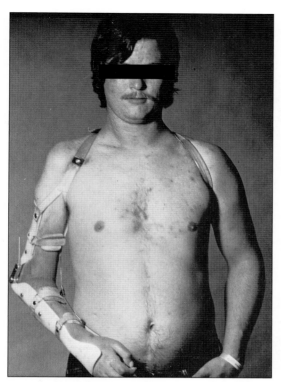

FIGURE 20-6 Some patients find an orthosis of help during the period of waiting for nerve regeneration after plexus injury; others refuse to wear either orthoses or prostheses with any consistency.

In cases where elbow flexion is restored but shoulder function has not been, shoulder fusion can improve function by placing the limb in a better position. For those with upper pattern loss, shoulder fusion may facilitate hand function, if elbow flexion is restored.[28,29,39,52] Shoulder fusion is most valuable if biceps/brachialis works or also can be substituted for, because provision of a more functional shoulder makes elbow flexion more useful. Some advocate shoulder fusion for patients with flail limbs.[20] It may also be useful to those who have undergone transhumeral amputation who use a prosthesis.

The optimal position for fusion remains controversial; many choose 30° abduction, 30° flexion, and 30° internal rotation. Various techniques have been described including external fixation, internal fixation (Fig. 20-7), and a combination of both.

Elbow flexorplasty

Restoration of elbow flexion is perhaps the highest priority in patients with brachial plexus lesions. For patients with incomplete lesions, several options exist for muscle or tendon transfer: pectoralis major[11,15] (Fig. 20-8) (± minor transfer), latissimus dorsi transfer (Fig. 20-9), triceps transfer (Fig. 20-10), and Steindler flexorplasty[4] (Fig. 20-11). Free functioning muscle transfer can be performed in incomplete and complete lesions (see Figs 20-12 to 20-16). All of these procedures have advantages and disadvantages, and proponents.

Substitution for absent and irrecoverable biceps/brachialis function is a possibility if either sufficient pectoralis major or latissimus dorsi is preserved and can be moved to the elbow region.[55] Unfortunately, most brachial plexus injuries severe enough to result in total loss of biceps are usually too extensive in regard to neural input to pectoralis major or latissimus dorsi to permit their transfer.

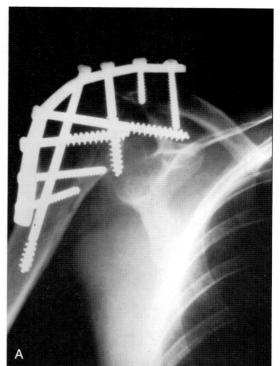
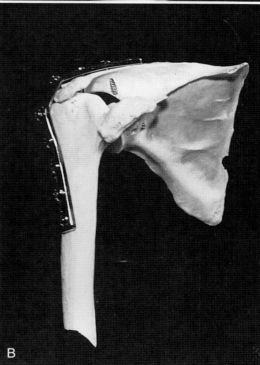

FIGURE 20-7 (A, B) Glenohumeral joint fusion can be useful in cases of poor abduction after irreparable or failed repair of outflow to axillary nerve. Patients obtain proximal control by way of trapezius, serratus anterior, and, if not part of the pattern of paralysis, latissimus dorsi and pectoralis major muscles. This procedure is especially useful if there is return of biceps or brachioradialis but not shoulder abduction, and especially if hand function is spared or recovers but proximal muscles do not.

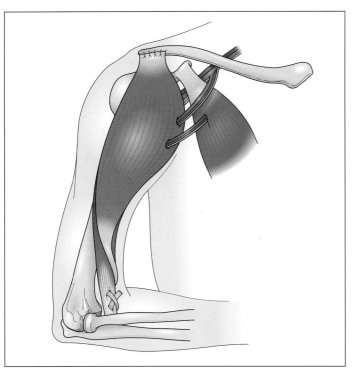

FIGURE 20-8 Pectoralis major transfer. (Copyrighted and used with the permission of Mayo Foundation for Medical Education Research)

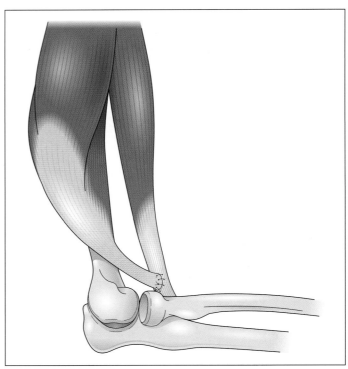

FIGURE 20-10 Anterior triceps transfer. (Copyrighted and used with the permission of Mayo Foundation for Medical Education Research)

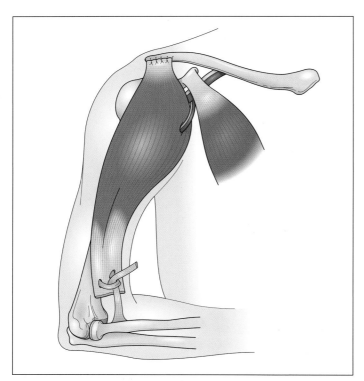

FIGURE 20-9 Latissimus dorsi transfer. (Copyrighted and used with the permission of Mayo Foundation for Medical Education Research)

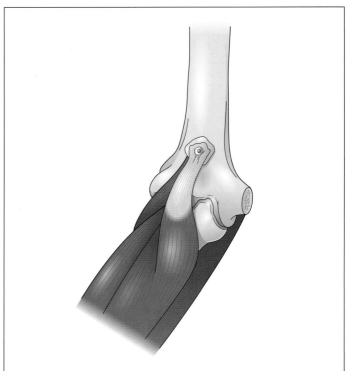

FIGURE 20-11 Steindler flexorplasty drawing. (Copyrighted and used with the permission of Mayo Foundation for Medical Education Research)

These transfers are technically demanding and are most commonly performed in a bipolar transfer. Use of the pectoralis major may diminish trunk prehension whereas functional loss from use of the latissimus dorsi is relatively limited. Transfer of the pectoralis major is cosmetically disfiguring to women. Both of these transfers have the potential for good strength, although the results are less predictable and somewhat inconsistent compared to the triceps transfer. The latissimus dorsi should not be considered as a potential source for a flexorplasty if external rotation is also considered a realistic goal as part of additional soft tissue reconstruction for

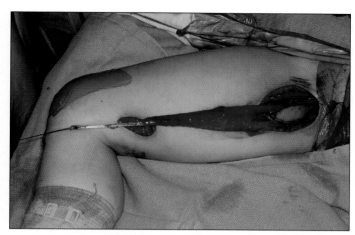

FIGURE 20-12 A gracilis muscle is being harvested. Note the long tendon which will allow distal connection. The neurovascular pedicle is located proximally. The skin paddle is useful to monitor the flap postoperatively.

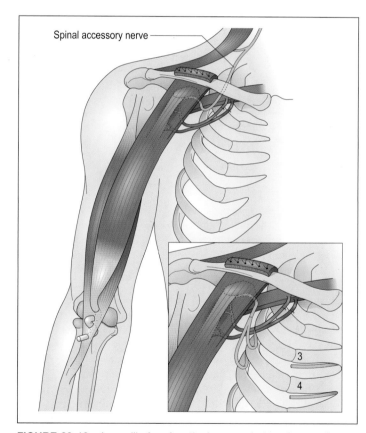

Spinal accessory nerve

FIGURE 20-13 A gracilis free functioning muscle transfer may be used to restore elbow flexion, even in late cases. It is neurotized by the spinal accessory nerve or intercostal nerves most commonly. The vascular repairs are done to the thoracoacromial vessels. (Copyrighted and used with the permission of Mayo Foundation for Medical Education Research)

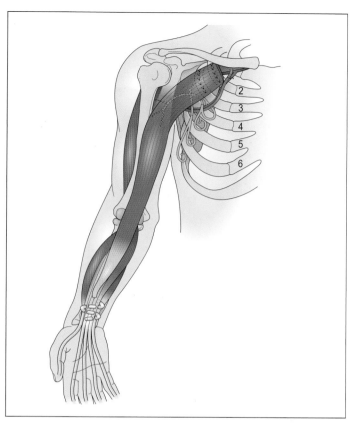

FIGURE 20-14 A gracilis free functioning transfer can be done to restore finger flexion as well. Here intercostal nerves neurotize the muscle and the vascular repair is done to the thoracodorsal vessels. (Copyrighted and used with the permission of Mayo Foundation for Medical Education Research)

which the latissimus dorsi might be transferred. The latissimus dorsi can also be transferred to allow soft tissue coverage as well as provide functional reconstruction.

Anterior triceps transfer can produce strong elbow flexion when triceps is strong. The procedure is relatively straightforward. When triceps function is strong, this elbow flexorplasty is reliable. The procedure is advantageous when biceps/triceps co-contraction exist. Loss of elbow extension is compensated by patient's use of gravity. Those patients with lower limb problems or who use assistive devices need triceps function.

A Steindler flexorplasty in which the flexor-pronator mass is moved proximal to the elbow can be effective if the flexor-pronator group of muscles are innervated, but this is often not the case in more severe injuries. An obvious exception is provided by the occasional C5–C6 stretch injury that does not result in useful elbow flexion from spontaneous reinnervation or after neural reconstruction. Technically, this flexorplasty is fairly simple to perform, and there is minimal donor deficit. When forearm flexors are spared or minimally involved, a flexorplasty may work well. Results are dependent on preoperative grip strength.[3] It seems to augment function better than restore function. It may result in a pronation and flexion contracture (Steindler effect). Ulnar nerve and median nerve compression have been described as complications of the procedure and these nerves should be protected.

Several other procedures have been described, including sterno-mastoid transfer, but are seldom performed.

Free functioning muscle transfer can be considered to reconstruct critical function when other options for conventional muscle/tendon transfer are unavailable.[14,33] It can be done late or early as part of a reconstructive scheme. Results are not time-dependent. It can be performed in adults and children.[24] Although technically demanding, a muscle with its neurovascular pedicle can be

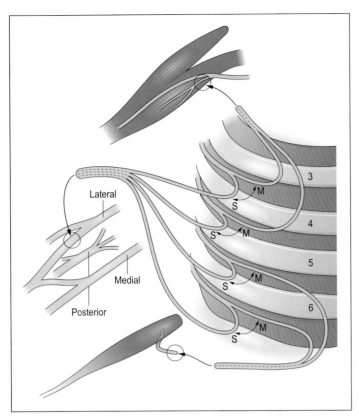

FIGURE 20-15 In a second-stage free functioning muscle transfer, motor intercostals supply the triceps and the free muscle and sensory intercostals are connected to the lateral cord contribution of the median nerve. (Copyrighted and used with the permission of Mayo Foundation for Medical Education Research)

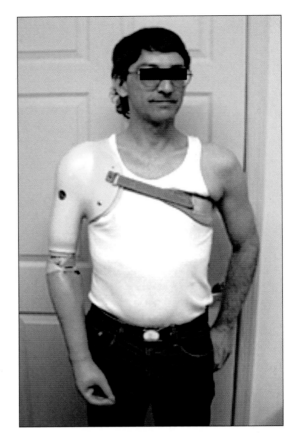

FIGURE 20-16 A transhumeral amputation was performed in this patient with a flail limb.

transferred to a new site to provide a new function. A requisite is an available motor nerve to innervate the free muscle and adequate arterial and venous supply. The gracilis muscle, among other muscles, has been used for this purpose. The design of the free functioning muscle transfer is based on the proximal neurovascular pedicle and the length of the muscle and distal tendon; these anatomic arrangements allow rapid reinnervation and restoration of more distal function (Fig. 20-13). Harvesting the muscle with a skin paddle allows monitoring of the flap postoperatively.

In the upper limb, free functioning muscle transfer is being used increasingly to supply elbow flexion (Fig. 20-12). The gracilis muscle is anchored to the clavicle and passed subcutaneously in the arm and connected to the biceps tendon in the antecubital fossa. In addition, the gracilis tendon can be passed more distally, allowing wrist extension combined with elbow flexion;[1] the ultimate strength may be diminished when the muscle is used to perform two separate functions.[2] The free functioning muscle transfer may be innervated by the spinal accessory nerve, intercostal nerves, or an ulnar nerve fascicular group.[25] The vascular repair is to the thoracoacromial vessels. Outcomes have been favorable in the reliable restoration of elbow flexion. Reinnervation usually begins by 3–6 months with maximal recovery achieved by 18 months.

Free functioning muscle transfer may also be performed to allow finger flexion (Fig. 20-14). The muscle is anchored to the second rib and passed subcutaneously down the arm and sutured to the flexor digitorum profundi and flexor pollicis longus in the forearm.

This free functioning muscle transfer is innervated by intercostals and supplied by the thoracodorsal vessels.

A double muscle transfer combining these two transfers may be done in a staged fashion. Doi has introduced and popularized combining two free muscle transfers for patients to achieve hand prehension, even in patients with 4 or 5 nerve root avulsions. Surgery must be performed by 6 months post injury.[18] This combination of procedures uses nerve grafts when there is a functioning proximal cervical root, nerve transfers, and free musle transfer to provide a stable shoulder,[19] elbow flexion and extension, hand prehension, and sensation. Nerve transfers may include the spinal accessory nerve, intercostal nerves, phrenic nerve, and contralateral C7. The first procedure entails brachial plexus exploration and nerve reconstruction of shoulder function. A free functioning muscle transfer is done for elbow flexion and finger extension neurotized by the spinal accessory nerve. At a second stage, four intercostal nerves are typically used. Two intercostal motor nerves power a free functioning muscle transfer to the finger flexors; two motor intercostals supply the triceps. Sensory intercostals are used to supply nerves in the hand (Fig. 20-15).

Elbow extension

Restoration of elbow extension with tendon transfer is performed relatively seldom in brachial plexus injuries. Techniques have been described using the latissimus dorsi or posterior deltoid as a tendon transfer (but associated shoulder weakness/paralysis limits its use), or occasionally, free functioning muscle transfer.

C5, C6, C7 pattern (C8, T1 spared)

In addition to shoulder and elbow reconstruction, which has been discussed, patients with sparing of C8 and T1 may have opportunities for tendon transfer: examples may include pronator teres (or flexor digitorum superficialis) to extensor carpi radialis brevis, flexor carpi ulnaris to extensor digitorum communis, and palmaris longus to extensor pollicis longus.

C8, T1 pattern loss

Judicious reconstruction may allow grasp and prehensile grip in patients with C8, T1 loss. Splinting may maintain position or correct the deformity. Some useful hand function can be provided with tendon transfer (brachioradialis, brachialis, and extensor carpi radialis longus are potentially available), tenodesis, and thumb fusion. Potential combinations include brachioradialis to flexor pollicis longus; extensor carpi radialis longus to flexor digitorum profundi (index through little fingers); thumb interphalangeal joint fusion, perhaps in combination with a Zancolli passive tenodesis. Free functioning muscle transfer can also be considered.

Amputation

Amputation is seldom performed. The question of amputation arises frequently with patients with severe neuropathic pain. Patients should be aware that neuropathic pain is not relieved by amputation, although it may help patients with some mechanical symptoms related to shoulder instability. Some other patients with severe, irreparable brachial plexus injuries, but with some proximal shoulder and upper arm sparing, may use a prosthesis (Fig. 20-16), but regular use of the prosthesis is typically poor. The more distal the amputation site, the more useful the prosthesis is and the more likely it is that the amputee will use it (Fig. 20-17). In general, even if the outlook is extremely poor for recovery, we usually wait for several years before having patients seriously consider amputation. Before this is done, every attempt should be made to restore shoulder and upper arm function so that the amputation can be as distal as possible.[52] Prior to the amputation, we encourage patients to meet with a reconstructive surgeon to ensure that all secondary procedures are considered as well as a prosthetist who specializes in amputees. By this time, it is clear to all, including the patient, that there is no hope for further recovery. Still some patients with flail arms opt for relatively early amputation of the limb, which they view as a useless impediment. Earlier amputation may be indicated if severe nerve injury is also associated with significant vascular, soft tissue, or bony injury or infection.[51]

Sequelae from obstetrical brachial plexopathy

Sequelae from obstetrical palsy include internal rotation contracture of the shoulder and weakness of shoulder external rotation and abduction. These deficits may result in significant functional limitations. Multiple surgical procedures have been described to improve active movement in the shoulder. Subscapularis muscle release or lengthening may improve the internal rotation contracture. Transfer of the conjoint tendon of the latissimus dorsi and teres major to the rotator cuff may improve abduction and external rotation (Fig. 20-18). Derotational humeral osteomy may also allow external rotation when other active methods are unavailable. Shoulder joint deformities and incongruence also need to be addressed, at times with bony procedures. Elbow deficiencies can be addressed with a variety of procedures, many of which have been previously described in this chapter. Forearm deformities are

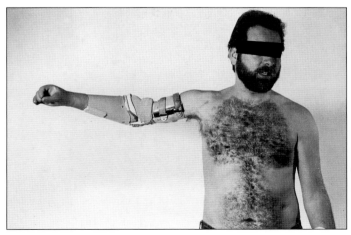

FIGURE 20-17 This patient with a flail arm had successful restoration of shoulder and biceps function by graft repair of the upper elements of the brachial plexus. Lower elements were torn out of their foramina and could not be repaired. As a result, he had a forearm-level amputation and was then fitted with a prosthesis.

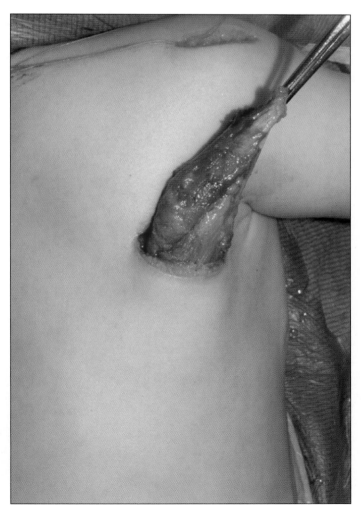

FIGURE 20-18 Latissimus dorsi/teres major tendon transfer performed as a secondary procedure in this child with sequelae from obstetrical brachial plexus palsy. This transfer can improve shoulder abduction and external rotation.

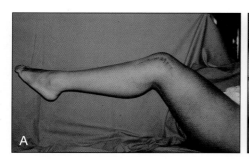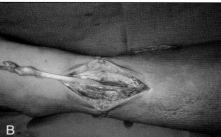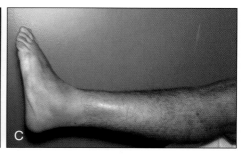

FIGURE 20-19 **(A)** Peroneal nerve palsy and footdrop. **(B)** Posterior tibialis tendon is harvested for anterior transfer. **(C)** Postoperatively, this patient regained foot dorsiflexion to neutral and did not require an ankle foot orthosis.

also common. Supination contracture may be treated with biceps rerouting, if the forearm is passively correctable. Similarly, pronation contracture may be treated by pronator rerouting. Fixed deformities can be corrected by forearm osteotomy. Restoration of grasp may be restored by tendon transfer, tenodeses, and free muscle transfers.

LOWER EXTREMITY NEURAL LOSS

Footdrop deformity results in gait abnormalities that are disabling. Some people function fairly well using a high-top shoe. Gait can be improved by patients' use of an ankle foot orthosis or a spring-loaded kick-up foot brace. Many patients function quite well with these orthoses and do not wish anything further to de done about their foot drop;[50] others, however, find these orthoses cumbersome, do not use them, and wish tendon transfer.

Several reconstructive procedures have been recommended to provide dorsiflexion of the foot for footdrop if this is lost due to peroneal palsy. The bridle procedure involves passing the tibialis posterior tendon through a split in the tibialis anterior to be inserted into the second cuneiform; the peroneus longus is rerouted anterior to the lateral malleolus. Unfortunately, anterior transfer of the posterior tibialis tendon is difficult to achieve in a balanced fashion and tends not to hold up in some patients who are large in stature and heavy in weight (Fig. 20-19).[5] Nonetheless, some workers with extensive experience with the lower extremity,[53] such as Birch or Millesi, have success with such a transfer and may even do this at the time of peroneal nerve repair if outlook for predicted neural recovery is limited. Unfortunately, this procedure can not be performed in many sciatic nerve or L5 lesions where footdrop is accompanied by weakness in posterior tibialis function.

Fusion at the ankle level also works better in small, light individuals than in the heavier-set persons. If both peroneal- and tibial-innervated muscles are lost, triple arthrodesis of the ankle is sometimes necessary to provide as stable a foot or base for walking as possible.

Substitution for tibial nerve loss is not satisfactory because provision of powerful enough plantar flexion to step off or walk more normally cannot be provided adequately by transfer of extensor tendons. With tibial sensory loss, great attention needs to be given to protection of the insensitive foot.[9] This may require a customized shoe or shoe insert. The major effort, though, must be directed toward educating the patient regarding the insensate foot, how to avoid injury to it, and how to inspect the foot for injury and skin changes. Tibial nerve reconstruction via nerve grafting or newer techniques of nerve transfer may restore protective sensation, even when performed late.

Reconstructive procedures available for patients with complete femoral nerve palsy are limited. Fusion of the knee in extension is not a very satisfactory substitute for a functional quadriceps. Similarly, braces to stabilize the knee and thigh are bulky, uncomfortable, and expensive and often are not worn by the patient. Some attempt at repair of the femoral nerve should be made whenever possible. The hamstrings may be transferred anteriorly for paralysis of knee extensors.

COMPLICATIONS

Complications can occur after these procedures. Infection, adhesion, and rupture may result. Tendon transfers may not function or may function suboptimally due to poor tensioning (under- or overtightening). Tendon transfers may produce awkward positioning which is deleterious. Nerve compression may result from the dissection, scarring, or tendon rupture.[45,46,48] Nerve injury has been reported after osteotomies. Nonunion, malunion, and fracture may occur after fusions. Flap failure is seen acutely in approximately 10% of free functioning muscle transfers.

CONCLUSION

The spectrum of secondary reconstruction is broad and offers patients many options to improve function. Successful surgery is dependent on the surgeon's understanding of anatomic and biomechanical principles and thoughtful rehabilitation. Results are often rewarding for the experienced surgeon, dedicated therapist, and the motivated patient.

REFERENCES

1. Akasaka Y, Hara T, and Takahashi M: Free muscle transplantation combined with intercostals nerve crossing for reconstruction of elbow flexion and wrist extension in brachial plexus injuries. Microsurgery 12:346–351, 1991.
2. Barrie KA, Steinmann SP, Shin AY, et al.: Gracilis free muscle transfer for restoration of function after complete brachial plexus avulsion. Neurosurgery Focus 16(5);E8, 2004.
3. Beaton DE, Dumont A, Mackay MB, et al.: Steindler and pectoralis major flexorplasty: a comparative analysis. J Hand Surg 20A:747–756, 1995.
4. Botte M and Wood MB: Flexorplasty of the elbow. Clin Orthop 245:110–116, 1989.
5. Bourrel P: Transfer of the tibialis posterior to the tibialis anterior, and of flexor hallucis longus to the extensor digitorum longus in peroneal palsy. Ann Chir 21:1451–1456, 1967.

6. Boyes JH: Bunnell's Surgery of the Hand, 5th edn. Philadelphia, JB Lippincott, 1970.

7. Brand P: Tendon transfers in the forearm. In: Flynn J, Ed: Hand Surgery. Baltimore, Williams & Wilkins, 1966:331–342.

8. Brand PW: Tendon transfers for median and ulnar nerve paralysis. Ortho Clin N Am 1:447–454, 1970.

9. Brand P and Ebner JD: Pressure sensitive devices for denervated hands and feet. J Bone Joint Surg 51A:109–116, 1969.

10. Burkhalter W, Christensen RC, and Brown P: Extensor indicis proprius opponensplasty. J Bone Joint Surg 55A:725–732, 1973.

11. Carroll RE and Kleinman WB: Pectoralis major transplantation to restore elbow flexion to the paralytic limb. J Hand Surg 4A:501–507, 1979.

12. Chammas M, Goubier JN, Coulet B, et al.: Glenohumeral arthrodesis in upper and total brachial plexus palsy. A comparison of functional results. J Bone Joint Surg 86B:692–695, 2004.

13. Chase RA: Atlas of Hand Surgery. Philadelphia, WB Saunders, 1984.

14. Chung DC, Carver N, and Wei FC: Results of functioning free muscle transplantation for elbow flexion. J Hand Surg 21A:1071–1077, 1996.

15. Clark JMP: Reconstruction of the biceps brachii by pectoral muscle transplantation. Br J Surg 34:180–181, 1946.

16. Cooney WP: Tendon transfer for median nerve palsy. Hand Clin 4:155–165, 1988.

17. Coessens BC and Wood MB: Levator scapulae transfer and fascia lata fasciodesis for chronic spinal accessory nerve palsy. J Reconstr Microsurg 11:277–280, 1995.

18. Doi K, Muramatsu K, Hattori Y, et al.: Restoration of prehension with the double free muscle technique following complete avulsion of the brachial plexus. Indications and long-term results. J Bone Joint Surg 82A:652–666, 2000.

19. Doi K, Hattori Y, Ikeda K, et al.: Significance of shoulder function in the reconstruction of prehension with double free-muscle transfer after complete paralysis of the brachial plexus. Plast Reconstr Surg 112:1596–1603, 2003.

20. Emmelot CH, Nielsen HK, and Eisma WH: Shoulder fusion for paralyzed upper limb. Clin Orthop 340:95–101, 1997.

21. Gelberman R, Ed: Operative Nerve Repair and Reconstruction. Philadelphia, JB Lippincott, 1991.

22. Goldner JL: Function of the hand following peripheral nerve injuries. American Academy of Orthopedic Surgeons Instruction Course Lectures 10. Ann Arbor, Michigan, JW Edmonds, 1953:268.

23. Green DP: Operative Hand Surgery. New York, Churchill Livingstone, 1988.

24. Hattori Y, Doi K, Ikeda K, et al.: Restoration of prehension using double free muscle technique after complete avulsion of brachial plexus in children: a report of three cases. J Hand Surg 30A:812–819, 2005.

25. Hattori Y, Doi K, and Baliarsing AS: A part of the ulnar nerve as an alternative donor nerve for functioning free muscle transfer: a case report. J Hand Surg 27A:150–153, 2002.

26. Jupiter J, Ed: Flynn's Hand Surgery. Baltimore, Williams & Wilkins, 1991.

27. Kettlekamp DB and Alexander H: Clinical review of radial nerve injury. J Trauma 7:424–432, 1967.

28. Leffert R: Brachial Plexus Injuries. London, Churchill Livingstone, 1985.

29. Leffert R: Reconstruction of the shoulder and elbow following brachial plexus injury. In: Omer GE and Spinner M, Eds: Management of Peripheral Nerve Problems. Philadelphia, WB Saunders, 1980.

30. Littler JW: Tendon transfer and arthrodesis in combined median and ulnar nerve paralysis. J Bone Joint Surg 31A:225–234, 1949.

31. Liu CT and Lewey FH: The effect of surging currents of low frequency in man on atrophy of denervated muscles. J Nerve Ment Dis 105:571–581, 1947.

32. Mackinnon SE and Dellon AL: Surgery of the Peripheral Nerve. New York, Thieme Medical Publishers, 1988.

33. Manktelow RT, Zuker RM, and McKee NH: Functioning free muscle transplantation. J Hand Surg 9A:32–39, 1984.

34. Narakas A: Thoughts on neurotization or nerve transfers in irreparable nerve lesions. Clin Plast Surg 11:153–159, 1984.

35. Omer GE: Evaluation and reconstruction of forearm and hand after acute traumatic peripheral nerve injuries. J Bone Joint Surg 50A:1454–1460, 1968.

36. Omer GE: Tendon transfers for the reconstruction of the forearm and hand following peripheral nerve injuries. In: Omer GE and Spinner M, Eds: Management of Peripheral Nerve Problems. Philadelphia, WB Saunders, 1980.

37. Omer GE: Tendon transfers for combined traumatic nerve palsies of the forearm and hand. J Hand Surg 17B:603–610, 1992.

38. Richards RR: Operative treatment for irreparable lesions of the brachial plexus. In: Gelberman R, Ed: Operative Nerve Repair and Reconstruction. Philadelphia, JB Lippincott, 1991.

39. Richards RR, Sherman RM, Hudson AR, et al.: Shoulder arthrodesis using a pelvic reconstruction plate: A report of 11 cases. J Bone Joint Surg 70A:416–421, 1988.

40. Riordan DC: Tendon transplantations in median nerve and ulnar nerve paralysis. J Bone Joint Surg 35A: 312–320, 1953.

41. Ruhmann O, Wirth CJ, and Gosse F: [Secondary operations for improving shoulder function after brachial plexus lesion]. Zeitschrift fur Orthopadie und Ihre Grenzgebiete 137:301–309, 1999.

42. Ruhmann O, Schmolke S, Bohnsack M, et al.: Trapezius transfer in brachial plexus palsy. Correlation of the outcome with muscle power and operative technique. J Bone Joint Surg 87B:184–190, 2005.

43. Seddon HJ: Surgical Disorders of the Peripheral Nerves. Baltimore, Williams & Wilkins, 1972.

44. Simard J and Sypert G: Closed traction avulsion injuries of the brachial plexus. Contemp Neurosurg 50:1–6, 1983.

45. Spinner RJ, Nunley JA, Lins RE, et al.: Median nerve palsy presenting as absent elbow flexion: a result of a ruptured pectoralis major to biceps tendon transfer. J South Ortho Assn 8:105–107, 1999.

46. Spinner, RJ and Spinner M: Superficial radial nerve compression following flexor digitorum superficialis opposition transfer. J Hand Surg 21A:1091–1093, 1996.

47. Steinmann SP and Wood MB: Pectoralis major transfer for serratus anterior paralysis. J Should Elbow Surg 12:555–560, 2003.

48. Tomaino NM and Wasko MC: Ulnar nerve compression following flexor digitorum superficialis tendon transfers around the ulnar border of the forearm to restore digital extension: case report. J Hand Surg 23A:296–299, 1998.

49. Tubiana R: The Hand, vol. 2. Philadelphia, WB Saunders, 1985.

50. White JC: The results of traction injuries to the common peroneal nerve. J Bone Joint Surg 40B:346–351, 1968.

51. Wilkinson MC, Birch R, and Bonney G: Brachial plexus injury: when to amputate? Injury 24:603–605, 1993.

52. Wynn-Parry CB: The management of traction lesions of the brachial plexus and peripheral nerve injuries to the upper limb: A study in teamwork. Injury 11:265–285, 1980.

53. Yeap JS, Birch R, and Singh D: Long-term results of tibialis posterior tendon transfer for drop-foot. Int Orthop 25:114–118, 2001.

54. Zancolli E: Structural and Dynamic Basis of Hand Surgery. Philadelphia, JB Lippincott, 1979.

55. Zancolli E and Mitre H: Latissimus dorsi transfer to restore elbow flexion. J Bone Joint Surg 55A:1265–1272, 1973.

21

Pain of nerve origin

David G. Kline and Ronald R. Tasker

GENERAL PRINCIPLES

Pain connected with peripheral nerve disease and/or injury is not always treatable by resection of the related nerve or by its repair even though the pain may have originated there.[11,41] Having said that, sometimes it is and that is one of the many challenges connected with nerve disorders, as selection of a case for either neurectomy or repair is not easy, and there is not a fail-safe recipe for such selections.[37,38,49,55,71] Those pain patterns more likely helped by a direct inspection and/or repair are usually associated with local findings. In this regard, some important questions need to be answered:

1. Is the pain in a peripheral nerve distribution?
2. Is there sensory motor, and/or autonomic loss associated with the pain? Are there spontaneous paresthesias or sensory symptoms in that distribution?[39,40]
3. Is there a Tinel sign when the nerve is percussed and does that Tinel sign give paresthesias in the distribution of the nerve?
4. Does anesthetic block of the nerve alleviate the pain?

If most of these criteria are met, then resection of the involved nerve, if it is a relatively small sensory one such as sural, saphenous, lateral femoral cutaneous or antebrachial cutaneous nerve, may alleviate the pain. If the nerve is larger and a mixed motor-sensory one, then neurolysis, nerve action potential (NAP) recordings, and repair if indicated by the latter may be of help for the pain.

Some other generalities about peripheral nerve pain can be cited.

- Identification of the source or potential source of the pain is very important and not always easy. Even surgical exploration of the potential pain source does not prove that it is the potential generator, unless its elimination or alteration gives long-standing pain relief. Put another way, at exploration there is no structure that "sends out signals" that say "I'm the source of the pain" for the peripheral nerve surgeon. This makes it especially important to try to localize the nerve or nerves involved in the pain problem.

- Milder pain problems can sometimes be satisfactorily treated by analgesics alone. However, if there is an element of neuritic or neuropathic pain with symptoms of burning paresthesias, electric shocks, and often some degree of allodynia, drugs more appropriate for these symptoms are necessary. Such medications include gabopentin (Neurontin), Mexitil, amitryptiline (Elavil), Keppra, and more recently Zymbalata developed for painful diabetic neuropathy. Important in the use of a medication such as gabopentin is to gradually increase its dosage. It is also important that the medication be used daily, and not as a p.r.n. dose. For an adult, a dosage of 1200–1800 mg/day is usually required. We usually begin with 300 mg b.i.d., and after 2 days increase that to t.i.d., and then after another 3 days to t.i.d. and h.s. We then hold the dose there for a few days to see if there is improvement in neuritic symptoms. If not, the dose is slowly increased to 1800–2400 mg/day. In this fashion, some of the side effects such as sedation, dizziness, and nausea may be reduced. These medications are particularly helpful for postoperative paresthesias, especially after tumor removal or internal manipulation of a nerve where a partial or split repair is done.

- There is usually no contradiction to using other analgesic medications in addition to the above antineuritic ones. Sometimes, however, the dosage of these or the other medications altogether can be reduced or eliminated as adequate levels of antineuritic medications are achieved.

- Must be kept in mind that the only true witness to pain is the patient himself of herself. Methods devised to measure pain are available but still rely heavily on each patient's description of it.[32,51,55,59]

- There is always the fear of addiction or its consequences even though a major responsibly for all physicians is the relief of pain and suffering. The physician treating pain of peripheral nerve origin must walk a fine line between effective pain control and too much sedation as well as addiction. In general I believe we err in favor of pain relief but readily admit that we are not uniformly successful in this since both the personality of the patient and the circumstances surrounding the disorder help to shape decisions about not only the medications to be used but also their dosages. The psychologic aspects of pain are immense and can mislead the unwary or inexperienced clinician. Although seen most obviously in patients with paralyzed limbs without an anatomic or physiologic etiology, conversion hysteria can have its concomitant in a painful disorder which is truly nonexistent.[56,67]

- The more severe patterns connected with pain of nerve origin usually require surgical answers. As pointed out by Birch and others where there is pain coupled with severe loss of function, and especially loss of motor movement, restoration of movement even in small amounts may help to reduce or eliminate pain.[4,5,73,74] This is perhaps best demonstrated by the patient with severe loss of upper extremity function due to a plexus stretch injury and also pain referred to the limb. Sometimes, restoration of a little shoulder or elbow motion and/or wrist motion appears to diminish the pain, presumably by providing increased afferent input from the otherwise paretic limb to compete centrally with painful impulses referred from the periphery or perhaps from circuits already set up centrally.[10,64,65]

NEUROMA PAIN

If pain is felt to originate from or be associated with an injured peripheral sensory nerve, neurectomy can sometimes help or even cure the pain. The alternative would be to repair such a lesion and hope that with regeneration the pain would be helped. The trouble is that such regeneration is often disordered and associated with axonal branching or division and a confusion of fiber regrowth which can result in a painful neuroma in continuity even though initially the pain is helped by the resection (Fig. 21-1).

The alternative is to resect the lesion and, since some sensory nerves do not supply important useful territories, not repair the nerve. This is a neurectomy. Our preferences under these circumstances are to:

1. Resect both a length of nerve to include not only the lesion or injury site but several inches of nerve proximally and distally. Removing a length of nerve distally may decrease the

neurochemical signaling which attracts proximal axons to regenerate and thus reduce the tendency for recreation of a neuroma.

2. By injection of a local anesthetic proximal to the resection site prior to resection, one may decrease the volley of peripheral to central firing associated with the secondary injury required to remove the primary injury. This may or may not help to decrease the possibility of setting up centrally another pain-oriented circuit.

3. The fine tipped bipolars forceps are used "to seal over" the exposed proximal fascicles. This step may decrease the tendency for a new neuroma to form and, if it does not, perhaps to increase the time it takes for this to occur.

4. It is important to place the residual proximal stump deep to the subcutaneous space, hopefully beneath a layer of muscle and/or fascia.[15,27]

This type of approach for sensory neuromas appears to work best for sural, saphenous, antebrachial cutaneous, dorsal cutaneous branch of the ulnar, and some distal superficial peroneal branch injuries as well as for some less superficial sensory radial and digital nerve injuries.

It should be kept in mind though that not all neuromas, whether in continuity or not, are painful. What factor(s) might make one painful and the other has not been a focus for research in our own unit in recent years.[16,21,22] Research concerning other neurochemical entities done elsewhere over the years has, of course, been extensive.[1,2,66] Much of this metabolic work has been nicely reviewed by Birch, Bonney, and Wynn Parry more recently in their excellent text.[5]

The importance of the balance of afferent feedback from the periphery to the central nervous system (CNS) and the role of disorder of that in not only producing pain but in setting up central pain-generating circuits has received widespread interest both in terms of potential pain mechanisms and also reference to treatment. This literature is immense.[12,13,18,31,47,58,65,69,70] The similarity of such disorders to pain of central origin has been noted for some time, and that fact is re-emphasized in the treatise by Tasker at the

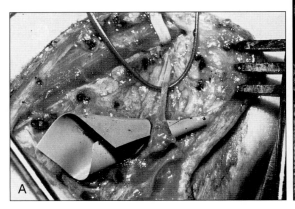
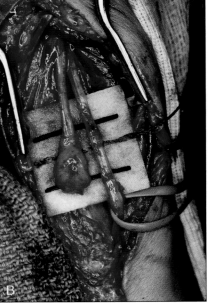

FIGURE 21-1 (A) Neuroma on a sensory portion of the cervical plexus due to a laceration. The patient had pain and paresthesias whenever this portion of the neck was bumped or stroked. **(B)** Neuroma on dorsal cutaneous nerve at the forearm level due to a lacerating injury. Remainder of ulnar nerve is to the right and is headed towards Guyon's canal. After resection, proximal nerve was trimmed sharply and fasciculi were grasped with fine-tip bipolar forceps and coagulated in an attempt to seal them shut. The freshly trimmed stump was left deep to the flexor carpi ulnaris.

end of the chapter.[10,43,45] Even the pathways for such pain transmission have received extensive reinvestigation [5,30]

In our experience, and that of others, methods to treat painful neuromas frequently fail.[41,63] Certainly a large number of diverse procedures have been recommended.[19,28,37,57,62] Some of these include placing the proximal stump after removal of the injury or neuroma into a drill hole in adjacent bone. Neuroma forms not at the tip of the implanted proximal stump but just proximal to the implanted stump and over a variable length of the nerve before it enters bone. Axoplasm can not escape well at the end of the implanted proximal stump but backs up into more proximal nerve. In addition, regenerative nerve fibers tend to "back up" and form a "new neuroma" more proximally. Other measures which are even more destructive to nerve such as ligation of the proximal stump with either resorbable or non-resorbable suture material, or injection of the proximal stump with formaldehyde or phenol, although of temporal value eventually lead to more rather than less neuroma. Even the idea of turning back and suturing the fascicles of the proximal stump to one another seems to fail frequently as does capping the proximal stump with silastic or other material. Harvest of veins that are closed at one end and then used to cap the nerve stump also can fail. Such procedures seem to introduce foreign material which the divided and newly regenerating nerve reacts to with an additional admixture of scar and confused axons.

NEUROMAS IN CONTINUITY

The situation is a bit more complicated with the mixed motor-sensory nerve which is usually a major nerve associated with pain and yet not capable of sacrifice without a great loss of important function. Here, every attempt should be made to thoroughly expose the nerve, do NAP recordings across the nerve and, based on these, either do an external or internal neurolysis or resection and repair. If there are positive NAPs across the lesion and yet pain is a major consideration, than the question is whether internal neurolysis will help the pain. It may or may not and, despite all care taken, it may be associated with more loss of function because of the manipulation of scarred, partially damaged fascicles. On the other hand, internal neurolysis despite a positive NAP across the lesion may be indicated if one portion of the circumference of the nerve appears more involved than another. With differential fascicular recordings, a portion of such a lesion may not conduct, and then resection and repair of those involved fascicles and neurolysis of the less involved ones may help not only the partial deficit but the pain. Such a split repair should be kept in mind for some cases although, most of the time, the recording of an NAP across even a painful peripheral lesion indicates regeneration or the potential for such, and then the usual indicated procedure is neurolysis only because with more time and more regeneration not only may the function increase but the pain may decrease or ameliorate enough to be manageable pharmacologically (Fig. 21-2).

USE OF STIMULATION THERAPY

A modality that has found some popularity for pain, particularly in an extremity, is nerve stimulation.[23–25] This can be tried proximally by small needle electrodes and if helpful be converted to an implanted, more permanent nerve stimulation device. Such systems require some manipulation of the nerve for their placement and, although well tolerated under most circumstances, can either fail or lead to scar which not only decreases their effectiveness but also

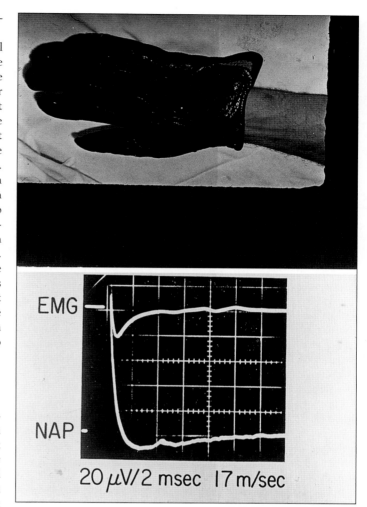

EMG

NAP

20 μV/2 msec 17 m/sec

FIGURE 21-2 Gunshot wound to forearm involving the median nerve one year before. Prior neurolysis of nerve had been done elsewhere because loss was incomplete with sparing of thenar intrinsic function. Patient had severe neuritic pain which had some elements of causalgic pain. He wore a glove over the hand, even in very hot weather (*upper inset*). Pain did not respond to sympathetic blocks. At exploration, a neuroma in continuity was found. This transmitted only a very small nerve action potential, and no motor function could be evoked by stimulating either above or below the lesion (*lower inset*). The lesion was resected, and an end-to-end repair was done with considerable improvement in pain and return of sensation to grade 3 or 4 over several years. Thenar function was not lost. In retrospect, this patient had a Martin-Gruber anastomoses with abductor pollicis brevis and opponens pollicis fibers traveling to hand in the ulnar nerve. Most of the pain was neuritic and due to an almost complete lesion in continuity which had regenerated poorly.

can result in a new locus for pain and sometimes disability. When they fail or need to be removed or changed, such systems are not always easy to extricate from the nerve without a good deal of manipulation and sometimes even damage to nerve. This is not to say such devices are bad, because they can help some people not helped by other surgical or pharmacologic means, but only to point out that the decision to use them usually depends on the failure of simpler steps. The same, of course, could be said for placement of morphine pumps, dorsal column stimulation (DCS), and cordotomy, or myletomy which should be reserved for patients who have failed earlier and usually simpler steps.[11,52] Despite these comments, a procedure such as DCS placement may rescue pain patients, especially if they have extremity pain, from an unacceptable day-to-day life.[11,33] One of the problems, of course, with injured or diseased nerves as opposed to pain of cancer origin is that the origin of pain and the secondary pathways produced, unless identified and corrected early on, can persist for a long time. Failing that, the pain itself must be successfully ameliorated by other measures for, if that is not accomplished, pain persists sometimes for many years or even the lifetime of the patient.

PAIN RESULTING FROM PLEXUS STRETCH/AVULSION

Most pain resulting from plexus stretch injuries improve or ceases altogether by a year or so post injury (Fig. 21-3). However, some pain resulting from such injuries can be persistent and extremely difficult to manage. It is more common in those with preganglionic as opposed to postganglionic lesions.[7,72] There is usually a rather constant pain, described as burning or throbbing, and then usually intermittent paroxysms of radicular electrical or shocking sensations. If the limb is totally paralyzed, which it often is in association with this pain, it may have a phantom limb-like nature. Such discomfort is much like that an amputee may experience, such as feeling that the hand was moving or had feeling even though it was not moving and was insensate.[55] There can be a feeling of great pressure, as if an "elephant was sitting on the hand" or it was "caught in a vice."

Plexus injury pain may sometimes be helped by direct repair or nerve transfers, especially if some function is recovered, but even this does not always ameliorate the symptoms.[8] Pain mediations including neuroleptics are often of little value. In addition, most peripheral and central pain-relieving procedures, including use of stimulation, usually fail.

In these cases, destruction of the dorsal root entry zone at multiple levels, whether by radiofrequency probe or by microsurgical technique, can be effective.[34,35,46,75]

This is not an easy procedure to accomplish and as a result should be left in the hands of those with more experience than just doing the occasional case.[17] When done well in carefully selected patients who have failed simpler steps, almost two-thirds of patients have at least what is described as a good result at 1 year postoperatively.[53] More sustained pain relief is not always achieved and complications can and do occur, especially to the corticospinal tract giving weakness and/or ataxia in the ipsilateral leg.[53,61] Contralateral sensory loss to pain and temperature can also result, as can some degree of respiratory insufficiency. The targets in the dorsolateral sulcus are not always obvious because of cord and residual root distortion by the traction injury as well as scar or gliosis in the area where the lesions need to be made.

At the present time we reserve selection of this procedure for patients refractive to most other pain-relieving steps and whose day-to-day life is obstructed by the pain. We then usually refer the patient to a center with a track record of experience with the technique.

Having said all of this, there may be some urgency in selecting the correct management for pain soon after its onset. This is because, with time, central mechanisms for maintenance or even increase in intensity of pain may be triggered.[5,51,55] Thus, pain specialists argue, and with reason we believe, that it is of utmost importance to provide adequate levels of pain medication as early as possible after onset of pain. This certainly seems to be so postoperatively, where our own pain specialists who are anesthesiologists will not infrequently make adjustments not only in the PCA pump medications but also in the supplemental drugs used for postoperative pain control.

SYMPATHETICALLY ORIGINATED OR MAINTAINED PAIN

There are some specialized pain syndromes that may require more specific or tailored treatment. Although infrequent, as pointed out

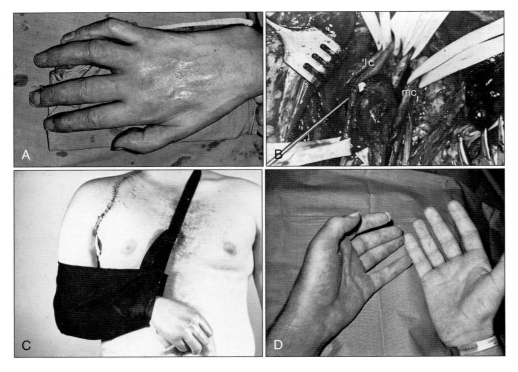

FIGURE 21-3 (A) Causalgic hand in patient who sustained a gunshot wound to the plexus nearly a year before. Loss in the distribution of each plexus element was incomplete, but severe hand pain prohibited effective use of the limb. **(B)** A moderate-sized pseudoaneurysm was found, involving axillary artery and stretching and displacing cord-to-nerve segments of plexus. The aneurysm was resected and a neurolysis of the plexus was done. This gave relief of the severe hand pain for 48 hours or so, but then this recurred, so a cervical sympathetic block was done which temporarily relieved the pain (lc, lateral cord; mc, medial cord). **(C)** As a result, a cervical sympathectomy was done through a supraclavicular approach, and this reversed the pain syndrome completely. The patient eventually made a nearly complete recovery. **(D)** In another patient, a post-sympathectomy hand to the left is compared with a more normal one to the right.

elsewhere in this chapter by Tasker, they do occur and need especial attention. These syndromes are felt to be either partially or greatly maintained by hyperactive sympathetic activity.[6,9,36]

TRUE CAUSALGIA

Every surgeon with experience with serious nerve injuries has seen patients with causalgia, or what we would term "true" causalgia.[3,42,44]

These patients usually have sustained a proximal, relatively severe injury to a major nerve, usually a mixed motor-sensory one. The injury is often a partial one to the nerve involved rather than a complete one. Penetrating wounds involving nerve(s), whether by glass, knife, or propeller or gunshot wound (GSW), are more likely to lead to causalgia than blunt injuries. These patients have a relatively acute onset of a severe, often burning, dysesthetic pain in the more distal portion of the extremity associated, usually with overresponse of sympathetic activity. This sympathetic activity takes the form acutely of coloration changes in the limb and excessive sweating but may trend in a relatively short period of time to a cool and blanched hand or foot. Very critical in our view is the fact that the limb cannot be manipulated even with distraction of the patient's attention. The patient will simply not permit the limb to be manipulated or touched at all.

Sympathetic block of the involved extremity should relieve or greatly improve the symptoms, including the autonomic ones, at least temporarily.[59] Repetitive blocks leading to temporary relief followed by recrudescence of symptoms will sometimes result in increased periods of relief and eventual nearly complete reversal of the pain.[42] If this is not the case, then surgical sympathectomy is the indicated procedure.[29,59] Irrespective of whether it is done in the thoracic or lumbar area, a length of the sympathetic chain needs to be removed for optimal results. Since ganglia as well as connecting fibers are removed, the sympathectomy will be preganglionic, and that seems to be the level of section necessary to achieve more lasting relief.

Sometimes, sympathetically related pain will be intermixed with neuritic or neuropathic pain and then the lesion involving nerve may need to be more acutely addressed than might otherwise be indicated. Even after delay, the situation can be more complicated, as illustrated by the following case.

CASE SUMMARY – CAUSALGIA

A 20-year-old college student was wounded in the right shoulder by a GSW from a relatively small-caliber rifle. The circumstances connected with this wounding were unclear. When he presented to his local university hospital there was an entry wound an inch or so below clavicle in the infraclavicular area and an exit wound in posterolateral shoulder. He had a partial plexus distribution loss, both motor and sensory, largely affecting the hand with relative sparing of more proximal arm- and forearm-innervated muscles and sensory territories. His partial loss was relatively mild even in hand-innervated muscles, all of which had some function. From the beginning he had severe pain and paresthesias in the hand, and the hand was ruborous, hyperhidrotic, and slightly swollen. He did not permit manipulation or close handling of the hand. Radial pulse was maintained, and an angiogram done some hours later was said to be normal. There was minimal bleeding from the entrance and exit sites. X-rays of the shoulder were normal but because of the severity and nature of his pain and his physical findings he had a sympathetic block done by anesthesia the day of the accident. There was some reduction in the sweating and rubor of the hand but only partial pain relief. Over the ensuing days to weeks, some 20 more blocks were done

but relief was partial. In retrospect, according to the patient, during this period of time there was a progressive increase in the severity of his pain and in the relative disuse of the hand. He was subsequently seen at several other centers and, because of the classic nature of his history and findings, had some 30 or more blocks without satisfactory resolution of his symptoms.

When seen nearly a year later at LSUMC in addition to a classic causalgia, we felt he had a somewhat tender axillary mass or fullness, a finding not previously noted. He kept his hand covered in Vaseline and wore over it a large rubber glove. He then enclosed that glove by an even larger cloth glove and liked to keep ice chips in between the two. Infraclavicular exploration revealed a pseudoaneurysm and scarred and somewhat stretched and displaced lateral and medial cords of the plexus. The pseudoaneurysm was resected and a neurolysis of the plexus was done. All elements conducted NAPs, although velocities were slow and amplitudes reduced. He awoke without a painful hand and was able to dispense with the Vaseline, gloves, and ice. However, 48 hours later his pain returned and he was back wearing his paraphernalia. A sympathetic block for the first time worked giving him excellent albeit temporary relief. As a result, the very next day he had a dorsal sympathectomy with more lasting relief. After several months of physical/occupational therapy he was able to return to college with a useful limb with only residual mild hand intrinsic weakness and mild sensory change in the ulnar and median distribution. Over the subsequent years he has had a useful but, of course, not completely normal limb and has had some neuritic symptoms, but not the severe pain he had in the first year or so post injury.

REFLEX SYMPATHETIC DYSTROPHY

Less satisfactory is both the diagnosis and management of reflex sympathetic dystrophy (RSD). Classically, such a disorder is much less frequent than is reflected by the number of patients sent to our clinics with that label. True RSD is associated with a more distal limb injury which usually does not directly involve a nerve, at least not a major nerve.[26,50] Often, the injury is a soft tissue one due to crush or contusion with or without fracture involving foot, hand, finger(s), or toe(s). Onset and initial findings are usually but not always somewhat delayed compared to true causalgia. Symptoms are similar to true causalgia, with a mix of a burning, dysesthetic pain and autonomic findings indicating either hypersympathetic function (usually acutely) or hyposympathetic function (usually subacutely or chronically). As with true causalgia, manipulation or stroking of the affected limb can be difficult to impossible to do without a relatively violent response on the part of the patient. Also, as with causalgia, use of adequate criteria for diagnosis including this clinical examination step are important.[54] Patients with symptoms similar to RSD, or what could be termed a "causalgia-like syndrome," and yet a limb that can be passively manipulated are much less likely to have RSD and are much less likely to respond favorably to sympathectomy or sympathetic block.

Some patients with RSD have the inexplicable spread of symptoms and disability to more proximal limb or contralateral upper or lower limb or even from lower limb(s) to upper limb(s). These patients are extremely difficult to treat and their symptoms difficult to reverse even with multimodality therapy and multiple specialists, including psychiatry's input.

The chronic patient with RSD affecting one limb can be almost as severely disabled as the acute one. The hand or foot with a shiny, thinned out, and tight-appearing skin which is often blanched and sometimes remains cool to the touch can be a fairly frequent outcome just as with unsuccessfully or incompletely treated true causalgia.[14] Nails may be elongated as well as distorted. It is often too painful for the patient to trim the nails or even have someone else trim them.

Unfortunately, the effect of sympathetic blocks and/or sympathectomy is less certain in this group of patients than in those with true causalgia or even more acute RSD. Nonetheless, these measures plus use of a neuroleptic as well as analgesic drugs are usually necessary for any degree of control.

Key to rehabilitation in both of these disorders, or for that matter any pain disorder related to nerve, is the absolute need to get the patient to move and then to use the limb. In the case of the foot or leg this means weight bearing. In the case of the hand or arm it means use of the limb at least for tasks of daily living, such as use of utensils for cooking and feeding, using the limb to dress, or to turn pages of a book.

There can be no substitute for motion where the limb is used repetitively despite the pain and the patient must be counseled in depth about the need for this. An understanding physical and occupational therapist can be a great help in this regard. Establishment of a daily routine of exercise as well as strategies to encourage use are, thus, extremely important.

CASE SUMMARY – REFLEX SYMPATHETIC DYSTROPHY

This 32-year-old woman sustained a work related crush injury to the digits of her left hand. One finger was fractured and required fixation by pin. The hand and fingers were, of course, both swollen and painful but several days later, despite lack of digital or other peripheral nerve involvement, she complained of paresthesias and a burning causalgia-like pain, and then over a period of several weeks developed cool, blanched-appearing fingers and hand. More acutely, her cast and bandages were adjusted but to no avail. A cervical sympathetic block a month after injury gave temporary relief but despite a series of such blocks relief was always temporary. Analgesic medications gave only partial relief of the pain. When seen several months after injury she still had a cool, somewhat swollen hand which she refused to use. The fracture had healed but use of the finger as well as the hand was minimal. Even with distraction, touching or manipulating the hand gave severe pain. Sensory testing showed no loss and if anything the fingers, including the one that had been fractured, were hyperesthetic. There was no obvious loss of motor function or hand intrinsic atrophy although it was difficult to elicit complete effort and cooperation on the part of the patient.

Since multiple sympathetic blocks had given good albeit temporary relief, a supraclavicular sympathectomy was done. This gave good pain relief. The patient had a partial but mild Horner syndrome and a phrenic palsy postoperatively but both resolved over time. With the help of physical/occupational therapy the hand eventually became useful even though workman's compensation and some legal issues surrounding the case slowed and made difficult to discern the outcome for a few years.

OTHER CAUSES OF PERIPHERAL NERVE PAIN

There are, of course, other disorders affecting nerve or the limbs that can be associated with pain.[68] These may or may not be helped by surgery on the nerve. Certainly, entrapments and tumors involving nerve are good examples of ones with pain that can be helped by surgery. Less certain and more controversial are the painful paresthesias associated with diabetes and some other presumed metabolic disorders such as alcoholic neuropathy. Here, the first order of business would seem to be a pharmacologic one unless

areas of entrapment of the nerve involved by neuropathy can be identified by electrophysiologic studies. Then, neurolysis of the metabolically involved nerve and release of an entrapment site may help the pain and paresthesias.

Pain associated with injury due to iatrogenic causation seems more frequent and more severe than due to injury of more spontaneous origin.[20] This makes it especially important to correct such medically induced lesions whenever possible and in as timely a fashion as possible.

Obviously, compressive lesions associated with trauma such as clots, pseudoaneurysms, and arteriovenous fistula should demand immediate attention and usually surgical intervention. Classically, the pain associated with them is not only severe but progressive in intensity, as are the deficits in function which may be mild to begin with but severe and sometimes permanent if early intervention is not carried out. The involved nerve or elements must be thoroughly cleared or neurolysed and the mass effect of the lesion either eliminated or markedly reduced.

A curious disorder associated with severe pain is that due to a glomus tumor. These patients have a severity of pain often equivalent to levels reported with true causalgia. In addition, the involved area of the limb is exquisitely tender and, like the causalgic limb, the involved area is kept away or withdrawn from the examiner.

Although glomus tumors are most common at subungual sites, particularly on a finger or thumb, they can occur at other sites including the leg or more proximal arm. We have had experience with several such lesions. They are difficult to completely excise without recurrence. Their histologic appearance is characteristic. There are few disorders with such a dramatic clinical picture and pathologic findings.

CASE SUMMARY – ANOTHER PAINFUL CONDITION – GLOMUS TUMOR

This teenager had sustained a ski boot injury to the lower shin of one leg due to a fall on a slope. The injury was unassociated with a fracture but involved soft tissues and required a number of weeks to resolve. She was left with a crease or indentation over the skin at this level. Some months later she developed severe pain at the level of the crease and began to complain of difficulty bearing weight with this limb. Motor and sensory function of the foot was normal as were EMG and conduction studies. X-rays and a bone scan were also negative. When seen in New Orleans, several years later, the area in the region of the soft tissue crease was exquisitely tender. Any attempt at palpation prompted tears as well as the patient pushing away the examiner, while manipulation of the more distal foot was not painful. The family and referring physicians had sought and obtained psychological help but that had not reversed the syndrome and, moreover, the youngster stopped going to college. Analgesic medication was of some but not completely helpful and she required sleeping pills to rest at night.

The patient was hospitalized and, with the approval of the family and the help of the nursing service, the area was palpated while she was asleep. She awoke immediately, complaining of severe pain localized to the anterior tibial area. As a result, the region was explored under general anesthesia the next day. A lesion of several centimeters, somewhat flat but firm and yet somewhat rubbery to palpation, was found. The lesion was attached to the periosteum of the tibia and was excised with good eventual relief of her pain. Histologic examination showed this to be a glomus tumor (see Chapter 23, Figs 23–46 and 23–47). Relief postoperatively was dramatic. She did well for 4.5 years and then the lesion recurred requiring re-operation. She did well for another 3–4 years but refused operation for a second questionable smaller recurrence.

PAIN DUE TO IMMOBILIZATION

The saddest painful condition the nerve surgeon has to deal with is that in a limb with denervation where most movement as well as proper physical and occupational therapy has been neglected. The stiff shoulder unassociated with fracture or capsular injury because of immobilization or fear on the part of the patient to have the shoulder joint mobilized and kept mobile epitomizes the problem. When institution of vigorous therapy does not reverse this joint's limited motion and attendant pain, definitive steps to do so are needed. This may include manipulation of the joint under anesthesia or capsular release when less invasive steps such as ultrasound or hydrotherapy and vigorous physical/occupational therapy failed. The establishment of an adequate level of patient analgesia is usually necessary before these steps can be instituted. This type of therapeutic conundrum might also apply to wrist, elbow, ankle, or knee. It is for this reason that we seldom immobilize a limb by cast or splint, especially for an extended period, unless an end-to-end nerve suture repair is under tension (and then we are more likely to do a graft repair anyway) or vascular or bony stabilization done at the time of the nerve repair requires this step. Even where end-to-end or epineurial nerve repair has been done, it is seldom necessary to immobilize the limb for more than 3–4 weeks.[60] We prefer with nerve repair almost immediate mobilization and if possible use of as much of the limb as the paralysis permits. As a result, even the lower limb with a femoral or sciatic nerve repair is moved on the first day postoperatively and, if the repair site permits it, the patient is gotten up and asked to bear at least partial weight with or without the help of crutches or a cane. An exception might be an operation on the ankle and especially the foot where, because of wound tensile strength considerations, full weight bearing might be delayed for a week or two.

The patient with a brachial plexus repair is usually placed in a non-Valpeau-type sling for a week or two. Even with that, some range of motion of elbow, wrist, and fingers is started right away to avoid painful contractures. In addition, the patient and family are instructed to have the patient make circular motions with the shoulder, either actively or passively, to begin on the first or second postoperative day so that a painful, stiff shoulder can be avoided or at least minimized. The tensile strength of most repairs of nerve will be maximal by 3 weeks and certainly by then more vigorous range of motion to the limb and physical therapy/occupational therapy can begin.

An issue that cannot be neglected is the fact that many insurance policies only reimburse or cover the patient for a finite period of physical and/or occupational therapy. Ideally, this period of physical therapy/occupational therapy will be best used if it coincides with the beginning or initiation of motor and sensory recovery rather than being expended just to maintain joints and to prevent ligament shortening. This means the nerve surgeon must be involved in instructing patient and family in frequent range of motion maneuvers for the involved limb once the tensile strength of any repair(s) is reached and until more structured physical therapy/occupational therapy can be optimally utilized.

SYMPATHECTOMIES FOR PAIN WITH SYMPATHETIC FIBER INPUT

An approach similar to that for thoracic outlet syndrome can be used for cervical sympathectomy. Ansae or small rootlets enter and leave T1 and lead the surgeon to the stellate ganglion and the caudal portion of the thoracic sympathetic chain. Another landmark is the vertebral artery, which can be found originating from the proximal portion of the subclavian and running upward and medially toward the transverse process of C6. By elevation of the proximal portion of the vertebral artery, the stellate ganglion can usually be found posterior to it; the rest of the thoracic sympathetic chain can be found inferior to it beneath the subclavian vessels and in the upper mediastinum. A long nerve hook is very helpful in pulling up the chain and displaying it as it runs inferiorly. One has to push the pleura forward to expose the chain, and this is easily done once the stellate ganglion is identified. Illumination and magnification are very helpful when one follows the chain down to the level of the third rib.

The usual cervical sympathectomy for upper extremity pain involves hemisection of the stellate ganglion. The lower half, along with the chain and ganglia at T1, T2, and T3 levels, is drawn superiorly. Then a vascular clip is placed on the distal portion of the chain, and the chain is sectioned proximal to this clip. This clip marks the most distal extent of the sympathetic chain removal. There are many important structures nearby (Figs 21-4, 21-5)

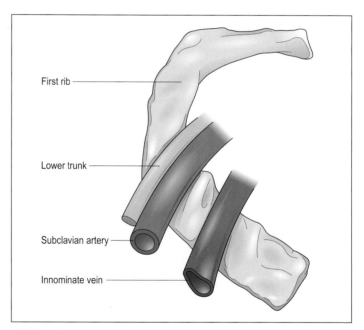

FIGURE 21-4 This is a downward-looking view of the right first rib. Like the anterior tubercles of the cervical spine and the coracoid process of the scapula, the medial border of the first rib is a characteristic landmark that is easily palpated. Note that the scalene tubercle, the inferior origin of the scalenus anticus, separates the vein lying anterior to it from the subclavian artery, which is hooking over the first rib to gain the axilla. Immediately posterior to the artery is the lower trunk, formed from the confluence of C8 and T1 spinal nerves. As the finger sweeps posteriorly, depressing the suprapleural membrane and pleura, a structure with the consistency of an India rubber eraser is encountered by the pulp of the fingertip. This is the stellate ganglion lying anterior to the neck of the first rib. The surgeon then identifies the thyrocervical trunk and the vertebral artery, which run superiorly from the upper border of the subclavian artery. Usually, the inferior attachment of scalenus anticus is divided once the phrenic nerve, which is adherent to its anterior surface, has been delineated, dissected away, and guarded. This enables the operator to move medially on the lower trunk to the foraminal exits of the C8 and T1 spinal nerves. The sharp medial border of the first rib can be a constant guide during these maneuvers. (From Atlas of Peripheral Nerve Surgery: Philadelphia, WB Saunders 2001, with permission.)

Labels in figure: First rib; Lower trunk; Subclavian artery; Innominate vein

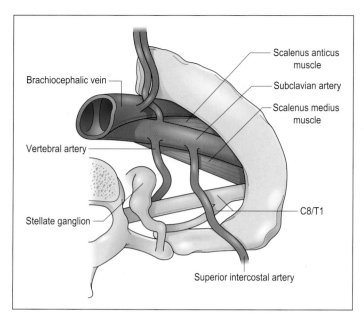

Brachiocephalic vein

Scalenus anticus muscle

Subclavian artery

Scalenus medius muscle

Vertebral artery

C8/T1

Stellate ganglion

Superior intercostal artery

FIGURE 21-5 This is a view of the left first rib and nearby structures as one looks up toward the neck from the thorax. Note that if the lower trunk is followed medially, it divides into T1 and C8 spinal nerves, which embrace the neck of the first rib. Seen from below, the T1 spinal nerve is running laterally and upward to join C8. T1 is in close relationship with the stellate ganglion. As a result, the T1 spinal nerve can be cut in error during a sympathectomy. Note the close relationship of these structures to the vertebral artery as it runs up to gain the foramen transversarium of the cervical spine. (From Atlas of Peripheral Nerve Surgery. Philadelphia, WB Saunders 2001, with permission.)

including lymphatic ducts and the great vessels. If chyle appears in the wound, the surgeon should stop long enough to identify the source and then either use the bipolar forceps to seal the leak or suture the opening shut. Today, many of these procedures are done endoscopically at a high thoracic level.[48]

LUMBAR SYMPATHECTOMY

The patient is anesthetized in a supine position using an endotracheal technique. A roll of sheets or several folded sheets are placed under the flank on the side to be operated. The hip and knee are partially flexed by placing a pillow beneath the ipsilateral knee. This tends to relax the psoas muscles somewhat. A skin incision is made in the flank obliquely from the tip of the lower ribs toward the inguinal region. The incision is usually 10–12 cm in length. External oblique muscle fibers are split in the direction they run and are kept apart by a self-retaining retractor. The internal oblique is then split in the direction of its fibers. Usually, the assistant holds these muscle edges apart with a small Richardson or Army-Navy retractor. Then the transversalis fibers are bluntly separated by the surgeon's gloved fingers in a lateral or inferior direction. This latter maneuver permits visualization of the extraperitoneal fat. The index and middle fingers are then inserted through the muscle-splitting incision, and their palmar surfaces are pressed against the transversalis muscle laterally. The fingers are used to dissect a plane of cleavage between the fat, posterior peritoneum, and the posterior abdominal wall. The gloved hand then slides over the inner surface of the quadratus lumborum to the lateral psoas muscle and up over this muscle group. In this fashion, peritoneal fat will lie on

the palmar surface of the hand, and the peritoneum will be above or superior to the back of the operator's hand. Either a cotton strip or a large cotton ball with an attached string can be held in place by the fingers while a Grant bladder or other curved retractor such as a Deaver is placed. This is used to elevate the peritoneum and its enclosed abdominal contents. This retractor is also used to help expose the lateral portion of the lumbar vertebrae. Another curved abdominal retractor can be inserted more cephalad, at or above the attachments of the crus of the diaphragm. The lumbar sympathetic chain is usually found lying in the gutter formed by the rounded portion of the belly of the psoas. The sympathetic chain can be elevated with a long-handled nerve hook so that rami, and then both ends close to the diaphragmatic crus and at the lumbosacral promontory, can be sectioned. The chain may lie beneath lumbar arterial branches on the left side, or lumbar bridging veins on the right side, and these may need to be tied off or coagulated before the chain is dissected out. In addition, on the right side, some of the vena cava may lie over the sympathetic chain, requiring gentle elevation of that vessel to expose the chain more completely.

After resection of a length of this chain, the muscle levels are closed in layers. Subcutaneous tissues and skin are tacked down to the external oblique muscle to avoid a dead space and thus a fluid collection in the flank.

CONCLUSION

1. An old sobriquet still remains true today: "The only witness we have for pain is the patient himself or herself." There is no other effective measure for its presence or severity.
2. As a somewhat final note, Sunderland[56] in a thoughtful essay published in 1991 stated: "While the injured segment of the nerve and the affected cutaneous tissues, particularly the former, are the loci generi of the pain mechanism in most nerve lesions, there is convincing evidence that in others, e.g. causalgia, the mechanisms responsible for the pain are located within the central nervous system and that these abnormal impulse generators can discharge spontaneously and quite independently of any peripheral influence."
3. "Because the mechanism [for pain] could be located in one or more [of these] sites, local, peripheral, and central, it is important in any individual case to determine which is at fault. Failure to do this means that therapy is likely to remain ill-directed and the outcome uncertain. Under these conditions it will be impossible to remove treatment from the thralldom of empiricism."
4. The next section is an especially thoughtful treatise on neuropathic pain by Ron Tasker.

REFERENCES

1. Anand P: Nerve growth factor and nociception. Br J Anesthesia 75:201–208, 1995.
2. Barbut D, Blah JM, and Wall PD: Substance P in spinal cord dorsal horn decreases following peripheral nerve injury. Brain Res 205:289–298, 1981.
3. Barnes R: Causalgia: a review of 48 cases. In: Seddon HJ, Ed: Peripheral Nerve Injuries. London, HMSO, 1954:156–185.
4. Berman J, Anand P, Chen L, et al.: Pain relief from preganglionic injury to the brachial plexus by later intercostal transfer. J Bone Joint Surg [Br] 78:759–760, 1996.
5. Birch R, Bonney G, and Wynn Parry CB: Surgical Disorders of the Peripheral Nerves. London Churchill Livinstone, 1988.

6. Bonica JJ: Causalgia and other reflex sympathetic dystrophies. In: Bonica JJ, Ed: The Management of Pain, vol. 2. Philadelphia, Lea & Febiger, 1990:220–243.

7. Bonnard C and Narakas A: Syndromes douloureux er lesions ost-traumatiques du plexus brachial. Helvetica Chirurgica Acta 52:621–632, 1985.

8. Bonney G: Prognosis in traction lesions of the brachial plexus. J Bone Joint Surg [Br] 41:4–35, 1959.

9. Bonney G: Causalgia. Br J Hosp Med 9:593–596, 1973.

10. Bowsher D: Central pain: clinical and physiological characteristics. J Neurol Neurosurg Psychiatry 61:62–69, 1996.

11. Burchiel KJ and Ochoa JL: Surgical management of posttraumatic neuropathic pain. Neurosurg Clin N Am 2(1):117–126, 1991.

12. Campbell JN and LaMotte RH: Latency to detection of first pain. Brain Res 266:203–208, 1983.

13. Campbell JN, Raja SN, and Meyer RA: Myelinated afferents signal the hyperalgesia associated with nerve injury. Pain 32:89–94, 1988.

14. Cooke ED, Steinberg MD, Pearson RM, et al.: Reflex sympathetic dystrophy and repetitive strain injury: temperature and microcirculatory changes following mild cold stress. J Roy Soc Med 86:690–693, 1993.

15. Dellon AL and Mackinnon S: Treatment of the painful neuroma by neuroma resection and muscle implantation. Plast Reconstr Surg 77:427–436, 1986.

16. England J, Happel J, and Kline D: Abnormal distribution of potassium channel activity in human neuromas. Neurosci Newsletters 255:37–40, 1998.

17. Friedman AH and Nashold BS Jr.: DREZ lesions for relief of pain related to spinal cord injury. J Neurosurg 65:465–475, 1986.

18. Gracely R, Lynch SA, and Bennett GJ: Painful neuropathy: altered central processing maintained dynamically by peripheral input. Pain 52:251–253, 1993.

19. Herndon JH, Eaton RG, and Littler JW: Management of painful neuromas in the hand. J Bone Joint Surg [Am] 58:364–373, 1976.

20. Horowitz SH: Brachial plexus injuries with causalgia resulting from trans-axillary rib resection. Arch Surg 120:1189–1191, 1985.

21. Kretchner T, Nguyen D, Beuerman R, et al.: Painful neuromas: A potential rule for structural transmembrane protein, Ankyrin G. J Neurosurg 97:1424–1431, 2002.

22. Kretschmer T, Happel L, England J, et al.: Accumulation of PN I and PN III sodium channels in painful human neuroma: evidence from immunochemistry. Acta Neurochir 144(8):803–810, 2002.

23. Laryea J, Schon L, and Belzberg A: Peripheral nerve stimulators for pain control. Semin Neurosurg 12(1):125–131, 2001.

24. Loeser J, Black R, and Christman A: Relief of pain by transcutaneous stimulation. J Neurosurg 43:308–314, 1978.

25. Long D: Neuromodulation for the control of chronic pain. Surg Rounds 5:25–34, 1982.

26. Low PA, Wilson PR, Sandroni P, et al.: Clinical characteristics of patients with reflex sympathetic dystrophy in the USA. Progress Pain Res Management 6:49–77, 1996.

27. Mackinnon S and Dellon A: Surgery of the Peripheral Nerve. New York, Thieme Medical Publishers, 1988.

28. Martini A and Fromm B: A new operation for the prevention and treatment of amputation neuromas. J Bone Joint Surg [Br] 71:379–382, 1989.

29. Mayfield F: Reflex dystrophies of the hand. In: Flynn JE, Ed: Hand Surgery. Baltimore, Williams & Wilkins, 1966:1095(see also 738–750).

30. Maynard CW, Leonard RB, Coulter JD, et al.: Central connections of ventral root afferents as demonstrated by the HRP method. J Comparative Neurol 172:601–608, 1977.

31. Melzack R and Wall PD: Pain mechanisms: A new theory. Science 150:971–979, 1965.

32. Melzack R: The McGill pain questionnaire. Pain 1:277–299, 1975.

33. Nashold BS and Friedman H: Dorsal column stimulation for control of pain. Preliminary report on 30 patients. J Neurosurg 36:590–597, 1972.

34. Nashold BS and Ostahl RH: Dorsal root entry zone lesions for pain relief. J Neurosurg 51:59–69, 1979.

35. Nashold BS: Current status of the DREZ operations. Neurosurgery 15:942–944, 1984.

36. Nathan PW: Pain and the sympathetic system. J Automic Nervous Sys 7:363–370, 1983.

37. Noordenbos W: Pain. Amsterdam, Elsevier, 1959.

38. Ochoa J: Pain in local nerve lesions. In: Culp WJ, Ochoa J, Eds: Abnormal Nerves and Muscles as Impulse Generators. New York and Oxford, Oxford University Press, 1982.

39. Ochoa J, Torebjörk H: Paresthesias from ectopic impulse generation in human sensory nerves. Brain 10(3):835–839, 1980.

40. Ochs G: Painful dysesthesias following peripheral nerve injury: A clinical and electrophysiological study. Brain Res 4:228–240, 1989.

41. Omer GE: The management of pain. In: Lamb DW, Ed: The Paralyzed Hand. Edinburgh, Churchill Livingstone, 1987:216–231.

42. Omer G and Thomas S: Treatment of causalgia: review of cases at Brook General Hospital. Texas Med J 67:93–96, 1972.

43. Pagni CA: Central pain due to spinal cord and brain stem damage. In: Wall PD, Melzack R, Eds: Textbook of Pain. Edinburgh,Churchill Livingstone, 1989:634–655.

44. Richards RL: Causalgia. A centennial review. Arch Neurol 16:339–350, 1967.

45. Richardson DE and Akill H: Pain reduction by electrical brain stimulation in man. J Neurosurg 47:178–187, 1977.

46. Richter HP and Sertz K: Dorsal root entry zone lesions for the control of deafferentation pain: experiences in ten patients. Neurosurgery 15:956–959, 1984.

47. Roberts WJ: A hypothesis on the physiological basis for causalgia and related pains. Pain 24:297–311, 1986.

48. Robertson DP, Simpson RK, Rose JE, et al.: Video-assisted endoscopic thoracic sympathectomy. J Neurosurg 79:238–240, 1993.

49. Scadding JW: Ectopic impulse generation in damaged peripheral axons in abnormal nerves and muscles as impulse generators. In: Ochoa J, Culp W, Eds: Abnormal Nerves and Muscles as Impulse Generators. Oxford, Oxford University Press, 1984.

50. Schwartzman RJ: Reflex sympathetic dystrophy and causalgia. In: Evans R, Ed: Neurology and Trauma. Philadelphia, JB Lippincott, 1996:496–510.

51. Seddon HJ, Ed: Surgical Disorders of the Peripheral Nerves. Baltimore, Williams & Wilkins, 1972.

52. Shealy CN, Mortimer JT, and Reswick JB: Electrical inhibition of pain by stimulation of the dorsal columns. Prelim Clin Report Anesth (Cleve) 46:489–491, 1967.

53. Sindou M, Blondet E, Emery E, et al.: Microsurgical lesioning in the dorsal root entry zone for pain due to brachial plexus avulsion: a prospective series of 55 patients. J Neurosurg 102:1018–1028, 2005.

54. Stanton-Hicks M, Jänig W, Hassenbusch S, et al.: Reflex sympathetic dystrophy: changing concepts and taxonomy. Pain 63:127–133, 1995.

55. Sunderland S: What can nerve trauma tell us about pain mechanisms? In: Nerve Injuries and their Repair: A Critical Appraisal. London, Churchill Livingstone, 1991:333–350.

56. Sunderland S: Conversion hysteria. In: Nerve Injuries and Repair. A Critical Appraisal. Edinburgh, Churchill Livingstone, 1991:327.

57. Swanson AB, Boeve NR, and Lumsden RM: The prevention and treatment of amputation neuromata by silicone capping. J Hand Surg 2:70–78, 1977.

58. Sweet WH: Deafferentation pain after posterior rhizotomy, trauma to a limb, and herpes zoster. Neurosurgery 15:928–932, 1984.

59. Sweet WH and Polette CE: Causalgia and sympathetic dystrophy. In: Aronoff GM, Ed: Evaluation and Treatment of Chronic Pain. Baltimore, Urban & Schwarzenberg, 1985:19–165.

60. Tarlov IM: How long should an extremity be immobilized after nerve suture? Ann Surg 126:336–376, 1947.
61. Thomas D and Kitchen ND: Long term follow-up of dorsal root entry zone lesions in brachial plexus avulsion. J Neurol Neurosurg Psychiatry 57:737–738, 1994.
62. Thomas M, Stirratt A, Birch R, et al.: Freeze thawed muscle grafting for painful cutaneous neuromas. J Bone Joint Surg [Br] 76:474–476, 1994.
63. Tindall S: Painful neuromas. In: Williams R and Regachary S, Eds: Neurosurgery. New York, McGraw Hill, 1985:1884–1886.
64. Torebjörk HE, Ochoa JL: Selective stimulation of sensory units in man. In: Bonica JJ, Lundblom H, and Iggo A, Eds: Advances in Pain Research and Therapy, vol 2. New York, Raven Press, 1983:99–104.
65. Torebjörk HE, Lundberg LER, and Lamotte RH: Central changes in processing of mechanoreceptor input in capsaicin induced sensory hyperalgesia in humans. J Physiol (London) 448:765–780, 1992.
66. Torebjörk E, Wahren LK, Wallin G, et al.: Noradrenaline evoked pain in neuralgia. Pain 63:11–20, 1995.
67. Tyrer P: Conversion hysteria. In: Classification of Neuroses. New York, Wiley, 1989:106, 107, 111–112.
68. Upton ARM and McComas AJ: The double crush in nerve entrapment syndrome. Lancet ii:359–361, 1973.
69. Wall PD: The gate control theory of pain mechanisms. A re-examination and re-statement. Brain 101:1–18, 1978.
70. Wall PD and Devor M: The effect of peripheral nerve injury on dorsal root potentials and on transmission of afferent signals into the spinal cord. Brain Res 209:95–111, 1981.
71. Wall PD and Gutnick M: The properties of afferent nerve impulses originating from a neuroma. Nature 248:740–742, 1974.
72. Wynn Parry CB: Pain in avulsion lesions of the brachial plexus. Pain 9:41–53, 1980.
73. Wynn Parry CB: Pain in avulsion of the brachial plexus. Neurosurgery 15:960–965, 1989.
74. Wynn Parry CB and Withrington RH: Painful disorders of peripheral nerves. Postgrad Med J 60:869–875, 1984.
75. Zorub D, Nashold BS, and Cook WA: Avulsion of the brachial plexus: I. A review with implications on the therapy of intractable pain. Surg Neurol 2:347–353, 1974.

A TREATISE ON NEUROPATHIC PAIN

Ronald R. Tasker

INTRODUCTION

Neuropathic pain is a much-to-be feared complication of injury, by whatever modality, to the somatosensory nervous system including sensory nerves and roots. The mechanism remains poorly understood and its occurrence appears to be idiosyncratic, since only about one person in five with identical injuries appears to develop pain. Gybels and Sweet[7] quote the incidence after peripheral nerve injury in wartime as 2–5%. Its occurrence appears to bear no relationship to the severity or completeness of the nerve injury and it may occur after injuries that leave no permanent clinically detectable sensory loss.

CLINICAL FEATURES

After nerve injury, the pain often develops immediately, although onset may be delayed and, once established, tends to persist.[1] In this author's opinion, there is little clinical difference in the quality of neuropathic pain caused by peripheral nervous injury compared with that from lesions of the spinal cord, usually the result of trauma, or the brain, usually the result of stroke,[15,17] other than the fact that in some cases of nerve injury, there appears to be sympathetic involvement. The pain usually appears within the distribution of the sensory loss or at least within the territory of the nerve injured, although there are exceptions, which will be discussed below.

The pain usually demonstrates three main features.[16] A steady burning or causalgic/dysesthetic element is the commonest feature.[3] As well, there may be allodynia or hyperpathia, or both (evoked pain), while some patients may also complain of a paroxysmal or intermittent, often lancinating, element to their pain.

IMPLICATION OF THE SYMPATHETIC NERVOUS SYSTEM

If these were the only puzzles of neuropathic pain to understand, it would be less of a problem, but in the case of pain resulting from peripheral nerve injury, the plot is even thicker, for the features of the pain may implicate, at least in some patients, the sympathetic nervous system[9] and a variety of terms have come into use to describe this: major causalgia, minor causalgia,[12] reflex sympathetic dystrophy (RSD), Sudeck's atrophy, sympathetically maintained pain (SMP)[4] and, most recently, chronic regional pain syndrome types I and II (CRPS I and II).[5] This author has, in his exclusively civilian practice over his lifetime, rarely seen these types of pain despite the fact that he has had a fairly extensive experience with neuropathic pain syndromes. The features that seem to incriminate the sympathetic nervous system include changes in skin temperature and color suggesting vasodilatation or vasoconstriction, edema, integumentary changes, motor effects, musculoskeletal changes including joint fixation, atrophy and osteoporosis, in addition to the pain itself. The pain is, at times, excruciating with striking allodynia, the patient evincing agony in response to footfalls on the floor, the sounds of television, and other auditory cues. The pain in these cases frequently expands to include the territory of nerves beyond those known to have been injured and the pain may include spread when the sensitive part is stimulated well beyond the area stimulated as well as temporal summation.

The term major causalgia (now CRPS II) came to be applied to the more dramatic cases, usually the result of partial injury from a low-velocity missile to a major nerve, particularly the median and sciatic as well as the brachial plexus. The term minor causalgia or RSD (CRPS I) was assigned to the rest where soft tissue injury appeared to be the cause. Although the terminology suggested that the sympathetic nervous system was at the bottom of the problem, possibly through its own hyperactivity through abnormal drive of the sympathetic system, through synapses or ephapses, antidromic release of substance P, abnormal sensitivity to norepinephrine or abnormal function of norepinephrine at the peripheral sympathetic terminals,[5] leading to extensive use of sympathetic blocks, sympathetic interruptions, or sympathicolytic drugs for treatment of the pain, unfortunately such it is not usually the case. Thus, before embarking on permanent sympathetic interruption, multiple trials of temporary blocking must be made leading to the recognition of the small subset of patients who seem to be suffering from SMP. In other than the SMP group of CRPS patients, there is no support for sympathetic hyperactivity as an etiological factor on the basis of Doppler studies, microneuronography or pathochemistry; central changes in cord or brain have been blamed for the symptoms.

Originally, various stages of progression of RSD were recognized; initially, there would be spontaneous and evoked pain, but then this would go on to be accompanied by integumentary and autonomic changes, eventually leading to joint fixation and musculoskeletal atrophy, but this staging is not felt by all workers to be valid.

PATHOPHYSIOLOGY

If we properly understood the mechanisms of neuropathic pain, we would be in a better position to treat it. It was only in the 1980s that it was recognized widely as an entity distinct from, say, the pain caused by cancer or inflammatory disease, broken bones, or tissue damage.[1] The invention of a number of neuropathic pain models has helped our understanding of its allodynic or hyperpathic elements,[2] but it is sometimes forgotten that we do not have a good animal model for the steady causalgic or dysesthetic element of the pain, for the study of which we need to be able to communicate with the sufferer. In this writer's opinion, this spontaneous steady pain is not dependent on transmission in pain pathways. After all, it can be caused by total section of the spinal cord or of a nerve and is never relieved by the most strenuous denervating procedures. When it follows a peripheral nerve injury, one can only conclude that is the result of abnormal activity in the central somatosensory structures in response to deafferentation; and the deafferentation need only be minimal or transient, as mentioned previously.

Better understood is allodynia and hyperpathia. Woolf[19] has shown that nerve injury can result in perverted processing of sensory information in the dorsal horn so that the activity in the hyperactive neurons there, whose normal activity is to pass on information to non-nociceptive pathways, now results in the spilling over of their activity into the spinothalamic tract. As a result, what is normally a non-noxious sensory stimulus now passes signals into the pain pathway and is experienced as pain.

The possibility has been advanced that the paroxysmal lancinating element mentioned above seen especially in brachial plexus or cauda equina lesions, is the result of the development of either ectopic impulse generation[13] or of false synapses, or ephapses[6,14] at the injury site, again allowing non-noxious input to spill over into the spinothalamic tract, signaling pain. Thus, both evoked and paroxysmal, but not steady dysesthetic, pain may be relieved by operations that interrupt the pain pathways (DREZ, cordotomy, and cordectomy).

THE ROLE OF THE SYMPATHETIC NERVOUS SYSTEM

But what about the possible role of the sympathetic nervous system in neuropathic pain? Various suggestions have been advanced to explain its implications:[5] aberrant healing, enhanced inflammatory response, protective immobilization, and dysfunction of the sympathetic nervous system. First, it must be remembered that pain in which the sympathetic nervous system may be involved is also an example of neuropathic pain for which the features discussed above apply.

Despite the fact that the sympathetic nervous system has been implicated in a wide range of pain syndromes, it is only in the subset of SMP that sympathetic modulation can be expected to be effective. The various proposed mechanisms in SMP include antidromic release of such compounds as substance P, sensitizing nociceptors, abnormal actions of norepinephrine on peripheral sympathetic receptors causing hyperpathia and hyperesthesia, and abnormal signaling of pain by norepinephrine through afferents of

uncertain identity. However, when it comes to treatment, sympathetic manipulation often fails in the cases that most suggest sympathetic hyperactivity and succeeds in patients with no clinical evidence to suggest sympathetic involvement, making SMP an elusive entity.

TREATMENT

Unfortunately, our understanding of these pain syndromes is incomplete so that attempts to treat them are imperfect.

MEDICAL THERAPY

When we come to understand the pathophysiology of neuropathic pain more accurately, being able to understand what neurotransmitters and other neuroactive agents are involved, we will hopefully be able to be more effective. At present, the drugs that have proven their worth in scientific trials in neuropathic pain are Amitriptyline and Nortriptyline. Certain anti-epileptic drugs such as Gabapentin or Neurontin are also used, as well as other medications, but the scientific basis for their use in less secure.[18]

NERVE BLOCKS

Although Livingston[10] felt that repeated local anesthetic blockade of the injured nerve in whose territory the pain occurred was effective treatment for neuropathic pain, this method of treatment has not been widely accepted and there is concern that temporary relief of neuropathic pain, so common with such blocks, may lead to unjustified permanent neural interruption of the same structure that was temporarily blocked, which may not only fail to relieved the pain permanently, but also may aggravate it by increasing the degree of deafferentation.

NEURAL INTERRUPTION

Interruption of pain transmission through nerve section, cordotomy, the DREZ operation, or cordectomy is usually ineffective for the relief of neuropathic pain except for the allodynic, hyperpathic, and the intermittent neuralgic components. Both of these latter types of pain, as we have mentioned, are dependent on transmission in the spinothalamic tract. The pain seen in brachial plexus avulsion and after injuries to the conus/cauda equina may respond well to the DREZ operation, for example. The much commoner burning, steady dysesthetic component is not relieved at all by these procedures, but may be by chronic stimulation that produces paresthesias in the area in which this steady pain is felt.[11]

Sympathetic nervous system manipulation

In those patients with proven SMP, various methods of manipulating the sympathetic pathway may be successful in treating the pain. Local anesthetic interruption of the sympathetic nervous system at various levels is a long-practiced and simple technique, or else drugs such as Phenoxybenzamine can be used to preferentially block postsynaptic alpha 1 sympathetic terminals. If used at full dosage for 6 weeks and then tapered off, irreversible blockade occurs. Intravenous regional blockade by Guanethidine[8] may replace norepinephrine, causing a sympathetic block, or else permanent surgical interruption at various levels may be tried, but only when evidence has been produced that SMP exists.

REFERENCES

1. Backonja M-M: Painful neuropathics. In: Loeser JD, Ed: Bonica's Management of Pain. Philadelphia, Lippincott Williams and Wilkins, 2001:371–387.
2. Bennett GJ and Xie YK: A peripheral mononeuropathy in rat that produces disorders of pain sensation like those seen in man. Pain 33:87–107, 1988.
3. Boureau F, Doubriere JF, and Luu M: Study of verbal description in neuropathic pain. Pain 42:145–152, 1990.
4. Campbell JN, Raja SN, and Meyer RA: Painful sequelae of nerve injury. In: Dubner R, Geghart GF, and Bond M. Pain Research and Clinical Management, vol. 3. Amsterdam, Elsevier, 1996:135–143.
5. Galer BS, Schwartz L, and Allen RJ: Complex regional pain syndrome – Type I: reflex sympathetic dystrophy, and Type II: causalgia. In: Loeser JD, Ed: Bonica's Management of Pain. Philadelphia, Lippincott Williams and Wilkins, 2001:388–411.
6. Granit R, Leksell L, and Skoglund CR: Fibre interaction in injured or compressed region of nerve. Brain 67:125–140, 1944.
7. Gybels JM and Sweet WH: Neurosurgical Treatment of Persistent Pain. Basel, Karger, 1989:237–281.
8. Hannington-Kiff JG: Intravenous regional sympathetic block with guanethidine Lancet 1(7865):1019–1020, 1974.
9. Leriche R: The Surgery of Pain. London, Baillière, Tindall and Cox, 1939.
10. Livingston WK: Pain Mechanisms. A Physiological Interpretation of Causalgia and Its Related States. New York, MacMillan, 1943.
11. Meyerson BA: Electrical stimulation of the spinal cord and brain. In: Bonica JJ, Ed: The Management of Pain, 2nd edn. Philadelphia, Lea and Febiger, 1990:1862–1877.
12. Mitchell SW: Injuries of Nerves and Their Consequences. Philadelphia, JB Lippincott,1872.
13. Nordin M, Nystrom B, Wallin U, et al.: Ectopic sensory discharges and paresthesiae in patients with disorders of peripheral nerves, dorsal roots and dorsal columns. Pain 20:231–245, 1984.
14. Raymond SA and Rocco AG: Ephaptic coupling of large fibres as a clue to mechanism in chronic neuropathic allodynia following damage to dorsal roots. Pain (Supple 5):S276, 1990.
15. Tasker RR: Central pain states. In: Loeser JD, Ed: Bonica's Management of Pain, 3rd edn. Philadelphia, Lippincott Williams and Wilkins, 2001:433–457.
16. Tasker RR, de Carvalho GTC, and Dolan EJ: Intractable pain of spinal cord origin: Clinical features and implications of surgery. J Neurosurg 77:373–378, 1992.
17. Tasker RR, Organ LW, Hawrylyshyn P: Deafferentation and causalgia. In: Bonica JJ, Ed: Pain. New York, Raven, 1980:305–329.
18. Watson CPN: Non-surgical considerations in neuropathic pain. In: Gildenberg PL and Tasker RR, Eds: Textbook of Stereotactic and Functional Neurosurgery. New York, McGraw Hill, 1998:1637–1643.
19. Woolf CJ: Evidence for a central component of post-injury pain hypersensitivity. Nature 306:686–688, 1983.

22 Anesthetic and positional palsies

David G. Kline

OVERVIEW

- The possibility of an anesthetic or positional palsy must be considered and as far as possible prevented before beginning an operation.
- Most likely palsies are those of brachial plexus and ulnar nerve but almost every nerve has been either reported or implicated in an anesthetic or positional palsy.
- Positions associated most frequently with such palsies are with arms extended in an airplane position at right angles to the body and in the prone position with arms extended in front as if sledding.
- Predisposing factors include diabetes, alcoholism, and hereditary entrapment neuropathies as well as a prolonged operation.
- Some patients, especially those with ulnar palsies postoperatively, may have preoperative asymptomatic conductive slowing at the elbow. When recovery does not begin in the early months, neurolysis of the involved nerve may be helpful, especially if the palsy localized to a site associated with entrapment.
- A variety of palsies can occur because of injection or cannulation injury; nerves most affected are median and ulnar.
- Even something as simple as a malpositioned automatic blood pressure cuff can result in a median or ulnar palsy.
- Although much of the literature reporting larger series of lower extremity cases is related to the lithotomy position, peroneal and even femoral palsy can also occur with other operative positions.
- Differential diagnosis should include disorders such as the Parsonage-Turner syndrome, more direct nerve damage due to the operation itself, and a preexisting neuropathy.

There is no lack or depth of published material on this subject but a periodic reminder about pathogenesis and prevention of operative palsies is seldom out of vogue.[14,33,34,42,44,50] This is important because the added deficit of such palsies not directly related to the pathology undergoing correction is most unwelcome. In addition, mechanisms of injury and pathogenesis are not always crystal clear. Although the surgeon is viewed as the "captain of the ship" and must ultimately be at least partially responsible for the position of the anesthetized patient and his or her limbs, the anesthesiologist also has important responsibilities in this regard, not only referable to positioning.[2,10] The anesthetist is the one individual usually placing intravenous and arterial lines.

Nonetheless, one worries that nothing new or more illuminating will be brought to the reader's attention. The only small advantage the authors may have in that regard is their age but because of that, no doubt, some prejudices regarding the topic may also exist.

It is obvious that operations on or close to nerves have the risk of injuring them. Mechanism of injury can include stretch, contusion, compression, and crush as well as partial or complete transection.[19] An understanding of how these types of iatrogenic injury comes about with certain operations, at specific sites, and thus their prevention, is important but not the subject of this paper. It is, however, equally important to recognize that such iatrogenic injuries may be a major differential diagnosis when considering positional or anesthetic induced palsies.

For convenience, we will discuss these palsies by nerve and the more common anatomic sites involving those nerves (Table 22-1).

ULNAR NERVE

This is one of the most frequently affected nerves, especially at the level of the elbow.[1,7,9,57] Referable to position as an etiology, one of two unfavorable positions is extension of the elbow, especially on a relatively hard surface, with the forearm and hand pronated rather than supinated. In this position, pressure is brought to bear on the nerve in the olecranon notch or groove.[24] Pressure on the nerve can be minimized by having the hand and forearm supinated so the tip of the elbow (olecranon) and its radial aspect rather than the olecranon groove receives the pressure.

Although less frequent in the operative setting, the second unfavorable position is prolonged full flexion of elbow, especially if there is any pressure on the olecranon notch area of the elbow. The nerve is under maximal tension when there is full flexion at the elbow. This is because nerve runs from a more volar locus at midarm level to a very posterior locus within the notch and then again takes a more volar course in the forearm to eventually reach the volar side of the palm of the hand. Thus, prolonged positioning of the arm in flexion should be minimized.

Of interest, many of the positional palsies involving ulnar nerve present days to several weeks after the operation and in some studies relate more frequently to those with conductive slowing across the elbow preoperatively.[29,41]

Less frequently, the nerve at wrist level is injured by intravenous line placement or on the rare occasion when radial artery cannot

Table 22-1 Injuries to the brachial plexus and peripheral nerves due to faulty positioning during surgery*

Nerve injury	No. of patients	Position during anesthesia
Brachial plexus	28	14 lateral decubitus 14 supine
Peroneal	15	6 lateral decubitus 5 supine 4 Bell fracture table
Radial	11	8 supine 2 lateral decubitus 1 prone
Ulnar	9	8 supine 1 lateral decubitus
Median	3	2 supine 1 lateral decubitus
Femoral cutaneous	3	2 prone 1 lateral decubitus

*Parks B: Postoperative peripheral neuropathies. Surgery 74:348–357, 1973.

be cannulated or is unavailable for arterial pressure measurement and percutaneous puncture of the ulnar artery is attempted. For example, a university professor who was diabetic had a hypoglycemic episode while lecturing and required resuscitation. Ulnar nerve was inadvertently punctured and an i.v. of glucose infused. After successful resuscitation, a severe distal ulnar palsy was found. Flexor carpi ulnaris and flexor profundus to the little finger graded 5/5 (LSUMC system) while there was complete loss of hypothenar, interossei, and lumbrical function for little and ring fingers. Hypoesthesia was present on little and ring finger and the hypothenar surface of the palm but not in the dorsal cutaneous innervational territory on the ulnar side of the dorsum of the hand. With no improvement clinically or electrically over a 4.5-month period, the nerve was surgically explored. A neuroma in continuity extending 1.5 inches proximal to the distal wrist crease was found. There was no nerve action potential (NAP) conduction across this lesion to superficial or deep ulnar branches. As a result, the neuroma had to be resected and a graft repair done. Recovery of hand intrinsic and ulnar sensory function was only partial.

Less frequent is injection injury due to needle, i.v. fluid, or drugs involving ulnar nerve at arm level although it can occur when the anesthetist finds no more distal veins at forearm or elbow level and a vein is searched for on the inner surface of the upper arm. Of course, the median nerve at arm level can have inadvertent injury in the same fashion. Such is much more frequent than an arm-level ulnar involvement due to injection.

MEDIAN NERVE

This nerve is actually more frequently involved secondary to injection injury while starting an i.v. or during fluid or drug delivery than it is by positioning of the patient during anesthesia.[8] Even if the palsy is minimal, pain and paresthesias in the median distribution can be bothersome to the patient and the managing physician. Such symptoms are not always helped by surgery unless the injection site leads to serious deficit and requires resection. In addition, extravasated i.v. fluids can compress the AIN branch of the median deep to both pronator teres and flexor superficialis and result in the classic loss of proper pinch involving flexor pollicis longus of the thumb and flexor profundus to the forefinger. Palmar- or wrist-level extravasation of fluid can also give a more distal palsy simulating a severe carpal tunnel syndrome.

We have also seen carpal tunnel like symptoms and median palsy after hand and wrist is placed in a hyperextended position by a splint, particularly if the surgeon or an assistant inadvertently leans on the wrist or a puncture for an arterial line is too close to or directly involves the nerve. Automatic cuff tourniquets for blood pressure determinations or tourniquets to prevent blood loss, if applied too close to the elbow, and used over a long period of time, can compress the median nerve by the lower edge of the cuff.[6,18,43,47] Of interest, both radial and ulnar palsy has been reported after use of an automatic blood pressure monitor.[5,53] Prolonged maintenance of the wrist and hand in a hyperflexed position can also lead to distal sensory and/or motor loss.

RADIAL NERVE

The classic site for operative positional compression is at the midarm level where nerve winds around the humerus and is in the humeral groove. The classic Saturday night or sleep palsy can lead to wrist drop, loss of finger extension, supination, and brachioradialis with sparing of triceps function. Operatively and with anesthesia, a radial palsy can be due to the head being laid on the arm when the patient is in a prone position, or if the patient is in a lateral decubitus position due to pressure on unprotected arm. A surgeon leaning on an upper arm hidden by drapes can also be responsible.[58] Less frequent is compression of the nerve at the axillary level due to a firm or hard bolster. In either case, this is analogous to a crutch paralysis in an unanesthetized patient. Thus, triceps as well as brachioradialis and more distal extensors may be paralyzed.

The second site of radial nerve compression is the posterior interosseous nerve (PIN) as it goes under volar supinator. Extravasation of i.v. fluid or an i.v. prompted hematoma can also be responsible for partial wrist extension weakness (ECU) and finger and or thumb drop due to lack of EC and EPL.[58] The superficial sensory radial nerve (SSR) can be injured at wrist or more proximal forearm level by overly tight restraints or by misdirected cannulation of the radial artery or a vein.

BRACHIAL PLEXUS

Anesthetic and/or positioning compression of the plexus is by no means rare or particularly unusual.[2,11,40,46] Direct injury can occur with attempted placement of a central line. It is amazing that such does not happen more frequently because of proximity of plexus to the major veins such as jugular and subclavian. Arterial injury with or without associated clot, although quite unusual, can also occur. A pseudoaneurysm or clot can compress plexus and lead to both severe pain and progressive loss of function.

More common is plexus loss due to compression or prolonged positioning with arm(s) in an "airplane-like position," i.e. extended and abducted when the patient is supine or extended in front in a diving or sled-like position when prone.[13] Other problematic factors are a Trendelenburg position with poorly padded and usually metal stops against posterior shoulder, or use of tape to pull down shoulders when the patient is in a sitting position, or the patient is in a reverse Trendelenburg position (Fig. 22-1).

A prolonged period of time in one position without the limb being moved or having its position changed appears to be an important factor in all positional palsies. Thus, prolonged procedures with either the arms abducted and extended or in a "dive-like" position are especially dangerous. For example, we have seen several patients with bilateral plexus palsies due to a prolonged prone position with the arms in a "dive" position associated with prolonged and complex spinal instrumentation procedures.

Compression of the shoulder can, less frequently, also result in accessory palsy and thus paresis or paralysis of the trapezius. Long thoracic nerve palsy can also result, especially if the shoulders are pulled down by tape or the arms are pulled down by restraints when the patient is sitting or in a reverse Trendelenburg position. In either case, a winged scapula can result and that interferes with shoulder abduction above the horizontal as well as also a smooth abductive motion. However, the exact stresses responsible for an isolated postoperative long thoracic palsy are not always evident (Fig. 22-2).[38]

Pulling the shoulders or arms down is more likely to result in upper (C5, C6) rather than lower (C8–T1) trunk palsy. Extension and abduction of the arms in an airplane position with the patient supine or with the patient prone and in a dive position is most likely to give lower C8–T1 palsy. If possible, the preferred position with the patient either prone or supine is with the arms at the sides with elbow, wrist, and hand well padded. Of course, if the upper extremity itself is to be operated upon, then one arm will need to have some abduction, but usually not 90 degrees or more. Plexus palsy can also result from a lateral decubitus position without a proper soft bolster under the axilla and arm on the lower side. Less frequently, the upper arm can have a paralysis if it is overstretched and poorly positioned on a "sled-like support" (Fig. 22-3).

Some plexus palsies associated with cardiac surgery can be related to opening and displacing laterally the sternum, in which case the first rib may rotate superiorly or even fracture to directly impact C8–T1 and/or lower trunk.[23,25,32,49,54]

LOWER EXTREMITY

SCIATIC NERVE

This nerve is less frequently involved by positional palsies than its branches such as the peroneal nerve.[39] Nonetheless, compression at a buttock level can occur in a somewhat lateral decubitus position with pressure between the ischial tuberosity and the operating table. Hyperflexion of the hip as well as knee in a leg holder for a lithotomy position can also be responsible for sciatic palsy. Actually, such is more likely if the knee is extended as well as the hip being hyperflexed since that places the nerve on maximum stretch. The sitting position for cranial or spinal procedures can also result in sciatic or peroneal palsy.[30,51] Good padding, mild rather than extreme flexion of the hips, and some flexion rather than full extension of the legs helps avoid this complication.[19]

PERONEAL NERVE

Once again, the lithotomy position with hips flexed and leg(s) in stirrup(s), especially if there is lateral compression on the knee or

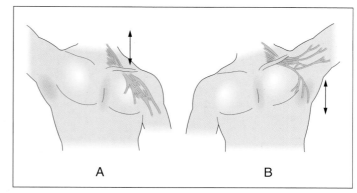

FIGURE 22-2 **(A)** Traction downward on the plexus which can result in upper plexus element damage which, if severe enough, can damage the entire plexus. **(B)** Hyperabduction of the arm can damage especially the lower plexus elements but, again if severe enough, can damage the entire plexus (see Chapter 16).

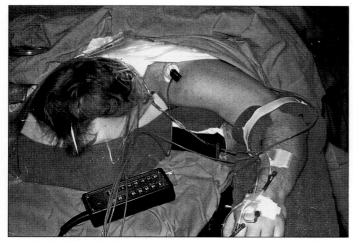

FIGURE 22-1 Prolonged positioning with arm(s) in the "dive" position can result in plexus palsy despite adequate padding of the axilla and elbow, as in this example.

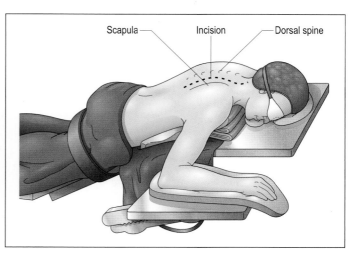

FIGURE 22-3 A more favorable position for the arm for an operation necessitating the prone position. In this case positioning is for parascapular paradorsal exposure for subscapular approach to the plexus (see Chapter 16).

if the knee is extended, can provide a mechanism for footdrop.[12,22] For the neurosurgeon or orthopedic surgeon, the lateral decubitus position, if not done carefully, can result in peroneal palsy involving the "down" leg. This is presumably due to pressure against the surgical neck of fibula, especially if the down leg is extended. Too much bolster or a firm object placed under the knee(s) with the patient supine for prolonged periods can be detrimental. Predisposing risk factors include a thin body habitus, use of tobacco by the patient, and a lengthy operative procedure (Fig. 22-4).[56,58]

Most of these peroneal palsies reverse over time but if function does not begin to recover in the early months, then surgical release or neurolysis of the nerve as it crosses the surgical neck of the fibula may be beneficial (Fig. 22-5).[56,58]

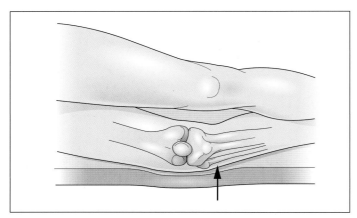

FIGURE 22-4   Placement in a lateral decubitus position, as in this case, can put the peroneal nerve at risk.

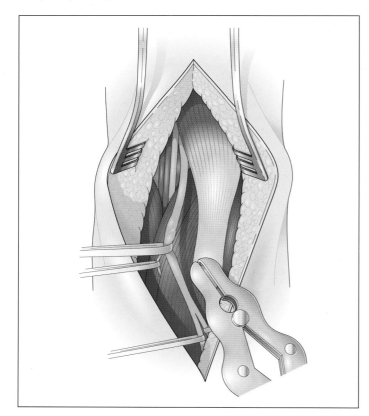

FIGURE 22-5   Neurolysis of the peroneal nerve and partial removal of the surgical neck of the fibula for a patient with persistent postoperative peroneal palsy due to operative malpositioning.

TIBIAL NERVE

This nerve is surrounded by fat and deep in the popliteal space, so seldom is it compressed behind the knee. Nerve is also deep in the lower leg between posterior tibia and gastrocnemius soleus so significant compression by positioning at that level is also rare. Compression, though, can occur at the level of the ankle near the medial malleolus, especially if the surgeon or his/her assistant leans on this area for a length of time.

FEMORAL NERVE

Although unusual, injury to this nerve can occur in the lithotomy position, especially if the thigh(s) is abducted too far and the hip(s) externally rotated.[26] What role if any, under these circumstances, angulation of the nerve as it passes beneath inguinal ligament provides is uncertain at this time. Although unusual, *lateral femoral cutaneous nerve* can be compressed by a laterally placed support bar for the lithotomy position or poorly padded lateral bolsters when the patient is in the prone position. Although not seen by ourselves, we could imagine that hyperextension of the hip in the prone position combined with pressure in the groin or inguinal area might stretch *and* compress the nerve.

OTHER NERVES

As can be imagined, saphenous nerve can be compressed on the inner side of the knee in the lithotomy position. Pressure over proximal mandible or excessive retraction of it can give facial palsy.[21] Recurrent laryngeal, lingual, and even hypoglossal palsies can result due to prolonged or malpositioned endotrachial intubation.[16,28,31,35]

PREVENTIVE STEPS

Knowing the propensity for certain nerves to have positional palsies related to special sites and different types of positions is helpful. In general, the nerve and nerve site should be padded with soft material and the position of the limb chosen should reduce as much as possible a stretched position for the nerve.

Some patients, such a diabetics and alcoholics, may have some predisposition to positional palsies as might the patient with multiple entrapment neuropathy or hereditary neuropathy with disability due to pressure palsies.[17,29] Monitoring nerve function during operative procedures can be used but there are limitations to its use for all operations.[25,36] Information on only one or two nerves can be accumulated and most procedures monitor the sensory system rather than the motor system. Nonetheless, in one series of scoliosis operations when both the spinal cord and the ulnar nerves were monitored, 18 of 500 patients had ulnar nerve conductive deficits.[48] When the involved limb was repositioned, this conductive abnormality disappeared and no deficit eventuated. As mentioned earlier, it should be stressed that a few studies have suggested that some patients have had a predisposition for ulnar palsy at the elbow having had preoperatively abnormal conduction studies across the elbow.

There is also some suggestion and evidence in the literature that operative palsies can occur in spite of diligent care in positioning the patient.[52,55] Nonetheless, it is one thing to have that happen, even though one took precautions to protect the subsequently involved nerve during positioning, and another when it happens under circumstances where one has not done that.

Closed claims studies by the American Society of Anesthesiologists published in both 1990 and 1999 support some of the above points.[2,15] From the files of medical liability insurance companies there were 1541 total cases and 178 (12%) involved one or more peripheral nerves, ulnar 77 (34%) and brachial plexus (23%) being the most common. Some 63% of nerve injury cases were judged to have met anesthetic level of care standards. Payments were made in 47% of nerve cases and the rate was the same whether care was judged to be standard or substandard. Some 18% of ulnar nerve positional palsies occurred despite data that strongly supported adequate intraoperative elbow padding. Results in the 1999 study were similar.[10] Again, quite a few of the palsies did not have, in retrospect, an obvious mechanism, so absolute prevention of perioperative nerve injury may not be possible.

DIFFERENTIAL DIAGNOSIS

In addition to direct nerve injury in the operative field, a major differential diagnosis is brachial plexitis or Parsonage-Turner syndrome.[3,27,45] This can present days to several weeks post surgery and can simulate positional brachial plexopathy or ulnar neuropathy.[37] Usually, several disparate parts of the upper extremity nervous system are involved, such as accessory or long thoracic nerve along with portions of the upper trunk or PIN or AIN. It is usually, but not always, reversible and very severe pain, often in the shoulder, is almost always present in the early days after onset. Then the pain dissipates and the patient is left with a disparate palsy. Etiology may be inflammatory or autoimmune but the palsies can also present after strenuous physical actively, usually involving the upper extremities, or injection for immunization.

Fortunately, most positional and anesthetic palsies improve, if recognized and managed with appropriate physical and occupation therapy and time.[4,50] There are, however, exceptions and the more severe palsies, if persisting for several months, may require surgery, operative recordings, and either neurolysis or resection and repair.

REFERENCES

1. Alvine FG and Schurrer ME: Postoperative ulnar-nerve palsy: are there predisposing factors? J Bone Joint Surg [Am] 69:255–259, 1987.

2. American Society of Anesthesiologists. Practice advisory for the prevention of perioperative peripheral neuropathies: a report by the American Society of Anesthesiologists Task Force on Prevention of Perioperative Peripheral Neuropathies. Anesthesiology, 93:1168–1182, 2000.

3. Arnason BG and Asbury AK: Idiopathic polyneuritis after surgery. Arch Neurol 18:500–507, 1968.

4. Ben-David B and Stahl S: Prognosis of intraoperative brachial plexus injury: a review of 22 cases. Br J Anaesth 79:440–445, 1997.

5. Bicker PE, Schapera A, and Bainton CR: Acute radial nerve injury from use of an automatic blood pressure monitor. Anesthesiology 73:186–188, 1990.

6. Bolton CF, McFarlane RM: Human pneumatic tourniquet paralysis. Neurology 28:787–793, 1978.

7. Britt BA and Gordon RA: Peripheral nerve injuries associated with anesthesia. Can Anaesth Soc J 11:514–536, 1964.

8. Butterworth J, Donofrio PD, and Hansen LB: Transient median nerve palsy after general anesthesia: does res ipsa loquitur apply? Anesth Analg 78:163–164, 1994.

9. Cameron MGP and Stewart OJ: Ulnar nerve injury associated with anaesthesia. Can Anaesth Soc J 22:253–264, 1975.

10. Cheney FW, Domino KB, Caplan RA, et al.: Nerve injury associated with anesthesia: a closed claims analysis. Anesthesiology 90:1062–1069, 1999.

11. Clausen EG: Postoperative "anesthetic" paralysis of the brachial plexus. Surgery 12:933–942, 1942.

12. Cooper DE: Nerve injury associated with patient positioning in the operating room. In: Gelberman RH, Ed: Operative Nerve Repair and Reconstruction, vol. 2. Philadelphia, Lippincott, 1991:1231–1242.

13. Cooper DE, Jenkins RS, Bready L, et al.: The prevention of injuries of the brachial plexus secondary to malposition of the patient during surgery. Clin Ortho Rel Res 228:33–41, 1988.

14. Dawson DM and Krarup C: Perioperative nerve lesions. Arch Neurol 46:1355–1360, 1989.

15. Dhuner K-G: Nerve injuries following operations: a survey of cases occurring during a six-year period. Anesthesiology 11:289–293, 1950.

16. Dziewas R and Ludemann P: Hypoglossal nerve palsy as complication of oral intubation, bronchoscopy and use of the laryngeal mask airway. Eur Neurol 47:239–243, 2002.

17. Earl CJ, Fulleton PM, Wakefield GS, et al.: Hereditary neuropathy, with liability to pressure palsies: a clinical and electrophysiological study of four families. Quart J Med 33:481–498, 1964.

18. Eckhoff NL: Tourniquet paralysis: plea for caution in extended use of pneumatic tourniquet. Lancet 2:343–345, 1931.

19. Edwards BN, Tullos HS, and Noble PC: Contributory factors and etiology of sciatic nerve palsy in total hip arthroplasty. Clin Ortho Rel Res 218:136–141, 1987.

20. Fowler TJ, Danta G, and Gilliatt RW: Recovery of nerve conduction after a pneumatic tourniquet: observations on the hind-limb of the baboon. J Neurol Neurosurg Psychiatry 35:638–647, 1972.

21. Fuller JE and Thomas DV: Facial nerve paralysis after general anesthesia. JAMA 162:645, 1956.

22. Garland H and Moorhouse D: Compressive lesions of the external popliteal (common peroneal) nerve. Br Med J 2:1373–1378, 1952.

23. Graham JG, Pye IF, and McQueen IN: Brachial plexus injury after median sternotomy. J Neurol Neurosurg Psychiatry 44:621–625, 1981.

24. Guardjian ES: Traumatic ulnar neuritis due to strapping of the elbow and forearm to the operating table. JAMA 96:944, 1931.

25. Hickey C, Gugino LD, Aglio LS, et al.: Intraoperative somatosensory evoked potential monitoring predicts peripheral nerve injury during cardiac surgery. Anesthesiology 78:29–35, 1993.

26. Hopper CL and Baker JB: Bilateral femoral neuropathy complicating vaginal hysterectomy: analysis of contributing factors in 3 patients. Obstet Gynecol 32:543–547, 1968.

27. James JL and Miles DW: Neuralgic amyotrophy: a clinical and electromyographic study. Br Med J 2:1042–1043, 1966.

28. Jones BC: Lingual nerve injury. A complication of intubation. Br J Anesthesia 43:730, 1971.

29. Jones HD: Ulnar nerve damage following a general anaesthetic: a case possibly related to diabetes mellitus. Anaesthesia 22:471–475, 1967.

30. Keykhah MM and Rosenberg H: Bilateral foot drop after craniotomy in the sitting position. Anaesthesiology 51:163–164, 1979.

31. King C and Street MK: Twelfth cranial nerve paralysis following use of a laryngeal mask airway. Anesthesia 49:786–787, 1994.

32. Kirsh MM, Magee KR, Gago O, et al.: Brachial plexus injuries following median sternotomy incision. Ann Thorac Surg 11:315–319, 1971.

33. Kroll DA, Caplan RA, Posner K, et al.: Nerve injury associated with anesthesia. Anesthesiology 73:202–307, 1990.

34. Lincoln JR and Sawyer HP: Complications related to body positions during surgical procedures. Anesthesiology 22:800–809, 1961.

35. Lloyd Jones FR and Hegab A: Recurrent laryngeal nerve palsy after laryngeal mask airway insertion. Anaesthesia 51:171–172, 1996.

36. Mahla ME, Long DM, Mckennett J, et al.: Detection of brachial plexus dysfunction by somatosensory evoked potential monitoring – a report of two cases. Anesthesiology 60:248–252, 1984.

37. Malamut RI, Marques W, England JD, et al.: Postsurgical idiopathic brachial neuritis. Muscle Nerve 17:320–324, 1994.

38. Martin JT: Postoperative isolated dysfunction of the long thoracic nerve: a rare entity of uncertain etiology. Anesth Analg 69:614–619, 1989.

39. Massey EW and Pleet AB: Compression injury of the sciatic nerve during prolonged surgical procedure in a diabetic patient. J Am Geriatr Soc 28:188–189, 1980.

40. Merchant RN, Brown WF, and Watson BV: Peripheral nerve injuries in cardiac anesthesia. Can J Anaesth 37:S152, 1990.

41. Neary D, Ochoa J, and Gilliatt RW: Sub-clinical entrapment neuropathy in man. J Neurol Sci 24:283–298, 1975.

42. Nicholson MJ and Eversole UH: Nerve injuries incident due to anaesthesia and operations. Anaesthesia Analg 36:19–32, 1957.

43. Ochoa J, Fowler TJ, and Gilliat RW: Anatomical changes in peripheral nerves compressed by a pneumatic tourniquet. J Anat 113:433–455, 1972.

44. Parks BJ: Postoperative peripheral neuropathies. Surgery 74:348–357, 1973.

45. Parsonage MJ and Turner WMJ: Neuralgic amyotrophy: the shoulder girdle syndrome. Lancet 1:973–978, 1948.

46. Posta AG, Allen AA, and Nercessian OA: Neurologic injury in the upper extremity after total hip arthroplasty. Clin Orthop Rel Res 345:181–186, 1997.

47. Rudge P: Tourniquet paralysis with prolonged conduction block. J Bone Joint Surg [Br] 56:716–720, 1974.

48. Schwartz DM, Drummond DS, Hahn M, et al.: Prevention of positional brachial plexopathy during surgical correction of scoliosis. J Spinal Dis 13:178–182, 2000.

49. Seyfer AE, Grammer NY, Bogumill GP, et al.: Upper extremity neuropathies after cardiac surgery. J Hand Surg 10A:16–19, 1985.

50. Slocum HC, O'Neal KC, and Allan CR: Neurovascular complications from malposition on the operating table. Surg Gynecol Obstet 86:729–734, 1948.

51. Standefer M, Bay JW, and Trusso R: The sitting position in neurosurgery: a retrospective analysis of 488 cases. Neurosurgery 14:649–658, 1984.

52. Stoelting RK: Postoperative ulnar nerve palsy – is it a preventable complication? Anaesth Analg 76:7–9, 1993.

53. Sy WP: Ulnar nerve palsy possibly related to use of automatically cycled blood pressure cuff. Anesth Analg 60:687–688, 1981.

54. Vander Salm TJ, Cereda J-M, and Cutler BS: Brachial plexus injury following median sternotomy. J Thorac Cardiovasc Surg 80:447–452, 1980.

55. Wadsworth TG: The cubital tunnel and the external compression syndrome. Anesth Analog 53:303–308, 1974.

56. Warner MA, Martin JT, Schroeder DR, et al.: Lower-extremity motor neuropathy associated with surgery performed on patients in a lithotomy position. Anesthesiology 81:6–12, 1994.

57. Wey JM and Guinn GA: Ulnar nerve injury with open heart surgery. Ann Thoracic Surg 39:358–360, 1985.

58. Winfree CJ and Kline DG: Intraoperative positioning nerve injuries. Surg Neurol 63(1):5–18, 2005.

23

Tumors involving nerve

Daniel H. Kim

OVERVIEW

Tumors involving nerve provide some of the most challenging and at times vexatious lesions to manage when dealing with a broad spectrum of peripheral nerve problems. Magnification, use of intra-operative recordings, and knowledge of the gross and microscopic pathology are important to the surgeon undertaking tumor resection.

An understanding of the tumor's disposition, with an awareness of the involved as well as spared fascicles, can improve the surgeon's ability to resect benign nerve sheath tumors.

Summarized in this chapter are the presentations, operative techniques used, and outcomes of a series of 397 benign nerve sheath tumors.

The success rate for excision without significant deficit for schwannomas in this series was almost 90%. This figure was 80% for solitary neurofibromas not associated with NF1 (von Reckling-hausen's disease), and that represents a departure from the stan-dard in most literature, especially where only biopsy is recommended for the majority of these lesions. Successful resection of NF1-associated neurofibromas has been 66%. On the other hand, it was difficult to gain any satisfactory results with plexiform tumors. Postoperative pain and the likelihood of functional deficit were less of a problem if the benign nerve sheath tumors had not been biopsied or undergone surgery at a previous time.

Malignant neural sheath tumors and neurogenic sarcomas of nerve require especially discriminating management. The operative experience at Louisiana State University Health Sciences Center (LSUHSC) and outcomes with 36 such lesions are presented. In recent years, an attempt at limb-sparing management has been studied, although amputation of the limb or forequarter amputa-tion was done in 13 of the 36 patients.

A relatively large operative experience with benign tumors or masses secondarily involving nerve is also presented. This subset included 33 ganglion cysts, 12 vascular tumors, 12 lipomas, and 11 desmoid tumors.

Although usually palliative, resection of secondary or metastatic cancer involving the plexus or nerve can help pain considerably and occasionally even reverse deficit in selected cases. Thirty-five such lesions, most of which involved the brachial plexus are discussed.

Less efficacious appears to be surgery for irradiation plexitis, either with or without associated metastatic disease.

An unusual surgical entity involving nerve, hypertrophic neu-ropathy or "onion whorl disease" is discussed based on the LSUHSC experience to date with 16 histologically verified samples.

INTRODUCTION

Two categories of tumors involve the peripheral nerve and include tumors derived from the neural sheath and those of non-neural sheath origin. Each category can be further subdivided into benign and malignant classifications.

The benign components of neural sheath tumors are the periph-eral neural sheath tumors (PNSTs). These tumors begin and grow within, and can project from, the nerve.[38,154] PNSTs include the schwannoma and neurofibroma whose differentiation has been clarified using electron microscopy and immunohistochemistry. These same techniques have resulted in a wide acceptance that the principle cell of origin of these tumors is the Schwann cell.[134] Malignant tumors of neural sheath origin include malignant schwannomas and malignant neurofibromas, which are indistin-guishable by histology and are together known as malignant PNSTs. Malignant PNSTs may arise from all elements of the neural sheath including Schwann cells, endoneurial fibroblasts, and perineurial cells.[133]

The second broad category of tumors involving nerve includes tumors of non-neural sheath origin. Its subdivisions are those of benign and malignant peripheral non-neural sheath tumors (PNNSTs).

Benign PNNSTs can behave aggressively and include ganglions, lipomas, desmoids, ganglioneuromas, hemangiomas, myoblastomas or granular cell tumors, lymphangiomas, and the rare hemangio-blastoma or meningioma.

Malignant PNNSTs arise from other tissue and involve the nerve by direct extension. For example, breast or pulmonary cancers often involve nerve and do so by infiltration or compression of the nerve, as exemplified by the Pancoast tumor. Osteogenic sarcoma or soft tissue sarcoma of non-nerve sheath origins also can involve nerve and extend to or encase the nerve.[7] Metastases from a distant origin such as lymphomas and melanomas can also secondarily spread to nerve.

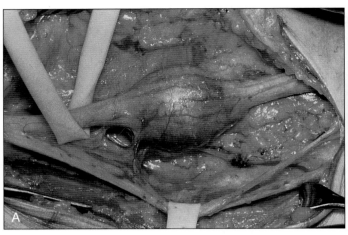

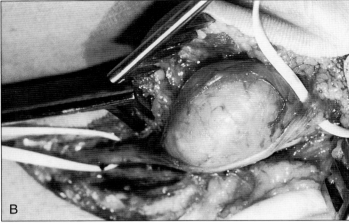

FIGURE 23-1 **(A)** This is the typical operative appearance of a neural sheath tumor, in this case a schwannoma of the tibial nerve in the popliteal fossa. Note that the surgical exposure has included a length of the involved nerve both proximal and distal to the lesion. **(B)** In a similar lesion, peripheral fascicles splayed around the mass, i.e. "basketing the mass," have been dissected away. Entering and exiting fascicles did not transmit a nerve action potential, so they were sectioned to permit total removal of the mass.

TUMORS OF NEURAL SHEATH ORIGIN

HISTORY OF CLASSIFICATION

Virchow described three types of peripheral nerve tumors in 1857: vascular, fatty, and fibrous, also called "Neuroma fibrillare amyelinicum," the tumor type subsequently described by von Recklinghausen.[2] Verocay is credited with first describing a nerve tumor as a separate entity in 1910.[158] He referred to its origin as the fibrous neural sheath, but did not describe a cell of origin. Verocay introduced the term "neurinoma" for these peripheral nerve tumors. Because this term translated into "nerve tumor" and did not allude to a cell of origin, however, most authors have recommended that it be discarded.[22,74,107,134] Mallory postulated that these tumors arose from the fibroblasts and coined the term "perineurial fibroblastoma."[105] This view was strongly supported by Penfield in 1930.[117] By 1935, Stout, the author of the first Armed Forces Institute of Pathology fascicle on peripheral nerve tumors, had introduced the term "neurilemoma" indicating the neuroectodermal origin of these tumors.[147] As Russell and Rubinstein pointed out later in 1959, however, this term refers to membranes, and not to the Schwann cell whose replication results in these tumors. In 1943, Ehrlich and Martin proposed "schwannoma" to indicate a Schwann cell origin for peripheral nerve tumors.[48] This latter term is now preferred for one of the subcategories of benign peripheral nerve tumors (Figs 23-1, 23-2).[134]

In 1968, Fisher and Vusevski demonstrated by electron microscopy that Schwann cells have a distinctive basement lamella that differentiates them from fibroblasts.[54] Fibroblasts form the epineurium of a nerve, which does not differ from mesenchymal tissue elsewhere in the body. The perineurial layer investing each nerve fascicle is formed of cells which, though appearing similar to fibroblasts using light microscopy, possess basement membranes by electron microscopy. In addition, these "perineurial fibroblasts" form tight junctions, accounting in part for the blood–nerve barrier properties representative of the peripheral nervous system.[79,134] Since Schwann cells have basement membranes, it may be that these perineurial fibroblasts are non-myelin-producing Schwann cells.

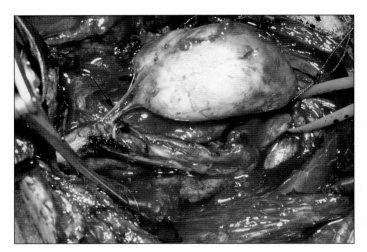

FIGURE 23-2 This is an intraoperative photograph of a schwannoma before sacrifice of several relatively small entering (*arrow*) and exiting fascicles. Most of the larger fascicles have been dissected away from the tumor and spared. This tumor was located in the vagal nerve and had produced hoarseness, but not paralysis of the vocal cord.

The differentiation of a solitary neurofibroma from a schwannoma is now straightforward using current histopathological techniques.[134] Controversy no longer exists as to whether the schwannoma and neurofibroma both arise from Schwann cells. Both tumors are thought to arise from Schwann cells primarily because electron microscopy has shown prominent basement membranes in each. There is a perineurial component of neurofibromas, however, which have been shown by ultrastructural studies.

The schwannoma and two main types of neurofibroma differ grossly from one another in the pattern of fascicular involvement (Fig. 23-3). The schwannoma grows extrinsic to its one or two parent fascicles. There are two variants of neurofibromas. The first is the fusiform: its few fascicles of origin become intertwined with tumor. A second type of neurofibroma is the plexiform neurofibroma, which consists of multiple nodular growths growing along a long segment of a major nerve trunk, and these growths may extend into the nerve branches.

Some of the immunohistochemical and electron microscopic features used to differentiate Schwann cells from perineurial cells and endoneurial fibroblasts are summarized in Table 23-1. These tests are helpful to differentiate individual cells, but not to identify a specific type of tumor. If they are used as a supplement to the histological criteria of light microscopy, they can be valuable, especially in making a decision as to the neural sheath origin of a tumor.[167]

The terminology for malignant peripheral neural sheath tumors (MPNSTs) has been confusing. Some neuropathologists have categorized them as either malignant schwannomas or malignant neurofibromas. These two tumor types usually are indistinguishable by microscopy, though the presence of mucopolysaccharide staining favors a malignant neurofibroma. Older terms used for MPNSTs include neurogenic sarcomas and neurofibrosarcomas.

Most malignant schwannomas arise de novo.[133] Harkin and Reed state that the malignant degeneration of solitary benign schwannomas rarely, if ever, occurs, except in the presence of von Recklinghausen's disease (NF1).[74] On the other hand, they believe that the malignant neurofibroma or neurofibrosarcoma is the most common type of malignancy in patients with NF1. There is general agreement that up to 50% of all malignant neurofibromas or neurofibrosarcomas arise within the context of NF1. The malignant neurofibroma or neurofibrosarcomas are complex tumors in which mesenchymal elements may be mixed with schwannian ones.[133]

Histologically, characteristics of malignancy such as pleomorphism and mitotic figures differentiate MPNSTs from their benign counterparts; however, distinctions between a MPNSTs and a variant of a benign and longstanding schwannoma exhibiting mitoses can still be difficult. Tumor assessment needs to be done by a pathologist experienced in this difficult and at times confusing field.

A major practical feature which distinguishes an MPNST from a mesenchymal fibrosarcoma is the former's origin within a nerve. Thus, our cases of malignant fibrosarcoma involving the brachial plexus and other nerves were differentiated by their gross appearance, since they did not seem to arise in the center of a plexus element or nerve.

BENIGN TUMORS OF NEURAL SHEATH ORIGIN

SCHWANNOMA

Schwannomas are the most common benign tumor of peripheral nerves, yet they account for fewer than 8% of all soft tissue tumors.[129] Schwannomas of the peripheral nerve reviewed in the literature over the past 20 years have consisted of case reports,[4,64,82,84,106] small series,[14,45,51,53,87,92,95,104,129,130,149] and large series.[8,10,94,108,124,143]

The incidence of benign schwannomas involving peripheral nerve tends to be higher in females than in males. These tumors can occur in patients with NF1; however, neurofibromas are much more common in this setting.[39]

Clinical presentation and examination

A benign schwannoma of peripheral nerve characteristically presents as a painless, eccentric, oval mass present for some time in a deep location in the course of a nerve or plexal element.[25] On palpation, they can be moved laterally, but not longitudinally in the

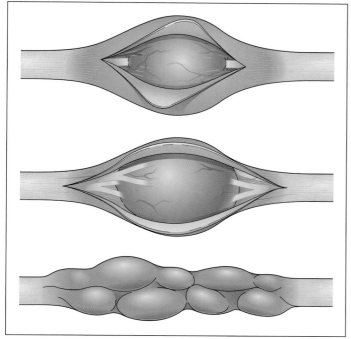

FIGURE 23-3 These drawings show the usual appearance of a schwannoma (*top*), a solitary neurofibroma (*middle*), and a plexiform neurofibroma (*bottom*). The schwannoma grows extrinsic to its parent fascicle, usually one or two in number, while the neurofibroma with usually more than two fascicles of origin become intertwined with these fascicles. Plexiform neurofibromas are characterized by multiple nodular growths along a long segment of a major nerve trunk and these growths extend into the nerve branches (From Donner T, Voorhies R, and Kline D: Neural sheath tumors of major nerves. J Neurosurg 81:362–373, 1994).

Table 23-1 Immunohistochemical and electron microscopic features of neural cells

	S-100 protein	EMA	Tight junctions	Pinocytotic vesicles	Basement membrane	Laminin	Type IV collagen	Fibronectin
Schwann cell	+	–	–	–	+	+	+	–
Perineurial cell	–	+	+	+	+	+	+	+
Endoneurial fibroblast	–	–	–	–	–	–	–	+

EMA, epithelial membrane antigen; +, present; –, absent.

Data collected by Voorhies RM from Theaker et al.: Histopathology 13:171–179, 1988; Ariza et al.; Am J Surg Pathol 12:678–683, 1988; Nakajima et al.: Am J Surg Pathol 6:715–727, 1982; Jaahola et al: J Clin Invest 84:253–261, 1989.

direction that the tumor runs. Percussion over the mass may produce a Tinel sign, i.e. paresthesias in the distribution of the involved nerve.[31]

Since the growth of peripheral nerve schwannomas usually occur over many years, large lesions slowly stretch and elongate the fascicles.[44,55] Thus, neurological function tends to be intact in these tumors. Loss of function from smaller benign schwannomas is rare, as well, unless a prior biopsy had injured the involved nerve or an unsuccessful attempt at tumor removal had been performed. Under these circumstances, the residual mass may be quite painful, motor loss in the distribution of the involved nerve can be severe, and sensation is markedly impaired or absent.

Microscopic appearance

The cell of origin of the schwannoma is the Schwann cell. The Schwann cell has a basement lamella and is more differentiated than, for example, the perineurial fibroblast.

The cells of the tumor are arranged in varying proportions of arrays of cells called Antoni type A and Antoni type B tissues (Fig. 23-4). The schwannoma's Antoni type A tissue is very cellular with a compact array of spindle-shaped cells. Some of these cells may palisade to form Verocay bodies. The Antoni type B pattern seen in some schwannomas, on the other hand, is less compact and has a loose-textured matrix.

If the schwannoma tissue is stained with Alcian blue, a mucopolysaccharide stain, or with reticular stains, these studies are less positive than those seen with a neurofibroma. In neurofibromas, connective tissue fibers, especially collagen, are conspicuous elements and nerve fibers within the tumor substance are more numerous and more obvious under the microscope than in the schwannomas.

Surgical approach

The removal of a schwannoma is straightforward; however, serious complications can occur if care is not taken with the dissection and preservation of involved plexal elements or nerves.[45,128,132]

Exposure of the nerve of origin well proximal and distal to the lesion itself is necessary. Other nerves or plexal elements and vessels are dissected away and spared. An area in the circumference of the capsule with few or no fascicles is then opened in a longitudinal fashion. The encapsulated tumor spreads or "baskets" the nerve fascicles apart, displacing them to its periphery.[163] These fascicles may be adherent to the outer capsular surface of the tumor, though they are seldom incorporated into the capsule itself.[66]

The capsule and accompanying "basketed" fascicles are gently dissected away and moved to one side or the other to expose the tumor itself (Fig. 23-5). This is carried out using a fine-tipped, double-ended or Rhoton dissector, a gauze-tipped "peanut," or the end of a Metzenbaum scissors. Some interfascicular dissection is then done at the proximal and distal poles of the tumor.

One, or sometimes two, small fascicles are seen entering and leaving the tumor and these are exposed and encircled with Vasoloops. Stimulation and recording across the fascicle(s) entering and the fascicle(s) leaving each pole of the encapsulated tumor is then performed (Fig. 23-6). Stimulation of the entering fascicle(s) usually does not produce distal muscle function, nor do these fascicles conduct a nerve action potential (NAP) through the tumor to distal elements or nerves. These mostly nonfunctional proximal or distal fascicles are sectioned and the tumor removed as a single mass (Fig. 23-7). One way to do this is to section one nonfunctional entering or leaving fascicle and to lift the tumor at that pole and to dissect it away from underlying and laterally reflected but retained fascicles. The opposite pole's nonfunctional fascicle is then sectioned to complete the removal.

An alternative approach sometimes used on large tumors is to open the capsule longitudinally and enucleate the homogenous or sometimes cystic tumoral contents using suction, forceps and scissors, or a Cavitron Ultrasonic Surgical Aspirator (CUSA).[26,114] The spared fascicles are teased away from the tumor capsule, which is then resected. The capsule is totally removed to reduce the chance of recurrence, although some surgeons disagree with this concept and leave the capsule.

Some schwannomas become quite large and extend beyond the immediate region of the nerve. These lesions are more difficult to remove, which increases the possibility of recurrence from the remaining tumor and/or capsule.[73]

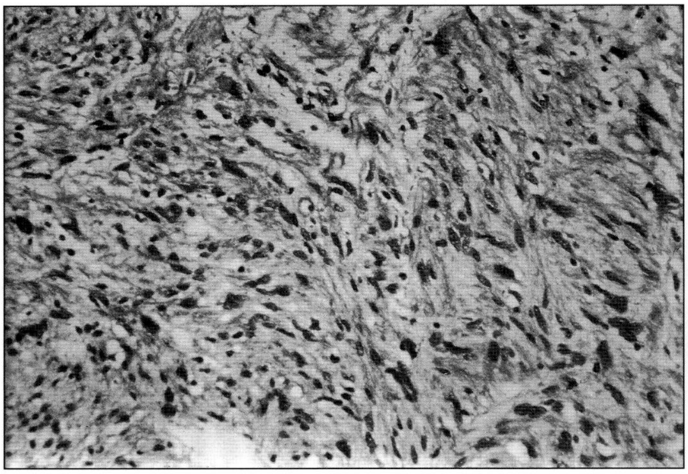

FIGURE 23-4 These are the photomicrograph findings of a schwannoma with its spindle-shaped neoplastic Schwann cells. Shown is an Antoni A area characterized by alternating areas of compact, elongated cells. A Verocay body is seen centrally; its nuclear palisades are formed by nearly parallel arrays of the nuclei of the tumor cells separated by compact, closely aligned cell processes and basement membranes. H & E, original magnification ×200.

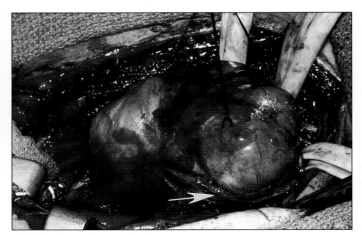

FIGURE 23-5 **(A)** An intraoperative photograph of a large schwannoma with its surrounding fascicles partially dissected away from it (*arrow*).

Results

Tables 23-2 through 23-4 show the distribution of 124 (34%) schwannomas of 361 benign PNSTs including schwannomas, solitary neurofibromas and NF1-associated neurofibromas resected at LSUHSC between 1969 and 1999 from the brachial plexus and various peripheral nerves. All tumor histologies were confirmed by a variety of studies.

There were 54 (38%) benign brachial plexus schwannomas of 141 brachial plexus PNSTs (Figs 23-8, 23-9). One hundred and ten PNSTs involved upper extremity peripheral nerves, of which 32 (29%) were benign schwannomas. One patient's median nerve schwannoma was a giant cell histologic variant and another patient with NF1 had an ulnar nerve tumor with the gross and microscopic appearance of a schwannoma. Graft repair of the originating peripheral nerve was required in two patients, both of whom had damage resulting from prior operations. Of 25 benign PNSTs of the pelvic plexus, six (24%) were schwannomas (Figs 23-10, 23-11). Of 85 PNSTs of the lower extremity, schwannomas were removed from 32 (38%) patients (Fig. 23-12).

All tumors except two large pelvic schwannomas were completely excised. One schwannoma of the pelvic plexus, thought to have been total excised at the first operation, recurred. This tumor was re-excised and has not subsequently recurred after 5 years of follow-up.

Examples of typical pre- and postoperative functional statuses, which can be expected from resections of schwannomas, are as follows. An analysis of 76 patients with schwannomas removed

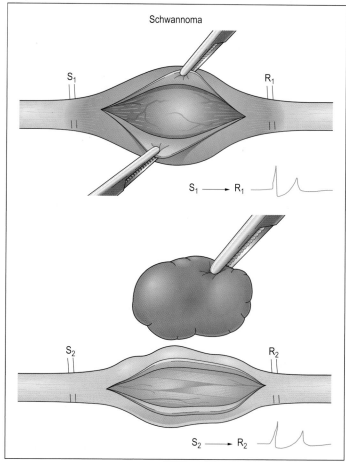

FIGURE 23-6 The usual steps in removal of a schwannoma are illustrated. A baseline nerve action potential (NAP) is recorded across the lesion. The entering fascicle is stimulated and a recording is taken from the exiting fascicle. A flat trace is usually seen. If a flat trace is obtained these fascicles are sectioned, and the tumor is usually removed as a solitary mass. In this example, the NAP recording after removal of the mass shows preservation of the potential. (Adapted from Lusk M, Kline D, and Garcia C: Tumors of the brachial plexus. Neurosurgery 21:439–453, 1987.)

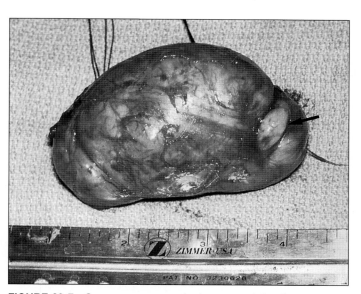

FIGURE 23-7 Gross appearance of a large neural sheath tumor. The entering fascicular structure, indicated by an arrow, was nonfunctional.

Table 23-2 Benign neural sheath tumors in the brachial plexus region (n=141)

	Schwannoma	Sporadic NF	NF–NF1	Totals
Supraclavicular brachial plexus	37	34	19	90
Infraclavicular brachial plexus	9	14	8	31
Axillary nerve	3	4	4	11
Musculocutaneous	3	2	1	6
Other	2	1	0	3
Totals	54	55	32	141

NF, neurofibroma; NF1, neurofibroma associated with NF1.

See also: Ganju A, Roosen N, Kline D, Tiel R: Outcomes in a consecutive series of 111 surgically treated plexal tumors: a review of the experience at LSUHSC. J Neurosury 95:51–60, 2001.

Table 23-3 Location of benign neural sheath tumors in the LSUHSC series – upper extremity (n=110)

	Schwannoma	Sporadic neurofibroma	Neurofibroma with NF1	Totals
Ulnar nerve				
Arm	5	10	8	23
Elbow/forearm	2	8	3	13
Wrist/hand	1	3	4	8
Median nerve				
Arm	7	10	5	22
Elbow/forearm	4	6	3	13
Wrist	6	3	3	12
Radial nerve				
Arm	5	2	3	10
Elbow	1	2	2	5
PIN/SSR	1	1	2	4
Totals	32	45	33	110

LSUHSC, Louisiana State University Health Sciences Center; NF, neurofibromatosis type I; PIN, posterior interosseous nerve; SSR, superficial sensory radial nerve.

Table 23-4 Location of benign neural sheath tumors in the LSUHSC series – lower extremity (n=110)

	Schwannoma	Neurofibroma	Neurofibroma with NF1	Totals
Pelvic plexus	6	10	9	25
Femoral nerve	5	7	2	14
Sciatic nerve				
Buttock	2	4	3	9
Thigh	8	9	6	23
Tibial nerve	10	5	5	20
Peroneal nerve	4	4	3	11
Saphenous nerve	2	1	0	3
Sural nerve	1	0	2	3
Obturator nerve	0	1	1	2
Totals	38	41	31	110

LSUHSC, Louisiana State University Health Sciences Center; NF1, neurofibromatosis type I.

from the brachial plexus and major nerves at LSUHSC was presented in a publication by Donner et al.[45] (Table 23-5; and see Table 23-8). Postoperative follow-up in this subgroup was 3–96 months (mean, 16.7 months). Sixty-eight (89%) schwannomas were excised without significant residual loss, i.e. had postoperative grades of 4 or 5, using the grading scale of 0 to 5 in use at LSUHSC.

Fifteen (20%) of 76 lesions had mild deficits or grade 4 function and eight (11%) had more serious deficits, i.e. grade 3 or less after resection.

Among 45 patients of the 76 patients studied who had intact strength preoperatively, 41 (91%) maintained full strength and four (9%) decreased to grade 4 postoperatively. Thirty-one (41%) of 76

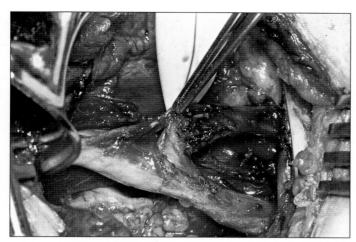

FIGURE 23-8 Plexus elements are shown after resection of a large schwannoma at a clavicular level. Forceps are grasping the entering fascicle, which was nonfunctional on stimulation and more distal recording. As a result, this fascicle and a similar exiting distal fascicle were sectioned.

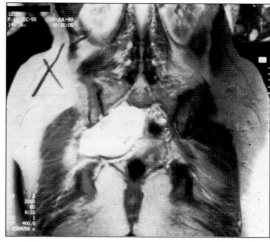

FIGURE 23-10 A magnetic resonance image of a schwannoma arising from the sacral plexus is seen. The tumor was approached transabdominally after mobilizing the bowel and bladder and identifying the ureter and great vessels. Fortunately, it could be "shelled out" away from the fascicles of the pelvic plexus elements with preservation of function.

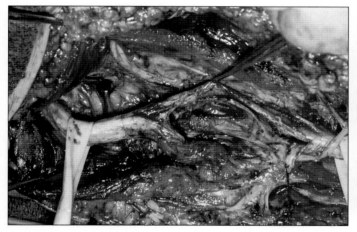

FIGURE 23-9 This is an intraoperative photograph of the bed of the brachial plexus after the removal of a large schwannoma involving the C7 to middle trunk. Despite a gross total resection, the tumor recurred 2 years later and was re-resected without deficit. The patient has had no new recurrence in over 4 years of further follow-up.

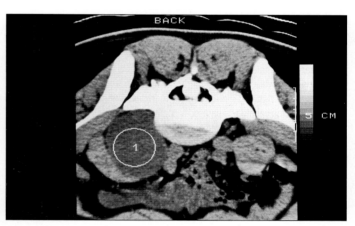

FIGURE 23-11 A magnetic resonance image of a large pelvic neural sheath tumor arising from lumbar roots and displacing the psoas muscle laterally is seen. The origin was the lumbar roots destined for the femoral nerve outflow.

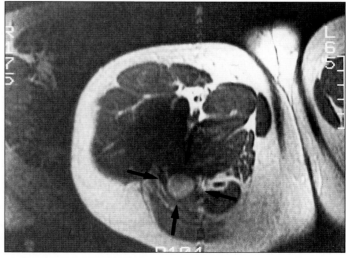

FIGURE 23-12 A magnetic resonance image of the thigh showing a neural sheath tumor involving the sciatic nerve (arrows).

patients with schwannomas involving the neural sheath had reduced preoperative functional grades from 0 to 4. Of these 31, 17 (55%) improved postoperatively, 10 (32%) were unchanged, and four (13%) had further reduction of functional status.

Of this same subset, 24 (32%) patients presented with pain syndromes (see Table 23-7). Twenty patients complained of purely radicular pain of which 15 (75%) had a resolution of this pain postoperatively, two (10%) had partial resolution, one (5%) had no change in the severity of pain and two (10%) patients had an increase in pain. Four patients presented with radicular pain plus a spontaneous pain component localized to the site of the tumor. All four had complete resolution of both components of pain postoperatively. Four (8%) of 51 patients who did not have preoperative pain had the new onset of a degree of pain postoperatively.

Postoperative grade	Preoperative grade					
	5	**4**	**3**	**2**	**1**	**0**
5	41	9	3			
4	4	6	3	1	1	
3		2	2			
2			2	1		
1					1	
0						

Table 23-5 Schwannoma (n=76)

The pre- and postoperative motor grades of the involved muscle groups in a group of patients with resected schwannomas. Overall, 17 patients improved, 8 worsened, and in 51, the grades remained the same. Of the 51 with no change, 41 had normal strength at presentation.

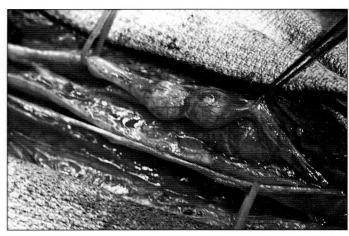

FIGURE 23-13 A plexiform neurofibroma is shown, which involved the tibial nerve in an "up-and-down" fashion. A partial decompression was performed because of severe neuritic pain. The lesions extended from the proximal thigh level of the tibial division of the sciatic nerve down to the ankle level of the posterior tibial nerve.

CASE SUMMARY – SCHWANNOMA

CASE 1

A 26-year-old female experienced pain radiating from behind the knee to the heel of her foot while riding a ski lift. She subsequently felt a lump behind her knee and noted that if it were bumped, a "shock-like" sensation radiated into her calf. Radiological studies showed a popliteal fossa mass. Function on clinical and electromyographic examination was normal in the leg.

At operation several months later, a 3 × 2.5 cm mass was found within the tibial nerve. Most of the fascicles could be dissected away from the tumor capsule. NAP testing was carried out on two smaller fascicles entering and leaving the tumor and they did not conduct. The tumor was removed as a single mass. Postoperatively, there was some decreased function of the toe flexors and intrinsic foot muscles, but good plantar flexion and inversion. Sensation on the sole of the foot was present. At follow-up 8 years later, there was full sciatic nerve including tibial nerve function.

The initial histopathology suggested the possibility of malignancy, since mitotic figures were seen in what was otherwise an "epithelial-like" schwannoma. A second opinion regarding the histopathology stressed that while the tumor was cellular and had mitotic activity, it was well differentiated. Spindle cells with Antoni A and B tissue were also described and the conclusion was that the tumor was most likely a benign schwannoma. There has been no recurrence over an 8-year period.

COMMENT

The diagnosis of a malignant nerve tumor necessitates radical treatment. The correct interpretation using light and electron microscopy, and at times histochemical studies, is therefore critical. In this case, the benign nature of the tumor was eventually discerned.

NEUROFIBROMA

There are two groups of neurofibromas. The first group includes the solitary tumor or non-NF1 neurofibroma, which is unassociated with other such tumors.[33] This tumor is most likely to be fusiform in appearance, i.e. tapered at each end.[40]

The second group of neurofibromas, the plexiform neurofibromas, are seen almost exclusively in conjunction with NF1. Plexiform neurofibromas exhibit multiple nodular growths along a long segment of a major nerve trunk and these growths extend into the nerve branches (Fig. 23-13). They result in the so-called "bag of worms" appearance on gross inspection and cross-sectional imaging. Fusiform lesions are more likely to be seen in patients with NF1, however, than are plexiform neurofibromas.

Cases presented in the literature have included case reports,[101,126] small series,[14,46,87,95,108,127] and large series.[10,94,108,124]

Clinical presentation and examination

Solitary neurofibromas occur more commonly in females than in males. Neurofibromas have a predilection for the right side of the body.

NF1-associated neurofibromas have a more equal distribution between the sexes and are also seen equally on both sides of the body. NF1-associated neurofibromas tend to present earlier than do the solitary neurofibromas (Fig. 23-14).

Neurofibromas are intraneural masses, which are more likely to be more painful than schwannomas. Percussion over a neurofibroma usually produces a dramatic Tinel sign.[37] Like schwannomas, these tumors, along with their nerve of origin, can be displaced from side to side, but cannot be moved in a proximal to distal direction and vice versa, and pain can become a very severe problem if there has been prior biopsy or attempted removal.[43]

NF1-associated neurofibromas are found in patients with other stigmata of that disease (Fig. 23-15).[136] The manifestations of NF1 are protean and include café au lait spots, multiple small spots of skin discoloration, skin tags or smaller subcutaneous tumors, Lisch nodules of the iris, and central nervous system tumors such as acoustic neurilemoma or tumors arising from the nerve roots of the spine (Fig. 23-16).

On occasion, larger neurofibromas, especially those associated with NF1, can undergo malignant transformation. Whether this is a change in the cell's potential for mitosis or whether cells with such potential are present from the beginning is not known.

A form of NF1 known as regionalized or segmental NF1 can occur in which multiple tumors affect one limb or one region of anatomy without the presence of tumors elsewhere (Fig. 23-17). The multiple tumors are frequently intrinsic to one or more nerves

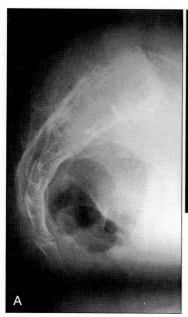

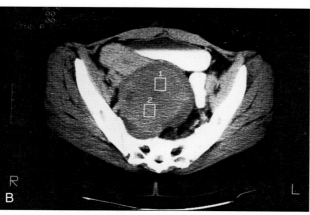

FIGURE 23-14 (A) A plain film of the sacrum showing posterior displacement and deformity by a large neurofibroma. (B) This computerized tomographic scan also shows the giant presacral neurofibroma. Removal required a pelvic exposure with mobilization of the bladder, identification of ureters and great vessels, and mobilization of the descending colon.

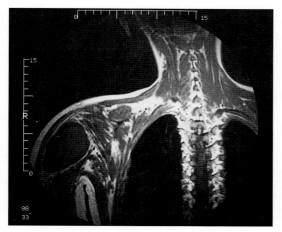

FIGURE 23-15 The magnetic resonance image shows a large neurofibroma of the axillary nerve in a patient with NF1.

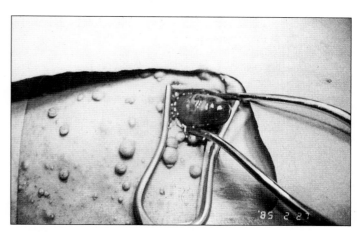

FIGURE 23-16 The cutaneous changes typical of NF1 are shown along with the surgical exposure of a partially removed neurofibroma located in the parascapular area.

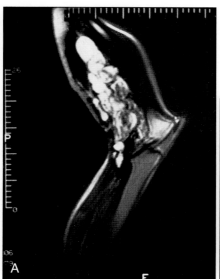

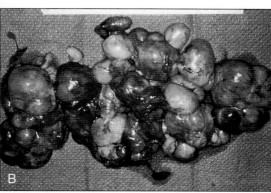

FIGURE 23-17 (A) A magnetic resonance image showing multiple extensive plexiform neurofibromas involving the sciatic nerve at the thigh and knee levels. Only a subtotal surgical removal was possible in this case of regionalized NF1 disease. (B) Some of the multiple tumors removed are seen in the surgical specimen. A painful recurrence later led to a second decompressive operation in this patient.

in a given region and on cross-section of nerve are shown to involve different quadrants of nerve at different levels. The usual systemic stigmata of NF1 are not present, except in the involved area. Thus, large café au lait lesions, multiple small spots of skin discoloration, skin tags, and even subcutaneous neurofibromas are confined to one limb or region of the body.

Microscopic appearance

The neurofibroma has a myxomatous matrix and exhibits a prominent mucopolysaccharide staining (Fig. 23-18). The neurofibroma's intense reticulum staining is due to the numerous collagen fibrils in its myxocollagenous background, while the schwannoma has a paucity of these collagen fibrils and, hence, stains poorly. As mentioned earlier, mucopolysaccharide and reticulum stains are more positive than those seen in the schwannoma. Unfortunately, the intensity of any stain can vary considerably according to the technique used, the technician performing the staining, and the preparation of the tissue.

The neurofibroma has fewer Schwann cells than a schwannoma and these cells are mixed together among distorted axon complexes with myelinated and unmyelinated axis cylinders. In the neurofibroma, the vasculature is less prominent and less likely to be thickened, hyalinized, or thrombosed than in schwannomas.

The tumor itself is histologically less compact than the Antoni type B tissue in a schwannoma.

Surgical approach

The necessary steps in the removal of a fusiform solitary neurofibroma are similar to those for a schwannoma. Fascicles need to be displaced away from the surface. Any capsule is opened and a subcapsular dissection of the tumor proceeds. The fascicular anatomy at both poles of the tumor needs to be dissected out. Neurofibromas are more likely than schwannomas to have fascicles adherent to the capsule or the tumor

The neurofibroma usually has two or more entering and exiting fascicles, which are larger than those seen in a schwannoma, and a capsule which is more adherent to the central mass of the tumor

than that of a schwannoma (Fig. 23-19). A large neurofibroma can sometimes be approached from above the inferiorly located fascicles or below fascicles located superiorly at the tumor's proximal or distal ends. The entering or exiting fascicles are then dissected free, sectioned, and used to elevate the tumor (Fig. 23-20). This maneuver allows the dissection of fascicular structures away from the tumor, beginning at one end until the opposite pole is reached.

Fascicles entering and exiting the tumor are tested by stimulating the proximal fascicles and recording NAPs from the distal ones. As with the schwannoma, if traces are flat, the entering and exiting fascicles can be sacrificed and the tumor removed as a solitary mass (Fig. 23-21). If NAPs are positive across these fascicles, the fascicles need to be traced into and out of the tumor and spared (Fig. 23-22). At times even these fascicles need to be sacrificed to achieve resection of the tumor. In these cases, fascicular defects can be replaced by grafts or, on occasion, partial fascicular graft repairs. Unfortunately, this may be difficult because of lengthy neural involvement in plexiform lesions or in other large and

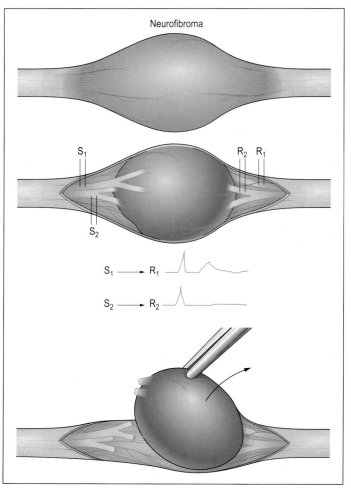

FIGURE 23-19 These are the steps in the exposure and resection of a solitary intraneural neurofibroma. The initial exposure is well proximal and distal to the tumor (*top*). The fascicles are dissected away from the periphery of the tumor and at both poles (*middle*). Intraoperative nerve action potential studies usually show flat traces from one or more fascicles entering and exiting the tumor, permitting their section. The tumor is elevated and dissected away from the fascicular bed (*bottom*). (Adapted from Lusk M, Kline D, and Garcia C: Tumors of the brachial plexus. Neurosurgery 21:439, 1987.)

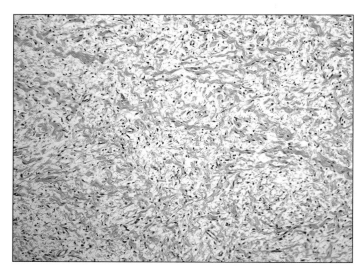

FIGURE 23-18 This is a photomicrograph of a neurofibroma showing the characteristic haphazardly arranged neoplastic Schwann cells, perineurial-like cells, and fibroblasts. These cells are present in a background of collagen fibers and mucosubstance. A "shredded carrots" appearance is noted in such tumors in which collagen formation is prominent.

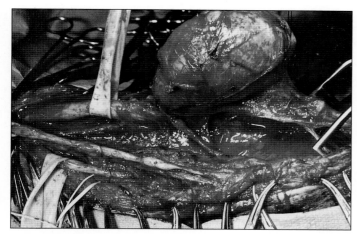

FIGURE 23-20 A large neurofibroma is seen intraoperatively. The distal exiting fascicles have been sectioned and, in this case, the distal end of the tumor was gradually elevated as the surrounding and primarily underlying fascicles were dissected away from it and spared.

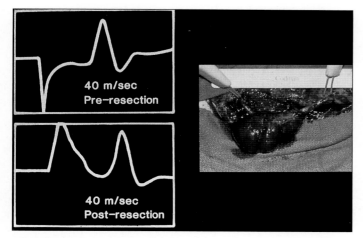

FIGURE 23-21 The pre-resection nerve action potential testing (*top left*) of a large neurofibroma of the tibial nerve associated with NF1 disease (*right*) is shown. Both the electrical conductivity (*bottom left*) and clinical function were maintained after tumor removal.

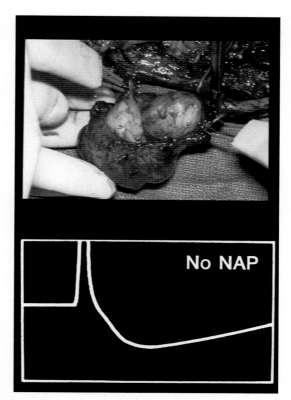

FIGURE 23-22 Nerve action potential (NAP) testing is shown intraoperatively. The entering fascicle (to the left) is stimulated and a recording is made from the exiting fascicle (to the right). There was no NAP (see recording below), so these fascicles could be sacrificed.

lengthy NF1-associated tumors. Even a large fusiform lesion can be associated with multiple smaller neurofibromas or neurofibromatous change in nerve both above and below the lesion, necessitating similar graft repair.

Removal of an NF1 neurofibroma is similar to that of a solitary neurofibroma. Often, there is a fine capsule between the fascicles and tumor, and dissecting down and through that is important before the tumor can be enucleated.

As with the schwannoma, an alternative approach is opening and evacuating the tumor contents, followed by dissecting away the fascicles, but this is seldom as satisfactory as removal of the mass as a whole.

The disposition of multiple tumors in regional or segmental NF1 makes satisfactory resection of the neurofibromas without significant deficit very difficult, especially if tumors are plexiform, rather than globular.

Results

Tables 23-2 through 23-4 show the distribution of 237 (66%) neurofibromas of a total of 361 benign PNSTs including schwanno-mas, solitary and NF1-associated neurofibromas. These are data from the recently updated series of PNSTs removed at LSUHSC between 1969 and 1999.

Most, or 87 (62%) of 141 PNSTs of the brachial plexus were neurofibromas, as were those of the upper extremity (78 of 110 tumors, 71%), the pelvic plexus (19 of 25, 76%) and the lower extremity (53 of 85 tumors, 62%).

SOLITARY OR NON-NF1 NEUROFIBROMA

Of 237 operative neurofibromas involving nerve, 141 tumors (59%) were solitary or non-NF1 neurofibromas. A solitary neurofibroma was the predominate tumor type removed from peripheral nerves in all locations. Thus, of neurofibromas involving the brachial plexus, 55 (63%) of 87 tumors were solitary neurofibromas (Fig. 23-23). Of tumors in the upper extremity, 45 (58%) of 78 tumors were solitary neurofibromas (Figs 23-24, 23-25). In the pelvic plexus and lower extremity, there was a preponderance of solitary tumors (10 of 19 tumors, 53%; and 31 of 53 tumors, 58%, respectively), as well.

In a subset of 99 LSUHSC patients with neurofibromas presented in the series by Donner et al.[45] available for follow-up, 58 (59%) presented with a motor deficit of some degree (Tables 23-6 to 23-8). Within this subgroup, 38 (66%) experienced improved long-term functional outcome, 14 (24%) did not change, and six (10%) had some further decrease in function noted at the last follow-up. Forty-one (41%) of the 99 patients had normal function at presentation. Thirty-two (78%) maintained normal function and nine (22%) had some degree of postoperative weakness.

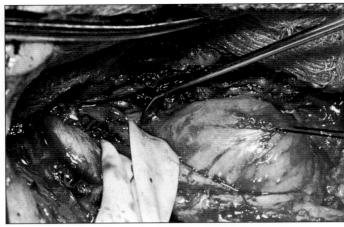

FIGURE 23-23 A large neurofibroma of the lower trunk of the plexus is seen. The upper and middle plexus trunks are retracted laterally by the Penrose drains. Most of the fascicular structure was inferior to the mass of the tumor itself. Entering and exiting fascicles were nonfunctional and the tumor could be excised without serious deficit, although the C8–T1 distribution sensation in the hand was grade 4 postoperatively.

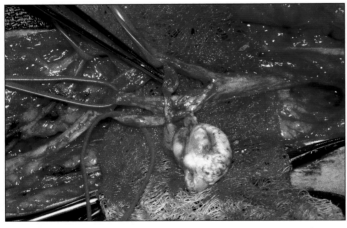

FIGURE 23-24 An intraoperative photograph of a small neurofibroma of the ulnar nerve at the elbow level, from which most of the fascicular structure has been separated.

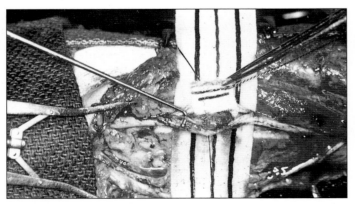

FIGURE 23-25 A small recurrent neurofibroma of the ulnar nerve at the level of the wrist is seen in this intraoperative photograph. The nerve hook is beneath the entering fascicles.

Table 23-6 Solitary neurofibroma (n=99)

Postoperative grade	Preoperative grade					
	5	4	3	2	1	0
5	32	16	6	2		
4	9	5	9		1	
3		2	5	2		1
2		1	2	1	2	
1				1	2	
0						1

The pre- and postoperative motor grades of the involved muscle groups in a group of patients with resected neurofibromas. Overall, 38 patients improved, 15 worsened, and in 46, the grades remained the same.

Table 23-7 NF1 neurofibroma (n=48)

Postoperative grade	Preoperative grade					
	5	4	3	2	1	0
5	10	8	2			
4	2	4	5	1		
3			2	2		
2		1		3	1	1
1			1	1	1	
0					1	2

The pre- and postoperative motor grades of the involved muscle groups in a group of patients with NF1. Overall, 18 patients improved, 8 worsened, and in 22, the grades remained the same.

Table 23-8 Benign neural sheath tumors* – resection without serious deficit

	Number of cases	Percentage good result
Schwannoma	76	89
Neurofibroma	99	80
NF1-neurofibroma	48	66
Total	223	

NF1, von Recklinghausen's disease.

*Includes 9 diffuse or "plexiform" tumors, 6 associated with NF1 and 3 without NF1, either subtotally or resected totally with repair. Prior attempted removal or biopsy decreased the chances of resection without added deficit and sometimes resulted in the need for repair.

Table 23-9 Resolution of pain after operation on benign neural sheath tumors

	Resolved (%)	Improved (%)	Unchanged (%)	Worse pain (%)	New pain (%)
Schwannoma	15/20 (75)	2/20 (10)	1/20 (5)	2/20 (10)	4/52 (8)
Solitary neurofibroma	29/46 (63)	11/46 (25)	3/46 (6)	3/46 (6)	7/53 (13)
NF1 neurofibroma	10/23 (43)	7/23 (31)	4/23 (17)	2/23 (9)	4/25 (16)

The outcome for patients with and without radicular pain syndromes preoperatively. The columns 2–5 represent results in patients who presented with pain syndromes. The column 6 represents the number of patients who had no pain preoperatively and yet developed pain after surgery.

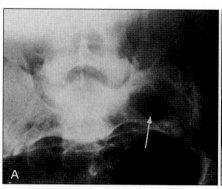
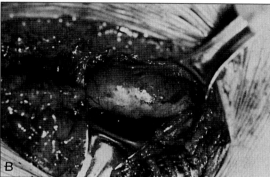

FIGURE 23-26 **(A)** Several sacral foramina were enlarged in this plain film of a patient with NF1 (*arrow showing an enlarged foramen*). **(B)** The intraoperative exposure of the sacral neurofibroma seen in (A) is shown here. The tumor was approached posterolaterally.

Forty-six of these patients presented with spontaneous pain syndromes (Table 23-9). The pain was radicular in all 46, and only two patients complained of additional pain at the site of the tumor. Postoperatively, the pain resolved completely in 29 (63%), partially in 11 (25%), not at all in three (6%) and was made worse in three (6%). New pain syndromes were encountered in seven (13%) of the remaining 53 patients, although all were mild.

NF1 NEUROFIBROMA

NF1-associated neurofibromas involving nerve followed solitary neurofibromas in number in the updated LSUHSC series. There were 96 (46%) such tumors of the 237 operative benign neurofibromas removed from nerve. Of 87 neurofibromas involving the brachial plexus, 32 (37%) were associated with NF1. One of the brachial tumors incompletely removed was a 25 cm tumor arising from the proximal brachial plexus, which extended deeply into the mediastinum. Of 110 operative neurofibromas removed from the upper extremity, there were 33 (42%) NF1-associated neurofibromas. The pelvic plexus had 19 neurofibromas of which nine (47%) were associated with NF1 (Fig. 23-26). One of the pelvic tumors, a 30 cm mass, was incompletely removed. Tumor left behind usually consisted of small fragments adherent or intrinsic to functional fascicles. The lower extremity, with 53 neurofibromas removed from nerve, had 22 (42%) associated with NF1.

Several patients with NF1-associated neurofibromas had plexiform tumors. Many patients had these multiple discrete tumors along the length of a single nerve. When this was encountered, smaller tumors, i.e. <1 cm, were left alone.

From the series by Donner et al.,[45] there were 48 patients with NF1-associated neurofibromas removed from nerve at LSUHSC, who were available for follow-up (Tables 23–7, 23–8). Twenty-three (48%) had presented with radicular pain syndromes (Table 23-9). Ten patients (43%) had complete resolution of pain, seven (31%) had partial resolution, and four (17%) had no change after surgery. In two patients (9%), pain was worse after operation. Of the 25 patients who presented without pain, four (16%) experienced new, but usually mild pain syndromes.

Thirty-six patients presented with weakness. Of these, 18 (50%) had improved at last follow-up, 12 (33%) had no change in their preoperative strength, and six (17%) worsened. Among the 12 patients who had normal strength at presentation, two (17%) experienced a decrease in function postoperatively.

MALIGNANT TUMORS OF NEURAL SHEATH ORIGIN

The majority of malignant PNSTs were solitary tumors not associated with NF1. Although malignant PNSTs can occur without a background of NF1,[35,141] their incidence was higher in NF1 patients than in the general population in which tumors were solitary. Those malignant PNSTs associated with NF1 tended to present at a younger age than those which were solitary. There was no gender preference in either group and these malignant PNSTs appeared to have no special laterality. Irradiation has occasionally been implicated as an inductive factor in the malignant PNSTs.[56]

These tumors are also rare. Stark et al. reported that malignant PNSTs accounted for 5–10% of soft tissue sarcomas, which represented relatively few cases.[146] Malignant tumors of nerve sheath origin have an incidence of 0.001% in the general population. There were single cases,[87,137] small series,[9,28,42] and a somewhat larger series in a review of the recent literature regarding these tumors.[8]

CLINICAL PRESENTATION AND EXAMINATION

Pain with or without progressive loss of function is the most common presenting complaint in patients with malignant PNSTs. Gradually worsening painful paresthesias in the distribution of the involved nerve prompts further medical, and eventually surgical, investigation.[159] In some cases, the patient notices a lump or mass that is painful upon palpation or upon being bumped (Fig. 23-27). In other cases, initial mild loss becomes more severe relatively rapidly. It is rare for these patients to present initially with metastasis to lung, bone, liver, or spleen. Other clinical findings that might suggest a malignant PNST include a rapid increase in size of a mass over a period of weeks to months and a large mass at the time of presentation.[80]

On examination, such malignant tumors are firmer and have an increased fixation to adjacent structures than their benign counterparts, the schwannomas or neurofibromas.[97] As with benign PNSTs, the mass can usually be moved from side to side, but not up and down. Palpation or percussion of the mass gives pain radiating distally and sometimes proximally in the distribution of the nerve or elements of origin.

MICROSCOPIC APPEARANCE

As stated, the differentiation of a malignant schwannoma and malignant neurofibroma (Fig. 23-28) often cannot be made (Fig. 23-29). It is still possible, at times, to distinguish between a neoplasm of pure schwannoma origin and the complex neurofibrosarcoma, most of which arise in the context of NF1.[134] The histological features of malignant schwannomas include increased cellularity with tumor cell polymorphism, spindle tumor cells arranged in a "herringbone pattern," and increased mitotic activity. There is neovascularization, which can occasionally result in intratumoral hemorrhage (Fig. 23-30).

Malignant neurofibromas or neurofibrosarcomas have mesenchymal mixed with schwannian elements. There is also an increased cellularity, and pleomorphism and abundant mitotic figures. Divergent differentiation may occur with metaplasia into cartilage, osteoid, bone and adipose tissue, and rhabdomyoblasts.

SURGICAL APPROACH

Despite some differentiating features on physical examination, the majority of malignant PNSTs are not suspected to be malignant until biopsy or attempted removal. Either procedure in inexperienced hands can lead to neural loss, which is more likely with malignant PNSTs than with PNSTs. This is because of the former's intrinsic relationship to the nerve or element of origin, and also because of the malignant PNSTs' adherence to adjacent neural structures and other soft tissues such as vessels, muscles, and bone. Malignant PNSTs presenting as rapidly growing, firm, and fixed lesions should have an open biopsy performed and if the presumed

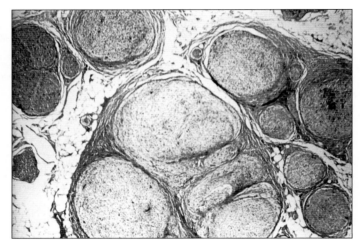

FIGURE 23-28 The malignant peripheral neural sheath tumor shown in this photomicrograph has spread throughout the fascicular structure of the nerve of origin, far proximal to the main mass of the tumor.

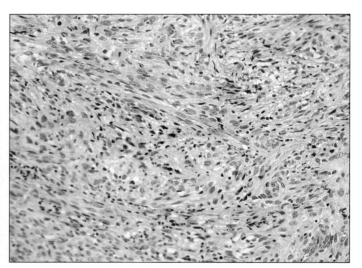

FIGURE 23-29 This photomicrograph depicts a malignant peripheral neural sheath tumor. Most arise from neurofibromas and rarely from schwannomas, the latter occurring in NF1. Mucopolysaccharide staining favors a malignant neurofibroma over a schwannoma. Note the fibrosarcoma-like growth pattern demonstrated as intertwined fascicles of tightly packed hyperchromatic spindle cells with tapered nuclei and faintly eosinophilic cytoplasm. Moderate-to-marked cytologic pleomorphism, atypical mitoses, and necrosis are usually identified. H & E, original magnification ×200.

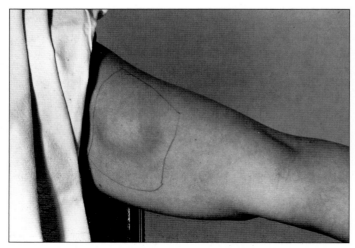

FIGURE 23-27 The photograph shows a painful mass in the medial arm, which was associated with a progressive sensorimotor loss. At operation, it was found to be a malignant peripheral neural sheath tumor arising from the median nerve.

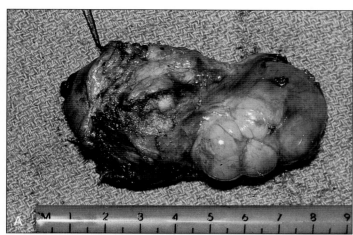

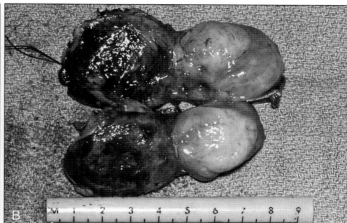

FIGURE 23-30   (A) This is a resected peripheral malignant neural sheath tumor. **(B)** On sectioning of the tumor, one nodule shows hemorrhagic change, as seen to the left in this photograph.

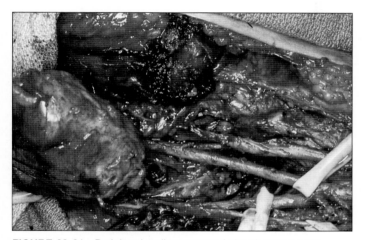

FIGURE 23-31   Peripheral malignant neural sheath tumor seen intraoperatively after being elevated away from the cords of the brachial plexus. The patient was elderly and did not wish to undergo a forequarter amputation. A recurrence at the skin level was treated successfully with radiation several years later, and the patient survived 8 years without other recurrences before succumbing to heart disease (see also Ganju A, Roosen N, Kline DG, Tiel RL: J Neurosurgery 95:51–60, 2001).

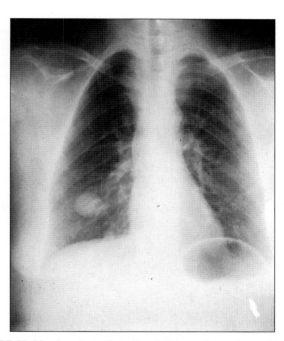

FIGURE 23-32   A metastasis to the right lower lung of a peripheral malignant neural sheath tumor is shown here. The primary tumor involved the sciatic nerve at a buttock level.

diagnosis is confirmed, a metastatic evaluation should be carried out, including chest X-ray, chest and abdominal computerized tomography (CT) or magnetic resonance imaging (MRI) and liver, spleen, and bone scans. Resection is then performed as follows.

Brachial plexus malignant PNSTs

Though total resection of a malignant PNST from the brachial plexus is the goal, this is often impossible without severe vascular and functional loss. Some loss occurs due to sacrifice of the element of origin. Simple biopsy sampling alone, without subsequent removal or substantial decompression of such a lesion, is seldom indicated, however (Fig. 23-31). Amputation is seldom carried out at the time of the initial operation, because it is necessary to obtain permanent specimen sections from multiple sites to confirm the diagnosis of malignancy and to assess the tumor's invasion of adjacent structures.

Extremity malignant PNSTs
Proximal limb malignant PNSTs

For malignant PNSTs involving a proximal limb, wide resection would remove vessels necessary for preservation of the limb or adjacent nerves. Amputation of the limb proximal to the lesion can be performed if the patient and the family wish, but only after the lesion has been verified on frozen section as malignant and has shown no evidence of distant spread on metastatic work-up (Fig. 23-32). When the diagnosis of malignancy is less certain because of less definitive pre- and intraoperative findings and frozen section results, only local total removal of the tumor is done. Further surgery is then dependent on permanent histological findings and patient and family wishes.

Distal limb malignant PNSTs

For distal limb malignant PNSTs, providing there is no evidence of metastatic disease, a wide local resection is carried out. This includes removal of the nerve of origin, adjacent adherent soft tissues, and a several-centimeter margin of entering and exiting nerve, all shown to be free of tumor on frozen and permanent sections. This regimen usually leads to a neural deficit. Depending on tumor morphology, further options include intraoperative placement of radioactive seeds in rods and postoperative external radiation and/or chemotherapy.

In patients who refuse further surgery beyond an attempt to remove the lesion and in those with metastatic disease, irradiation of the limb with or without adjuvant chemotherapy is undertaken. In recent years, an attempt at limb-sparing surgery has been favored whenever possible for sarcomas involving the extremities, but sometimes amputation or forequarter amputation is still done.[19]

ADJUNCTIVE TREATMENT

Radiation therapy and/or chemotherapy have a variable and unpredictable effect on these malignancies. Casanova et al. presented a review of 24 pediatric patients with malignant PNSTs treated during a 20-year period. Primary radical surgery without adjuvant therapy was performed in 10 patients. Postoperative radiotherapy (RT) alone was administered in 12 cases and only postoperative adjuvant chemotherapy in 19. Eight patients were alive without evidence of disease, six in first complete remission and two in a new complete remission after a median follow-up of 230 months. The 10-year event-free survival was 29% in those undergoing only postoperative RT and 41% in those who had adjuvant chemotherapy after surgery. Survival at 10 years was 80% for the patients who underwent complete resection and 14% for the others undergoing subtotal resection. With regard to tumor size, the 10-year survival was 71% for patients with tumors smaller than 5 cm and 29% for those with tumors 5 cm or larger. Complete surgical excision remained the most effective treatment for malignant PNSTs and was the main prognostic factor along with tumor size. Radiotherapy seemed to play a role in achieving local control, whereas the role of chemotherapy was uncertain.[28]

A study by Wanebo et al. of 28 cases of malignant PNSTs found a median disease-free survival time of 11 months and the median overall survival time of 44 months. Their approach included aggressive surgery with wide surgical margins combined with adjuvant radiation therapy. Chemotherapy was thought possibly to have a role for treatment failures.[161]

Stark et al. reported eight cases of malignant PNSTs. All patients underwent surgery with curative intent, but total resection defined by negative surgical margins was achieved in only three cases. All developed local recurrences with a mean disease-free survival time of 10.6 months. In five cases adjuvant radiation was given. Three patients developed distant metastases and five of eight patients died during follow-up with a mean survival time of 11.6 months after diagnosis. The authors concluded that the prognosis in malignant PNSTs remains dismal in spite of multimodal therapy encompassing surgical resection and adjuvant radiotherapy including brachytherapy.[146]

RESULTS

Of 36 patients with malignant PNSTs of the brachial and pelvic plexi and major peripheral nerves, removed at LSUHSC between 1969 and 1999, 28 (78%) were malignant PNSTs and eight (22%) were other sarcomas, such as fibrosarcoma and spindle cell, synovial, and perineurial sarcomas. Of the 28 malignant PNSTs, 16 (57%) were solitary tumors in patients without NF1 and 12 (43%) were in patients with NF1 (Table 23-10).

The brachial plexus was the location of the majority of malignant PNSTs (Fig. 23-33). Of 21 brachial plexus malignant PNSTs including other sarcomas, 13 (62%) were those not associated with NF1 and eight (38%) were associated with NF1.

Twenty of 36 (56%) patients with malignant PNSTs including other sarcomas had a local resection. Sixteen (44%) of 36 had a local resection with margins. Ten (28%) of 36 had forequarter amputation of the shoulder and arm or hip disarticulation and three (8%) of 36 patients with malignant PNSTs had more distal amputations.

Twenty (56%) of 36 patients with malignant PNSTs had radiation therapy and four (11%) of 36 had placement of radioactive seeds in rods. There were 22 deaths (61%) out of 36 patients and these had survived an average of 25 months before succumbing to their tumors.

CASE SUMMARY – MALIGNANT PNST

CASE 1

This 40-year-old physician had noticed paresthesias in the right hand for a few months, followed by weakness of the right shoulder, wrist, and hand. Computed tomography and MRI of the neck revealed a large supraclavicular brachial plexus mass. Needle biopsy suggested a malignant tumor, most likely a neurogenic sarcoma.

Upon examination, partial dysfunction in the distribution of the C5- and C6-innervated muscles was noted. Loss was severe in the distribution of the C7, C8, and T1 elements.

An operative procedure was undertaken. The lesion was approached by a posterior subscapular operation with resection of the first rib. After excision of the posterior scalene muscle, the posterior portion of a mass 8 cm in diameter was revealed. The tumor was then dissected circumferentially with maintenance of its capsule. A plane of dissection was found posteriorly, superiorly, and laterally, but inferiorly and medially the tumor was more adherent and the capsule had to be entered to remove tumor from the superior and medial pleura and

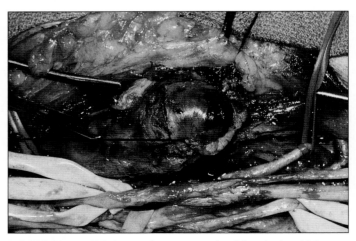

FIGURE 23-33 This is a malignant tumor involving the brachial plexus at a cord level. Most of the cords of the plexus have been dissected away and are encircled by Penrose drains. The axillary artery is encircled by a plastic loop to the right.

Table 23-10 Malignant neural sheath tumors in the LSUHSC series (n=36)

	NS sporadic cases	Cases with NF1	LR	LRM	RT	Rods	Amp	4 Qtr	Average follow-up	No. of deaths**
Neurogenic sarcomas										
Brachial plexus	10	7	11	6	8	0	1	6	52	14 (25)
Ulnar	2	0	0	2	1	1	0	0	52	1 (37)
Sciatic	2	2	2	2	1	1	0	3	32	2 (16)
Femoral	1	1	0	2	1	1	1	0	46	1 (16)
Peroneal	1	1	0	2	2	0	0	0	48	0
Tibial	0	1	1	0	1	0	1	0	50	0
Other sarcomas* (excluding Ewing's sarcoma)										
Brachial plexus	3	1	4	0	4	0	0	0	47	2 (40)
Sciatic	2	0	2	0	1	0	0	0	27	1 (12)
Femoral	1	0	0	1	1	0	0	1	18	1 (18)
Peroneal	1	0	0	1	0	1	0	0	28	0
Totals	23	13	20	16	20	4	3	10	46	22 (25)

*Includes fibro-, spindle cell, synovial, and perineurial sarcomas.

**( ), averaged postoperative survival (months).

LSUHS, Louisiana State University Health Sciences Center; NS, neurosarcoma; NF1, neurofibromatosis type I; LR, local resection; LRM, local resection with margin; AMP, amputation; 4 Qtr, fore-quarter amputation of the shoulder and arm or hip disarticulation; RT, radiation therapy.

deeper mediastinal structures. The tumor was relatively soft in consistency and moderately vascular. Removal of some tumor from the C5, C6, and C7 roots and upper and middle trunk was necessary, as well as removal of a moderate portion attached to the C8 and T1 roots and lower trunk. The tumor was also attached to the subclavian vessels, first rib, apical pleura, and anteromedial mediastinum. A section of pleura 4 cm in diameter was resected and replaced by a graft of fascia lata.

Tumor was seen to enter widened foramina at the C6–C7 and C7–T1 levels. The foramina were entered for tumor removal, but a small amount within the spinal canal was not removed.

After tumor dissection, NAP recordings were performed. There were large NAPs from C5 and C6 to upper trunk, moderate-sized NAPs from C7 to middle trunk, but only a trace of an NAP from C8 or T1 to lower trunk.

At the end of the surgical procedure, a chest tube was placed at the fifth intercostal space. Permanent histologic sections confirmed the diagnosis of malignant PNST.

The chest tube was removed on the fifth postoperative day. The patient gained good pain relief and, surprisingly, recovered some C8 and T1 spinal nerve function and in the ipsilateral hand intrinsic function improved. This occurred over an 8-month period, during which he underwent radiation therapy and chemotherapy. The patient survived a little over 4 years postoperatively and then died from disseminated disease.

COMMENT

Local control of the tumor was obtained by an extensive but palliative operation. Thus, this operation was not curative, and neither radiation nor chemotherapy could halt the spread of the disease.

BENIGN TUMORS OF NON-NEURAL SHEATH ORIGIN

Benign peripheral nerve tumors of non-neural sheath origin are uncommon tumors. In the literature over the last three decades there is a paucity of case reports or small series of patients for each type. An exception is the more common ganglion cyst of the peroneal nerve, about which many reports have been published.

Benign peripheral non-neural sheath tumors (PNNSTs) secondarily involve nerve and tend to produce symptoms because of nerve compression, rather than actual origination in nerve (Fig. 23-34).[24,121,140] There are exceptions, however, and these include the desmoids, myoblastomas, lymphangiomas, or the rare extraspinal meningioma, all of which can be quite adherent to epineurium and difficult to remove, with a high incidence of recurrence.[167] Some ganglions are extraneural and can compress nerve, while others either dissect down to or originate at an intraneural level. As a result, removal of these lesions can be either incomplete or accompanied by a deficit. Hemangiomas or hemangiopericytomas can envelop nerve or elements of the brachial plexus, but the extremely rare hemangioblastoma can arise in nerve, as can rare tumors of congenital origin such as a triton tumor of the plexus.

The benign PNNSTs are summarized in Table 23-11. The presentation of both the table and the text are arranged in order of frequency, from most to least prevalent, with some exceptions, such as the tumors involving bone and the vascular tumors, which are subgrouped together.

Table 23-11 Location and number of benign peripheral non-nerve sheath LSUHSC tumors (n=111)

Tumor	Locations of tumors							
	Brachial plexus region		U.E. nerves		Pelvic plexus		L.E. nerves	
Ganglion cyst (33)	Suprascapular nerve	4	Median	4			Femoral	2
			Radial-PIN	3			Obturator	1
			Ulnar-Guyon's canal	2			Sciatic	1
							Peroneal	15
							Posterior tibial	1
LHN (16)	Brachial plexus	3	Median	4			Sciatic complex	6
			Radial	2				
			Ulnar	1				
Lipoma (12)	Brachial plexus	2	Median	4			Sciatic	1
	Musculocutaneous	1	PIN-radial	1				
	Axillary	1	Ulnar	2				
Lipofibrohamartoma (4)			Median	4				
Desmoid (11)	Brachial plexus	6	Median	1			Sciatic complex	2
			Radial	1			Peroneal	1
Osteochondroma (4)	Brachial plexus	1	Radial	1			Peroneal	2
Myositis ossificans (4)	Brachial plexus	2	Median	1				
			Radial	1				
Ganglioneuroma (4)	Brachial plexus	3			Pelvic plexus	1		
Hemangioma (3)			Ulnar	2			Peroneal	1
Venous angioma (4)			Median	1			Sciatic	1
							Femoral	1
							Tibial	1
Hemangiopericytoma (2)	Brachial plexus	1	Median	1				
Hemangioblastoma (1)			Median	1				
Glomus tumor (2)			Digital	1			Peroneal	1
Meningioma (2)	Brachial plexus	2						
Cystic hygroma (2)	Accessory	2						
Myoblastoma or granular cell tumor (2)	Brachial plexus	2						
Triton tumor (2)	Brachial plexus	2						
Lymphangioma (2)	Brachial plexus	1	Median/ulnar	1				
Epidermoid cyst (1)							Sciatic	1
Totals		33		39		1		38

LHN, localized hypertrophic neuropathy; No., number; U.E., upper extremity; L.E., lower extremity.

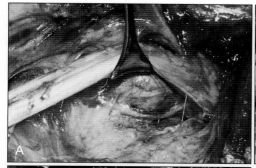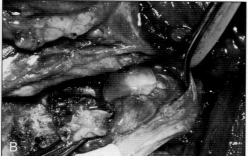

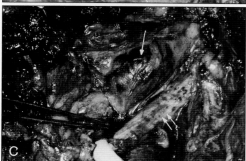

FIGURE 23-34 **(A)** Shown is a sciatic notch ganglion cyst. The cyst is compressing the sciatic nerve, which is being retracted superiorly with a vein retractor. **(B)** A sciatic notch epidermoid tumor is shown, which is displacing the sciatic nerve laterally to the right. **(C)** An aneurysmal dilatation of the vein (*single arrow*) is seen in juxtaposition to the sciatic nerve (*double arrow*) just distal to the sciatic notch.

GANGLION CYSTS

Most ganglion cysts arise near joints. These are thought to occur at the site of a small tear in the ligament overlying a tendon sheath or joint capsule. Ganglion cysts tend to be present in areas that do not involve nerves, such as the dorsum of the hand or wrist.[140]

Many ganglia, however, involve the peripheral nerves, and at LSUHSC have been found at the elbow and forearm levels compressing the posterior interosseous nerve (PIN). They also can occur at the wrist level and compress the median nerve or its thenar sensory branch, the ulnar nerve or its superficial and deep branches in Guyon's canal and the superficial sensory radial branches. Ganglion cysts can occasionally be found to cause femoral or sciatic compression at the hip level, and one has been found at the ankle level. A ganglion cyst involving the peripheral nerve is thought to arise from the adjacent synovial joint and then to track back along a small articular nerve branch to reach its final position within a major nerve trunk.[144]

More difficult to explain in terms of origin are ganglion cysts at the suprascapular notch, which compress the suprascapular nerve (Fig. 23-35). In the LSUHSC patients with cysts in this region, the ganglia did not appear to arise from the shoulder joint.

There is a third type of ganglion cyst, though, which may arise de novo within the nerve and does not appear to have a discernible connection to a joint or can arise from a joint and grow into the nerve. This type of cyst most frequently occurs in the peroneal nerve behind the head of the fibula (Figs 23-36, 23-37), but can also occur at the wrist or ankle levels, and less frequently at the level of the hip (see Fig. 23-34A). In the recent literature, the peroneal nerve was the most frequently involved nerve, with 40 cases reported at this site in a review in 2001 by Coleman et al.[30]

Clinical presentation

Ganglion cysts usually present as a tender mass with pain and paresthesias in the distribution of the involved nerve or its branches. In the suprascapular region, ganglion cyst compression usually presents similarly to a spontaneous suprascapular neuropathy. Occa-

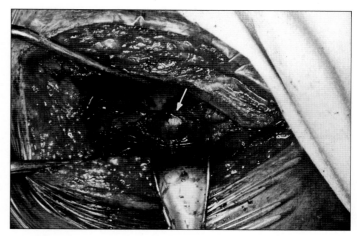

FIGURE 23-35 A ganglion cyst (*arrow*) involving the suprascapular nerve near the scapular notch. Exposure was gained by splitting apart and retracting the supraspinatus muscle. In some cases these lesions extended through and below the scapular notch and required dissection of the infraspinatus muscle away from the scapula.

sionally, however, for ganglia in this area there is an initiating history of heavy lifting or trauma to the shoulder.

Microscopic appearance

The cysts contain a mucoid material (Fig. 23-38). The cyst wall of ganglion cysts is composed of compressed collagen fibers and occasional flattened cells (Fig. 23-39) there is an associated mucoid degeneration of the surrounding fibrous tissue. There is an absence of inflammatory cells, a lack of mitotic activity, and there is no synovial or epithelial lining of the single or multiloculated cysts.

Surgical approach

For a ganglion cyst which is extrinsic to and causes compression of a nerve, the involved nerve is protected while the cyst is dissected away, then dissection is performed around the cyst itself. The cyst's

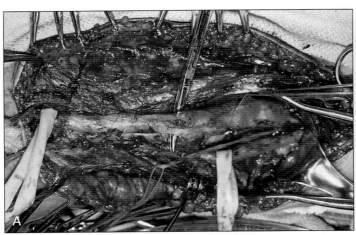
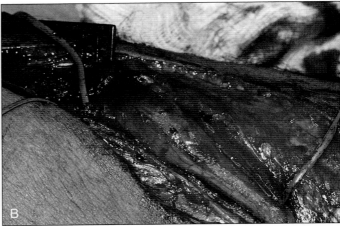

FIGURE 23-36 **(A)** A ganglion cyst of the peroneal nerve near the head of the fibula is shown. This lesion had no obvious connection with the knee joint and could be dissected out by exposing the fascicles above and below and dissecting them off the cyst. **(B)** Another ganglion cyst of the peroneal nerve, which was totally intraneural, is shown.

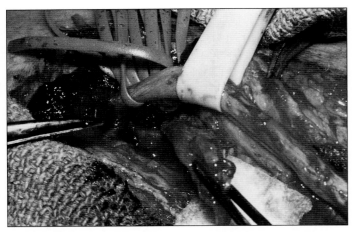

FIGURE 23-37 An extraneural ganglion is being teased away from beneath the peroneal nerve at the head of the fibula (proximal is to the right and distal is to the left). The origin of this lesion was from the knee joint.

neck and then the origin of the cyst from the joint is identified and ligated. For example, the tibiofibular joint branch, the usual origin of a cystic lesion compressing the peroneal nerve, is ligated close to the joint to reduce the risk of recurrence. Most ganglia, which are extrinsic to nerve, can be resected in this fashion with preservation of neurological function.

An intraneural ganglion, however, requires a different approach, i.e. an interfascicular one. The ganglion cyst is usually dissected out and an internal neurolysis of the involved nerve is performed in the process. As in the extrinsic ganglia, the entry point is isolated and ligated to reduce recurrence. For larger intraneural cysts, the synovial-like contents of the cyst are evacuated and then the capsule dissected away from the decompressed and split-apart fascicles. A larger lesion sometimes requires several operations before obliteration.

Results

In the LSUHSC series of 33 ganglion cysts involving nerve, most ganglion cysts arose from the lower extremity (20 of 33, 61%). The peroneal nerve was the most frequently involved nerve, representing 15 (75%) of 20 lesions in the lower extremity. One of the peroneal ganglion cysts recurred 2.5 years after the first operation and required a second removal. Two others were extensive and could not be totally removed since doing so would have caused a severe deficit: these were only decompressed. A fourth patient was a 12-year-old girl, who presented with a cystic mass behind the knee and an accompanying ipsilateral footdrop. At operation, the intraneural ganglion extended proximally into the thigh as well as the buttock levels of the sciatic nerve. Only a decompression could be performed and as was expected there has been no reversal of the footdrop. A tibial distribution loss has not developed, however.

The other sites of origin in the leg for 20 ganglion cysts included the femoral nerve, which was involved by two (10%) ganglia, followed by one lesion each (5%) in the obturator nerve, the sciatic nerve near the sciatic notch, and the ankle level involving the posterior tibial nerve. The ankle-level cyst had recurred three times: the first after a prior partial decompression done elsewhere, the second after a procedure at LSUHSC which included removal of the capsule, and the third 5 months later, again at LSUHSC. At the time of the third procedure, the cyst was re-evacuated, the capsule again removed and this time several fascicles were resected and replaced by sural nerve grafts. There was no recurrence after this procedure.

Ganglion cysts were next most common in the upper extremity (nine of 33, 27%). Ganglion cysts arising from upper extremity joints were extraneural and caused compression of the median nerve or the median nerve's thenar sensory branch at the wrist (four of nine, 44%) and the PIN (three of nine, 33%). Cysts in this series were also found to compress the ulnar nerve or its superficial and deep branches in Guyon's canal at the wrist (two of nine, 22%).

Of 33 ganglion cysts, there were four cysts arising from a nerve from the brachial plexus (12%). These four cysts originated near the shoulder in this series, though they did not appear to arise from the shoulder joint and involved the suprascapular nerve near the suprascapular notch or the scapular notch. In both cases, presentation was similar to a spontaneous suprascapular entrapment neuropathy.

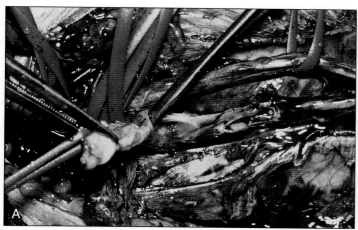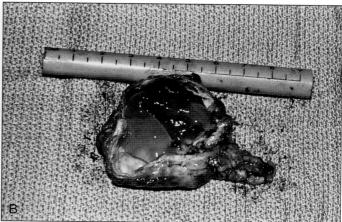

FIGURE 23-38 **(A)** The wall of a ganglion cyst is shown being teased from the fascicles of the peroneal division of the sciatic nerve. The nerve superior to the ganglion cyst is the tibial portion of the sciatic nerve. **(B)** The resected ganglion cyst has been opened to show the typical mucoid contents.

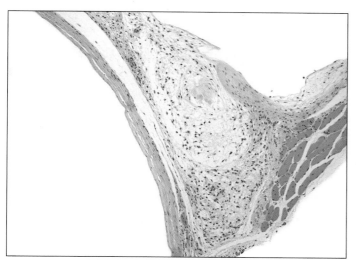

FIGURE 23-39 This is a photomicrograph of a ganglion cyst, which shows the cyst to be fibrous-lined with associated mucoid degeneration of the surrounding fibrous tissue. No chondroid differentiation of multinucleated giant cells is seen. H & E, original magnification ×100.

LIPOMAS

There are four lipomatous conditions that can affect nerve: a solitary lipoma; "macrodystrophia lipomatosa," which produces an overgrowth of the hand or fingers can both cause neural compression; an encapsulated lipoma; and a lipofibromatous hamartoma. The latter two lipomas can both have growth which begins within the nerve (Fig. 23-40).[140]

In the recent literature there is a preponderance of reports of lipomas involving nerve. Most involve the upper extremity, with Babins and Lubahn[11] presenting five palmar lipomas compressing the median nerve. Goldstein et al.[67] presented a perineural lipoma causing nerve compression when postoperative edema developed after vascular graft placement. Three lipomas were presented involving the PIN branch of the radial nerve, two by Nishida et al.[113] and one by Hashizume et al.[76] One lipoma reported by Zvijac et al.[171] compressed the suprascapular nerve, while two compressed

the peroneal and posterior tibial nerves, as reported by Resende et al.[125]

There is a small group of patients who may develop a lipohamartomatous condition in which there is a significant fatty, fibrous mass within the nerve. There were six radial, four median, and one ulnar nerves involved by lipofibromatous hamartomas presented in five recent publications.[12,72,90,109,166]

Clinical presentation

The usual fatty tumors are benign, subcutaneous, and globose or ovoid, and they usually do not involve nerves. Exceptions occur when a large subcutaneous lipoma envelops or compresses nerve, or originates at a deeper level in the limb and entraps and compresses a nerve. Both presentations produce symptoms specific to the involved nerve.

Microscopic appearance

Lipomas have a fine capsule and are composed entirely of adipose tissue. Lipohamartomas present as a significant fatty, fibrous mass within nerve.

Surgical approach

The removal of large lipomas is not easy, and neural damage can result. These lipomas can grow quite large and can lie atop or adjacent to the nerve, sometimes surrounding the nerve. Removal is difficult if the lipoma occurs at a plexus level, especially if there has been a prior unsuccessful surgical attempt with resulting scar tissue.

The usual management for removal of lipohamartomas, which tend to involve the median nerve at the palmar and sometimes wrist level, is section of the transverse carpal ligament and decompression rather than an attempt to remove lipomatous tissue. When serious loss of median function occurs, more extensive surgery is required. An internal neurolysis can be performed, with reduction of the bulk of the tumor from around individual fascicles, or in the case of a more focal lipohamartoma, resection and repair.

Results

In the LSUHSC series, the upper extremity was the site of seven (58%) of 12 lipomas, with four (33%) of the upper extremity lesions involving the median nerve, two (17%) the ulnar, and one

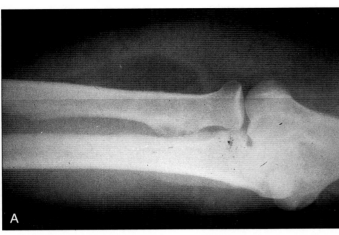
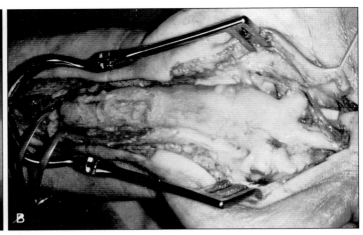

FIGURE 23-40 **(A)** A plain film of the elbow region with an area of hypodensity seen over the radius. This radiographic appearance is pathognomonic of a lipoma. At surgery, the lesion was found to be compressing the posterior interosseous nerve. **(B)** The exposure of a lipohamartoma (lipofibromatous hamartoma) involving the median nerve at the level of the wrist and palm is shown intraoperatively. The patient presented with symptoms of a carpal tunnel syndrome. At the time of carpal tunnel release, diffuse, fatty infiltration of the nerve was found (From Hudson A, Gentilli F, Kline D: Peripheral nerve tumors. In: Schmidek and Sweet W, Eds: Operative Neurosurgical Techniques, 2nd edn. New York, Grune & Stratton, 1988).

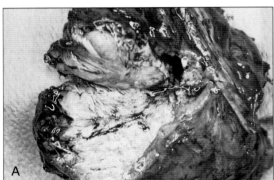
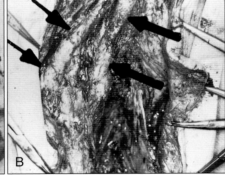

FIGURE 23-41 **(A)** A gross specimen of a large desmoid tumor is shown resected from the sciatic complex at a thigh level. **(B)** The sciatic complex just proximal to the popliteal space is seen to be relatively clear of the removed desmoid tumor shown in (A). The neural elements are scarred and thickened.

(8%) the radial nerve. Four (25%) lipomas arose in the brachial plexus region, of which two (50%) were removed from the brachial plexus itself and one (25%) each involved the musculocutaneous and axillary nerves. One lipoma involved the sciatic nerve.

There were four fatty, fibrous lipohamartomas in the LSUHSC series, each found within the median nerve. Three of the four lipohamartomas were managed by section of the transverse carpal ligament and decompression rather than removal of lipomatous tissue. A fourth patient had progressive neuritic pain and severe paresthesias, despite two decompressive operations. This patient thus required a third operation with internal neurolysis of fascicles, as well as digital branches. A mixture of scar and lipoma was resected, but a portion of the nerve complex was severely involved and no longer transmitted NAPs. Partial resection of the median and several digital branches led to their replacement with sural grafts and eventually to incomplete recovery of both thenar sensation and function.

In two cases the lipomas appeared to arise in nerve. These two tumors could be teased from the nerve with most of the nerves' function preserved.

Several cases of solitary lipomas causing neural compression that were treated elsewhere and had the nerve inadvertently resected required repair at LSUHSC. Cases of macrodystrophia lipomatosa have been seen at LSUHSC, but have not undergone surgical

intervention. There has been one case of an encapsulated lipoma located entirely inside the nerve.

DESMOID TUMORS

Desmoid tumors involving nerve or plexus can occur, but are infrequent. Brachial plexus involvement by desmoid tumors is reported in the recent literature in six case reports,[61,62,123,135,169] one report of seven patients and another of four patients.[68,136] Fuchs et al.[58] also presented one case involving the sciatic nerve. Ferraresi et al.[52] published a report of a patient who had radial nerve involvement by a desmoid tumor and Bregeon et al.[19] had two cases of sciatic nerve involvement.

Clinical presentation

Although desmoids are benign, they tend to be invasive of soft tissues, and if close to nerve, such a tumor can envelop and be quite adherent to it and other structures connected to muscle (Fig. 23-41).[103]

The most frequent site of origin is the abdominal musculature, but desmoids can originate in the neck, shoulder, and upper and lower extremities, where they can involve soft tissue and can compress, incorporate, or adhere to major nerves.

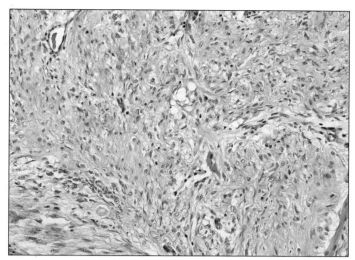

FIGURE 23-42 This is a photomicrograph of a desmoid tumor with pale eosinophilic fibroblasts and myofibroblasts with variable tapering or plump vesicular nuclei arranged in fascicles. These fascicles infiltrate the surrounding residual muscle fibers. Individual cells are well separated by collagen. No atypical mitoses are present. H & E original magnification ×200.

Microscopic appearance

Desmoids are of mesenchymal origin. These tumors are composed of well-collagenized, uniform fibroblasts with rare mitoses. The tumor has pale eosinophilic fibro- and myoblasts, which have a variable tapering appearance or plump vesicular nuclei arranged in fascicles. These fascicles infiltrate the surrounding residual muscle fibers. Individual cells are well separated by collagen (Fig. 23-42).

Surgical approach

The operative treatment involves a wide exposure of the lesion and identification of nerve(s) or plexus element(s) involved. The tumor is sharply dissected, as far as possible, away from the nerve or plexus elements. The involved epineurium requires resection. Since the desmoid is usually adherent to nerves, as well as vessels and other structures, an extensive and lengthy operation is required.

Desmoid tumors have poorly delineated surgical margins.[60] Despite what would appear to be gross total excision, recurrence is common, especially if wide resection is difficult because of contiguous important neural or vascular structures. Tumors removed at LSUHSC in the region of the plexus have been difficult to completely eliminate and have tended to recur. Despite this, several have been successfully re-resected. One extensive lesion at the axillary level, however, led to progressive neural loss, required two resections, recurred a third time and finally, because of an almost flail arm and severe pain, required a forequarter amputation.

Surgical excision is the treatment of choice for these tumors. Gross total excision with microscopically negative margins has been reported to produce recurrence rates of 5–50%, while positive microscopic margins produce recurrence rates as high as 90%.[1,21,50,60,93,120]

Adjunctive treatment

Radiation therapy may control low-grade growth, and external beam radiation (55 Gy) improves local control in patients with positive margins.[60,71,100,120] Some series have shown a significant injury to the brachial plexus in patients receiving as little as 40 Gy to tumors in this region, however.[60,111]

Tamoxifen has been used as a chemotherapeutic adjunct to surgery mainly in locations other than the peripheral nerve for desmoids. The reduced recurrence rates that have been documented,[15,60,85,155,164] however, are variable and there have also been late recurrences in some cases.[57,60,122] Cytotoxic therapy with vincristine, actinomycin D, and cyclophosphamide are known to have an effect and corticosteroids have been shown to cause tumor regression, though rarely.[60]

Results

The majority of the 11 desmoid tumors removed at LSUHSC (six of 11, 55%) involved the brachial plexus. The lower extremity had the next most frequent number of desmoid tumors involving nerve (three of 11, 27%) of which the sciatic complex was the site of two tumors (18%) followed by the peroneal nerve, which had one (9%). The upper extremity (two of 11, 18%) was the site of one tumor each (50%) removed from the median and radial nerves.

CASE SUMMARY – DESMOID TUMOR

CASE 1

A 12-year-old girl presented to her pediatrician with a large buttock mass. A desmoid tumor was removed from the buttock musculature. Within 2 years, there was a recurrence which had extended to the thigh level. This required an extensive dissection at both the buttock and thigh levels to free the sciatic nerve of tumor and to remove tumor from the buttock and from the hamstring muscles. Most sciatic function could be preserved.

In a few years, however, tumor was at the popliteal and proximal calf levels with adherence to the popliteal vessels, as well as to the tibial and peroneal nerves. This required another extensive operation, which was followed over the next 2 years by several procedures at a midcalf level. The tumor seemed to move progressively down the limb.

Later, the patient required a number of procedures for recurrent tumor at the level of the ankle, dorsum of the foot, and more recently in relation to the toes and their web spaces. Fortunately, there is no sign of recurrence at the buttock, thigh, or calf levels. Because of determination, and an active exercise program, she completed college and even had a successful career as a television newscaster. It has now been more than 30 years since the discovery of her disease.

COMMENT

During dissection, it may be difficult to determine where a desmoid ends and more normal tissues begin, because the latter are often infiltrated by the tumor. The pattern of centrifugal growth seen in this case is most unusual.

OSTEOCHONDROMA

Osteochondromas are also tumors with major calcification. Published cases of osteochondromas involving nerve documented eight cases over the last 10 years. The peroneal nerve was involved in seven cases[27,59] and the musculocutaneous nerve in one.[89]

Microscopic appearance

The microscopic picture is that of a cartilage-capped bony projection, i.e. normal cartilage covering normal bone. The cartilage cap resembles layers of the normal growth plate; however, the cartilage is more disorganized than normal. There are binucleate chondrocytes in the lacunae. The mass is covered with a thin layer of periosteum.

Results

Four osteochondromas involved nerve in the LSUHSC series. One patient had a large brachial plexus region osteochondroma, which had arisen spontaneously in a paraspinal location and was associated with a thoracic outlet syndrome. Symptoms included pain and paresthesias in the upper arm and forearm with arm abduction or use of the arm above a horizontal level. A posterior subscapular approach was used for resection of both the tumor and the posterior portion of the first rib followed by neurolysis of the brachial plexus.

In the upper extremity, one tumor involved the humerus in a middle-aged male, resulting in a preoperative severe radial distribution deficit. After removal of the tumor and neurolysis of the radial nerve the patient slowly regained function over a 2-year period.

In the lower extremity, two of these tumors were removed from the region of the peroneal nerve. One of these tumors arose from the proximal fibula and had to be dissected free not only from the peroneal nerve, but also from the proximal portions of the superficial and deep branches. A similar problem arose in a young man who had a bony proliferation of both fibular heads and bilateral entrapment of the peroneal nerves.

MYOSITIS OSSIFICANS

Myositis ossificans is a mass related to prior trauma or surgery. Myositis ossificans has major amounts of calcification within it and usually produces a hard mass of tissue which surrounds adjacent nerves, vessels, muscles, and tendons and occasionally bone. Although the origin is different, an occasional lipoma can also become calcified after trauma or prior surgery

There have been no myositis ossificans cases reported in the literature from the last 10 years, but rather "neuritis ossificans" has been described, in which the ossifying process was intraneural.[63,162,170]

Clinical presentation

The tumor can be symptomatic owing to neural involvement. Vascular involvement by the tumor can indirectly result in symptoms, as well.

Microscopic appearance

The histological appearance of myositis ossificans consists of immature bone, cellular proliferation, and a "zoning" pattern consisting of three distinct zones. The zones include a central portion in which there is fibroblastic proliferation which can vary markedly in cellularity, pleomorphic characteristics, and numbers of mitotic figures; an intermediate portion of collagen and osteoid deposition among proliferating spindle cells, with early trabeculation of ossifying areas; and a peripheral zone of osteoid trabeculae rimmed by osteoblasts, with bone surrounded by loose fibrous tissue and atrophic fat.

Surgical approach

Removal of these masses can be technically difficult. Mobilizing the nerve away from the mass and neurolysis often dramatically improves the patient's symptoms. Complete resection of these masses, although sometimes possible, is usually not indicated.

Results

In the LSUHSC series, four cases of myositis ossificans were encountered, two of which involved the brachial plexus. One of two patients with a brachial plexus ossified mass was a 32-year-old male, who underwent partial resection of a large area of axillary fibromyositis and had reoperation for resection of residual tumor and exploration of the brachial plexus. Grafts were placed at this time from the lateral and medial cords to both median and ulnar nerves. At follow-up 4 years later, there was no recurrence. Most of the median nerve function had returned, as had function of the flexor carpi ulnaris and flexor digiti minimi profundus III and IV muscles. There was no recovery of the ulnar-innervated hand intrinsic function.

The other patient with a brachial plexus mass was a 30-year-old man who had sustained a severe left brachial plexus stretch injury as a result of a motorcycle accident. The left limb was flail and the patient had a Horner sign. Attempt at operative repair elsewhere had been unsuccessful and was terminated due to severe bleeding from the axillary artery. He presented to LSUHSC with a large, partially calcified mass incorporating the brachial plexus at the supra- and infraclavicular levels. In exposing the residual portions of the plexus elements in this large calcified mass, the axillary artery was re-injured in several places and had to be sutured. A graft repair of the infraclavicular plexus elements was finally accomplished; however, the grafts were 7.5–15 cm in length. On the second postoperative day, embolization to the radial artery occurred and the limb had to be subsequently amputated at an upper arm level. Recovery would probably not have occurred due to the length of the grafts necessary to restore continuity and the severe scarring causing neural injury which was encountered.

Two tumors were removed from the upper extremity, specifically one involving the median and one the radial nerve. The radial nerve tumor presented as a large calcified mass arising in the triceps, the location of a prior contusion of the lateral upper arm. The tumor compressed the nerve as it came around the humerus in the radial groove and was adherent to the nerve, but had not invaded it. As the mass grew, the patient developed a partial radial palsy. Triceps function was spared, but that of the brachioradialis and extensor digitorum communis muscles was grade 2, the extensor pollicis longus grade 3, and the wrist extensors were grade 2 to 3. The fibrotic, calcified mass was removed in this case and neurolysis was carried out. Function in the muscles innervated by the radial nerve improved dramatically and at 1.5 years postoperatively were excellent.

An example of a lipoma which had become calcified and had hemangiomatous changes after prior partial removal occurred behind the knee of a teenage girl. It involved the peroneal nerve and required an extensive dissection for removal. Most of the peroneal function was preserved, with postoperative function in the anterior compartment muscles averaging grade 4.

HEMANGIOMAS

Hemangiomas are tumors of vascular origin, which can compress or envelop nerve or, less frequently, arise within it. One hemangioma involving the median nerve was presented by Ergin et al.[49] in 1998 and one each of the PIN and posterior tibial nerves by Busa et al.[23] and Vigna et al.,[160] respectively, in the recent literature. Peled et al. published a hemangioma of the median nerve in 1980[116] and Losli presented two cases in 1952.[102]

Microscopic appearance

The hemangioma consists of many variously sized, endothelium-lined vascular channels, some of which are filled with blood (Fig. 23-43). Various microscopic presentations of the neoplasm may consist of proliferating capillaries without lumina, opening of the lumina beginning at the periphery, increasing interstitial fibrosis, and thrombosis of vessels.

Surgical approach

The operative technique for hemangiomas involves isolating and ligating vessels at the periphery of the lesion, if they are not the major supply to an extremity. Nerves are dissected away from the lesion. Occasionally, a hemangioma directly involves the nerve or appears to originate within it; a careful interfascicular dissection is necessary to remove each fascicle or group of fascicles containing abnormal vascular tissue.

Results

The LSUHSC cases of hemangiomas included two hemangiomas removed from the ulnar nerve. These tumors had also been resected elsewhere and the resections had led to neural loss. In one instance, a large hemangioma of the forearm had been resected, leading to ulnar loss. On secondary exploration, a 12.7 cm gap was found in the forearm involving the ulnar nerve. Five centimeters were gained by an ulnar transposition at the elbow and the remaining gap was closed by sural nerve grafts. Only partial recovery of ulnar function occurred; however, NAPs could be transmitted through the grafts several years later. One tumor was removed from the peroneal nerve.

VENOUS ANGIOMAS

There has been only one case of a venous angioma involving a peripheral nerve previously reported. This has been recently published by Maniker et al.[106] and was a case of a traumatic venous varix of the inferior gluteal vein which caused a compression sciatic neuropathy.

Microscopic appearance

The vessels comprising a venous angioma contain smooth muscle and elastic tissue, but to a lesser extent than in normal arterial walls. Hyalinization and thickening of the vessel walls are common. Neural tissue is found between the vascular elements of this malformation.

Results

In the LSUHSC experience, there were four venous angiomas and the majority (three of four tumors, 75%) was in the lower extremity and one was removed from the median nerve.

In two cases, enlargement of the lesion occurred whenever the involved limb was placed in a dependent position. The first patient's job involved stocking shelves in a food store. If he stocked shelves above the waist, he was asymptomatic, but if he worked on the lower shelves, he developed a tender swelling at the wrist and experienced paresthesias in the median distribution of the hand. He gradually developed atrophy of the thenar eminence. A venous angioma was found to involve the median nerve at a distal forearm-to-wrist level (Fig. 23-44). The angioma was intrinsic to nerve and seemed to be fed proximally by small arterioles and was partially drained by veins distally. An internal neurolysis was performed and angioma was removed from the fascicles under magnification. He did well for 3 years, although there was no reversal of thenar atrophy. The thenar mass recurred and numbness redeveloped in the median distribution. Resection and replacement with grafts was necessary 4.5 years after his initial presentation. There has been no recurrence. He has had partial sensory, but not motor recovery. The lesion was sinusoidal and its wall had more of a venous than arterial structure. Enlargement with dependency could be readily demonstrated at the operating table and the contained blood had a bluish tinge.

A similar lesion was seen in a 22-year-old woman, but it involved the posterior tibial nerve behind the knee. Branches of this nerve were incorporated in a venous aneurysm-like structure proximal to their entry into and deep to the gastrocnemius soleus muscle.

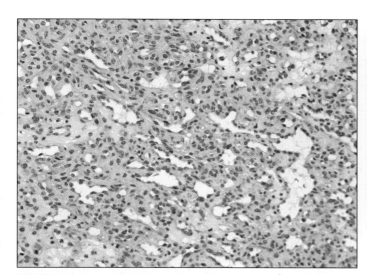

FIGURE 23-43 A photomicrograph of a hemangioma is seen. It has a collection of bland capillaries with well-developed lumina. Various states of the neoplasm may consist of proliferating capillaries without lumina, opening of lumina beginning at the periphery, increasing interstitial fibrosis, and thrombosis of vessels. H & E, original magnification ×200.

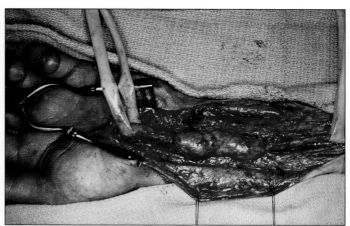

FIGURE 23-44 This is a venous angioma involving the distal forearm-level median nerve, as seen intraoperatively. The patient stocked shelves in a store and, while stocking the lower shelves, he experienced painful paresthesias in a median distribution that dissipated when he worked on higher shelves. The lesion was resected by clearing individual fascicles of vessels and scar. Five years later this venous angioma recurred and required resection and a sural nerve graft repair of the median nerve.

Involved branches were dissected proximally and cleared of the aneurysmal investment. This dissection included an internal neurolysis of the distal tibial nerve. Resection was accomplished without loss of function, and there has been no recurrence over a 15-year period.

Two additional patients had nerve compression without deficit, accompanied by paresthesias as a result of each having a venous angioma extrinsic to nerve. One case involved the sciatic nerve near its exit from the sciatic foramen. Another patient with a history of venous insufficiency had a saphenous vein angioma involving the femoral sensory branches.

HEMANGIOBLASTOMAS

Hemangioblastomas are much more common in the central rather than in the peripheral nervous system. The recent literature has reports of only two peripheral nerve hemangioblastomas, one each of the sciatic nerve at midthigh level[65] and the radial nerve.[20]

Microscopic appearance

The histology of the peripheral nerve hemangioblastoma is similar to that seen in central nervous system lesions. The tumor is cellular and multinodular with areas of microcystic degeneration. The hemangioblastoma of nerve involves primarily the epineurium, but invasion of the fascicles by tumor cells (called "stromal cells") is often seen. Stromal cells have round nuclei and vacuolated, lipid-rich cytoplasm, and fill the interstices between innumerable capillaries.

Results

The single hemangioblastoma in this series involved the median nerve at an elbow level and required an interfascicular dissection to clear the fascicles of tumor (Fig. 23-45). Some years later it recurred and total resection of the involved segment of nerve followed by graft repair was necessary.

HEMANGIOPERICYTOMAS

Hemangiopericytomas can arise in mediastinum and grow superiorly to envelop or become adherent to brachial plexus. These tumors sometimes behave in a malignant fashion and metastasize to other sites, even the brain. A hemangiopericytoma of the sciatic notch presenting as sciatica was documented by Harrison et al.[75] in 1995.

Microscopic appearance

Histologically, the tumor is composed of basophilic spindle-shaped mononuclear cells that appear similar to smooth muscle cells. There are irregular vascular channels of varying sizes arranged in what is often described as a "staghorn" pattern. Perivascular hyalinization is often present.

Surgical approach

Hemangiopericytomas cannot usually be removed entirely from the plexus. Complete removal is difficult even if plexus is not involved.

Results

In the LSUHSC series one hemangiopericytoma was removed from the brachial plexus and one from the median nerve.

The thoracic surgery service approached one case by splitting the mediastinum and removing the mediastinal portion by dissecting it away from the intrathoracic paraspinal structures, including the arch of the aorta and its superior vessels. We then proceeded to dissect the remaining tumor away from the lower elements of the brachial plexus.

GLOMUS TUMORS

Two cases of glomus tumors involving digital nerves have been reported to date. These included one each by van der Lei et al.[156] and Wong et al.[166] in 1997 and 2001, respectively.

Microscopic appearance

These unusual tumors are thought to arise from glomeruli where a small arteriole connects to an adjacent vein by way of a tiny canalicular system.[147] These microscopic structures may relate to local changes in blood flow, perfusion pressure, and regulation of heat exchange.

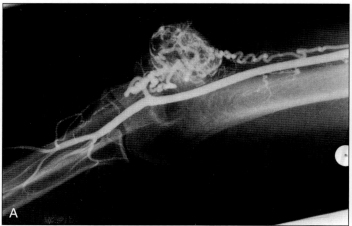
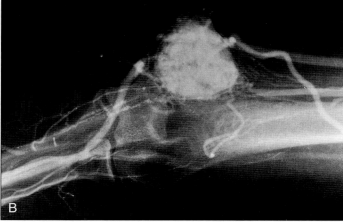

FIGURE 23-45 **(A)** The arterial phase of a brachial angiogram of a vascular tumor involving the median nerve just proximal to the elbow is seen. A prior attempt at biopsy had led to a profuse amount of bleeding, which suggested the need for angiography. The patient presented with a partial median nerve deficit. This deficit was made slightly worse by operation and then slowly reversed over several years. **(B)** A later phase in the same angiogram showing a relatively early venous filling is seen here. Histologically, this vascular mass proved to be a hemangioblastoma.

Glomus tumor histology shows endothelium-lined vascular spaces surrounded by clusters of so-called glomus cells in a canaliculus-like arrangement (Fig. 23-46). Glomus cells are monomorphous round or polygonal cells with plump nuclei and scant eosinophilic cytoplasm.

Surgical approach

The glomus tumors in this series required wide local excision. This wide local excision was carried out to minimize recurrence.

Results

Despite the tendency to arise in the area of the nail bed or subungual region, there were two patients who underwent glomus tumor resections at LSUHSC, one each from an upper extremity digital nerve and a lower extremity peroneal nerve.

The peroneal lesion was in a 14-year-old girl, who presented with severe pain and tenderness over the lower anterior tibia. She had seen many physicians and was considered to be hysterical or to have an excessive degree of emotional overlay. She would ward off all attempts to palpate this area; however, when palpation was performed it documented a slight, smooth fullness there, but no actual mass. The area was exquisitely tender, but light percussion did not give a Tinel sign. There were mild dysesthesias in the superficial peroneal sensory distribution. Foot function was otherwise normal, although when walking she did not wish to bear full weight on the involved leg. She was hospitalized and with her parent's consent while asleep, the area was repalpated; she awoke, shrieking with pain. As a result, the area was surgically explored with the patient under general anesthesia. A reddish-brown mass adherent to the anterior periosteum of the tibia was found and it was excised along with the tibial periosteum in that area (Fig. 23-47). Sensory branches of the peroneal nerve were not directly involved, but were present over the mass. These branches were mobilized and displaced to either side of the mass. The mass proved to be a glomus tumor and the histology was characteristic (see Fig. 23-46).

Postoperatively, she was free of pain and had a normal gait for 4.5 years. A painful lump recurred in that area and was re-excised when she was 19 years of age. She did relatively well, until the age of 22 when she returned with a possible recurrence. No specific mass was palpable and tenderness was not as severe as it had been in the past. She declined further surgery at that time.

Tumors formed from such cells can recur. Depending on the locus, these tumors can invade peripheral nerve branches, as in this case.

MENINGIOMAS

A recent report of a peripheral nerve meningioma was presented by Anderson et al.[5] This tumor involved the radial nerve.

Microscopic appearance

Meningiomas are grouped into two main divisions. The first is the classic meningioma, which consists of the meningothelial, fibrous, and transitional types. This group also includes the psammomatous, angiomatous, microcystic, secretory, clear cell, chordoid, and lymphoplasmacyte-rich types as classified by the World Health Organization. The second category is composed of the atypical and malignant meningiomas.

Results

Two meningiomas involving the brachial plexus were removed at LSUHSC. One small meningioma involved the C7 spinal nerve. An intraspinal component had been successfully removed elsewhere. Residual intraforaminal scar and tumor were subsequently removed by a posterior subscapular approach to this spinal nerve.

The other large peripheral nerve meningioma was difficult to remove (Fig. 23-48). This tumor involved the supraclavicular plexus from the spinal nerve to divisional level of the trunks. There had been four prior attempts at removal. Using an extensive anterior approach, the tumor was resected and we performed a partial graft repair of the C6 to upper trunk divisions and C7 to the middle trunk of the plexus. Postoperative functional loss occurred in the upper and middle trunk distributions. Some of this function was recovered over time and the main deficit that has persisted is poor shoulder abduction. Follow-up magnetic resonance imaging (MRI) done 2 years later indicated recurrence along the paraspinal portions of the lower roots and plexus trunks to divisions beneath the clavicle and over the pleural apex. Irradiation, rather than further operation, was advised, but further follow-up is lacking.

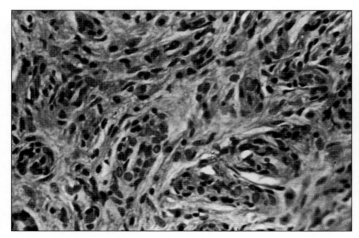

FIGURE 23-46 A hematoxylin and eosin stain is seen of a glomus tumor resected from the periosteum of the lower tibia. The microscopic section shows endothelium-lined vascular spaces surrounded by glomus cells in a caniculus-like arrangement.

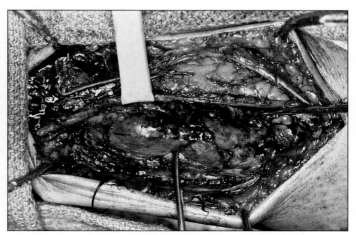

FIGURE 23-47 This intraoperative photograph shows the gross appearance of a fairly sizeable glomus tumor located over the lower tibia. The lesion has been partially elevated from the periosteum. The superficial peroneal branch is being retracted by a Penrose drain.

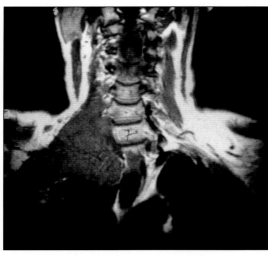

FIGURE 23-48 A very large meningioma involving the right brachial plexus is seen. This unusual lesion was associated with severe functional loss and had had several resections with a recurrence after each procedure.

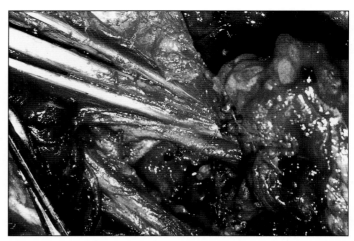

FIGURE 23-49 A lymphangioma is shown undergoing dissection away from cords of the plexus. The mass of the tumor is pulled up and to the right.

MYOBLASTOMA OR GRANULAR CELL TUMOR

There were three case reports in the recent literature for myoblastomas involving nerve. Two cases involved the ulnar nerve and the third, the sural nerve.[3,34,36,168]

Clinical presentation

Myoblastomas very rarely involve nerve. Common sites of occurrence of this tumor which do not involve nerve include the skin, breast, tongue, larynx, bronchi, and the submucosal layer of the gastrointestinal tract. Though this tumor is categorized here as benign, myoblastomas can occasionally assume malignant characteristics.

Microscopic appearance

These tumors are formed of a mixture of plump, angular cells with a cytoplasm containing eosinophilic granules, which represent a large number of lysosomes.[13] The cells have small, regular, hyperchromatic nuclei. Cells tend to be rather compactly arranged. Mitotic figures are few in number and these tumors are classified as benign, but occasionally the tumor takes on an invasive behavior.[22] This tumor tends to spread as a sheet of tumorous tissue. Groups of lymphoid cells occur at the periphery of most lesions.

Surgical approach

These tumors rarely involve nerve, but when they do, they are adherent and require careful dissection for their removal. Treatment involves a wide surgical exposure to determine normal anatomy distal and proximal to the lesion before skeletonizing the involved nerve and moving it away from the lesion.

Results

The current LSUHSC series includes two myoblastomas, each involving elements of the brachial plexus. Both tumors were firmly attached and involved the plexus trunks, as well as the extraforaminal portions of the spinal nerves. One tumor could be removed using careful dissection under magnification. The second patient initially had had surgery elsewhere and had severe functional loss

in the distribution of the lower elements. This patient required a posterior approach with resection of scar and recurrent tumor from the upper mediastinum, as well as from the plexus. Because the immediate preoperative deficit was severe and pain was a problem since the lower roots to trunks were involved over a length, the latter elements were resected along with recurrent tumor and scar. This tumor had some mitotic figures, and a small recurrence was treated with chemotherapy 2 years later. There has been no further recurrence after another 3 years of follow-up. Pain relief has been good, despite loss of hand-intrinsic function.

LYMPHANGIOMAS

There are only two reports of lymphangiomas involving nerve in the recent literature. One case involved the ulnar nerve[151] and the other, the posterior tibial nerve.[165]

Clinical presentation

When these tumors involve nerve, they have many of the same characteristics as myoblastomas.[32] The cells tend to spread as a sheet of tumorous tissue enveloping structures, rather than forming a true mass lesion (Fig. 23-49).

Microscopic appearance

Lymphangiomas are focal proliferations of well-differentiated lymphatic tissue that present as multicystic accumulations. They are subdivided into three categories. Capillary lymphangiomas are thin-walled lymphatic channels that occur as small, well-circumscribed cutaneous lesions. The second category is that of the cavernous lymphangiomas, which are also thin-walled lymphatic channels; however, these tumors have an associated stroma. Cystic lymphangioma, the third category, has large, well-circumscribed, multiloculated cystic spaces lined by endothelium that contain a significant connective tissue component. Cavernous and cystic lymphangiomas can coexist within the same lesion.

Surgical approach

The surgical excision for these tumors is the same as that described for the myoblastoma.

Results

Two lymphangiomas were removed at LSUHSC. One lymphangioma was contiguous with brachial plexus elements and was removed by a posterior subscapular approach. The first rib was resected and tumor was successfully removed from the C7, C8, and T1 spinal nerves and the middle and lower trunks of the brachial plexus. The other tumor involved the medial upper arm and enveloped the proximal median and ulnar nerves, which required neurolysis.

NON-TUMORAL MASS LESIONS INVOLVING NERVE

PSEUDOANEURYSMS

Clots, especially those associated with trauma or, less frequently, with anticoagulation, can compress nerves and lead to serious neurological deficits. An example of these lesions is the pseudoaneurysm. Pseudoaneurysms occur because of a penetrating injury to a vessel, which permits dissection of blood into the vessel wall. The vessel expands and a sizable encapsulated mass forms.

These vascular masses usually occur due to injury to the axillary artery. Presentation and behavior at that site are discussed in the chapter concerning the brachial plexus and gunshot wounds (Chapter 15).

Clinical presentation

The delayed onset of pain and paresthesias after a penetrating injury near a major vessel and nerve and an expanding mass with or without a palpable thrill or bruit heard on auscultation should suggest the possibility of a pseudoaneurysm. Neural loss may be progressive and unless the lesion is resected in a timely fashion the deficit may become permanent.

Results

Pseudoaneurysms managed at LSUHSC have included not only those of the axillary artery, but also those of the femoral artery caused by femoral angiography and those on the popliteal vessel resulting from severe penetrating injury behind the knee.

In the three pseudoaneurysms due to femoral angiography, neural involvement was severe and the markedly stretched nerves required replacement by grafts extending from the pelvis to the thigh. In the pseudoaneurysm involving the popliteal artery, neurolysis of the tibial and peroneal nerves and resection of the mass sufficed.

A pseudoaneurysm can cause a partial injury to a nerve or plexus elements to extend, resulting in a more severe and complete loss. This lesion is thus one of the few mechanisms producing a progressive loss of nerve function after the original injury.

ARTERIOVENOUS FISTULAE OR MALFORMATIONS

Arteriovenous (AV) fistulae or arteriovenous malformations can occur close enough to the nerve so as to directly involve it. At times, the fistula is only in the vicinity of the injured nerve and yet the patient develops progressive neural symptoms. The lesion is caused by the same, usually penetrating, wound that involved the nerve. The penetrating injury to nerve usually does not result in progressive neural loss, but the additional presence of a fistula often does.

Surgical approach

In the first case at LSUHSC, neurolysis of the ulnar and median nerves was performed after coagulating or ligating arterial feeders to the fistula. The ulnar nerve was then transposed volar to the elbow and buried beneath the flexor carpi ulnaris and pronator teres muscles.

In the second case, the fistula was obliterated and the median nerve was unroofed from the upper arm to the forearm by sectioning the lacertus fibrosis and a portion of the overlying pronator teres.

Results

A classic example of an AV fistula was provided by a case at LSUHSC in which a 14-year-old boy sustained an accidental rifle wound to the left elbow and developed a pulsatile enlargement of the arm around the elbow as well as a progressive ulnar palsy. Ulnar arterial to venous connections had formed a fistula just proximal to the elbow. The feeding artery also had an aneurysm in it proximal to the fistula site.

A similar fistula involving the median nerve at the elbow was seen in another patient, but was related to a knife wound. The origin of the fistula was from the brachial artery.

Both cases had excellent outcomes after the fistulae were obliterated.

MALIGNANT TUMORS OF NON-NEURAL SHEATH ORIGIN

TUMORS METASTATIC TO NERVE

Malignant peripheral non-neural sheath tumors (PNNSTs) are uncommon, but do occur. Publications regarding malignant PNNSTs over the last 10 years include one from LSUHSC of a primary lymphoma metastatic to the radial nerve[157] and one case each of primary non-Hodgkin's lymphoma metastatic to the sciatic nerve reported by Kanamori et al.[91] and Roncaroli et al.[131] Fifteen patients with brachial plexus malignant fibrosarcoma or desmoid tumors were presented by Gaposchkin et al.[60] and an intraneural synovial sarcoma of the median nerve at the wrist was published by Chesser et al.[29]

Malignant PNNSTs usually involve brachial plexus elements or peripheral nerves by direct extension from a primary site, but they may occasionally metastasize from the primary site via the bloodstream to the nerve or to tissue adjacent to nerve, the latter resulting in nerve compression or ultimately in its invasion. Management of these tumors must be individualized due to this variability in presentation and extent of involvement, both of which in turn are related to each type of cancer's individual behavior. Metastasis to the brachial plexus and less frequently the peripheral nerve can occur from skin, breast, thyroid, thymus, pancreas, lung, bladder, and prostate cancers and a host of non-organ tumors.

The supraclavicular brachial plexus is commonly involved by metastasis from tumors invading nearby lymph nodes and is exemplified by breast cancer, which represented the largest category of metastasis to nerve in the LSUHSC malignant non-nerve tumors. Metastasis to the axillary level infraclavicular brachial plexus, on the other hand, usually presents by direct extension from the primary tumor.

Surgical approach

If a mass is palpable and/or is visualized on a scan in a patient with a history of primary cancer, then decompression of involved neural elements is undertaken. En bloc removal of tumor and adjacent tissues is not indicated for malignant non-nerve tumors involving the plexus, although it is for malignant PNSTs.

Nerves involved by metastasis from breast (Fig. 23-50), melanoma, or other metastatic cancer can usually be treated with external neurolysis and careful removal of tumor from involved nerve. As much of the adjacent mass as possible is also removed. Accompanying scar secondary to irradiation if present makes dissection more difficult, but not impossible. Usually this type of cancer does not invade nerve beyond the epineurial level; however, exceptions exist, especially with breast cancer.

Patients with intraneural lesions require excision of the element(s) or nerve involved. If pain is a problem, resection of the involved neural element is palliative in some cases. This is especially so with pulmonary carcinoma where decompressive procedures sometimes include the spinal canal as well as nerve roots, spinal nerves, and plexal trunks and yet some nerve elements may require excision.

With melanomas involving the plexus, removing the tumor from any epineural attachment usually suffices and is followed by local irradiation. A similar approach is also appropriate, at least for palliative treatment, for lymphomas.

Another type of cancer involving nerve, especially the plexus, is pulmonary metastatic disease. Lung cancer may involve the brachial plexus by direct extension and often produces a Pancoast syndrome. This syndrome sometimes occurs due to local extension of a pulmonary apical tumor to involve the C8, T1, and T2 nerves and there is usually shoulder pain radiating down the arm in the ulnar distribution. Radiologic destruction of the first and second ribs is also seen. If pain is a severe problem, a palliative approach

consists of a posterior subscapular resection of the first rib and subtotal resection of the apical tumor to decompress the lower elements of the plexus. This procedure is combined with cervical laminectomy for associated epidural metastatic disease. A high contralateral open cervical cordotomy can also be carried out to control the pain associated with a Pancoast syndrome. The main focus of this palliative operation is to decompress the spinal cord, as well as the compressed or entrapped plexal elements, to improve pain relief.

Results

Thirty-five patients presented to LSUHSC between 1969 and 1999 with carcinomas involving nerve and underwent operations for these metastatic tumors (Table 23-12). The largest category of metastatic tumor was breast carcinoma (15 of 35 tumors, 43%) and this usually involved the brachial plexus or one of its outflows in the majority (14 of 15 tumors, 93%) of patients.

In the case of a lymphoma metastatic to the radial nerve, a physician with central nervous system lymphoma presented 3 years after craniotomy and cranial irradiation with a complete radial palsy at the midhumeral level (Fig. 23-51). At exploration, lymphoma was found within the substance of the radial nerve. No other sign of lymphoma, either residual in the brain or elsewhere was found for 5 years, and then the patient succumbed with extensive pulmonary lymphoma.

The nine cases of pulmonary metastatic disease involved the brachial plexus and in most cases were caused by direct extension of the tumor, rather than by true metastasis (Figs 23-52, 23-53). Occasionally, a benign nerve sheath tumor involving a lower plexus element can indent the apex of the lung and mimic a Pancoast tumor (Fig. 23-54).

Ewing's sarcoma involving the brachial plexus was removed from one patient. Occasionally, a malignancy arising from blood vessels such as an angiosarcoma can secondarily involve nerve, but we have not had experience with such a sarcoma.

Two patients with metastatic melanoma had large lesions, one involving plexus at the C8 to lower trunk level and the other the

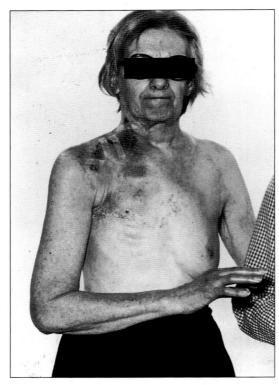

FIGURE 23-50 This patient is status-post mastectomy and radiation for breast carcinoma. She developed subsequent pain, paresthesias, and progressive loss in a brachial plexus distribution and underwent neurolysis of the plexus for irradiation plexitis. She is shown here a few days postoperatively.

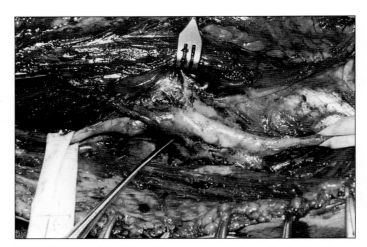

FIGURE 23-51 A lymphoma is seen metastatic and intrinsic to the radial nerve. There was total loss of function distal to the triceps branch. After a resection, a graft repair was performed. Subsequent radiation of this area most likely contributed to a lack of radial recovery. (From Van Bolden A, Kline D, Garcia C, et al.: Isolated radial nerve palsy from primary malignant lymphoma of brain. Neurosurgery 21:905–909, 1988.)

Table 23-12 Operative carcinomas involving nerve (n=35)

	No. of cases	LR	LRM	Repair/RT*	Improved pain	Maintained function	Avg. f/up (mon)	Deaths
Breast								
Brachial plexus	14	14	0	0/0	11	10	17	5 (16 mon)
Radial	1	0	1	0/0	1	1	18	0
Lung								
Brachial plexus	9	7	0	1/0	7	7	18	5 (8 mon)
Melanoma								
Brachial plexus	2	2	0	0/2	2	2	27	1 (18 mon)
Bladder								
Brachial plexus	1	1	0	0/0	1	1	14	0
Rectum								
Pelvic plexus	1	1	0	0/0	1	1	12	0
Skin (squamous)								
Ulnar	1	1	0	1/1	1	0	14	1 (18 mon)
Ewing sarcoma								
Brachial plexus	1	1	0	0/1	1	1	72	0
Osteosarcoma								
Brachial plexus	1	1	0	0/0	1	1	13	0
Lymphoma								
Radial	1	0	1	1/1	1	0	60	1 (60 mon)
Head and neck								
Brachial plexus	1	1	0	0/1	1	0	4	1 (4 mon)
Thyroid								
Brachial plexus	1	1	0	0/1	1	0	42	0
Chordoma								
Brachial plexus	1	1	0	0/0	1	0	30	0
Totals	35	31	2	3/7	30	24	20	14 (15 mon)

Avg. f/up, average follow-up; LR, local resection of tumor; LRM, local resection with margins; ( ), average postoperative survival.

*Repair was by grafts; RT, radiation therapy by external beam from a cobalt source.

lateral cord to musculocutaneous outflow (Fig. 23-55). Gross total excision was possible, but other metastatic lesions appeared in lung and bone 2 and 3.5 years later, even though both the original and the metastatic sites were thought to be adequately treated by irradiation.

Complications

Expected complications resulting from operations on all tumors, both benign and malignant PNSTs and tumors of non-nerve sheath origin, included postoperative neural loss and new pain (Fig. 23-56). Several patients with plexus tumors approached anteriorly had transient phrenic paralysis and two approached posteriorly had scapular winging, which was also transient. There were two patients with plexus tumors who required thoracenteses postoperatively and one who required a chest tube for 3 days. There were two wound infections; both were superficial and responded to antibiotic and local wound care.

RADIATION-INDUCED BRACHIAL PLEXUS LESIONS (ACTINIC PLEXITIS)

A common dilemma in patients with new functional loss in the distribution of muscles innervated by the involved plexus elements or, rarely, peripheral nerve is the nature of the lesion. For example, in a patient who has undergone prior mastectomy for removal of primary breast carcinoma, a lesion in the brachial plexus causing functional loss may be due to radiation fibrosis, recurrent carcinoma with invasion of the plexus, or both of these entities.[96] The specific etiology of the brachial plexus lesion often cannot be resolved without operation and biopsies at multiple sites.

Several criteria suggest carcinomatous compression or invasion, including: (1) rapid progression of motor and/or sensory loss in the distribution of specific plexus elements, especially lower trunk, medial cord, or its outflows, accompanied by severe pain in the distribution of specific plexus elements; (2) onset in the months to early years after the original diagnosis of breast cancer, with some exceptions; (3) a localized mass seen on CT or MRI; (4) evidence of metastasis elsewhere in the body; (5) neoplastic tissue obtained by needle biopsy; and (6) no fasciculations/myokimia on electromyography. Unfortunately, in a few cases, we have seen intraneural breast carcinoma occur in the plexus many years after the patient was felt to be cured.

Less definite but also suggestive of carcinoma are severe pain, especially in the distribution of specific plexus elements, and absence of lymphedema.[153]

Features favoring irradiation plexitis include: (1) the slow progression of motor and/or sensory loss accompanied by pain with paresthesias, often the dominant symptom; (2) onset tending to

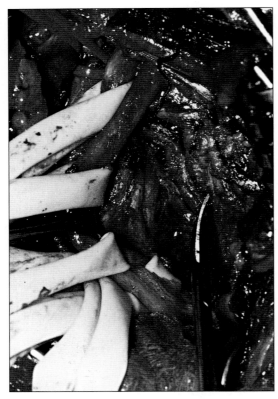

FIGURE 23-52 Metastatic pulmonary carcinoma (*arrow*) attached to the proximal humerus and compressing the plexus at a cord level. Plexus elements and major vessels have been dissected away from the tumor and are retracted medially (to the left) by Penrose drains.

occur years after the diagnosis of breast cancer, with some exceptions; (3) neuroimaging showing plexal thickening, without a discrete mass; (4) no evidence of metastasis elsewhere in the body; (5) no neoplastic tissue and a marked degree of scarring seen on the histology obtained from needle biopsy; and (6) electromyography showing fasciculations and/or myokimia.[99] Unfortunately, we have also seen the onset of irradiation plexitis symptoms within only a few months of completion of radiation therapy in a few cases.

There may be both carcinomatous invasion and irradiation plexitis present concomitantly, in which case the dichotomy described for the two lesions above becomes indistinct.

Other criteria favoring carcinoma involving the brachial plexus, rather than radiation fibrosis includes: (1) a history of a radiation dose less than 6000 rads and (2) the presence of a Horner syndrome.[99] At LSUHSC, as well as at other institutions, cases of irradiation plexitis without carcinoma may present, however, with one or more of these latter features.[103]

We have also seen other exceptions to all these criteria. For example, in addition to the several women described above who have presented to LSUHSC many years, i.e. 15 or more years, after the initial treatment of breast carcinoma with evidence of neoplastic tissue found within one or more brachial plexus elements, there is another exception. The time of onset of radiation plexitis is also quite variable and can begin as early as 6 months or as long as 18–20 years after the course of radiation therapy.

CASE SUMMARY – RADIATION-INDUCED BRACHIAL PLEXUS LESION (ACTINIC PLEXITIS)

CASE 1

This 39-year-old, right-handed woman had a simple mastectomy in 1982 for breast cancer. Postoperatively, she received 23 radiation treatments and 6 months of chemotherapy. She underwent reconstructive surgery with an attempted placement of a breast prosthesis, but developed a skin infection and had to have a skin graft. She had noticed progressive hand and forearm weakness and severe arm and hand pain for several years. Subsequently, she underwent a first-rib resection through a transaxillary approach but believed that her hand weakness and pain increased postoperatively.

On examination, the hand and forearm were swollen and somewhat stiff. In the supraclavicular area, there was a mild fullness and the skin was thickened and had telangiectasia. Tapping on this area elicited a Tinel sign with an "electrical shock" sensation radiating down to the fingers. Supra- and infraspinatus

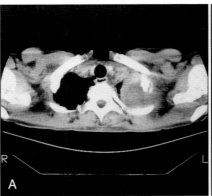
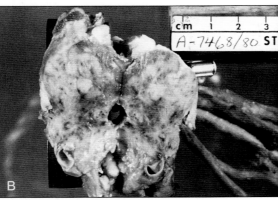

FIGURE 23-53 **(A)** This is a Pancoast tumor involving the left brachial plexus as seen on an axial section of a computerized tomographic scan of the superior lung fields. **(B)** A pathologic specimen of a large Pancoast tumor involving the brachial plexus elements, the latter of which are seen to the right.

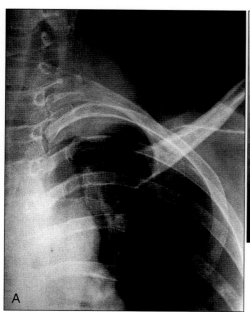

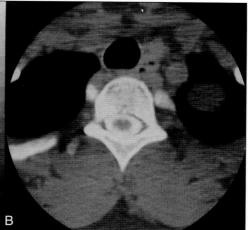

FIGURE 23-54 A chest X-ray **(A)** and computerized tomographic scan **(B)** of two different apical lung tumors, which required and could be removed by a plexus dissection, rather than thoracotomy. Both lesions were schwannomas. These studies should be compared to the malignancy seen in Figure 23-53A.

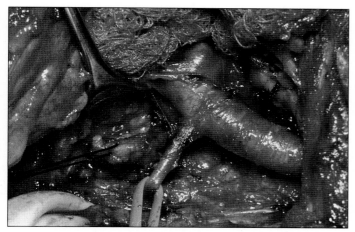

FIGURE 23-55 A nodule of a metastatic melanoma (held by a traction suture) is seen lying next to the subclavian artery and proximal to the origin of the vertebral artery, which is retracted downward by a plastic loop. The tumor was adherent to, but not invasive of, the C8 to lower trunk junction of the plexus.

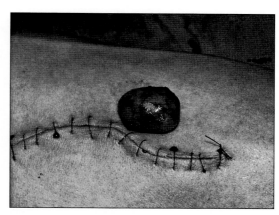

FIGURE 23-56 This is a neural sheath tumor after removal via the long curvilinear incision shown. A generous up-and-down exposure to resect even a small tumor is required; unless this is done, the nerve of origin or adjacent nerves can be damaged.

muscles were found to have grade 5 strength; deltoid, biceps and brachioradialis muscles were grade 4; and triceps had only a trace strength, i.e. grade 1. There was no wrist flexion or extension, no thumb or finger flexion or extension, and no hand-intrinsic muscle function. These findings were consistent with a complete actinic plexopathy in the outflows of the C7, C8, and T1 roots or spinal nerves.

The patient underwent a posterior subscapular approach to the plexus. The residual first rib was removed, as was an elongated C7 transverse process. The plexus demonstrated an anatomical variation, being post-fixed with a contribution from the T2 nerve root. A large amount of scar tissue was removed from the lower elements. Histological examination of tissue from this area revealed not only dense fibrocollagenous tissue, but also metastatic carcinoma of breast origin. Following neurolysis, NAP recording gave no electrical response from C8, T1, or T2 to the lower trunk and none from C7 to the middle trunk. The postoperative course was uneventful. Neurological function remained the same as preoperatively; however, good pain relief was achieved.

COMMENT

Direct operation on the plexus may give some pain relief in carefully selected cases. It is difficult to improve function, particularly of the hand. This patient succumbed to metastatic carcinoma 2 years later.

THE POSTERIOR SUBSCAPULAR APPROACH FOR BRACHIAL PLEXUS TUMORS

The posterior approach is used to operate on the brachial plexus,[47] specifically for tumor involvement of (1) spinal nerves at an intraforaminal level (Figs 23-57, 23-58), (2) C7, C8, and T1 roots, (3) the lower brachial plexus trunk, or (4) if the patient had undergone tumor resection and/or radiation therapy with consequent substantial scarring anterior to the plexus. The posterior subscapular approach is also useful in exposing both the intra- and extraforaminal part of the dumbbell-shaped neural sheath tumors, most of which are neurofibromas.

LOCALIZED HYPERTROPHIC NEUROPATHY ("ONION WHORL DISEASE")

This uncommon disorder results in thickening of a peripheral nerve. Localized hypertrophic neuropathy (LHN) of a peripheral nerve results from hyperplasia of Schwann and/or more likely perineurial cells in an "onion bulb" fashion leading to fascicular enlargement. There is a moderate length of localized cylindrical or fusiform swelling in the course of one and sometimes two major peripheral nerves in a limb (Fig. 23-59). The lesion does not spread to other nerves or to other sites in the body.

Unfortunately, the term LHN has been used in the literature to denote two distinct unrelated lesions: (1) a rare, non-hereditary localized Schwann cell proliferation characterized by "onion bulb" formation, now solely referred to as LHN and (2) a more common intraneural tumor composed of perineurial cells with "pseudo-onion bulb" formation, now called perineurioma.

Johnson and Kline[88] observed the perifascicular perineurium of LHN, as now defined, to be defective, attenuated, fibrotic, or hyalinized due to a postulated damage to perineurium with breakdown of the perfusion barrier as the primary event in the lesion's pathogenesis. Gruen et al.,[70] in a relatively large series of cases, however, found no history of significant trauma for most LHN cases or, for that matter, in those previously reported in the literature. They proposed that the pathophysiological proliferative response in LHN may be a reaction to an unknown chemical, toxic, or compressive mechanical injury, or a neoplastic process.

In the English literature from the last 10 years, Simmons et al.[138] reported one case of LHN each for the brachial plexus, radial, femoral, and sciatic nerves. Stumpo et al.[148] reported bilateral LHN involvement of brachial plexi in a patient, while Isaac et al.[83] reported a radial nerve involved by LHN, and Takao et al.,[152] a femoral nerve with LHN enlargement. The tumor was also found in the tibial division of the sciatic nerve by Suarez et al.,[150] and common peroneal nerve as reported by Heilbrun et al.[78] Earlier literature presented case reports or presentations of a few cases.[17,69,77,86,115,142] LHN probably occurs more frequently than these sporadic case reports suggest, however.

LHN can affect children. A number of our patients were young adults and some were even middle-aged.

MICROSCOPIC APPEARANCE

Histologically, there is a striking proliferation of perineurial cells in a whorl formation surrounding each individual axon with marked endoneurial fibrosis and also fibrotic replacement of the perineurium. Myelin is either lost or greatly diminished in thickness. This characteristic histologic feature of the disease has led to the term "onion whorl disease." Compartmentation, in which the axon is surrounded by fibrous tissue and also seems to be encircled by its own perineurium, is also characteristic. This produces hypertrophic fascicles.

Studies using S-100 protein as an immunocytochemical marker, as well as other histologic characteristics, suggest that the whorls of fibrous tissue around the fibers originate from perineurial cells.[88,110,118,145]

Intraneural tumors and other nontumorous and nontraumatic causes of nerve enlargement should be in the differential diagnosis.[41,98,115] They include amyloidosis, Hansen's disease, Charcot-Marie-Tooth disease, and Dejerine-Sottas disease (Fig. 23-60).[6,112]

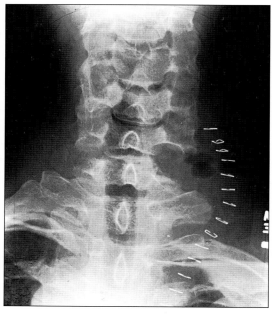

FIGURE 23-57 A postoperative anteroposterior plain film of the cervical spine is seen after a posterior subscapular removal of a relatively large intraforaminal neurofibroma involving the C7 spinal nerve. Note the extent of the bone removal and placement of skin staples.

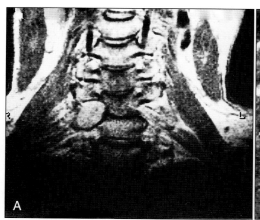
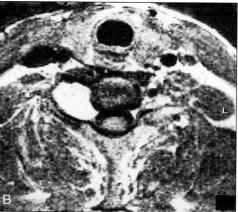

FIGURE 23-58 Magnetic resonance images of two different intraforaminal spinal nerve tumors as viewed in a coronal **(A)** and an axial plane **(B)**.

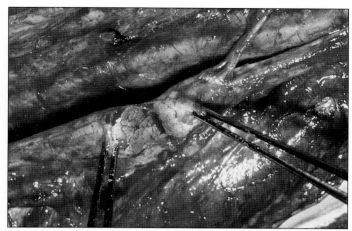

FIGURE 23-59 This shows an intraoperative section through a nerve involved by hypertrophic neuropathy. The nerve was swollen and firmer than usually and, as can be seen, had enlarged fascicles. A histologic study confirmed "onion-whorl" changes with connective tissue proliferation around each fiber.

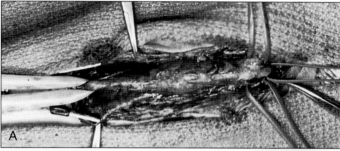

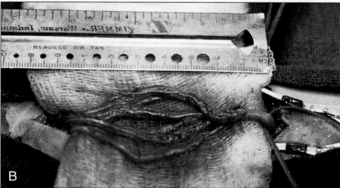

FIGURE 23-60 **(A)** Exposure of the median nerve at a palmar level in a 4-year-old child with Dejerine-Sottas disease. Preoperative symptoms included pain, local tenderness, paresthesias, and an enlarging mass at the palmar level. **(B)** A carpal tunnel release and an internal neurolysis were done.

SURGICAL APPROACH

External neurolysis alone or with additional internal neurolysis was usually performed on an LHN lesion in the past. Manipulation of the lesion, particularly by internal neurolysis, at times produced additional or even complete loss of function, despite the fact that neurolysis was less invasive than resection. As a result, later encounters with this unusual entity have led to an alternative which was to proceed with resection, despite the attendant loss. The lost

segment was replaced with autologous grafts in nine LSUHSC patients, using interposed sural or antebrachial cutaneous nerves and 7–0 or 8–0 monofilament suture. Because the disease commonly involved a significant segment of nerve, the grafts were usually lengthy. There has been a limited number of reported cases and functional outcomes using this approach.[16,41,81,88,119,139]

Intraoperative NAP recording was performed in all cases of LHN undergoing surgery at LSUHSC. Potentials were recorded proximal to the lesion, and the NAP was traced through and distal to the lesion. The lesion was resected if no NAP or one of poor amplitude requiring a large amount of amplification was recorded across the lesion. Before resecting any portion of nerve, frozen section analysis was obtained confirming that the "onion whorls" of LHN were present. Uninvolved margins proximal and distal to the lesion were then obtained, i.e. normal fascicular structure was observed at both ends of all resected segments. Exceptions to resection have been lengthy lesions in nerves such as the proximal ulnar or peroneal nerve, in which resection of the lesion and lengthy graft repair seldom yield significant return. On the other hand, more focal lesions have been resected and replaced with grafts and have had some recovery.

RESULTS

Sixteen LHN lesions were removed at LSUHSC. Sciatic nerve lesions represented six of 16 LHN tumors (38%) and six of 38 lower extremity tumors (16%). Seven were resected from the upper extremity (seven of 16 LHN tumors, 44%) and represented seven of 39 upper extremity tumors (18%). The median, radial, and ulnar nerves were the sites of four (four of seven tumors, 57%), two (29%) and one tumor (14%), respectively. The brachial plexus region was involved by three of 16 LHN tumors (19%) or three of 33 non-neural sheath brachial plexus region tumors (9%).

CASE SUMMARIES – LOCALIZED HYPERTROPHIC NEUROPATHY

CASE 1

A 12-year-old boy presented with a painless but slowly progressive footdrop which began 3 years earlier. In addition to both clinically severe weakness and denervational change in the peroneal-innervated evertor, anterior tibialis and extensor hallucis longus muscles, there was mild weakness and electromyographic changes in the tibial-innervated muscles. At surgical exploration, an 8-cm fusiform swelling of the sciatic nerve was found just proximal to its bifurcation and extending into both the tibial and peroneal nerves (Fig. 23-61). An NAP could be recorded from the proximal sciatic to tibial nerve, but only a small response to the peroneal nerve beyond its enlargement could be recorded. An internal neurolysis of both divisions of the sciatic nerve was done. Postoperatively, peroneal-innervated muscle function loss was nearly complete and tibial nerve-innervated muscle function was reduced further from its preoperative status. Follow-up over a 7-year period showed full recovery of function of the muscles innervated by the tibial nerve, but no significant return of those innervated by the peroneal nerve. Fragments of fascicles removed were characteristic of hypertrophic neuropathy.

Comment

Unfortunately, loss in the distribution of a nerve involved by this disease is usually progressive. Loss is neither reversed nor slowed by neurolysis alone.

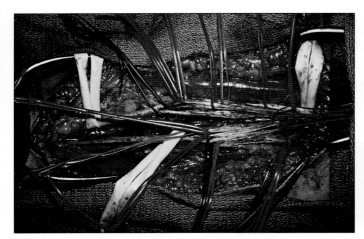

FIGURE 23-61 An internal neurolysis on the sciatic complex is shown being performed; both divisions were involved by hypertrophic neuropathy.

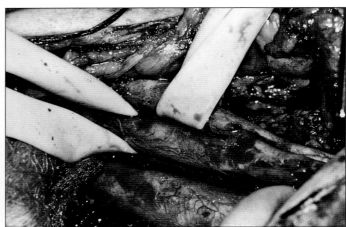

FIGURE 23-62 Hypertrophic neuropathy or "onion-whorl" change is shown involving the C5 and C6 to upper trunk and C7 to middle trunk. The elements were swollen and firm. After nerve action potential recording, most of the involved plexus was resected and replaced by grafts.

CASE 2

A 9-year-old boy had a 1.5-year history of footdrop without a definite history of trauma; however, he had been involved in a number of sports-related activities including football and soccer. Exploration was done at the buttock level because of the weakness and denervational changes in the lateral (short) head of the biceps femoris muscle. The sciatic nerve was swollen at the level of the buttocks over a 5-cm distance. The tibial division was split away from the peroneal division, and the latter was resected and replaced with sural grafts. Over a 5-year period, function of muscle innervated by the tibial nerve was maintained, but peroneal-innervated muscle function only partially returned and a shoe-insert foot brace was still necessary for a normal gait. The resection of segments of the peroneal division of the sciatic nerve, as was carried out in this case, were characteristic of LHN.

Comment

The sciatic nerve was evaluated and repaired in a split fashion. It remains difficult to obtain good results with a proximal peroneal division repair.

CASE 3

A 16-year-old girl had a history of progressive weakness of the left foot and ankle and trouble walking on her heels. There was a family history of diabetes mellitus, but the patient had been tested repeatedly for this and had no known diabetes. On examination, there was anterior compartment atrophy in the left leg, and the function of the peroneal muscle was grade 4, anterior tibialis grade 1, the extensor hallucis longus was grade 0, and the extensor digitorum communis of the feet grade 1. Electromyography showed severe denervation in the distribution of the deep branch of the peroneal nerve with less change in that of the superficial branch.

At operation, hypertrophy of the nerve was found in a segment of the peroneal nerve over the head of the fibula extending into the deep branch of the nerve. The deep branch fascicles were split away from the superficial branch fascicles, and each was individually tested by NAP recording. The superficial branch fascicles and their distal branch conducted, but the deep branch did not conduct. Testing of the adjacent sural branch showed good NAP conduction. As a result, the deep branch fascicles and more distal branch were resected and replaced with three sural grafts, each slightly greater than 4 cm in length.

By 4 years postoperatively, the strength of toe extension, including the extensor hallucis longus muscle, was grade 3 to 4, eversion was grade 5, but the anterior tibialis was only grade 1 to 2. The patient was able to walk without a brace, went swimming, and was able to do most activities. The resected tissue showed a well-established and prominent hypertrophic neuropathy, or "onion-bulb" neuropathy.

Comment

Results in this patient were good, even though the junction of the nerve and the graft was imperfect. Despite incomplete recovery, the patient's performance of daily activities was unimpeded.

CASE 4

Another 16-year-old girl had a 4-year history of a painless progressive loss of function in the C5, C6, C7 distribution of the left brachial plexus. Severe shoulder and upper arm atrophy ensued. At exploration, fusiform enlargement of the upper three plexus roots and the upper and middle trunk was found (Fig. 23-62). An NAP could be evoked to the anterior and posterior divisions of the upper trunk by stimulation of C5, but not by simulation of C6. Conduction from C7 to the middle trunk was absent. C6 and its contribution to the upper trunk were resected, and an attempt was made to preserve some of the C5 input by splitting it away from the C6 input to upper trunk. The C7 through middle trunk was resected and the resected segments were replaced by five 8 cm sural grafts. Again, the resected segments proved to be characteristic of "onion whorl disease." Follow-up over 3.5 years showed recovery of the deltoid muscle to grade 3 to 4, the biceps to grade 2 to 3, and the triceps to grade 3. There was no recovery of the brachioradialis or supinator muscles. Shoulder and upper arm atrophy had reversed only partially.

Comment

Recovery of proximal plexus outflow of C6 to the biceps and C7 to the triceps was partial but good. Recovery of more distal outflow to the brachioradialis and supinator muscles did not occur.

REFERENCES

1. Acker JC, Bossen EH, and Halperin EC: The management of desmoid tumors. Int J Radiat Oncol Biol Phys 26:851–858, 1993.
2. Ahn MS, Jackler RK, and Lustig LR: The early history of the neurofibromatosis. Evolution of the concept of neurofibromatosis type 2. Arch Otolaryngol Head Neck Surg 122:1240–1249, 1996.

3. Al-Qattan MM, Thomson HG, and Becker LE: A granular cell tumor of the digital nerve. An unusual occurrence. Can J Plast Surg 27:177–178, 1994.

4. Amano H, Shinada J, Miyanaga S, et al.: Case report of surgically treated dumbbell-type schwannoma arising in the right brachial plexus with von Recklinghausen disease. Nihon Kokyuki Gakkai Zasshi 39:71–74, 2001.

5. Anderson SE, Johnston JO, Zalaudek CJ, et al.: Peripheral nerve ectopic meningioma at the elbow joint. Skeletal Radiol 30:639–642, 2001.

6. Appenzeller O and Kornfeld M: Macrodactyly and localized hypertrophic neuropathy. Neurology 24:767–771, 1974.

7. Ariel I: Current concepts in the management of peripheral nerve tumors. In: Omer G and Spinner M, Eds: Management of Peripheral Nerve Lesions. Philadelphia, WB Saunders, 1986.

8. Ariel I: Tumors of the peripheral nervous system. Semin Surg Oncol 4:7–12, 1988.

9. Arpornchayanon O, Hirota T, Itabashi M, et al.: Malignant peripheral nerve tumors: a clinicopathological and electron microscopic study. Jpn J Clin Oncol 14:57–74, 1984.

10. Artico M, Cervoni L, Wierzbicki V, et al.: Benign neural sheath tumours of major nerves: characteristics in 119 surgical cases. Acta Neurochir (Wien) 139:1108–1116, 1997.

11. Babins DM and Lubahn JD: Palmar lipomas associated with compression of the median nerve. J Bone Joint Surg [Am] 76:1360–1362, 1994.

12. Ban M, Kamiya H, Sato M, et al.: Lipofibromatous hamartoma of the median nerve associated with macrodactyly and port-wine stains. Pediatr Dermatol 15:378–380, 1998.

13. Bataskis JG: Tumors of the Head and Neck: Clinical and Pathological Considerations. Baltimore, Williams & Wilkins, 1974:231–240.

14. Benzel EC, Morris DM, and Fowler MR: Nerve sheath tumors of the sciatic nerve and sacral plexus. J Surg Oncol 39:8–16, 1988.

15. Berk T, Cohen Z, McLeod RS, et al.: Management of mesenteric desmoid tumours in familial adenomatous polyposis. Can J Surg 35:393–395, 1992.

16. Bilbao JM, Khoury NJ, Hudson AR, et al.: Perineurioma (localized hypertrophic neuropathy). Arch Pathol Lab Med 108:557–560, 1984.

17. Baker DK, Schonberg F, and Gullotta F: Localized hypertrophic neuropathy – a rare, clinically almost unknown syndrome. Clin Neuropathol 3:228–230, 1984.

18. Bolton JS, Vauthey JN, Farr GH Jr, et al.: Is limb-sparing applicable to neurogenic sarcomas of the extremities? Arch Surg 124:118–121, 1989.

19. Bregeon C, Renier JC, Pidhorz L, et al.: An unusual cause of sciatica: soft tissue desmoid tumor. Apropos of 2 cases. Rev Rhum Mal Osteoartic 50:427–434, 1983.

20. Brodkey JA, Buchignani JA, and O'Brien TF: Hemangioblastoma of the radial nerve: case report. Neurosurgery 36:198–200; discussion 200–201, 1995.

21. Brodsky JT, Gordon MS, Hajdu SI, et al.: Desmoid tumors of the chest wall. A locally recurrent problem. J Thorac Cardiovasc Surg 104:900–903, 1992.

22. Burger PC and Vogel FS: Surgical Pathology of the Nervous System and Its Coverings. New York, John Wiley & Sons, 1982.

23. Busa R, Adani R, Marcuzzi A, et al.: Acute posterior interosseous nerve palsy caused by a synovial haemangioma of the elbow joint. J Hand Surg [Br] 2:652–654, 1995.

24. Byrne JJ: Nerve tumors. In: Gelberman R, Ed: Operative Nerve Repair and Reconstruction. Philadelphia, Lippincott, 1991.

25. Byrne JJ and Cahill JM: Tumors of major peripheral nerves. Am J Surg 102:724–727, 1961.

26. Campbell R: Tumors of peripheral and sympathetic nerves. In: Youmans J, Ed: Neurologic Surgery, 3rd edn. Philadelphia, WB Saunders, 1990.

27. Cardelia JM, Dormans JP, Drummond DS, et al.: Proximal fibular osteochondroma with associated peroneal nerve palsy: a review of six cases. J Pediatr Orthop 15:574–577, 1995.

28. Casanova M, Ferrari A, Spreafico F, et al.: Malignant peripheral nerve sheath tumors in children: a single-institution twenty-year experience. J Pediatr Hematol Oncol 21:509–513, 1999.

29. Chesser TJ, Geraghty JM, and Clarke AM: Intraneural synovial sarcoma of the median nerve. J Hand Surg [Br] 24:373–375, 1999.

30. Coleman SH, Beredjeklian PK, and Weiland AJ: Intraneural ganglion cyst of the peroneal nerve accompanied by complete foot drop. A case report. Am J Sports Med 29:238–241, 2001.

31. Cravioto H: Neoplasms of peripheral nerves. In: Wilkins R and Rengachary E, Eds: Neurosurgery. Baltimore, Williams & Wilkins, 1988.

32. Curtis RM and Clark G: Tumors of the blood and lymphatic vessels. Philadelphia, JB Lippincott, 1991.

33. Cutler EC and Gross R: Neurofibroma and neurofibrosarcoma of peripheral nerves. Arch Surg 33:733–779, 1936.

34. Daentzer D, Schmidinger A, and Boker DK: Atypical granular cell tumour of the sural nerve mimicking a Schwannoma. Acta Neurochir (Wien) 145:1019–1020; discussion 1020, 2003.

35. D'Agostino AN, Soule EH, and Miller RH: Primary malignant neoplasms of nerves (malignant neurilemomas) in patients without manifestations of multiple neurofibromatosis (von Recklinghausen's disease). Cancer 16:1003–1014, 1963.

36. Dahlin LB, Lorentzen M, Besjakov J, et al.: Granular cell tumour of the ulnar nerve in a young adult. Scand J Plast Reconstr Surg Hand Surg 36:46–49, 2002.

34. Dart LH Jr, MacCarty CS, Love JG, et al.: Neoplasms of the brachial plexus. Minn Med 53:959–964, 1970.

38. Das Gupta TK: Tumors of the peripheral nerves. Clin Neurosurg 25:574–590, 1978.

39. Das Gupta TK, Brasfield RD, Strong EW, et al.: Benign solitary Schwannomas (neurilemomas). Cancer 24:355–366, 1969.

40. DaSilva AL and deSouza RP: Neurofibroma solitario do plexobraquial. Hospital (Rio) 65:853–859, 1964.

41. de los Reyes RA, Chason JL, Rogers JS, et al.: Hypertrophic neurofibrosis with onion bulb formation in an isolated element of the brachial plexus. Neurosurgery 8:397–399, 1981.

42. deCou JM, Rao BN, Parham DM, et al.: Malignant peripheral nerve sheath tumors: the St. Jude Children's Research Hospital experience. Ann Surg Oncol 2:524–529, 1995.

43. deSouza FM, Smith PE, and Molony TJ: Management of brachial plexus tumors. J Otolaryngol 8:537–540, 1979.

44. Dodge HW Jr and Craig WM: Benign tumors of peripheral nerves and their masquerade. Minn Med 40:294–301, 1957.

45. Donner TR, Voorhies RM, and Kline DG: Neural sheath tumors of major nerves. J Neurosurg 81:362–373, 1994.

46. Duba M, Smrcka M, and Lzicarova E: Effect of histologic classification on surgical treatment of peripheral nerve tumors. Rozhl Chir 82:138–141, 2003.

47. Dubuisson AS, Kline DG, and Weinshel SS: Posterior subscapular approach to the brachial plexus. Report of 102 patients. J Neurosurg 79:319–330, 1993.

48. Ehrlich H and Martin H: Schwannomas (neurilemomas) in the head and neck. Surg Gynecol Obstet 76:577–583, 1943.

49. Ergin MT, Druckmiller WH, and Cohen P: Intrinsic hemangiomas of the peripheral nerves: report of a case and review of the literature. Conn Med 62:209–213, 1998.

50. Faulkner LB, Hajdu SI, Kher U, et al.: Pediatric desmoid tumor: retrospective analysis of 63 cases. J Clin Oncol 13:2813–2818, 1995.

51. Feliciotti F and Boi A: Peripheral schwannomas: a case report. Chir Ital 34:393–403, 1982.

52. Ferraresi S, Garozzo D, and Bianchini E: Aggressive fibromatosis (desmoid tumor) of the radial nerve: favorable resolution. Case report. J Neurosurg 95:332–333, 2001.

53. Fierro N, Gallinaro LS, D'Ermo G, et al.: Neurinoma of the brachial plexus: 2 case reports. G Chir 23:209–211, 2002.

54. Fisher ER and Vuzevski VD: Cytogenesis of schwannoma (neurilemoma), neurofibroma, dermatofibroma, and dermatofibrosarcoma as revealed by electron microscopy. Am J Clin Pathol 49:141–154, 1968.

55. Fisher RG and Tate HB: Isolated neurilemomas of the brachial plexus. J Neurosurg 32:463–467, 1970.

56. Foley KM, Woodruff JM, Ellis FT, et al.: Radiation-induced malignant and atypical peripheral nerve sheath tumors. Ann Neurol 7:311–318, 1980.

57. Fong Y, Rosen PP, and Brennan MF: Multifocal desmoids. Surgery 114:902–906, 1993.

58. Fuchs B, Davis AM, Wunder JS, et al.: Sciatic nerve resection in the thigh: a functional evaluation. Clin Orthop 382:34–41, 2001.

59. Gallagher-Oxner K, Bagley L, Dalinka MK, et al.: Case report 822: Osteochondroma causing peroneal palsy – imaging evaluation. Skeletal Radiol 23:71–72, 1994.

60. Gaposchkin CG, Bilsky MH, Ginsberg R, et al.: Function-sparing surgery for desmoid tumors and other low-grade fibrosarcomas involving the brachial plexus. Neurosurgery 42:1297–1301; discussion 1301–1303, 1998.

61. Garant M, Remy H, and Just N: Aggressive fibromatosis of the neck: MR findings. AJNR Am J Neuroradiol 18:1429–1431, 1997.

62. Gehman KE, Currie I, Ahmad D, et al.: Desmoid tumour of the thoracic outlet: an unusual cause of thoracic outlet syndrome. Can J Surg 41:404–406, 1998.

63. George DH, Scheithauer BW, Spinner RJ, et al.: Heterotopic ossification of peripheral nerve ("neuritis ossificans"): report of two cases. Neurosurgery 51:244–246; discussion 246, 2002.

64. Ghaly RF: A posterior tibial nerve neurilemoma unrecognized for 10 years: case report. Neurosurgery 48:668–672, 2001.

65. Giannini C, Scheithauer BW, Hellbusch LC, et al.: Peripheral nerve hemangioblastoma. Mod Pathol 11:999–1004, 1998.

66. Godwin JT: Encapsulated neurilemoma (schwannoma) of the brachial plexus; report of eleven cases. Cancer 5:708–720, 1952.

67. Goldstein LJ, Helfend LK, and Kordestani RK: Postoperative edema after vascular access causing nerve compression secondary to the presence of a perineuronal lipoma: case report. Neurosurgery 50:412–413; discussion 414, 2002.

68. Goubier JN, Teboul F, and Oberlin C: Desmoid tumors and brachial plexus. Chir Main 22:203–206, 2003.

69. Grossiord A, Lapresle J, Lacert P, et al.: Apropos of a localized form of hypertrophic neuritis. Rev Neurol (Paris) 119:248–252, 1968.

70. Gruen JP, Mitchell W, and Kline DG: Resection and graft repair for localized hypertrophic neuropathy. Neurosurgery 43:78–83, 1998.

71. Gunderson LL, Nagorney DM, McIlrath DC, et al.: External beam and intraoperative electron irradiation for locally advanced soft tissue sarcomas. Int J Radiat Oncol Biol Phys 25:647–656, 1993.

72. Guthikonda M, Rengachary SS, Balko MG, et al.: Lipofibromatous hamartoma of the median nerve: case report with magnetic resonance imaging correlation. Neurosurgery 35:127–132, 1994.

73. Gyhra A, Israel J, Santander C, et al.: Schwannoma of the brachial plexus with intrathoracic extension. Thorax 35:703–704, 1980.

74. Harkin JC and Reed RJ: Tumours of the peripheral nervous system. In: Atlas of Tumor Pathology, Fascicle 3. Washington, DC: Armed Forces Institute of Pathology, 1969.

75. Harrison MJ, Leis HT, Johnson BA, et al.: Hemangiopericytoma of the sciatic notch presenting as sciatica in a young healthy man: case report. Neurosurgery 37:1208–1211; discussion 1211–1212, 1995.

76. Hashizume H, Nishida K, Nanba Y, et al.: Non-traumatic paralysis of the posterior interosseous nerve. J Bone Joint Surg [Br] 78:771–776, 1996.

77. Hawkes CH, Jefferson JM, Jones EL, et al.: Hypertrophic mononeuropathy. J Neurol Neurosurg Psychiatry 37:76–81, 1974.

78. Heilbrun ME, Tsuruda JS, Townsend JJ, et al.: Intraneural perineurioma of the common peroneal nerve. Case report and review of the literature. J Neurosurg 94:811–815, 2001.

79. Hudson A and Kline D: Peripheral nerve tumors. In: Schmidek H and Sweet W, Eds: Operative Neurosurgical Techniques, 2nd edn. New York, Grune & Stratton, 1993.

80. Hutcherson RW, Jenkins HA, Canalis RF, et al.: Neurogenic sarcoma of the head and neck. Arch Otolaryngol 105:267–270, 1979.

81. Imaginario JDG, Coelho B, Tome F, et al.: Nevrite interstitielle hypertrophique monosymptomatique. J Neurol Sci 1:340–347, 1964.

82. Inoue M, Kawano T, Matsumura H, et al.: Solitary benign schwannoma of the brachial plexus. Surg Neurol 20:103–108, 1983.

83. Isaac S, Athanasou NA, Pike M, et al.: Radial nerve palsy owing to localized hypertrophic neuropathy (intraneural perineurioma) in early childhood. J Child Neurol 19:71–75, 2004.

84. Isenberg JS, Mayer P, Butler W, et al.: Multiple recurrent benign schwannomas of deep and superficial nerves of the upper extremity: a new variant of segmental neurofibromatosis. Ann Plast Surg 33:659–663, 1994.

85. Itoh H, Ikeda S, Oohata Y, et al.: Treatment of desmoid tumors in Gardner's syndrome. Report of a case. Dis Colon Rectum 31:459–461, 1988.

86. Iyer VG, Garretson HD, Byrd RP, et al.: Localized hypertrophic mononeuropathy involving the tibial nerve. Neurosurgery 23:218–221, 1988.

87. Jarmundowicz W, Jablonski P and Zaluski R: Brachial plexus tumors – neurosurgical treatment. Neurol Neurochir Pol 36:925–935, 2002.

88. Johnson PC and Kline DG: Localized hypertrophic neuropathy: possible focal perineurial barrier defect. Acta Neuropathol (Berl) 77:514–518, 1989.

89. Juel VC, Kiely JM, Leone KV, et al.: Isolated musculocutaneous neuropathy caused by a proximal humeral exostosis. Neurology 54:494–496, 2000.

90. Kameh DS, Perez-Berenguer JL, and Pearl GS: Lipofibromatous hamartoma and related peripheral nerve lesions. South Med J 93:800–802, 2000.

91. Kanamori M, Matsui H, and Yudoh K: Solitary T-cell lymphoma of the sciatic nerve: case report. Neurosurgery 36:1203–1205, 1995.

92. Kang HJ, Shin SJ, and Kang ES: Schwannomas of the upper extremity. J Hand Surg [Br] 25:604–607, 2000.

93. Karakousis CP, Mayordomo J, Zografos GC, et al.: Desmoid tumors of the trunk and extremity. Cancer 72:1637–1641, 1993.

94. Kehoe NJ, Reid RP, and Semple JC: Solitary benign peripheral-nerve tumours. Review of 32 years' experience. J Bone Joint Surg [Br] 77:497–500, 1995.

95. Kokin GS and Tyshkevich TG: Benign tumors of the peripheral nerve trunks. Vopr Onkol 33:24–28, 1987.

96. Kori SH, Foley KM, and Posner JB: Brachial plexus lesions in patients with cancer: 100 cases. Neurology 31:45–50, 1981.

97. Kragh LV, Soule EH, and Masson JK: Benign and malignant neurilemmomas of the head and neck. Surg Gynecol Obstet 111:211–218, 1960.

98. Lallemand RC and Weller RO: Intraneural neurofibromas involving the posterior interosseous nerve. J Neurol Neurosurg Psychiatry 36:991–996, 1973.

99. Lederman RJ and Wilbourn AJ: Brachial plexopathy: recurrent cancer or radiation? Neurology 34:1331–1335, 1984.

100. Leibel SA, Wara WM, Hill DR, et al.: Desmoid tumors: local control and patterns of relapse following radiation therapy. Int J Radiat Oncol Biol Phys 9:1167–1171, 1983.

101. Lesoin F, Bouasakao N, Bousquet C, et al.: Tumors of the brachial plexus. Apropos of 2 cases. J Chir (Paris) 121:171–173, 1984.

102. Losli EJ: Intrinsic hemangiomas of the peripheral nerves, a report of two cases and a review of the literature. Arch Pathol 53:226–232, 1952.

103. Lusk MD, Kline DG, and Garcia CA: Tumors of the brachial plexus. Neurosurgery 21:439–453, 1987.

104. Maiuri F, Donzelli R, Benvenuti D, et al.: Schwannomas of the brachial plexus – diagnostic and surgical problems. Zentralbl Neurochir 62:93–97, 2001.

105. Mallory F: The type cell for the so-called dural endothelioma. J Med Res 41:349–364, 1920.

106. Maniker AH, Padberg FT Jr, Blacksin M, et al.: Traumatic venous varix causing sciatic neuropathy: Case report. Neurosurgery 55: E1236–E1239, 2004.

107. Masson P: Experimental and spontaneous schwannomas. Am J Pathol 8:384–417, 1932.

108. Matejcik V, Benetin J, and Danis D: Our experience with surgical treatment of the tumours of peripheral nerves in extremities and brachial plexus. Acta Chir Plast 45:40–45, 2003.

109. Meyer BU and Roricht S: Fibrolipomatous hamartoma of the proximal ulnar nerve associated with macrodactyly and macrodystrophia lipomatosa as an unusual cause of cubital tunnel syndrome. J Neurol Neurosurg Psychiatry 63:808–810, 1997.

110. Mitsumoto H, Wilbourn AJ, and Goren H: Perineurioma as the cause of localized hypertrophic neuropathy. Muscle Nerve 3:403–412, 1980.

111. Mondrup K, Olsen NK, Pfeiffer P, et al.: Clinical and electrodiagnostic findings in breast cancer patients with radiation-induced brachial plexus neuropathy. Acta Neurol Scand 81:153–158, 1990.

112. Neary D and Ochoa J: Localized hypertrophic neuropathy, intraneural tumour, or chronic nerve entrapment? (letter). Lancet 1:632–633, 1975.

113. Nishida J, Shimamura T, Ehara S, et al.: Posterior interosseous nerve palsy caused by parosteal lipoma of proximal radius. Skeletal Radiol 27:375–379, 1998.

114. Ott W: The surgical treatment of solitary tumors of the peripheral nerves. Texas State J Med 20:171–175, 1924.

115. Peckham NH, O'Boynick PL, Meneses A, et al.: Hypertrophic mononeuropathy. A report of two cases and review of the literature. Arch Pathol Lab Med 106:534–537, 1982.

116. Peled I, Iosipovich Z, Rousso M, et al.: Hemangioma of the median nerve. J Hand Surg [Am] 5:363–365, 1980.

117. Penfield W: Tumors of the sheaths of the nervous system: Section 19. In: Cytology and Cellular Pathology of the Nervous System, vol 3. New York, Paul B Hoeber, 1932.

118. Perentes E, Nakagawa Y, Ross GW, et al.: Expression of epithelial membrane antigen in perineurial cells and their derivatives. An immunohistochemical study with multiple markers. Acta Neuropathol (Berl) 75:160–165, 1987.

119. Phillips LH 2nd, Persing JA, and Vandenberg SR: Electrophysiological findings in localized hypertrophic mononeuropathy. Muscle Nerve 14:335–341, 1991.

120. Plukker JT, van Oort I, Vermey A, et al.: Aggressive fibromatosis (non-familial desmoid tumour): therapeutic problems and the role of adjuvant radiotherapy. Br J Surg 82:510–514, 1995.

121. Posch J: Soft tissue tumors of the hand. In: Jupiter J, Ed: Flynn's Hand Surgery. Baltimore, Williams & Wilkins, 1991.

122. Posner MC, Shiu MH, Newsome JL, et al.: The desmoid tumor. Not a benign disease. Arch Surg 124:191–196, 1989.

123. Press JM, Rayner SL, Philip M, et al.: Intraoperative monitoring of an unusual brachial plexus tumor. Arch Phys Med Rehabil 73:297–299, 1992.

124. Prokop A and Pichlmaier H: Peripheral neurogenic tumors – surgical therapy of nerve sheath tumors. Review and personal results. Zentralbl Chir 118:665–675, 1993.

125. Resende LA, Silva MD, Kimaid PA, et al.: Compression of the peripheral branches of the sciatic nerve by lipoma. Electromyogr Clin Neurophysiol 37:251–255, 1997.

126. Richardson RR, Siqueira EB, Oi S, et al.: Neurogenic tumors of the brachial plexus: report of two cases. Neurosurgery 4:66–70, 1979.

127. Rinaldi E: Neurilemomas and neurofibromas of the upper limb. J Hand Surg [Am] 8:590–593, 1983.

128. Rizzoli H and Horowitz N: Peripheral nerve tumors. In: Horowitz N and Rizzoli H, Eds: Postoperative Complications of Extracranial Neurological Surgery. Baltimore, Williams & Wilkins, 1987.

129. Rockwell GM, Thoma A, and Salama S: Schwannoma of the hand and wrist. Plast Reconstr Surg 111:1227–1232, 2003.

130. Romner B, Nygaard O, Ingebrigtsen T, et al.: Large peripheral cystic schwannomas. Two case reports and a review. Scand J Plast Reconstr Surg Hand Surg 28:231–234, 1994.

131. Roncaroli F, Poppi M, Riccioni L, et al.: Primary non-Hodgkin's lymphoma of the sciatic nerve followed by localization in the central nervous system: case report and review of the literature. Neurosurgery 40:618–621; discussion 621–622, 1997.

132. Rosenberg AE, Dick HM, and Botte MJ: Benign and malignant tumors of peripheral nerve. In: Gelberman R, Ed: Operative Nerve Repair and Reconstruction. Philadelphia, JB Lippincott, 1991.

133. Rubinstein LJ: The malformative central nervous system lesions in the central and peripheral forms of neurofibromatosis. A neuropathological study of 22 cases. Ann NY Acad Sci 486:14–29, 1986.

134. Russell DS and Rubenstein LJ: Pathology of Tumours of the Nervous System, 6th edn. New York, Oxford University Press, 1998.

135. Sakamoto K, Okita M, Takeuchi K, et al.: Desmoid tumor of the chest wall infiltrating into the brachial plexus: report of a resected case. Kyobu Geka 54:160–163, 2001.

136. Seinfeld J, Kleinschmidt-Demasters BK, Tayal S, Lillehei KO: Desmoid-type fibromatoses involving the brachial plexus: treatment options and assessment of c-KIT mutational status. J Neurosurg 104:749–756, 2006.

137. Sharma RR, Mahapatra AK, Doctor M, et al.: Sciatica due to malignant nerve sheath tumour of sciatic nerve in the thigh. Neurology India 49:188–190, 2001.

138. Simmons Z, Mahadeen ZI, Kothari MJ, et al.: Localized hypertrophic neuropathy: magnetic resonance imaging findings and long-term follow-up. Muscle Nerve 22:28–36, 1999.

139. Simpson DA and Fowler M: Two cases of localized hypertrophic neurofibrosis. J Neurol Neurosurg Psychiatry 29:80–84, 1966.

140. Smith R and Lipke R: Surgical treatment of peripheral nerve tumors of the upper limb. In: Omer G and Spinner M, Eds: Management of Peripheral Nerve Lesions. Philadelphia, WB Saunders, 1980.

141. Snyder M, Batzdorf U, and Sparks FC: Unusual malignant tumors involving the brachial plexus: a report of two cases. Am Surg 45:42–48, 1979.

142. Snyder M, Cancilla PA, and Batzdorf U: Hypertrophic neuropathy simulating a neoplasm of the brachial plexus. Surg Neurol 7:131–134, 1977.

143. Spiegl PV, Cullivan WT, Reiman HM, et al.: Neurilemoma of the lower extremity. Foot Ankle 6:194–198, 1986.

144. Spinner RJ, Atkinson JL, Scheithauer BW, et al.: Peroneal intraneural ganglia: the importance of the articular branch. Clinical series. J Neurosurg 99:319–329, 2003.

145. Stanton C, Perentes E, Phillips L, et al.: The immunohistochemical demonstration of early perineurial change in the development of localized hypertrophic neuropathy. Hum Pathol 19:1455–1457, 1988.

146. Stark AM, Buhl R, Hugo HH, et al.: Malignant peripheral nerve sheath tumours – report of 8 cases and review of the literature. Acta Neurochir (Wien) 143:357–363; discussion 363–364, 2001.

147. Stout AP: Tumors featuring pericytes; glomus tumor and hemangiopericytoma. Lab Invest 5:217–223, 1956.

148. Stumpo M, Foschini MP, Poppi M, et al.: Hypertrophic inflammatory neuropathy involving bilateral brachial plexus. Surg Neurol 52:458–464; discussion 464–465, 1999.

149. Sturzenegger M, Buchler U, and Markwalder R: Microsurgical and histological observations in schwannoma of peripheral nerves. Handchir Mikrochir Plast Chir 24:304–309, 1992.

150. Suarez GA, Giannini C, Smith BE, et al.: Localized hypertrophic neuropathy. Mayo Clin Proc 69:747–748, 1994.

151. Sun JC, Maguire J, and Zwimpfer TJ: Traumatically induced lymphangioma of the ulnar nerve. Case report. J Neurosurg 93:1069–1071, 2000.

152. Takao M, Fukuuchi Y, Koto A, et al.: Localized hypertrophic mononeuropathy involving the femoral nerve. Neurology 52:389–392, 1999.

153. Thomas JE and Colby MY Jr.: Radiation-induced or metastatic brachial plexopathy? A diagnostic dilemma. JAMA 222:1392–1395, 1972.

154. Thomas JE, Piepgras DG, Scheithauer B, et al.: Neurogenic tumors of the sciatic nerve. A clinicopathologic study of 35 cases. Mayo Clin Proc 58:640–647, 1983.

155. Tsukada K, Church JM, Jagelman DG, et al.: Noncytotoxic drug therapy for intra-abdominal desmoid tumor in patients with familial adenomatous polyposis. Dis Colon Rectum 35:29–33, 1992.

156. van der Lei B, Damen A, and van Valkenburg E: Compression of the lateral cutaneous nerve of the forearm by a glomus tumour. J Hand Surg [Br] 22:71–72, 1997.

157. vanBolden V 2nd, Kline DG, Garcia CA, et al.: Isolated radial nerve palsy due to metastasis from a primary malignant lymphoma of the brain. Neurosurgery 21:905–909, 1987.

158. Verocay J: Zur Kenntnis der Neurofibrome. Beitr Pathol Anato Allg Pathol 48, 1910.

159. Vieta JO and Pack GT: Malignant neurilemmomas of peripheral nerves. Am J Surg 82:416–431, 1951.

160. Vigna PA, Kusior MF, Collins MB, et al.: Peripheral nerve hemangioma. Potential for clinical aggressiveness. Arch Pathol Lab Med 118:1038–1041, 1994.

161. Wanebo JE, Malik JM, VandenBerg SR, et al.: Malignant peripheral nerve sheath tumors. A clinicopathologic study of 28 cases. Cancer 71:1247–1253, 1993.

162. Wasman JK, Willis J, Makley J, et al.: Myositis ossificans-like lesion of nerve. Histopathology 30:75–78, 1997.

163. Whitaker WG and Droulias C: Benign encapsulated neurilemoma: a report of 76 cases. Am Surg 42:675–678, 1976.

164. Wilcken N and Tattersall MH: Endocrine therapy for desmoid tumors. Cancer 68:1384–1388, 1991.

165. Winterer JT, Laubenberger J, Berger W, et al.: Radiologic findings in lymphangioma of the posterior tibial nerve. J Comput Assist Tomogr 22:28–30, 1998.

166. Wong CH, Chow L, Yen CH, et al.: Uncommon hand tumours. Hand Surg 6:67–80, 2001.

167. Woodruff JM: The pathology and treatment of peripheral nerve tumors and tumor-like conditions. CA Cancer J Clin 43:290–308, 1993.

168. Yasutomi T, Koike H, and Nakatsuchi Y: Granular cell tumour of the ulnar nerve. J Hand Surg [Br] 24:122–124, 1999.

169. Yoshida S, Kimura H, Iwai N, et al.: A surgical case of aggressive fibromatosis. Nippon Kyobu Geka Gakkai Zasshi 45:2016–2020, 1997.

170. Yoshida S, Taira H, Kataoka M, et al.: Idiopathic heterotopic ossification within the tibial nerve. A case report. J Bone Joint Surg [Am] 84:1442–1444, 2002.

171. Zvijac JE, Sheldon DA, and Schurhoff MR: Extensive lipoma causing suprascapular nerve entrapment. Am J Orthop 32:141–143, 2003.

24

Iatrogenic injury to peripheral nerve

Robert J. Spinner

OVERVIEW

- Iatrogenic injury to nerve, while under-reported, is a relatively common occurrence that physicians and surgeons will ultimately face either directly or indirectly in their practice.
- All healthcare deliverers are at risk, although certain subspecialists, techniques, and procedures are more frequently associated with nerve-related complications than others.
- Information on avoidance, diagnosis, and management of these injuries is lacking in the literature, and education and experiences are necessary to heighten one's awareness of the potential problem.
- Timely intervention is often associated with improved outcomes.
- Delay in diagnosis and treatment is as concerning as the initial injury and negatively impacts long-term results.

INTRODUCTION

Simply stated, in an effort to do well, physicians may inadvertently do harm. Although the prevalence of iatrogenic injury to peripheral nerve is not known, it is not rare. Several referral centers have estimated rates as high as 20% of traumatic injuries to nerve. Still, these values are probably underestimates. Knowledge about these injuries is important in the treatment of patients being treated with other medical conditions (potentially at risk for iatrogenic injuries) or those with iatrogenic injuries.

Iatrogenic injuries have a broad spectrum.[4] While many of them may be preventable, others are not. Peter Blum has implemented an informal classification[6] to subdivide these types of iatrogenic injuries. Firstly, there are those injuries that directly or indirectly affect the nerve. Some of these are "potentially preventable" (i.e. lymph node biopsy injuring the spinal accessory nerve[25] or injection injury to the sciatic or radial nerve) or "probably unavoidable" (e.g. sciatic nerve after total hip arthroplasty[43] or peroneal nerve after total knee arthroplasty[2,18,21,24,28,40,42]); rarely "sheer stupidity" or "carelessness" is involved (using the median nerve rather than palmaris longus as a tendon graft). Secondly, neglect or delay of referral or treatment not uncommonly adversely affects the quality of treatment.

This is a broad topic.[4,8,24,27,29,55] The purpose of this chapter is not to be encyclopedic but rather to provide readers with a broad, balanced overview as to the nature of the injury, and how best to diagnose, manage, and avoid these injuries. Other chapters in this textbook will discuss specific injury patterns affecting individual nerves and treatments in more detail. Only through education, exposure, and experience will people learn these principles.

WHO CAUSES IATROGENIC INJURIES?

Every healthcare deliverer who treats patients is effectively at risk.

Technicians, nurses and physicians may cause iatrogenic injury. Technicians may injure nerves when performing venipuncture[17] or obtaining intravenous access, and nurses when administering intramuscular injections. Anesthesiologists are at risk when positioning patients, placing arterial lines, or performing peripheral nerve blocks;[10] radiologists, performing catheterizations; oncologists, prescribing radiation or chemotherapy; physicians, initiating anticoagulation therapy.[59]

Surgeons, however, are the most vulnerable. Nonoperative therapy or operative intervention may place nerve(s) at risk. Steroid injection,[32] immobilization, etc. may result in nerve injury. Every operation places at least one nerve, often more, at risk. The adage "If you operate, you will have complications" is true, especially as it applies to iatrogenic complications. While surgeons of all subspecialties experience iatrogenic injury, certain specialists seem to cause iatrogenic injuries most commonly, namely: orthopedists, general surgeons, neurosurgeons, vascular surgeons, obstetricians, gynecologic surgeons, and plastic surgeons.

WHICH OPERATION?

Any operation can cause nerve-related injury. In fact, certain minor operations, e.g. lymph node biopsy, ganglia resection, or trigger digit releases, are well known to cause nerve injury. No operation – large or small; open or endoscopic – is free from nerve-related risks. Quite simply, there are no "trivial" operative procedures. With new operations, come new complications. For example, increasing use of lengthening procedures has unveiled relatively high rates of nerve complications;[35,60] however, critical analysis of these procedures has taught us about important thresholds and indications (and outcomes) for surgical interventions. Similarly, advances in arthroscopic and endoscopic techniques have also introduced other nerve injury patterns.

Specific procedures, done where important nerves are located in the same operative field, seem to be associated with nerve injuries. Other relatively common examples include arthroplasty and diagnostic arthroscopy or arthroscopic repair of any joint,[14,22,31,33,38,39,44,50,51] osteosynthesis or plate removal (especially of the humerus or proximal radius), osteotomy (especially of the proximal fibula),[26,41,45,58] bone grafting (from the anterior iliac crest), and shoulder stabilization by orthopedists[7,37] (Fig. 24-1); hernia repair, varicose vein ligation, first rib resection by general or thoracic surgeons.[23]

Operations on nerves themselves (i.e. for injury, entrapment, and tumor) may also be associated with iatrogenic injuries and are discussed further in individual chapters. Dissection of traumatized nerves, such as neural elements of the brachial plexus in a post-ganglionic C5–C6 lesion, makes nerves vulnerable during the exposure. These may include nerves that may be completely non-

functional or incompletely functioning (such as the upper trunk) as well as others that are functioning normally that may be in the operative field (e.g. phrenic or long thoracic, not to mention nerve branches of the cervical plexus). Scarring directly or indirectly involving these functioning nerves may place these nerves at some added risk during their identification and mobilization.

The management of entrapment neuropathy is known for its diagnostic and therapeutic errors.[5] Failed surgery should be thought of in terms of: persistent symptoms, recurrent symptoms, and new symptoms. Surgery can expose the compressed nerve and neigh-boring nerves (some mixed, some cutaneous nerves) to iatrogenic injury. For example, even carpal tunnel surgery, the most commonly performed surgery for entrapment neuropathy, while generally safe and effective, can have significant neurovascular injuries when done using either open or endoscopic techniques;[49] injuries to the median nerve occur as do those to the palmar cutaneous branch, thenar branch, digital nerves, ulnar nerve and its branches, and the super-ficial palmar arch. Surgery for ulnar nerve entrapment has the same spectrum of complications.[20]

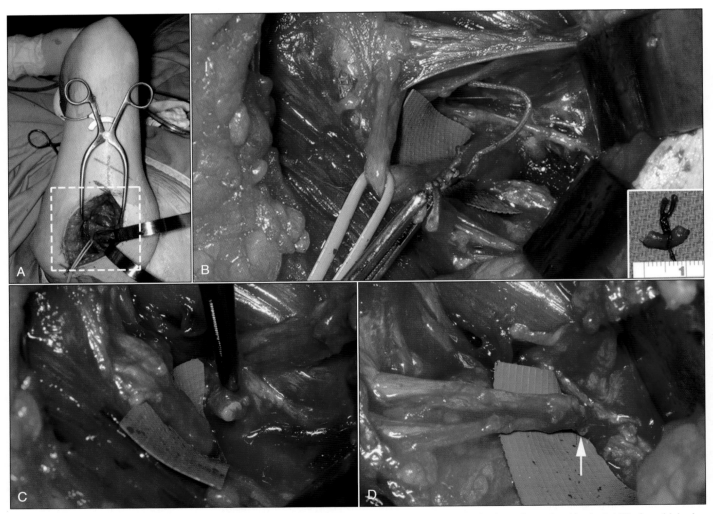

FIGURE 24-1 Axillary nerve paralysis after shoulder stabilization procedure. This young woman had previous shoulder instability for which she underwent capsular shift procedure done through a deltopectoral incision. She awoke with significant shoulder pain and subsequently noted impairment in shoulder abduction. The pain resulted in further shoulder stiffness. **(A)** Exploration through the anterior infraclavicular approach did not reveal any pathology to the axillary nerve. A posterior approach was then done. **(B)** Sutures used in the stabilization procedure were found around the axillary nerve. No nerve action potentials were recorded. Inset demonstrates resected neuroma encircled by suture. **(C)** Good fascicular structure was seen after the neuroma was resected. **(D)** A direct repair was accomplished (*arrow*). The patient obtained good recovery of the deltoid and some improvement in the pain syndrome.

Tumor surgery is a frequent source of iatrogenic injury to nerve.[47] Not uncommonly, entire segments of nerve are unnecessarily resected with extraneural masses (Fig. 24-2). For example, lipomas or extraneural ganglia which may be compressing a nerve are excised along with the major nerve; these masses usually can be dissected away from the nerve (Fig. 24-3). Benign lesions located in the upper chest have been resected with the lower trunk, though there was no evidence of compression. Benign nerve sheath tumors (specifically schwannomas) which intrinsically involve nerve not infrequently are resected en bloc although they can often be removed at a fascicular level, sparing other fascicles (the majority of the nerve) by surgeons experienced with this technique. In many cases, surgeons mistakenly believe that the nerve sheath tumor is a simple soft tissue mass (typically without adequate preoperative imaging or intraoperative dissection and identification of the nerve). In other cases, they are not aware of this technique for tumor resection.

WHICH NERVE?

Any nerve may be at risk for iatrogenic injury, although some seem predisposed due to their anatomic location. Nerves within the operative field are frequently affected, including those that are identified and protected, blindly retracted, or not identified. Even nerves remote from the surgical field may be injured. Mixed nerves and cutaneous nerves may be injured.

When major nerves, including elements of the brachial plexus, are injured, a significant neurologic deficit is typically present. The

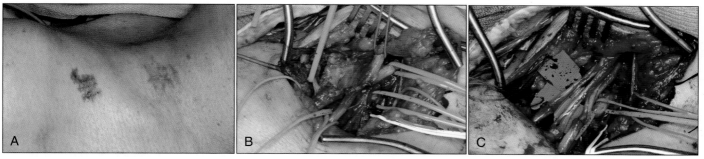

FIGURE 24-2 Upper trunk paralysis after schwannoma resection. **(A)** This patient underwent resection of a presumed lymph node in the neck through a small incision. The patient awoke with an upper trunk paralysis. Pathology demonstrated a schwannoma and large peripheral nerve segments. **(B)** Only a fascicle connected C5 and C6 with upper trunk. **(C)** Interpositional nerve grafting was performed from C5 to suprascapular nerve and posterior division and from C6 to anterior division. The patient made useful recovery but had functional limitations. (With permission, Spinner RJ: Complication avoidance. Neurosurg Clin N Am 15:193–202, 2004.)

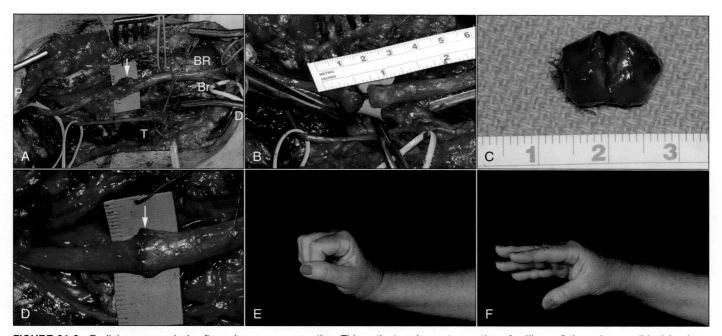

FIGURE 24-3 Radial nerve paralysis after schwannoma resection. This patient underwent resection of a "lipoma" through a small incision in the midarm by a general surgeon. During the procedure the wrist jumped, the patient awoke with a complete radial nerve lesion (distal to the triceps branches) and pathology confirmed a schwannoma. Timely referral led to re-exploration, direct repair (after resection of a neuroma that did not conduct a nerve action potential), and good functional recovery. **(A)** The radial nerve neuroma was identified (arrow) after exposing the nerve in the interval between the brachioradialis (Br) and the triceps (T) at the elbow joint and the brachialis (BR) and triceps (T) in the distal and midarm (P, proximal; D, distal). **(B)** The neuroma did not conduct a nerve action potential and was resected. **(C)** The resected specimen. **(D)** Despite the nerve gap, mobilization of the radial nerve allowed direct repair (arrow). **(E)** The patient obtained strong wrist dorsiflexion within 6–9 months and then good finger extension **(F)** which allowed her to play piano again at her pre-injury level.

most common nerve injured is largely dependent on referral practice, but include the spinal accessory, brachial plexus, radial, sciatic, and the peroneal nerves. For example, the spinal accessory nerve most commonly is injured during posterior cervical lymph node biopsies (Figs 24-4, 24-5)[25] but may also be injured during ventriculoperitoneal or ventriculojugular shunt placement, carotid endarterectomy, internal jugular vein cannulation, or following cosmetic facial surgery.

In contrast, with relatively minor cutaneous nerves, when injured, surprising (and alarming) degrees of dysfunction may result from neuropathic pain. Commonly injured cutaneous nerves include the superficial radial, sural, saphenous,[33,50] digital, and intercostobra-

chial, not to mention those in the groin[34] (i.e. ilioinguinal [Fig. 24-6], iliohypogastric, genitofemoral, and lateral femoral cutaneous nerves [Fig. 24-7]). For example, superficial radial nerve injuries are well known following surgery for de Quervain's tendonitis, wrist ganglia, distal radius fractures,[16] and the like. Problematic sural neuromas may result from a routine ankle fracture fixation or a casual nerve biopsy.

Certain types of operations or surgical approaches seem to place specific nerves at risk. One example is cervical lymph node biopsies in the posterior triangle where the spinal accessory nerve is positioned and vulnerable. Posterior approaches during hip replacement are known to be associated with sciatic nerve injuries

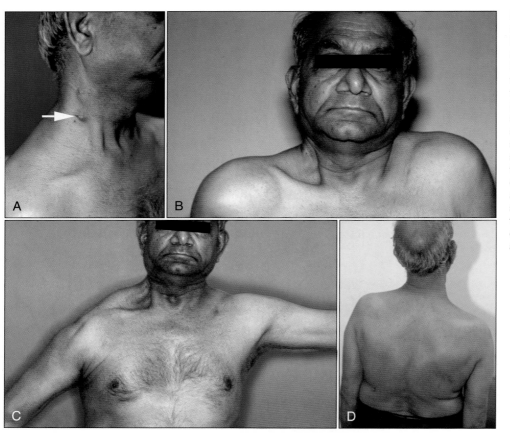

FIGURE 24-4 Clinical appearance of a patient with a spinal accessory nerve injury. **(A)** This man sustained a spinal accessory nerve lesion following biopsy for presumed tuberculosis through a short transverse incision in the posterior aspect of the neck (*arrow*). **(B)** While the trapezius does supply the patient with the ability to shrug one's shoulder, this function still is carried out well by the levator scapulae which is preserved. **(C)** The functional loss is due to destabilization of the scapula which impairs shoulder abduction. **(D)** The shoulder sags. In some cases, this drooped posture of the shoulder may even lead to thoracic outlet-type symptoms in the ulnar aspect of the hand.

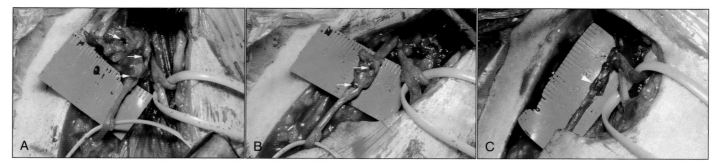

FIGURE 24-5 Operative appearance of a different patient with a spinal accessory nerve lesion. This woman underwent biopsy of an enlarged posterior cervical lymph node through a small incision in the posterior cervical region. The biopsy proved benign. However, she noted atrophy of the trapezius and the inability to position her hand overhead. **(A)** A suture was found in a neighboring lymph node (*arrow*) and two were seen in the spinal accessory nerve itself (*arrows*). A Vasoloop encircles the great auricular nerve and a branch of the cervical plexus. **(B)** The nerve and the sutures (*arrows*) are seen after the lymph node was resected. A nerve action potential was not obtained across the lesion. **(C)** The neuroma was resected and a direct repair (*arrow*) was accomplished.

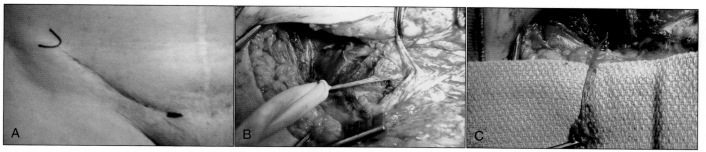

FIGURE 24-6 Ilioinguinal neuroma after open hernia repair. **(A)** This patient developed significant groin pain after an elective open inguinal hernia repair was peformed. **(B)** At surgery, an ilioinguinal neuroma was identified and resected **(C)** with a good surgical outcome.

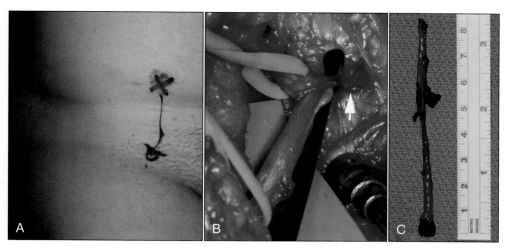

FIGURE 24-7 Lateral femoral cutaneous nerve lesion after an endoscopic hernia repair. This patient had an endoscopic hernia repair and awoke with excruciating pain radiating into the lateral thigh. **(A)** Percussion tenderness was present more medial to the anterior superior iliac crest than was typical for the presumed location of the lateral femoral cutaneous nerve. **(B)** At surgery, a staple was seen tethering the nerve in a medial location. **(C)** Resection of the neuroma led to cure at long-term follow-up.

more commonly than anterior approaches to the hip. The median nerve has been injured during carpal tunnel releases done through palmar (limited open, standard, or extended) incisions, transverse wrist incisions, or two-portal or one-portal endoscopic techniques.[49]

MECHANISMS OF INJURY

Different mechanisms exist for nerve injury from nonoperative and operative treatment. Nonoperative causes include injection injuries,[15,46] compression (from casts, splints, bands, dressings, orthotics, etc.). Injuries from venipuncture, injections, and arteriography may result from compression or direct injury. For example, extraneural injury (from hematoma, fibrosis, pseudoaneurysm, for example) or intraneural (extra- or intrafascicularly) from direct injury can occur from the penetrating sharp object or, from effects of the agent administered, compression can occur. Operative causes span the gamut including compression, stretch, transection/resection, ligation, thermal, ischemia, tourniquet,[12,36] and other mechanisms. Operative nerve injuries typically occur abruptly at the time of surgery; occasionally, they may occur in a more delayed fashion, such as after a hematoma.

Intraoperative positioning[57] can result from excess pressure (external compression) against an unprotected or insufficiently protected body part by hard surfaces or straps (e.g. ulnar neuropathy at the elbow[52]). Alternatively, stretch/traction from extremes of body positioning may result in injury (e.g. femoral nerve palsy from lithotomy position[53]). Both of these mechanisms are exacerbated by the use of muscle relaxants and general anesthesia. Intraopera-

tive peripheral nerve injuries occur in approximately 1 per 1000 operative cases; the ulnar nerve has been found to be most commonly affected. Patients with subclinical evidence of neuropathy (whether from common conditions such as diabetes mellitus, or rare ones such as hereditary neuropathy with liability to pressure palsy [HNPP]), may be predisposed to developing symptoms perioperatively.

At surgery, iatrogenic injury may result from compression (from plates, cerclage wires, etc.) or retraction (lower trunk injury is a known complication from sternal retraction during cardiac bypass surgery). Direct injury to nerves in the field may result in their transection or ligation (e.g. the ilioinguinal nerve in inguinal hernia repair, the peroneal nerve following ligament reconstruction (Fig. 24-8) or meniscal repair; the recurrent laryngeal nerve in thyroid surgery. Nerves may be penetrated by sutures, needles, pins, wires, screws, etc. In addition, the operative field may extend beyond that which is immediately obvious to the surgeon. We have seen several cases of transection to the distal sciatic nerves, tibial or peroneal nerves related to arthroscopic knee repairs where surgeons were convinced that they could not have caused the injury as the injured nerves are not located in the "vicinity" of where they were operating. Heat generated from a cautery or from polymerizing cement can injure nerves. Hypothermic damage may result in phrenic nerve dysfunction following cardiac surgery.[48] Ischemia may present itself in monomelic neuropathy[54] such as after vascular surgery or placement of vascular access (fistula) for renal dialysis; in our experience, many of these fistula-related nerve injuries are due to more direct problems to nerves in the neighborhood. Tourniquet palsy may result from compression or ischemia. Prolonged

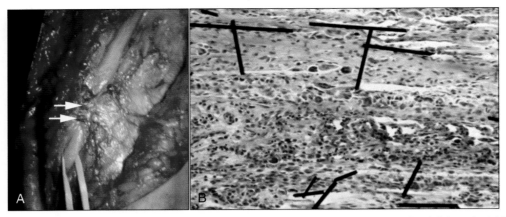

FIGURE 24-8 Peroneal nerve injury lateral collateral ligament reconstruction. This man had a longstanding left knee instability from a lateral collateral ligament injury. Following reconstruction of this ligament, he awoke with a complete peroneal nerve paralysis. He was referred several months later and underwent re-exploration. **(A)** Two carbon fibers (*arrows*) from the ligament repair were seen penetrating the common peroneal nerve. The carbon fiber sutures were removed. With microdissection and microrecordings, the injury only involved a 1-cm long segment of two fascicular groups of the nerve which were repaired directly (split repair). Neurolysis was performed of the remainder of the nerve. By 2 years, he regained grade 5 tibialis anterior and peronei, grade 4+ extensor digitorum longus, and grade 4 extensor hallucis longus function. Sensation was normal in his foot and first web space. He was not using an orthotic and had returned to work in an automobile assembly plant. **(B)** Resected specimen shows carbon fibers with an inflammatory giant cell reaction.

ischemia can lead to compartment syndrome and Volkmann's contracture.

Postoperatively, iatrogenic injuries can occur as well. These are usually related to compression from hematomas (especially when they occur at sites of fibro-osseous tunnels), extrinsic compression in bed (patients may still be anesthetized), from bandages, assistive devices, or crutches. Another condition, Parsonage-Turner syndrome, which is thought to be immune-mediated or inflammatory in nature, may present in the perioperative period.[29,30]

MANAGEMENT

Healthcare providers need to be careful at all times and express humility. Iatrogenic complications can occur and do occur, even under the best of circumstances. A concerted effort can decrease errors in judgment, diagnosis, and treatment, which ultimately will improve outcomes.

AVOIDANCE

Avoidance of injury during procedures, positioning, and surgery is based on a few key principles: displaying knowledge of normal, variant anatomy, and nerves "at risk;"[13,19] preparing before any intervention; possessing good technique for simple and complex procedures; and having good luck. Ultimately, avoidance is dependent on education and experience.

Some simple strategies should be employed preoperatively, intraoperatively, and postoperatively. Preoperatively, operative anatomy should be reviewed in detail, and procedures should be rehearsed in a step-by-step fashion.

At operation, vulnerable nerves should be protected and padded judiciously. Awkward positions should be avoided. Limbs should not be stretched.[1] Lighting should be optimized and loupe magnification can assist visualization. Surgeons should operate in a bloodless field when possible. A bipolar coagulator allows immaculate hemostasis. Neuromuscular blockade should be avoided, whenever possible.

Incisions should be long enough to allow surgeons to feel comfortable about the safe visualization or protection of nerves. Minimally invasive or endoscopic techniques demand rigorous training; "learning curves" are well described to diminish complications. New techniques should be practiced in courses on cadavers. Surgeons should have a low threshold to extend incisions or convert an endoscopic to an open procedure. Surgeons should be familiar with "safe zones" and "danger zones" that have been described when performing certain procedures.[3,4,41]

Cutaneous nerves and mixed motor nerves and branches in the operative field should be anticipated based on one's knowledge of anatomy, identified, and protected.

A portable electrical stimulator may help identify motor nerves. Cutting boldly should be avoided. Nerves should be handled gently and retracted carefully and briefly. In cases of scarring, especially in revision surgery, nerves should be identified proximally and distally in normal territory. Only then should they be traced into the zone of pathology.

Aggressive cutting instruments should be used cautiously, and should not be used in close proximity to nerves (unless the nerves have been identified). Nerve monitoring may help preserve neurologic function when surgeons are doing procedures that place selected nerves at risk – whether elective surgery such as joint arthroplasty (e.g. hip or knee) or fixation of fractures (e.g. acetabular).[51]

Hemostasis should be obtained at the end of the operation with tourniquets deflated. Surgical drains should be considered. While circumferential postoperative dressings are often applied, they should not be overly compressive. Pressure points should be adequately padded. Care should be taken to ensure that the limbs in all patients, but especially those who are anesthetized or paralyzed, are not subjected to injury.

EARLY RECOGNITION

Occasionally, intraoperatively, ends of a transected nerve with sprouting fascicles may be seen and/or a muscle may have contracted vigorously. While rarely is the case so obvious, if it is, it should be addressed intraoperatively, if possible. The majority of the time, if a nerve is severed, it is not seen, lying deep, hidden in the wound. Alternatively, an injured nerve may be beneath a retractor blade[9] or even in a Vasoloop.

The diagnosis of a neurologic problem should be made in a timely fashion.

The diagnosis then is dependent on listening to and examining patients thoroughly. The nurse should understand the particulars of the neurologic examination. Any new neurologic complaint or deficit deserves attention and must be taken seriously. Weakness or sensory abnormality may not be immediately apparent based on a cursory neurologic examination; in fact, it may not be apparent to those without experience and expertise in the subtleties of the assessment. Furthermore, deficits may be eclipsed by a dressing or an immobilizer. In addition, as all nerves have some elements of pain fibers, pain is a relatively consistent feature. Pain should not be ignored, especially when it appears disproportionate to the procedure performed. Neuropathic pain can be masked by analgesics; it should not be assumed or misinterpreted to be "incisional" or musculoskeletal pain. The absence of pain, however, should not be taken as a sign that a nerve is not injured.

Careful neurologic examination can typically still be done, even when the limb is immobilized. Electrodiagnostic studies can be helpful after nerve injury. Nerve conduction studies performed within several days of the injury (before Wallerian degeneration occurs) can help confirm injury to a nerve. After several days, nerve conduction studies may show conduction block suggestive of a neurapraxia. Denervational changes on electromyogram typically appear 2–3 weeks after injury and do not distinguish reliably between differing grades of severity of nerve injury. Ultrasound is a radiographic modality that may be used increasingly in the future to help visualize continuity of a nerve.

Parsonage-Turner syndrome (also known as brachial plexitis, neuralgic amyotrophy, or brachial neuropathy) is a relatively uncommon condition; it is under-recognized and under-diagnosed.[4] It may occur after surgery and should be considered in patients who present with a delayed neurologic deficit in this setting (Fig. 24-9). In some cases, this may be part of a hereditary component. Although the pathogenesis is not fully understood, the stress of surgery is thought to induce the condition in some individuals. Patients typically have pain in the shoulder girdle that is noted immediately after surgery or within the first week postoperatively; the pain lasts for days to weeks. Within days or several weeks, shoulder and/or limb weakness is noted, characteristically when the pain resolves. Parsonage-Turner syndrome typically affects various combinations of certain peripheral nerves (e.g. long thoracic, axillary, suprascapular, anterior interosseous nerve, radial) often in a patchy manner, although occasionally it may affect a single nerve in isolation. Bilateral findings may be seen. Electrodiagnostic studies demonstrate denervational changes. Magnetic resonance imaging of the shoulder region demonstrates denervation atrophy of affected muscles and excludes other musculoskeletal conditions that are in the differential diagnosis (such as shoulder pathology, including rotator cuff disease).

TIMELY AND APPROPRIATE REFERRAL

Once an iatrogenic peripheral nerve injury is diagnosed, efforts need to be made to ensure that the patient is evaluated and managed by a surgeon trained in peripheral nerve surgery. The initial treating physician should know his or her own limitations.

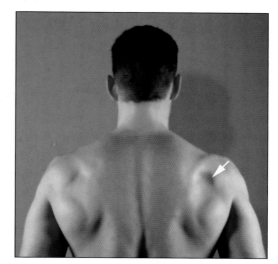

FIGURE 24-9 Perioperative Parsonage-Turner syndrome. This rodeo star awoke from an uncomplicated anterior cruciate ligament reconstruction with shoulder pain which lasted several weeks. At that time, when his pain resolved, he discovered new shoulder weakness which was manifested in his spinati (*arrow shows infraspinatus atrophy*) and deltoid. This neural deficit was thought to be due to positioning, but was in fact, due to Parsonage-Turner syndrome. His mother also had experienced a perioperative nerve complication from Parsonage-Turner syndrome many years earlier.

If a referral is deemed desirable, it should be timely, as there is an important timeframe for nerve repair or reconstruction. Babies with obstetric birth palsy should be referred to an interdisciplinary brachial plexus clinic within several months.

APPROPRIATE TREATMENT

The timing of intervention is critical and depends largely on the suspected injury mechanism. The goals of surgery are to improve function, pain, and cosmesis.

If a nerve is known to be sharply transected, it should be repaired early (within days), at the initial operation whenever possible. Early surgery in this setting allows direct end-to-end repair.

Often, the continuity of the nerve is not known. If a new neurologic deficit is detected in the recovery room, simple measures can be taken should a compressive etiology be suspected. Bandages can be loosened. Limbs can be gently flexed.

Surgeons should maintain a high index of suspicion for a transected nerve (neurotmesis), especially if a deficit follows certain operations (such as a spinal accessory nerve palsy after a cervical lymph node biopsy). Additional information can sometimes be ascertained by reviewing pathology (a large nerve may be seen with the tumor resection) or by speaking directly with the referring surgeon.

Patients who are observed for signs of clinical recovery should have their pain addressed. Physical therapy should be instituted to maintain range of motion in the limb and strengthen other functioning muscles. Splints should be provided where necessary to maintain the limb in good position and to prevent contracture.

Any patient who has a perioperative neurologic lesion worsen while under one's observation should be considered for surgery; a hematoma should be evacuated promptly; a pseudoaneurysm should be resected.

The majority of patients with other types of lesions thought to be in continuity should be followed for 3 months to see if there is clinical or electrophysiologic recovery. Surgery is indicated for failure of recovery from a presumed axonotmetic lesion.

As explained in other chapters in this book, our surgical approach at this time should be guided by intraoperative nerve action potentials. If a lesion is in continuity, nerve action potential can help predict whether or not functional recovery can be anticipated. If a nerve action potential is obtained, then neurolysis alone is performed. If a nerve action potential is not obtained, then the neuroma is resected. Healthy stumps with good fascicular structure should be seen. The nerve gap should be minimized. If the two stumps can be repaired directly (without tension), that is preferable. If interpositional grafting is necessary, this should be accomplished. Split repair with microelectrophysiologic recording can also be done in selected cases.

Surgery is also indicated in the treatment of patients with persistent, refractory pain. In these cases, neurolysis or neurectomy can improve pain in selected cases and should be considered in the management of patients with pain syndromes. Some surgeons prefer to perform nerve repair or reconstruction for cutaneous neuromas.

Patients referred late, or who have made incomplete recovery, might be well served with non-nerve-related operative interventions. They may benefit from tendon transfers or other soft tissue or bony procedures. Appropriate referral might be necessary in these cases if these procedures are outside of one's surgical armamentarium.

Patients with perioperative Parsonage-Turner syndrome should be managed nonoperatively. Their pain can be treated with analgesics. Physical therapy should be employed. No trials have supported the routine use of steroids or IVIG. Patients should be observed periodically for clinical recovery with clinical and electrophysiologic testing over months to 2 years. Sequelae can be treated with other measures.

COMMON PITFALLS TO AVOID

FAULTY TECHNIQUE

- Inappropriate attention to detail during patient positioning and operative dissection.
- Operating beyond one's comfort or skill level.
- Misinterpreting a response obtained by a surgeon intraoperatively with a nerve stimulator from a nerve distal to an injury; this observation may provide an inexperienced surgeon who does not comprehend that Wallerian degeneration has not occurred with a false sense of security.

"Failure to make the diagnosis of a nerve injury, and failure to treat that complication of the first surgery, the iatrogenic nerve injury, is as much a cause for concern as the initial injury to the peripheral nerve."[11]

DELAY IN DIAGNOSIS

- Not detecting a neurologic deficit due to inadequate neurologic assessment.
- Not appreciating the apparent deficit and thinking it is due to postoperative discomfort.
- Adopting a "head in the sand" position or denying the complication.

DELAY IN REFERRAL OR TREATMENT

- Failing to diagnose the depth, nature, and extent of injury.
- Assuming all nerve lesions are "neuropraxias" without accurate electrophysiologic evidence of conduction block.
- Delaying surgery, being overly or unrealistically optimistic about spontaneous recovery.
- Inaccurately assessing clinical recovery.
- Not referring patients to surgeons experienced in the management of iatrogenic injuries.

OUTCOMES

Specific outcomes are discussed elsewhere in the book. A few generalizations can be made. Patients with positioning-related nerve injuries and those with incomplete lesions recover approximately 90% of time, although recovery may take months to years.

When indicated, microsurgical solution is often helpful. Results of surgery, of course, depend on many factors – specific nerve, type of injury, degree of damage, timing of surgery, age of patient, etc. Repairs by peripheral nerve experts fare better than those done by novices. The early diagnosis of iatrogenic injury leads to earlier surgery and improved outcomes. Still, even timely surgery does not always result in satisfactory results. Delayed diagnosis subsequently delays intervention. Nerve surgery beyond 9 months has been associated with poorer outcomes. Unfortunately, some people with iatrogenic injury have an impaired quality of life. Patients involved in litigation may magnify symptoms and treatment of them may be disappointing.

Patients with perioperative Parsonage-Turner syndrome share a good prognosis with nonoperative measures. They may have some residua, especially with scapular winging. Recovery may take several years.[30,51]

MEDICOLEGAL IMPLICATIONS

Iatrogenic injuries have inherent medicolegal implications. There are large numbers of claims of alleged negligence, verdicts, and high indemnity payments. Iatrogenic injuries represent a sizeable proportion of medical liability cases. These injuries have contributed to increased malpractice rates, a shortage of physicians in certain high-risk geographic locations, and an uncomfortable medicolegal climate. Of the cases of iatrogenic injury, we believe that many are unavoidable and only a small minority represents true negligence. In these uncommon cases, one can usually identify problems that have occurred at several stages in the medical process including lack of informed consent, failure to diagnose, and failure to treat, as well as surgical misadventures.

There are essential steps that surgeons should take to minimize risks. First, a detailed discussion regarding informed consent must take place with the patient, and this ideally in the presence of another medical professional. This discussion should include: the risks and benefits of a procedure; potential injuries to nerve(s), and unanticipated loss of function (the single most common cause of litigation). Patients with potential predispositions to nerve injury (e.g. hip dysplasia, leg length discrepancy, previous surgery during primary or revision total hip arthroplasty) should be counseled about their predictive risks. Review of risks and benefits and alternatives should take place no matter how minor the surgical procedure. However, even exhaustive informed consent does not release the surgeon from his or her responsibilities.

Second, detailed neurologic assessments must be performed before and after any intervention. These are especially important prior to discharging patients undergoing same-day surgery.

Finally, accurate documentation is critical preoperatively, intraoperatively, and postoperatively. "If it's not documented, it wasn't done." If meticulous documentation regarding the steps taken to protect nerve from injury is not present in the record, the inference could be drawn that this was not done. On the other hand, if this information is carefully documented suggesting that all necessary steps were taken, then this action by itself would support the fact that not only was the surgeon well aware of the risks, but also that adequate actions were taken to protect the patient from these.

If, despite taking all these steps, iatrogenic injury does occur, the treating physician should rule out potential causes. A systematic review of potentially reversible causes which can result in the complication should be carried out. Carefully document what measures are taken to correct it. These perioperative steps taken to protect the patient can be helpful to protect the surgeon against litigation – either in defending a lawsuit or preventing it from being filed initially.

Fear of legal process must not compromise appropriate treatment. Prompt referral also provides good care and instills confidence. Surgeons caring for patients who have had an iatrogenic injury should also document their findings carefully, with photographs and pathologic specimens, as they are not immune from the legal process either.[11,56]

Despite risk management and thoughtful treatment, ultimately, good rapport and communication are most important.

REFERENCES

1. American Society of Anesthesiologists: Practice advisory for the prevention of perioperative peripheral neuropathies: a report by the American Society of Anesthesiologists Task Force on Prevention of Perioperative Peripheral Neuropathies. Anesthesiology 92:1168–1182, 2000.
2. Asp JP and Rand JA: Peroneal nerve palsy after total knee arthroplasty. Clin Orthop 261:233–237, 1990.
3. Bennett WF and Sisto D: Arthroscopic lateral portals revisited. A cadaveric study of the safe zones. Am J Orthop 24:546–551, 1995.
4. Birch R, Bonney G, and Wynn Parry CB, Eds: Surgical Disorders of the Peripheral Nerves. Edinburgh, Churchill Livingstone, 1998:293–333.
5. Blair SJ: Avoiding complications for nerve compression syndromes. Orthop Clin N Am 19:125–130, 1988.
6. Blum PW: Iatrogenic nerve injuries – 1990 to 2000. World Federation of Neurological Surgeons meeting, Sydney, Australia, September 2001.
7. Boardman ND 3rd and Cofield RH: Neurologic complications of shoulder surgery. Clin Orthop Rel Res 368:44–53, 1999.
8. Bonney G: Iatrogenic injuries of nerves. J Bone Joint Surg [Br] 68:9–13, 1986.
9. Brash RC, Bufo AJ, and Kreienberg PF: Femoral neuropathy secondary to the use of a self-retaining retractor. Dis Colon Rectum 38:1115–1118, 1995.
10. Cheney FW, Domino KB, Caplan RA, et al.: Nerve injury associated with anesthesia: a closed claims analysis. Anesthesiology 90:1062–1069, 1999.
11. Dellon A: Invited discussion: management strategies for iatrogenic peripheral nerve lesions. Ann Plast Surg 54:140–142, 2005.
12. Denny-Brown D and Brenner C: Paralysis of nerve induced by direct pressure and by tourniquet. Arch Neurol Psychiat 51:1–26, 1944.
13. Deutsch A, Wyzkowski RJ, and Victoroff BN: Evaluation of the anatomy of the common peroneal nerve. Defining nerve-at-risk in arthroscopically assisted lateral meniscus repair. Am J Sports Med 27:10–15, 1999.
14. Ferkel RD, Health DD, and Guhl JF: Neurological complications of ankle arthroscopy. Arthroscopy 12:200–208, 1996.
15. Gentili F, Hudson AR, and Hunter D: Clinical and experimental aspects of injection injuries of peripheral nerves. Can J Neurol Sci 7:143–151, 1980.
16. Hochwald NL, Levine R, and Tornetta P III: The risks of Kirschner wire placement in the distal radius. A comparison of techniques. J Hand Surg [Am] 22:580–584, 1997.
17. Horowitz SH: Peripheral nerve injury and causalgia secondary to routine venipuncture. Neurology 44:962–964, 1994.
18. Idusuyi OB and Morrey BF: Peroneal nerve palsy after total knee arthroplasty. Assessment of predisposing and prognostic factors. J Bone Joint Surg 78:177–184, 1996.
19. Jackson DW, Proctor CS, and Simon TM: Arthroscopic assisted PCL reconstruction: a technical note on potential neurovascular injury related to drill bit configuration. Arthroscopy 9:224–227, 1993.
20. Jackson LC and Hotchkiss RN: Cubital tunnel surgery. Complications and treatment of failures. Hand Clin 12:449–456, 1996.
21. Johanson NA: Neurovascular complications following total knee replacement: causes, treatment and prevention. Instr Course Lect 46:181–184, 1997.
22. Jurist KA, Greene PW 3rd, and Shirkhoda A: Peroneal nerve dysfunction as a complication of lateral mensicus repair: a case report and anatomic dissection. Arthroscopy 5:141–147, 1989.
23. Kauppila LI and Vastamäki M: Iatrgoenic serratus anterior paralysis: long-term outcome in 26 patients. Chest 109:31–34, 1996.
24. Khan R and Birch R: Iatropathic injuries of peripheral nerves. J Bone Joint Surg [Br] 83:1145–1148, 2001.
25. Kim DH, Cho YJ, Tiel RL, et al.: Surgical outcomes of 111 spinal accessory nerve injuries. Neurosurgery 53:1106–1112, 2003.
26. Kirgis A and Albrecht S: Palsy of the deep peroneal nerve after proximal tibial osteotomy. J Bone Joint Surg [Am] 72:1180–1185, 1992.
27. Kömürcü F, Zwolak P, Benditte-Klepetko H, et al.: Management strategies for peripheral iatrogenic nerve lesions. Ann Plast Surg 54:135–139, 2004.
28. Krackow KA, Maar DC, Mont MA, et al.: Surgical decompression for peroneal nerve palsy after total knee arthroplasty. Clin Orthop 292:223–228, 1993.
29. Kretschmer T, Antoniadis G, Braun V, et al.: Evaluation of iatrogenic lesions in 722 surgically treated cases of peripheral nerve trauma. J Neurosurg 94:905–912, 2001.
30. Malamut RI, Marques W, England JD, et al.: Postsurgical idiopathic brachial neuritis. Muscle Nerve 17:320–324, 1994.
31. Marshall PD, Fairclough JA, Johnson SR, et al.: Avoiding nerve damage during elbow arthroscopy. J Bone Joint Surg [Br] 75:129–131, 1993.
32. McConell JR and Bush DC: Intraneural steroid injection as a complication of carpal tunnel syndrome. A report of three cases. Clin Orthop 250:181–184, 1990.
33. Mochida H and Kikuchi S: Injury to infrapatellar branch of saphenous nerve in arthroscopic knee surgery. Clin Orthop 320:88–94, 1995.
34. Nahabedian MY and Dellon AL: Outcome of the operative management of nerve injuries in the ilioinguinal region. J Am Coll Surg 184:265–268, 1997.
35. Nogueira MP, Paley D, Bhave A, et al.: Nerve lesions associated with limb-lengthening. J Bone Joint Surg [Am] 85:1502–1510, 2003.

36. Ochoa J, Fowler TJ, and Gilliat RW: Anatomical changes in peripheral nerves compressed by a pneumatic tourniquet. J Anat 113:433–455, 1972.

37. Richards RR, Hudson AR, Bertoia JT, et al.: Injury to the brachial plexus during Putti-Platt and Bristow procedures. A report of eight cases. Am J Sports Med 15:374–380, 1987.

38. Rodeo SA, Forster RA, and Weiland AJ: Neurological complications due to arthroscopy. J Bone Joint Surg [Am] 75:917–926, 1993.

39. Rodeo SA, Sobel M, and Weiland AJ: Deep peroneal-nerve injury as a result of arthroscopic meniscectomy. J Bone Joint Surg [Am] 75:1221–1224, 1993.

40. Rose HA, Hood RW, Otis JC, et al.: Peroneal-nerve palsy following total knee arthroplasty. J Bone Joint Surg [Am] 64:347–351, 1982.

41. Rupp RE, Podeszwa D, and Ebraheim NA: Danger zones associated with fibular osteotomy. J Orthop Trauma 8:54–58, 1994.

42. Schinsky MF, Macaulay W, Parks ML, et al.: J Arthroplasty 16:1048–1054, 2001.

43. Schmalzried TP, Amstutz HC, and Dorey FJ: Nerve palsy associated with total hip replacement. Risk factors and prognosis. J Bone Joint Surg [Am] 73:1074–1080, 1991.

44. Small NC: Complications in arthroscopy: the knee and other joints. Arthroscopy 2:253–258, 1986.

45. Slawski DP, Schoenecker PL, and Rich MM: Peroneal nerve injury as a complication of pediatric tibial osteotomies: a review of 255 osteotomies. J Pediatr Orthop 14:166–172, 1994.

46. Small SP: Preventing sciatic nerve injury from intramuscular injections: literature review. J Adv Nurs 47:287–296, 2004.

47. Spinner RJ: Complication avoidance. Neurosurg Clin N Am 15:193–202, 2004.

48. Swan H, Virtue RW, Blount SG Jr, et al.: Hypothermia in surgery: analysis of 100 clinical cases. Ann Surg 142:382–400, 1955.

49. Thoma A, Veltri K, Haines T, et al.: A meta-analysis of randomized controlled trials comparing endoscopic and open carpal tunnel decompression. Plast Reconstr Surg 114:1137–1146, 2004.

50. Tifford CD, Spero L, Luke T, et al.: The relationship of the infrapatellar branches of the saphenous nerve to arthroscopy portals and incisions for anterior cruciate ligament surgery. An anatomic study. Am J Sports Med 28:562–567, 2000.

51. Unwin AJ and Thomas M: Intra-operative monitoring of the common peroneal nerve during total knee replacement. J Roy Soc Med 87:701–3, 1994.

52. Warner MA, Warner ME, and Martin JT: Ulnar neuropathy. Incidence, outcome, and risk factors in sedated anesthetized patients. Anesthesiology 81:1332–1340, 1994.

53. Warner MA, Martin JT, Schroeder DR, et al.: Lower-extremity motor neuropathy associated with surgery performed on patients in a lithotomy position. Anesthesiology 81:6–12, 1994.

54. Wilbourn AJ, Furlan A, Hulley W, et al.: Ischemic monomelic neuropathy. Neurology 33:447–451, 1983.

55. Wilbourn AJ: Iatrogenic nerve injuries. Neurol Clin N Am 16:55–82, 1998.

56. Wilbourn AJ: Re: Iatrogenic peripheral nerve lesions. Ann Plast Surg 55:112, 2005.

57. Winfree CJ, Kline DG: Intraoperative positioning nerve injuries. Surg Neurol 63:5–18, 2005.

58. Wooton JR, Ashworth MJ, and MacLaren CA: Neurological complications of high tibial osteotomy – the fibular osteotomy as a causative factor: a clinical and anatomical study. Ann Roy Coll Surg Engl 77:31–34, 1995.

59. Young MR and Norris JW: Femoral neuropathy during anticoagulant therapy. Neurology 26:1173–1175, 1976.

60. Young NL, Davis RJ, Bell DF, et al.: Electromyographic and nerve conduction changes after tibial lengthening by the Ilizarov method. J Pediatr Orthop 13:473–477, 1993.

1 Summarizing clinical data

There are many disadvantages to summarizing clinical data, including the fear of misleading the reader based on averaged rather than individual cases results. Despite this observation, one possible advantage is an opportunity to compare results among different nerves, operations done on them, and the influence of level of injury. Examples of this type of comparison can be seen throughout the book and in Tables 1 and 2 in this addendum.

As expected, results with management of radial or median nerve injuries were substantially better than those for the ulnar nerve. On the other hand, the majority of patients with ulnar nerves

Table 1 LSUMC operative results based on 378 serious upper extremity lesions*

Nerve involved/operation	Lesion level		
	Upper arm	**Elbow**	**Forearm or wrist**
Radial nerve/neurolysis^			
Grade 3 or better	100	90	94
Grade 4 or better	90	83	89
Radial nerve/repair~			
Grade 3 or better	72	81	79
Grade 4 or better	60	62	60
Median nerve/neurolysis			
Grade 3 or better	90	93	93
Grade 4 or better	78	87	90
Median nerve/repair			
Grade 3 or better	68	75	81
Grade 4 or better	45	64	68
Ulnar nerve/neurolysis			
Grade 3 or better	90	92	100
Grade 4 or better	79	83	92
Ulnar nerve/repair			
Grade 3 or better	41	69	56
Grade 4 or better	15	31	40

*Percent with functional return using LSUMC grading system. Does not include brachial plexus lesions, peripheral nerve tumors, or nerve entrapment cases.

^Neurolysis was usually based on a positive nerve action potential transmitted across a lesion in continuity.

~Repair category included end-to-end repairs, graft repairs, and split or partial repairs.

Table 2 LSUMC operative results based on 378 serious upper extremity lesions irrespective of level and method of injury*

Type of injury	Percentage with grade 3 or better return
Transections	
Primary suture	78
Secondary suture	70
Grafting	63
In continuity	
Neurolysis – Based on a positive nerve action potential	92
Suture – Based on a negative nerve action potential	75
Grafting – Based on a negative nerve action potential	66

*LSUMC grading system for whole nerve used. Does not include brachial plexus lesions, peripheral nerve tumors, or nerve entrapment cases.

repaired at either the elbow or wrist level recovered significant useful function, and this was a pleasant surprise. Not unexpectedly, those numbers dropped considerably when only grade 4 or better results were tabulated. Patients with median repairs also fared better than might have been predicted, and this even included lesions at either the arm or elbow levels. Recovery of function in both grade 3 and grade 4 categories was not as good as that of the radial at an arm level, but came close to it, and elbow-level scores were quite comparable.

If neurolysis rather than repair was done on lesions in continuity because of a positive nerve action potential across the lesion, average results in 90–100% of cases achieved a grade 3 recovery, irrespective of nerve involved or level of injury. These values reduced for grade 4 recoveries but did not fall to less than 80%, except for median and ulnar lesions at an arm level.

If figures for repair of each of the three upper extremity nerves are averaged, there is a gradation for results. Outcomes were superior for primary repair (which were also done for the less serious and sharper transecting injuries), next best for secondary repair (usually the more severe lesions having an element of stretch or contusion that required resection).

As subsets of data relating type of injury to level and operation are reviewed, there may be reasons why outcomes for median injuries were nearly comparable to those of the radial:

1. Gunshot wounds did well in either series, but there were fewer of those involving radial at an arm level than median. Conversely, not all fracture-associated lesions in the radial series had successful recovery, but most in the median did.
2. On the other hand, median lesions of most types had a higher incidence of associated vascular injuries, especially at arm and elbow level, than did radial lesions.
3. The elbow-level median series included a number of injection injuries, usually caused by venipuncture, and loss was usually partial to begin with in these nerves. The fact that median injuries at an elbow level did slightly better than radial in the neurolysis category is somewhat misleading because more of the radial injuries having a transmitted nerve action potential at this level had a complete distal loss of function than did the median lesions in continuity. As a result, it was harder for the radial series at this level to recover as extensively after having a neurolysis, even based on a transmitted nerve action potential, than the median series.

This type of analysis emphasizes the importance of the demography for individual subsets of injury and the need to deal with detail when attempting to predict outcomes with any type of nerve operation. Other considerations, such as time interval between injury and operation, patient age, effect of other associated nerve injuries, and the individual operative experience need to be factored in as well.

2

Additional muscle testing procedures

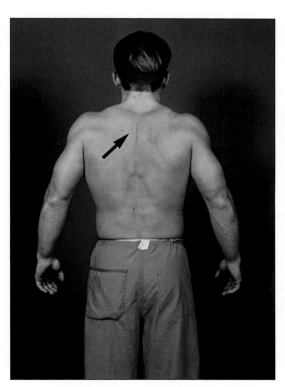

FIGURE 1 The back should not be neglected as a site for inspection and grading of muscle function. In this instance, the model is bracing the shoulders backward as if at military attention. The arrow points to contraction of the left rhomboid. This muscle receives input from C5 to dorsal scapular nerve. Grading is difficult but can be done by comparing both sides: 0 = absent, 1 = trace, 3 = contraction present but not full, 4 = reduced bulk but good contraction, and 5 = full contraction with normal bulk.

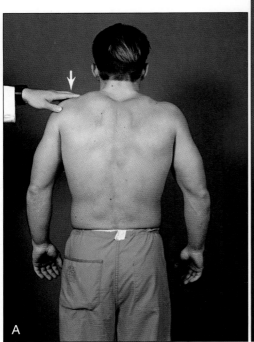

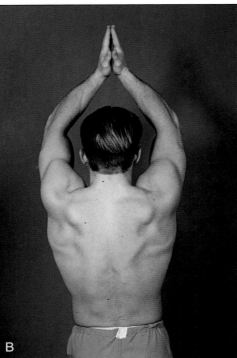

A

B

FIGURE 2 **(A)** Trapezius function is tested in a number of ways. In this photograph, the subject is shrugging the shoulder up against pressure from the examiner's hand *(arrow).* Contraction of the superior portion of the muscle can be observed and palpated. **(B)** The lower or thoracic portion of the trapezius helps to hold the scapula against the chest wall and helps rotate it to permit full and smooth shoulder abduction. Thus, scapular function can be observed as the shoulder is abducted. The function of lower trapezius can also be checked by having the subject push forward or across the chest with the partially flexed arm and observing whether or not the scapula protrudes or "wings." Degree of elevation of shoulder against resistance, amount of scapular winging, and shoulder abduction ability can be combined to provide a grade for trapezius and thus accessory nerve function.

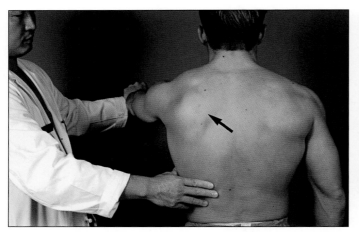

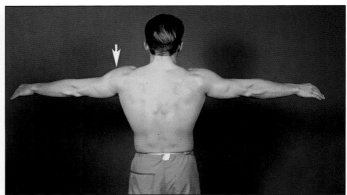

FIGURE 4 Deltoid contraction as observed from behind. The bulk of the muscle *(arrow)* can be observed and palpated and resistance offered by the examiner as the subject attempts abduction. Posterior and anterior shoulder abduction can be observed, although we have used a grading scale based on lateral abduction.

FIGURE 3 In this healthy subject, the examiner is testing the subject for winging of the scapula with the shoulder flexed or abducted forward and the subject pushing forward with the arm fully extended at the elbow. Scapular winging under these circumstances is caused by serratus anterior palsy. This muscle is the sole destination for fibers carried in the long thoracic nerve. Loss of this muscle's function also affects smooth abduction of the arm, especially above the horizontal. Degree of winging in region of arrow and secondary difficulty in shoulder abduction can be used to define a grading system.

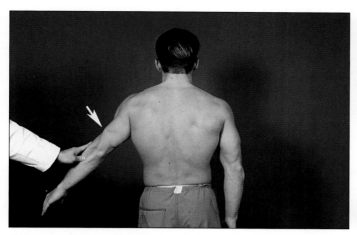

FIGURE 5 The first 30 degrees or so of shoulder abduction is provided by supraspinatus located superior to the spine of the scapula. The arrow indicates the direction for counter-pressure used to test the supraspinatus. This muscle receives input from suprascapular nerve, which receives fibers primarily from C5 but also from C6. This muscle can be readily graded against gravity.

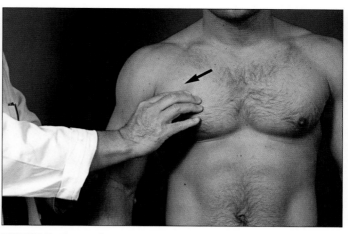

FIGURE 7 Pectoralis major serves as an adductor, but its clavicular head also provides a downward thrust to the shoulder and arm. Pectoralis can be palpated (arrow) and observed as the shoulder is adducted in different positions.

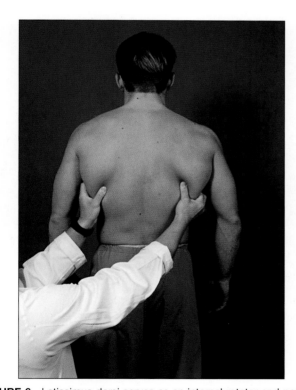

FIGURE 6 Latissimus dorsi serves as an internal rotator and partial adductor of shoulder and arm. For example, the muscle contracts and plays a major role during climbing by adducting the shoulder to help pull the individual up. The muscle is most readily tested by having the patient cough and palpating its mass in the posterolateral lower chest as the muscle contracts. Grading is by comparison to the contralateral and usually normal muscle.

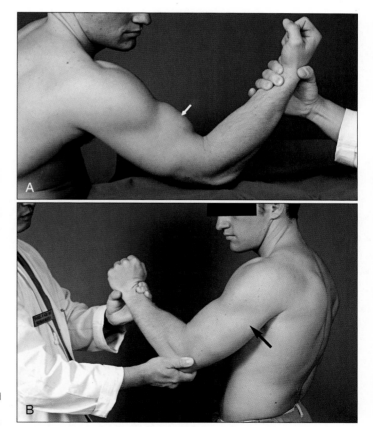

FIGURE 8 (A) Biceps (arrow) is easily tested. Elbow is placed on a flat surface, and forearm is flexed upward against resistance. Strength can be compared to contralateral biceps. (B) Testing triceps muscle (arrow). Subject extends forearm against the examiner's resistance at a forearm level or, as in this example, at a wrist level. Muscle can be observed and palpated as it contracts and it can be readily graded.

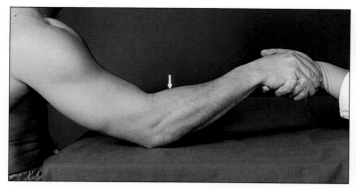

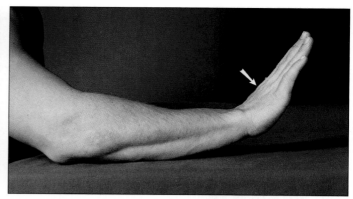

FIGURE 9 Testing pronator teres *(arrow)*. The subject has grasped the examiner's hand, and he is attempting to place the hand palm down against resistance.

FIGURE 10 Dorsiflexion of the wrist is observed in this photograph. Dorsiflexion against resistance can be tested by applying pressure at the point indicated by the arrow. The two muscles primarily responsible for this function are the extensor carpi radialis and the extensor carpi ulnaris. The functions of these muscles can be readily differentiated and graded.

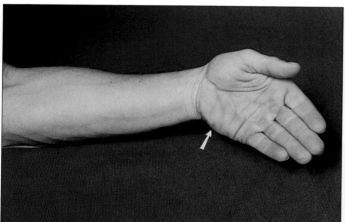

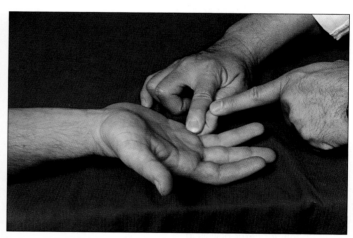

FIGURE 12 Testing flexor profundus of the little finger. The proximal phalanges are stabilized by one of the examiner's forefingers while the patient flexes the distal little finger phalanx against the examiner's other forefinger.

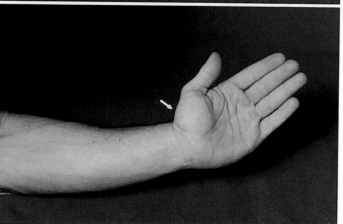

FIGURE 11 Flexor carpi ulnaris **(A)** and flexor carpi radialis **(B)** are easily examined and graded by asking the patient to flex against resistance at the points shown by the arrows.

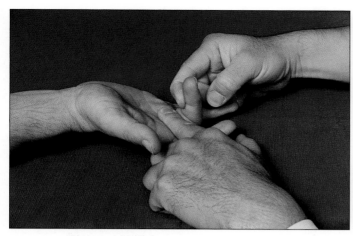

FIGURE 13 Testing flexor superficialis, in this instance of the ring finger. Metacarpal phalangeal joint is fixed by downward pressure of the examiner's left forefinger, and the opposite forefinger is used to resist and grade flexion of the first and second phalanges.

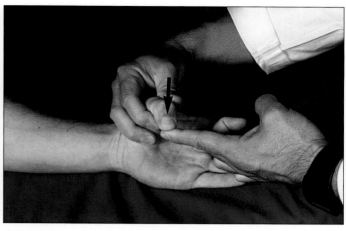

FIGURE 14 Flexor pollicis longus is tested by "suspending" and fixing the thumb's metacarpal phalangeal joint. The distal phalanx is then flexed downward in the direction of the arrow and against the examiner's forefinger and its strength is graded.

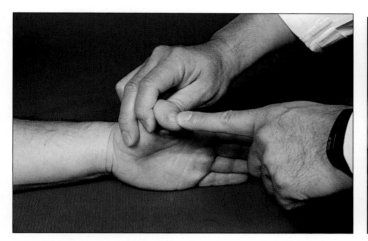

FIGURE 15 Positioning for testing the extensor pollicis longus is similar to that for flexor pollicis longus. The examiner's forefinger resists extension of the thumb's distal phalanx.

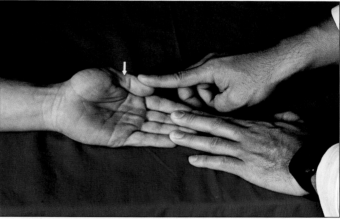

FIGURE 16 Attempt to abduct thumb away from palm at right angles and against the examiner's resistance *(arrow)*. This maneuver tests abductor pollicis brevis.

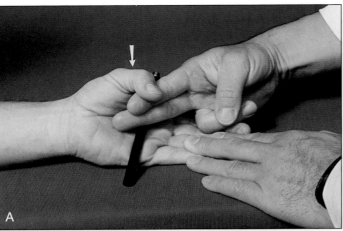

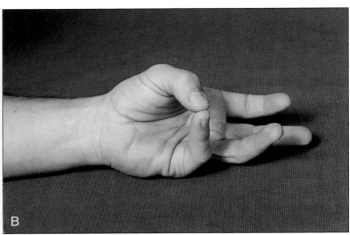

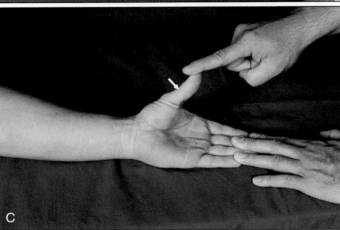

FIGURE 17 **(A)** Opposition of thumb by median-innervated opponens pollicis. With full opponens function, the examiner (to the right) will have difficulty separating his or her forefinger from long finger as the subject presses down *(arrow)* with the thumb. **(B)** Opposition of thumb (by opponens pollicis) and little finger (by opponens digiti quinti minimi). **(C)** Abductor pollicis brevis is supplied by the recurrent branch of the median nerve in the hand; it is one of the more distal muscles innervated by the median. It is tested by asking the subject to pull the thumb upward and at right angles to the palm of the hand *(arrow).*

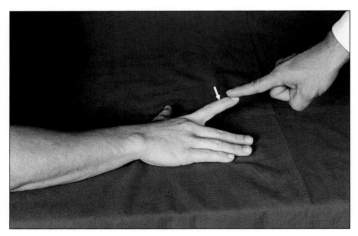

FIGURE 18 Testing, extensor communis input to forefinger. The palm and fingers have been placed flat on the table. The subject is asked to lift the forefinger upward against gravity and, as in this case, some pressure. Arrow shows direction of resistance against this motion.

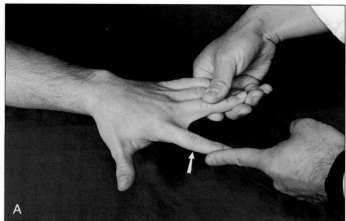

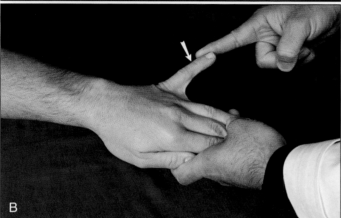

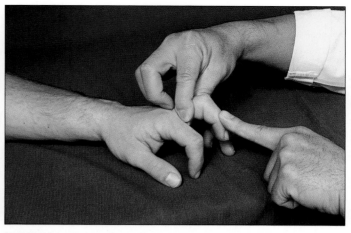

FIGURE 20   One method of testing for lumbrical function. In this example, the metacarpophalangeal joint has been extended by the examiner. The subject is attempting to extend the second phalanx against gravity and some pressure.

FIGURE 19   (A) Proper method for testing interosseous function (in this case, the first dorsal interosseous). The subject is given a target (the examiner's forefinger) which is placed volar to the palmar plane. If this spatial consideration is ignored, and the target is at the plane of the palm or more dorsal, then extensor communis will contribute to the abduction motion provided by the interosseous. **(B)** If target is dorsal to palmar level, as in this example using little finger, then extensor digiti minimi is tested. Arrows indicate direction of resistance applied against these motions.

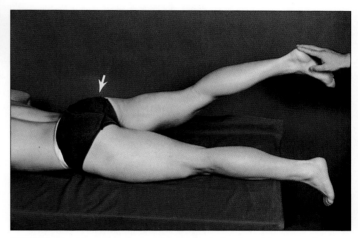

FIGURE 21   Hip extension and lateral rotation by gluteus maximus *(arrow)* can be tested with the patient placed prone. With the knee extended, the patient is asked to lift the leg posteriorly, in this case against pressure provided by the examiner's hand on the heel. Hip abduction provided by gluteus medius can also be tested in this position.

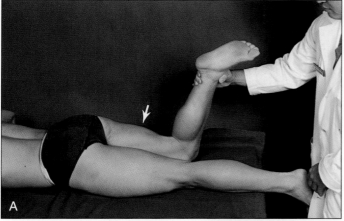

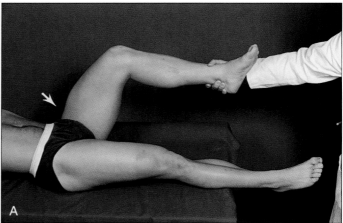

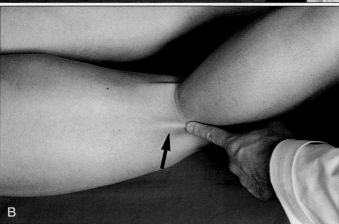

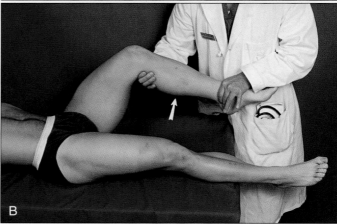

FIGURE 22 **(A)** Hamstring function can also be tested with the patient prone. Leg is flexed back on thigh, and hamstring muscle *(arrow)* is observed and palpated. **(B)** Short or lateral head of biceps femoris, which is innervated by peroneal division of the sciatic, can be readily palpated. Loss of this function implies a proximal peroneal division lesion. The examiner is palpating this tendon *(arrow)* just proximal to its insertion into the head of the fibula as the patient flexes the knee against resistance.

FIGURE 23 **(A)** Hip flexion provided by the iliopsoas is tested with the patient supine. Arrows indicate direction of resistance against this muscle. **(B)** The next step is to have the patient extend or straighten out the leg or the thigh so that quadriceps can be assessed. The examiner inspects and palpates the muscle as the patient attempts to extend the knee against resistance. Arrow indicates the direction in which leg extension occurs as quadriceps is tested.

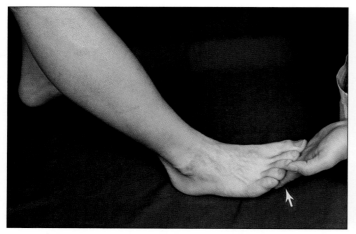

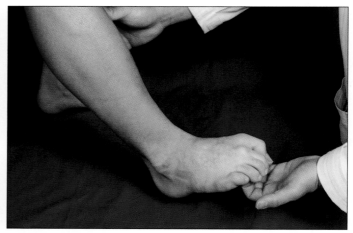

FIGURE 24 Plantar flexion provided by gastrocnemius-soleus can be tested by having the patient place his or her heel flat on the floor and push down with the sole of the foot on the examiner's hand *(arrow)*. To eliminate the effect of gravity, the patient can be placed supine with leg extended. Patient is then asked to push the foot down or to plantar flex. The calf muscle can be readily palpated by the examiner.

FIGURE 25 Toe flexion can be assessed by asking the patient to grasp the examiner's fingers with his or her toes. This function is best tested by matching it against the contralateral toe flexors.

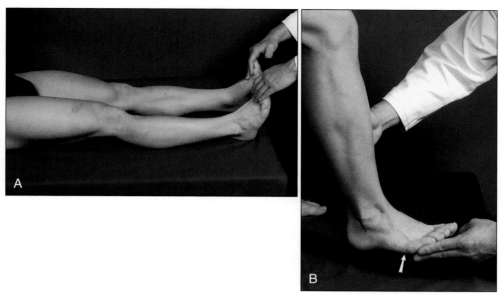

FIGURE 26 **(A)** In this photograph, dorsiflexion of the toes and feet with patient supine is assessed by the examiner, who is providing resistance with one hand on each foot for comparison. **(B)** Eversion provided by peronei is readily tested by having the patient dorsiflex and flare the foot laterally. This proximal anterolateral compartment muscle can also be readily observed and palpated. Arrow indicates direction of resistance on foot to test eversion.

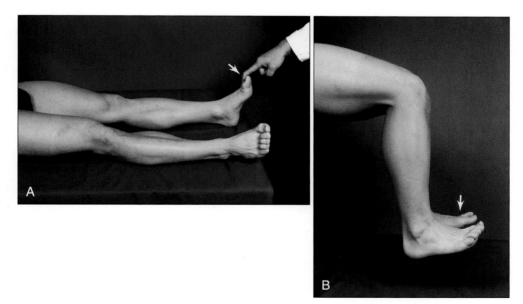

FIGURE 27 **(A)** The patient's left extensor hallucis longus is being tested with resistance provided by the examiner's forefinger *(arrow)*. **(B)** Poor toe extension against gravity is noted in patient's left foot *(arrow)* compared with excellent contraction against gravity in the right foot.

3

"Thirteen years down the track" by Sir Sydney Sunderland

(Read posthumously before The Sunderland Society, Seattle, September 1993, by Edward Almquist, MD, and George Omer, MD)[1]

It is a little more than 13 years since this group first met at the Harrison Conference Center of Glen Cove, Long Island, New York, on 17 and 18 July 1980. If we use the creation of this society as a useful point of reference, we are now 13 years down the track, which brings to mind the words that enlightened British philosopher-surgeon, Wilfred Trotter, when he wrote that "even the most assiduous workman will from time to time stand back to get a more general view of his work and to contemplate its wider relations. Indeed, such intermissions are necessary if he is to escape the tyranny of detail."

As I reflect back over past events, I find that I am asking questions to which, in my autumn years and in my present circumstances, I am no longer capable of providing answers. It is perhaps not surprising that I should use the occasion of this Seattle meeting in an attempt to satisfy my curiosity. This presentation, then, has been designed solely to stimulate discussion and debate.

My first two questions relate to axon regeneration.

QUESTION 1:

What is the greatest distance that a neuron, originally supporting a short axon, can be expected to regenerate a new and functionally effective axon?

This is relevant to the planning and undertaking of some cross-innervations. Are we demanding too much of the provider neuron in these cases?

And here a note of caution. Beware of experiments on small animals, where the distances involved are too short to provide an acceptable experimental model.

QUESTION 2:

My second difficulty concerns the vexing question of neurotropism as a factor assisting useful functional regeneration after nerve repair. If neurotropism, which now appears to be back in business, is doing what it is supposed to do, how are we to explain the following facts?

1. Great importance is assigned to correct axial alignment of the nerve ends during repair. Experience tells us that neurotropism does not compensate for malalignment.
2. Neuromas form at suture lines because regenerating axons grow just as readily into the interfascicular connective tissue as into fasciculi.
3. It has been demonstrated experimentally that motor regenerating axons will enter and grow down sensory endoneurial tubes, and this obviously occurs in autografting.

It seems to me that neurotropism as an aid to functional regeneration remains seriously flawed, although others may think differently.

QUESTION 3:

Despite the wealth of information that has accumulated in recent years, are the results of nerve repair today consistently better and more predictable than in the past? I suspect that the answer must be only marginally so, largely because of our inability to exploit the mass of information that is now available to the surgeon. We now appear to be in an unfortunate position in which much detailed information is available on the factors adversely affecting functional regeneration but little can be done in the way of corrective measures to offset their pernicious influences.

Let us take a closer look at only three of these unfriendly factors.

1. If a length of nerve has been destroyed and the fascicular patterns at the nerve ends in no way correspond, correct alignment of the nerve ends still remains largely a matter of guesswork. Malalignment during the repair remains a potential source of error until we have a foolproof method for ensuring correct coaptation of the nerve ends. Are we any closer to a solution to this problem?
2. As yet nothing can be done to prevent the loss of those regenerating axons that enter functionally unrelated endoneurial tubes and the interfascicular epineurium. This leaves reinnervation both imperfect and incomplete.

---

[1]Permission to publish this address was given by Lady Gwen Sunderland, George Omer, MD, and Edward Almquist, MD, in the spring of 1994.

3. Scarring at the site of coaptation of the nerve ends remains in variable and unpredictable quantity in regard to both its density and the manner in which it obstructs and misdirects the passage of regenerating axons across the nerve end interface. Will it ever be possible to control and standardize the behavior of fibroblasts and healing at that site in order to provide a framework that will facilitate the orderly passage of regenerating axons? The dilemma here, of course, is to achieve this without threatening the integrity and strength of the union.

After a searching audit of all known possible sources of error, one can only conclude that unexpected shortfalls in recovery will be inevitable and should be expected. It seems that the outcome after any nerve repair continues to carry an element of doubt and uncertainty.

QUESTION 4:

We come now to the question of plasticity of neural mechanisms within the central nervous system and the role that it plays in bringing about that further improvement that continues long after it can be attributed to any peripheral phenomena. Clearly this late improvement in response to remedial training must involve re-adjustments to, and the reorganization of, flexible central mechanisms, enabling the motivated patient to compensate for incomplete and imperfect patterns of peripheral reinnervation.

There is much supporting clinical evidence to favor the existence of such central mechanisms and their far greater potential in the very young than in the adult. This evidence throws no light on their nature or modus operandi.

The question then becomes "would knowing more about these central mechanisms inevitably lead to further and substantially improved recoveries?" Here one suspects that it will be well into the future before speculation has been replaced by reality.

QUESTION 5:

My fifth and last question goes to the core of evaluating and recording motor and sensory recovery after nerve repair. Historically, the method currently in use for doing this is a continuum of that adopted and later published in 1954 in the postwar British Medical Council Report on peripheral nerve injuries. Faced with a rapid influx of war injuries in large numbers in the early 1940s, a standard method of evaluating and grading recovery was established to meet the clinicians' needs for one that was simple, clear, precise, and easily and quickly obtained; one that could be used to quantify recovery so that, ultimately, the data collected could be used for comparing the recovery of one nerve with that of another, and the recovery of one nerve under different circumstances. All this was planned in the interest of determining management policy for the treatment of large number of patients with the least possible delay.

To cut through the detail, there finally emerged from the deliberations an M0 to M5 grading for motor recovery and one of S0 to S5 for sensory recovery, each representing recognizable steps in recovery and with defined criteria for each of the five grades. With minor modifications over the years, this method has become entrenched in clinical practice and in the literature.

My question is, should we be satisfied with this method of recording recovery?

In response to this question, it seems to me that there are good grounds for subjecting it to a search audit. In the first place, it lacks a useful functional basis and is, at the same time, flawed and inadequate in other respects.

When the method was introduced, it was emphasized that it was to be limited to testing and that the sensory grading was to be confined exclusively to the primary sensory elements of pain (using graded pin prick and spring algesiometers), tactile sensibility (using a standardized series of Von Frey hairs), thermal sensibility (using recording techniques ranging from the simple to the complex), two-point sensory discrimination (using the points of a compass), position sense, and localization. Moving two-point discrimination and vibration sense were added at a later date. Despite the fact that the restoration of function is the central objective of nerve repair, it was specifically stated at that time that usefulness as a criterion of recovery was to be rejected and that testing useful functional recovery was to be avoided because of the complexities involved and, presumably, because this would add to the delay in finalizing management policy.

These were serious omissions, and in their absence it is difficult to accept the claim that the results gave a clear picture of the ultimate outcome. On the contrary, because restoration of function is the name of the game, published results leave the reader with a totally inadequate picture of the ultimate outcome, limited as it is to individual movements and the primary elements of sensibility. To the patient, this information is meaningless. What is important to the patient is what can be done with, for example, the affected hand and digits when they are called upon to perform the wide range of both simple and complex tasks that are required in the course of conducing daily activities.

Again, not only does the method fall short of what is required, but it may easily lead to misleading reporting. In my own experience, repeated testing at short intervals often gave conflicting results.

Turning now to the motor grading of M0 to M5, this relates to individual reinnervated muscles acting solely as prime movers. This, however, is an oversimplistic approach to the evaluation of useful motor function. Concentrating solely on its action as a prime mover in this way neglects the muscle's important role as an antagonist, synergist, and fixator in the execution of a wide range of movements to give them refinement and precision. A residual paresis, therefore, not only impairs a muscle's function as a prime mover but also, and importantly, destabilizes the actions of other normally innervated muscles. The latter is not covered by the test for motor recovery.

Furthermore, this method of grading and recording recovery disregards the importance of sensory mechanisms in motor performance and of motor functions in sensory discrimination and stereognosis. The latter is not possible in the absence of movement. Though a variety of tests is now available for testing and evaluating tactile discrimination, the recording of sensory recovery is still based on the primary elements of sensory function.

Despite these deficiencies, the method remains entrenched in clinical practice. Persisting confidence in it is also evidenced by the reporting of new devices and techniques to facilitate testing and by the efforts taken, in the belief that measurement brings respectability, to provide, in exact numerical terms, values for each of the primary sensory components. No great accuracy can be claimed for these measurements because they relate to functions with fluctuating fortunes, and as one who has spent hours engaged in this practice, it soon became clear that it was a fruitless attempt to quantify the unquantifiable. As Trotter reminded us 52 years ago, "The affectation of scientific exactitude in circumstances where it has no meaning is perhaps the fallacy of method to which medicine is not most exposed."

Finally, we return to the original claim that the method of coding recovery, as originally introduced, gave a "good picture" of the ultimate outcome. It is difficult to decide whether this is a statement of fact or just an expression of expectation because, to the best of my knowledge, the claim has never been subjected to a searching examination in an attempt to ascertain if the code did in fact equate with the restoration of useful function. Too much has to be inferred in order to make the method as decisive as some writers over the years have claimed.

In other words, when you read of a recovery grading, for example, of M4S4, what does it really tell you about the ability of the patient to use the affected digits and hand in a purposeful way to provide for a wide range of selected manual tasks and skills of a type required for the performance of his or her daily activities? End results as currently recorded are capable of grave misrepresentation.

There is, I believe, good reason for concluding that the coding system of M0 to M5 and S0 to S5 fails to cover modern requirements as these relate to complex motor and sensory functions. Despite the fact that it represents an attempt to bring objectivity into what are essentially subjective events, and no matter how useful it may be for monitoring the progress of recovery, the system is totally inadequate for recording a meaningful end result assessment. For the latter it needs to be amended and extended.

Moberg was absolutely correct in directing attention to the flaws inherent in the use of oversimplistic procedures, but even his criticism did not go far enough. Nevertheless, his "pick up" testing method represented a distinct improvement.

In recent times, the pick up test has admittedly undergone considerable modification, elaboration and improvement, and a variety of tests is now available for evaluating tactile discrimination. However, if the literature is any guide, much of what is currently written on the subject indicates that the main thrust of their use is to follow the progress of recovery as this occurs during a regime of motor and sensory re-education directed to restoring function to the hand. In this respect, it is important to distinguish between recording an end result assessment and monitoring the progress of recovery during re-educational therapy.

If medical records and published papers on this subject are to be kept within reasonable limits, then it becomes necessary to convert end result information on assessment. Needed is a coding scale that can convey to the reader, elsewhere and at a later date, a clear picture of the residual function of the hand and digits as this is reflected in the performance of the patient's daily activities. Furthermore, each grade in the scale would need to be based on clearly defined criteria, so that each grade represents clearly defined differences in the ultimate outcome of the repair, and each grade conveys to both recorder and reader the same clear and precise picture of the status of the recovery for that grade. Only in this way could the scale be used with confidence for comparing one set of results with another, one technique with another and one management policy with another.

Briefly, this would, of course, call for the selection of suitable tasks that would need to be standardized and approved by some international body for universal acceptance and use. Clearly, there are problems in such an undertaking, but it should not be beyond the wit of man to reduce the type of tests required to achieve this to manageable proportions and to convert them to some reliable and practical coding system.

Clearly, this list of questions could be extended, but I believe I have said sufficient to indicate that the saga of nerve injury, nerve regeneration and nerve repair is still far from complete, and it is imperative not only that research should be continued but, even more importantly, that it should be specifically directed to meeting the needs of those faced with the management of nerve injuries.

Index

Page numbers in italic refer to tables

499